ANTLER, BONE & SHELL ARTIFACTS

IDENTIFICATION & VALUE GUIDE

Lar Hothem

COLLECTOR BOOKS
A Division of Schroeder Publishing Co., Inc.

Front Cover:

Large item, top right corner: Shell-face mask gorget, Chicamauga style, 5⁹⁄₁₆" x 7¹⁄₁₆". This large marine shell gorget came from an island in the Tennessee River. Marion County, Tennessee. Jim Maus collection, North Carolina. Museum grade.

Upper left: Hairpin(?), double shafts, 4⅝" long. This piece is nicely carved and in fine condition. Limestone County, Alabama. Robin Fiser collection. **$125.00.**

Center, far left: Bone spear point, historic period (ca. AD 1750), 3¼" long. It came from Morton County, North Dakota. Private collection. Museum grade.

Center: Snowshoe needle, bone, ¹³⁄₁₆ x 3⅛", ⅛" thick. Historic, it is decorated with incised lines and a turtle figure. Michigan. Michael F. Slasinski collection, Michigan. **$250.00.**

Below snowshoe needle: Hide-working tool, bison or elk bone, 7" long. One end has a toothed edge and is decorated with incised lines. Four Corners area, Arizona. Don Casto collection. **$50.00.**

Bottom right: Cup and pin game set, historic, bone cups ⅝" x ⅞" and bone pin 5 inches long. It has a decorative leather flap and a glass trade bead. Well made, this unusual set is Chippewa, from Michigan. Michael F. Slasinski collection, Michigan. **$400.00.**

Back Cover:

Cover design by Beth Summers
Book design by Allan Ramsey

COLLECTOR BOOKS
P.O. Box 3009
Paducah, Kentucky 42002-3009

www.collectorbooks.com

The current values in this book should be used only as a guide. They are not intended to set prices, which vary from one section of the country to another. Auction prices as well as dealer prices vary greatly and are affected by condition as well as demand. Neither the author nor the publisher assumes responsibility for any losses that might be incurred as a result of consulting this guide.

Searching For A Publisher?

We are always looking for people knowledgeable within their fields. If you feel that there is a real need for a book on your collectible subject and have a large comprehensive collection, contact Collector Books.

Proudly printed and bound in the United States of America

CONTENTS

INTRODUCTION

Antler, bone, shell, and ivory artifacts were once highly important for tools, weapons, and ornaments in North America. These materials were used in all prehistoric time-periods, and evidence suggests that uncounted millions of artifacts once existed. They were an integral part of ancient lives. Enough examples have survived to provide artifacts for collectors and archaeologists to study, and to offer a more complete picture of what life was like long ago.

Organic materials, once part of living things, were readily and widely available in most regions. They came from animals and birds normally hunted and gathered for food and clothing. Once the animals and birds were consumed, the skeletons (bone), antlers and horns, and exo-skeletons (shell) remained as a sort of side benefit. Antlers could be taken from deer or wapiti (elk) or caribou carcasses, and horns from antelope and bison. Freshwater and marine mollusks could be retrieved from water or found on banks of rivers or shores of lakes and oceans.

Bone was strong, somewhat elastic, lightweight, already about tool-size, and easily shaped using standard prehistoric manufacturing techniques. Antler tines were already suitable for making awls and projectile points. Large shells became dishes and dippers, while small shells were ideal for beads, pendants, and gorgets. Bone polished easily because of the existing smooth surface, and had a near-white color that was attractive.

Unlike Indian artifacts made of more durable substances (flint, chert, hardstone, and glacial slate) organic materials are relatively soft. They have a tendency to deteriorate along with the more delicate tissues when an animal, bird, or shellfish dies. The majority of artifacts made of organic material has disappeared, not even leaving a trace of what they once were. Microorganisms of many kinds treat these materials as a food source, and over the years, the artifacts are literally eaten away. This is why forest floors and meadows are not carpeted with bones of many kinds.

Special conditions, however, can protect and preserve antler and bone artifacts, and these conditions prevent bacteria from attacking the material. In the far North, low temperatures in permafrost (soil below freezing, year-round) preserve bone and ivory. Near-zero moisture in dry and dusty rock shelters across the southern United States and elsewhere provides the same benefit. Kitchen middens (household trash heaps) with much shell debris create an alkaline soil that preserves bone, especially when little moisture is present. Sometimes sloped earth above a midden is sufficient to divert water and protect the contents.

At the opposite extreme, a permanent water environment can also protect organic material. Many artifacts have been recovered from Southern rivers. There they were buried for centuries in riverbed mud and silt, which excluded oxygen, and prevented the growth of certain bacteria. Time itself is a factor. Sites four or five hundred years old generally have more bone awls, antler projectile points, and bone fishhooks than sites thousands of years old.

Antler, bone, and shell were fairly easy to shape into desired artifacts. These could be broken with hammerstones, cut and carved with flint knives, and given a final shaping with sandstone abraders. Some artifacts, like hairpins, were even engraved and polished, and the polishing step was probably done with leather, grease, and fine grit. Generally, like other classes of Indian artifacts, tool and weapon parts of organic materials were designed for long use.

Today's collectors and students of prehistory sometimes overlook artifacts made of organic materials. The artifacts are not typical field-finds, at least in many areas. It is true that some of these artifacts lack the dramatic impact of chipped points and knives, or the obvious utility of celts and axes, or the artistic and esoteric beauty of bannerstones. Yet, these mundane awls, points, and scrapers once helped make survival possible. Today they offer a more complete perspective of what North American prehistory was all about.

Awls

Awls are pointed tools for making or enlarging holes. They were used to perforate skins and leather for sinew and fiber threads, and for domestic tasks that included making and repairing clothing, footwear, and equipment like bags and quivers. There is even a suggestion that the pointed tools were used as meat-skewers or forks when cooking and eating.

Other than bone bits and scraps from tool-making, awls are the most common surviving bone artifact class. They are found across North America and are known to be from the Archaic period (8000 – 1000 BC) through the Mississippian period (AD 800 – 1500). Awl use continued in some places into the early historic period, at which time they were largely replaced by more durable and longer lasting iron and steel awls. In sewing, awls made the initial hole and stiff sinew (dried and twisted strips of animal tendon) was inserted and drawn tight.

The most widely used material for this most widely used tool was deer bone. While awls were also made from the bones of other large regional birds and animals, deer ranged most of the contiguous United States. The whitetail was in the eastern two-thirds of the country while the mule deer covered the western half, and there was some overlap of range. Awls were often made from long bones that might be modified in only two ways. Cut near a joint, that section was then sharpened to a working tip. The remaining bone served as a handle, making the awl a one-piece tool.

Awls can be from barely 2" to over 8" long, depending on the original bone length and the amount of resharpening done to the awl. Shaft thickness varies, again depending on the original bone size and how much taper is present after grinding, smoothing, sharpening, and resharpening. Most awls have some polish, and it is not always clear how much of the polish is the result of original finishing and how much is mainly use-wear.

The frequency with which such little-modified awls were made and used probably depended on how available deer were in any single hunting or trapping region. However, such awls were also made from the bones of other animals, including wapiti (elk), antelope, bear, bison, cougar, wildcats, and wolves.

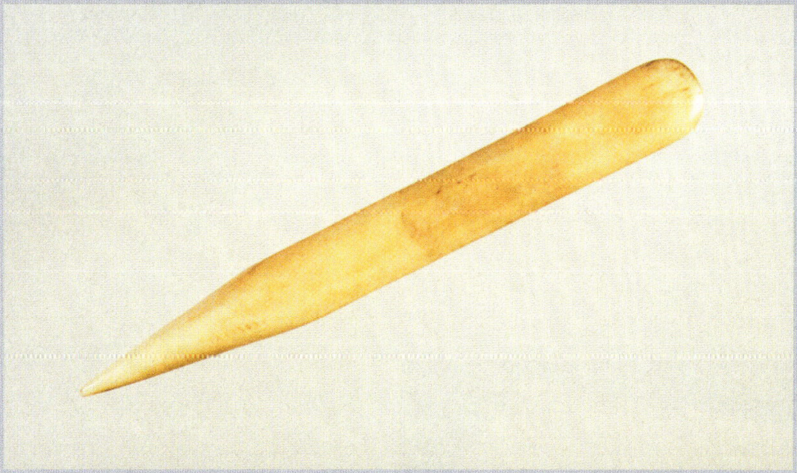

Awl, thick bone with high polish, 3¼" long. It is rectangular in cross-section and is ex-collections Copeland and Hooks. Southern Ohio. Fred Winegardner collection. **$45.00.**

Awls

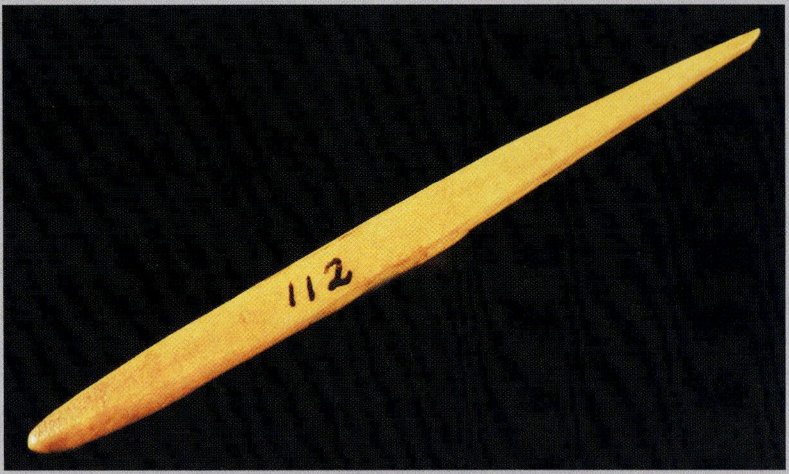

Awl, thick split deer bone, $3\frac{15}{16}$". This is a typical example of a split bone awl, well-made and polished. Southern Ohio. Private collection. **$15.00.**

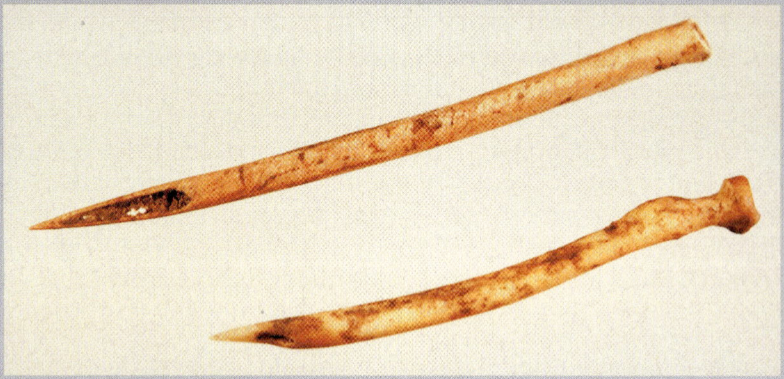

Awls, radial bones from large birds, both from southern Indiana. Private collection. Top, 4" long, cut off at thicker end, longitudinal hairline crack. **$20.00.** Bottom, $3\frac{1}{32}$", very pointed tip. **$15.00.**

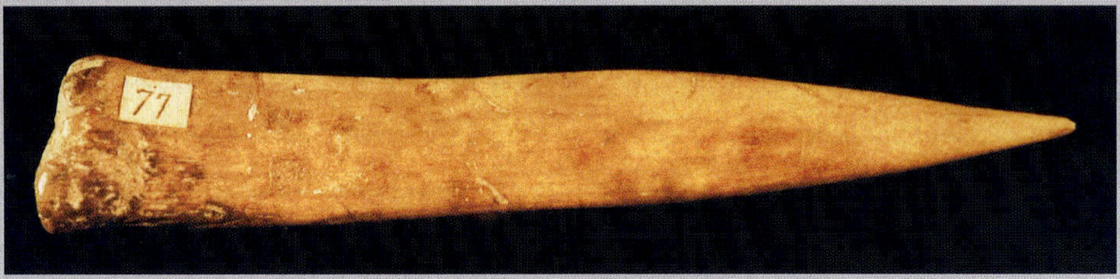

Awl, well-shaped, smoothed base end, gray-brown patination. Polished, the awl measures $3\frac{7}{8}$" and came from southern Ohio. Private collection. **$25.00.**

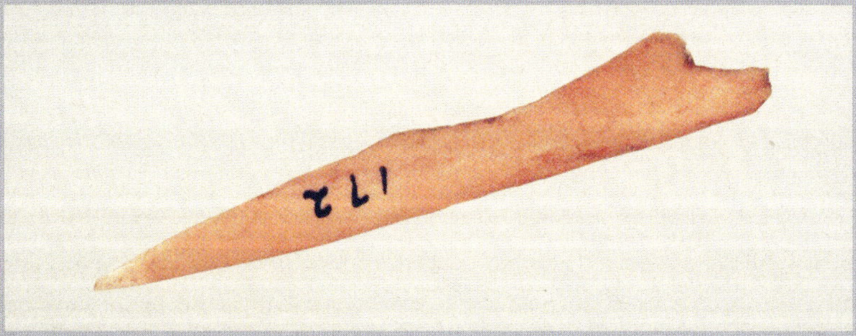

Perforator, bone from large bird, chemically treated. This artifact, $2\frac{7}{8}$" long, is from Kentucky or Tennessee. Private collection. **$7.00.**

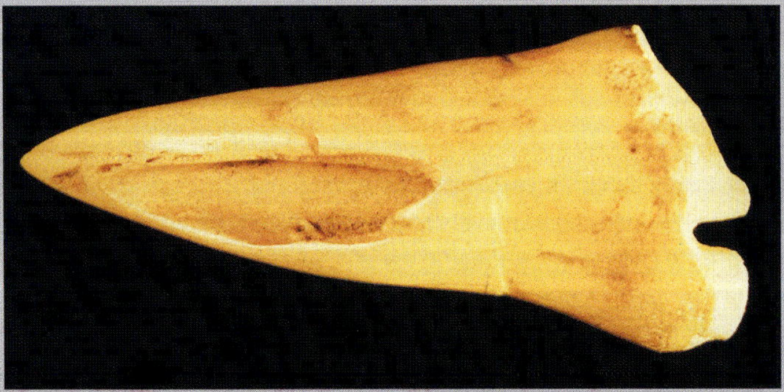

Awl, cut section of large bone, much use-polish, $3\frac{3}{8}$". Cutting and smoothing flattened the tip and shaft. Lar Hothem collection. Southeastern Illinois. **$40.00.**

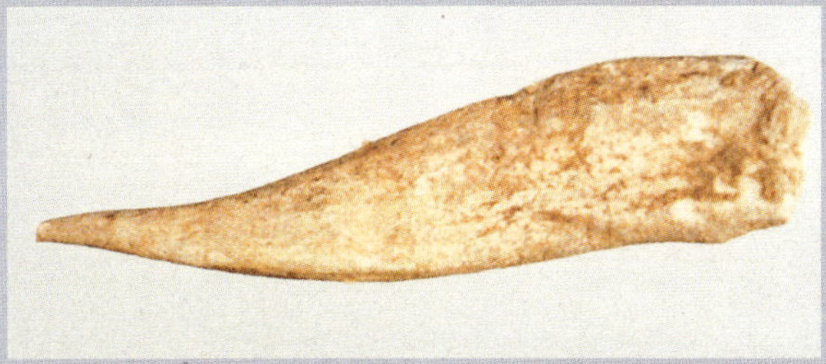

Awl, antler, 2⅝". Still retaining the original antler outline, the awl is from Kentucky. Fred Winegardner collection. **$12.00.**

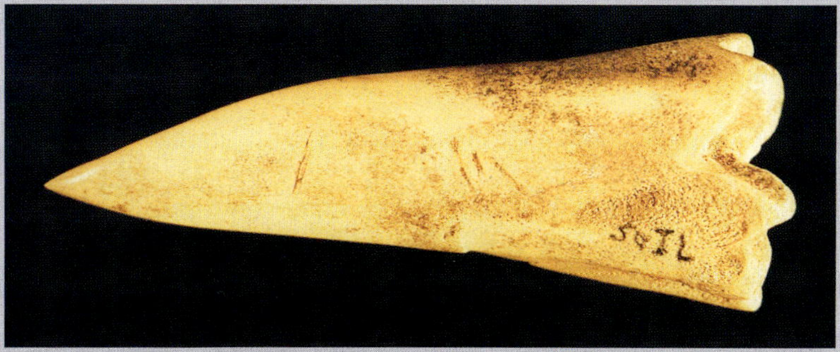

Awl, heavy bone, 3¼". This awl is probably made from the radius bone of an elk. Southeastern Illinois. Private collection. **$40.00.**

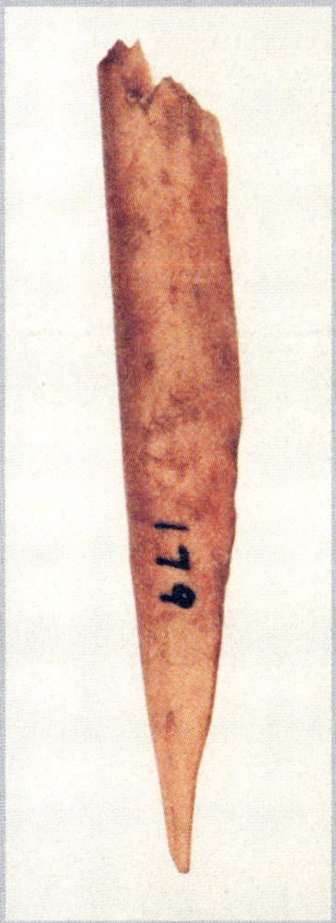

Awl, thin-walled bird bone, 2½" long. This piece was not suited for any kind of heavy work. Kentucky or Tennessee. Private collection. **$12.00.**

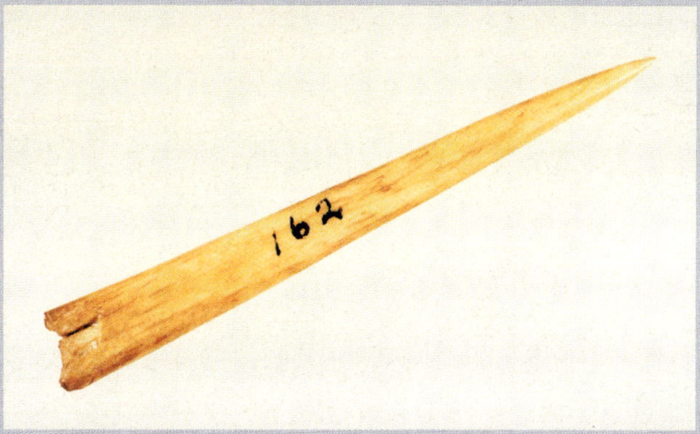

Awl, deer bone, broken, highly polished. It is Fort Ancient in time, 2⅝" long. Southern Ohio. Private collection. **$12.00.**

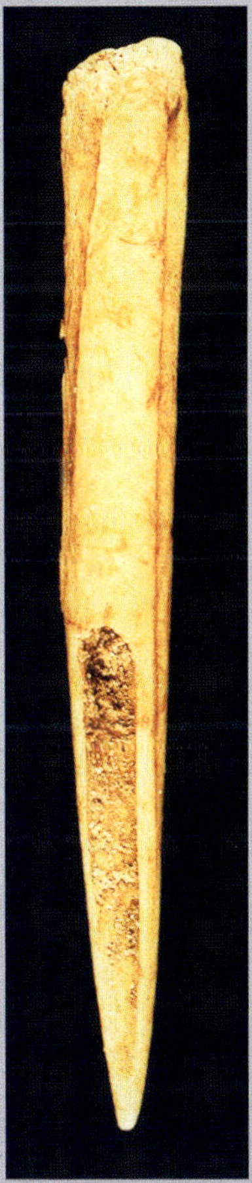

Awl, bone from large bird, shellac coating. The awl is 3¾" long and came from a Fort Ancient site. Southern Ohio. Private collection **$15.00.**

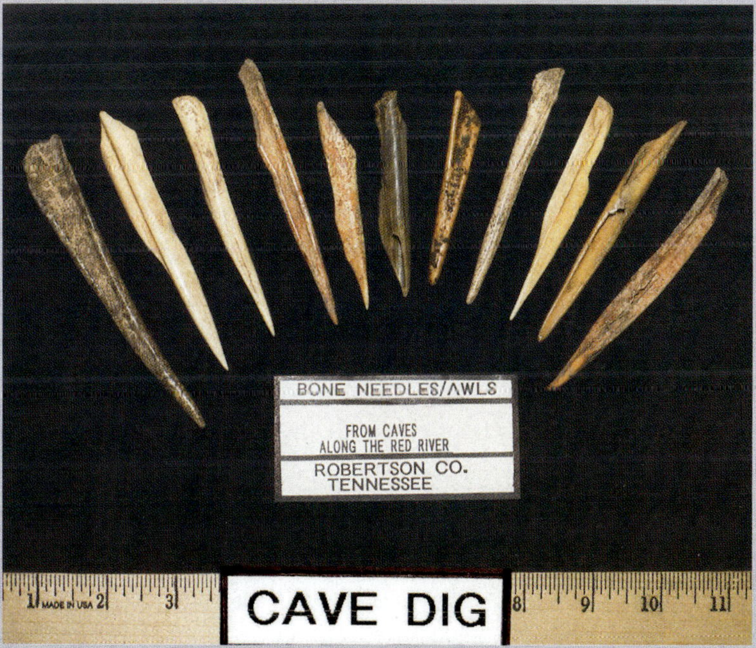
BONE NEEDLES/AWLS
FROM CAVES
ALONG THE RED RIVER
ROBERTSON CO.
TENNESSEE
CAVE DIG

Bone awls, mainly split bone, frame size 8 x 12". These were found in rock shelters. Robertson County, Tennessee. Back to Earth. Frame, **$195.00.**

Awls

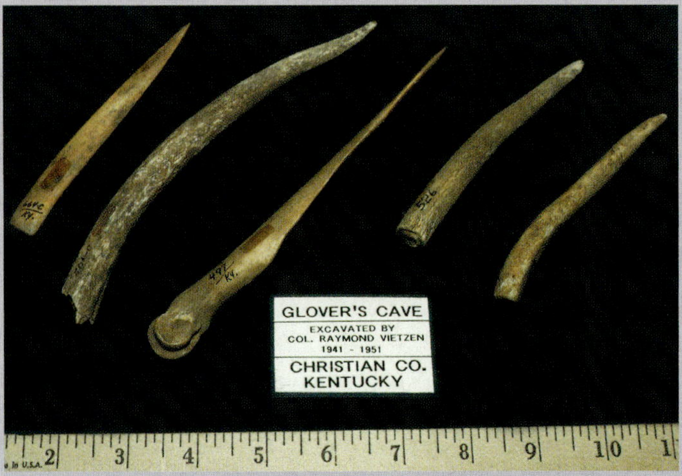
GLOVER'S CAVE
EXCAVATED BY
COL. RAYMOND VIETZEN
1941 - 1951
CHRISTIAN CO.
KENTUCKY

Bone tools, found by Col. Vietzen in the period 1941 – 1951. Christian County, Kentucky. Back to Earth. Unlisted.

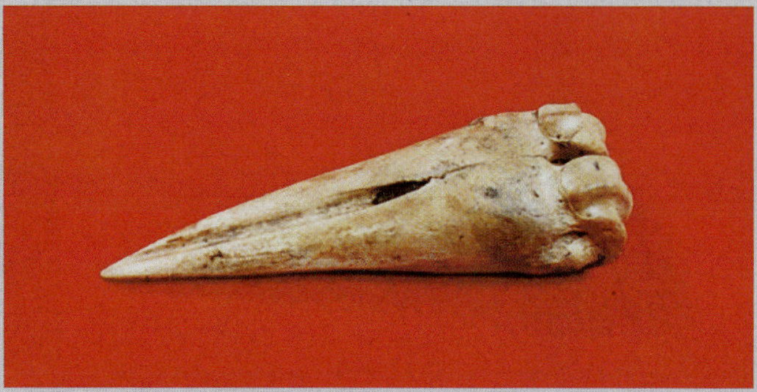

Awl, Late Archaic to Woodland, deer bone, 4¼". Formerly in the Vietzen collection, the awl has good polish and length. Christian County, Kentucky. Pete Timoch collection. **$100.00.**

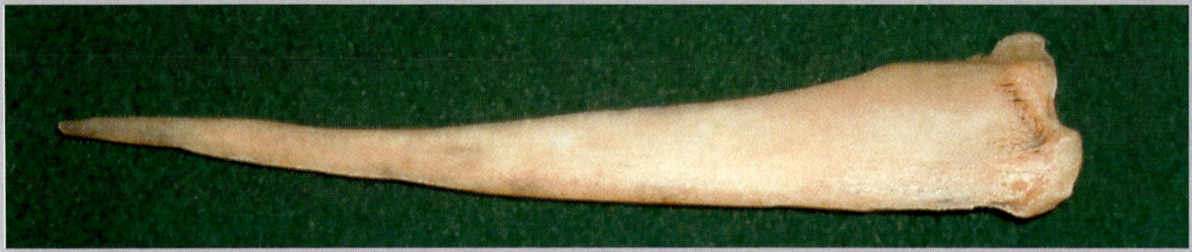

Bone awl, 5½" long, deer bone. The awl is ex-collection Noel and was found in Casey County, Kentucky. Keith and Rhonda Dodge collection, Michigan. **$85.00.**

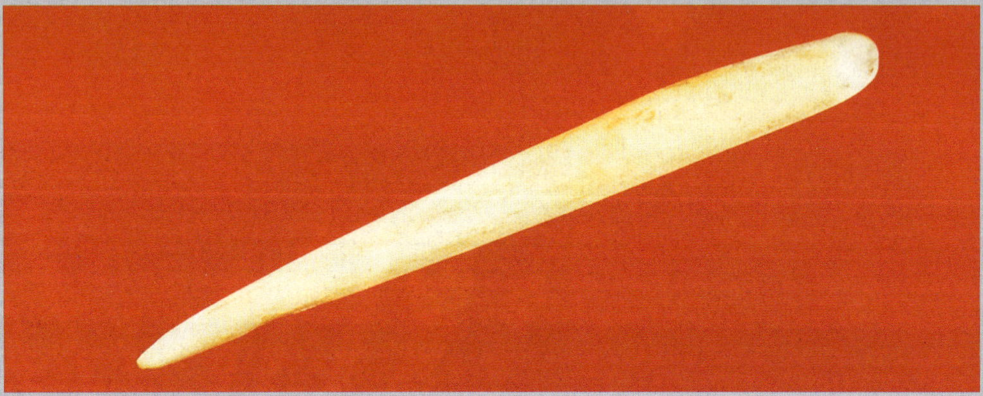

Awl or pin, bone with rounded cross-section, 3⅝". This artifact is highly polished and was found in Kentucky. Private collection. **$20.00.**

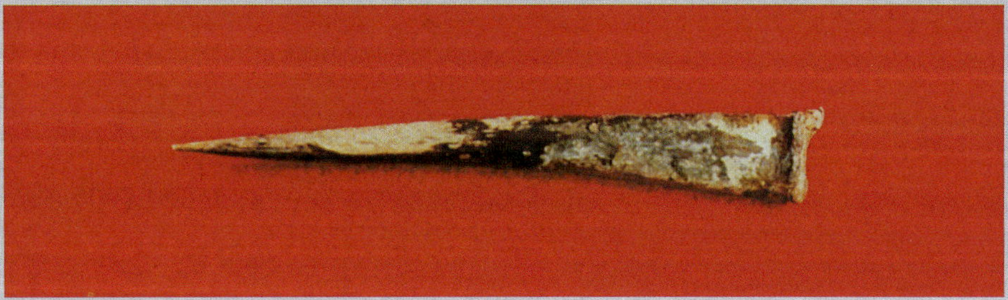

Hairpin or awl, bone, pointed tip, 2¾". From Woodland or Mississippian times, this solid example is ex-collection Vietzen. Ohio-Kentucky region. Pete Timoch collection. **$100.00 – 150.00.**

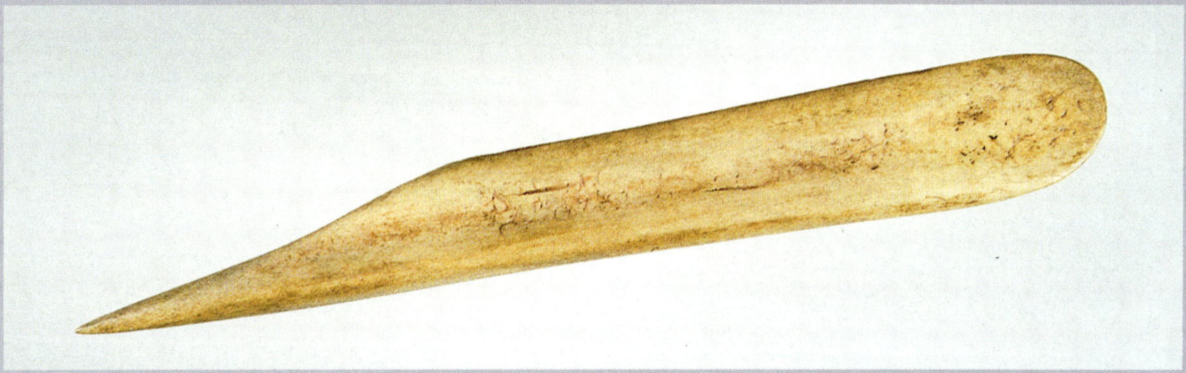

Awl or spatula tool, Mississippian period, 5¹¹⁄₁₆". The bone is solid and heavy, with high overall polish. Kentucky. Fred Winegardner collection. **$100.00.**

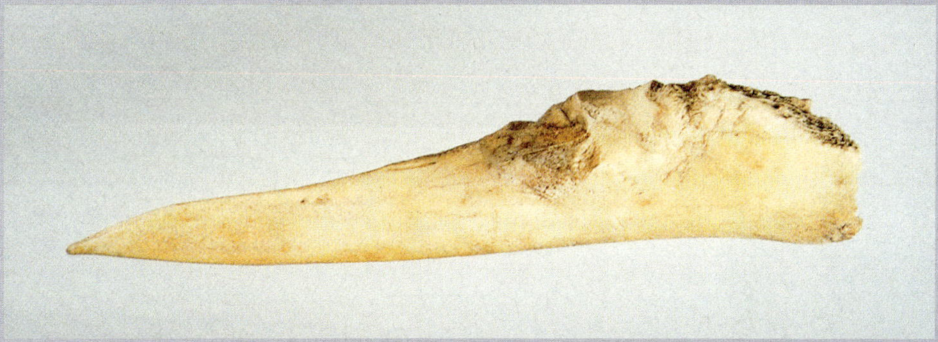

Awl, deer bone, good polish along shaft, 4 ⅜" long. Made from an ulna, the trigger portion was removed. Ohio. Fred Winegardner collection. **$40.00.**

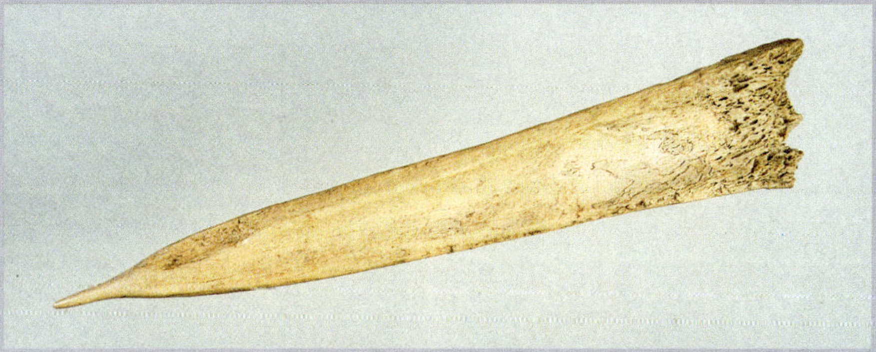

Awl, split deer bone, 3⅞". The tip has an abrupt taper, and the Fort Ancient artifact was found in southern Ohio. Fred Winegardner collection. **$30.00.**

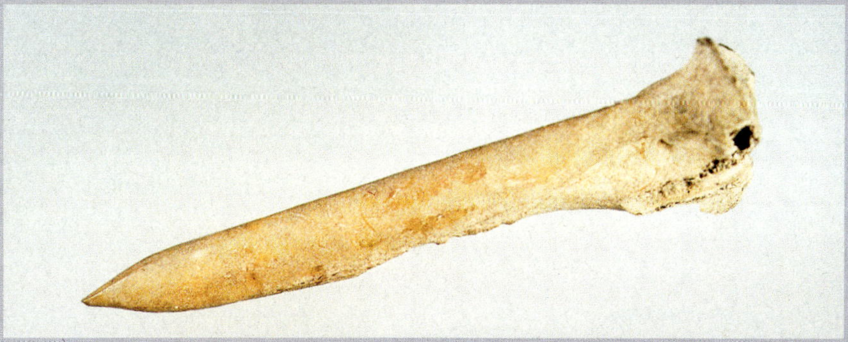

Awl, probably wild turkey bone, 3⁷⁄₁₆". Mississippian (Whittlesey) in time, the awl is from Tuscarawas County, Ohio. Fred Winegardner collection. **$20.00.**

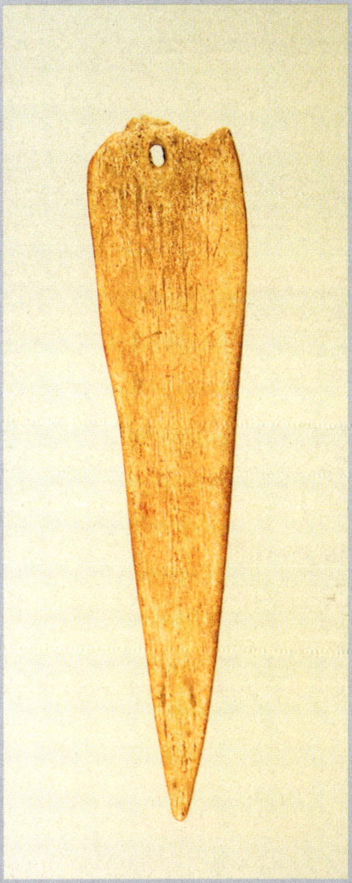

Awl or needle, with small, elongated eye, wide and flat bone, 3⅛". Made of deer bone, it was found in Kentucky. **$20.00.**

Awls

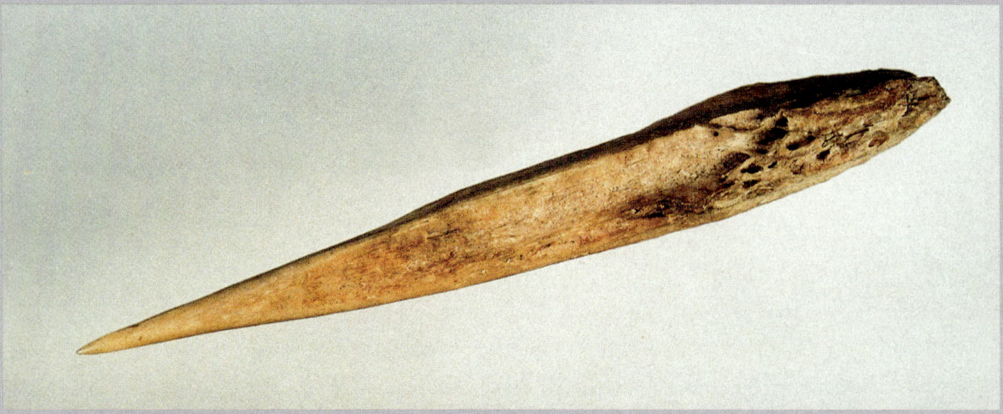

Awl, split deer bone, polished shaft. It is 4½" long, from a Fort Ancient site in southern Ohio. Fred Winegardner collection. **$30.00.**

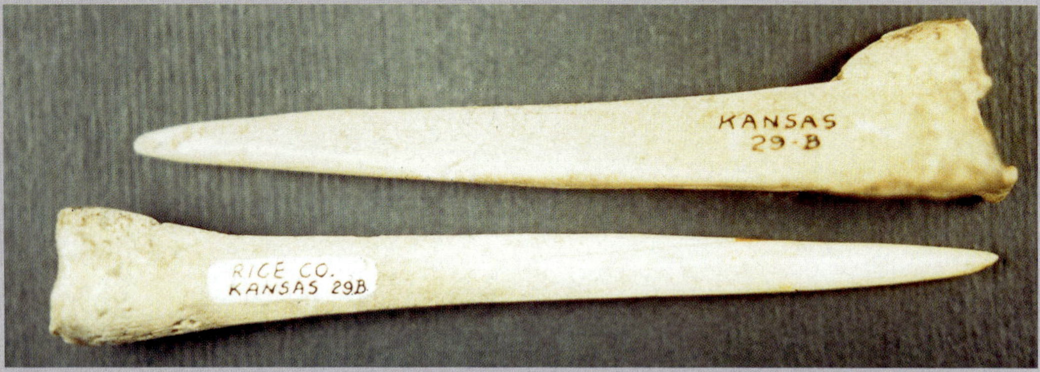

Bone daggers or large awls, probably buffalo (bison), fine condition. They were found in Rice County, Kansas. Lee Hallman collection, Pennsylvania. Top, **$50.00.** Bottom, **$65.00.**

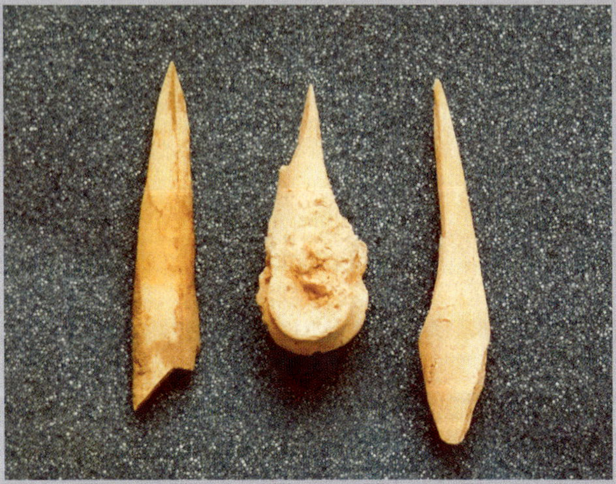

Bone splinter awls, Lamoka phase of the Middle Archaic (3000 – 2500 BC), 1⅞ to 2½" long. Schuyler County, New York. Dave Summers collection, Victor, New York. Each, **$20.00.**

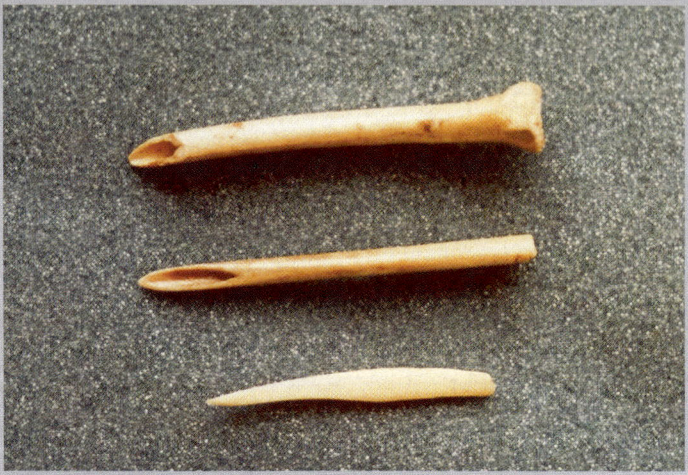

Round bone awls, highly polished surfaces, 2¼ to 3⅛" long. They are Brewerton phase of the Late Archaic, ca. 1600 BC. Cayuga County, New York. Dave Summers collection, Victor, New York. Each, **$15.00 – 35.00.**

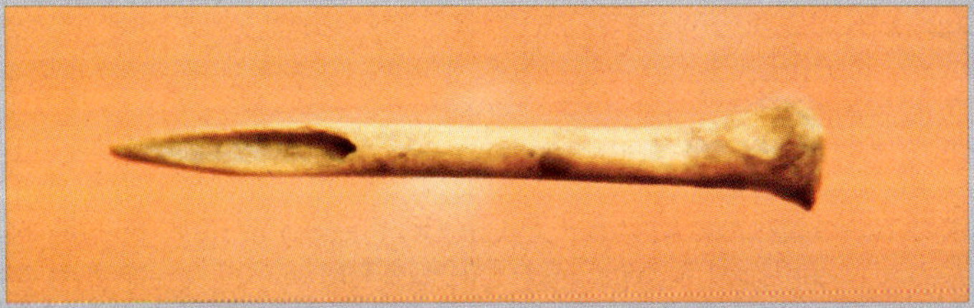

Awl, lynx tibia, 3⅛" long. It is Lamoka phase from the Middle Archaic and came from near Tyrone, Schuyler County, New York. Dave Summers collection, Victor, New York. **$65.00.**

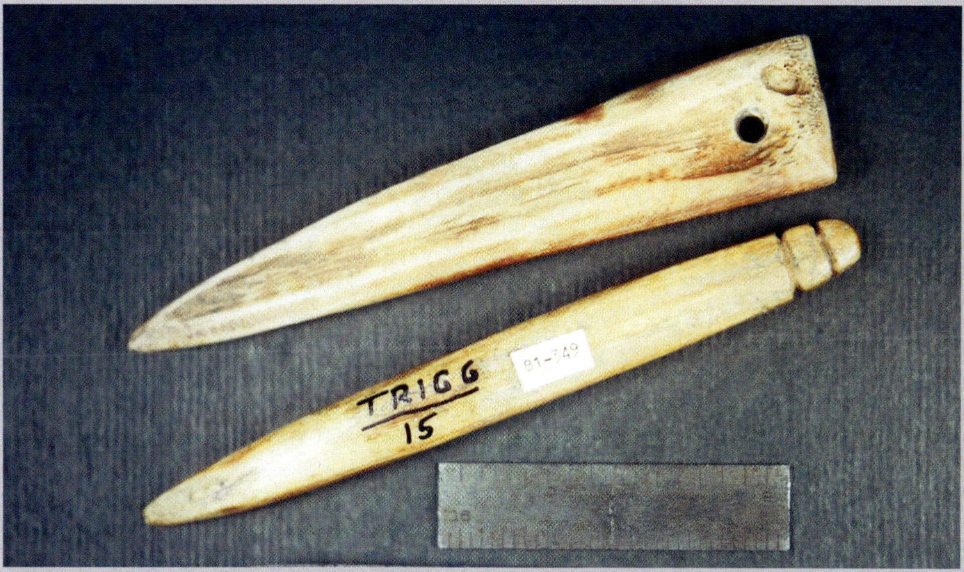

Bone artifacts, both from Trigg County, Kentucky. Upper, wide awl or dagger; Lower, decorative bone awl or pin. Lee Hallman collection, Pennsylvania. Dagger, **$125.00;** pin, **$150.00.**

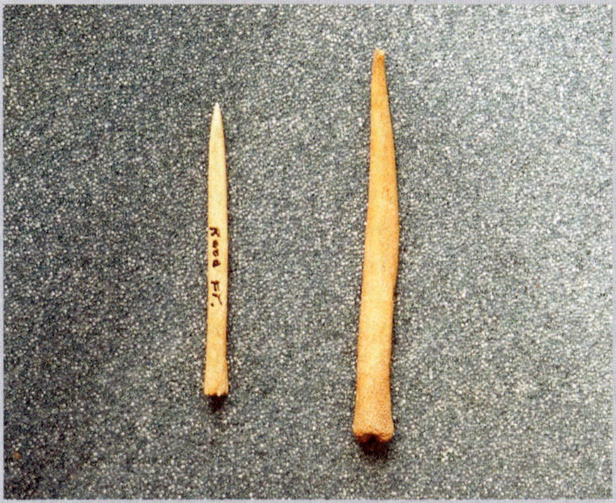

Awls, narrow joint bones. Iroquois phase, ca. AD 1540–1560. They are 2 and 2⅝" long, respectively, and were found near Richmond Mills, Ontario County, New York. Dave Summers collection, Victor, New York. Each, **$20.00.**

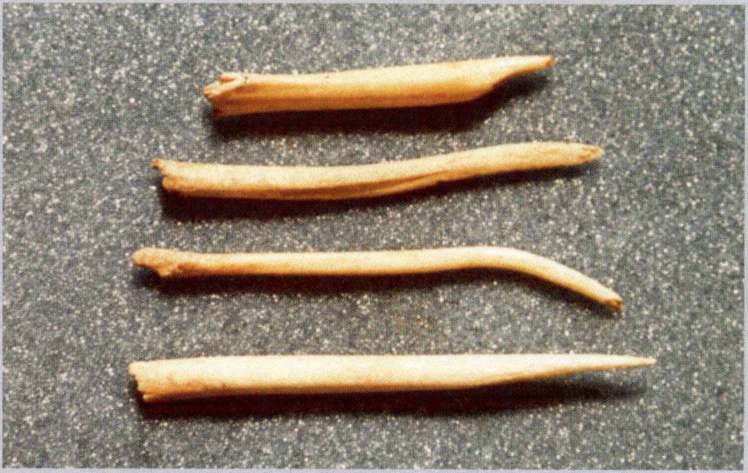

Bone awls, 3½ to 4¾", historic Iroquois (Seneca), ca. 1650 – 1675. Found near Honeoye Falls, they are from Monroe County, New York. Dave Summers collection, Victor, New York. Each, **$20.00 – 40.00.**

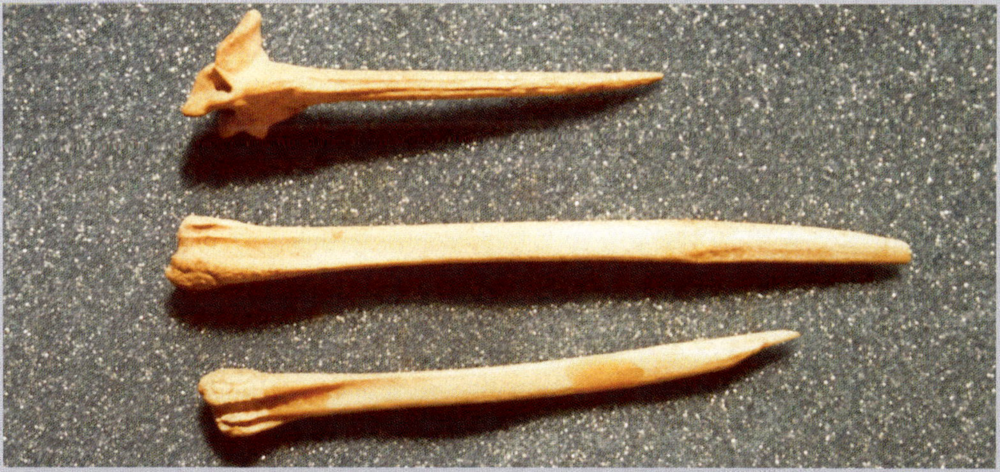

Joint bone awls or punches, 3¼ to 5⅛" long, historic Iroquois (Seneca), ca. AD 1650 – 1675. These artifacts came from near Honeoye Falls, Monroe County, New York. Dave Summers collection, Victor, New York. Top, **$45.00;** middle, **$60.00;** bottom, **$55.00.**

Awls

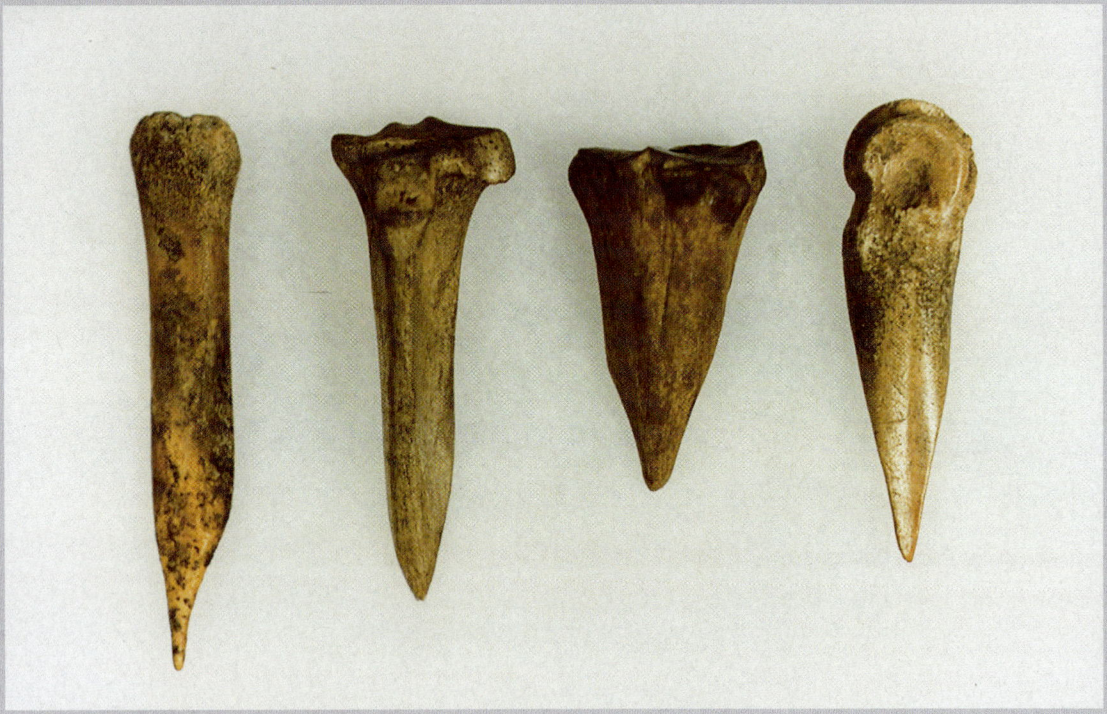

Awls, probably Late Woodland, animal leg bones, longest is 3¼". The bone joints have been left intact to form part of the handle. Ex-collection Vietzen. The left specimen is from Christian County, Kentucky, while the remainder are from northern Ohio. Pete Timoch collection. Each, **$50.00.**

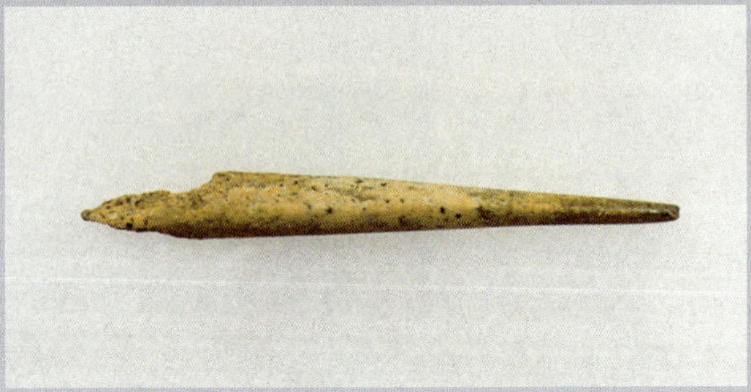

Awl, split animal bone, Late Archaic to Woodland, highly polished and spotted with age. It is 3¼" long and the wider end was gnawed by a rodent for nutrients in the material. The awl was in the Vietzen collection and came from Christian County, Kentucky. Pete Timoch collection. **$20.00.**

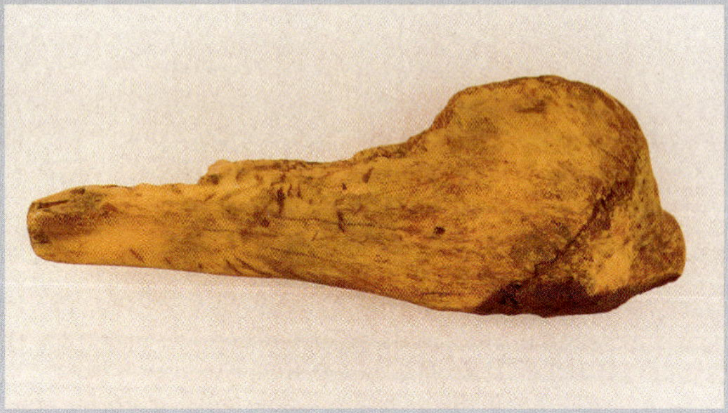

Awl, Late Archaic to Woodland, deer bone that has been ground to shape. Well-used and with blunted tip, it is 3¼" and ex-collection Vietzen. Christian County, Kentucky. John Timoch collection. **$25.00.**

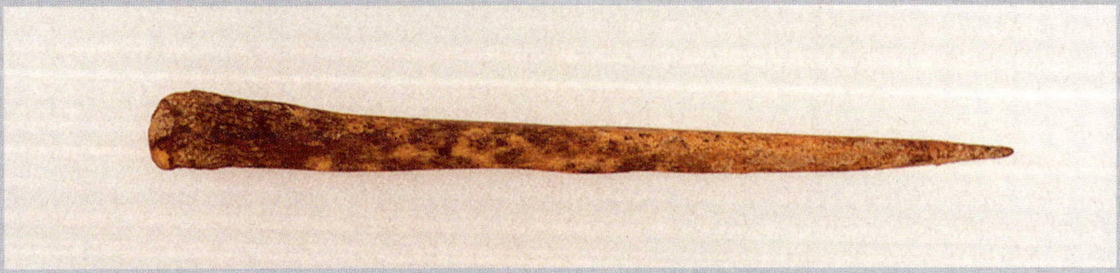

Awl, split bone, 4⅞", pointed tip and gray spotting over brown patination. Ex-collection Vietzen, the awl is Late Archaic to Woodland in time. Christian County, Kentucky. Pete Timoch collection. **$100.00.**

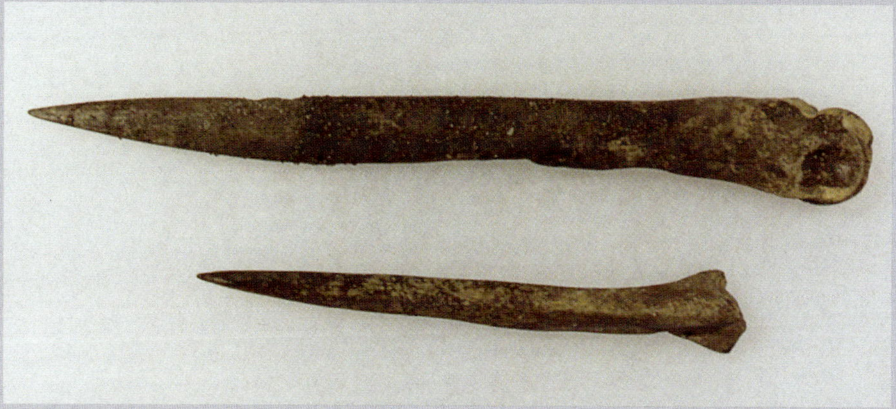

Awls, split deer leg bones, from the Ohio-Kentucky region. Large, 7", bone split full-length, tabular cross-section, reverse with bone groove. **$100.00.** Smaller, 4⅝", most of length polished, bone groove ground away and polished to a black and brown marbled finish. Both are ex-collection Vietzen. Pete Timoch collection. **$100.00.**

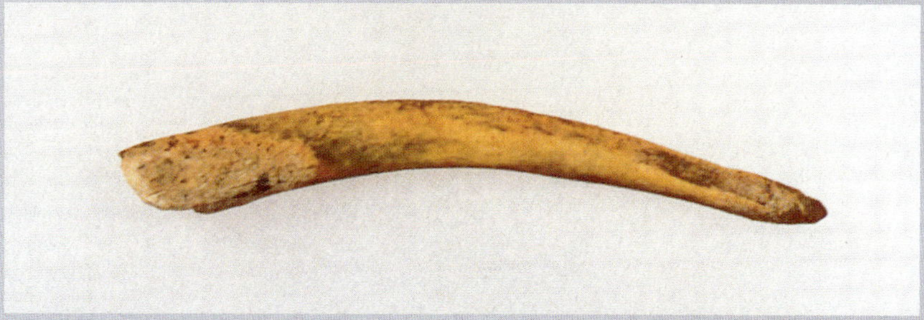

Awl, made from the rib bone of a large animal, 3⅝" along the outside curve. Late Archaic to Woodland, it is ex-collection Vietzen. Christian County, Kentucky. Pete Timoch collection. **$50.00.**

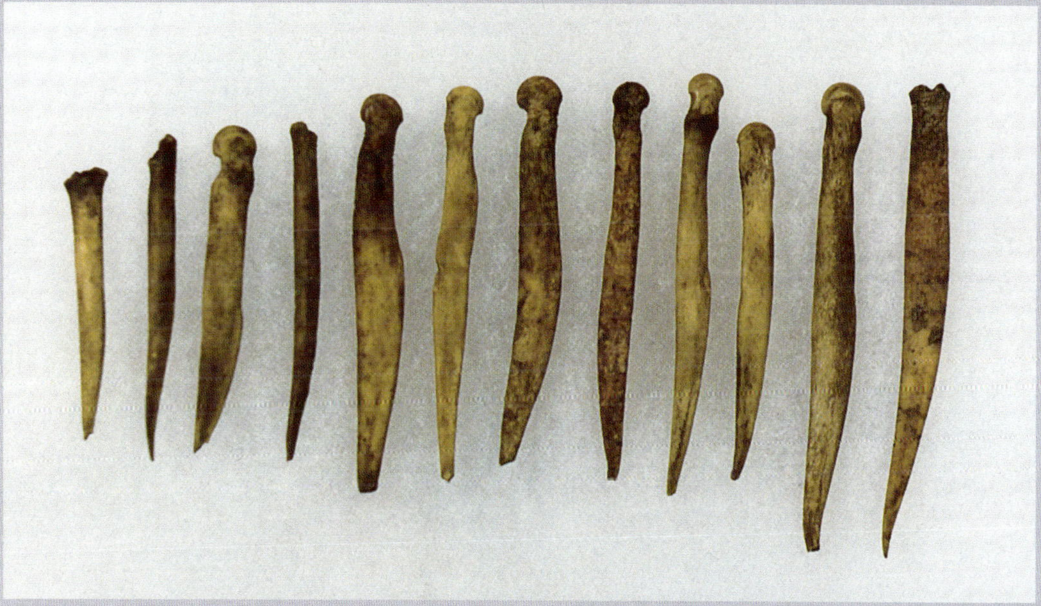

Awls, irregular to rounded ends, longest is 3". The natural contours of the bones were largely followed, making these multi-purpose tools that could be used as pins, perforators, or toothpicks. At least one account suggests use as skewers for removing food from the fire or pottery vessels. Once owned by Col. Vietzen, they are from the Ohio-Kentucky region. Pete Timoch collection. Each, **$20.00 – 40.00.**

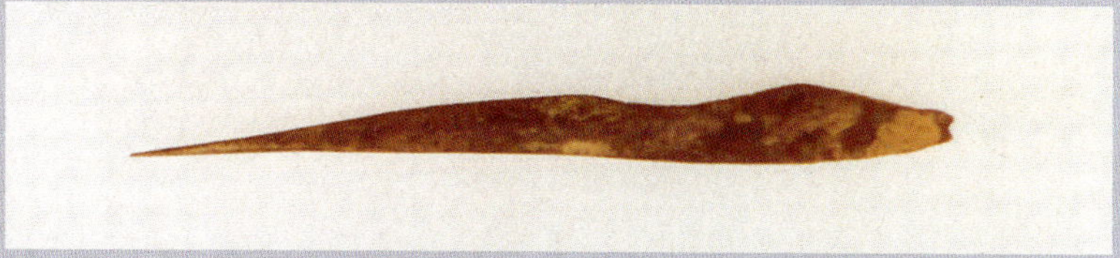

Needle awl, split bird bone, Late Woodland. It is 3½" long and ex-collection Vietzen. The artifact is pictured in Vietzen's book *The Saga of Glover's Cave*, page 181. A fine piece, it is surprising the tip is still intact. Lost City region, Kentucky. Pete Timoch collection. **$200.00.**

Awls

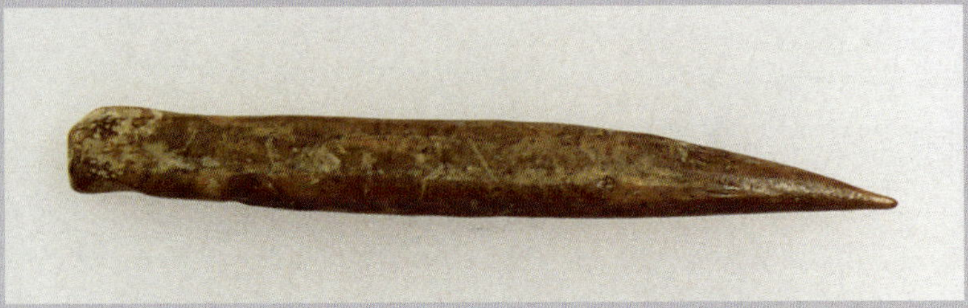

Pin or awl, split deer leg bone, Woodland period, 3⅝". It is entirely polished and has a brown and tan marble-like finish. Owned by Col. Vietzen, it came from Christian County, Kentucky. Pete Timoch collection. **$50.00 – 75.00.**

Awl, bird bone, 3¾" long. Well-shaped, the lower portion is polished from use. Midwestern. Don Casto collection. **$25.00.**

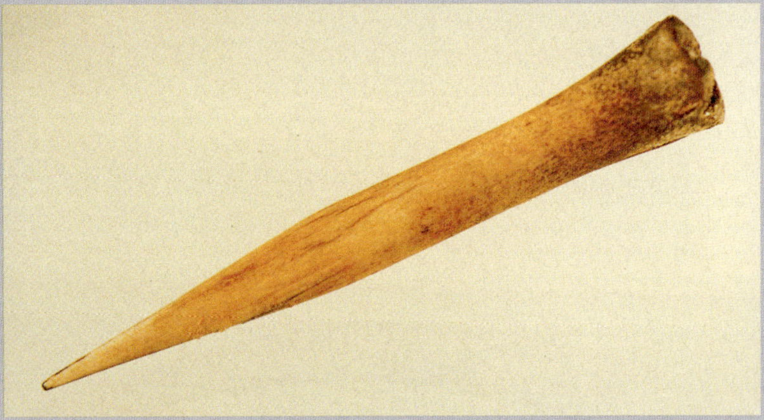

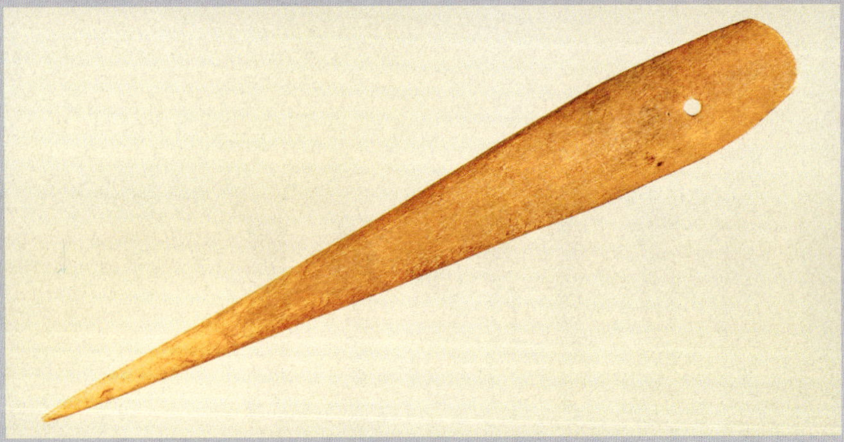

Awl, lower shaft region near tip (off-white color) with high polish. The small hole near the wide end was made by a previous collector, who had this and other bone artifacts attached by a string loop. This well-shaped awl is 4" long and came from Kentucky. Private collection. **$25.00.**

Awl, short and thick with a very pointed tip, 3⁷⁄₁₆". This piece, with high lower shaft polish, has been chemically stabilized. Kentucky. Private collection. **$20.00.**

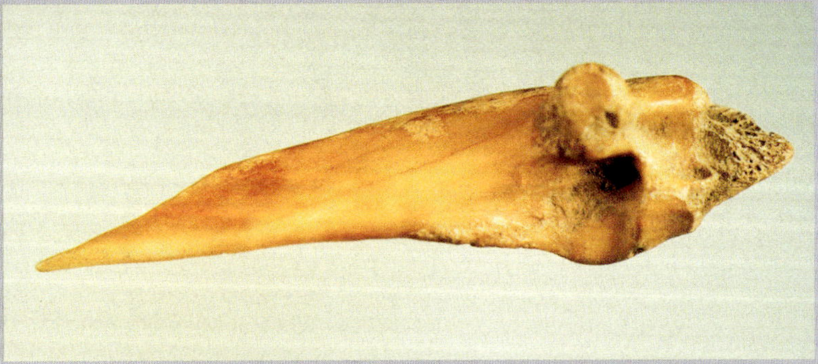

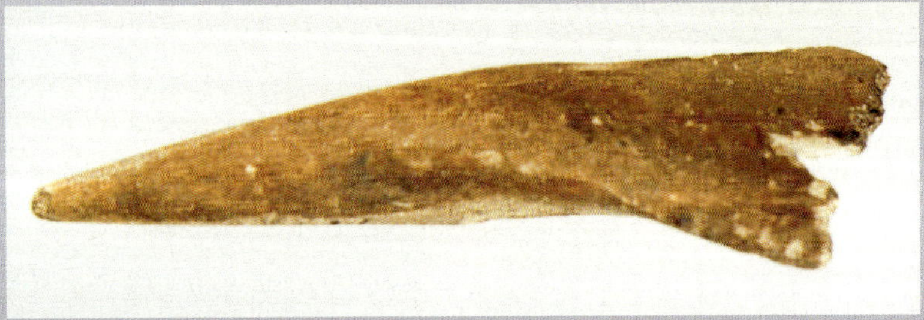

Awl, Mississippian period, split deer bone, 3⅝". This particular example is patinated a rich medium brown. Southern Ohio. Private collection. **$12.00.**

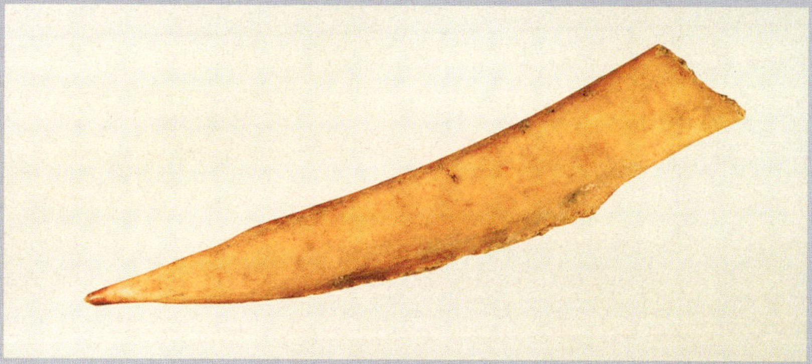

Awl or perforator, probably deer rib bone section, 3⁵⁄₁₆". It has considerable use-polish, especially near the tip. Kentucky. Private collection. **$12.00.**

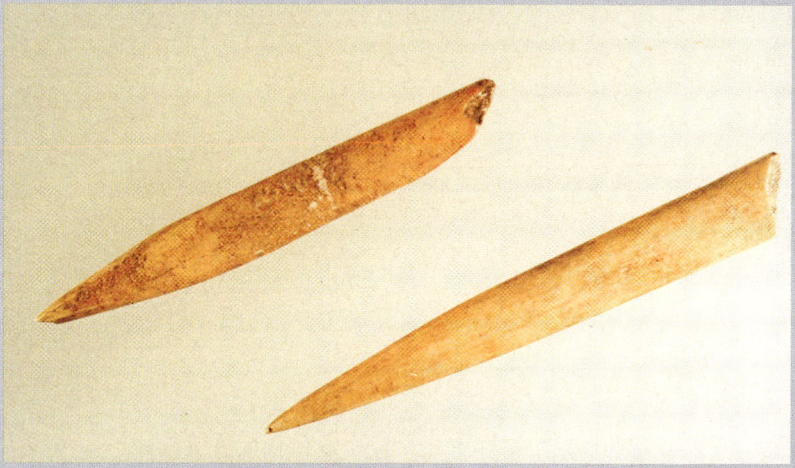

Awls, bone splinters, longest with polish, both Midwestern. Don Casto collection. Long, 3⅝". **$15.00.** Shorter, weathered, **$10.00.**

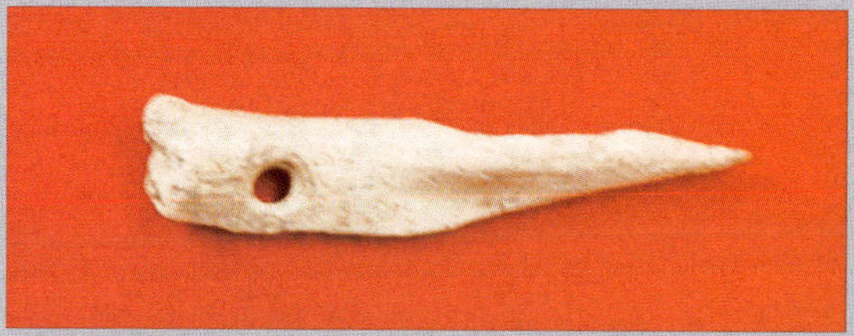

Needle or awl, Woodland period, bone or antler, 2½" long. Such artifacts could be used as wide needles, or, the hole may have been used for cord attachment so that relatively small awls like this did not become lost. Kentucky. Pete Timoch collection. **$75.00.**

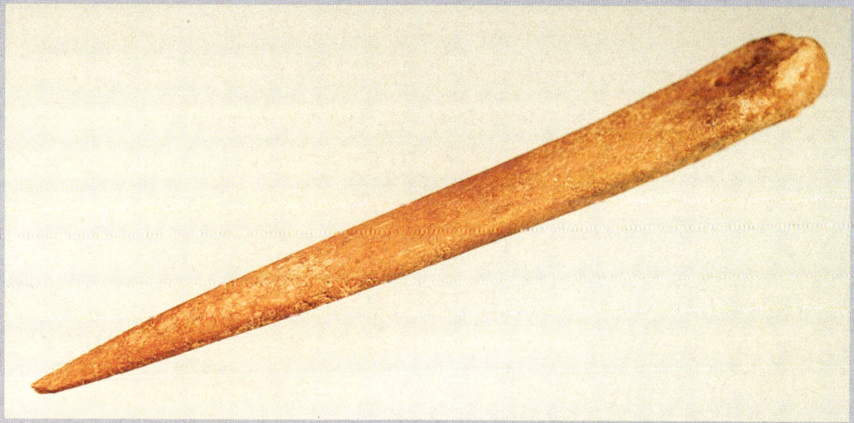

Awl, deer bone, good taper, 4¾". The surface of this artifact is weathered, giving it a checked and rough texture. Kentucky Private collection. **$20.00.**

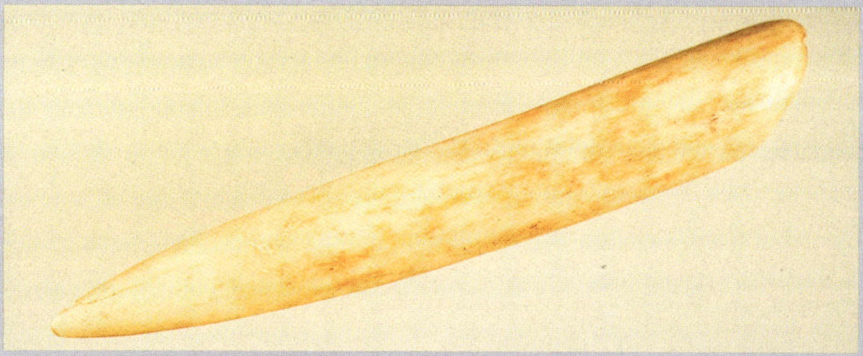

Awl, ivory-like finish on section of deer bone, high wear/use polish. The awl is 3¹⁵⁄₁₆" long and was found in Kentucky. Private collection. **$15.00.**

Awls

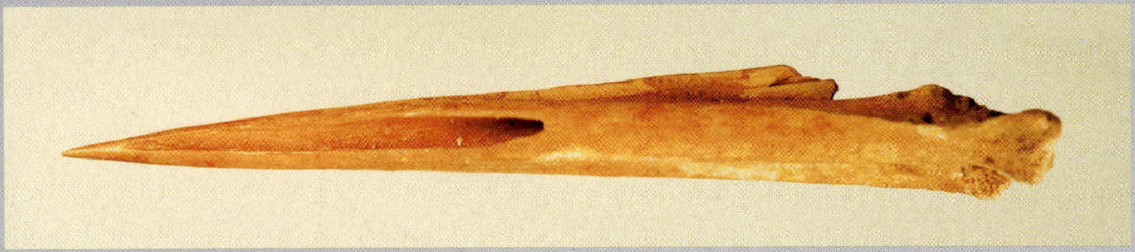

Awl, made from a large bird bone, length is 5 7/16". The lower shaft portion has heavy use-polish. This fine example came from Kentucky. Private collection. **$40.00.**

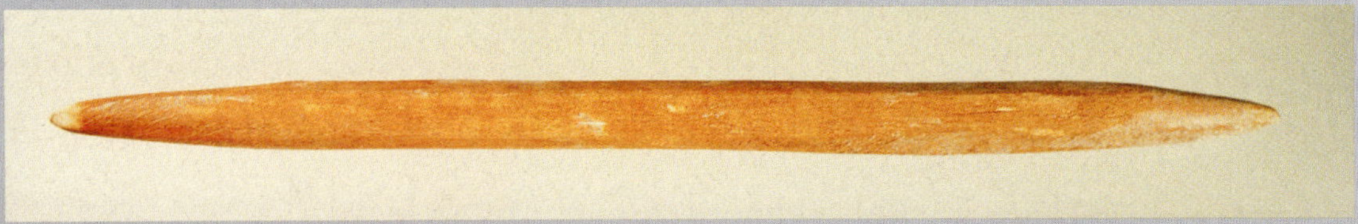

Awl or pin, double-tipped, probably deer bone, lower left tip reshaped recently as indicated by color change (patina disturbance) and more abrupt taper. Modern work lowers the value. It is 5 11/16" long, solid, and heavy. Private collection. **$12.00.**

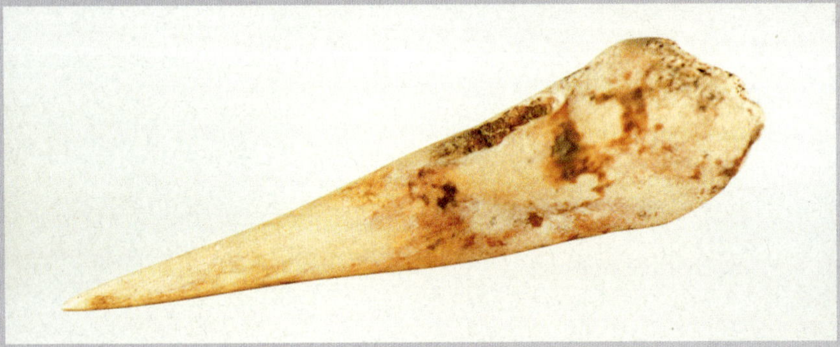

Awl, polished bone, Fort Ancient people of the late prehistoric. The awl is 3¾", from southern Ohio. Private collection. **$30.00.**

Awl, large hollow bird bone, highly polished from use, gray patina. This is probably a wild turkey leg bone (see Smith's *Prehistoric Ethnology of a Kentucky Site*, plate XXXIV nos. 3 and 4). The awl is 3⅞" long and Fort Ancient in origin. Southern Ohio. Private collection. **$45.00.**

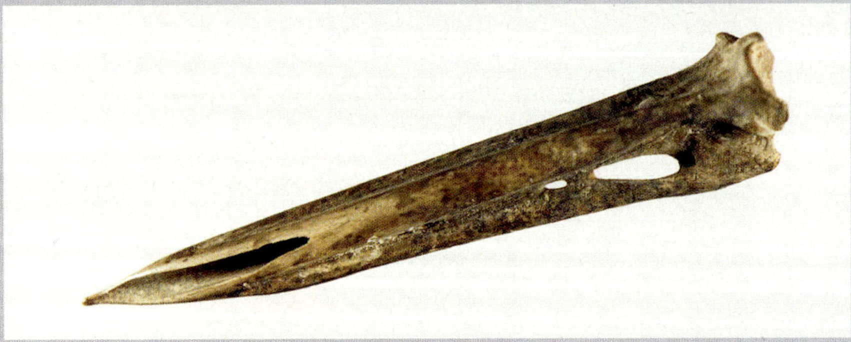

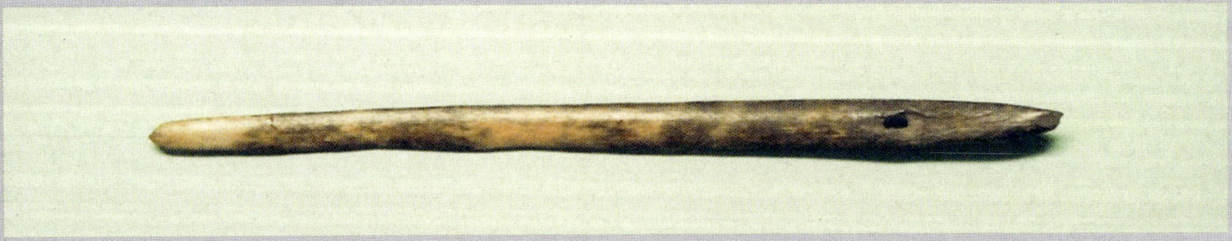

Weaving shuttle, mammal rib bone, 5/16 x 5¼" long, 1/16 inch thick. The shuttle is highly polished and the base has an oblong hole. The artifact came from Weber County, northern Utah. Dann Russell collection, Utah. **$50.00.**

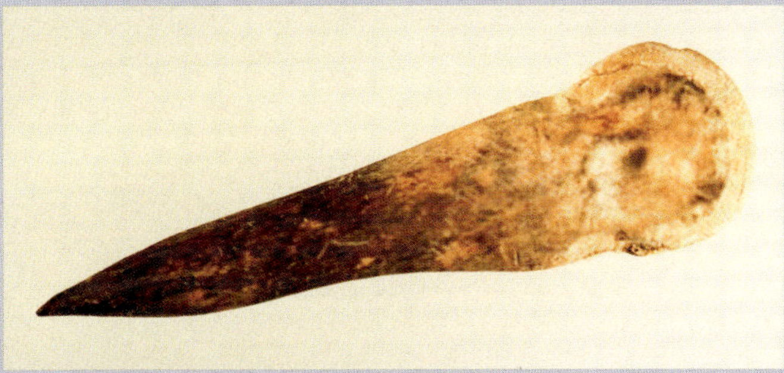

Awl, large animal bone, 3" long. The darkened color is probably fire-scorching, and most of the shaft is polished. Midwestern. Don Casto collection. **$20.00.**

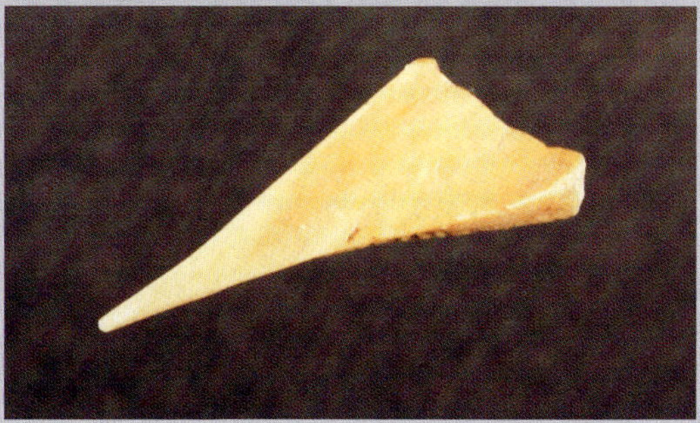

Awl, thick bone chip with polished tip, 1½" long. The awl is Fort Ancient and was found in southern Ohio. Private collection. **$10.00.**

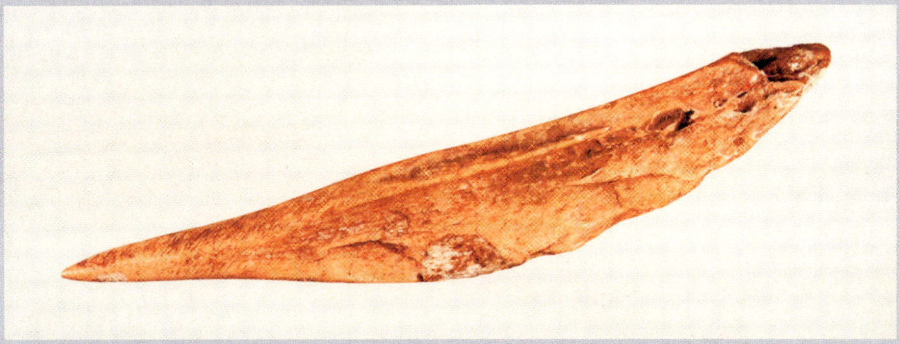

Awl, bone splinter from large animal, 4¼" long. The bone wall is about 5⁄16 inch thick and may be from an elk. Tennessee. Private collection. **$25.00.**

Awl or hairpin, polished deer bone with an ivory-like yellowish sheen, 3 11⁄16". It is from the Midwest. Don Casto collection. **$45.00.**

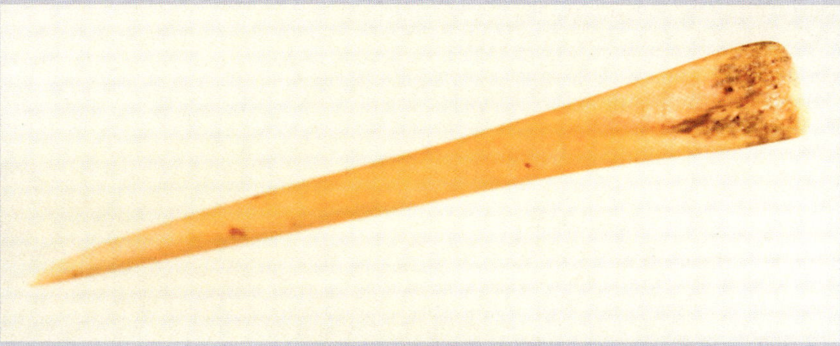

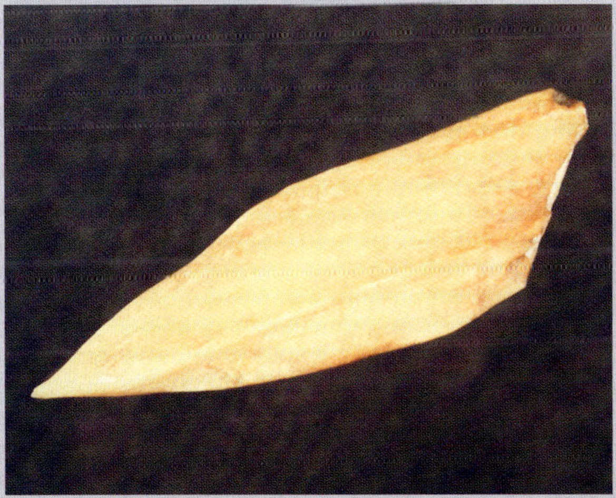

Awl, thin chip of animal bone, 2⅝" long. Chemically stabilized, it is Fort Ancient in origin. Southern Ohio. Private collection. **$10.00.**

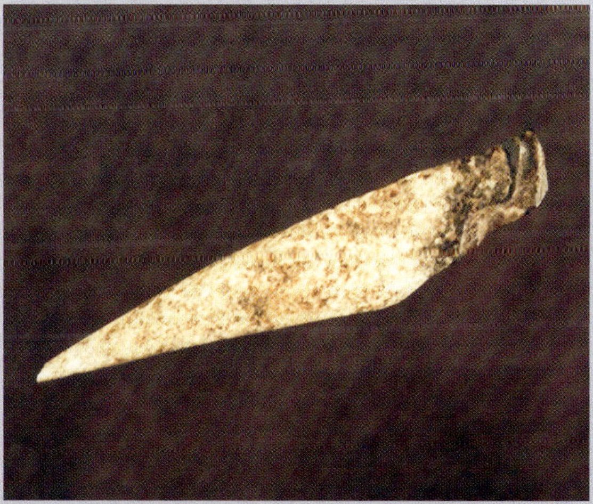

Awl, splinter of thick bone, gray and near-black patination, 2⅜". It came from a Fort Ancient site in southern Ohio. Private collection. **$6.00.**

Awls

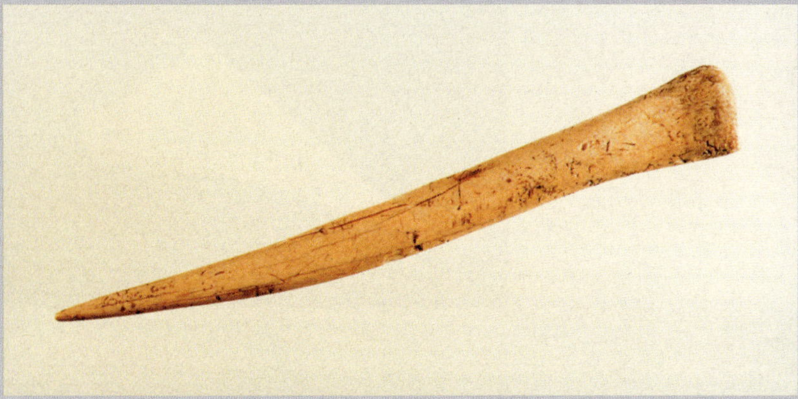

Awl, curved and polished bone with rounded base. It is 3¾" long, from the Midwest. Don Casto collection. **$25.00.**

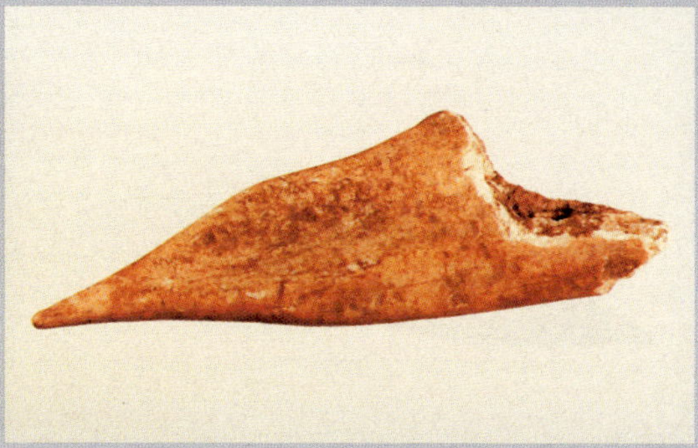

Awl or perforator, salmon-pink patination and tapered tip, 2¼" long. It was picked up in Kentucky. Private collection. **$10.00.**

Awls, large animal bone broken and glued, 3¾". The shorter awl is a small animal bone, lightly weathered, 2⅝" long. Kentucky. Private collection. Each, **$7.00.**

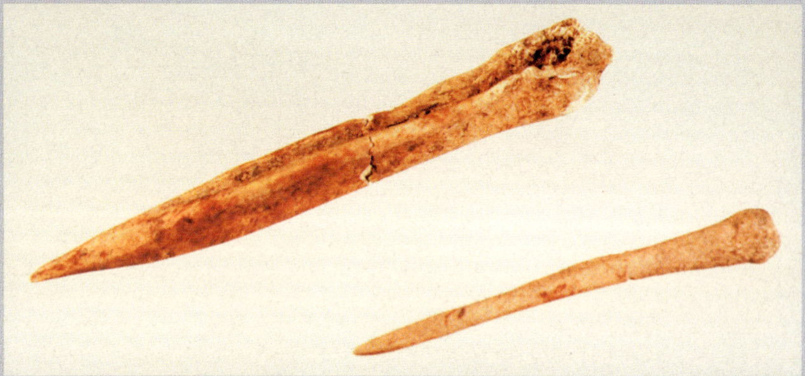

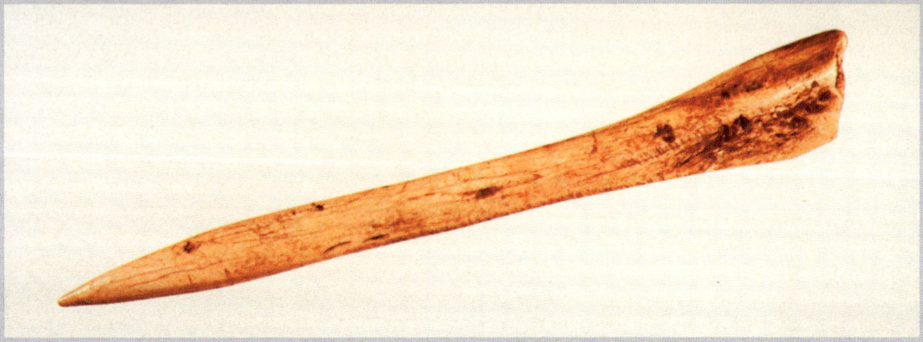

Awl, thick and heavy bone, well-polished shaft and tip, 4¼" long. It was found in Tennessee. Private collection. **$20.00 – 25.00.**

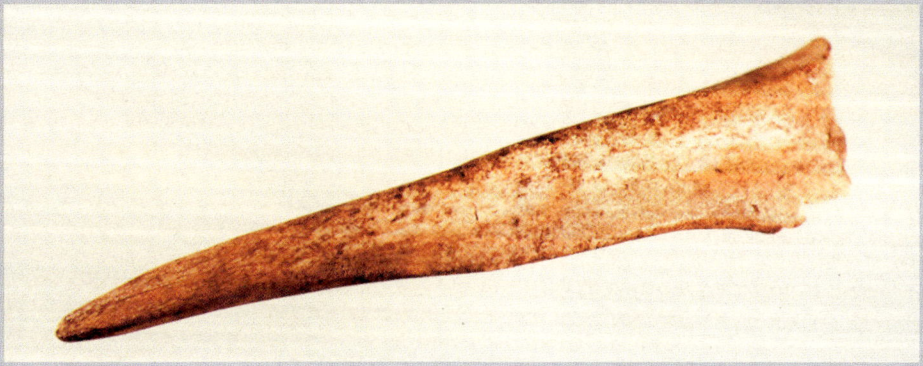

Awl or punch, weathered antler, brownish-gray patination. The example is 4¼" long and has had little modification. Tennessee. Private collection. **$8.00.**

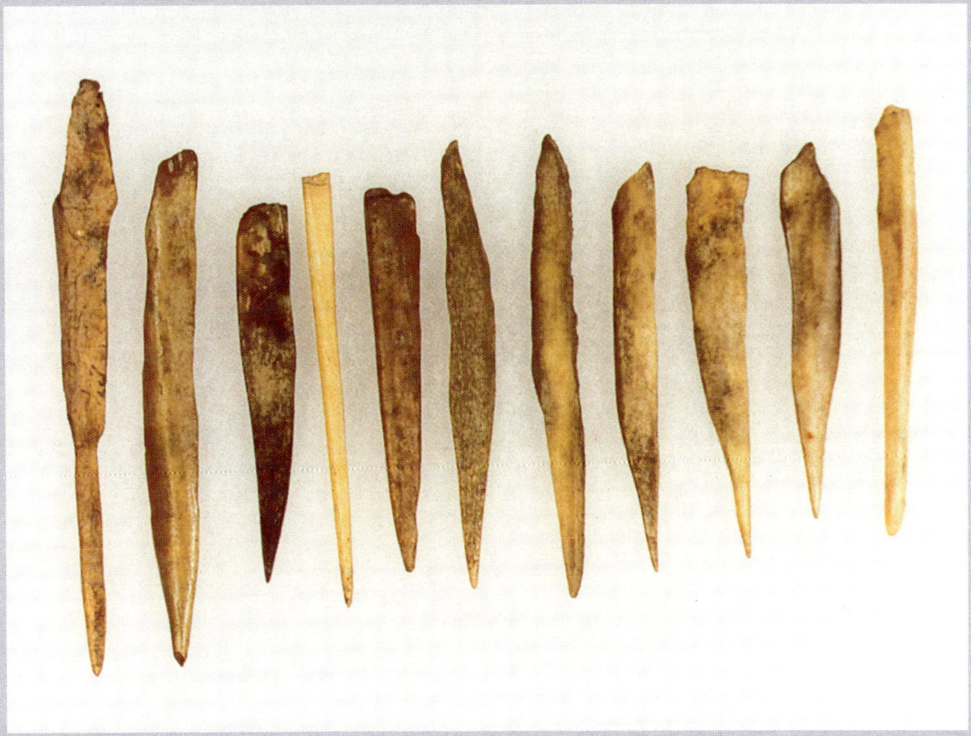

Awls, split animal bone, longest is 4¹¹⁄₁₆". This is an instructive grouping that illustrates the wide range of shapes for a fairly simple tool form. All have careful tip treatment and are from the Vietzen collection. They were found on sites in Ohio and Kentucky. Pete Timoch collection. Each, **$25.00 – 50.00.**

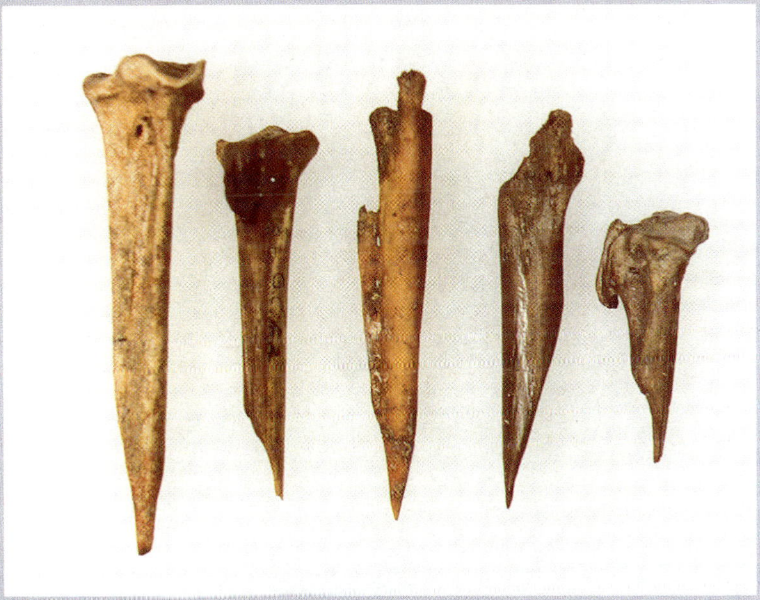

Awls, made from the leg bones of large birds, longest is 3½". Ex-collection Vietzen, origin is as follows: Left three awls, Kentucky, probably Woodland; right two awls, northern Ohio, Sandusky or Whittlesey peoples. Pete Timoch collection. Each, **$25.00 – 80.00.**

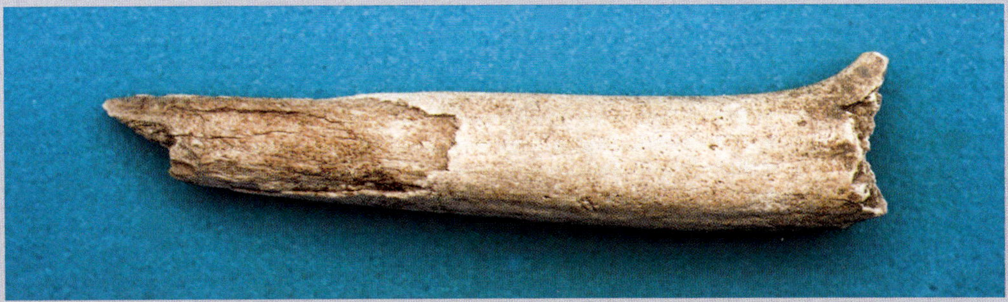

Awl fragment, Archaic or later, 1⅛ x 5". Harwood found it, and find-location is unknown. Collection of, and photograph by, Gary Henry, North Carolina. **$5.00.**

Awls

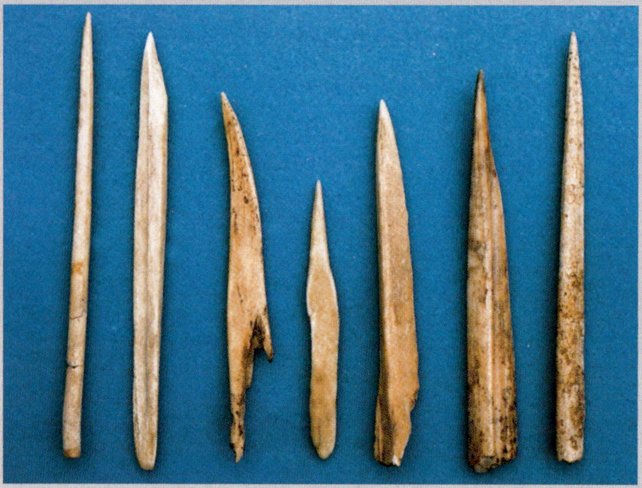

Group of seven awls, longest (far left) is ¼ x 5". Archaic or later, these are ex-collection Snyder. Meigs County, Tennessee. Collection of, and photograph by, Gary Henry, North Carolina. Each, **$8.00 – 30.00.**

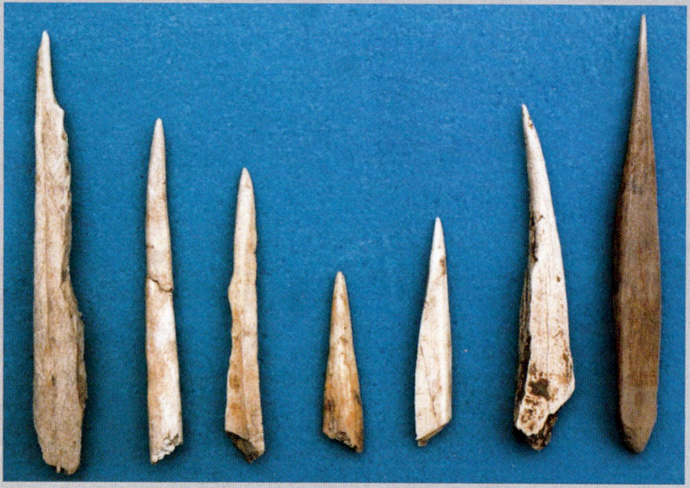

Group of seven awls, Archaic or later, longest (far right) is 7⁄16 x 3 11⁄16". Ex-collection Snyder, the awls came from Meigs County, Tennessee. Collection of, and photograph by, Gary Henry, North Carolina. Each, **$8.00 – 15.00.**

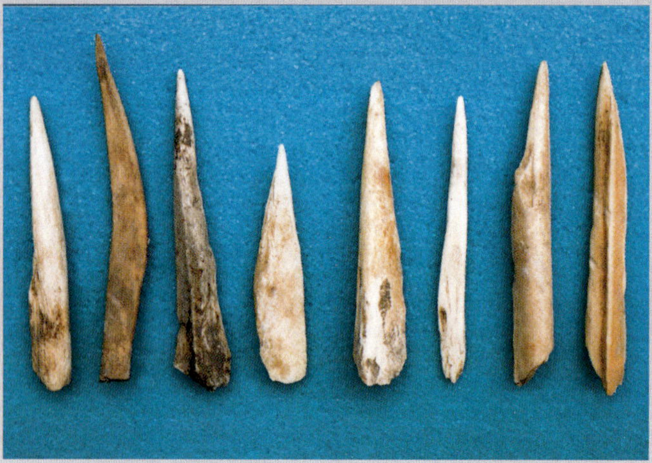

Group of eight bone awls, Archaic or later, longest (second from left) is 5⁄16 x 2½". These are ex-collection Snyder and were found in Meigs County, Tennessee. Collection of, and photograph by, Gary Henry, North Carolina. Each, **$8.00 – 15.00.**

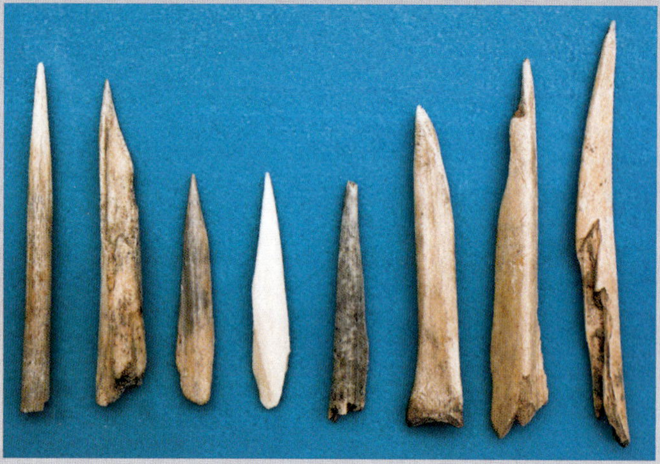

Group of eight bone awls, longest (far right) is 7⁄16 x 4¼". Archaic or later, they are ex-collection Snyder and were picked up in Meigs County, Tennessee. Collection of, and photograph by, Gary Henry, North Carolina. Each, **$8.00 – 15.00.**

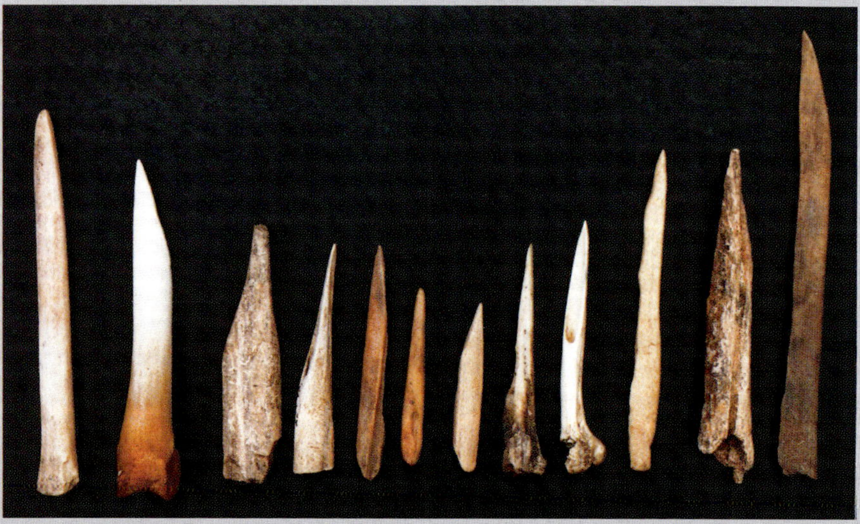

Group of awls, various bone materials, longest (far right) is ⅝ x 6⅝". Archaic period or later, these are ex-collection Snyder and came from Talladega County, Alabama. Collection of, and photograph by, Gary Henry, North Carolina. Each, **$8.00 – 65.00.**

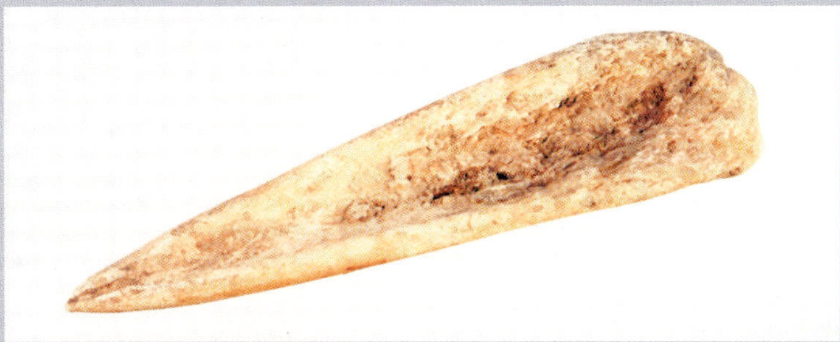

Awl, split deer bone, 3¼". Ex-collection Vietzen, it was found on a Fort Ancient site in southern Ohio. Fred Winegardner collection. **$20.00.**

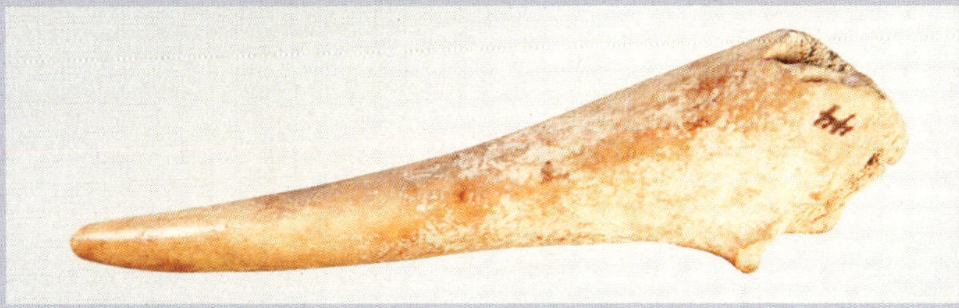

Tool, 3⅞" long, high polish for about one-half of length. It came from Kentucky. Fred Winegardner collection. **$15.00.**

Bone awls, Woodland period, 3 and 3½" long respectively. These awls were found in southwestern Iowa. Richard Krueger collection, Iowa. Sandra Krueger photograph. Each, **$20.00.**

Antler flaker, Woodland period, 5½" long. Well-shaped and polished, the flaker is from southwestern Iowa. Richard Krueger collection, Iowa. Sandra Krueger photograph. **$65.00.**

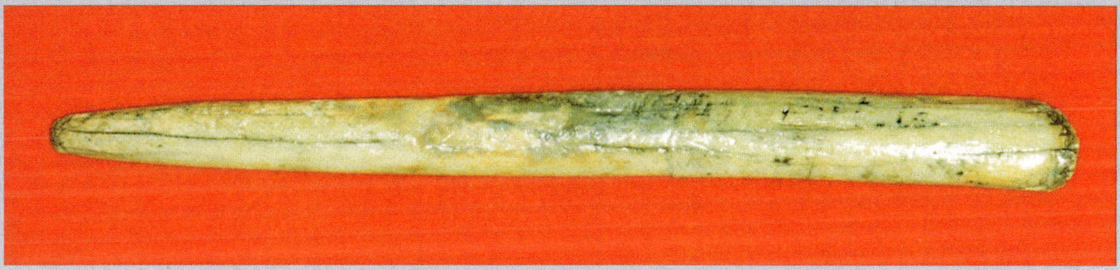

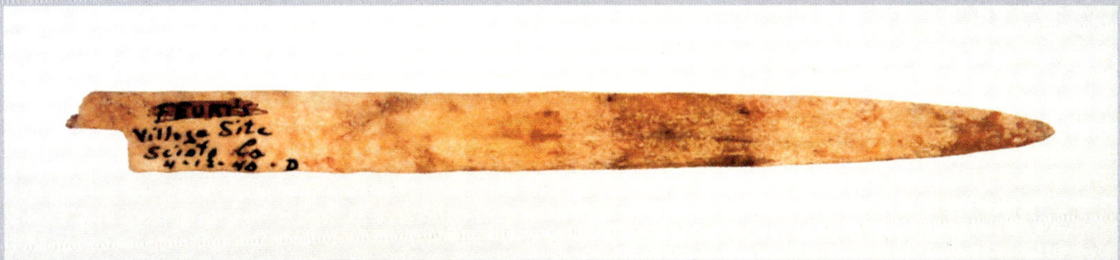

Bracelet or anklet strip, deer bone, 4¹⁵⁄₁₆". Extremely thin, it was collected in 1940. Southern Ohio. Fred Winegardner collection. **$75.00.**

Bone awl, highly polished overall, ⁵⁄₁₆ x 3¾" long. It has been cut at the basal end and was found in Weber County, northern Utah. Dann Russell collection, Utah. **$40.00.**

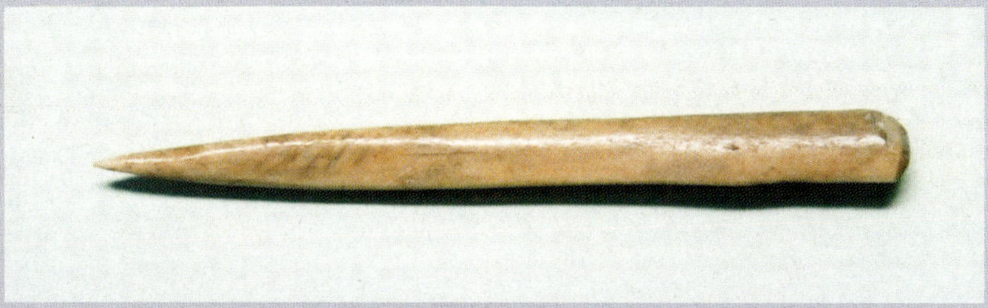

Awls

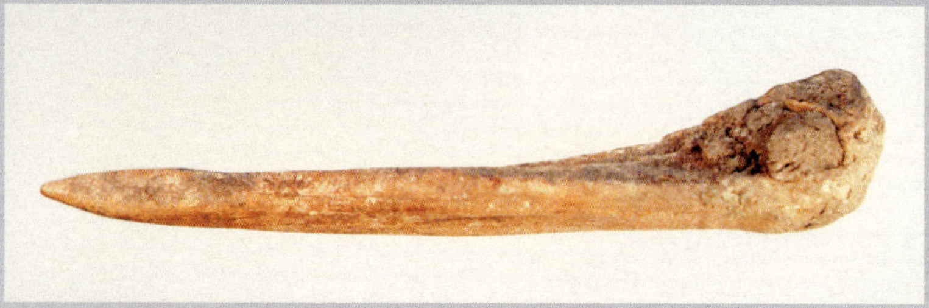

Awl, deer bone, ex-collection Vietzen. The awl, 3⅝" long, is from southern Ohio. Fred Winegardner collection. **$20.00.**

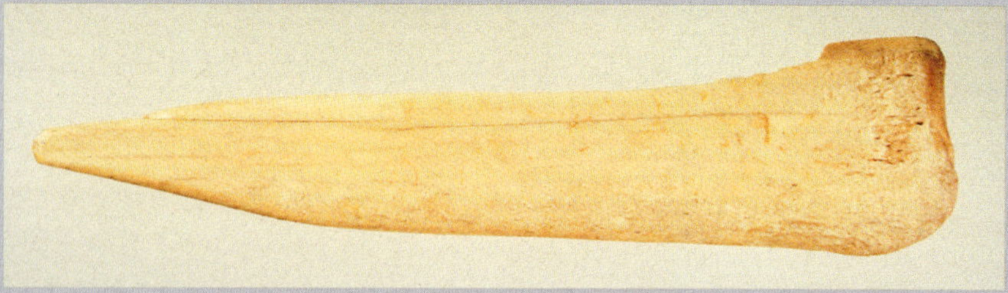

Splinter awl, wide animal bone, 4⅓₂" long. Found in Tennessee. Robin Fiser collection. **$25.00.**

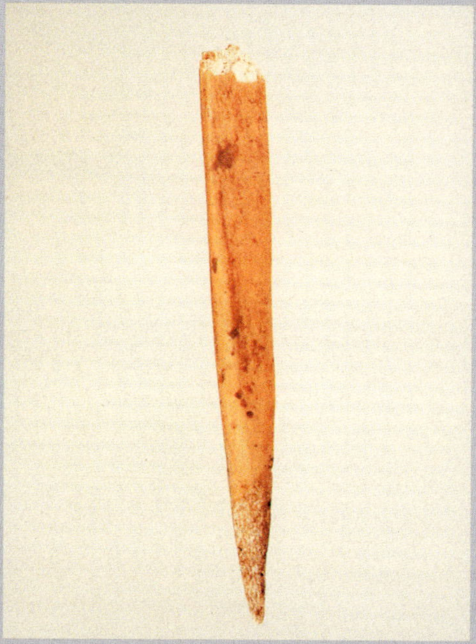

Bone awl, tip and lower shaft colored gray and orange-tan, bone interior is creamy white. Broken, the remainder is 2¾" long. Kentucky. Private collection. **$8.00.**

Awl or perforator, antler tine with hollowed base, 3½" long. This artifact is of special interest because it has many rodent teeth marks. Eastern Midwest. Fred Winegardner collection. **$15.00.**

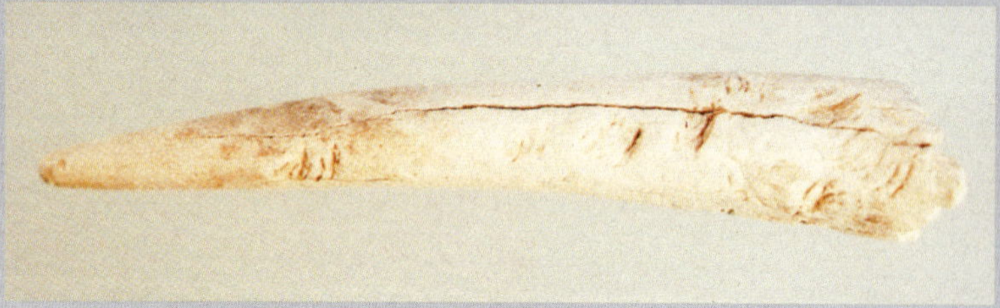

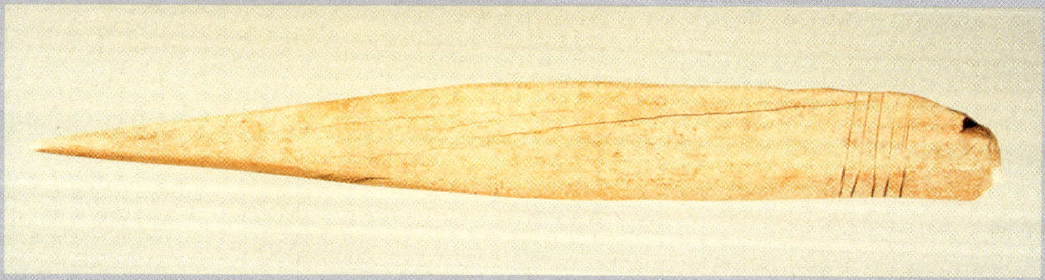

Awl, five incised decorative lines on the wide end, 4⅞" long. Such touches on awls are not common. Frankfort County, Alabama. Robin Fiser collection. **$85.00.**

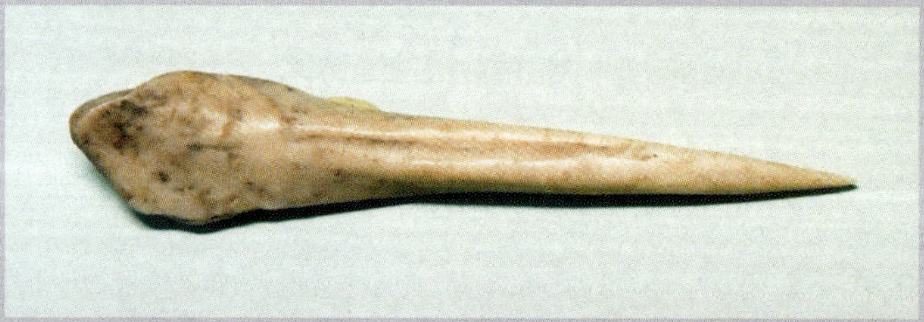

Awl, mammal bone, high polish and sharp tip. The maximum diameter is 5⁄16 inch and the awl is 3" long. It came from Box Elder County, northern Utah. Dann Russell collection, Utah. **$40.00.**

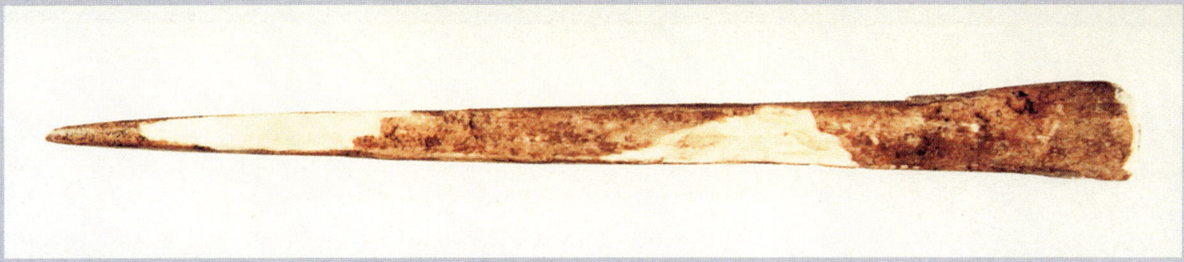

Awl, exfoliated bone surface, 5¾" long. This awl came from Kentucky. Robin Fiser collection. **$45.00.**

Awl, solid and ivory-like, 3⅝". This fine example came from Alabama. Robin Fiser collection. **$50.00.**

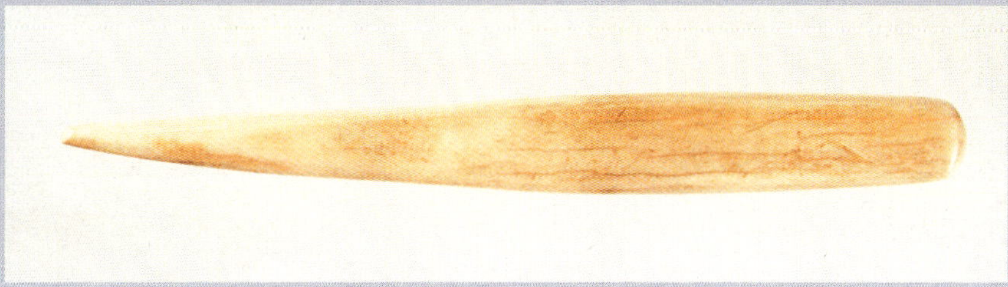

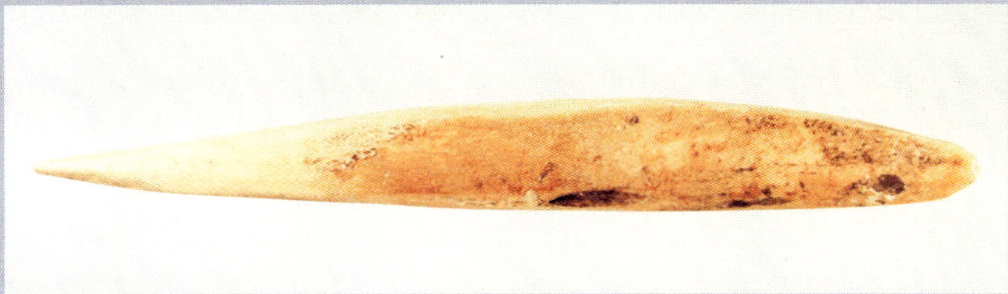

Awl, thick bone, 4⅛" long. The lower portion is well-polished and the artifact came from the Nashville area, Tennessee. Robin Fiser collection. **$50.00.**

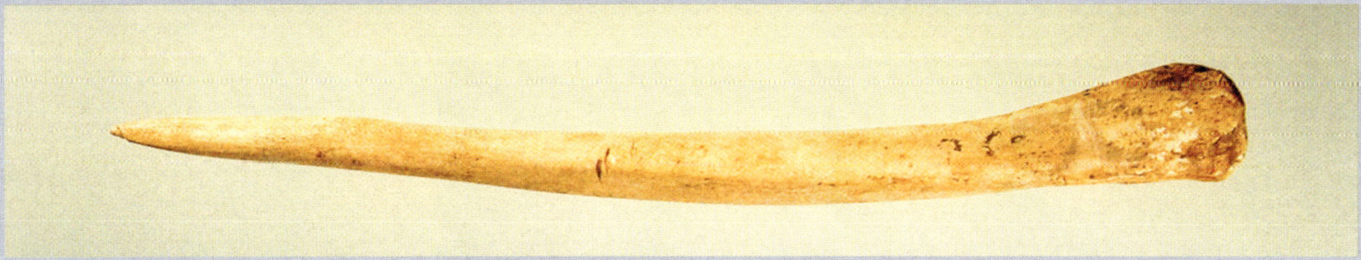

Hairpin or dagger, bear penis bone, 6½" long. This is a rare material for artifacts of any kind, and this example came from the Augusta area, Kentucky. Robin Fiser collection. **$150.00 – 200.00.**

Awl, base is rounded and smoothed, 3½" long. Made of split deer bone, this polished example is from Kentucky. Fred Winegardner collection. **$45.00.**

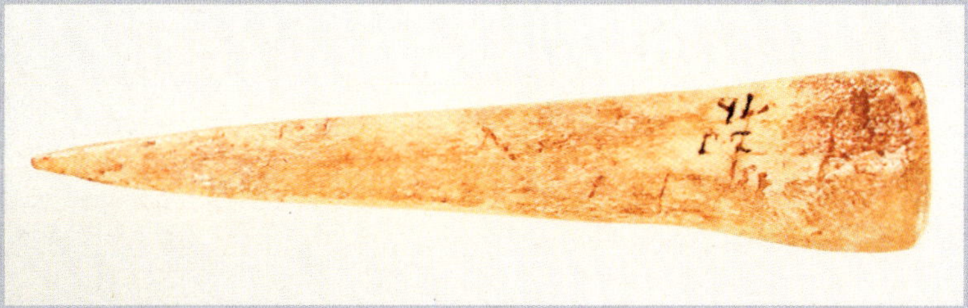

Awls

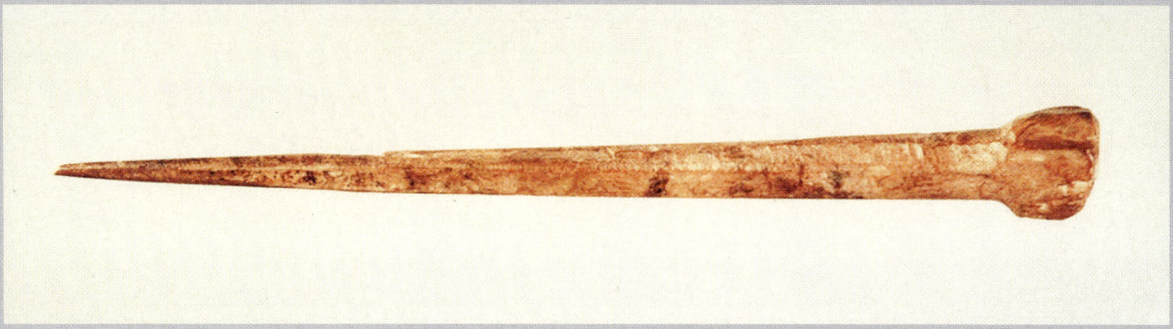

Hairpin, decorative terminal knob, 5¾" long. It has a mixed brown patina and came from the northwest coast of Alaska. Robin Fiser collection. **$75.00.**

Needle, hollow bird bone, 4" long. Needles of this type, having the cord run through the bone, are commonly found in Kentucky and Tennessee. They are probably also found elsewhere. Tennessee. Robin Fiser collection. **$35.00.**

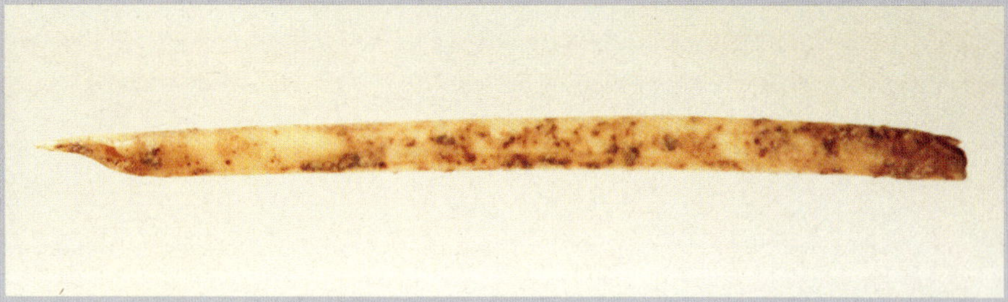

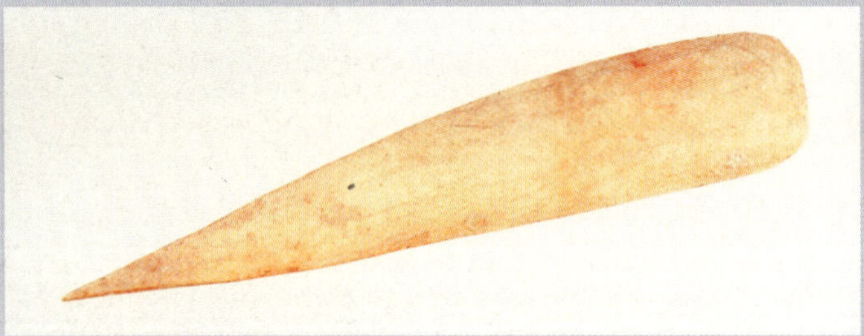

Awl, bird bone, polished for length, 3". From the Vietzen collection, it is from Ohio or Kentucky. Fred Winegardner collection. **$25.00.**

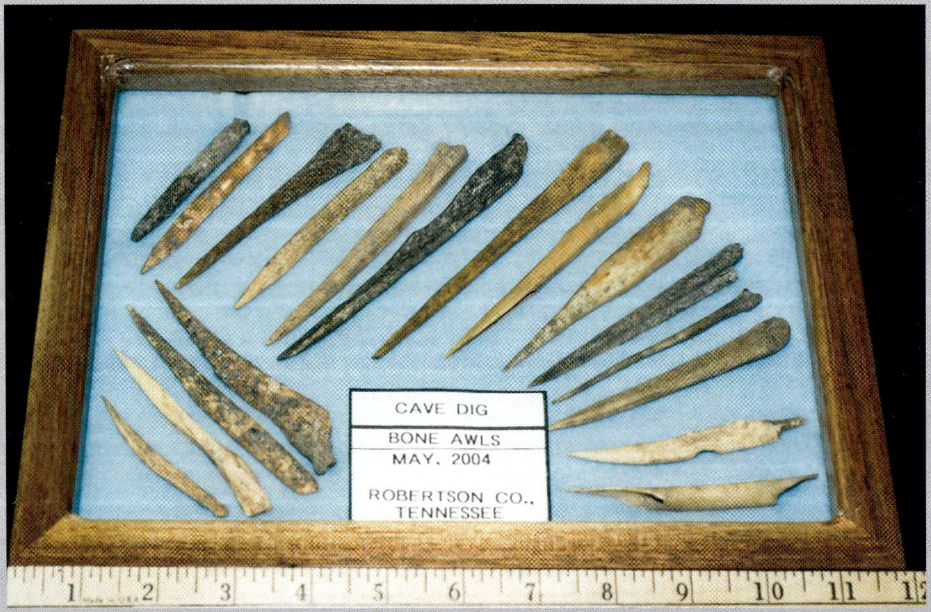

Bone awl collection, from a rock shelter, longest artifact is 5⅝". These 18 pieces were found in May of 2004 in Robertson County, Tennessee. Back to Earth. Group, **$375.00.**

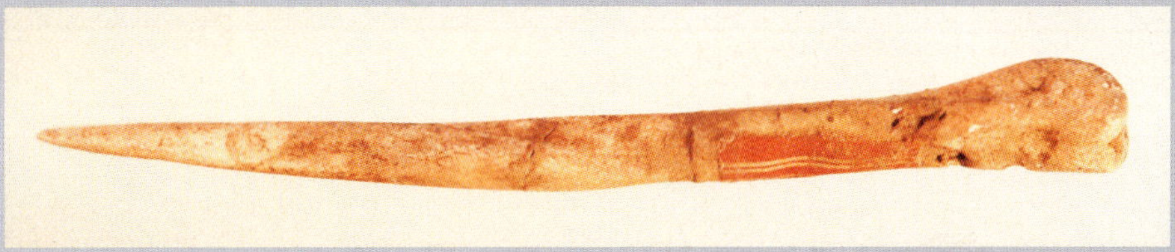

Awl, bird bone, 4¼" long. This example was once in the Vietzen collection and came from Kentucky. Fred Winegardner collection. **$30.00.**

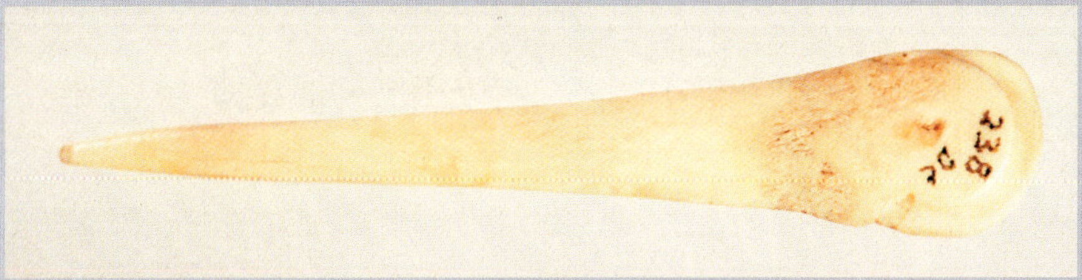

Awl or pin, highly polished bone, 4⅛" long. This well-made example was found in Kentucky. Fred Winegardner collection. **$45.00.**

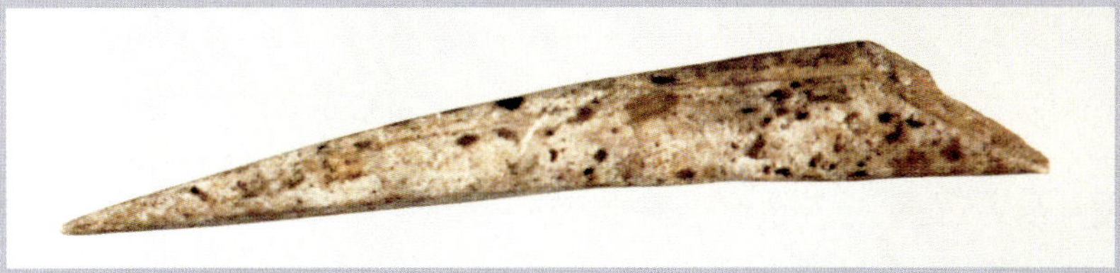

Awl, polished, gray patina with black spots, 3⅝" long. It is ex-collection Hall, from Wayne County, Kentucky. Private collection. **$10.00.**

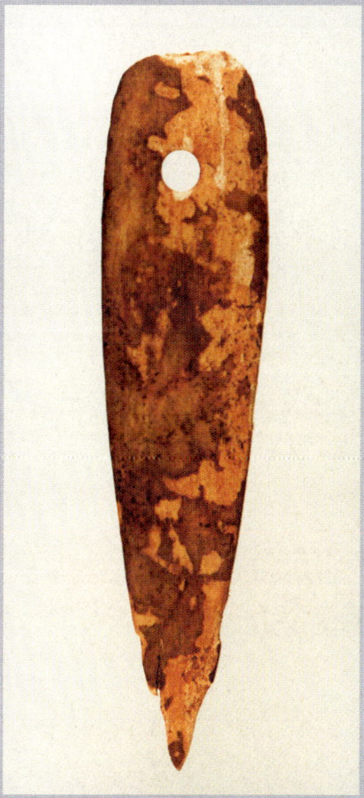

Bone pendant or awl, very thin, weathered surface. It measures 3½" long and is Eskimo (Inuit) in origin. Don Casto collection. **$25.00.**

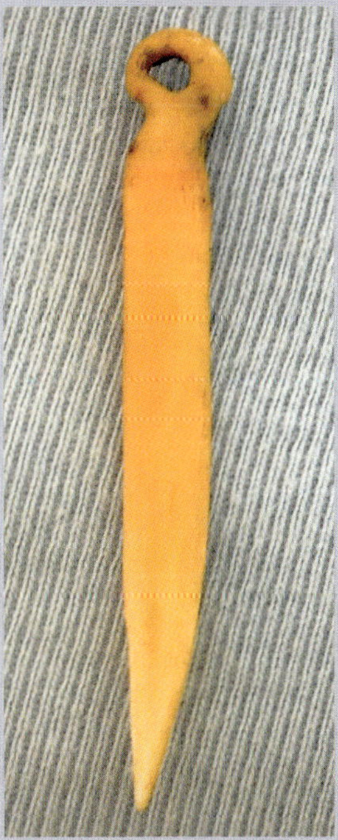

Needle with large eye, 2½" long. Made from a bone splinter, it came from Preble County, Ohio. Rod Fuller collection, Nebraska. **$75.00 – 100.00.**

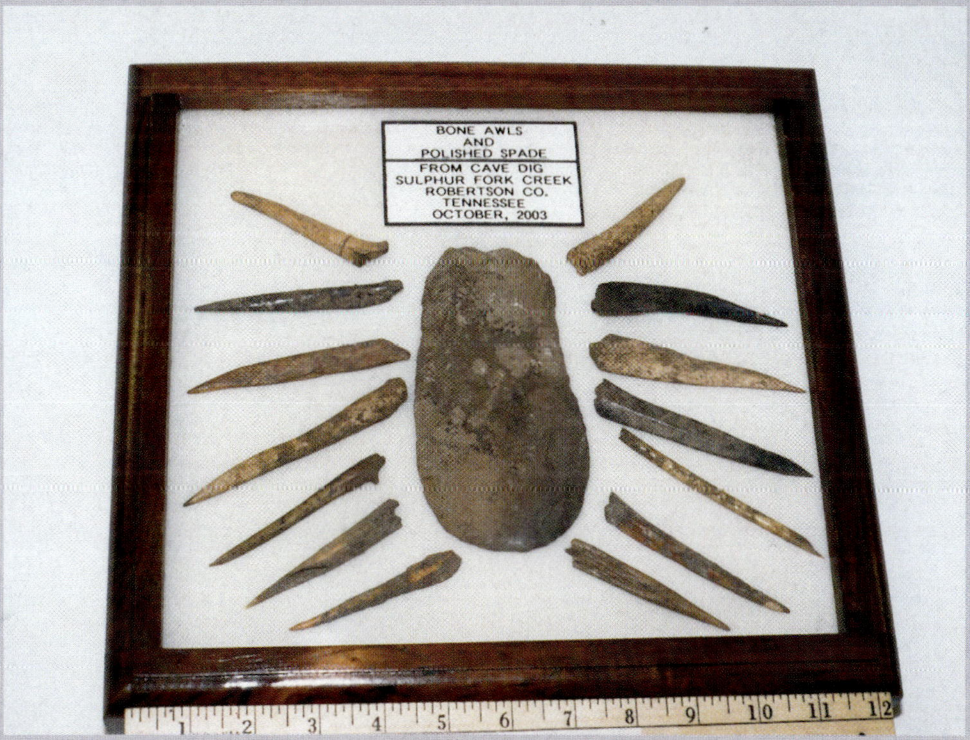
BONE AWLS
AND
POLISHED SPADE
FROM CAVE DIG
SULPHUR FORK CREEK
ROBERTSON CO.
TENNESSEE
OCTOBER, 2003

Awls, bone and antler, with a polished spade, all found together in 2003. The presence of the spade suggests the artifacts are from the Woodland or Mississippian period. Robertson County, Tennessee. Back to Earth. Frame, **$300.00 – 325.00.**

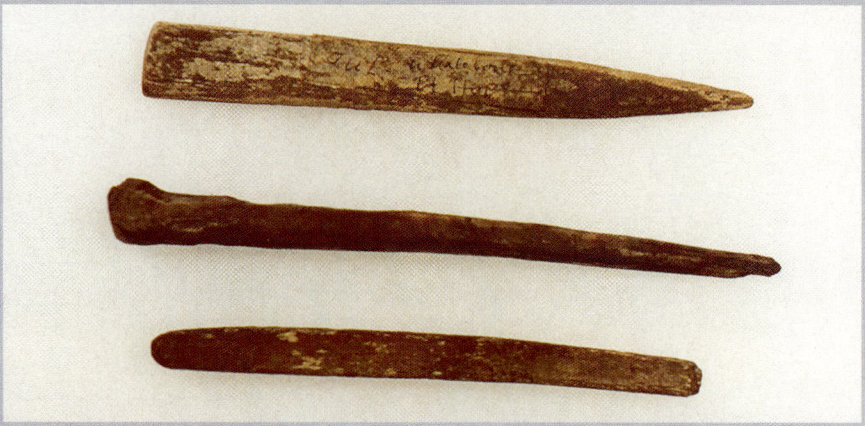

Awls or pins, the longest is 6⅞". The top example is made of split whalebone, while the middle awl is a polished antler spike. With a spatulate end, the bottom has a flattened cross-section. All are from Point Hope, Alaska. John Timoch collection. Each, **$50.00 – 75.00.**

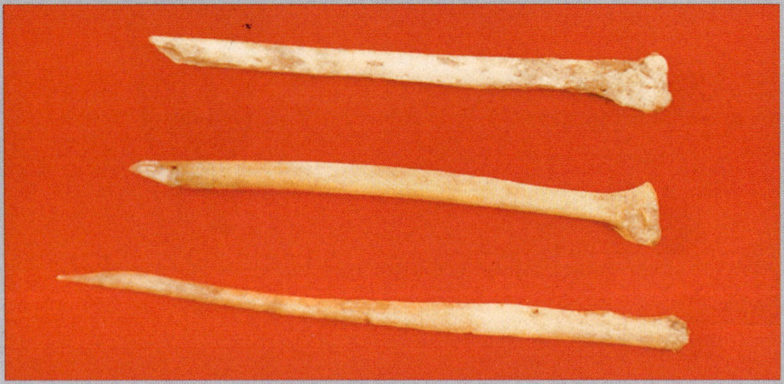

Awls or hairpins, bird bones, Late Archaic to Woodland. The longest specimen is 3⅜" and is ex-collection Vietzen. Christian County, Kentucky. Pete Timoch collection. Each, **$30.00.**

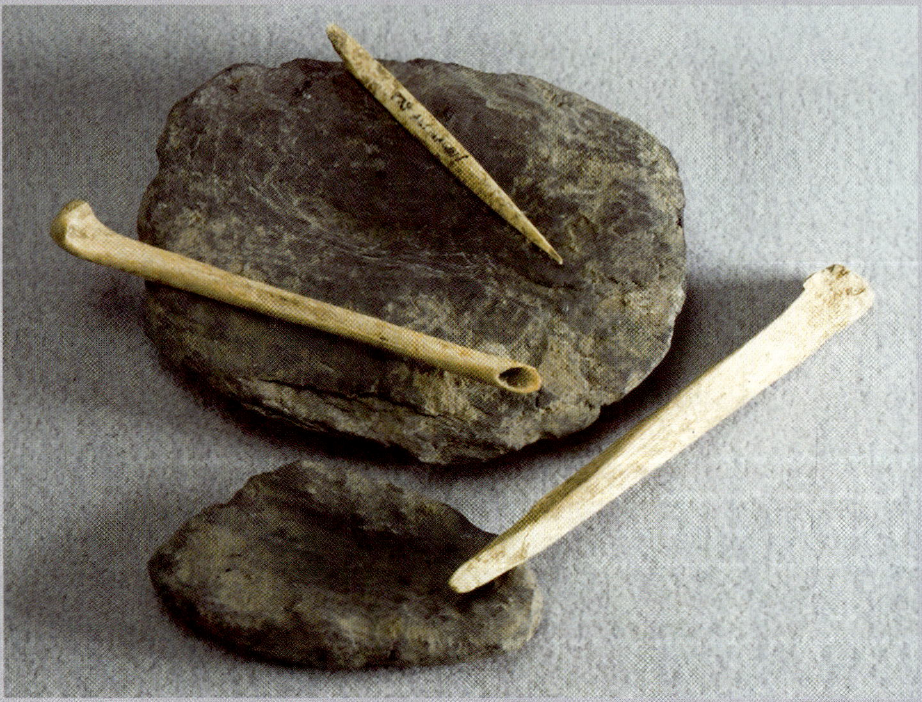

Slate whetstones or sharpening stones for bone or antler tools, longest tool shown is 11 cm long. There are three awls or piercing tools, with a bird bone splinter awl (top), a sharpened wing bone (center), and a heavily worn deer bone (at right). Private collection. Bone artifacts, each **$10.00 – 25.00;** whetstones, each **$25.00 – 45.00.**

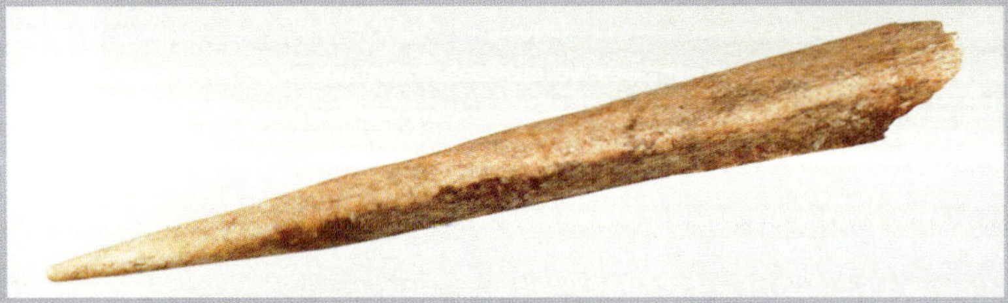

Awl, animal bone splinter, triangular cross-section, 3½" long. It has a pinkish-orange patina and came from Wayne County, Kentucky. Private collection. **$10.00.**

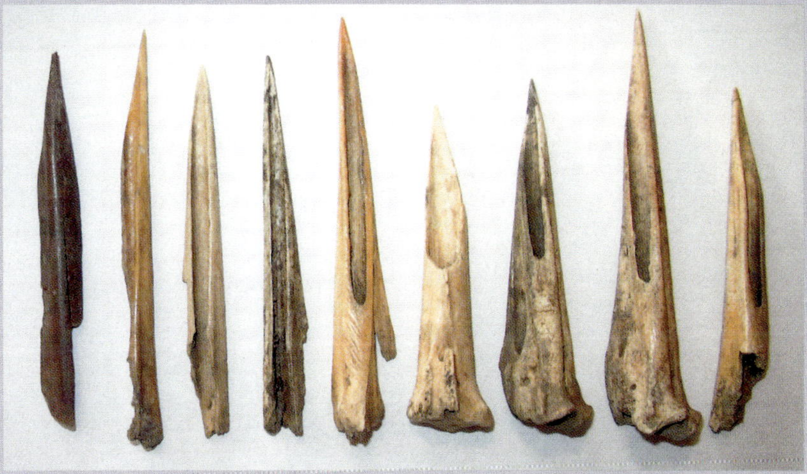

Awls, wild turkey leg bones, Mississippian period, largest is 4½" long. These were found on a site along the Ohio River. Mason County, West Virginia. Private collection. Rodney Roberts photograph. Each, **$15.00 – 60.00.**

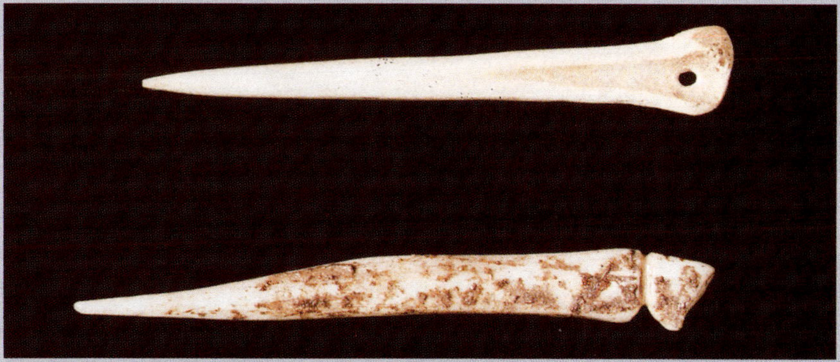

Needles, turkey bone needle (top) mainly drilled from the reverse face, 7 cm long. The bottom needle is a deer bone splinter, notched for a sewing cord. Private collection. Drilled needle, **$75.00;** notched needle, **$45.00.**

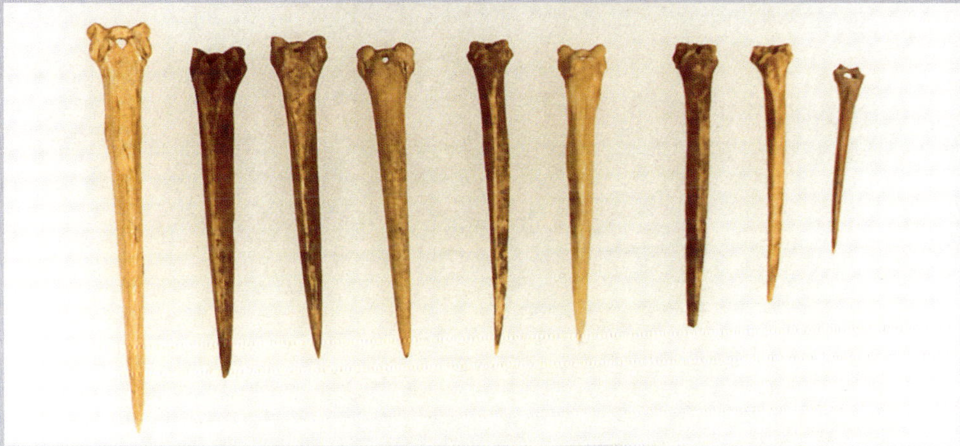

Necklace components, Mississippian period, sizes range from 1$\frac{1}{16}$ to 2⅜" long. The natural shape of the catfish barbs is close to that of awls, and the bones could be strung on necklaces. Values are based on size, polish, and condition. These are ex-collection Vietzen, from Ohio and Kentucky. Pete Timoch collection. Each, **$10.00 – 50.00.**

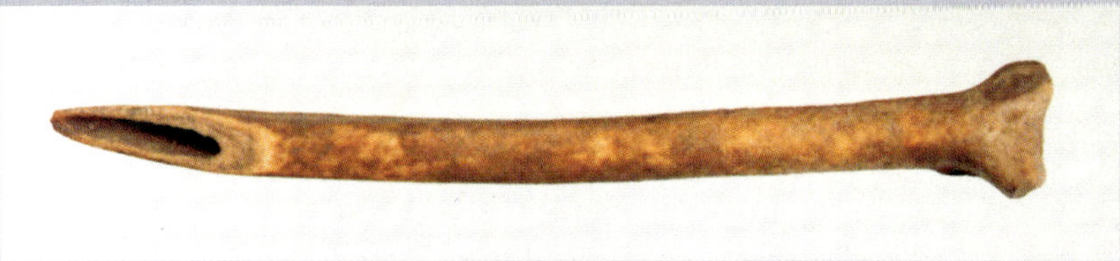

Awl or pin, bird bone, angle-ground tip, 3⅜" long. This piece, ex-collection Hall, is from Wayne County, Kentucky. Private collection. **$15.00.**

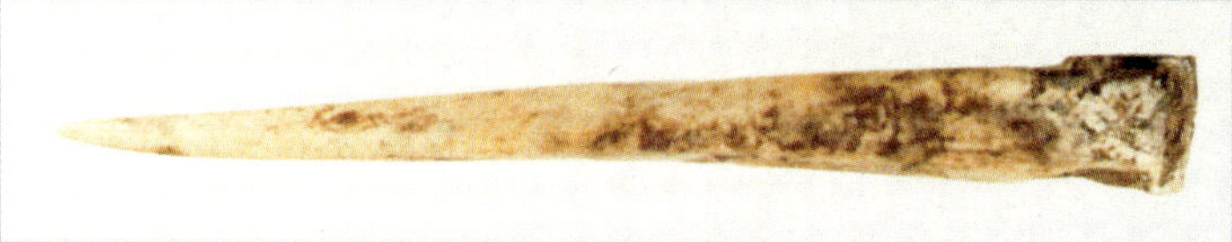

Awl, animal bone splinter, polished, 3¼" long. It is ex-collection Hall, from Wayne County, Kentucky. Private collection. **$10.00.**

Awls

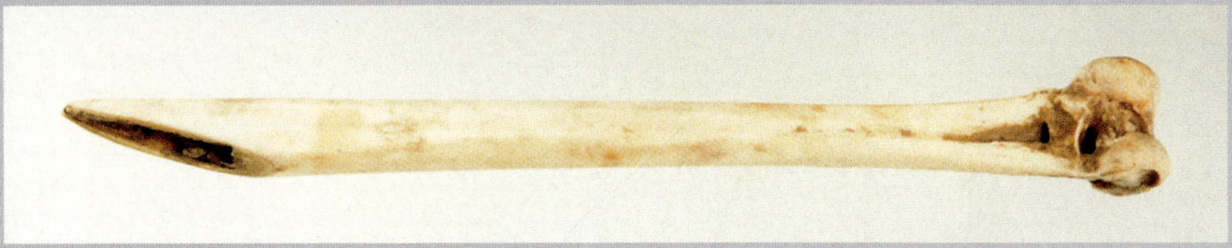

Awl, bird bone, tip ground at an angle, artifact is 5⅞" long. This piece is ex-collection Hall, from Wayne County, Kentucky. Private collection. **$30.00.**

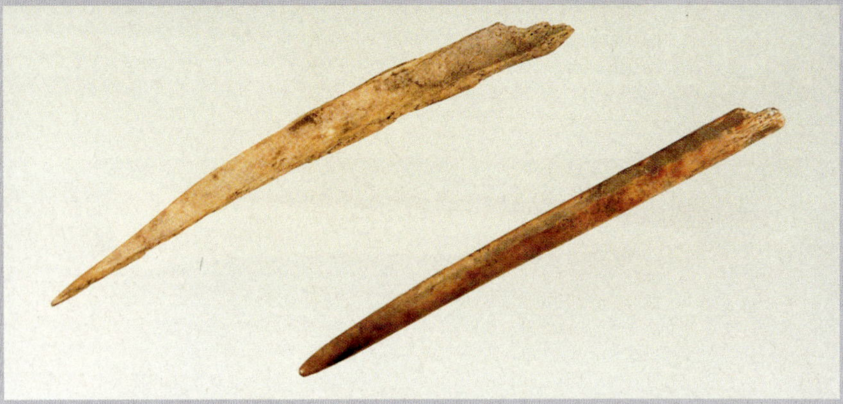

Awls, bone splinters, longest is 3⅞". The lower awl is rounded in cross-section and polished. They are ex-collection Hall, from Wayne County, Kentucky. Private collection. Each, **$4.00 – 6.00.**

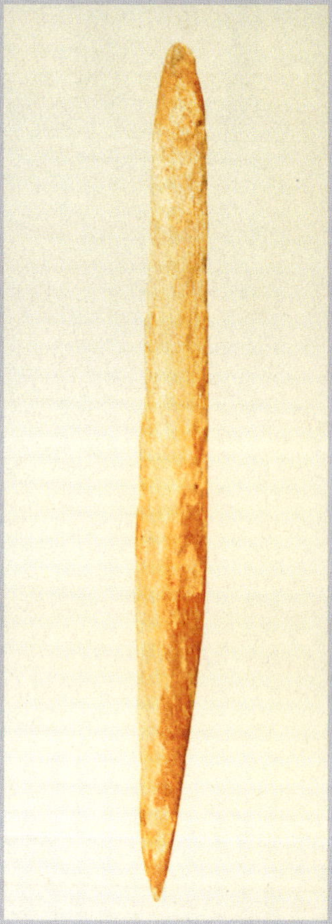

Pin or double-tipped awl, thick bone splinter, 3⅞". This pin has moderate surface deterioration, probably from acid soil and weathering. Kentucky. Private collection. **$8.00.**

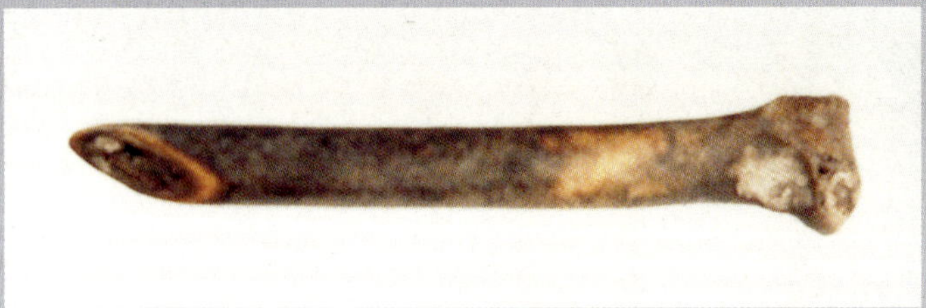

Tool, bird bone, tip formed by grinding at an angle, 2½" long. It has a glossy dark patina and is ex-collection Hall. Wayne County, Kentucky. Private collection. **$10.00 – 12.00.**

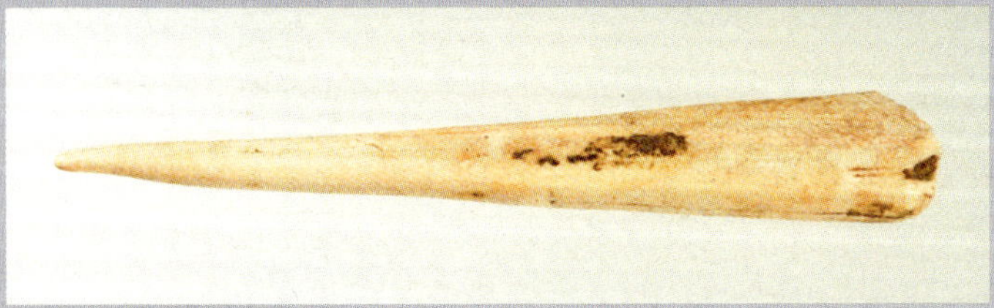

Awl, polished shaft, longitudinal wear striations, 2⅞". This piece is ex-collection Hall, Wayne County, Kentucky. Private collection. **$7.00.**

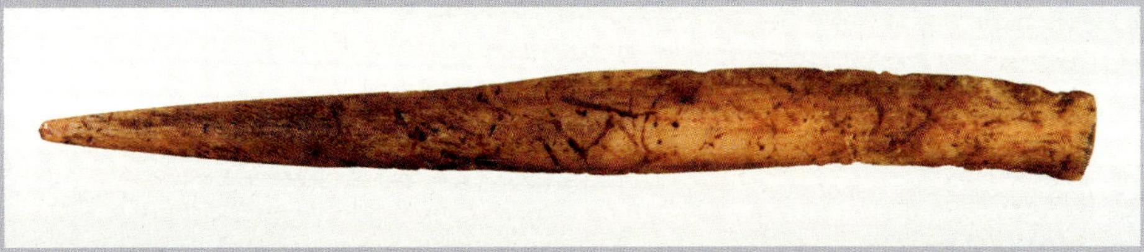

Awl, bird bone splinter, golden brown patina. Found in the 1950s, this example is 4⅜" long. Pulaski or Wayne County, Kentucky. Private collection. **$15.00.**

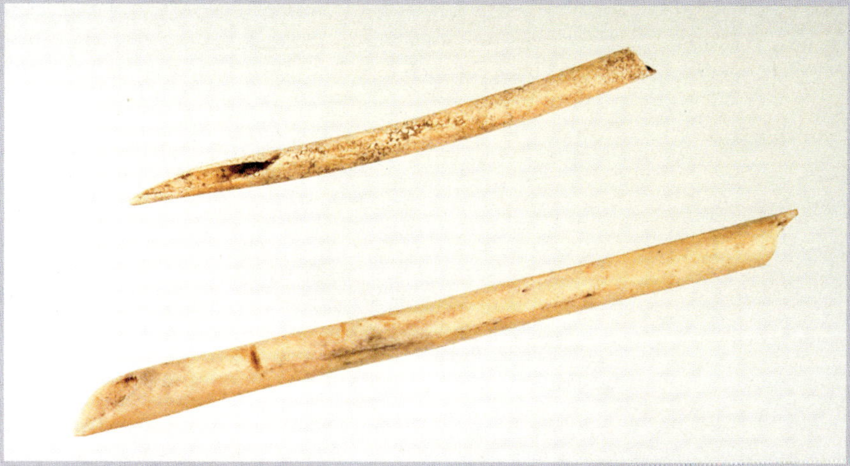

Bird bone sections, broken along shaft, longest is 4". Both have tips that are ground at an angle. These may be needles that had sinew thread in the hollow interior. Ex-collection Hall, Wayne County, Kentucky. Private collection. Each, **$10.00 – 15.00.**

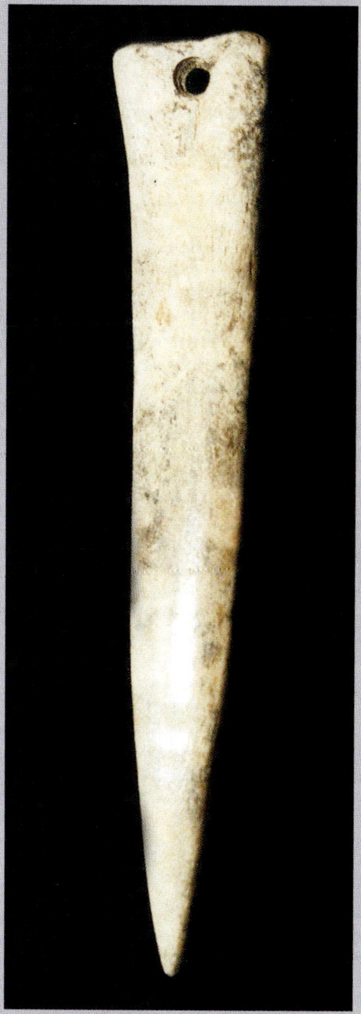

Awl or pendant, drilled bone, 4⅛" long. Well-polished, the artifact was found in Mississippi County, Arkansas. Garvin collection. **$85.00.**

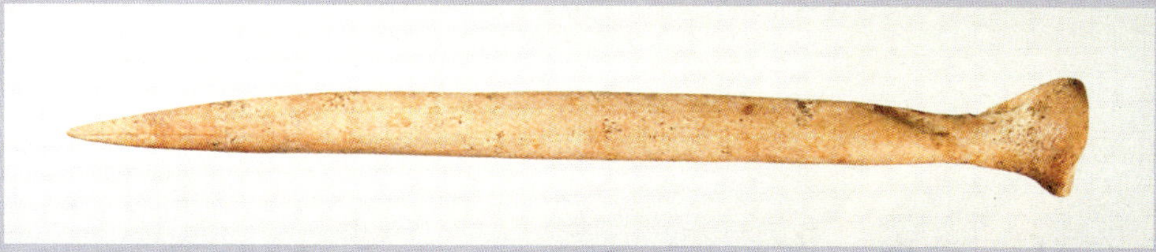

Pin or hairpin, wide and oblong head, bird bone. This piece is 4⅜" long and was picked up in Wayne County, Tennessee. Private collection. **$20.00 – 25.00.**

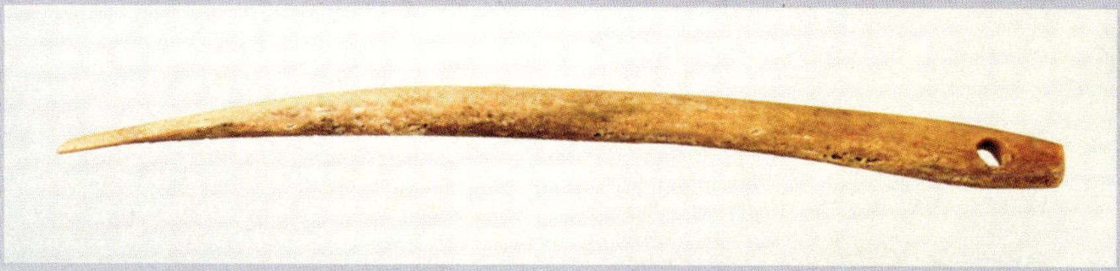

Needle, curved, split animal bone, 4¹⁄₃₂" long. It was found in Wayne County, Tennessee. Private collection. **$40.00.**

Awl, saw-marks on the surface in four places, 4¹⁄₁₆" long. This awl came from Wayne County, Kentucky. Private collection. **$20.00.**

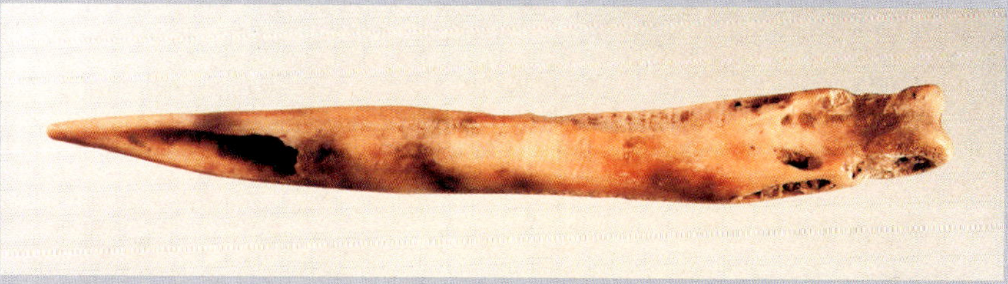

Awl, tapered bird bone, 3⅞" long. The example is ex-collection Selb, from West Virginia. Doug Hooks collection. **$20.00.**

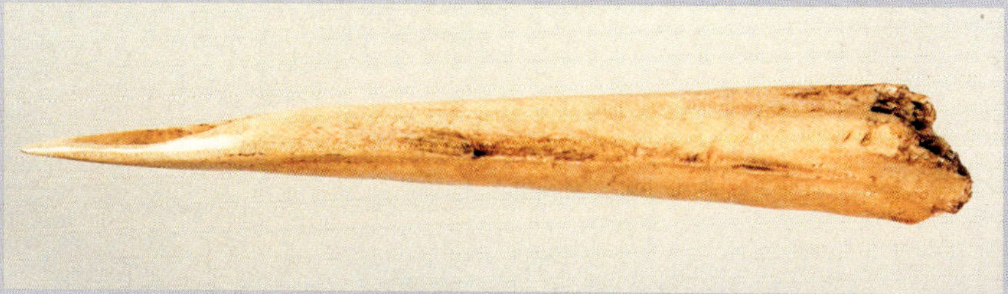

Awls

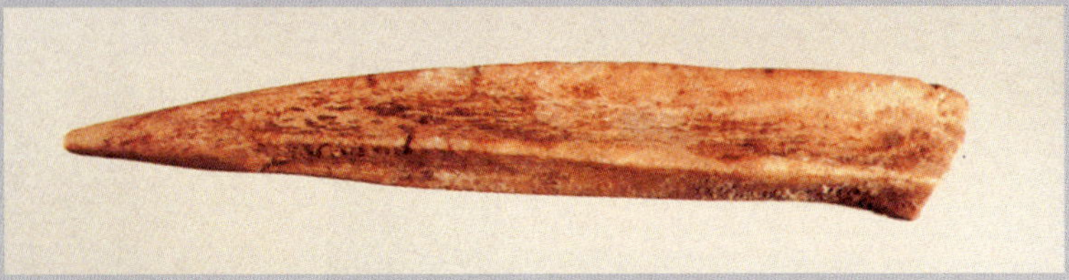

Awl, thick animal bone splinter, 3$\frac{3}{16}$" long. The surface of this piece has been smoothed through long use. Wayne County, Kentucky. Private collection. **$10.00 – 12.00.**

Needles or awls, splinter bone, grooved at rounded ends for cord, longest is 3¼". They are ex-collection Selb, from West Virginia. Doug Hooks collection. Each, **$20.00 – 30.00.**

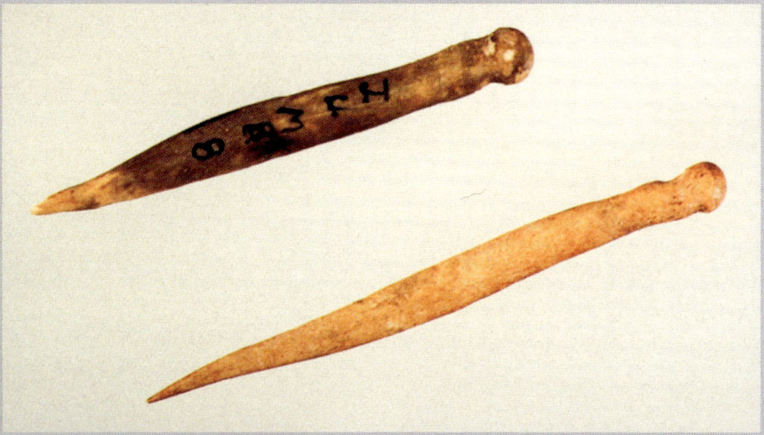

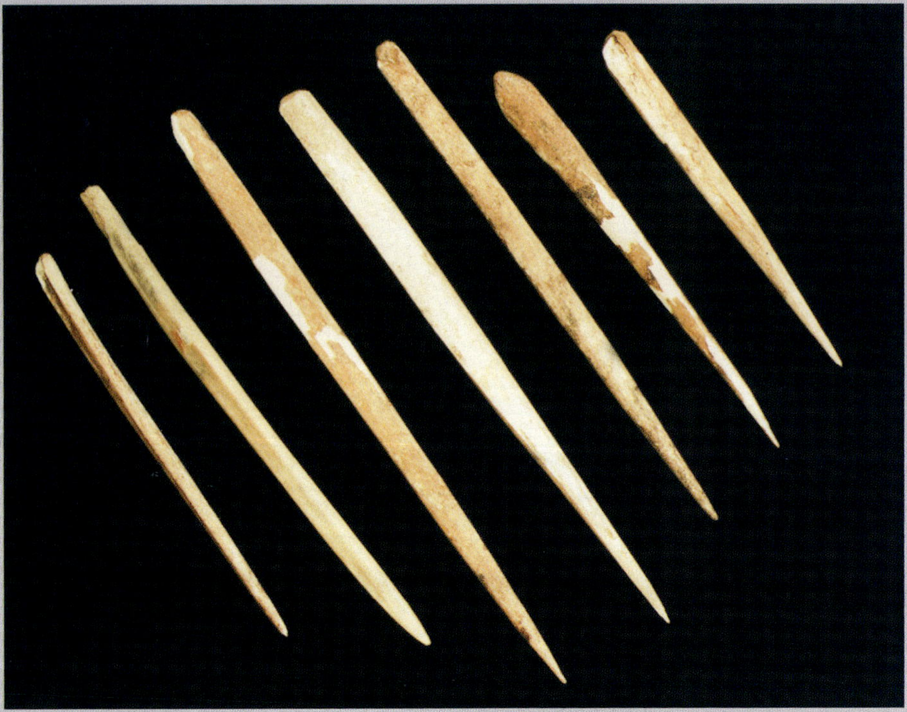

Awls, bone, all fine examples, 3¾ to 6¼" long. They were found in rock shelters in Parke and Fountain Counties, Indiana. First Mesa, Indiana. Each, **$20.00 – 85.00.**

Tool, rounded tip, small animal bone, chocolate-brown patina. The artifact is 2⅜" long, from Wayne County, Kentucky. Private collection. **$10.00 – 12.00.**

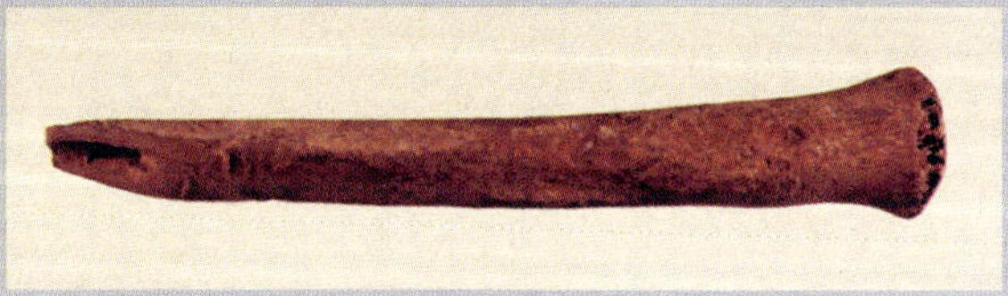

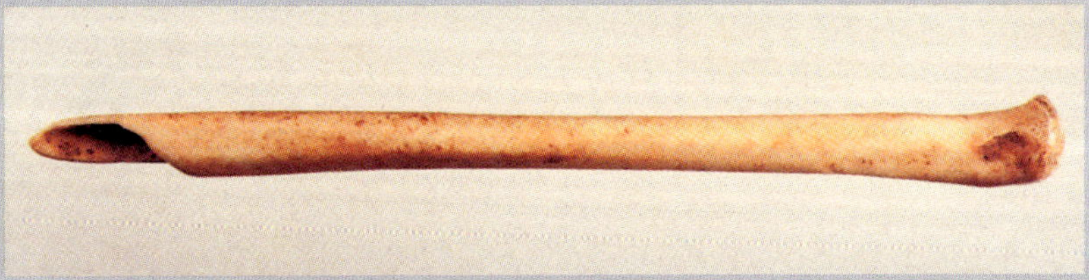

Awl or pin, bird bone, 3¾". The small end was broken rather than cut, and was smoothed and pointed at the break area. Wayne County, Kentucky. Private collection. **$12.00.**

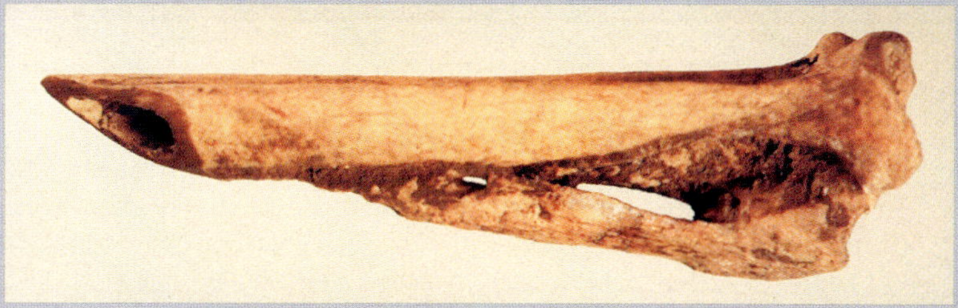

Awl, heavy bird bone, angled working tip, 3⅜" long. It was found in Wayne County, Kentucky. Private collection. **$20.00.**

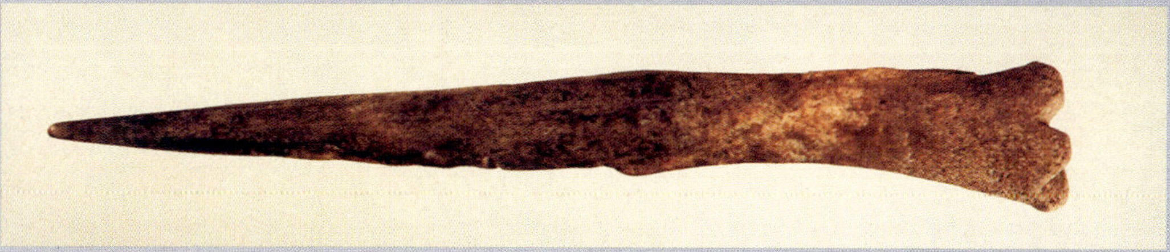

Awl, deer bone splinter, ⅘ of length with use polish. It is 4⅞" long and the reverse has an incised straight line from near the base to near the tip. Wayne County, Kentucky. Private collection. **$25.00.**

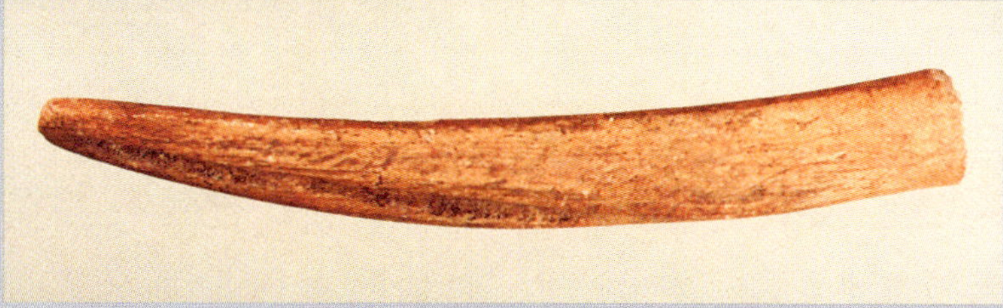

Tool, rib bone, broken, rounded smaller end, 3⅜" long. It has overall polish, and came from Wayne County, Kentucky. Private collection. **$12.00.**

Bone chisel, blade ground at an angle, 3⅜" long. This artifact was found in Wayne County, Kentucky. Private collection. **$20.00 – 25.00.**

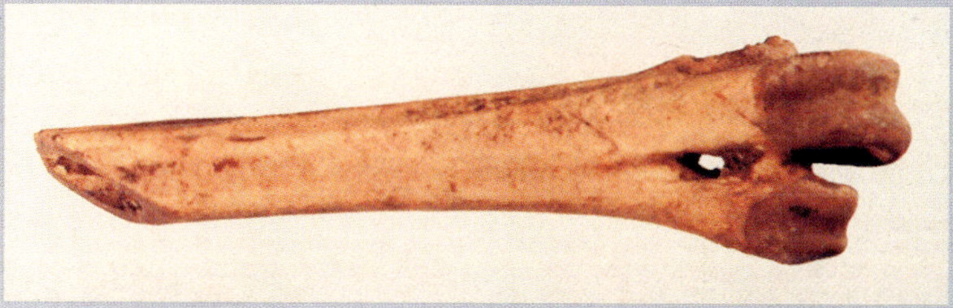

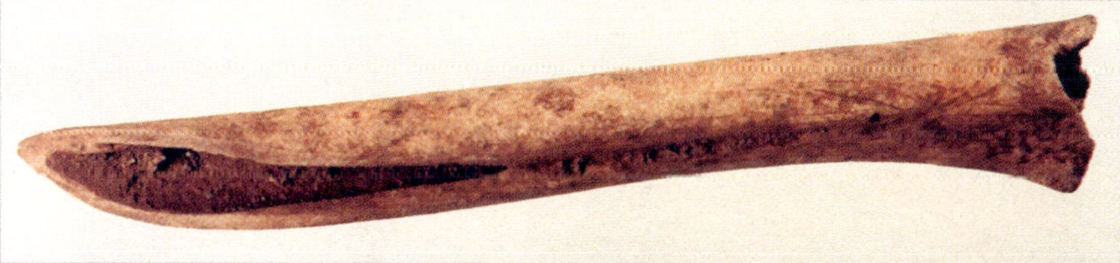

Tool, large for an awl but actual use unknown, 4⅛". The bone is partially hollowed and the tip is ground at an angle. This artifact has a light brown patina. Wayne County, Kentucky. Private collection. **$25.00 – 30.00.**

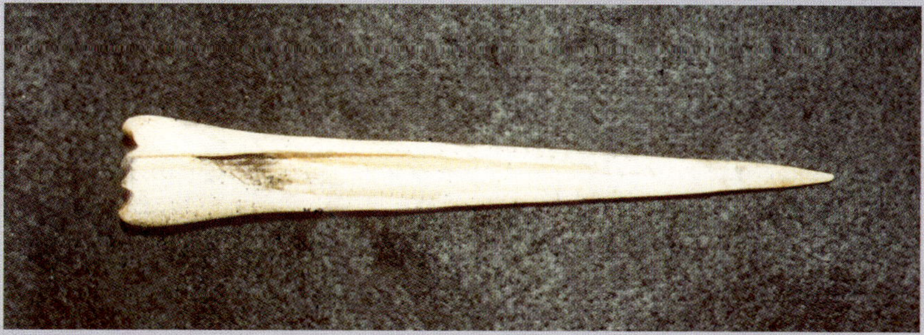

Dagger, heavy animal bone, 7½" long. This is a fine piece, with a straight blade and good lines. Northwestern Arkansas. Kenneth Hamilton collection, Arkansas. **$250.00.**

Awls

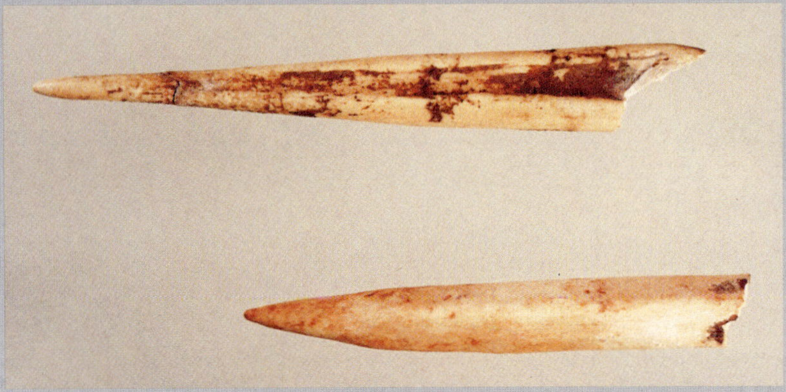

Awl tip sections, longest is 3⅜". It has a recent break, which exposed the lighter-colored interior. Wayne County, Kentucky. Private collection. Each, **$5.00.**

Awl, ivory-like bone splinter, 3¹⁵⁄₁₆" long. This heavy piece has wear polish on all edges. Wayne County, Kentucky. Private collection. **$20.00 – 25.00.**

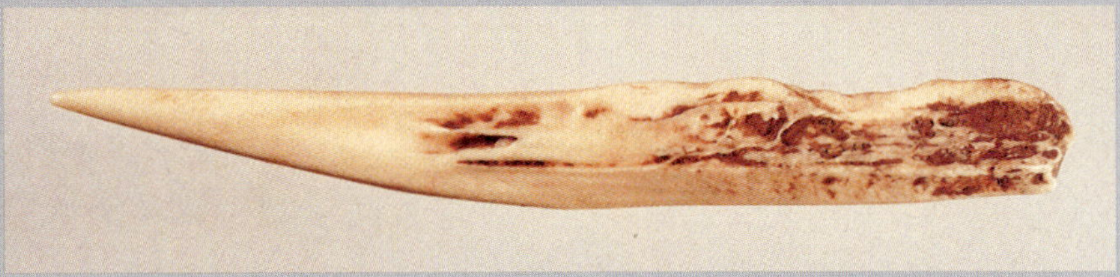

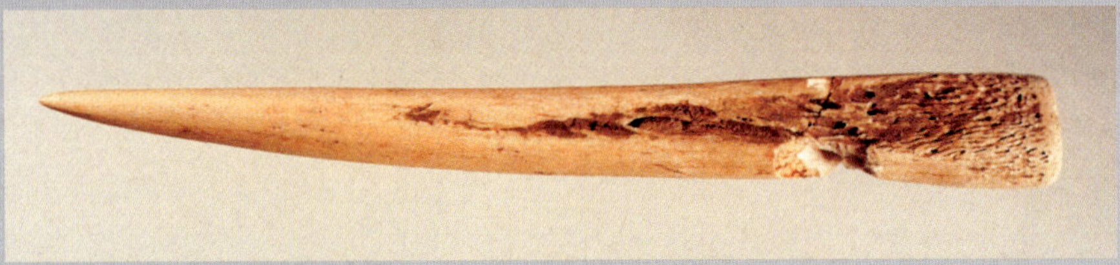

Awl or hairpin, thick animal bone, broken and glued. This example is 4⅛" long. From Wayne County, Kentucky. Private collection. **$10.00 – 12.00.**

Awls, catfish barbs, longest is 2½". They are naturally pointed and required little additional work. Fulton County, Illinois. Fred Smith collection, Illinois. Each, **$10.00 – 15.00.**

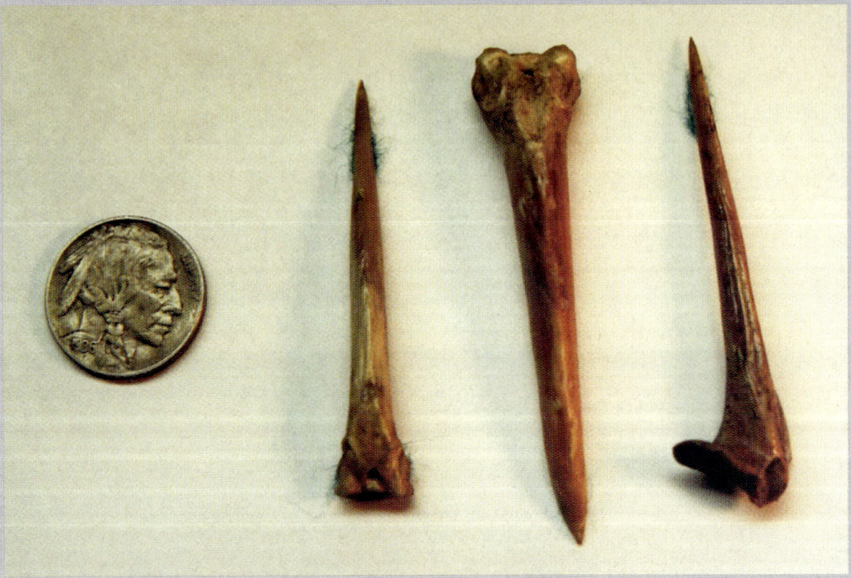

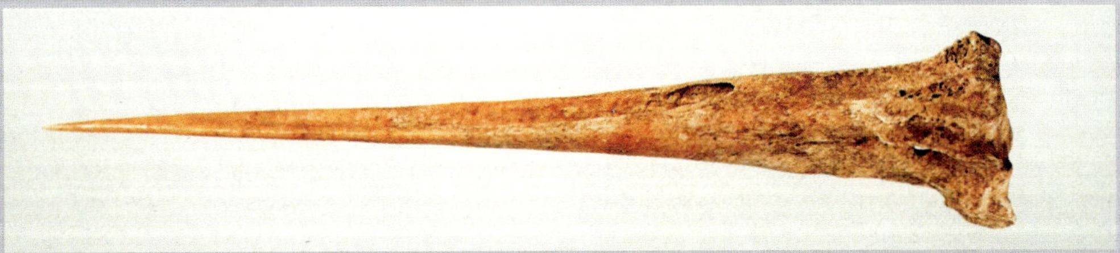

Awl, wild turkey bone, extremely long and polished needle-tipped shaft, 4¾". Ex-collection Miller, southern Tennessee. Lar Hothem collection. **$150.00.**

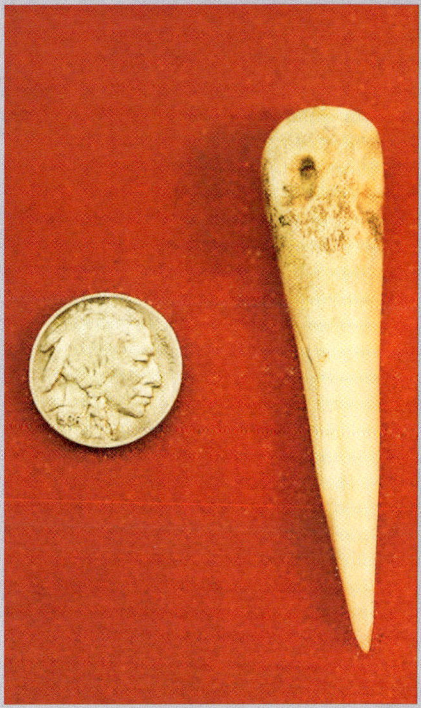

Awl, deer bone, 3⅞" long, polished shaft. It was found at a Mandan village site in South Dakota. Fred Smith collection, Illinois. **$75.00.**

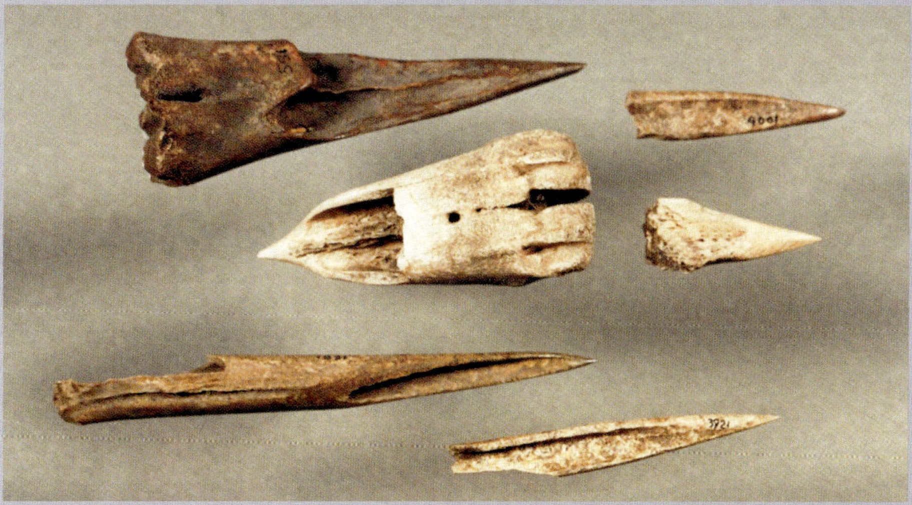

Bone awls, Riverton culture of Late Archaic times, sizes range from 1¼ to 4½" long. The awls are often found on major village sites, which consist mainly of deep mussel shell ridges beside major rivers. As with many organic material artifacts, values often depend on condition. Crawford County, Illinois. John Smith collection, Illinois. Each, **$5.00 – 20.00.**

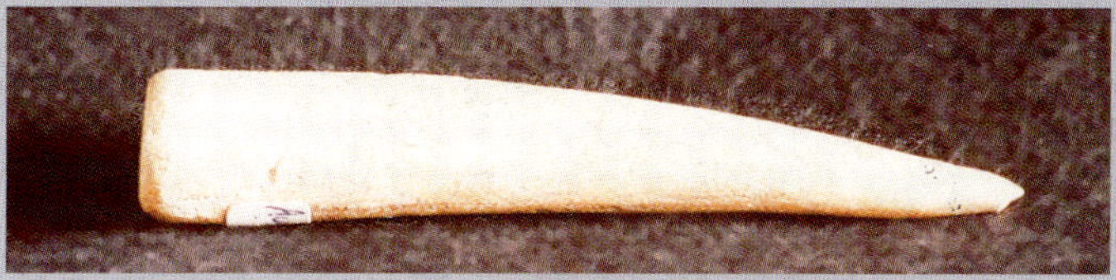

Antler projectile point, 3⅜" long. It was found in the Augusta area, Kentucky. John F. Wubker collection, Illinois. **$45.00.**

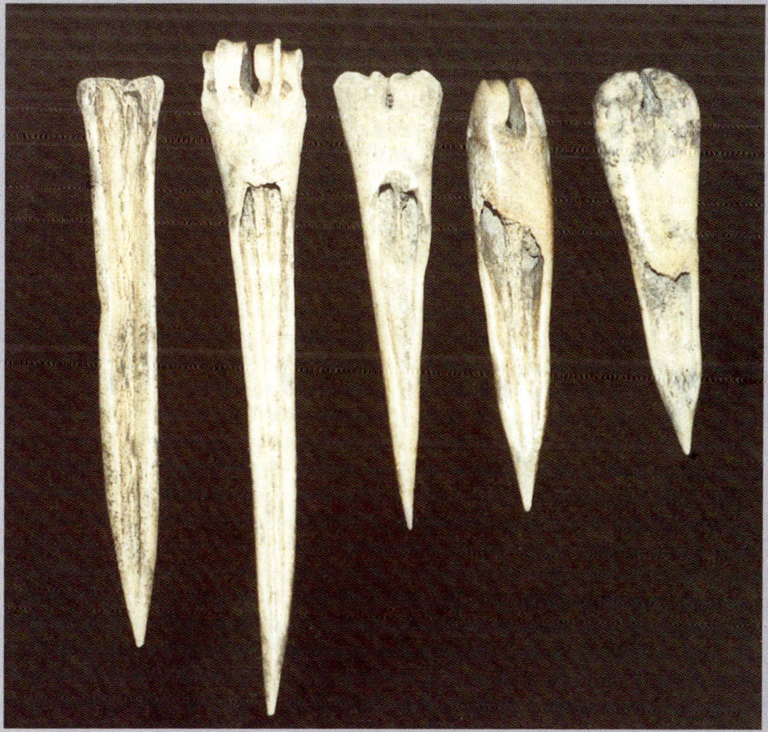

Daggers or wide awls, longest is 8½". These are fine specimens made of heavy animal bones. Northwestern Arkansas. Kenneth Hamilton collection, Arkansas. Each, **$75.00 – 200.00.**

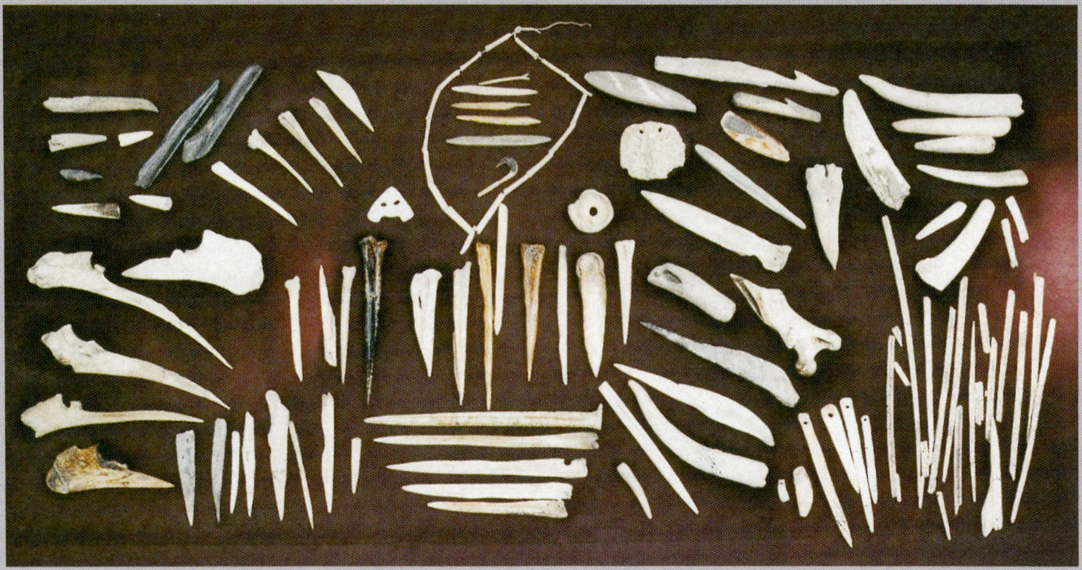

Bone tool collection, awls or daggers from 2½ to 7½" long. There are bone beads, two probable Atl-atl hooks, trigger awls, split bone awls, daggers, and needles (both with and without eyes). This is a nice regional grouping. Northwestern Arkansas. Kenneth Hamilton collection, Arkansas. Each, **$10.00 – 200.00;** Atl-atl hooks, each **$200.00 – 300.00.**

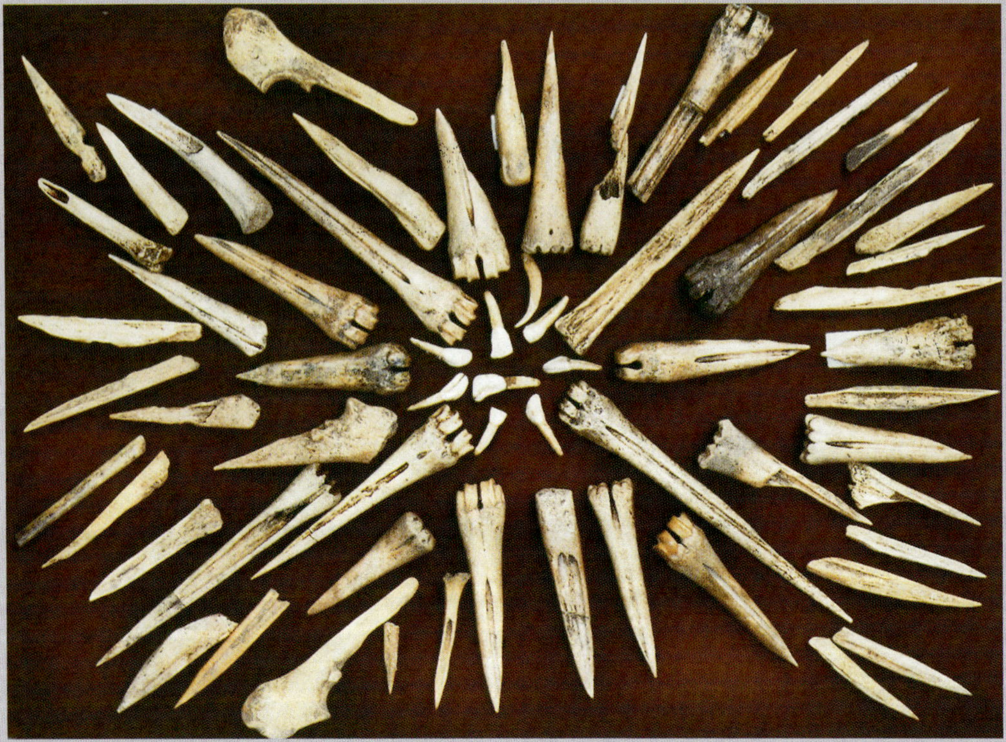

Bone awls, split bone awls, and daggers, sizes range from 2½ to 8½". While there is an obvious sameness to the artifacts, there are also minor differences. All were found in northwestern Arkansas. Kenneth Hamilton collection, Arkansas. Each, **$10.00 – 200.00.**

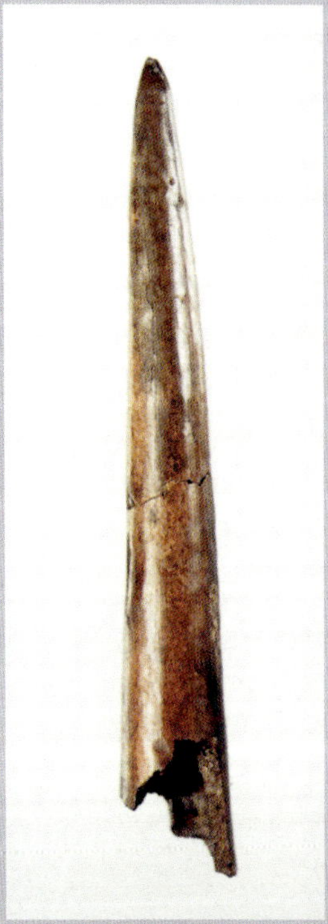

Antler projectile point, drilled base, well-shaped, and polished. Broken about mid-length and with part of the base missing, the point has also been burned. Value of this piece would be five times as much if it were in fine condition. It is 3¼" long, from southern Tennessee. Private collection. **$20.00.**

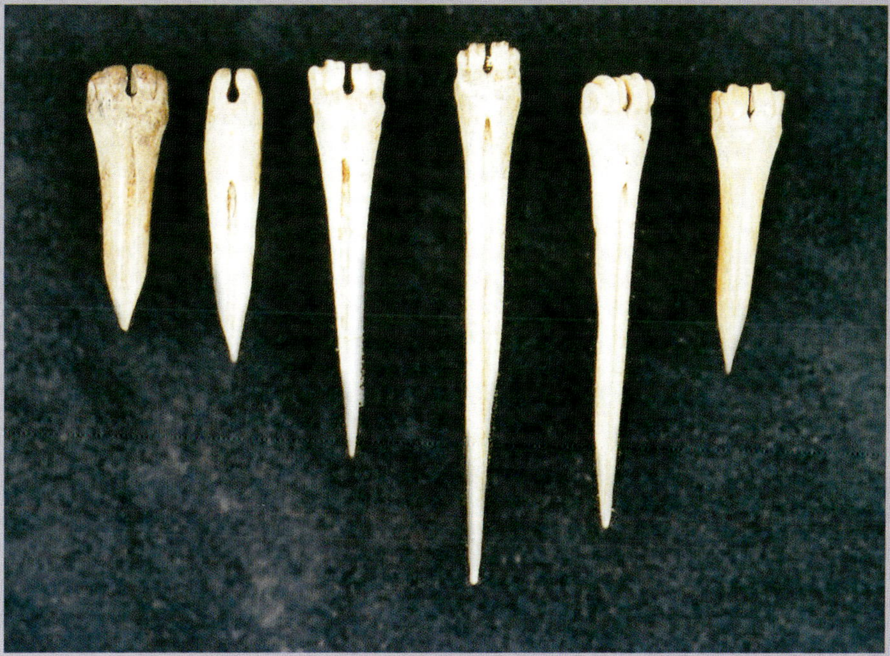

Daggers or wide awls, lengths range to 8½". All are from northwestern Arkansas. Kenneth Hamilton collection, Arkansas. Each, **$25.00 – 150.00.**

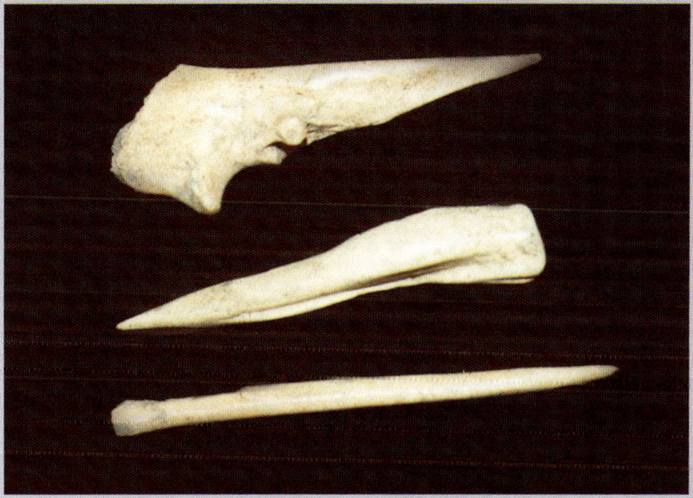

Bone artifacts, worn trigger awl at top. The central awl is 3½" long and bottom needle is 4½". Northwestern Arkansas. Kenneth Hamilton collection, Arkansas. Trigger awl, **$30.00;** awl, **$25.00;** needle, **$40.00.**

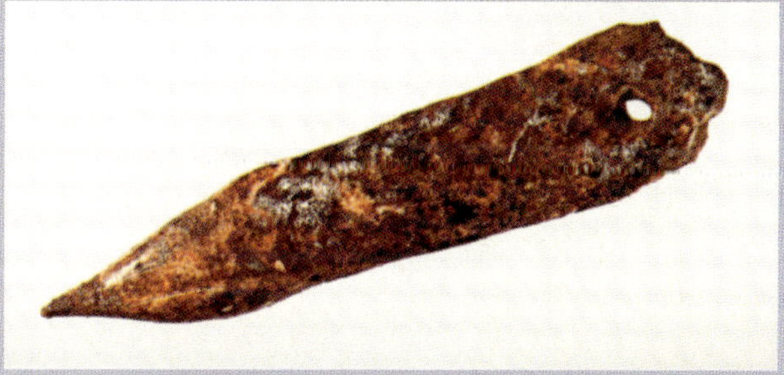

Awl or needle, small eye, deer bone splinter, 2½" long. It is heavily coated with rock shelter deposits. Southern Tennessee. Private collection. **$20.00.**

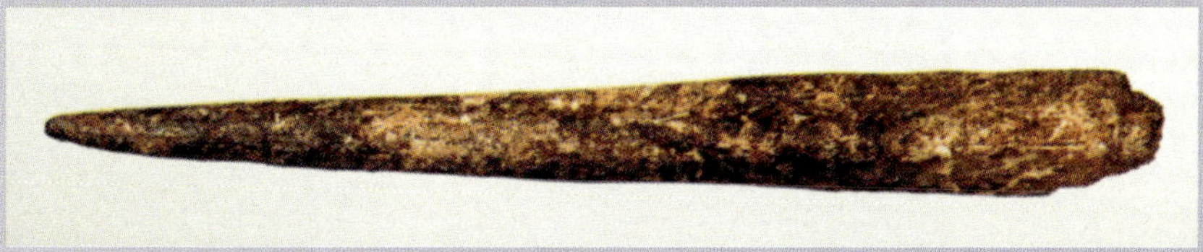

Awl, deer bone, triangular cross-section near base, 3⅝" long. It has rock shelter deposits and was found in southern Tennessee. Private collection. **$20.00.**

Awls

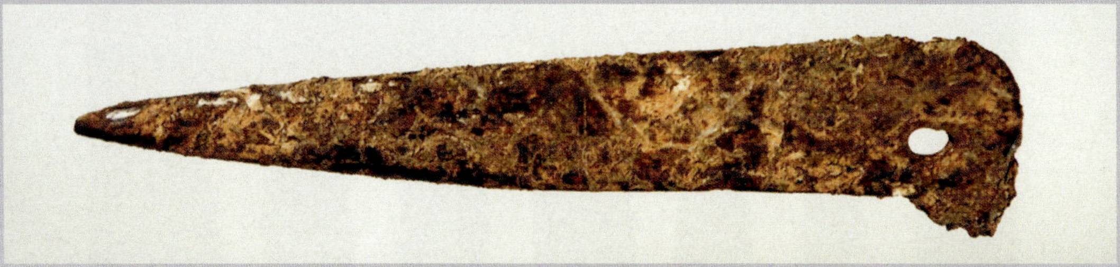

Awl, drilled deer bone splinter, heavy rock shelter deposits. The shaft obverse (shown) has light incised lines around part of the drill-hole and there are several dozen lines along the shaft at right angles to it. Ex-collection Miller, it is from southern Tennessee. Lar Hothem collection. **$75.00.**

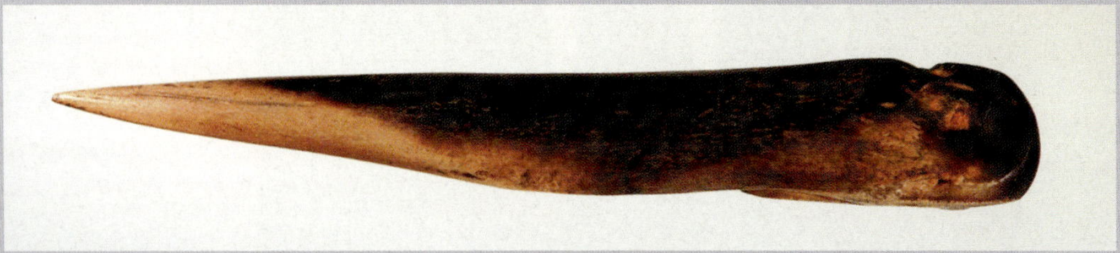

Awl, deer bone ground flat on reverse, 4⅞" long. This interesting piece has high overall polish including the base. The original bone was fire-darkened, then worked afterward; sharpening reveals the original and lighter bone color. Ex-collection Hooks, origin is unknown. Lar Hothem collection. **$90.00.**

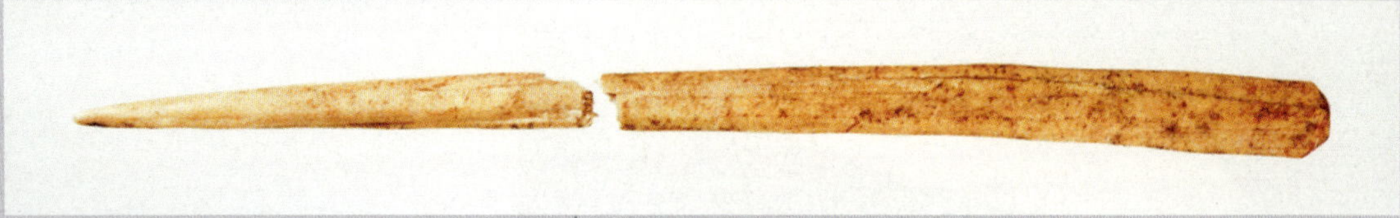

Hairpin, recent complete break, well-shaped and polished. Assembled length is 5" exactly. Examples like these are often restored or at least glued at the break area. Southern Tennessee. Private collection. **$20.00.**

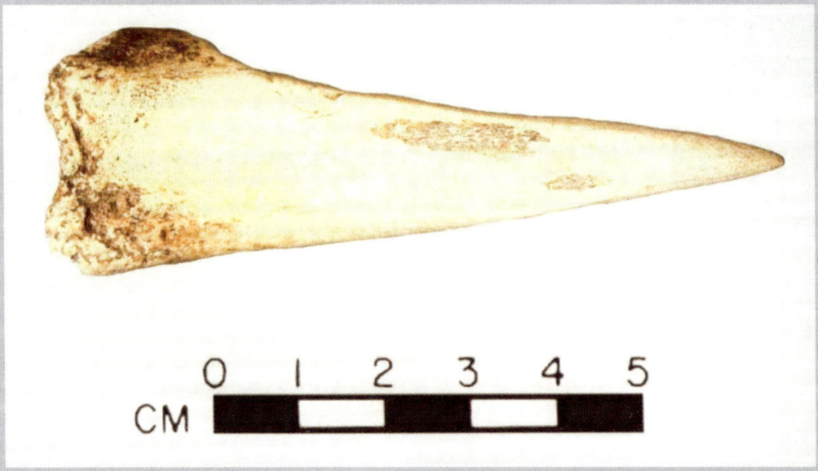

Awl, deer bone, size as indicated by scale. Part of a late prehistoric cache, this artifact was reported in the *Ohio Archaeologist*, Vol. 50 No. 4, Fall 2000. Imaged by Thomas R. Pigott. Sofsky Archives. Unlisted.

Needle, bone, with eye, 3" long. Slightly curved, the needle came from the Great Basin, Nevada. Victor T. Trujillo collection, Nevada. **$40.00 – 50.00.**

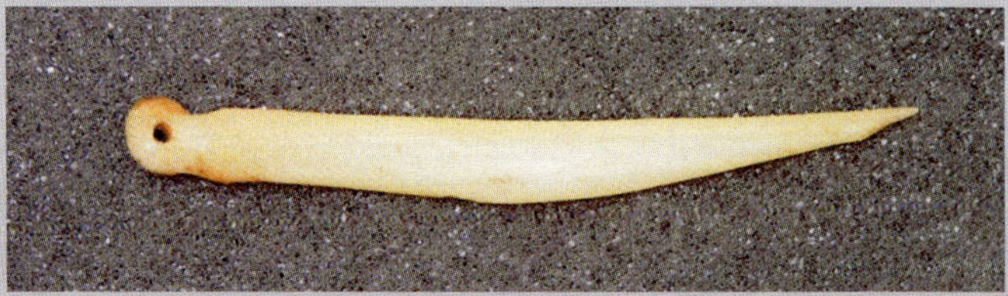

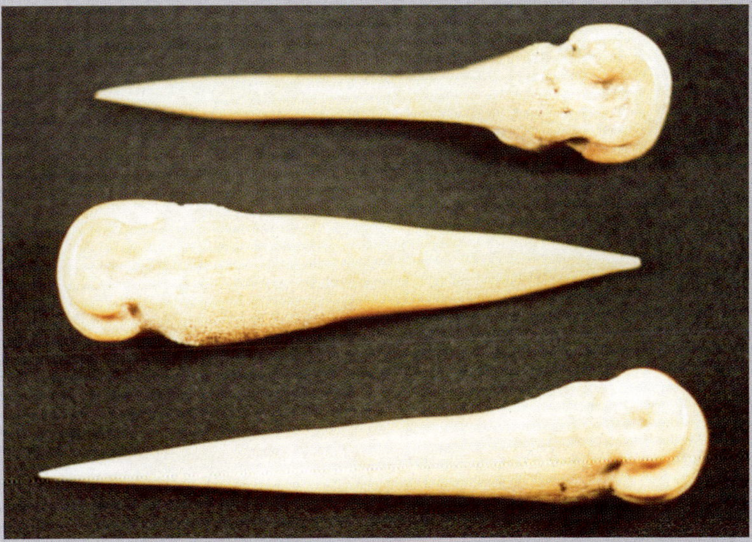

Awls, joint bones, longest is 4", different degrees of shaft reworking. The three were found near Mobridge, South Dakota. Mike Fox collection, Iowa. Each, **$35.00 – 65.00.**

Hairpins or bodkins, longest example (on far left) is 8¼". These are Shell Mound Archaic and most have incised decorations on the thick end. Southern Georgia. Robert Palmer collection, Georgia. Longest example, **$2,000.00;** others, each, **$500.00.**

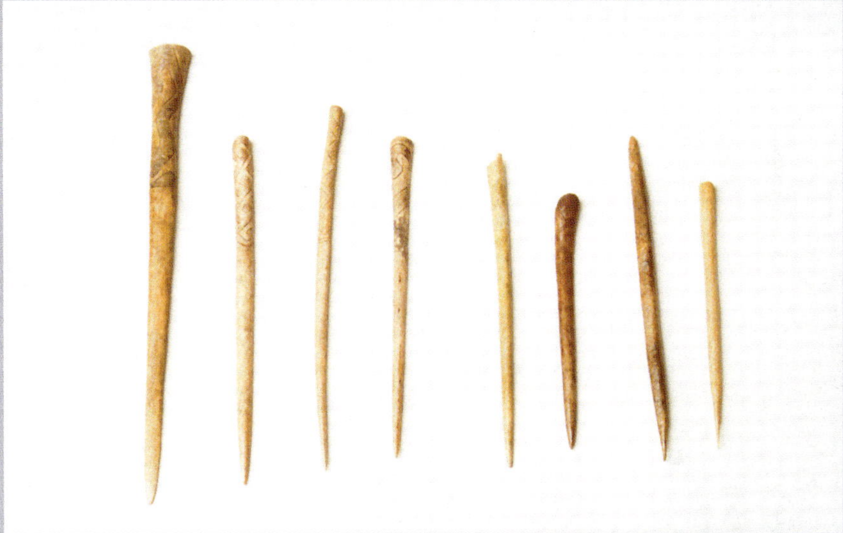

Bone awl, 4⅜" long, well-shaped and highly polished. This fine example is from the Buffalo area, New York. John F. Wubker collection, Illinois. Museum grade.

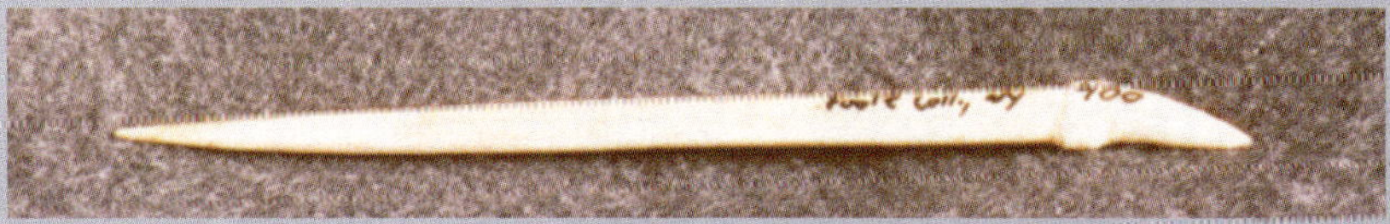

Needle or pin, bone, 5⅝" long. This piece is well-shaped and has high polish, with a small drilled hole. Find-site unknown. John F. Wubker collection, Illinois. **$200.00.**

Awl, large bird bone, length 3¾". It is marked "Sevier / 1704." The awl came from a rock shelter in southern Tennessee. Private collection. **$15.00.**

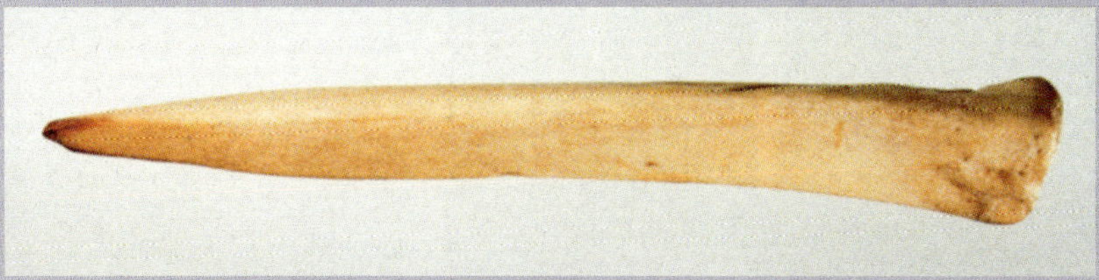

Awls

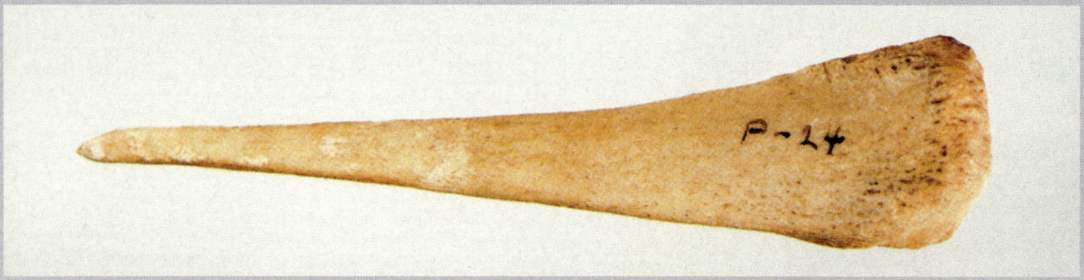

Awl, deer bone, 4¾" long. A common awl type, it has a portion of the joint remaining. Southern Tennessee. Private collection. **$20.00.**

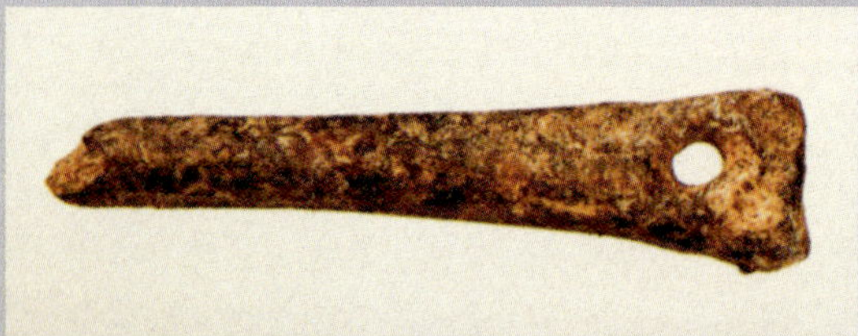

Awl or needle, ancient break, heavy rock shelter coating, 2¼" long. From southern Tennessee. Private collection. **$7.00 – 10.00.**

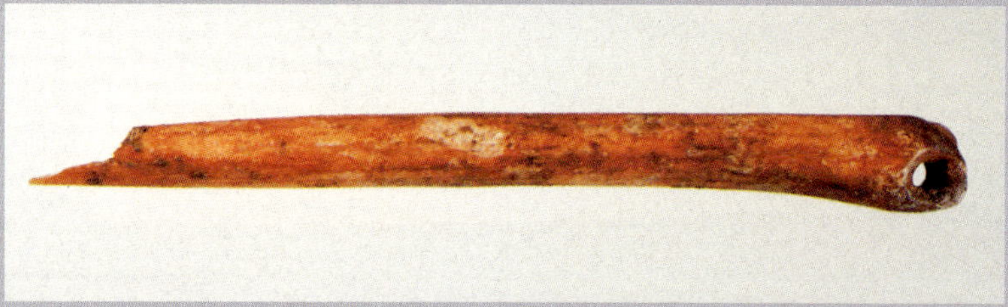

Needle or awl, rounded bone splinter, 3⅝" long. This piece was broken in prehistoric times. Southern Tennessee. Private collection. **$15.00.**

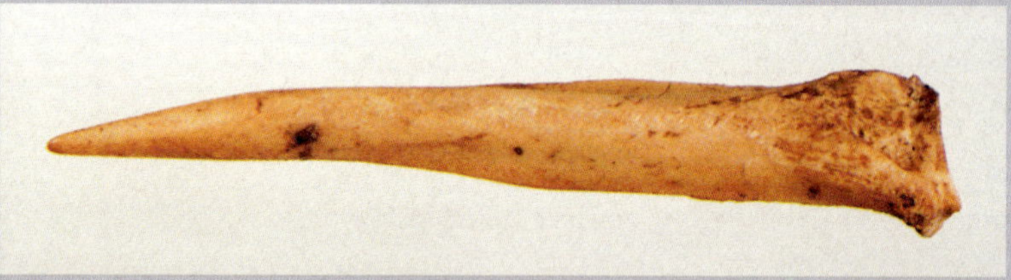

Awl, small animal bone, 3¼". The tip of the awl is rounded and polished from long use. A rock shelter find, this piece is from southern Tennessee. Private collection. **$15.00 – 20.00.**

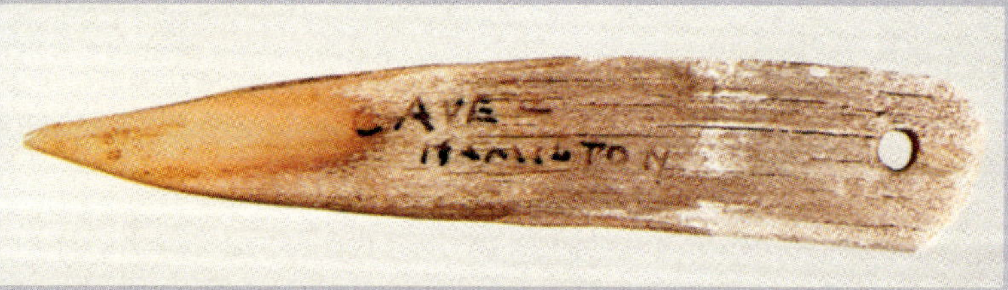

Drilled awl or needle, rock shelter find, 3⅜" long. This is a strange artifact, bleached and weathered like a piece of driftwood. Also, the smaller third of the awl is highly translucent. It is a rock shelter piece, from southern Tennessee. Lar Hothem collection. **$45.00.**

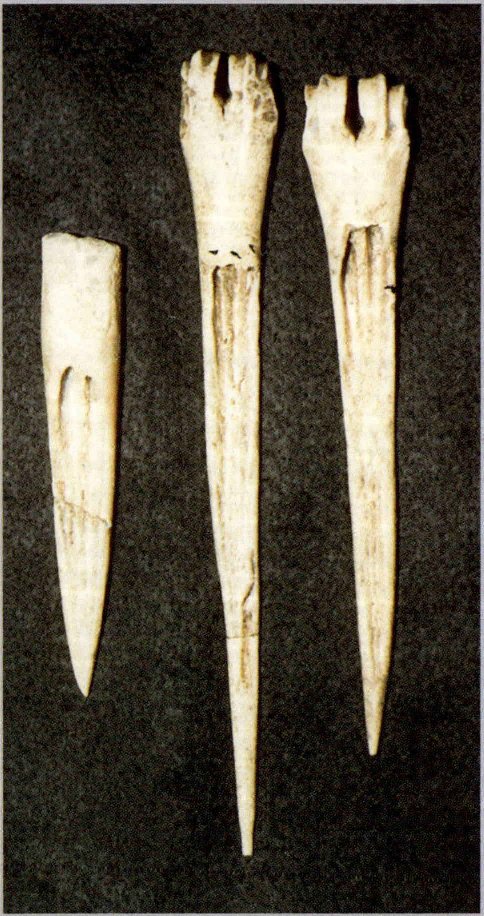

Daggers or wide awls, large animal bones, longest is 8½". Left and center examples are broken and glued, right example is intact. All are from northwestern Arkansas. Kenneth Hamilton collection, Arkansas. Left, **$30.00;** center, **$90.00;** right, **$125.00.**

Splinter Awls

While awls are indeed the largest bone tool class, the most plentiful types (or subtypes) within the class are splinter awls made from broken bones. Again, deer provided most of the raw material. For splinter awls, whole bones were broken into pieces, and this breaking was likely done at least initially with a club or hammerstone. The bones apparently were carefully broken (not smashed) so that long sections remained intact. At times this might have been more than half of the bone shaft, or a fourth, or mere slivers.

Broken bone sections were then treated in the usual manner, being ground or smoothed on the sharp broken edges and then given a pointed tip.

The base or butt end of splinter awls, depending on where the section was located on the main shaft, might have part of the joint remaining or none at all. The end itself might be rather narrowed or pointed, but most ends are irregular and without extensive reworking.

Splinter awls offered three advantages for the prehistoric maker and user. The maker could obtain several awl blanks from a large bone, thus conserving a resource. Often the bone splinters could be made long and narrow, with less work in turning them into the finished product. And the maker often had a small-based, slender awl that could readily be fitted into a bone, wood, or antler handle. This made actual use easier. A custom-fitted handle could be retained and a fresh awl inserted when the old awl broke or wore out and was discarded.

There may also have been a special need for slender awls that could be given more pointed tips. Some splinter awls have such long and delicate, even break-prone, tips that they must have been used for special tasks. Tattooing needles and toothpicks are possible, just as pins and needles today serve other purposes. Splinter awls may be from a little over 1" to 6" or longer, and vary in width depending on how the bone was broken. Thickness relates to the animal from which they came.

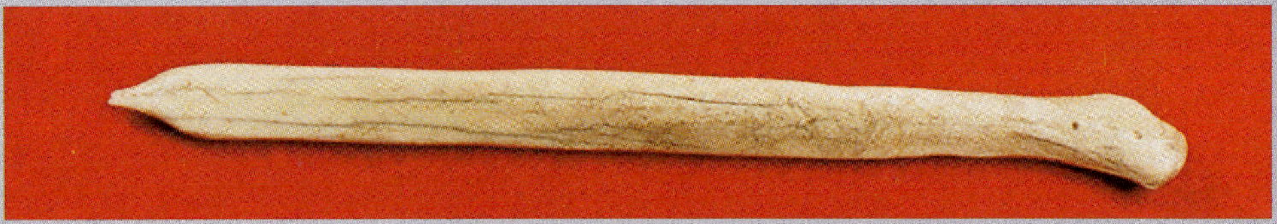

Awl or hairpin, split animal bone, Mississippian period, 5³⁄₁₆". Triangular in cross-section, there is very high polish and the unusual tip suggests a special purpose. The bone, with age cracks, is ex-collection Vietzen and from Ohio. Pete Timoch collection. **$100.00.**

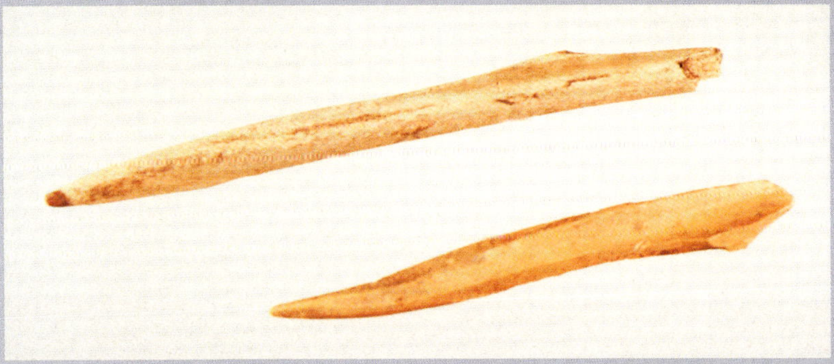

Awls, deer bone splinters, longer one is 3½". The tips of the awls are polished and both were found in Kentucky. Private collection. Each, **$7.00 – 10.00.**

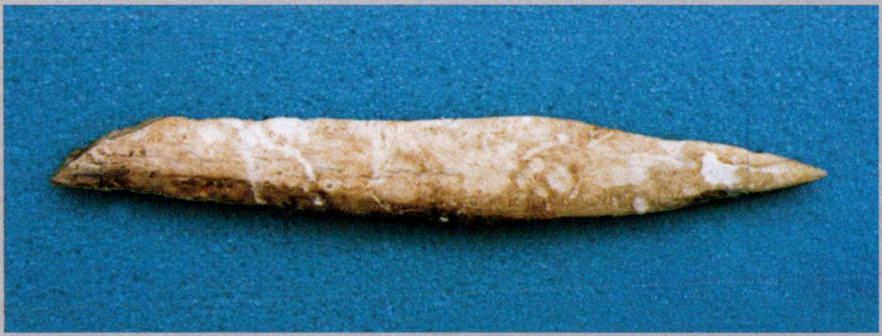

Awl, bone splinter, Archaic or later, ⅞ x 3³⁄₁₆". Ex-collection Snyder, it is from western Tennessee. Collection of, and photograph by, Gary Henry, North Carolina. **$10.00.**

Splinter Awls

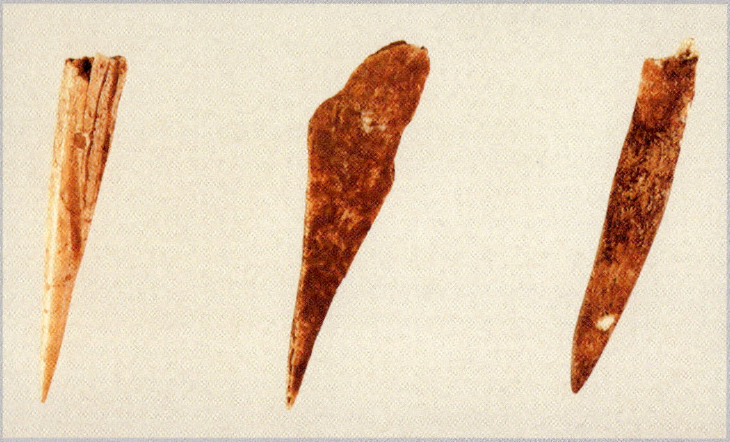

Awls or perforators, all made of splintered animal bone, center example is 1⅞". These were found in Kentucky. Private collection. Each, **$5.00 – 10.00.**

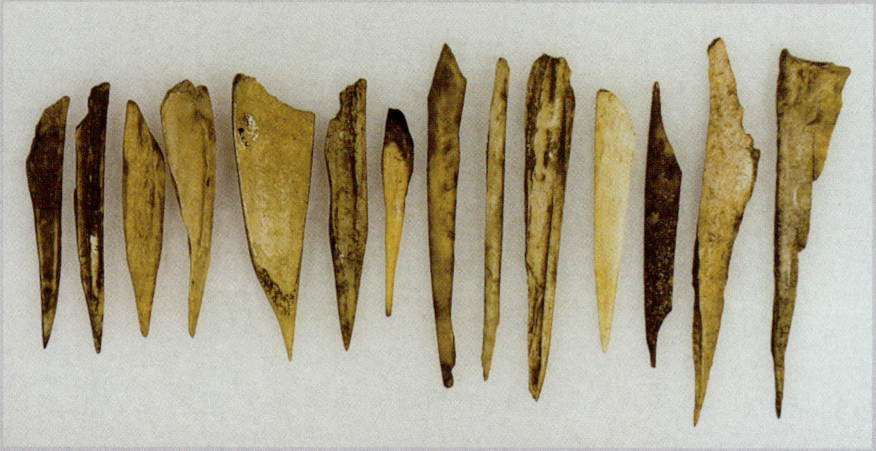

Awls, split animal bones, longest is 5¼". The group indicates various levels of use-wear, individual craftsmanship and perhaps style development over the centuries. All are ex-collection Vietzen, from Ohio and Kentucky. Pete Timoch collection. Each, **$20.00 – 50.00.**

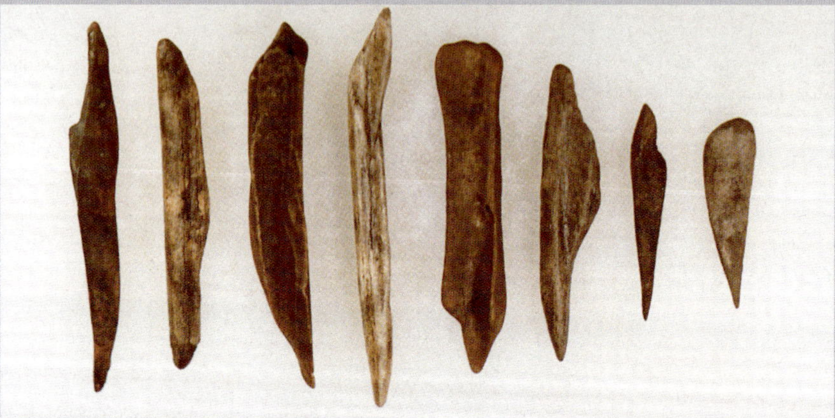

Awls, split bone, Woodland to Mississippian periods, longest is 4¼". They were all found in eastern Missouri. Pete Timoch collection. Each, **$10.00 – 20.00.**

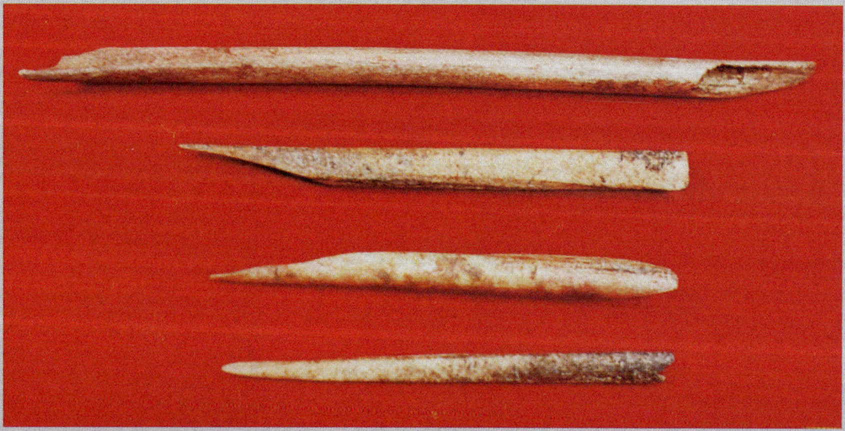

Awls or pins, Late Archaic to Woodland, bird bones. The longest bipointed example at top is 8$\frac{5}{16}$" and may be from a trumpeter swan. The second example down has the end cut and ground. Ex-collection Vietzen, Christian County, Kentucky. Pete Timoch collection. Each, **$75.00.**

Awl, Archaic or later, bone splinter, polished tip. This example is ½ x 3⅛", ex-collection Snyder. Christian County, Kentucky. Collection of, and photograph by, Gary Henry, North Carolina. **$15.00.**

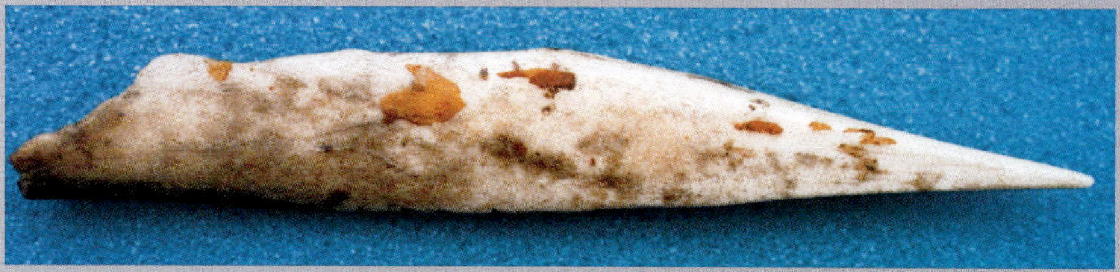

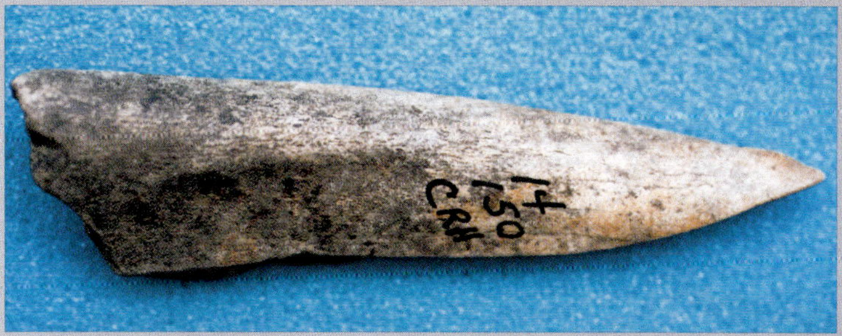

Awl, bone splinter, Archaic or later. This example, found by Harwood in 1958, measures ⅞ x 3³⁄₁₆". Morgan County, Alabama. Collection of, and photograph by, Gary Henry, North Carolina. **$10.00.**

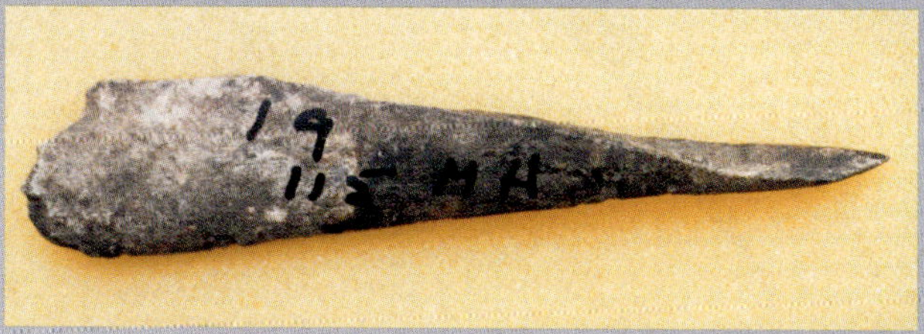

Awl, Archaic or later, ⁹⁄₁₆ x 2¾". Harwood found the bone splinter awl in 1954 or 1961. Limestone County, Alabama. Collection of, and photograph by, Gary Henry, North Carolina. **$10.00.**

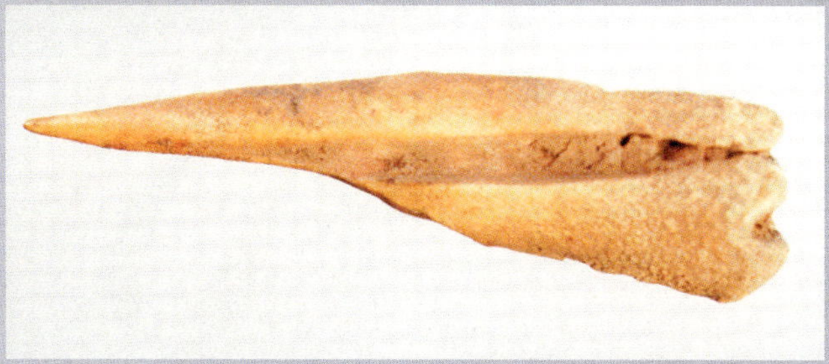

Awl, deer bone splinter, 2¾" long. It is ex-collection Vietzen, from southern Ohio. Fred Winegardner collection. **$20.00.**

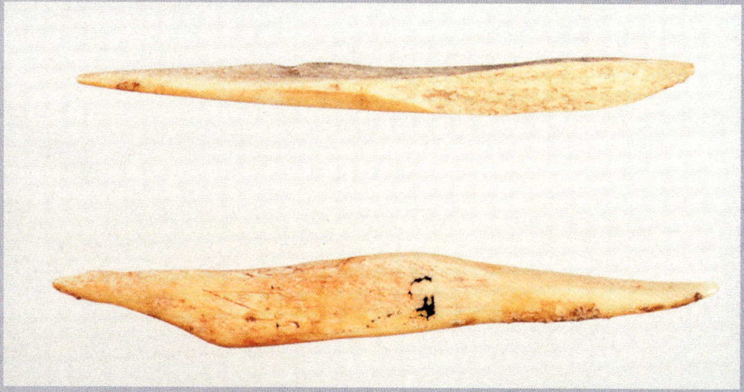

Awls, deer bone splinters, longest is 3⅛". Both are well-polished and the double-tipped examples came from Tuscarawas County, Ohio. Fred Winegardner collection. Each, **$10.00 – 15.00.**

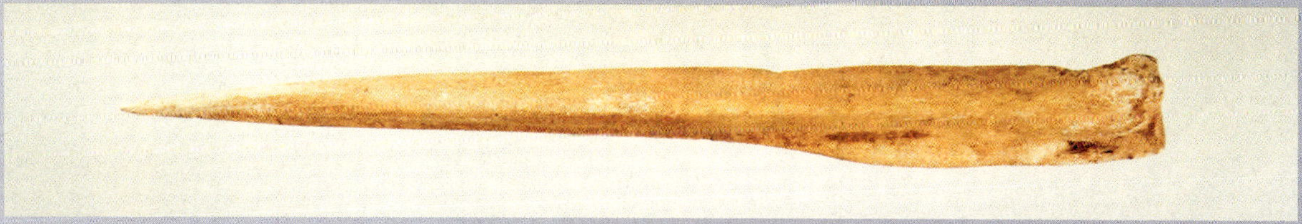

Pin or awl, animal bone, polished lower tip. This large example, 7⅛" long, came from the Nashville area, Tennessee. Robin Fiser collection. **$60.00.**

Awl, deer bone splinter, 4³⁄₁₆". It is from the huge collection once owned by Col. Vietzen, and came from Ohio or Kentucky. Fred Winegardner collection. **$12.00.**

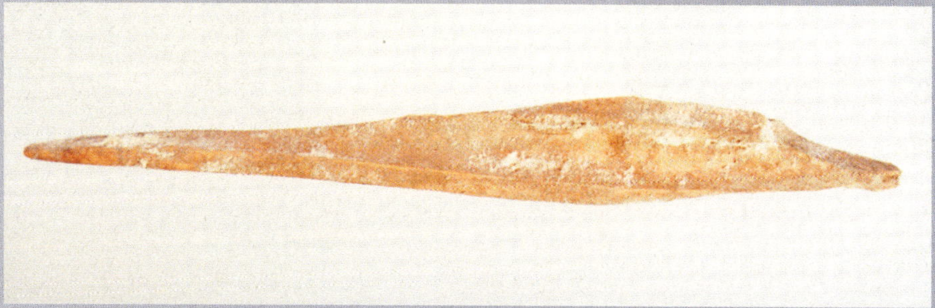

Splinter Awls

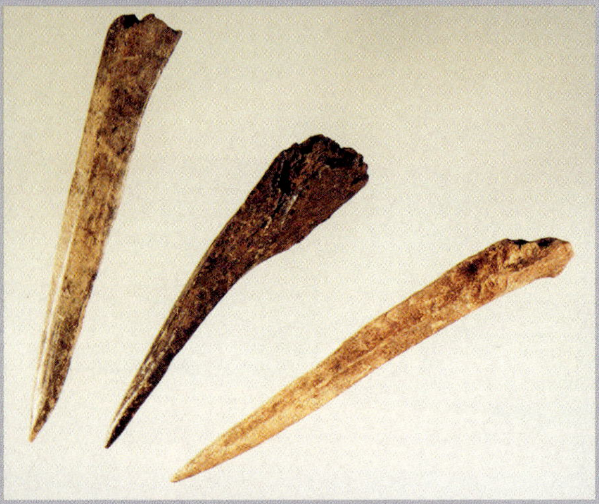

Awls, split animal bones, longest is 4¼". All were found along Sulphur Fork Creek, Robertson County, Tennessee. Robin Fiser collection. Each, **$12.00 – 15.00.**

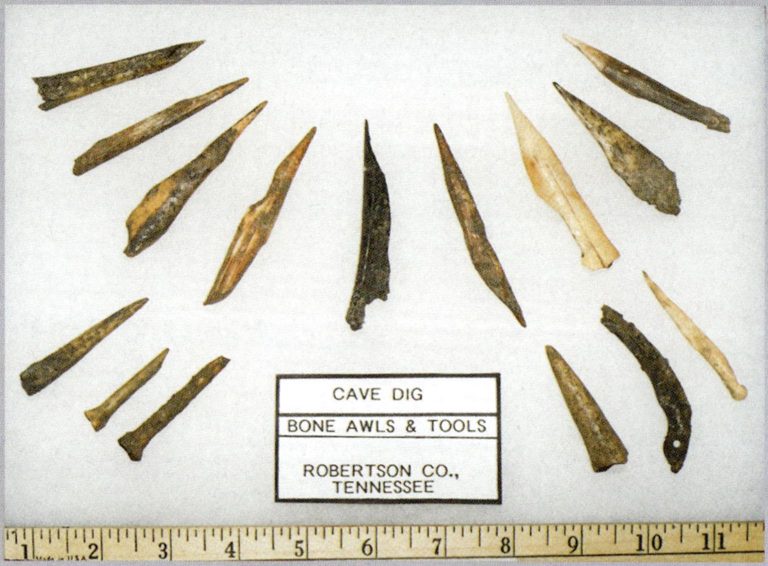

Bone awls and tools, longest example is 3¼". These came from a rock shelter site in Robertson County, Tennessee. Back to Earth. Group, **$85.00.**

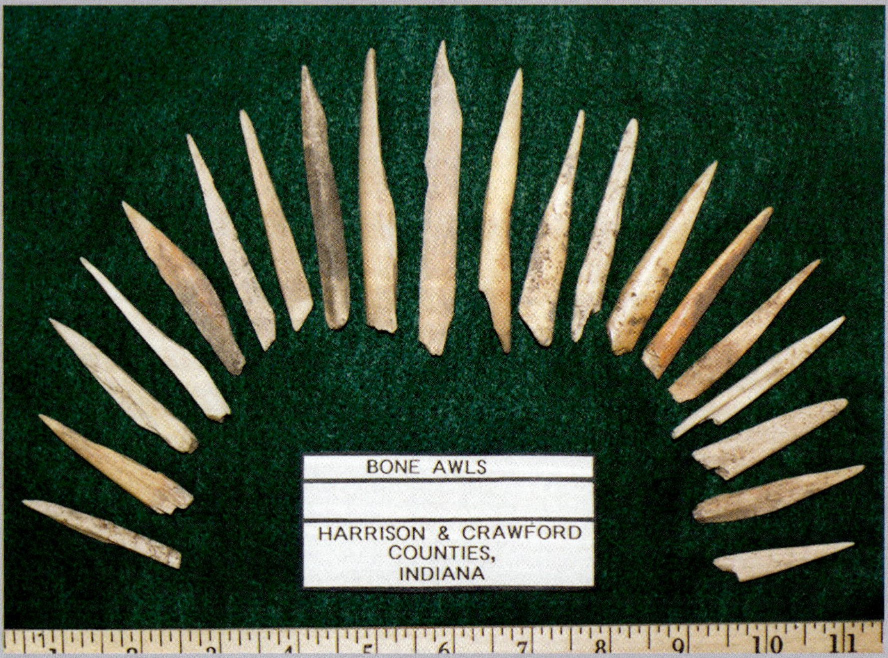

Awls, most examples are split bone or splinter types, sizes are as indicated. These came from Harrison and Crawford Counties, Indiana. Back to Earth. Group, **$120.00.**

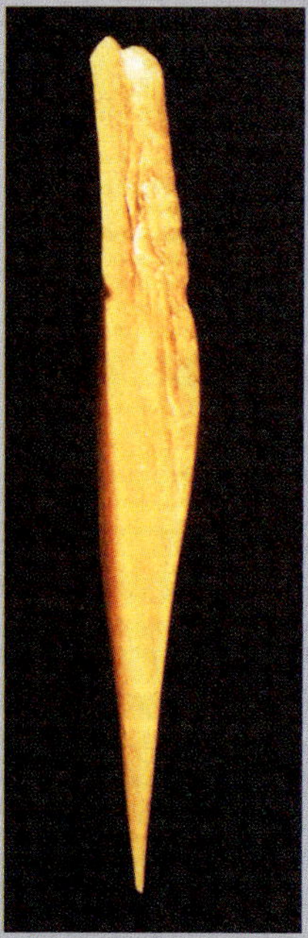

Awl, deer bone splinter, very pointed tip, 2¹¹⁄₁₆". The upper shaft is contracted as if for a handle on this awl. Found in southern Ohio. Private collection. **$12.00.**

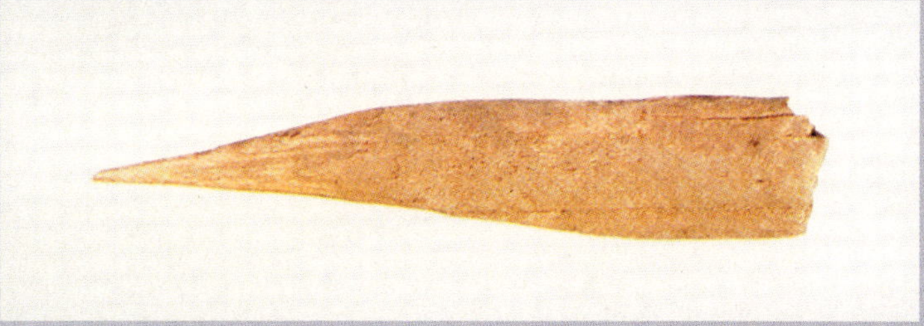

Awl or perforator, split deer bone, 2⅜" long. It is ex-collection Vietzen, from Ohio or Kentucky. Fred Winegardner collection. **$12.00.**

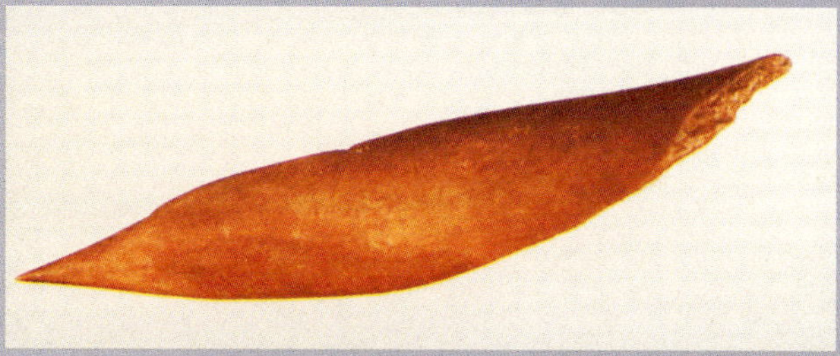

Awl, split deer bone, 2⅞" long. Coated with shellac, it was once in the Vietzen collection. Ohio or Kentucky. Fred Winegardner collection. **$15.00.**

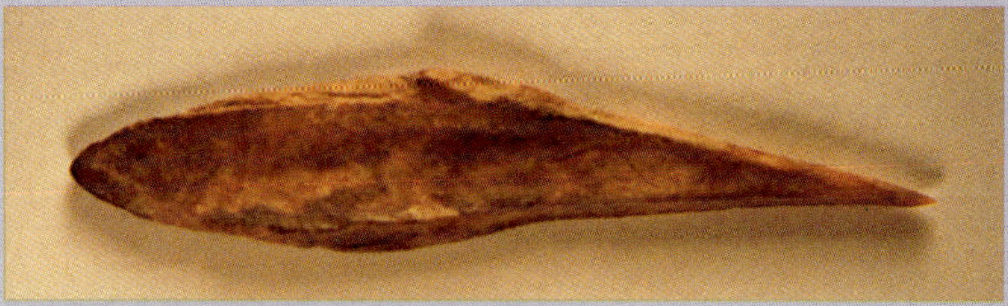

Awl, bone splinter, ⅝ x 3⅝". It is Mississippian in time, and was found along a stream that joins the Ohio River. Private collection. Rodney Roberts photograph. Cabell County, West Virginia. **$20.00.**

Awl, large split bone, high polish on lower shaft. It is 4¾" long. Ex-collection Hall. Wayne County, Kentucky. Private collection. **$20.00.**

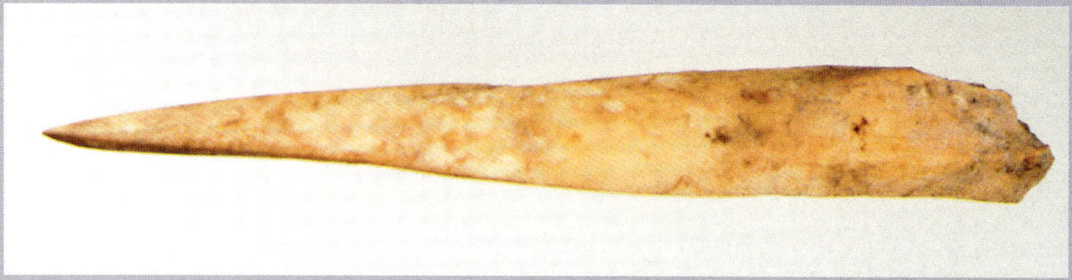

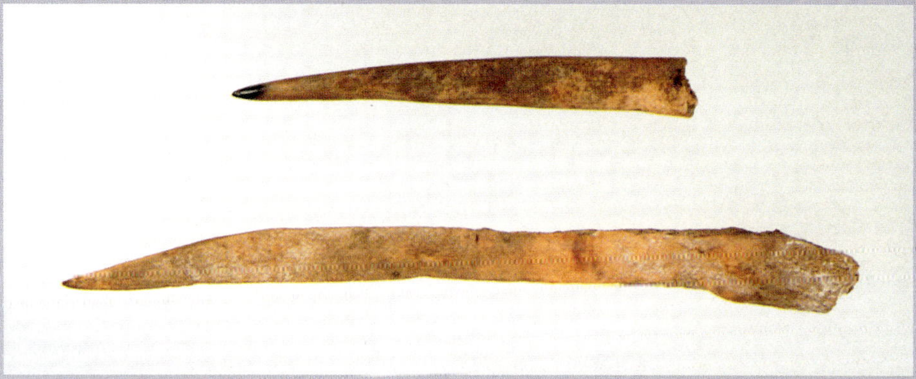

Splinter awls, bone, longest is 4⅜". The shorter awl evidences much wear and use-polish. Ex-collection Hall, Wayne County, Kentucky. Private collection. Each, **$4.00 – 6.00.**

Awl, ivory-like bone splinter, shaft heavily polished for entire length. It is 3½" long, and ex-collection Hall. Wayne County, Kentucky. Private collection. **$15.00.**

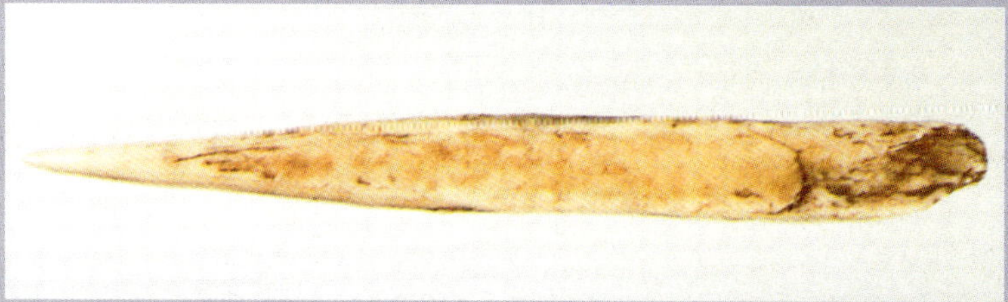

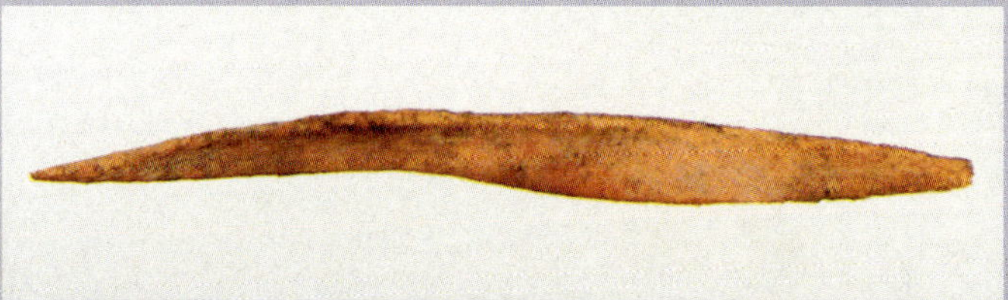

Awl or perforator, thin bird bone, 2[15]⁄16" long. It is from Pulaski or Wayne County, Kentucky. Private collection. **$7.00.**

Splinter Awls

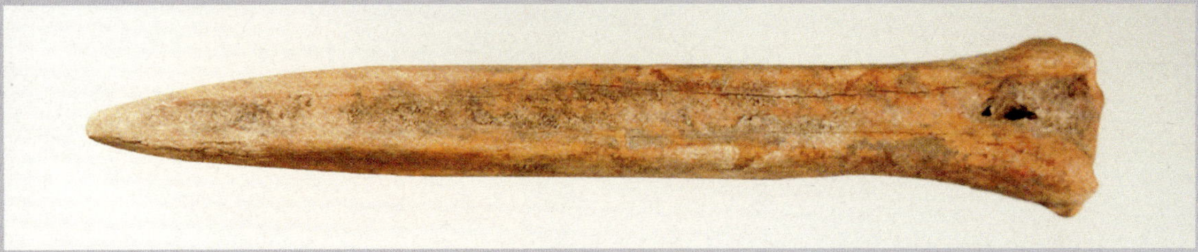

Dagger(?), pale orange patina, split animal bone, 5⅜" long. It is ex-collection Hall, from Wayne County, Kentucky. Private collection. **$30.00.**

Awl, bone splinter, translucent tip, 4½" long. This example, with pointed base, may originally have had a bone or antler handle. Ex-collection Hall, Wayne County, Kentucky. Private collection. **$12.00 – 15.00.**

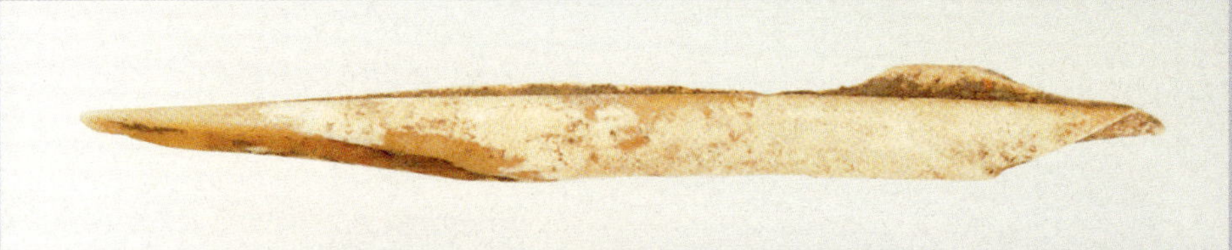

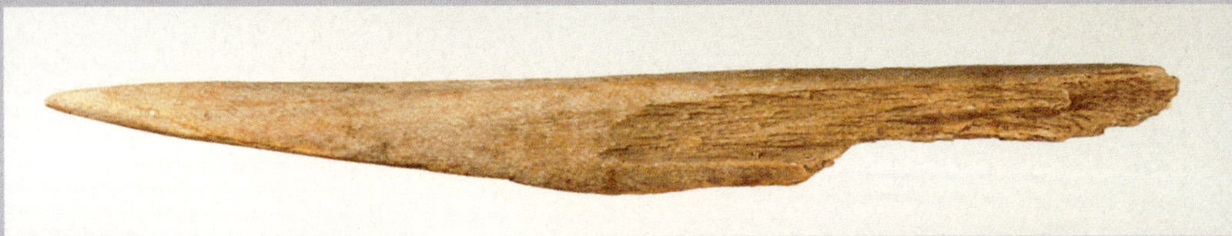

Awl, bone splinter, worn lower shaft portion, 5⅛" long. It is ex-collection Hall, from Wayne County, Kentucky. Private collection. **$12.00. – 15.00.**

Awl or perforator, animal bone splinter, 4 31/32" long. It was found in the 1950s and came from Pulaski or Wayne County, Kentucky. Private collection. **$15.00 – 20.00.**

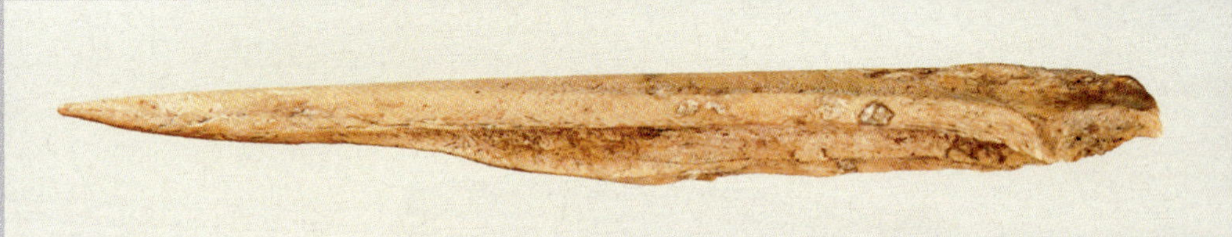

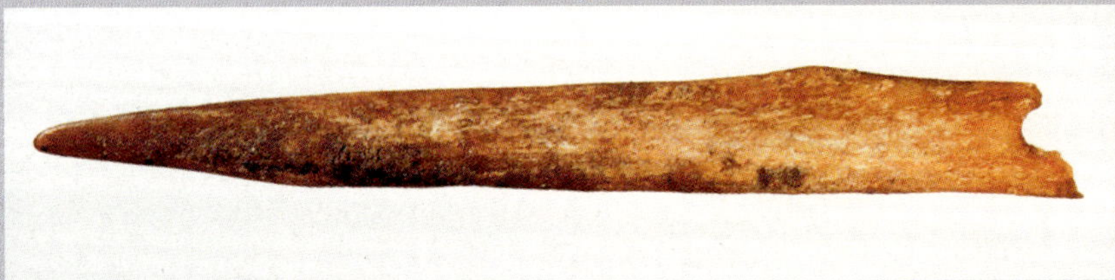

Awl or needle, broken at the wide end eye, 3¾" long. With a combination light brown and dark brown patina, the artifact was found in the 1950s. Pulaski or Wayne County, Kentucky. Private collection. **$10.00.**

Awl, bone splinter, high polish on lower shaft, 3¾" long. Found in the 1950s, it came from Pulaski or Wayne County, Kentucky. Private collection. **$12.00.**

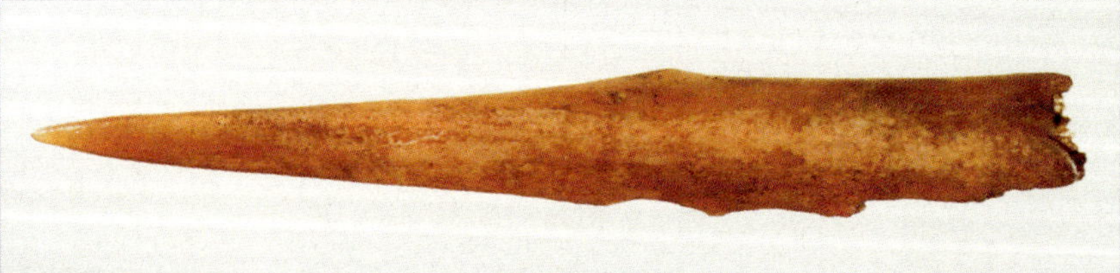

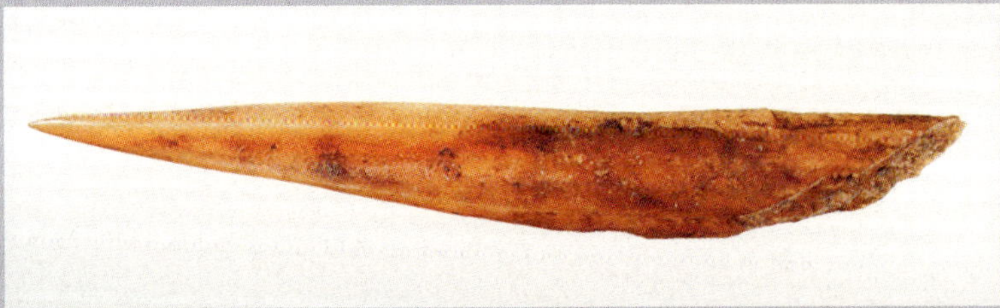

Awl, polished animal bone splinter, translucent lower half of shaft. It is 3½" long and was found in the 1950s. Pulaski or Wayne County, Kentucky. Private collection. **$15.00.**

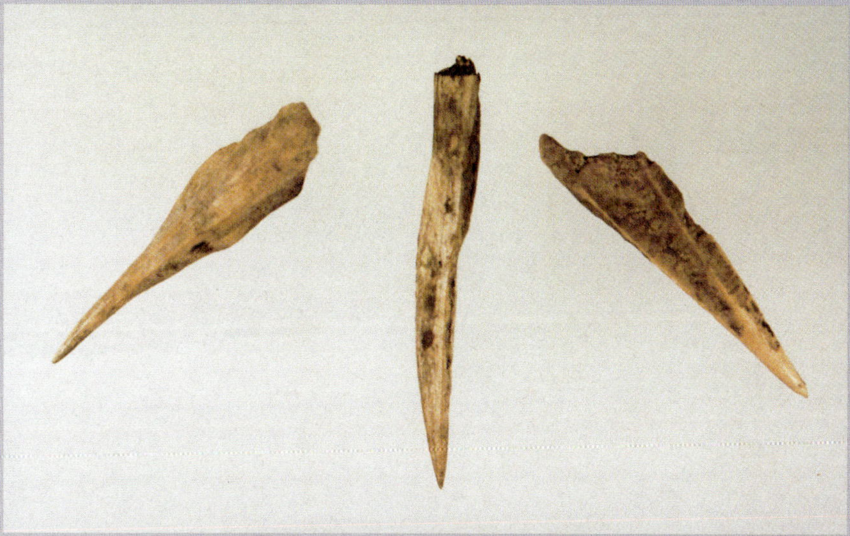

Awls, split animal bones, center example is 2¼". These were made on short sections of bone and indicate that (on the site where found) even small bone pieces were utilized. Wayne County, Kentucky. Private collection. Each, **$4.00 – 6.00.**

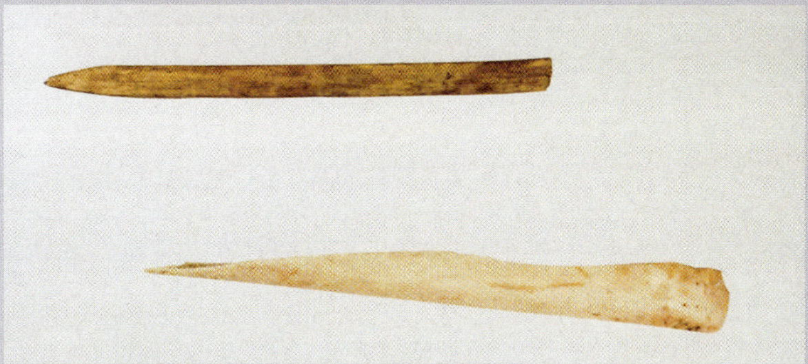

Awls or perforators, thin-walled bird bone splinters, longest is 2½". Both are quite delicate and could not have been used for heavy-duty work. Ex-collection Hall, Wayne County, Kentucky. Private collection. Each, **$4.00 – 7.00.**

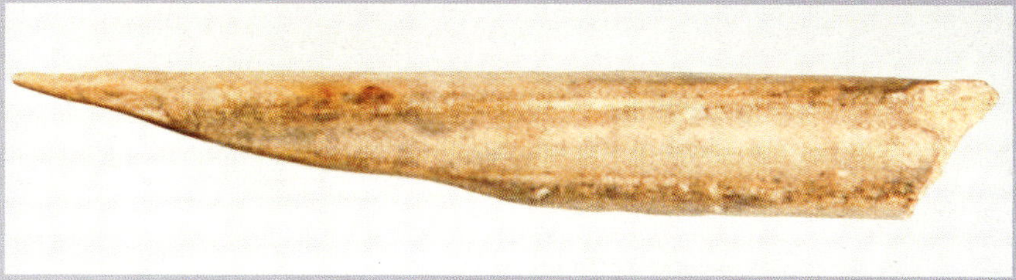

Awl, thick bone splinter, polished surface, 3⅞" long. Found in the 1950s, it is from Pulaski or Wayne County, Kentucky. Private collection. **$15.00.**

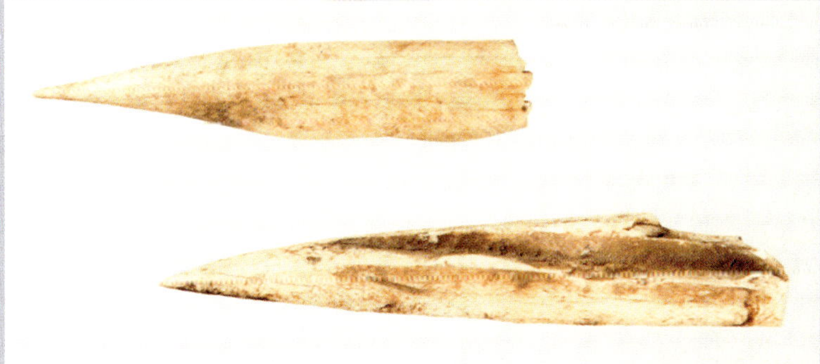

Awls, bone splinters, longest is 2¾". Both have worn and polished shafts. Ex-collection Hall, they are from Wayne County, Kentucky. Private collection. **$7.00 – 10.00.**

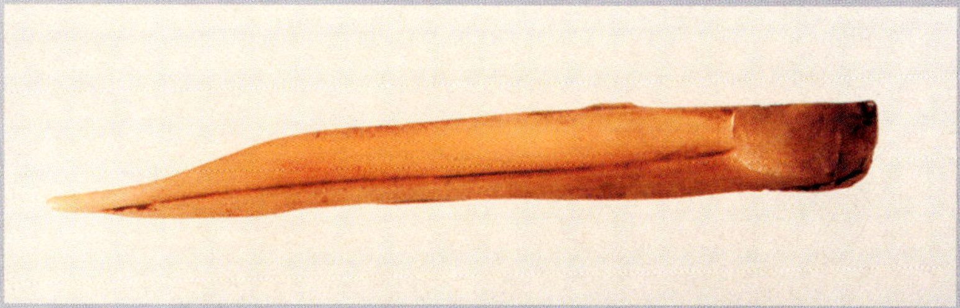

Awl, thick splinter of animal bone, 3¼" long. This artifact is very translucent for the entire length. Wayne County, Kentucky. Private collection. **$15.00.**

Splinter Awls

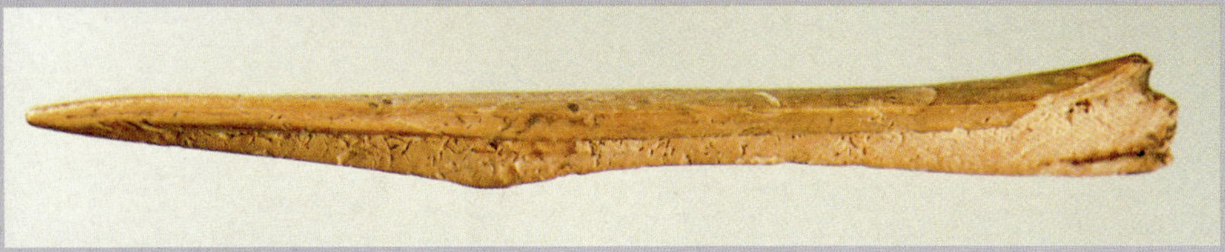

Awl, bone splinter, worn shaft edges, 4⅝". It was found in the 1950s and came from either Pulaski or Wayne County, Kentucky. Private collection. **$15.00.**

Awl, split animal bone, weathered surface, 4⅜". This example is ex-collection Hall, from Wayne County, Kentucky. Private collection. **$8.00.**

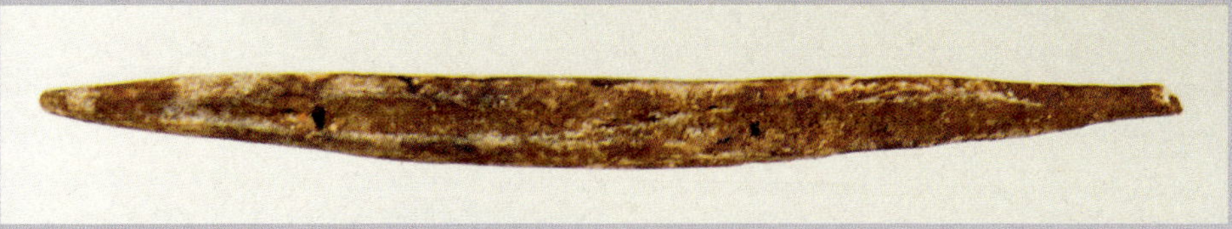

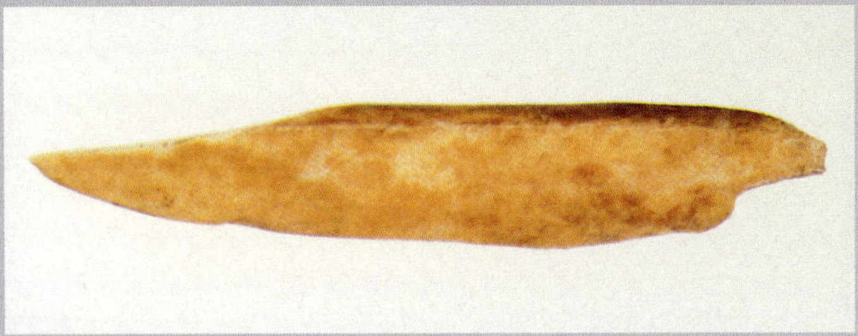

Awl or perforator, splintered bird bone, 3" long. It has a pleasing brown patina and the lower awl edges are polished. Ex-collection Hall, it is from Wayne County, Kentucky. Private collection. **$10.00.**

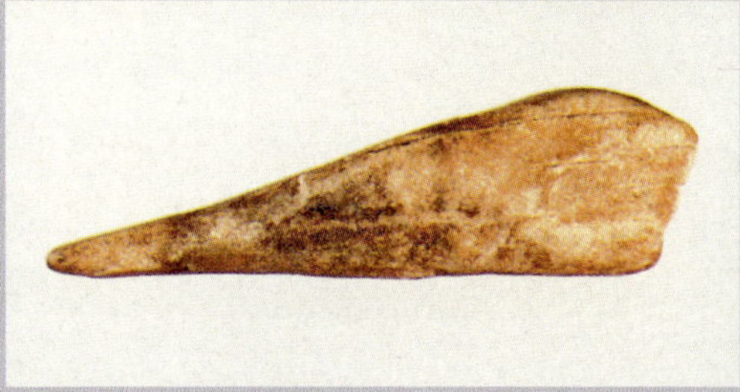

Awl, short and wide for type, animal bone, worn tip and lower shaft. It is 2⅛" long. From Wayne County, Tennessee. Private collection. **$7.00.**

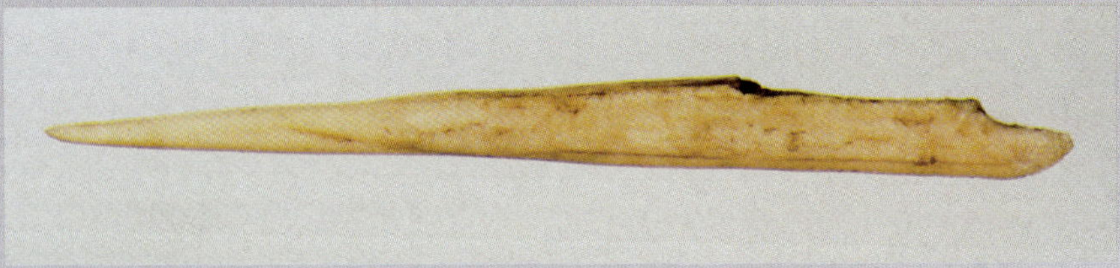

Awl, split bird bone, thin walls, polished shaft. This awl is 4" long and came from Wayne County, Tennessee. Private collection. **$12.00 – 15.00.**

Awl, split animal bone, polished lower shaft, 4⅛" long. Found in the 1950s, it is from Pulaski or Wayne County, Kentucky. Private collection. **$15.00.**

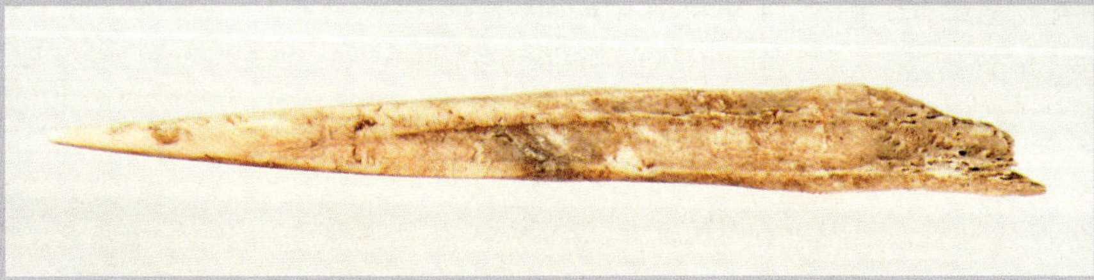

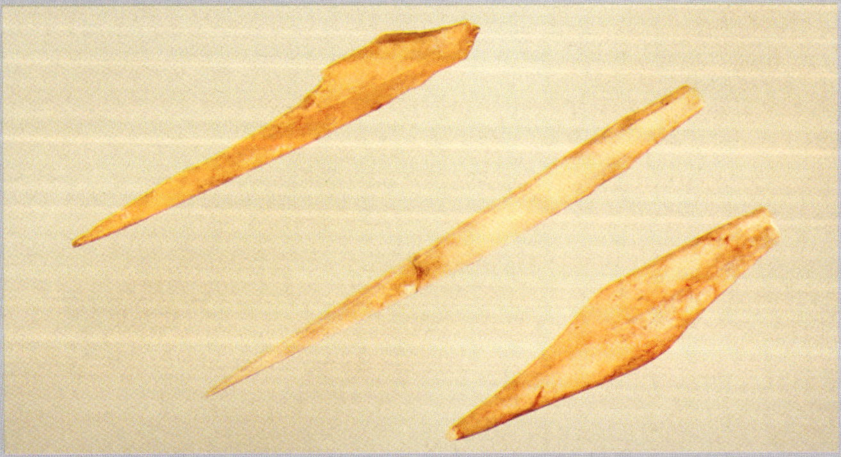

Splinter awls, animal bones, longest bird bone example (broken and glued) at center is 3⅝". Ex-collection Selb, West Virginia. Doug Hooks collection. Each, **$10.00 – 15.00.**

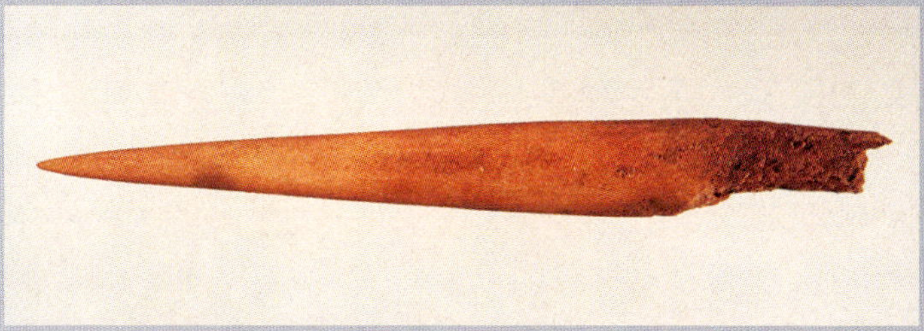

Awl, thin bone splinter, translucent for most of length, 3⅛" long. Wayne County, Kentucky. Private collection. **$15.00.**

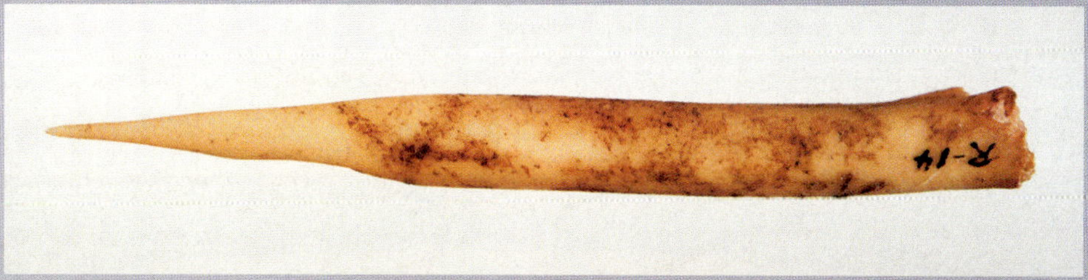

Awl, bone from large bird, 4⅜" long. This awl is translucent for most of the length. It came from a rock shelter in southern Tennessee. Private collection. **$20.00.**

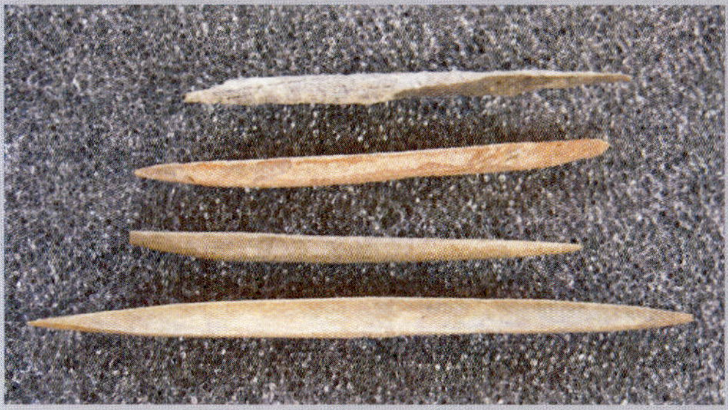

Bone fishing tools or gorge hooks, averaging 2" long. They came from Pyramid Lake in the Great Basin of Nevada. Victor T. Trujillo collection, Nevada. Each, **$10.00 – 20.00.**

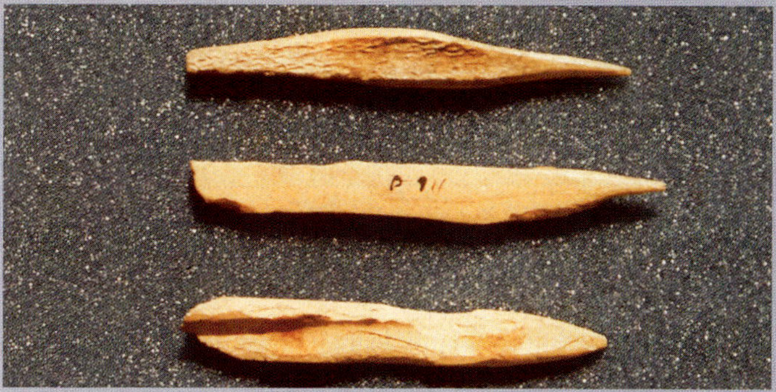

Splinter bone awls, 2¾ to 3" long, historic Iroquois (Seneca), ca. AD 1650 – 1675. Probably made of deer bone, the awls are from near Honeoye Falls. Monroe County, New York. Dave Summers collection, Victor, New York. Each, **$20.00.**

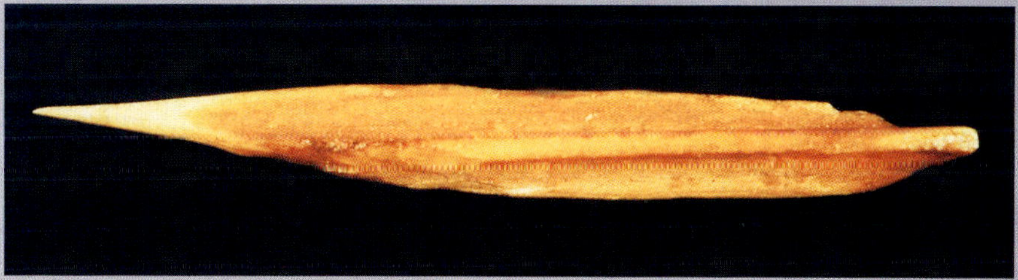

Awl, deer bone splinter, chemically stabilized, 4⅛". It has a polished tip and is Mississippian in time. Southern Ohio. Private collection. **$20.00.**

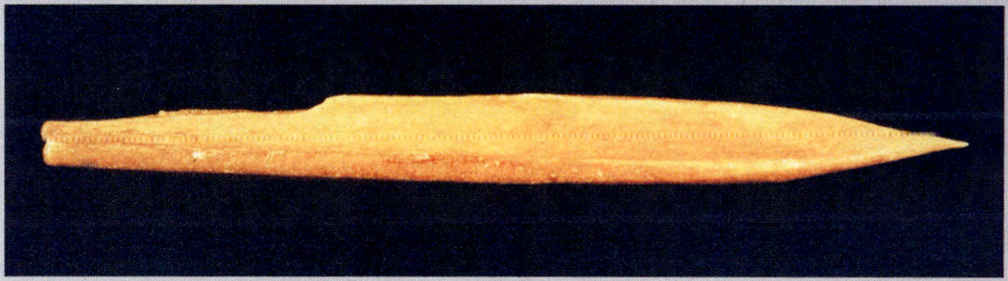

Awl, bone splinter, needle tip, medium brown patination. It is coated with shellac and measures 3¹⁵⁄₁₆". Southern Ohio. Private collection. **$15.00.**

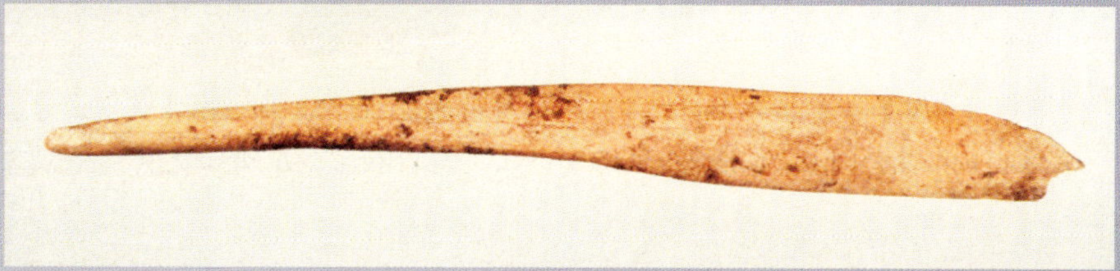

Awl, thin-walled animal bone splinter, coated with preservative, 4⅛". This typical awl is from Kentucky or Tennessee. Private collection. **$10.00.**

Splinter Awls

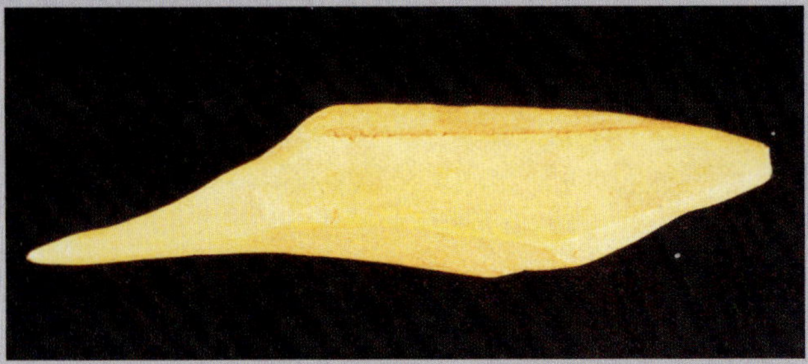

Awl, heavy bone chip, pale orange patination, $2\frac{11}{16}$". There is much wear polish on all edges for this piece. Fort Ancient and from southern Ohio. Private collection. **$15.00.**

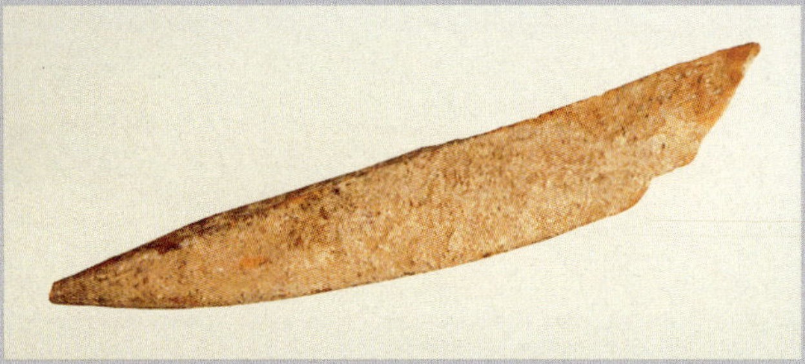

Awl, bone splinter, $2\frac{3}{4}$". This typical awl has a gray-brown patina and came from Kentucky. Fred Winegardner collection. **$12.00.**

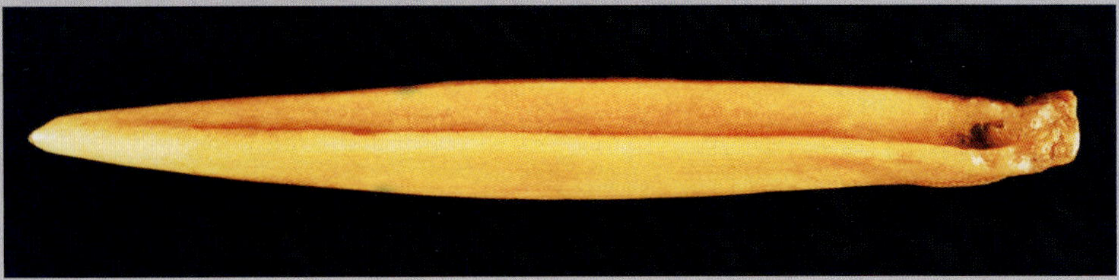

Awl, split deer bone, $4\frac{1}{2}$" long. It is chemically stabilized, and the particular process used provides a slightly translucent coating, uniform smoothness and texture, plus a bit more weight than is usual. Fort Ancient, southern Ohio. Private collection. **$30.00.**

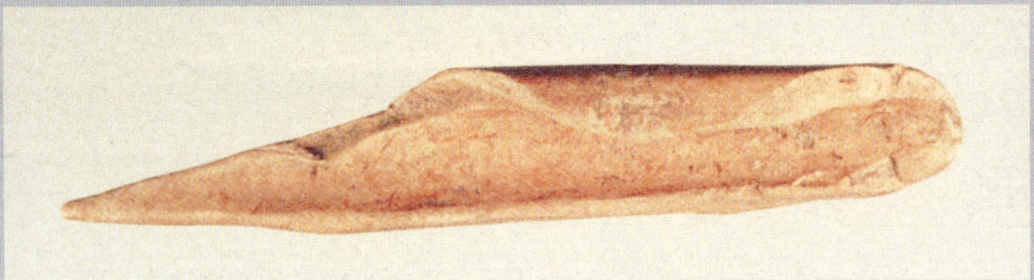

Awl, split heavy bone, yellowish patina, $3\frac{7}{8}$" long. It is from Kentucky or Tennessee. Private collection. **$12.00.**

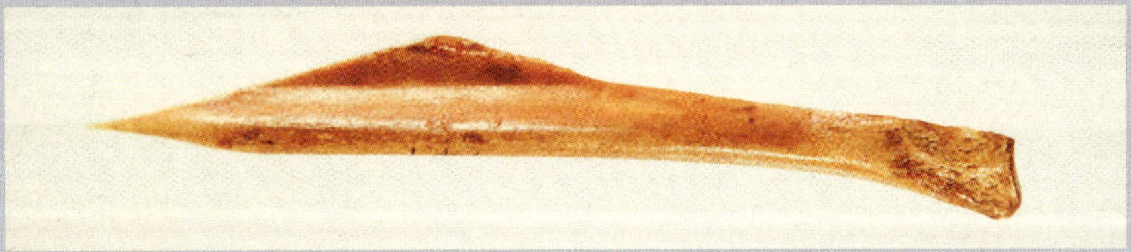

Awl, split deer bone, very pointed tip and with use polish on edges. It is $3\frac{15}{16}$" long and has a golden brown patination. Coated with shellac, the piece came from southern Ohio. Private collection. **$15.00.**

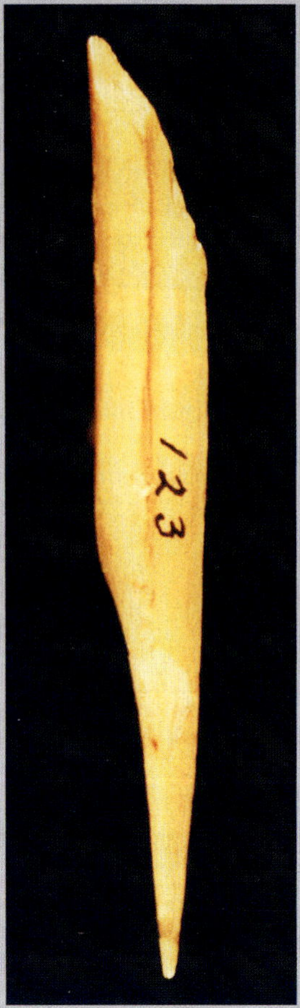

Awl, deer bone splinter, $3\frac{3}{4}$". It was found on a Fort Ancient site (late prehistoric) in southern Ohio. Private collection. **$12.00.**

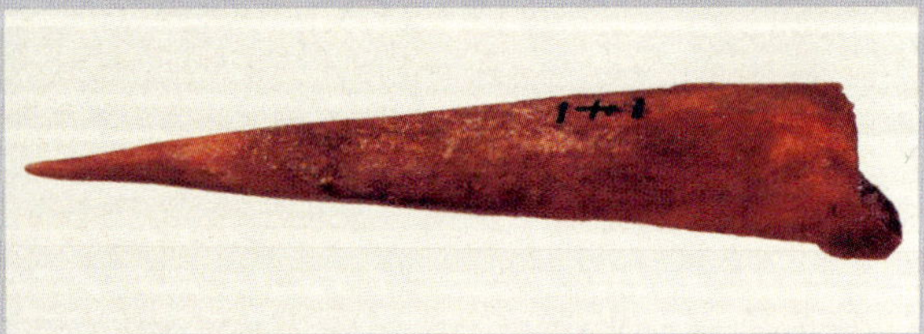

Awl, bone splinter, patinated to a deep amber-brown color. It is $2\frac{1}{2}$" long and the tip is polished. Kentucky or Tennessee. Private collection. **$12.00.**

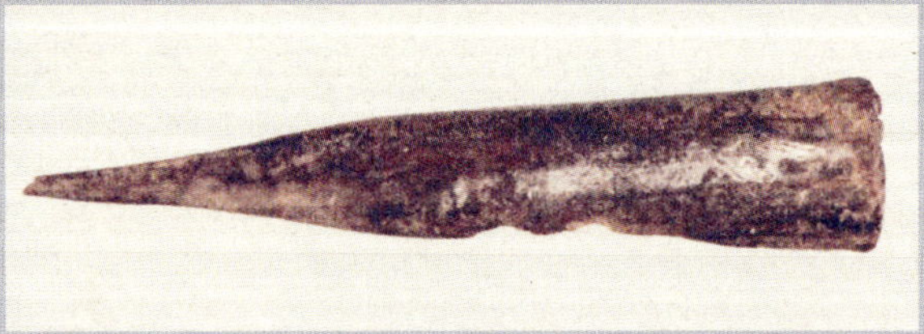

Awl, bone splinter, chemical coat over dark patina, $2\frac{1}{2}$". It was found in 1974 and came from southern Ohio. Private collection. **$8.00.**

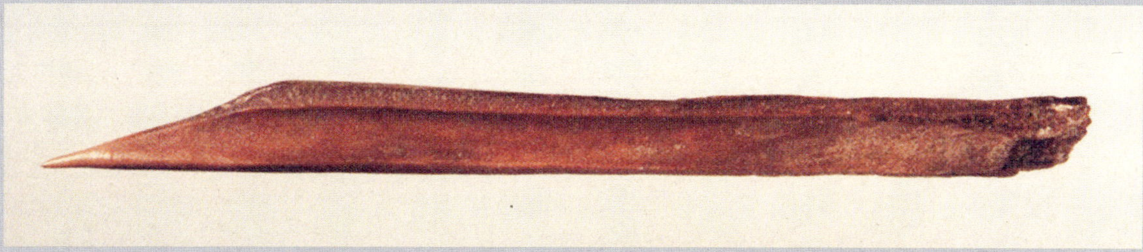

Awl or perforator, split bone, 5½". It is unusually long and the tip and lower shaft have much use-polish. Kentucky or Tennessee. Private collection. **$20.00.**

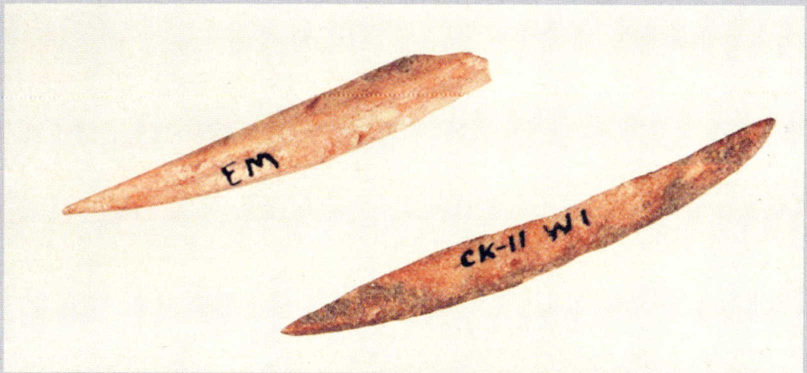

Awls, bone splinters. Longer awl is double-tipped and 2⅞"; the shorter one is thick for its size. Both are from Kentucky or Tennessee. Private collection. Each, **$5.00.**

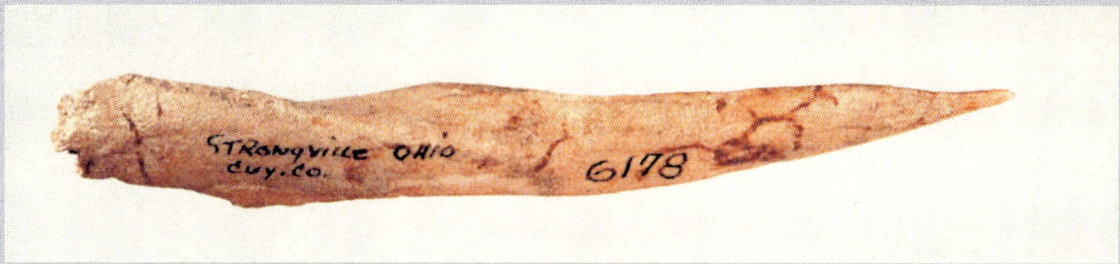

Awl, splintered animal bone, 4¼". Found near Strongville in Cuyahoga County, this part of the state had both Sandusky and Whittlesey peoples in Mississippian (AD 800 – 1500) times. Ohio. Private collection. **$15.00.**

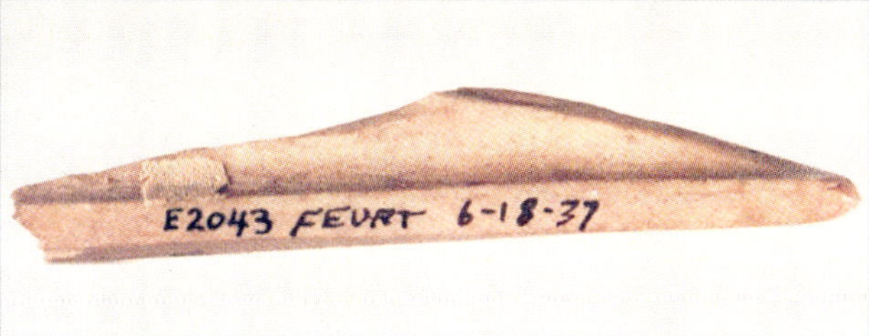

Awl, blunt tip, splint made from large animal bone, 2¾" long. For a common artifact like this, provenance information (owner, site, and date) helps value. Ex-collection Copeland. Found in 1937, it is from southern Ohio. Private collection. **$15.00.**

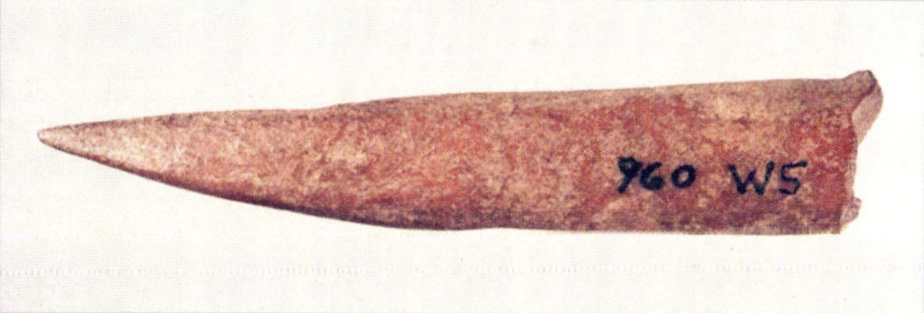

Awl, split animal bone, reddish patina, 3¼". Well-used, the awl is from Kentucky or Tennessee. Private collection. **$12.00.**

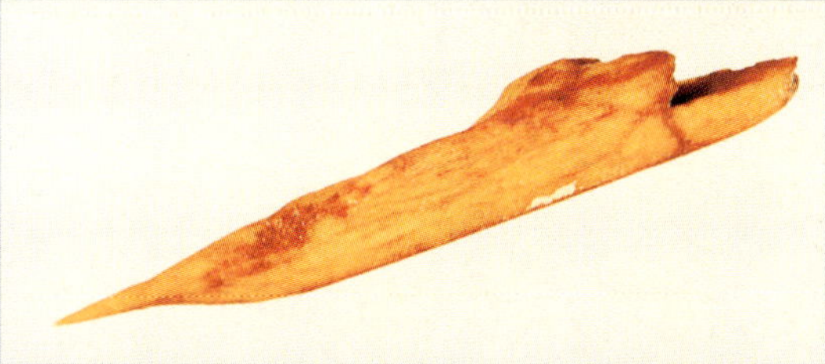

Splinter awl, with needle tip, 2⅛" long, coated with shellac. It is Fort Ancient, Mississippian period, southern Ohio. Private collection. **$12.00.**

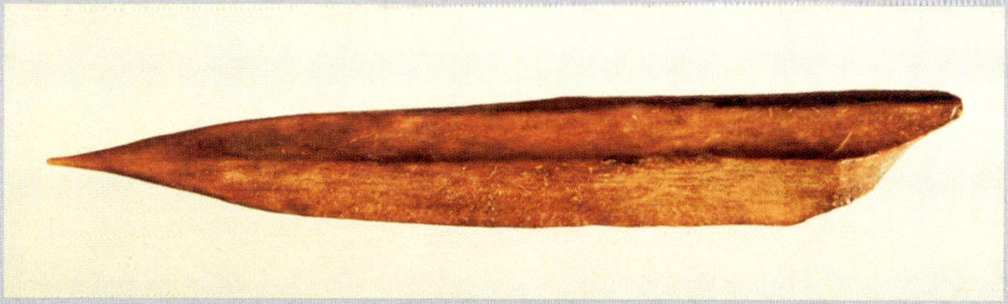

Awl, heavy bone splinter with amber-brown patina. Coated with shellac, it is 3¾" long and came from southern Ohio. Private collection. **$20.00.**

Splinter Awls

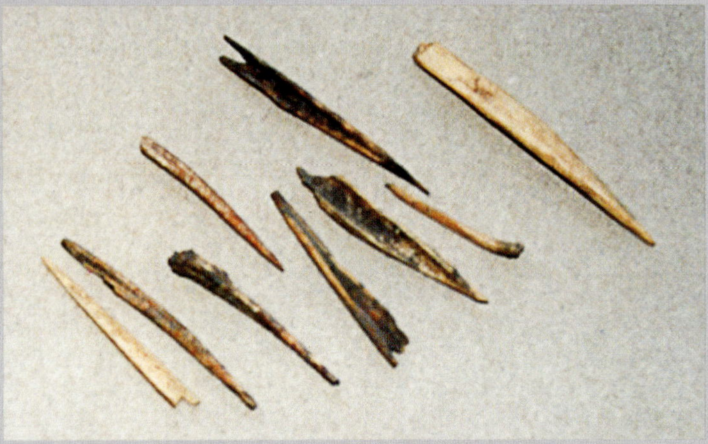

Awls, made from bird bones, 1½ to 3" long. All were found in Florida. Wilfred Dick collection, Mississippi. Each, **$5.00 – 25.00.**

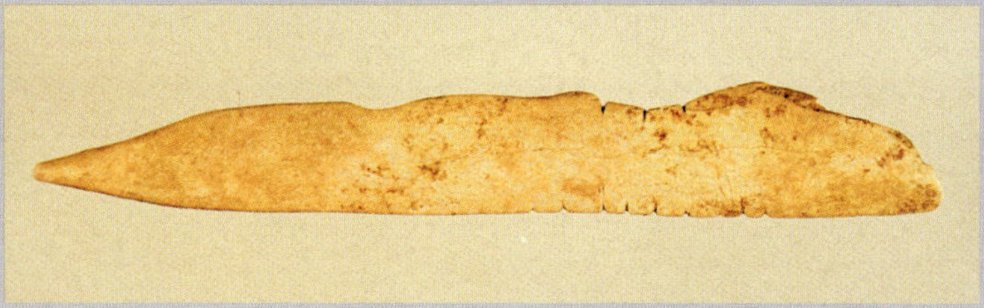

Awl, deer bone splinter, 3⅜". It has tally marks on the upper shaft, three on one side and nine on the other. These narrow notches, judging by location, may have been a hafting aid for fastening to a handle. Southern Ohio. Private collection. **$30.00.**

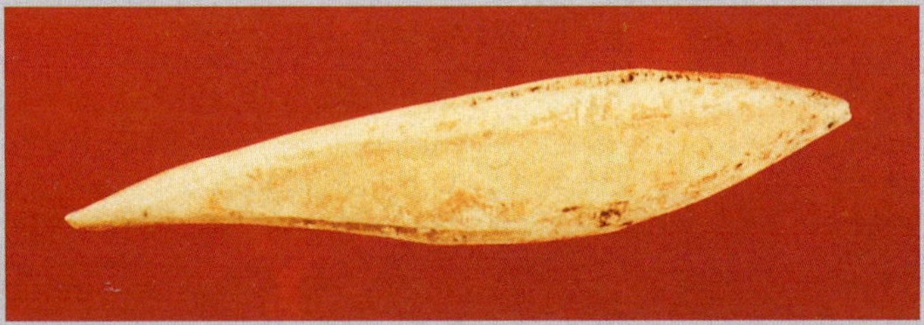

Awl, probably made from a section of deer bone, 2¹³⁄₁₆". This example is double-tipped and came from Kentucky. Private collection. **$12.00.**

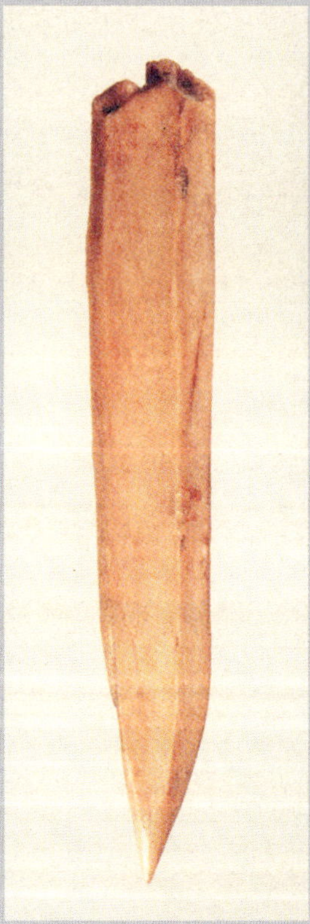

Awl, bone splinter, chemically stabilized. The awl is 3½". From Kentucky or Tennessee. Private collection. **$10.00.**

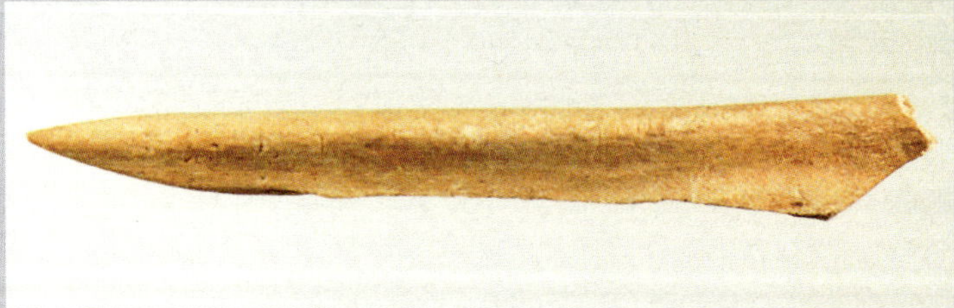

Awl, deer bone splinter, polished tip, 3¼". It was found in southern Ohio. **$10.00.**

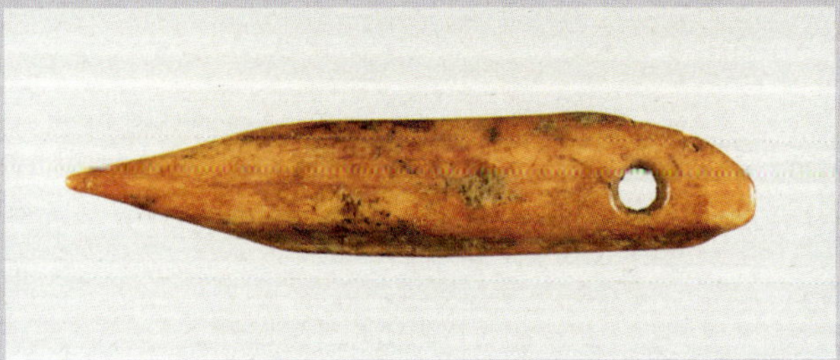

Needle or eyed awl, bone splinter with high polish, 2⅜". It has a golden brown patina and came from a rock shelter. Fairfield County, Ohio. Lar Hothem collection. **$30.00.**

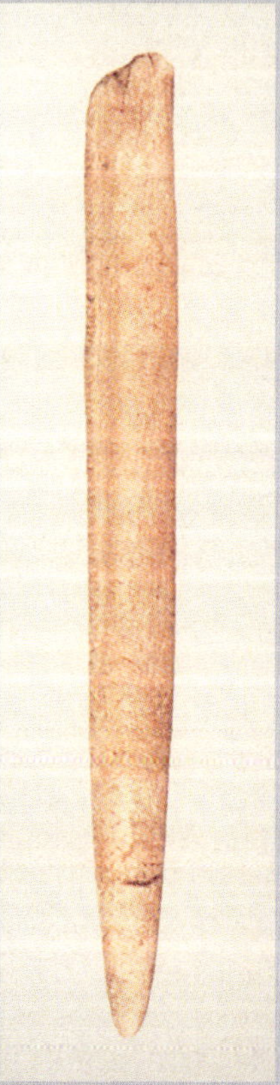

Awl, thick-walled bone splinter, rounded at tip, 3⅝" long. From Kentucky or Tennessee. Private collection. **$10.00.**

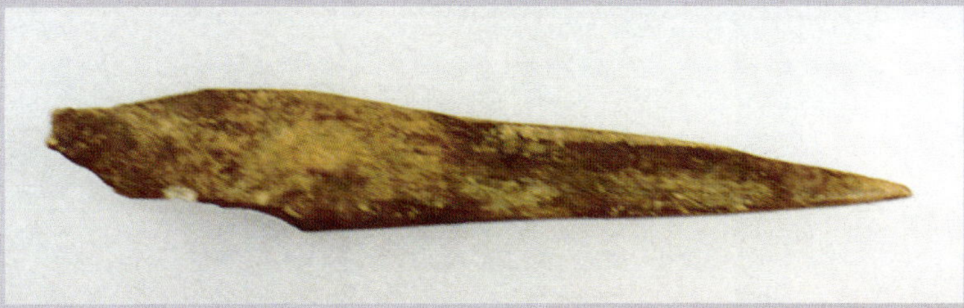

Awl, split animal bone, 3½", lower one-third with good polish. The awl has a weathered finish and is Late Archaic to Woodland. Ex-collection Vietzen, it came from Christian County, Kentucky. Pete Timoch collection. **$50.00.**

Awl or point, split bone, Mississippian period, 4⅜" long. Ex-collection Vietzen, the wider end has been narrowed as if to fit into a handle socket. Northern Ohio. John Timoch collection. **$50.00.**

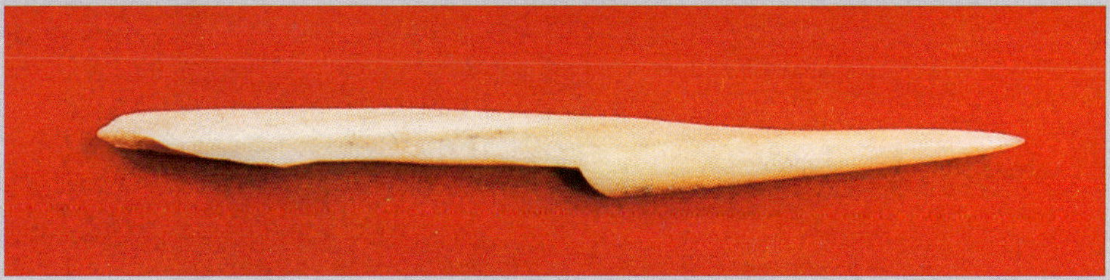

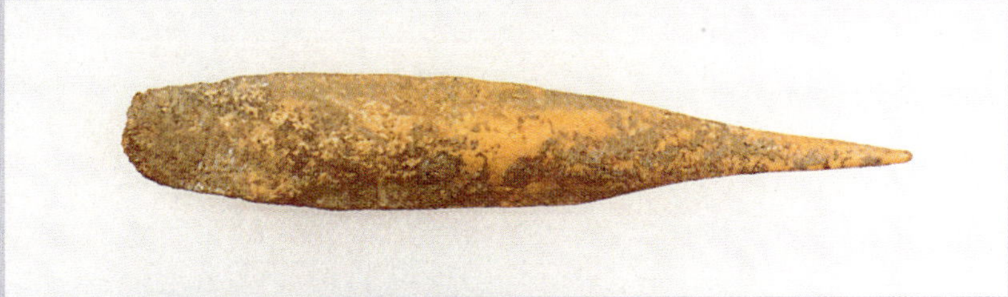

Awl, split bone, 3¾", surface with good wear and polish. The lower portion is nicely tapered on this awl. Once owned by Col. Vietzen, Christian County, Kentucky. Pete Timoch collection. **$60.00.**

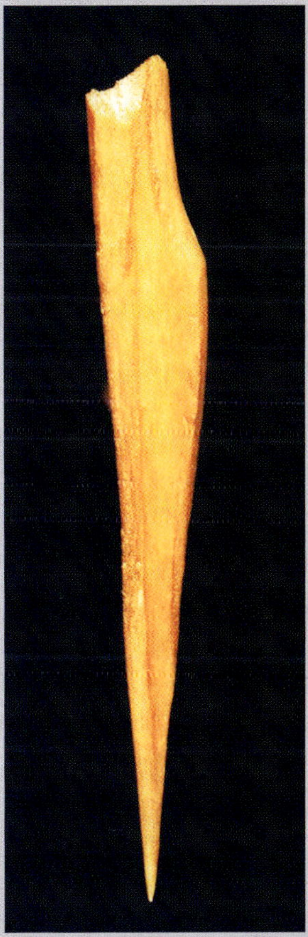

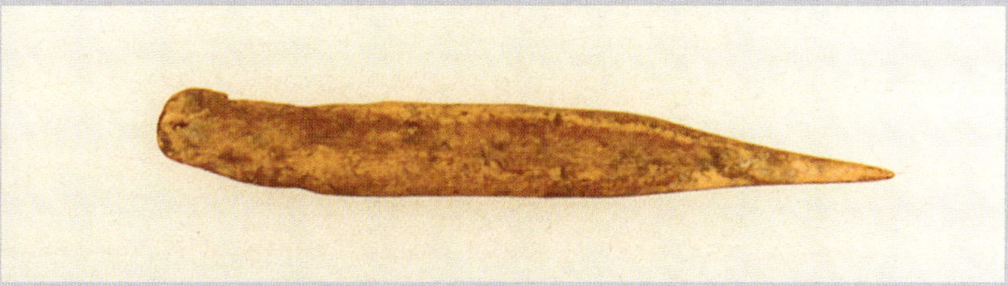

Awl, split bone, Late Archaic to Woodland, 3¹⁵⁄₁₆". The lower one-third of the length has polish around the shaft. This is a classic and very representative split awl. Ex-collection Vietzen, Christian County, Kentucky. Pete Timoch collection. **$75.00.**

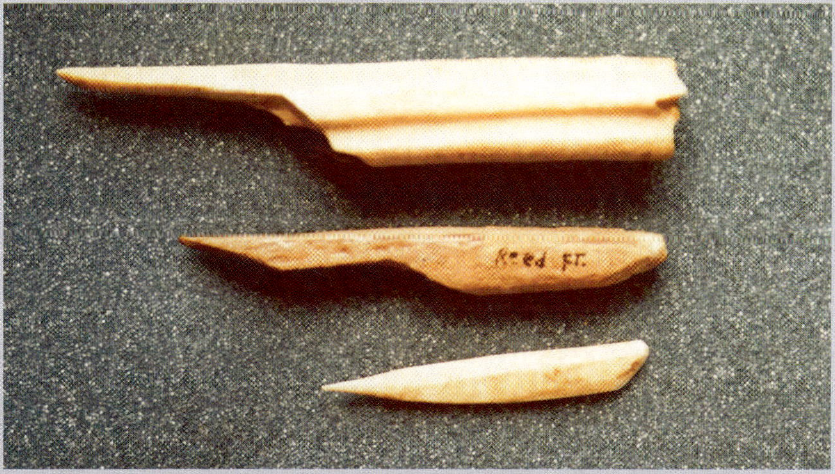

Awl, deer bone splinter, thin, 4" long. Chemically stabilized, it has a very pointed tip and is from southern Ohio. Private collection. **$15.00.**

Splinter awls, Iroquois phase, ca. AD 1540-1560. They range in length from 2¼ to 4⅛" and came from near Richmond Mills, Ontario County, New York. Dave Summers collection, Victor, New York. Each, **$15.00 – 25.00.**

Splinter Awls

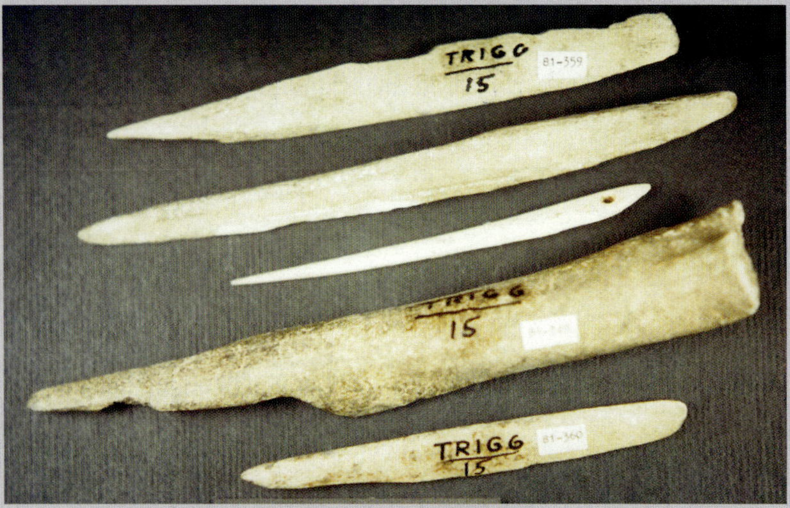

Split and splinter awls and one needle (center), these came from a rock shelter in Trigg County, Kentucky. Lee Hallman collection, Pennsylvania. Awls, each **$15.00 – 25.00;** needle, **$75.00.**

Awl, bone splinter, 3⅞". Nicely tipped, the size and thickness identify this as a deer bone. Southern Ohio. Fred Winegardner collection. **$20.00.**

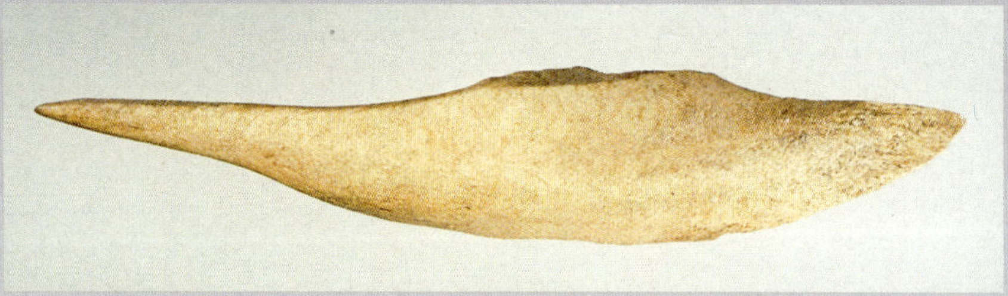

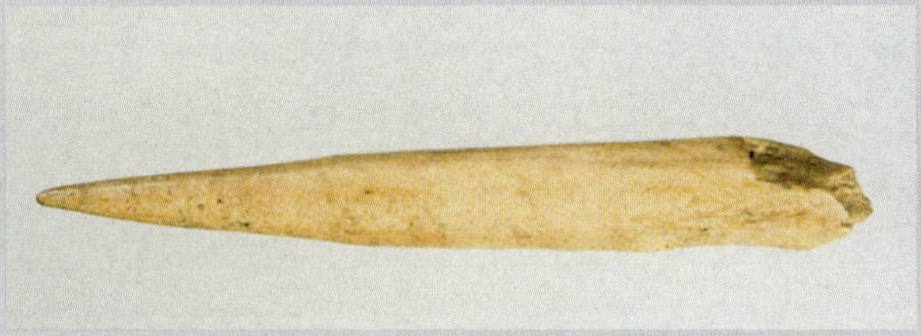

Awl, split bone, polished for length, 2⅝". Rounded in cross-section, the awl was found in Tuscarawas County, Ohio. Fred Winegardner collection. **$15.00.**

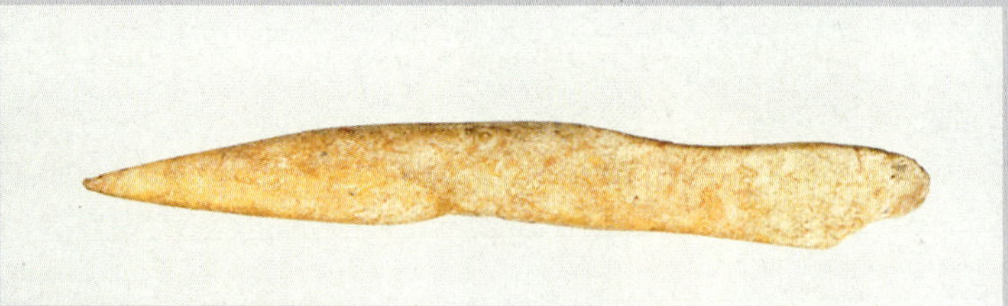

Awl, deer bone splinter, 2¾". It has some polish, and was found in Ohio. Fred Winegardner collection. **$15.00.**

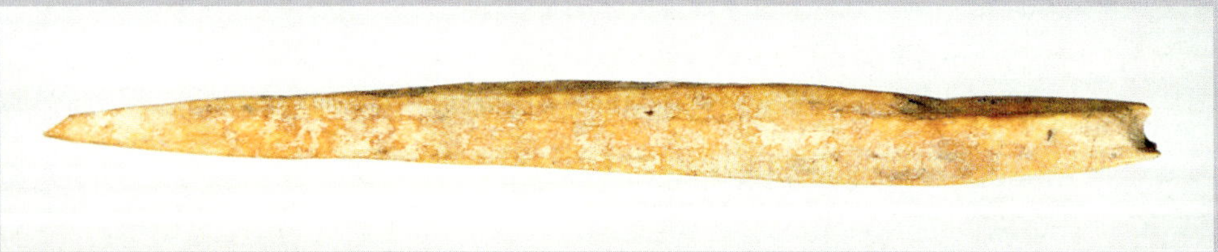

Awl, long and narrow deer bone splinter, 4⅝". Early investigators reported that the original bones were probably broken with a twisting action rather than being struck directly. Ohio. Fred Winegardner collection. **$20.00.**

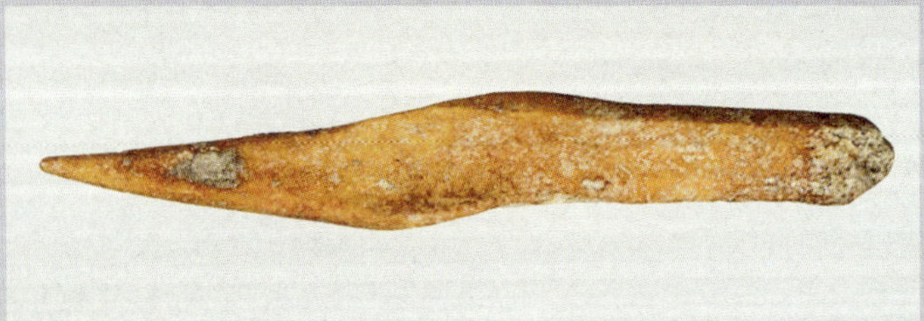

Awl, bone splinter, orange-tan patination, 3⅛". This awl was found in Ohio. Fred Winegardner collection. **$15.00.**

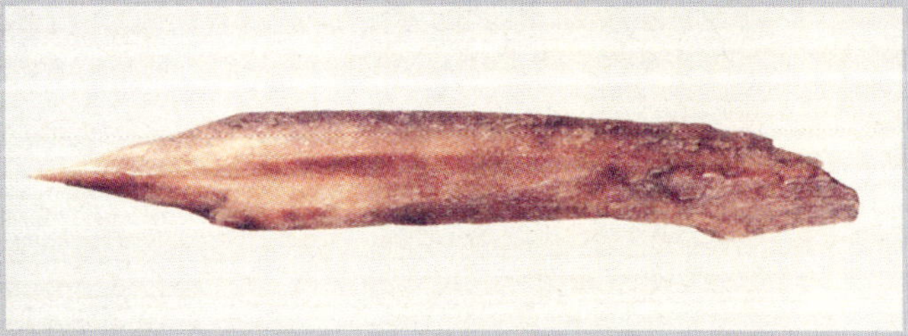

Tattooing(?) instrument, deer bone splinter, short and very pointed tip, overall length is 2½". Chemically stabilized and with a brown patina, the artifact is from Kentucky or Tennessee. Private collection. **$15.00.**

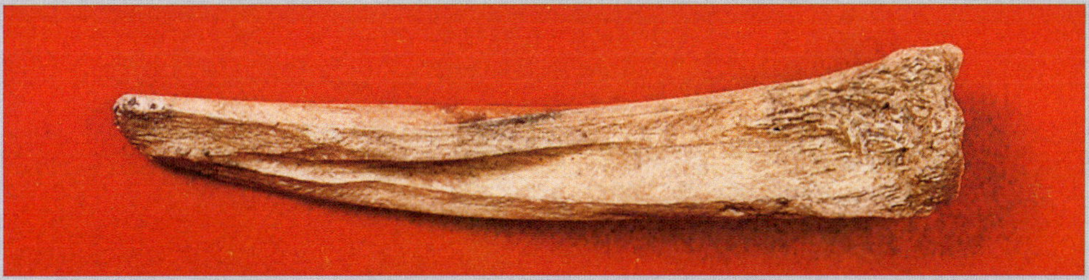

Knife, Mississippian period, split leg bone of a large animal, 4$\frac{5}{8}$" long. It was in the Vietzen collection and came from northern Ohio. Pete Timoch collection. **$75.00.**

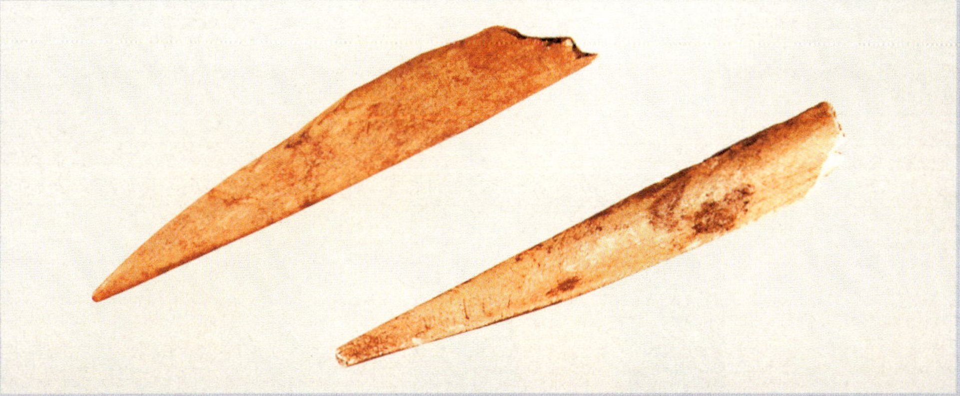

Awls, bone splinters, both from Kentucky. Private collection. Upper, 3$\frac{11}{16}$", **$10.00.** Lower, broken tip, **$5.00.**

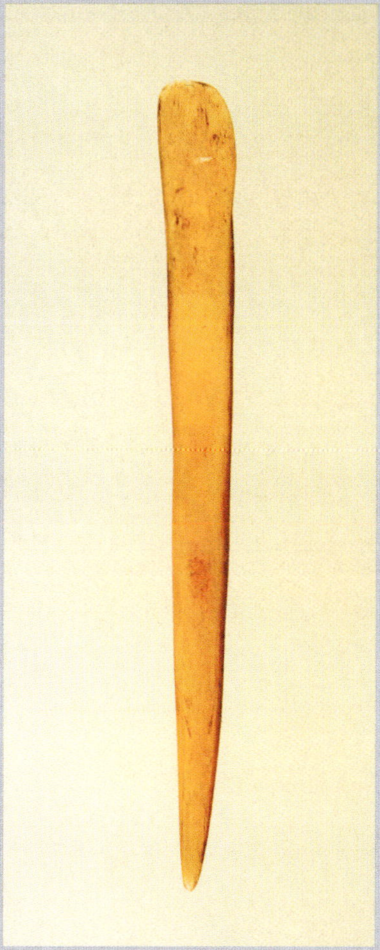

Awl, deer bone splinter, 3$\frac{3}{4}$". Nicely tapered and with smooth finish, the awl came from Kentucky. Private collection. **$15.00.**

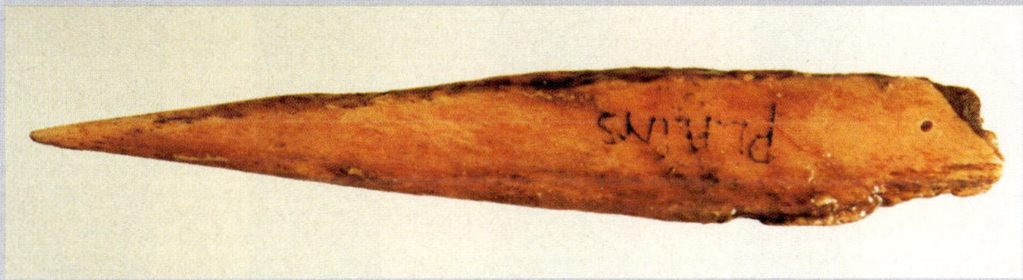

Awl, bone splinter, 4$\frac{1}{8}$" long. This artifact has no other information than that it came from the Plains region. Don Casto collection. **$30.00.**

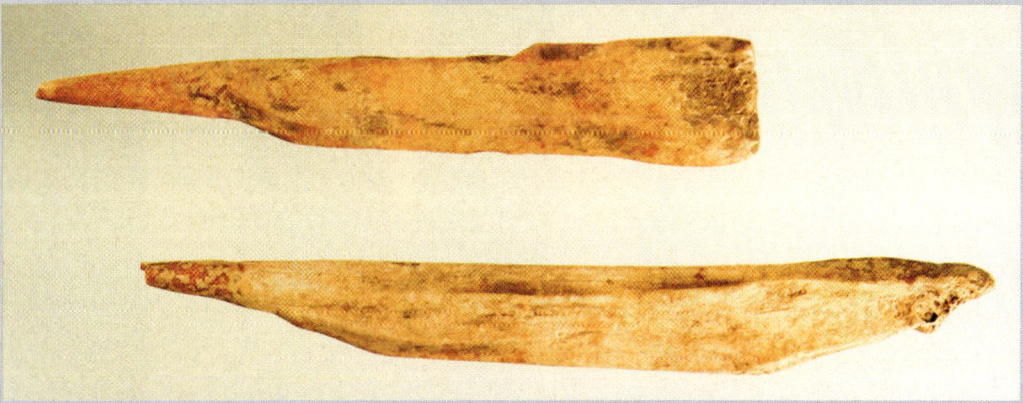

Awls, polished splinters of heavy bone, longer one is 4$\frac{3}{4}$". Midwestern. Don Casto collection. Longer, **$15.00.** Shorter, **$10.00.**

Splinter Awls

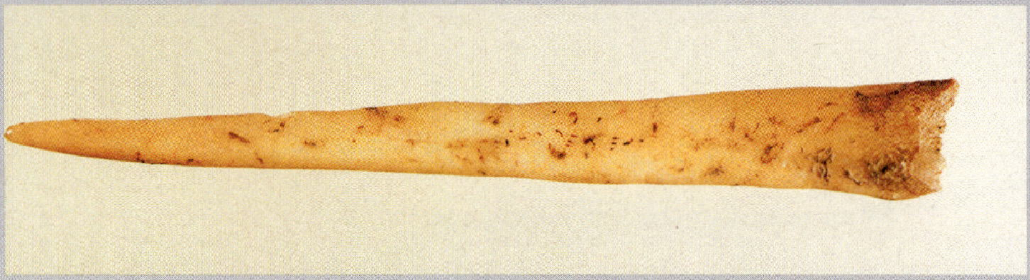

Awl, polished bone splinter, 4 1/16" long. Nicely shaped, it is from the Midwest. Don Casto collection. **$35.00.**

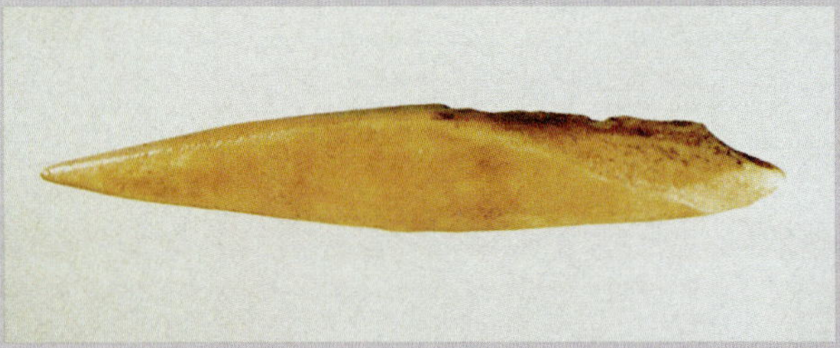

Awl, deer bone splinter, polished tip, 2 5/8" long. Tuscarawas County, Ohio. Fred Winegardner collection. **$12.00.**

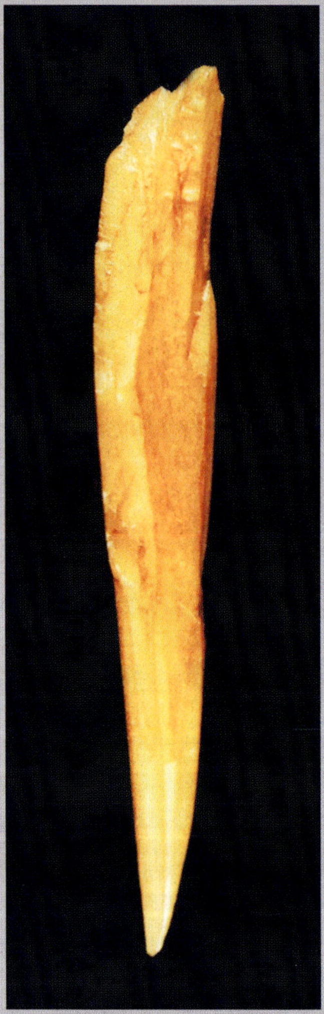

Awl, probably elk bone (judging by wall thickness), 4 9/32". It has chemical stabilization and is Fort Ancient in origin. Southern Ohio. Private collection. **$25.00.**

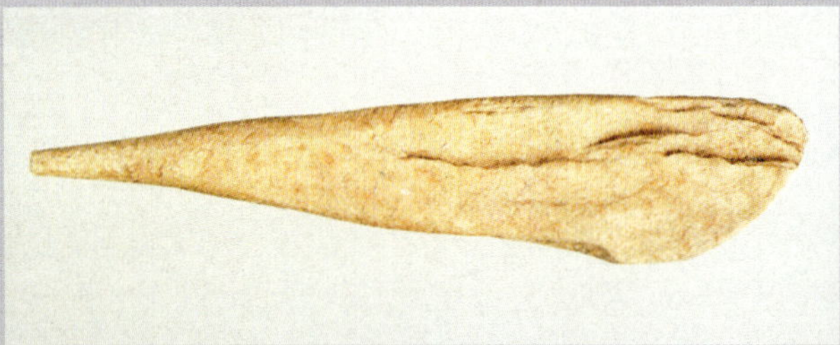

Awl, bone splinter, wide end ground smooth, 2 3/4". This example is from a Whittlesey (Mississippian) site in Tuscarawas County, Ohio. Fred Winegardner collection. **$15.00.**

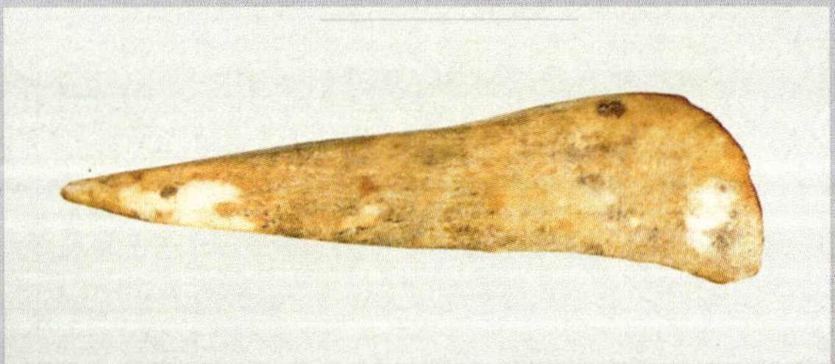

Awl, deer bone, 2 3/8". The small white patches indicate portions where weathering or micro-organisms have removed the gray-tan patina. Ohio. Fred Winegardner collection. **$10.00.**

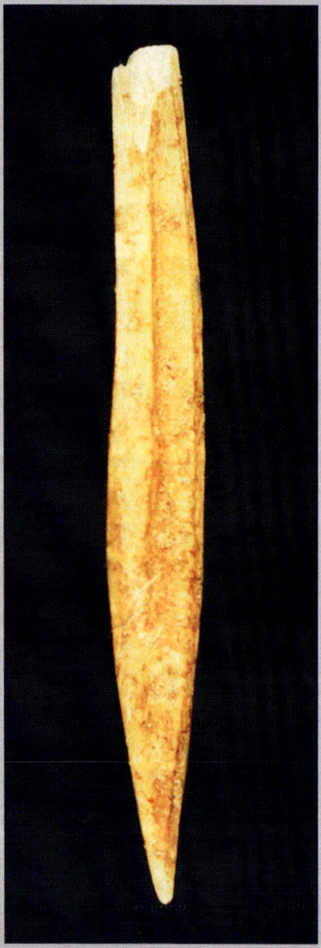

Awl, deer bone splinter, shellac coating. The awl is 4 1/4" and came from southern Ohio. Private collection. **$12.00.**

Trigger Awls

The easiest awl to recognize is undoubtedly the "trigger" awl, which can easily be assigned to the skeletal part and usually to the animal that provided it. The animal is most often the deer and the bone is the ulna, which along with the radius, makes up the bony structure of the lower forelimb.

The common name itself comes from the curved trigger-like concavity on one side, somewhat giving the appearance of a handgun. The widest portion of the base makes up the gun mass and the shaft extension equates to the barrel. As mentioned, most of these awls came from deer, and length range is about 3½" to 6". The elk is also represented sometimes, and its bone is much larger and thicker, more massive. Even comparing a large deer ulna and a small elk ulna should not be confusing. Elk trigger bone awls can be 8" to 10" long.

It is not surprising that these particular awls were favorite prehistoric tools. The average trigger awl can be comfortably held (and presumably used) in three positions: Tip up when held in a fist; tip down, same; and, tip projecting forward when held so that the middle finger passes over the trigger curve. There are other possible positions as well, and use-purpose may have dictated how the tool was positioned. This is an awl type that is one-piece, with awl and handle as a single unit.

The presence of polish on the edges of tools like trigger awls poses some questions. Some areas may be the original smooth bone surface, or polish purposely done, or polish from the hand, or polish from the work. Depending on the condition of the bone (and degree of polish), surface striations may be present. These are the marks of shaping by grinding. Trigger awls also tend to have an abrupt taper on the shaft near the tip, which leaves a wider shaft and gives great strength for this tool form.

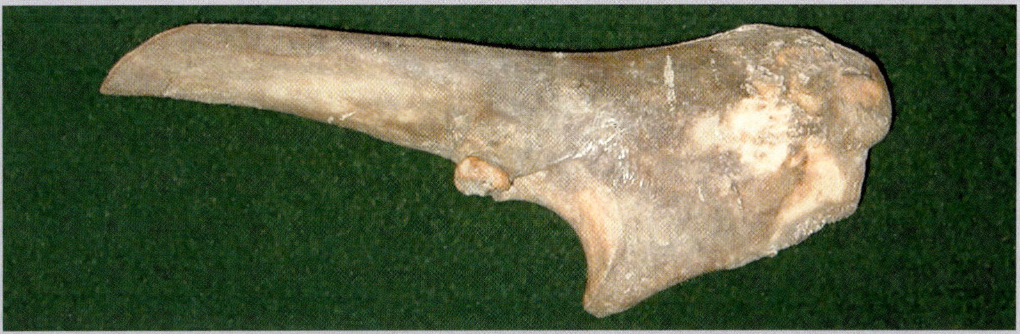

Bone trigger awl, deer ulna, 5⅜" long. Ex-collection Noel, it came from Kentucky. Keith and Rhonda Dodge collection, Michigan. **$35.00.**

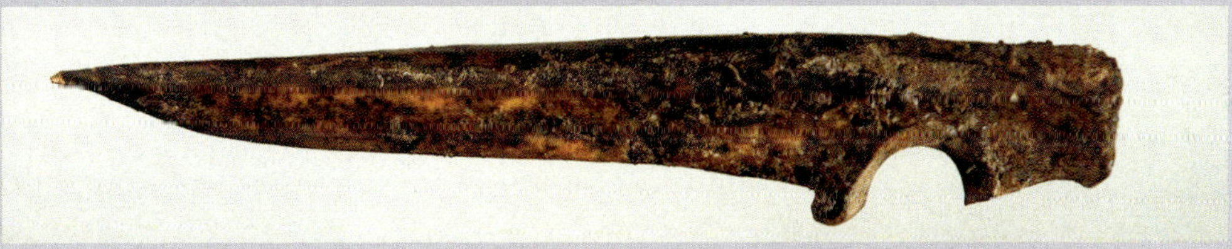

Bone awl, ulna, probably bobcat, rock shelter deposits, 4¾" long. Cleaning might uncover the extent of shaft polish, which appears to be high. Ex-collection Miller, it is from southern Tennessee. Lar Hothem collection. **$65.00.**

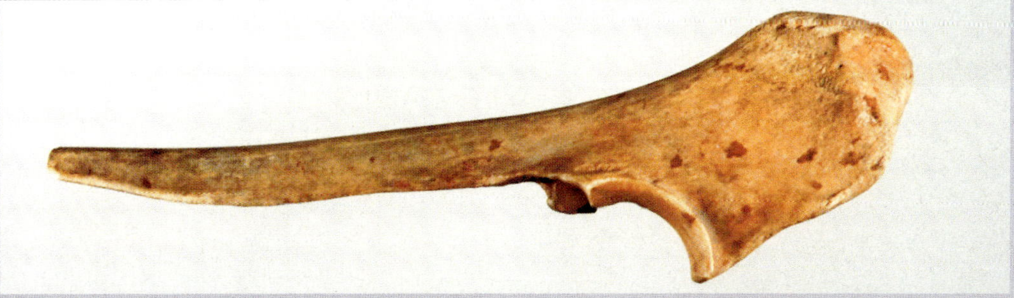

Tool, deer ulna, smaller end flattened and with spatulate tip, much wear on excurvate edge of shaft. It is 5¼" long and may be a specialized knife form. Southern Tennessee. Lar Hothem collection. **$50.00.**

Trigger Awls

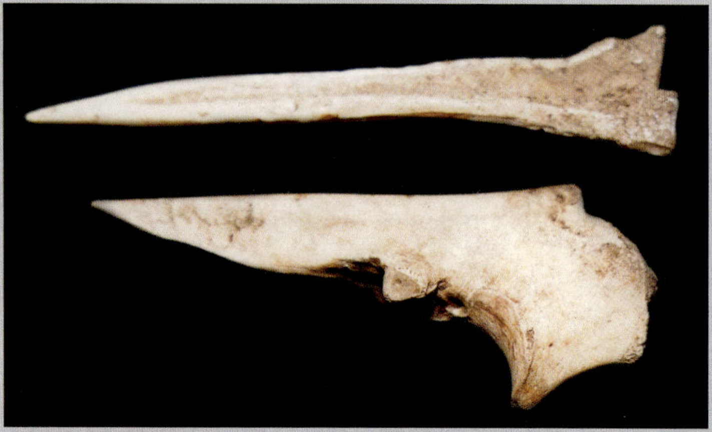

Trigger awls, bottom, 3¼" long, worn working tip. Top, polished awl, 4¼" long, irregular base. Both are from Russell County, Kentucky. Back to Earth. Bottom, **$45.00;** top, **$40.00.**

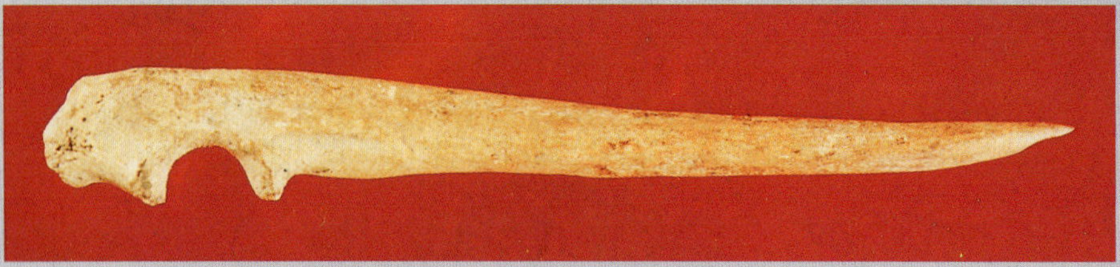

Trigger awl, probably raccoon bone, 4" long. Weathered tan, the awl came from Kentucky. Private collection. **$30.00.**

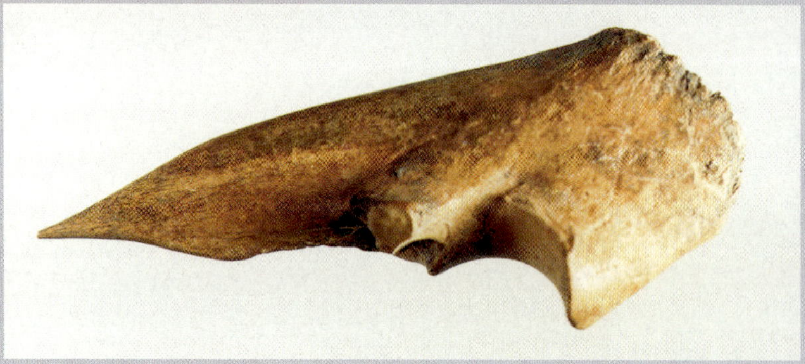

Trigger awl, deer bone, 4¼", patinated a uniform brown. It has good surface polish and the tip is shortened from long-term use. Fort Ancient, ca. AD 800 – 1500, it is from southern Ohio. Private collection. **$45.00.**

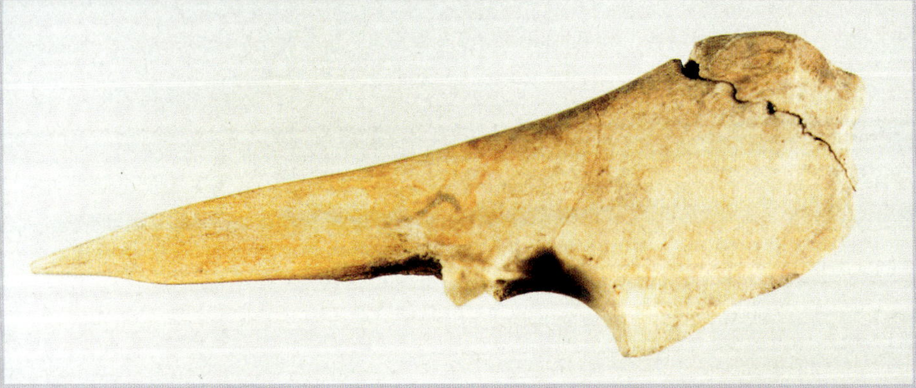

Trigger awl, deer bone, some cracking and bone separation, 5¼". It was found on a Fort Ancient site in southern Ohio. Private collection. **$35.00.**

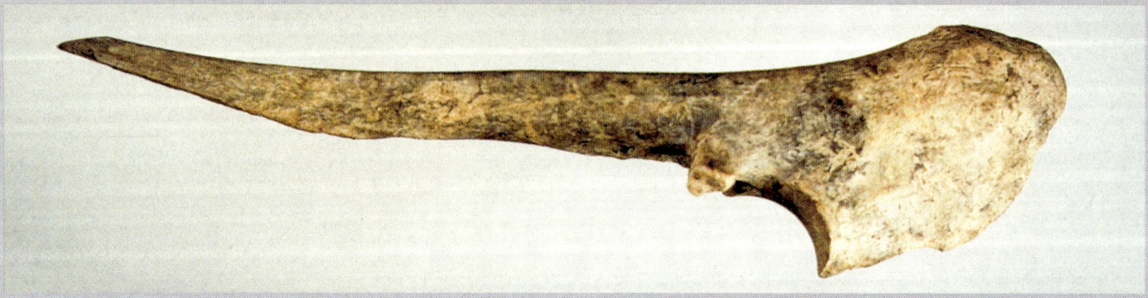

Bone trigger awl, deer ulna, 6⅝" long. The artifact was found in Lawrence County, Ohio. Fred Winegardner collection. **$45.00.**

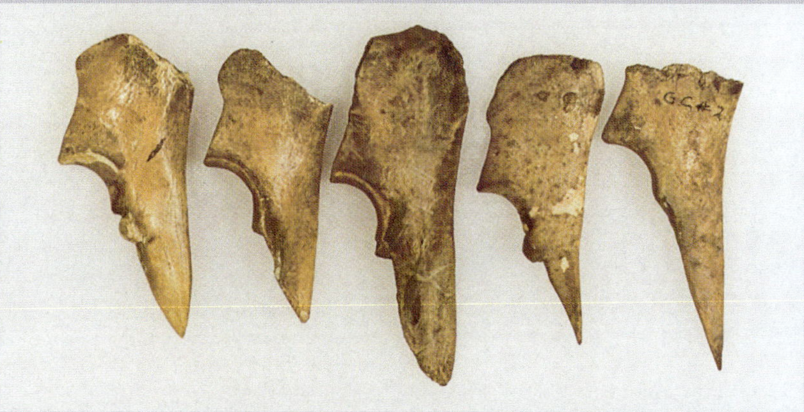

Trigger awls, well-used sizes, center example is 4¼". Ex-collection Vietzen, they are Late Archaic to Woodland in time. These have high polish and two examples have very pointed tips. Christian County, Kentucky. Pete Timoch collection. Each, **$40.00 – 50.00.**

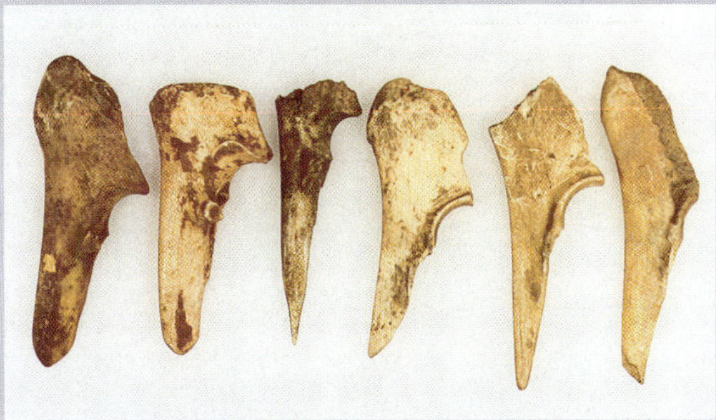

Trigger awls, Late Archaic to Woodland, deer ulna bones. From the Vietzen collection, the longest example is 5⅛". All were excavated in the 1930s and 1940s in Ohio and Kentucky. Pete Timoch collection. Each, **$50.00 – 70.00.**

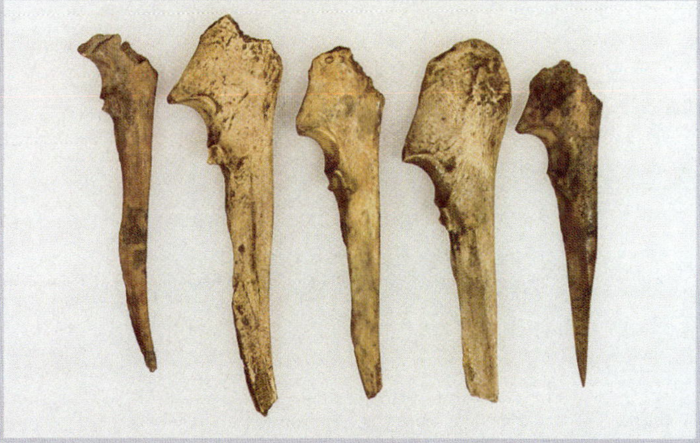

Trigger awls, deer ulna bones, Late Archaic to Woodland periods. The longest example is 6¼" and all came from the Vietzen collection. These show various degrees of resharpening. Christian County, Kentucky. Pete Timoch collection. **$25.00 – 40.00.**

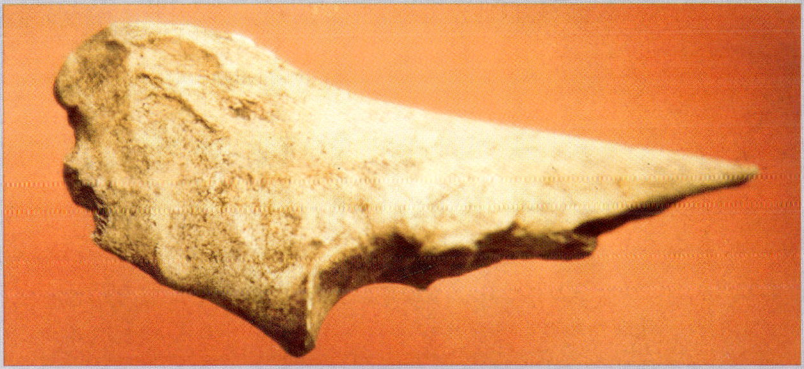

Trigger awl, large deer bone, 4⅞" long, Middle Archaic period, Lamoka phase. It came from near Tyrone, New York. Dave Summers collection, Victor, New York. **$40.00.**

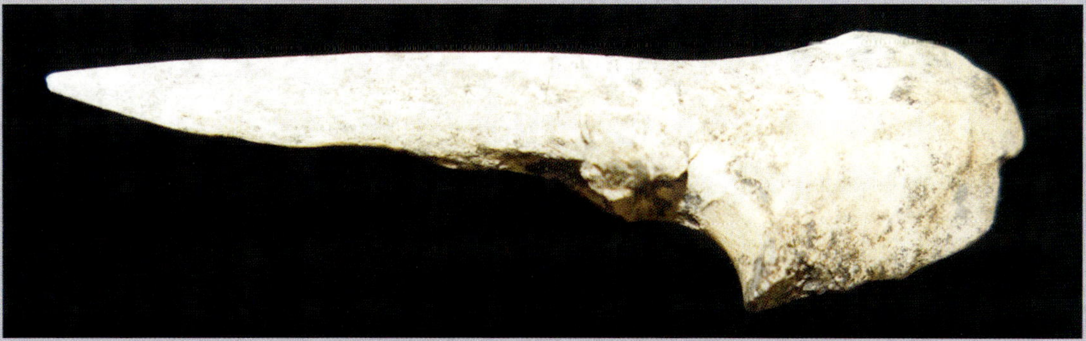

Trigger awl, 5¾" long, a personal find by the owner. Mississippi County, Arkansas. Garvin collection. **$45.00.**

Trigger Awls

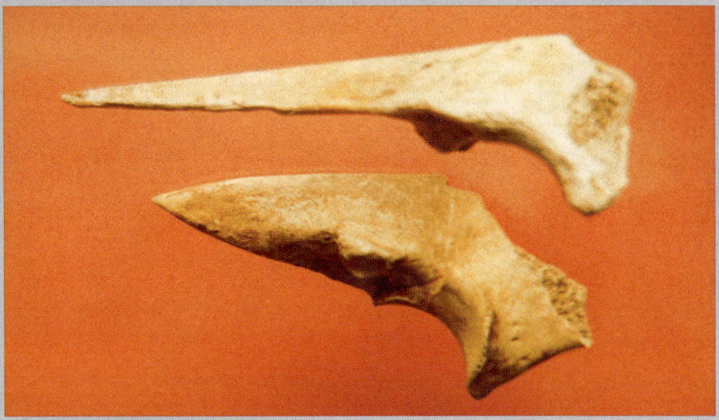

Trigger awls, deer ulna bones, top piece is 3½" long, bottom piece is 2¾". Lamoka phase, these Archaic pieces were found near the town of Tyrone, New York. Dave Summers collection, Victor, New York. Upper, **$30.00;** lower, **$25.00.**

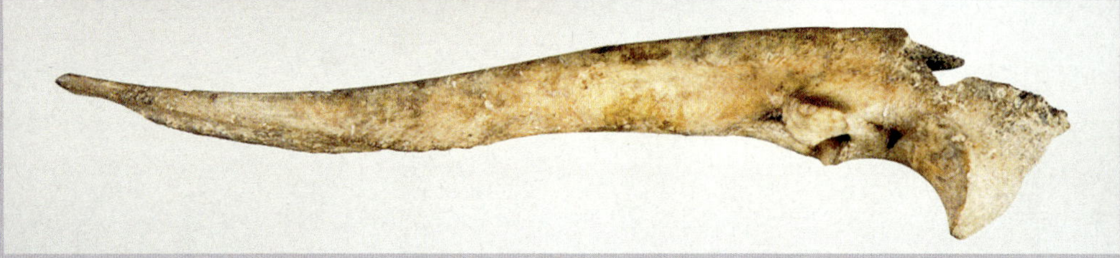

Awl, deer ulna, 6¼" long. Though the base is missing, size and general shape make the bone easy to identify. Lawrence County, Ohio. Fred Winegardner collection. **$35.00.**

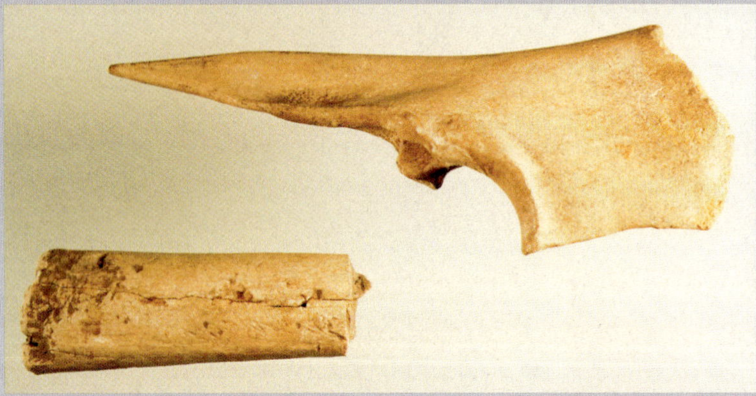

Artifacts, bone trigger awl (top) is 4¼" long and made from a deer ulna. The bottom artifact is a cut section of antler. Both are from Arkansas and in the Don Casto collection. Awl, **$35.00;** antler section, **$10.00.**

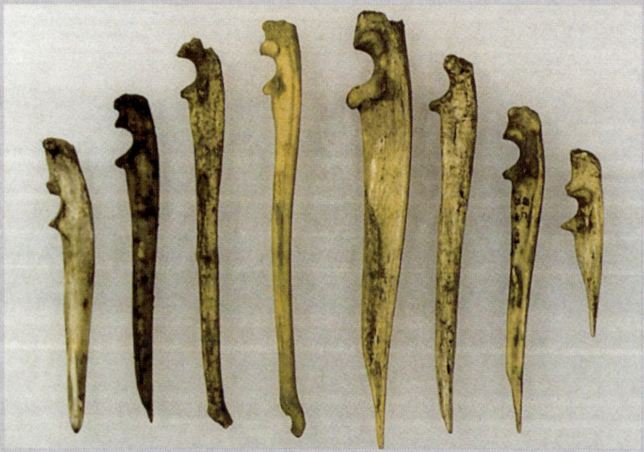

Awls and hairpins, ulna bones from various animals, Late Archaic to Woodland, longest is 4⁹⁄₁₆". All were once in the Vietzen collection. Col. Vietzen was a well-known archaeologist, collector, and author in Ohio and Kentucky. Christian County, Kentucky. Pete Timoch collection. Each, **$40.00 – 75.00.**

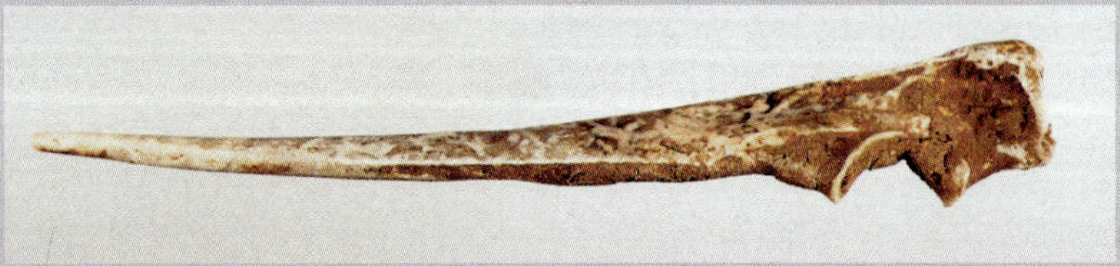

Trigger awl, fox(?) ulna, 3½" long. This is a tapered and graceful artifact, found in Kentucky. Fred Winegardner collection. **$30.00.**

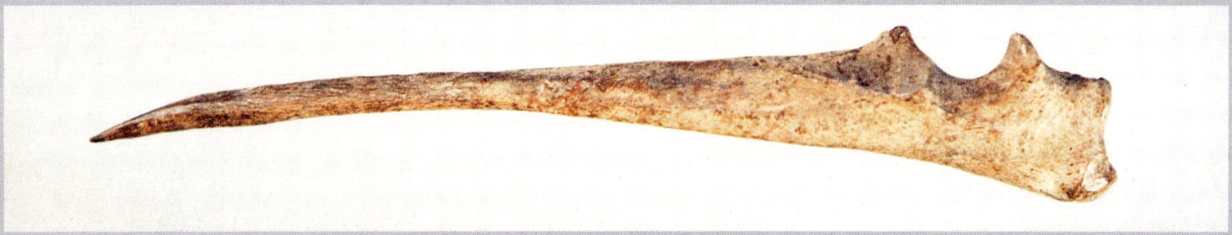

Hairpin or awl, 6⅓₂". Size indicates this could be either a wolf or coyote ulna, but the distribution range of the animals suggests it is that of a wolf. (See Gilbert, *Mammalian Osteology*, pp 143, 330, and 336.) Ex-collection Vietzen, southern Ohio. Fred Winegardner collection. **$125.00.**

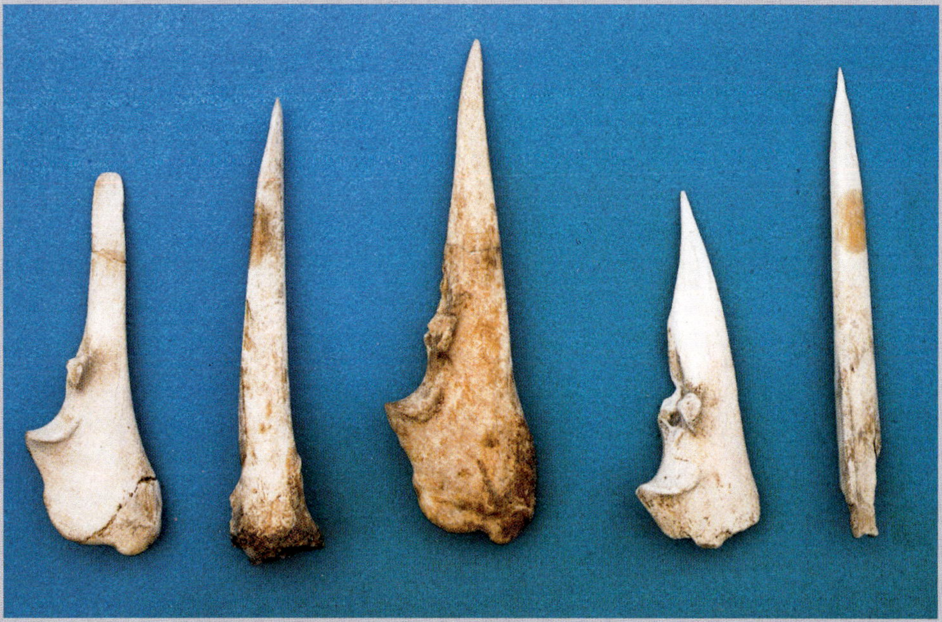

Group of five bone awls, resharpened to average length of 3½". This example is from a rock shelter in southern Tennessee. Private collection. **$25.00.**

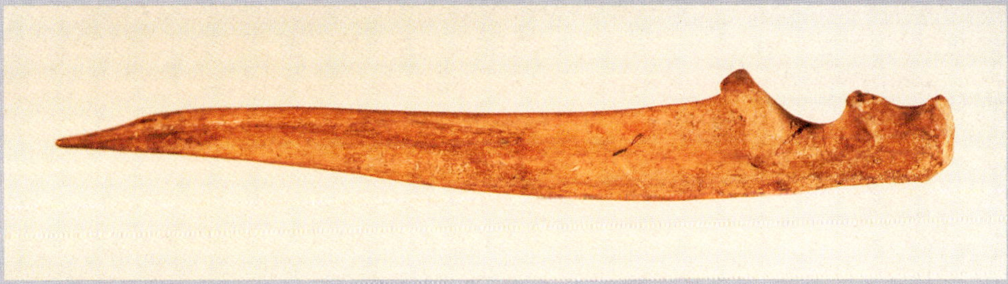

Trigger awl, probably from a bobcat judging by size, width, and configuration, 4⅝" long. (See Gilbert's *Mammalian Osteology*, page 335.) Found in 1940, it is from southern Ohio. Fred Winegardner collection. **$100.00.**

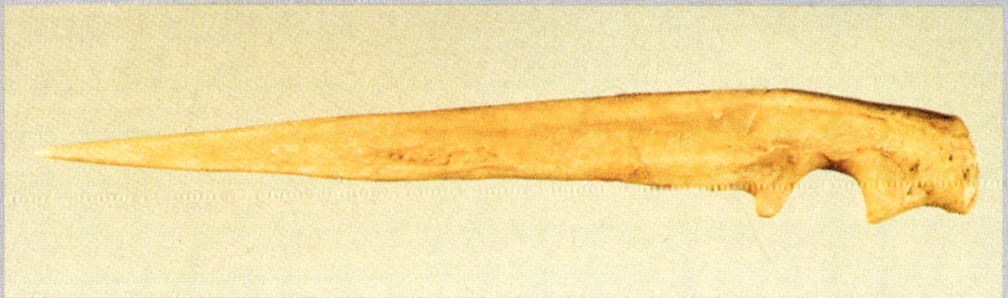

Trigger awl, probably raccoon bone, 3½" long. This well-shaped example came from Hamilton County, Ohio. Robin Fiser collection. **$45.00.**

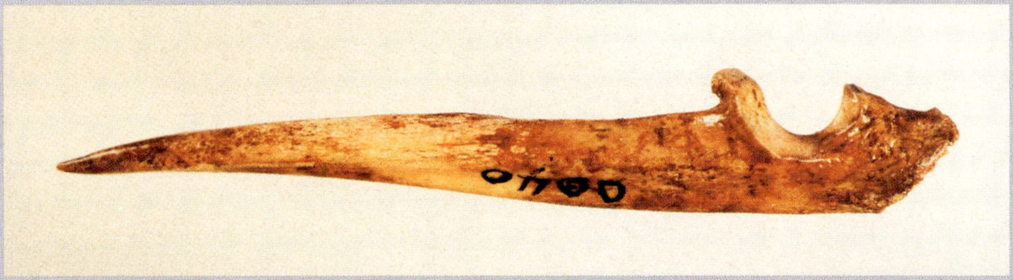

Trigger awl, probably a bobcat ulna, 4⁷⁄₁₆" long. This example is ex-collection Vietzen and came from a Fort Ancient site in southern Ohio. Fred Winegardner collection. **$100.00.**

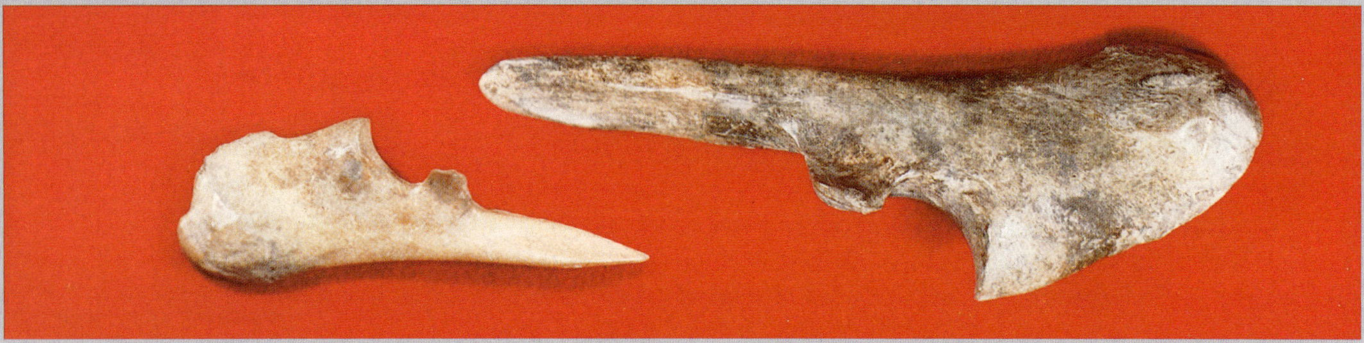

Trigger awls, smaller is 4¼" and larger is 7½". Both have about 100% polish and the elk ulna has a mirror-like sheen. The darkened color was probably caused by contact with midden wood ashes. This is a very instructive photograph, showing typical deer and elk bone size differences. They have a differing amount of wear in the trigger area from finger placement. Mississippian, southern Ohio. Pete Timoch collection. Smaller, **$60.00**; larger, **$200.00.**

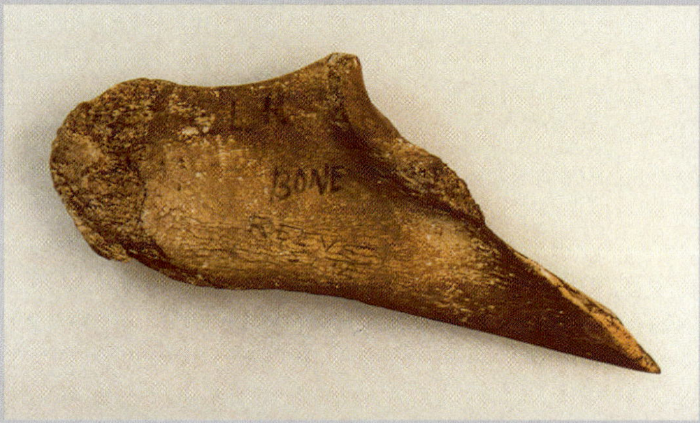

Awl, elk trigger bone, 7¼" long. This is a large and heavy bone, from the Mississippian period. Ex-collections Hovan and Sauer, it is from Ohio. Pete Timoch collection. **$200.00.**

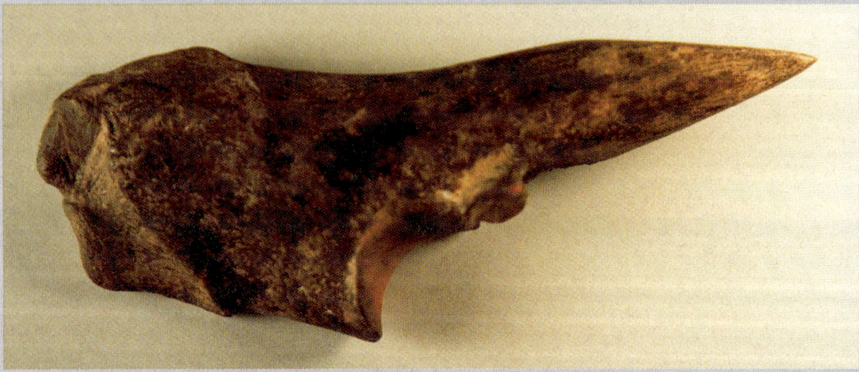

Trigger awl, bone, Mississippian, 1½ x 4½". This well-polished example was found along a stream that runs into the Ohio River. Cabell County, West Virginia. Private collection. Rodney Roberts photograph. **$40.00.**

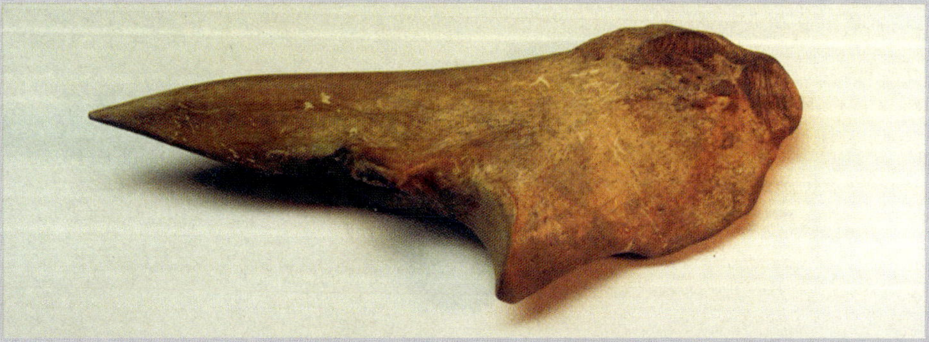

Trigger awl, deer ulna, a much-used example. Fulton County, Illinois. Fred Smith collection, Illinois. **$25.00 – 30.00.**

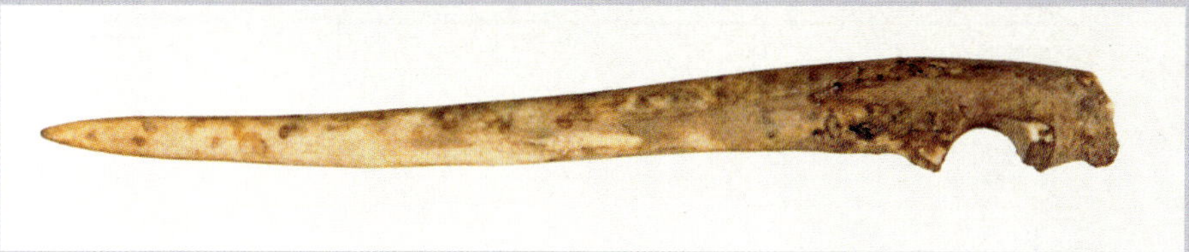

Trigger awl, ulna, probably from a raccoon, 3⅞" long. This artifact is ex-collection Hall, from Wayne County, Kentucky. Private collection. **$20.00.**

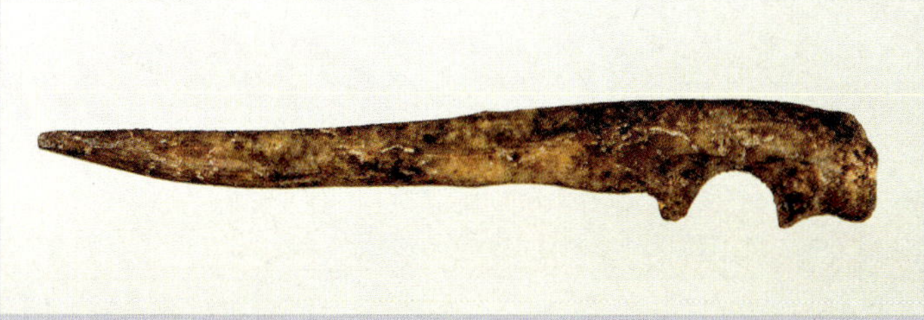

Awl, small animal and possibly a raccoon, 3⅛" long. The shaft is polished and the awl has rock shelter deposits. Southern Tennessee. Private collection. **$25.00.**

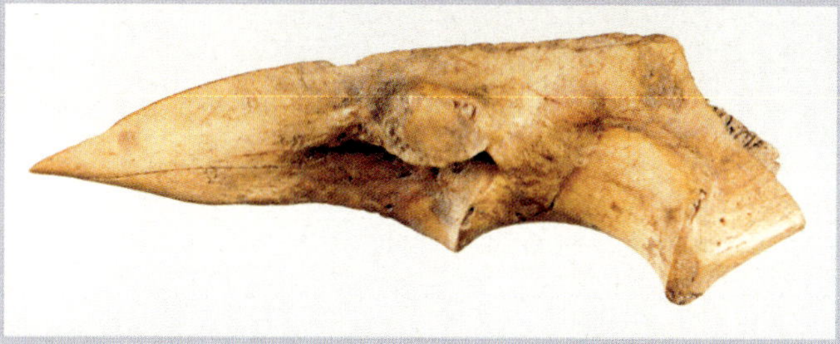

Trigger awl, deer ulna, polished edges and worn to a shortened length, 2⅞" long. Ex-collection Hall. Wayne County, Kentucky. Private collection. **$20.00.**

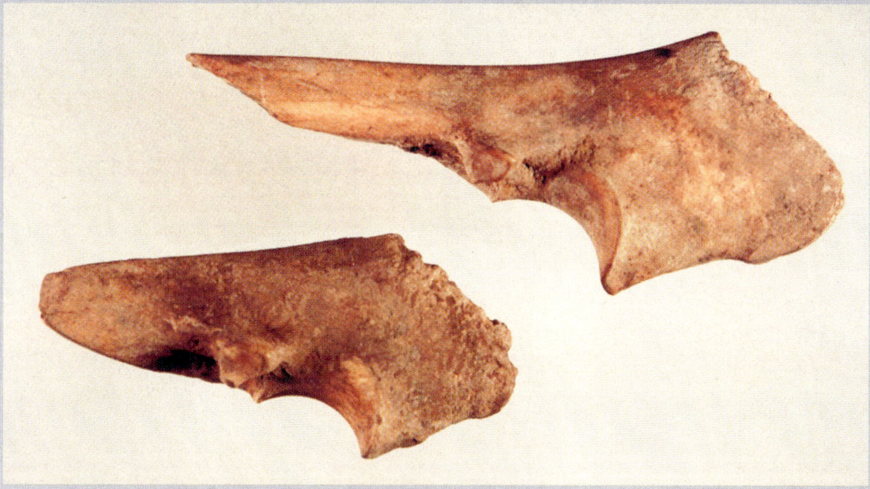

Trigger awls, deer bone, top well-worn example is 4⅛" long. The bottom trigger awl is in worn-out or exhausted condition. Both are from Wayne County, Kentucky. Private collection. Top, **$15.00 – 20.00;** bottom, **$10.00 – 12.00.**

Trigger awl, deer ulna, 3⅝" long. Compared to typical trigger awls, the shaft on this piece has been heavily worked and narrowed. This example came from West Virginia. Doug Hooks collection. **$45.00.**

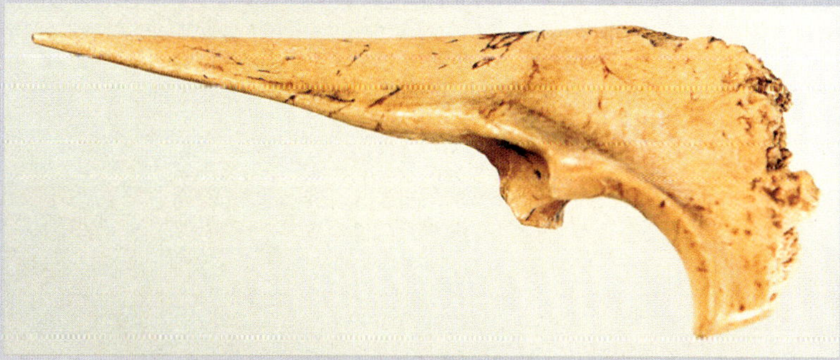

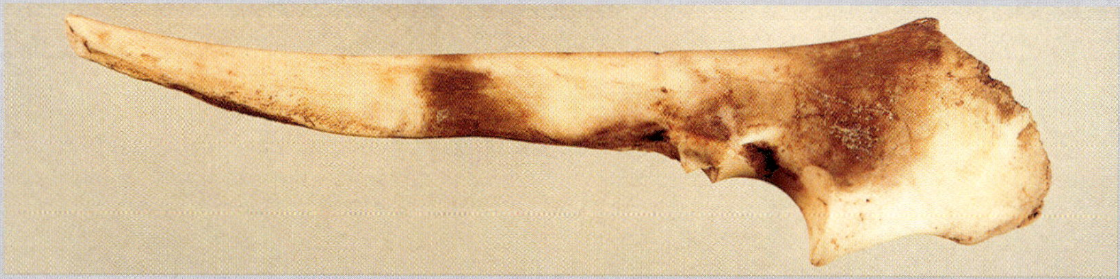

Tool, deer ulna, blunt working end, smoothed and polished shaft. It is 6½" long and was found in Wayne County, Kentucky. Private collection. **$35.00.**

Trigger Awls

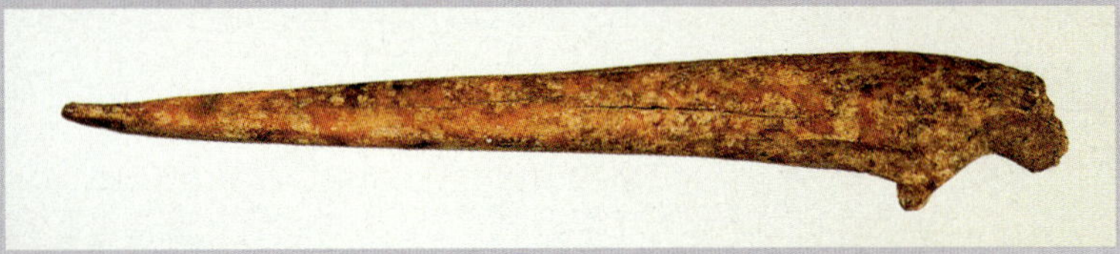

Awl, ulna, may be young fox, base heavily worked and reshaped by maker. It is 3½" long and was found in a rock shelter. Southern Tennessee. Lar Hothem collection. **$30.00.**

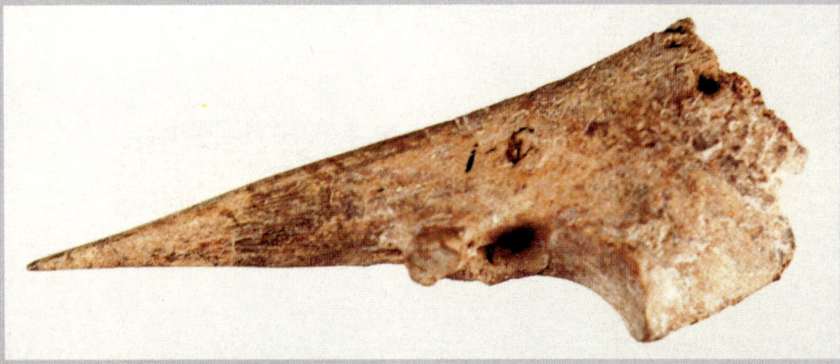

Awl, deer ulna, resharpened to present length of 3½". This example is from a rock shelter in southern Tennessee. Private collection. **$25.00.**

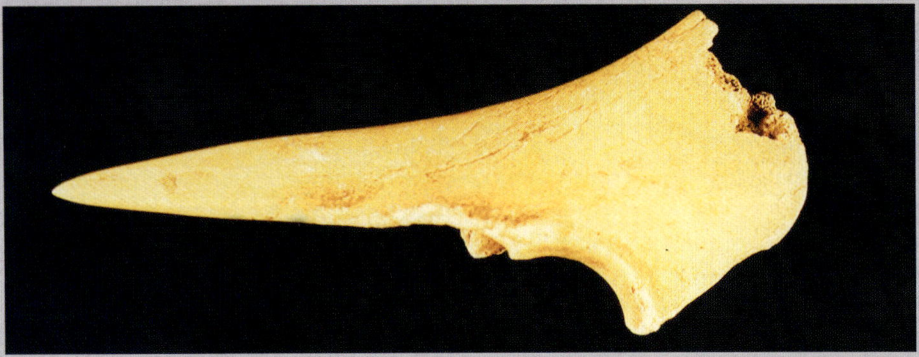

Trigger awl, deer ulna, pinkish patination. The awl is 4⅝" long and came from southeastern Illinois. Private collection. **$35.00.**

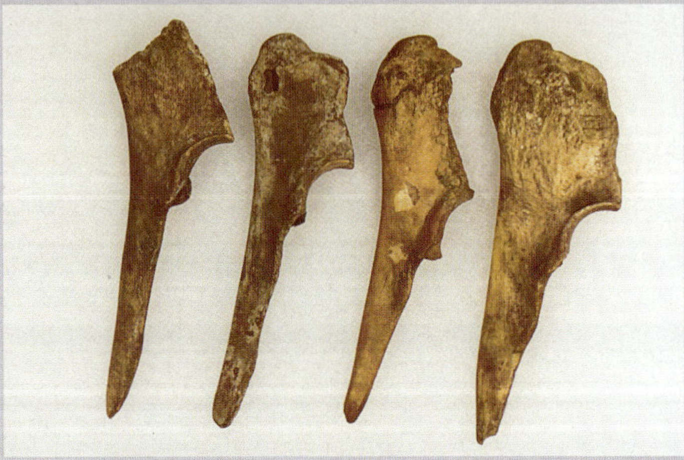

Trigger awls, deer ulna bones, Late Archaic to Woodland periods. These are classic examples and the longest is 5¼". The far right awl has incised lines or cut-marks that encircle the artifact at the polished trigger groove, and there are a few cuts or tallies on the handle portion. These were in the Vietzen collection and came from Christian County, Kentucky. Pete Timoch collection. Each, **$75.00.**

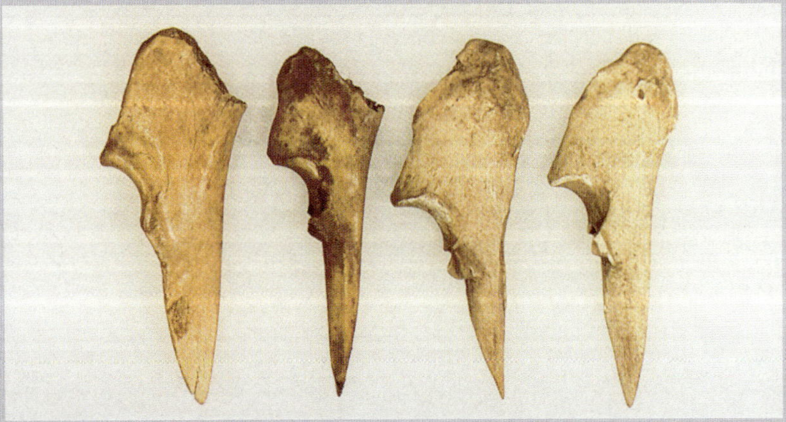

Trigger awls, Late Archaic to Woodland times, longest is 4⅞". The deer ulna artifacts are from the Vietzen collection and have classic shapes and good polish. All are from Ohio, except the second example from left, which is from Kentucky. Pete Timoch collection. Each, **$60.00 – 75.00.**

Projectile Points

Antler and bone projectile points have played an important role in all of North American prehistory. While some were duo-tipped or double-pointed, the majority were cylindrical and had a pointed tip at one end. The base was either hollowed to fit around a shaft or designed to be inserted into a shaft or foreshaft. The shaft, in turn, is thought to have changed, early to late, from spear (hand-held), to javelin (atl-atl thrown), to arrow (bow-propelled). Of course, the methods were not always exclusive to the times, since the Atl-atl persisted into historic times in a few places.

Paleo (12,000 – 8000 BC) bone points are large and heavy, rounded, and tapered. Often one end is beveled or cut at an angle and the interior surface of the cut is incised with crisscrossed lines. Two beveled ends were likely fastened together to make an extra-long "pin spear" point.

Archaic (8000 – 1000 BC) bone points were often made of antler tips. At the Late Archaic site of Indian Knoll in Kentucky, antler points were the most common antler artifacts. The base of a cut tine was drilled, and the tine was shaped to make a symmetrical point. Some projectile points at Indian Knoll were made of bone splinters and pointed at each end, while others had wide and shallow side notches. Some bone points were discolored by heat as if in an attempt to fire-harden them.

Woodland (1000 BC – AD 800) points were sometimes double-pointed, and a few point-like artifacts of flat bone with rounded to irregular bases are known. While a few projectile points have been found in mounds, many more have been recovered from village sites.

Mississippian (AD 800 – 1500) points exist in large numbers, partly because it is the most recent of the four great prehistoric eras. Also, the various peoples made a wide variety of points to tip arrows. Antler was the preferred material, with tine bases drilled to receive the arrow shaft, and some points had a basal extension that served as a barb. Deer toe bones were sometimes worked for arrow points.

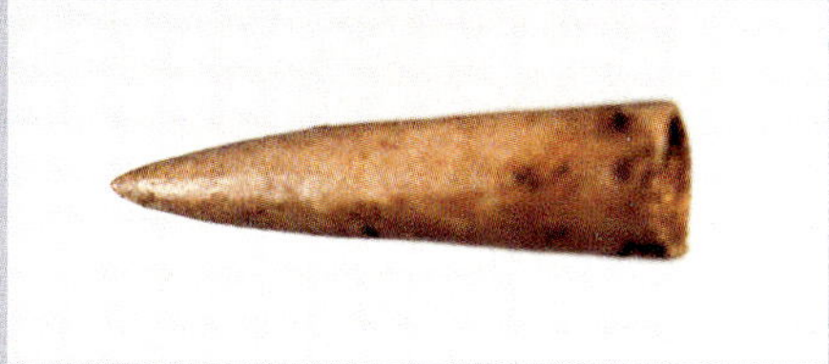

Arrowpoint, interior hollowed, 1¾" long. The interior sides have drill striations present. Ex-collections Copeland and Hooks, the point is from southern Ohio. Fred Winegardner collection. **$20.00.**

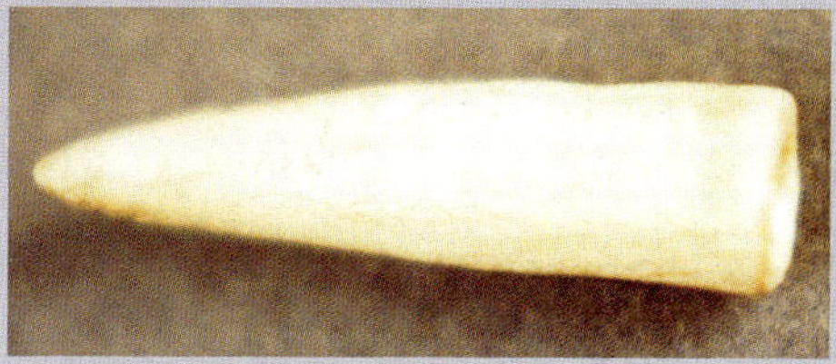

Antler projectile point, drilled and hollowed at base center, 1⅞" long. It was found in Mississippi County, Arkansas. Back to Earth. **$20.00.**

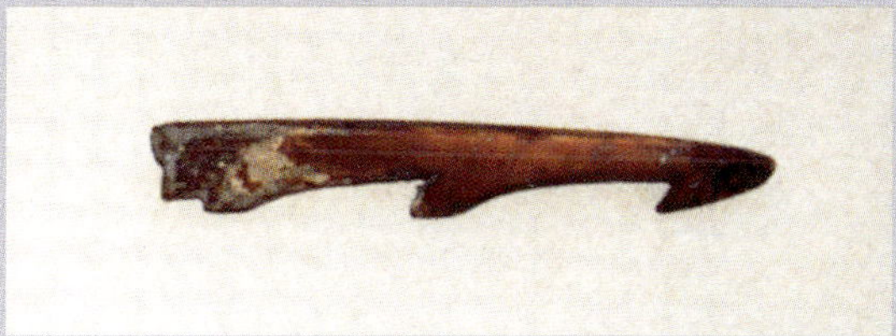

Harpoon tip, three unilateral barbs, bone section 2" long. This piece was found in the Pacific Northwest. Wilfred Dick collection, Mississippi. **$40.00.**

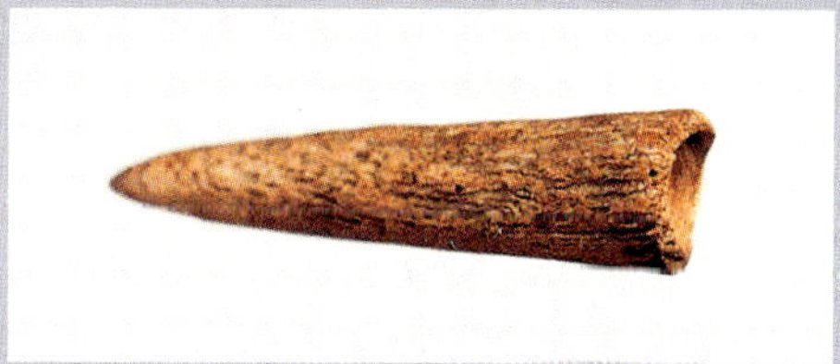

Arrowpoint, antler, drilled at base, surface darkened and weathered, 1⅝" long. It is from Kentucky. Fred Winegardner collection. **$20.00.**

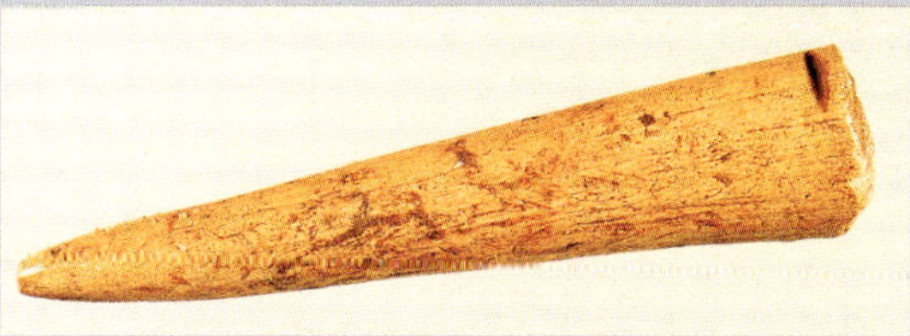

Arrow tip, antler with drilled-out base, shallow cut-mark near base. The point is 2¼" and was found in southern Ohio. Private collection. **$15.00.**

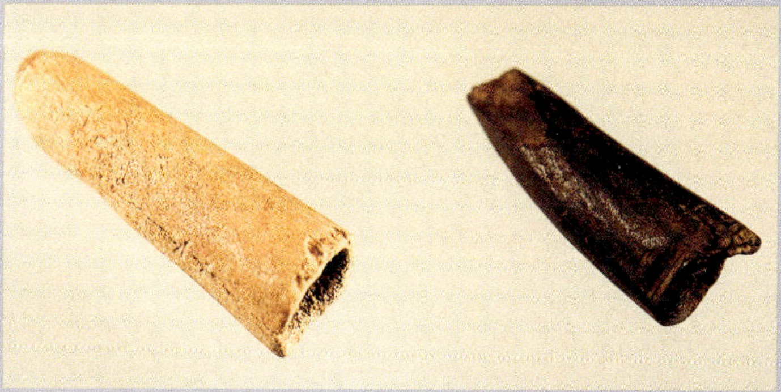

Antler projectile points, both found in Kentucky. Left piece has a blunt tip and is 1$\frac{13}{16}$" long. Right piece is stained brownish-black, tip has flaked off, and is barbed at base in Fort Ancient style. Private collection. Left, **$15.00;** Right, **$10.00.**

Projectile Points

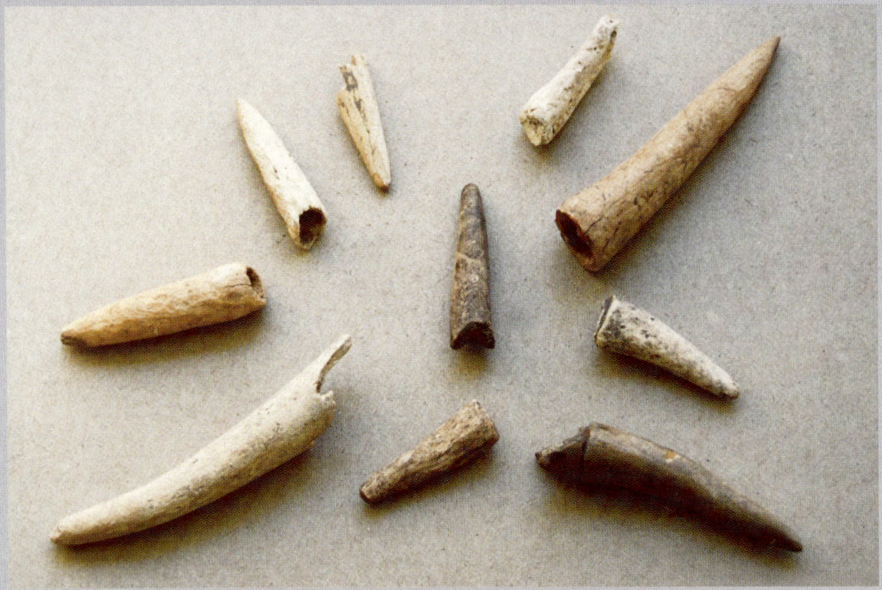

Projectile points, all made of deer antler tines, bases of most are hollowed to receive a wooden shaft. These were found in Mississippi and Arkansas. Wilfred Dick collection, Mississippi. Each, **$5.00 – 30.00.**

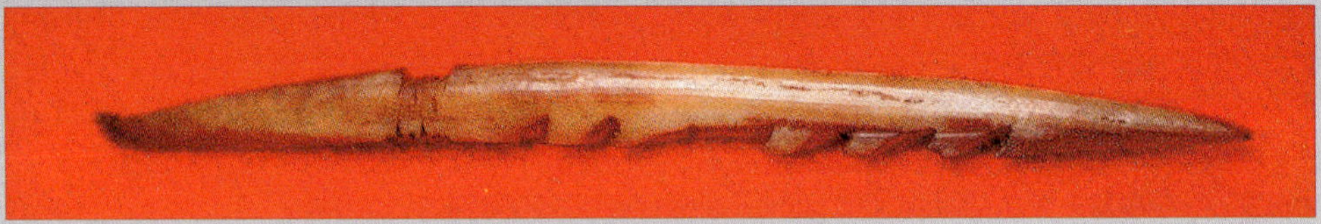

Harpoon tip, antler or bone, ⅜ x 5⅜", ¼" thick. Well-made and in good condition, the origin is unknown. Michael F. Slasinski collection, Michigan. **$350.00.**

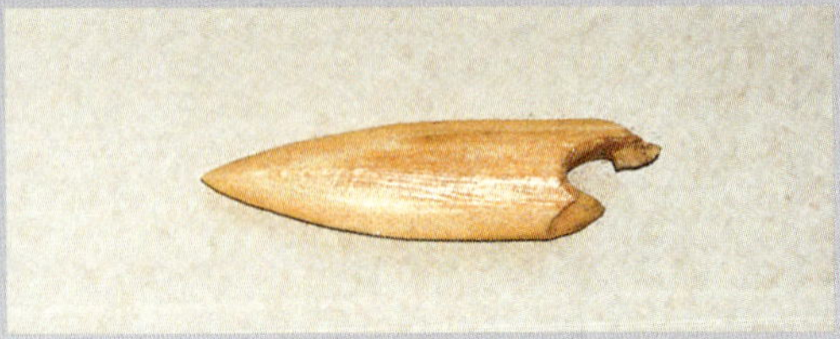

Harpoon tip, broken at cord-attachment hole, remaining length is 2". This example in ivory or bone is from the Pacific Northwest. Wilfred Dick collection, Mississippi. **$20.00.**

Blunt projectile point, bone, ⅝ x 1¼". This carved and decorated piece is quite unusual, and was found in Saginaw, Michigan. Michael F. Slasinski collection, Michigan. Museum grade.

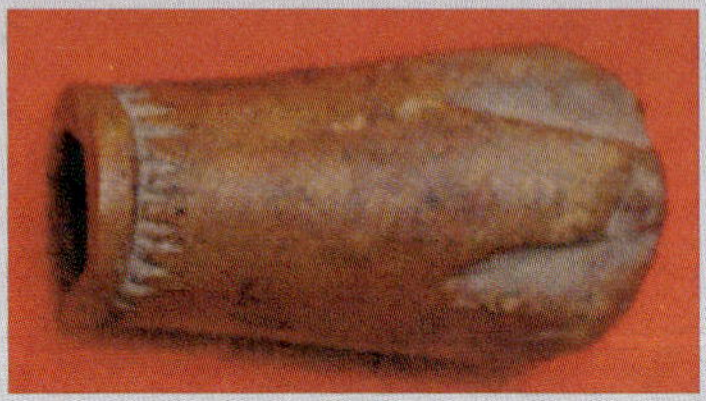

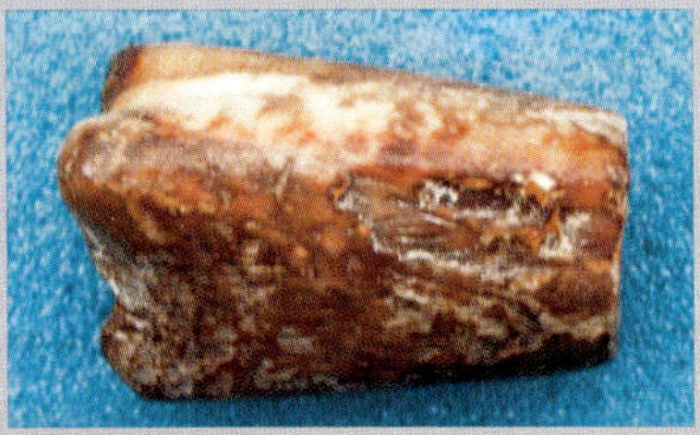

Blunt projectile tip, ivory, prehistoric(?), 1$^{3}/_{16}$ x 1$^{3}/_{16}$" long. It is ex-collection Cantrell, from Alaska. Collection of, and photograph by, Gary Henry, North Carolina. **$35.00.**

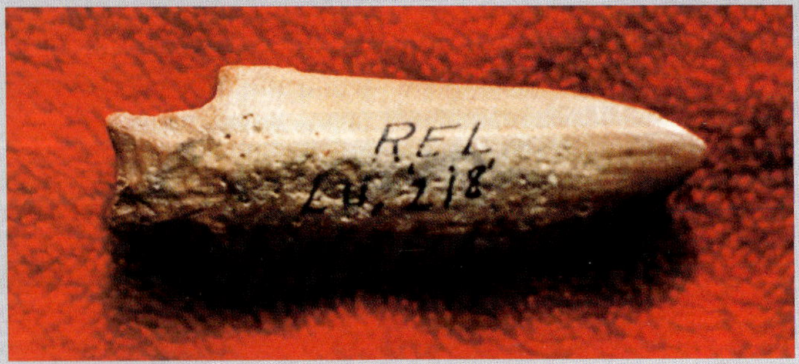

Bone projectile point or knife, made from a deer ulna, 1$^{3}/_{16}$ x 3⅛". It is ex-collection Goldberg and has a Berner COA. Pemiscot County, Missouri. Brandon Trivette collection, North Carolina. **$125.00.**

Projectile point, hollowed bone, ¾ x 2" long. It dates to about 2500 BC and came from an island in the Savanna River near Augusta, Georgia. H. B. Greene II collection, Naples, Florida. **$30.00.**

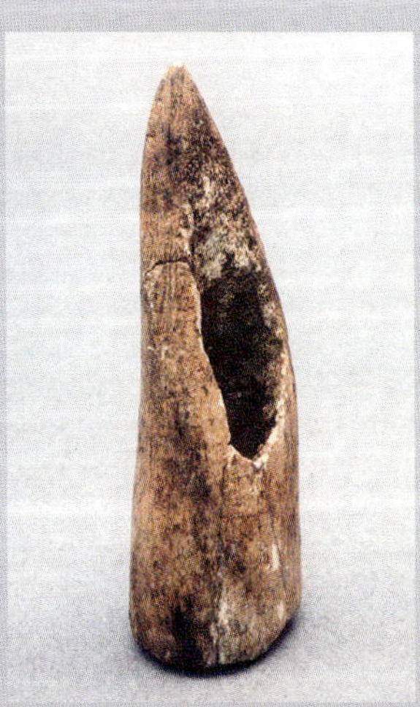

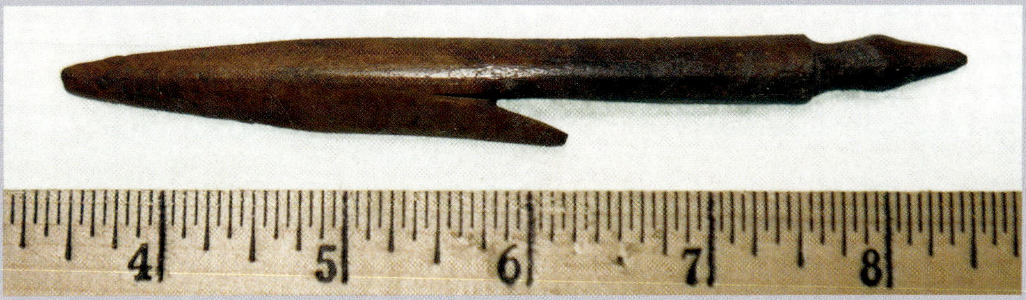

Bone harpoons, Upper Chinook group, Perino COA. This piece was found in Sherman County, Oregon. Back to Earth. Unlisted.

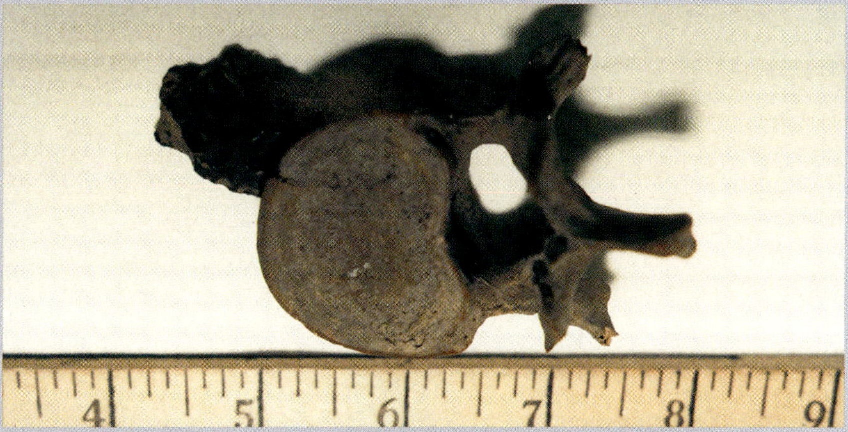

Bison vertebra, with embedded projectile point. Probably Plains region. Back to Earth. Unlisted.

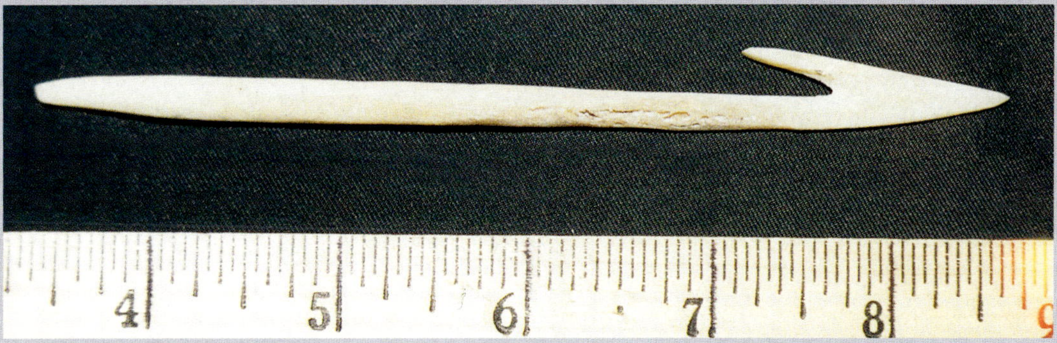

Bone harpoon, 5½" long, single barb. This example was found in Adams County, Illinois. Back to Earth. **$125.00.**

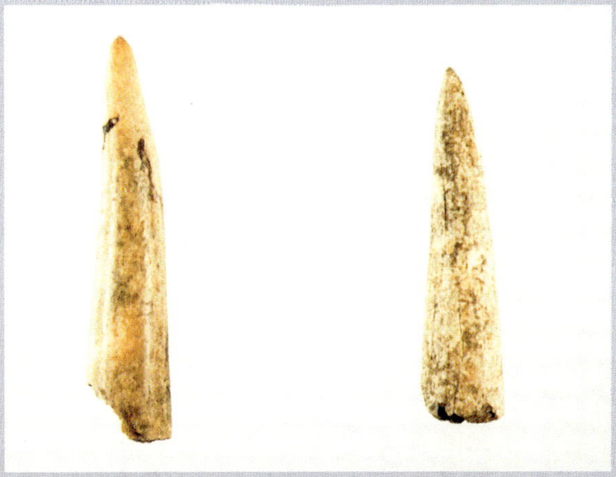

Antler tips, longer piece is 1¾", polished. Both were broken from the antler branch, and the size indicates they were for projectile points. Eastern Ohio. Private collection. Each, **$3.00.**

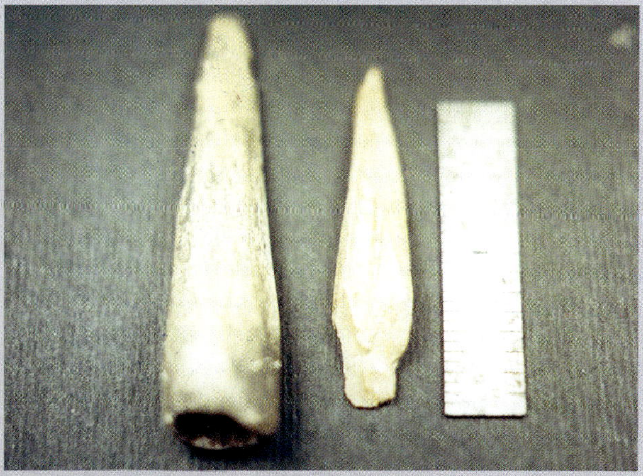

Projectile points, both from Monroe County, Pennsylvania. Left, arrow or Atl-atl point; right, bone point. Lee Hallman collection, Pennsylvania. Conical point, left, **$30.00;** right, **$15.00.**

Projectile Points

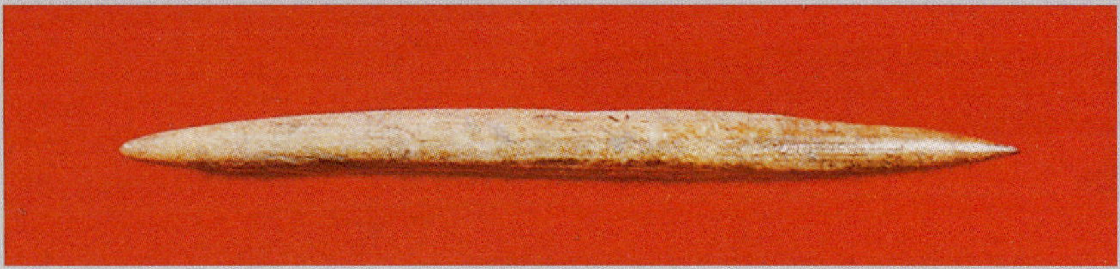

Point or awl, double-tipped, 4⅛". It is difficult to determine whether this is bone or antler because of the high polish and absence of identifying characteristics. Ex-collection Vietzen, the artifact is from the Ohio-Kentucky region. Pete Timoch collection. **$125.00.**

Point, bone, double-tipped, Archaic to Woodland. The split bone is 3⅜" long. Such examples may have been socketed into long shafts (as projectile points) or shorter handles (as awls or perforators). Once in the Vietzen collection it is from the Ohio-Kentucky region. Pete Timoch collection. **$70.00.**

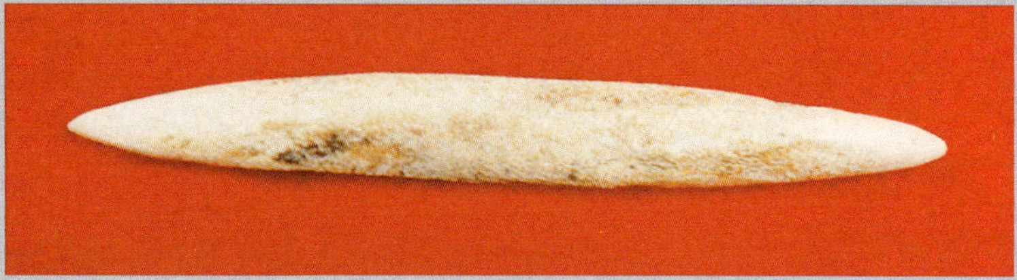

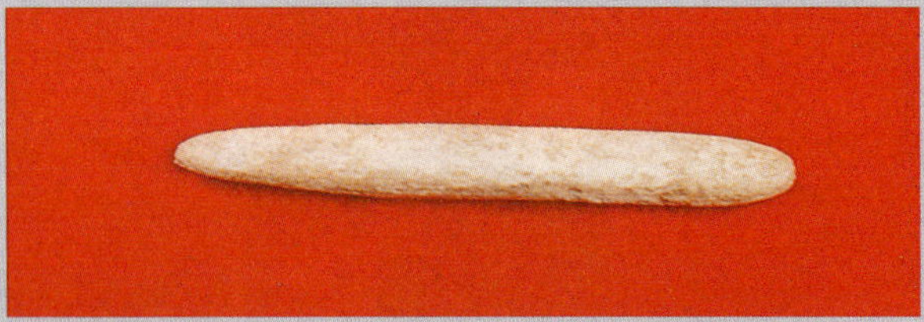

Point, double-tipped, Archaic to Woodland period, 2⅝". The split bone was ground to shape and the surface is smooth. Ex-collection Vietzen, it is either from Ohio or Kentucky. Pete Timoch collection. **$50.00.**

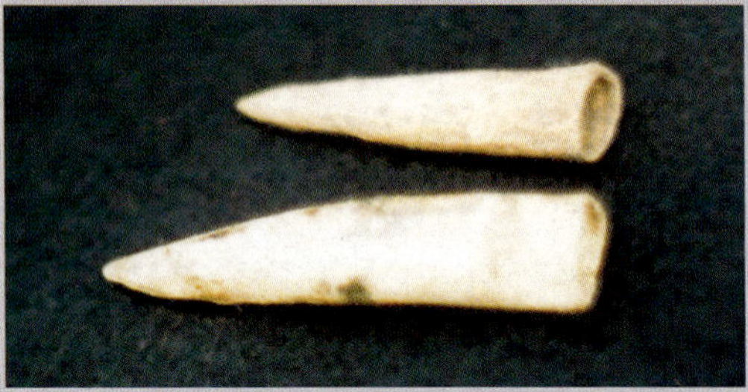

Projectile point, antler, Archaic or later, 5/16 x 1 5/16". Harwood found it between 1954 and 1982. Greene County, Tennessee. Collection of, and photograph by, Gary Henry, North Carolina. **$50.00.**

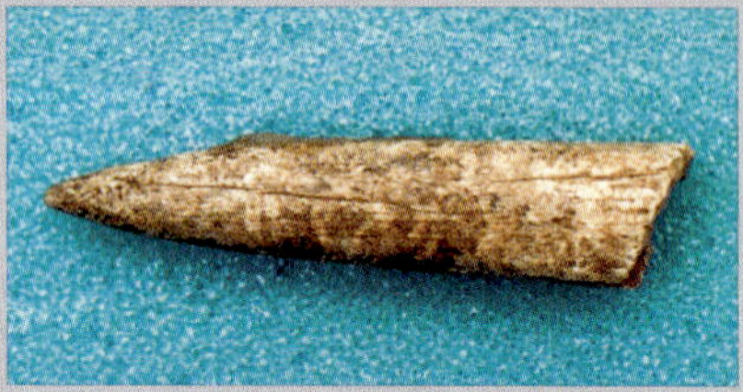

Projectile points, antler, bases hollowed. They are 1½ and 2" long respectively, and were found in Missouri. Bob Hess collection, Indiana. Each, **$20.00 – 30.00.**

Projectile point, deer antler tine, Middle Woodland, 1½" long. From this time-period, the point could have either tipped an Atl-atl dart or an arrow. It was found near Van Buren, Onondaga County, New York. Dave Summers collection, Victor, New York. **$80.00.**

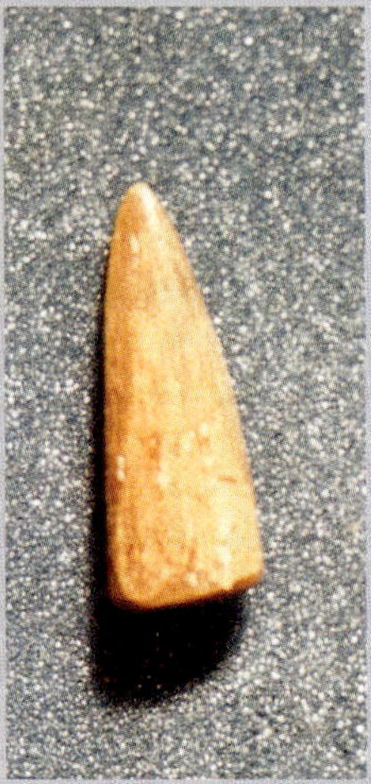

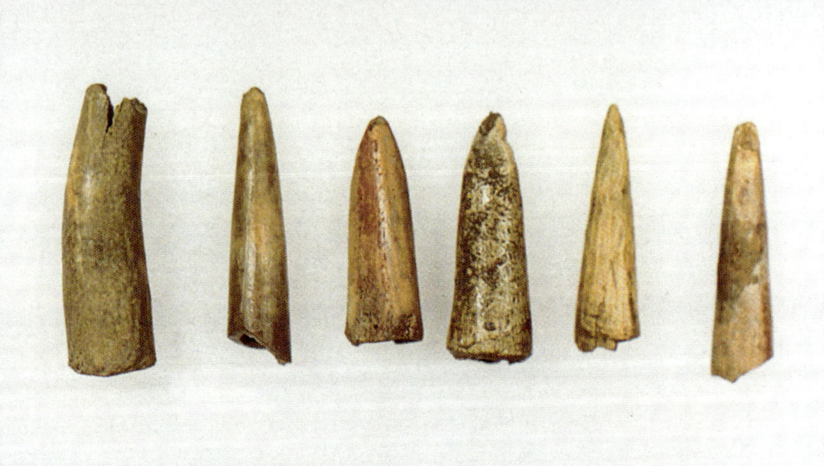

Socketed projectile tips, antler, Late Woodland to Mississippian, longest is 2⅛". Col. Vietzen found them in the late 1930s, and the third example from right is pictured in his book *The Saga of Glover's Cave*. All were found at Lost City, Kentucky. Pete Timoch collection. Each, **$10.00 – 20.00.**

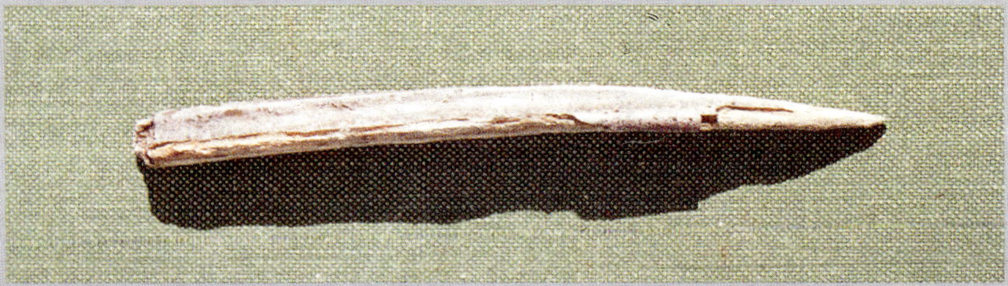

Pleistocene (ice age) projectile point, made of deer rib, 4¼" long, from the Caloosahatchee River. Such artifacts from Paleo times are extremely scarce. Lee County, Florida. Dave Summers collection, Victor, New York. **$125.00.**

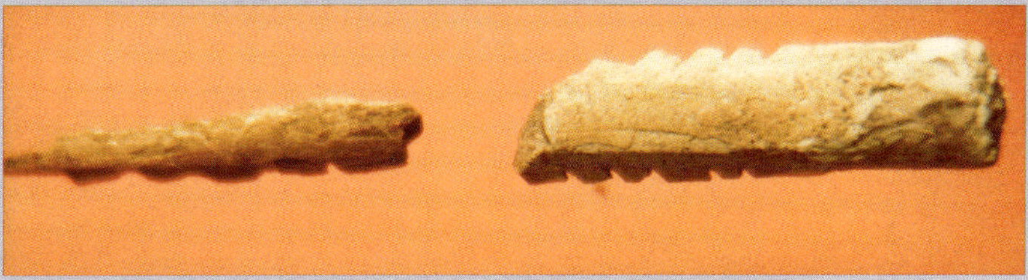

Bone harpoon sections, with multiple barbs, Late Archaic, Frontenac phase, 2⅛" and 2⅜" long, respectively. They are ex-collection Wray. They are from Cayuga County, New York. Dave Summers collection, Victor, New York. Each, **$70.00.**

Projectile points, antler, Woodland and Mississippian periods (1000 BC – AD 800), longest specimen is 3⅛". Ex-collection Vietzen, these came from various sites in Ohio and Kentucky. Pete Timoch collection. Each, **$5.00 – 15.00.**

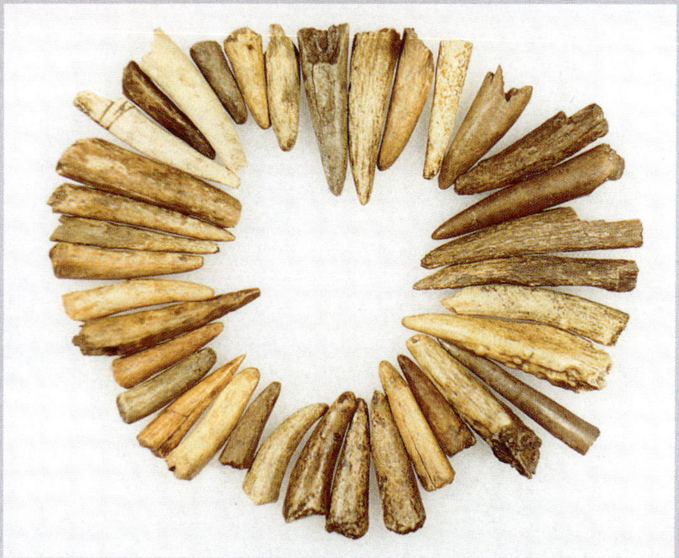

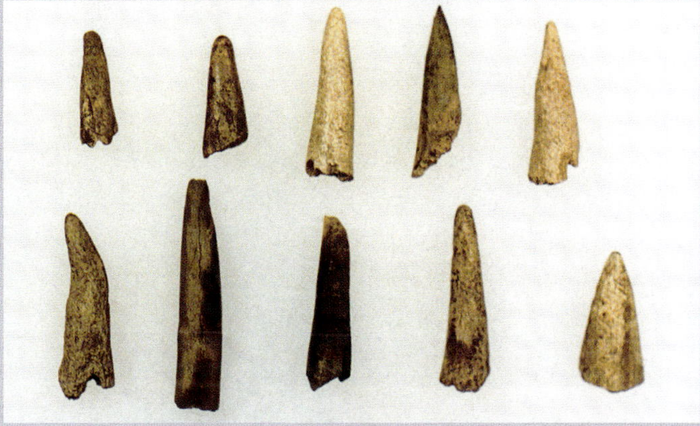

Socketed antler projectile tips, Fort Ancient (Mississippian), longest is 2". The arrowpoints were found in 1937 by Col. Vietzen and are from his collection. Ohio. Pete Timoch collection. Each, **$5.00 – 10.00.**

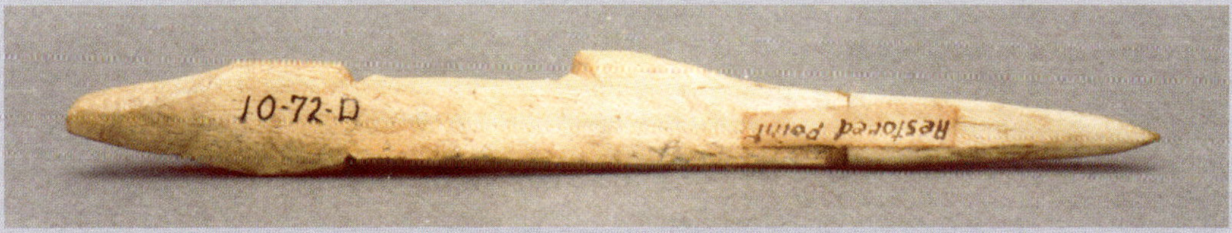

Harpoon head, bone, 5" long. With a replaced point, this is an historic piece, ca. AD 1600 – 1800. It was found near Richmond Mills, New York. H. B. Greene II collection, Naples, Florida. **$100.00.**

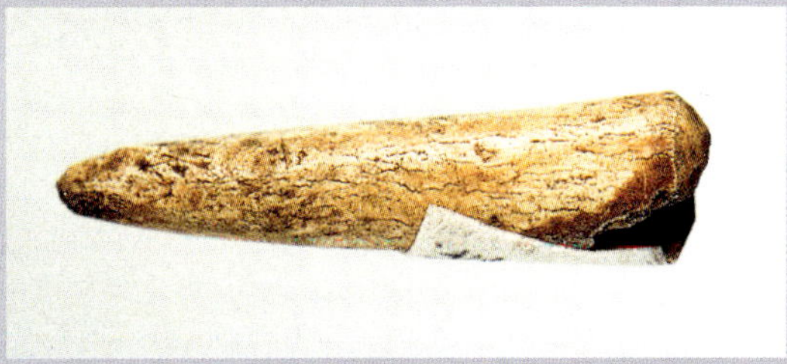

Projectile point, 1¾", polished surface. It was found in the Portland area, Indiana. Dwight Wolfe collection. **$25.00.**

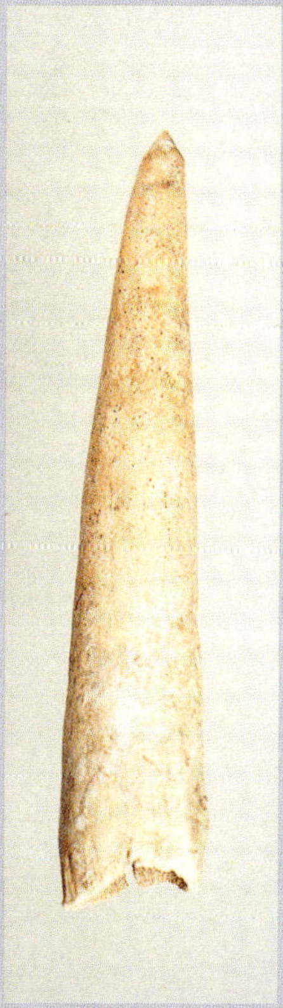

Projectile point, possibly a spearpoint (judging by size), 3½". This antler point has a hollowed base and was found in Kentucky. Fred Winegardner collection. **$20.00.**

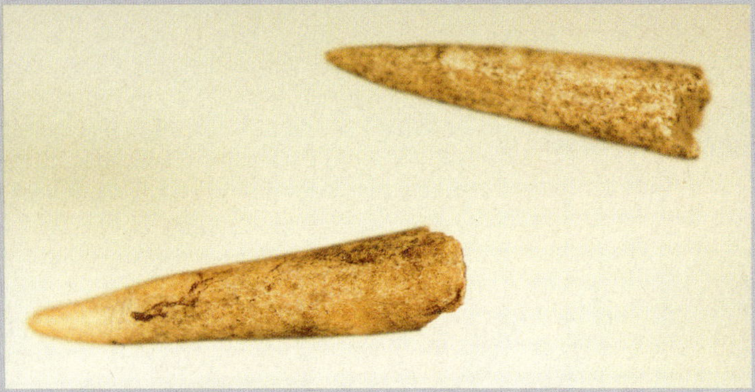

Projectile points, antler tines, longer one is 1¾". These were broken from larger antler sections, and the bases are still irregular and not finished for points. Fort Ancient, they are from Kentucky. Private collection. Each, **$5.00.**

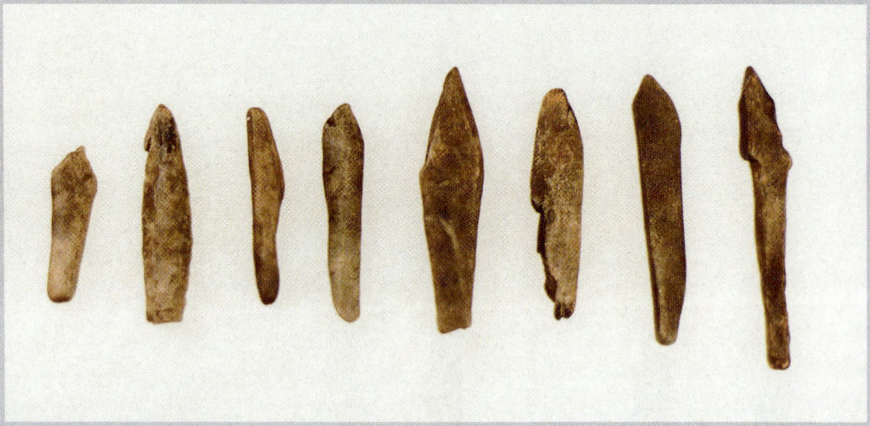

Bone projectile points, stemmed, longest is 2½". The second example from left has a small barb cut in the upper left side, and all have reduced stems for possible fitting in socketed shafts. Eastern Missouri. Private collection. Each, **$25.00 – 50.00.**

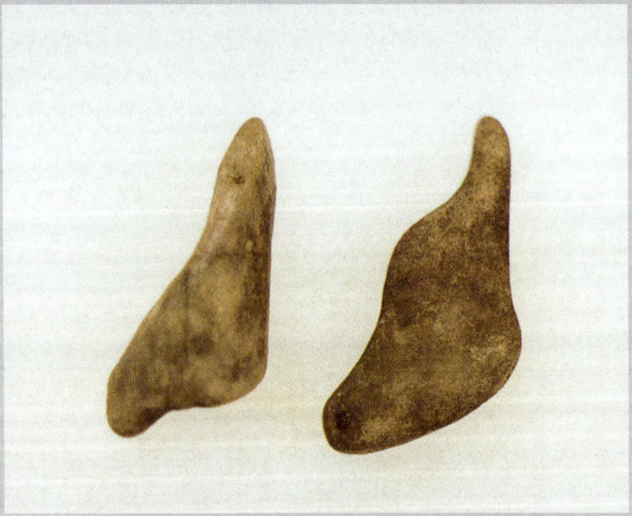

Harpoon heads, Woodland to Mississippian periods. The longer piece is 2¼" and they are made of polished bone. These are similar to some Alaskan forms. Eastern Missouri. Private collection. Each, **$25.00.**

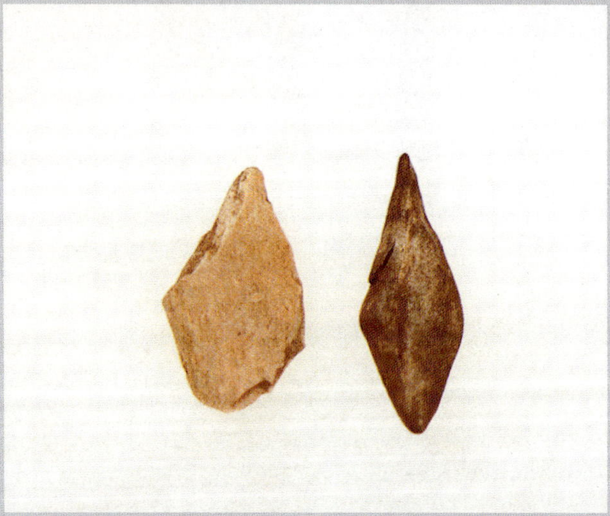

Bone projectile points, Woodland to Mississippian periods, longer piece is 1½". The left example has the basal area ground thin for a haft and the right has a narrow cut which forms a shallow barb. Eastern Missouri. Private collection. Each, **$20.00 – 40.00.**

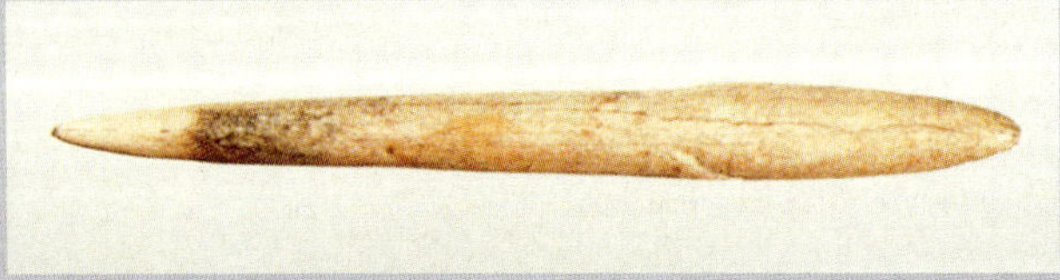

Projectile point or pin, animal bone, rounded cross-section. It is $2^{11}/_{16}$" long, from Wayne County, Tennessee. Private collection. **$20.00.**

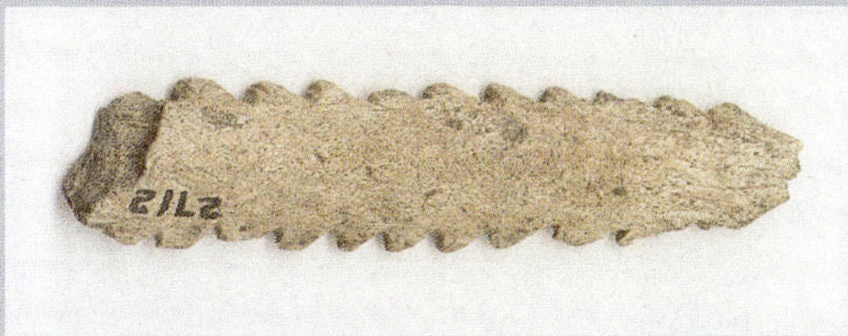

Bone harpoon tip, serrated or barbed on both sides. It was found near the Seneca River, New York. Kirk Spurr collection. Unlisted.

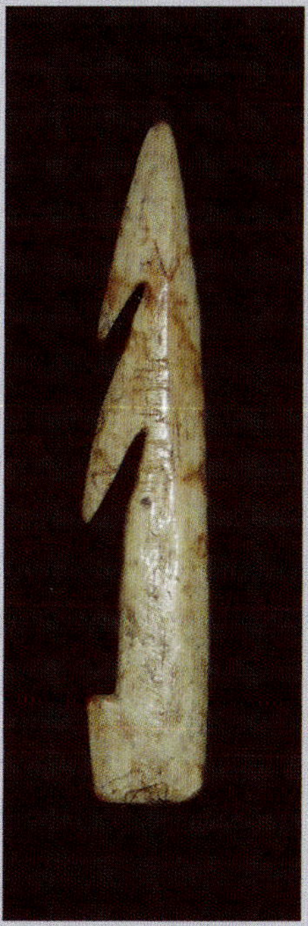

Antler harpoon head, high polish, two unilateral barbs, head is ½" wide and 2⅞" long. This fine piece was found in southcentral Pennsylvania. Private collection. Museum grade.

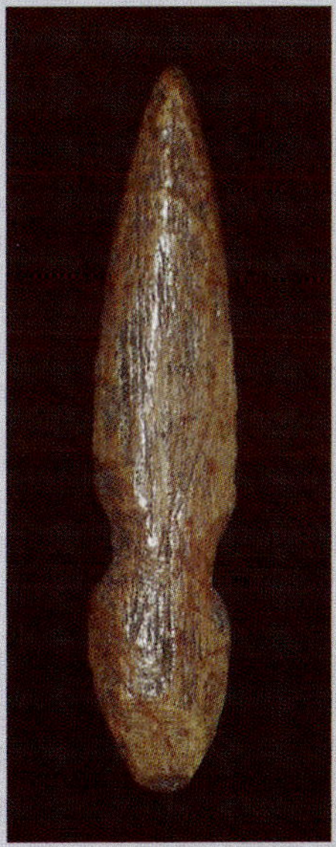

Antler projectile point, ½" wide and 2¼" long. The point is polished and provenance is unlisted. Private collection. Museum grade.

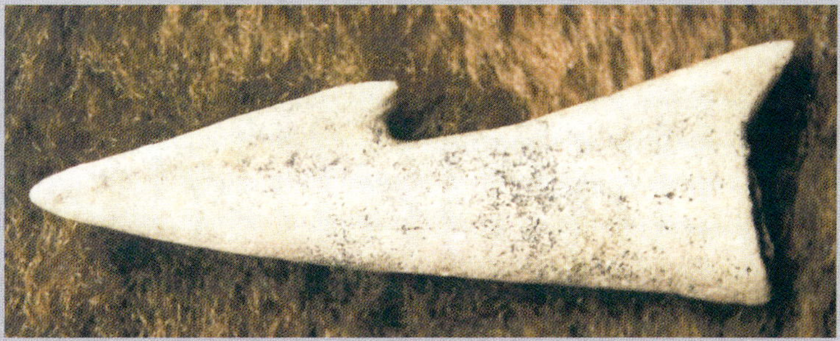

Bone harpoon, two barbs, 2⅝" long. This example was found by the owners and is the only known harpoon from the area. Scotland County, Missouri. Dale and Betty Roberts collection, Iowa. **$325.00.**

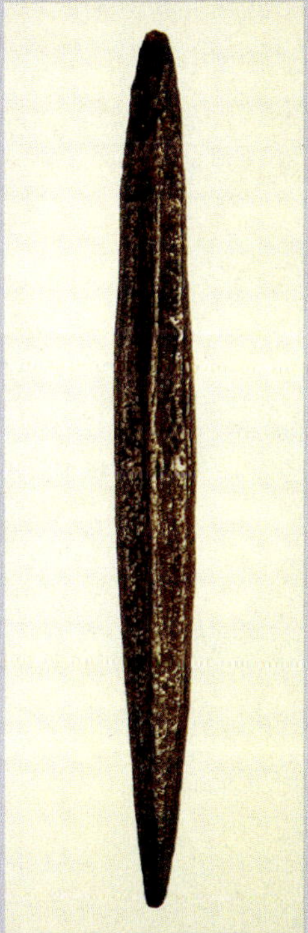

Projectile point or pin, split deer bone, double-tipped, mineralized and stained black. It is 3 3/16" long and was found years ago in a Florida river. Private collection. **$20.00.**

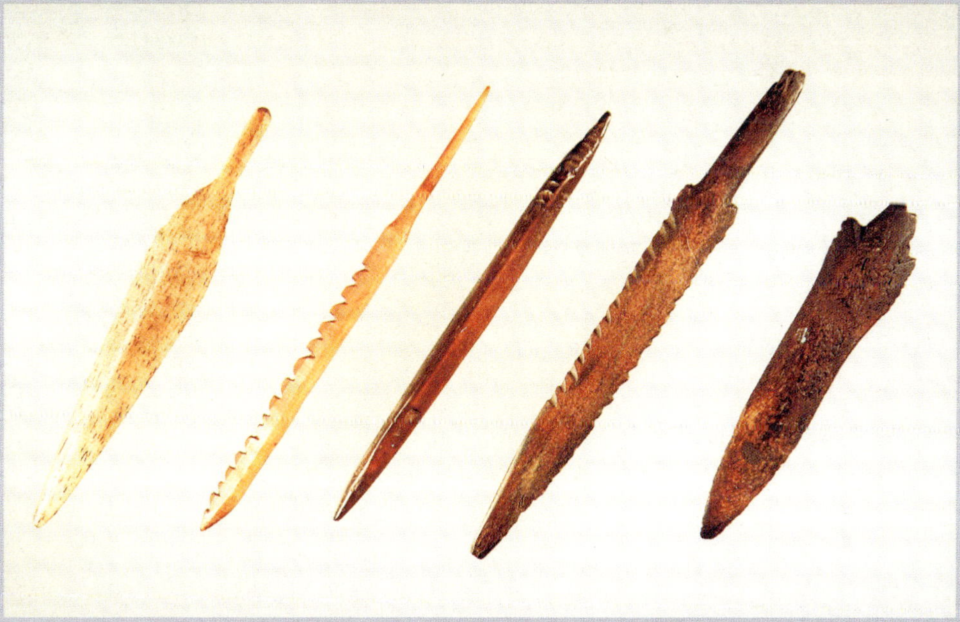

Arrowheads, five different stemmed styles, left to right: leaf-shape, barbed one side, duo-tipped, barbed two sides, and standard. The longest example shown is 4" long. These are Eskimo, from Alaska. Robin Fiser collection. Each, **$25.00 – 40.00.**

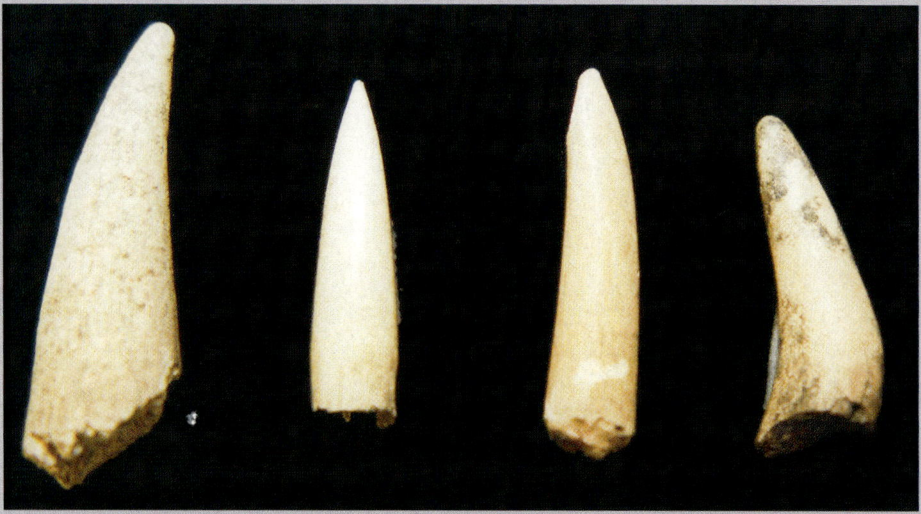

Arrow points and tools, antler tines, lengths range from 1⅜ to 1⅝". All were personal finds by the owner in Mississippi County, Arkansas. Garvin collection. Each, **$10.00 – 15.00.**

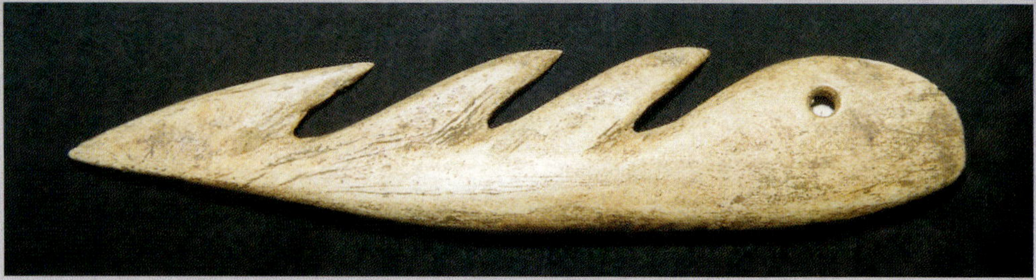

Harpoon, three barbs and drilled attachment hole, 4¾" long. This is an exceptional Fort Ancient piece. Mason County, Kentucky. Garvin collection. **$275.00 – 300.00.**

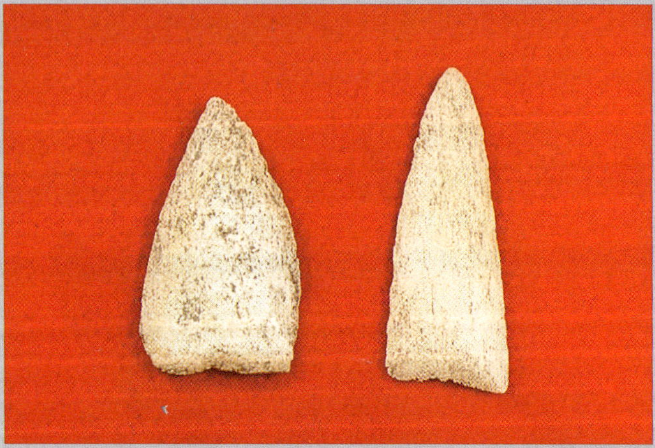

Projectile points, flattened bone, probably late prehistoric. Northwest Coast. Pete Timoch collection. Left, 1½". **$40.00.** Right, 1¾". **$60.00.**

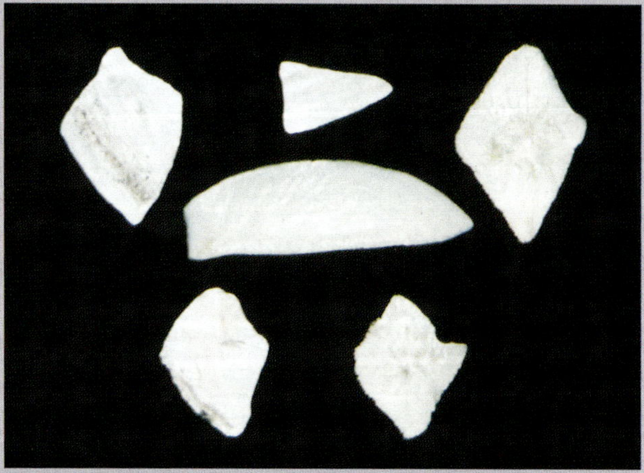

Shell arrowpoints, shown actual size, all found along the Fox River. Such points are rare, and these are the only examples found by the owner in ten years of surface hunting. Kane County, Illinois. Joseph Sulka collection, Illinois. Unlisted.

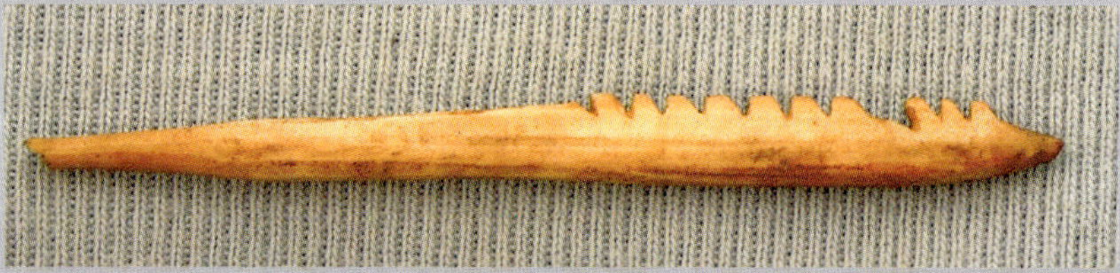

Ivory arrowpoint, unilaterally barbed, 2⅞" long. This piece is Eskimo, from Eek, Alaska. Rod Fuller collection, Nebraska. **$75.00.**

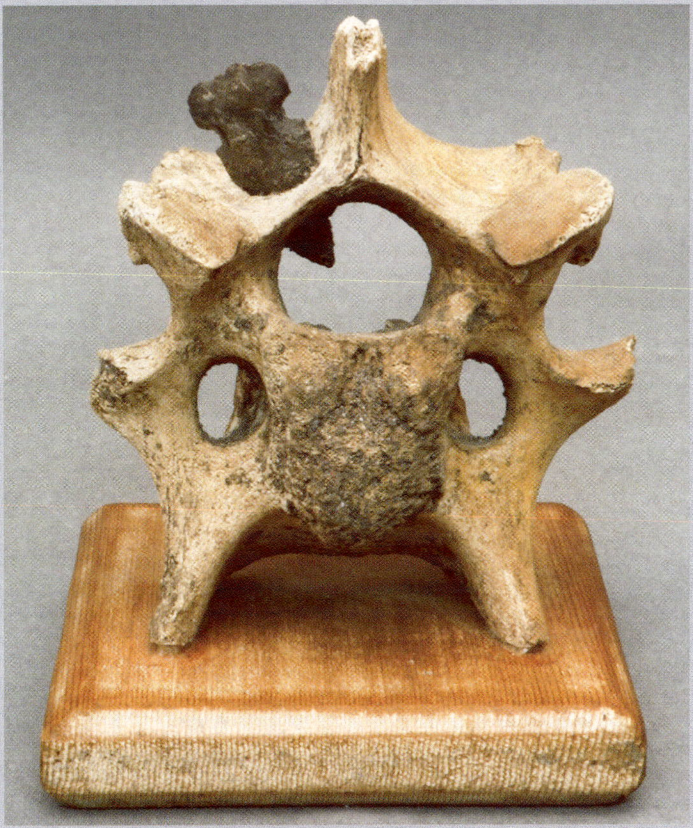

Bison vertebra with arrowhead, bone, 3½ x 4". Late prehistoric or early historic, the piece was probably found in Montana. H. B. Greene II collection, Naples, Florida. Unlisted.

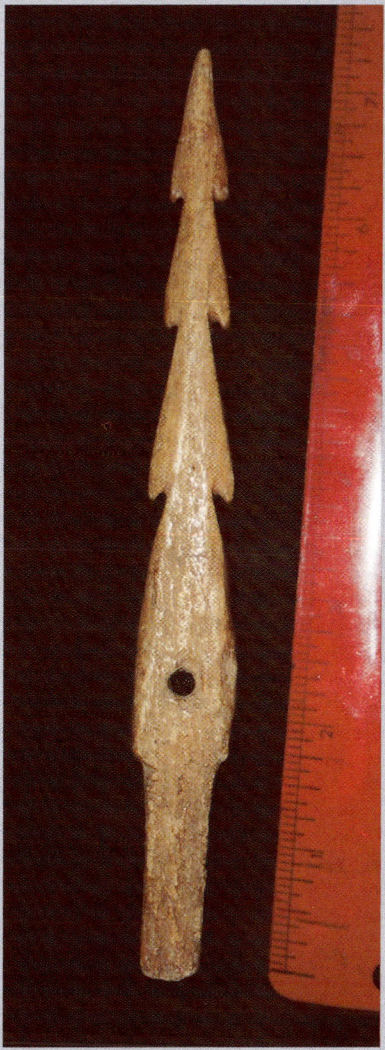

Antler harpoon, ¾" wide and 7⅜" long. This is an extraordinary harpoon tip, complete with paired barbs, cord hole, and shaft socket. It was found in southcentral Pennsylvania. Private collection. Museum grade.

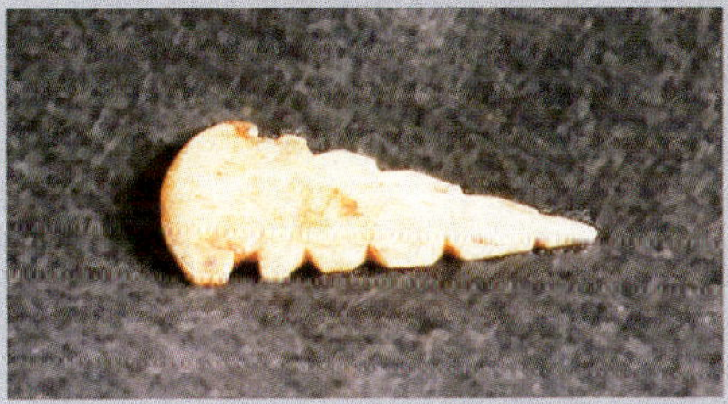

Bone projectile point, notched sides, 1⅝" long. Atypical, it is ex-collection Liehr and was found in Pike County, Illinois. John F. Wubker collection, Illinois. Unlisted.

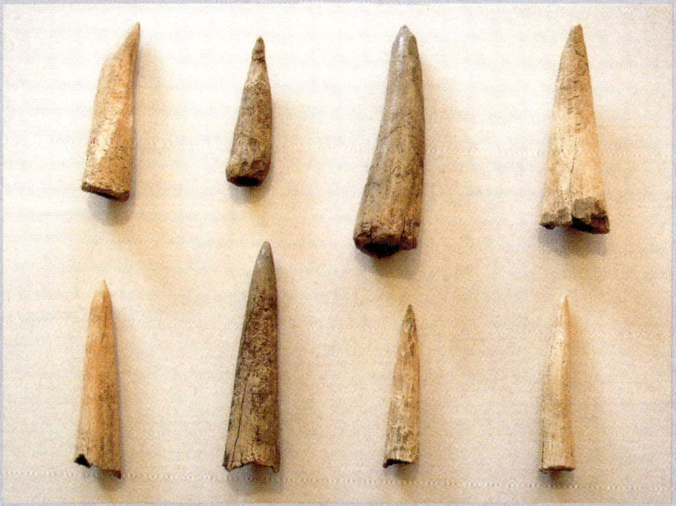

Antler projectile points, all drilled from wide bases, Mississippian period. They are from 1½ to 2½" long. The owner found them, and when the bottom right point was cleaned it was found to contain part of the original wooden arrow shaft. Ohio River area, Mason and Cabell Counties, West Virginia. Private collection. Rodney Roberts photograph. Each, **$12.00 – 25.00.**

Projectile Points

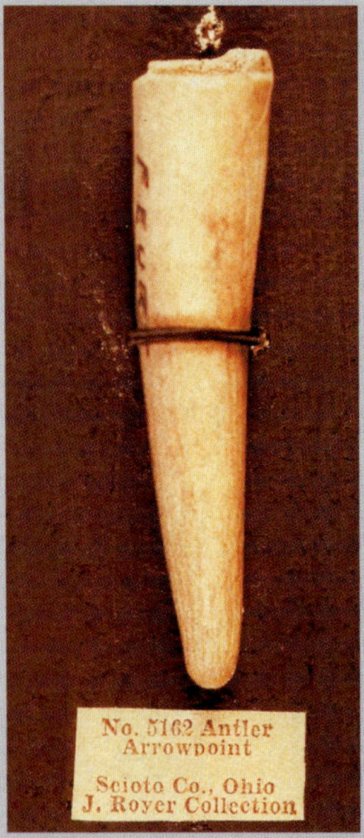

Antler projectile point, 2¼" long, hollowed base. It was collected long ago in Scioto County, Ohio. Fred Winegardner collection. Unlisted.

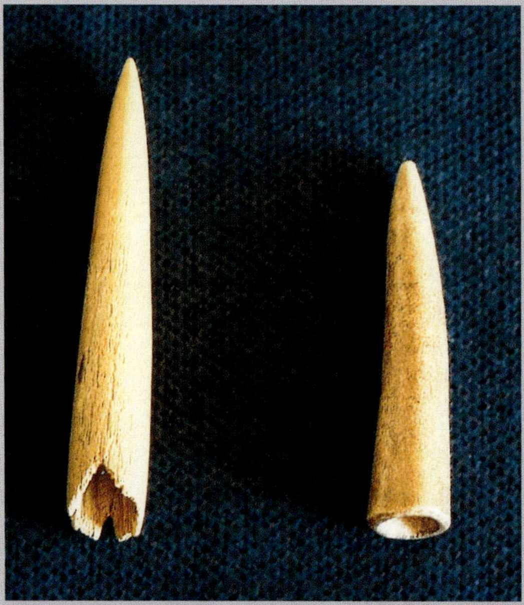

Arrowpoints, deer antler tines, 2⅜ and 2" long respectively. They are both hollowed at the base for arrowshaft insertion. North Platte area, Nebraska. Rod Fuller collection, Nebraska. Each, **$40.00 – 55.00.**

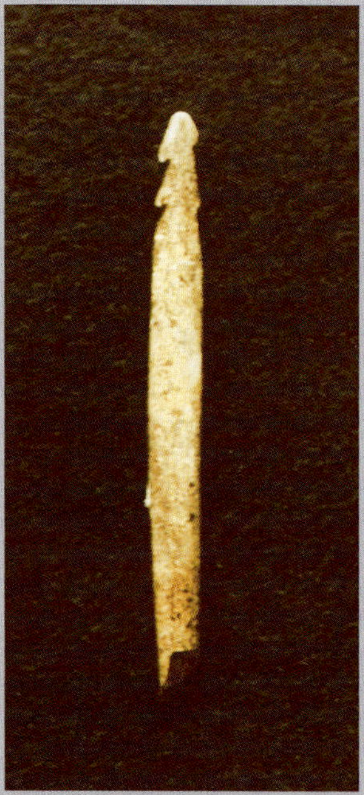

Barbed bone harpoon, 2¾" long, Middle Woodland period, ca. AD 1 – 1000. It was found near the town of Van Buren, Onondaga County, New York. Dave Summers collection, Victor, New York. **$85.00.**

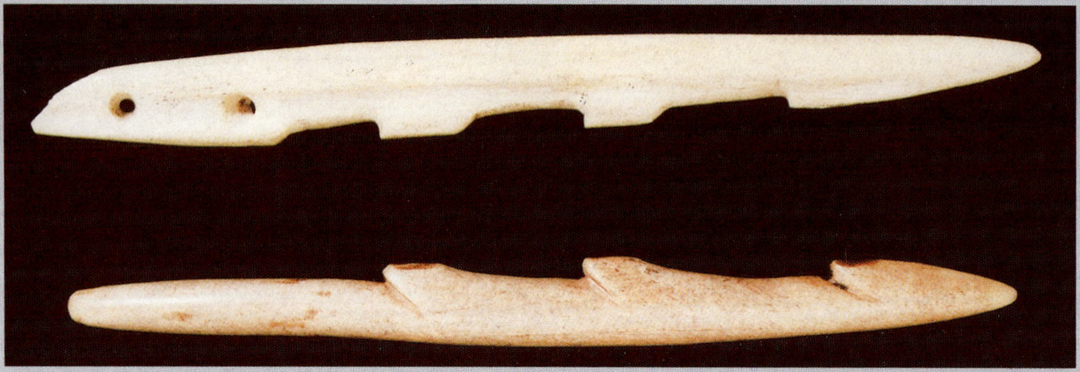

Harpoons, top example found in a shell heap, 5¼" long. The base has been reworked in ancient times and attachment holes are drilled from both sides, but at an angle. The bone material is quite thick. It was found near Corea, Maine. Bottom harpoon, also 5¼" long, is possibly polished antler or more likely a deer ulna. The material is very dense, and it came from Tennessee. Private collection. Top, drilled example, **$400.00;** bottom, tapered base, **$300.00.**

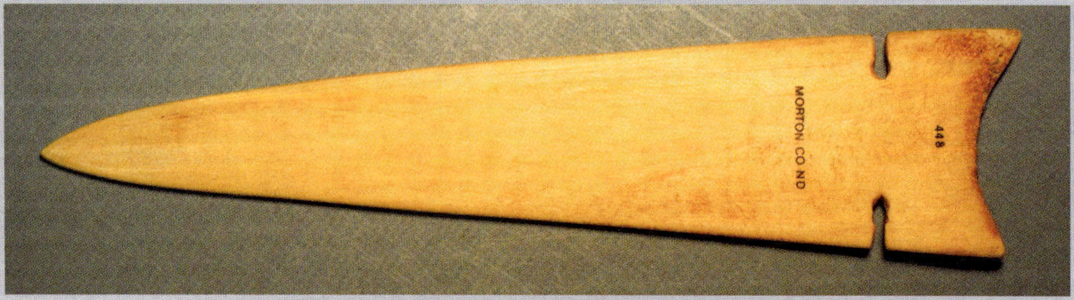

Bone spear point, rare, named by Gregory Perino as the "Boley Spear" and sketched in his *Selected Preforms, Points and Knives,* Volume 2, p 30. It was found on the Boley site in the late 1970s and is ca. AD 1750. This superb piece is 8½" long. Morton County, North Dakota. Private collection. Museum grade.

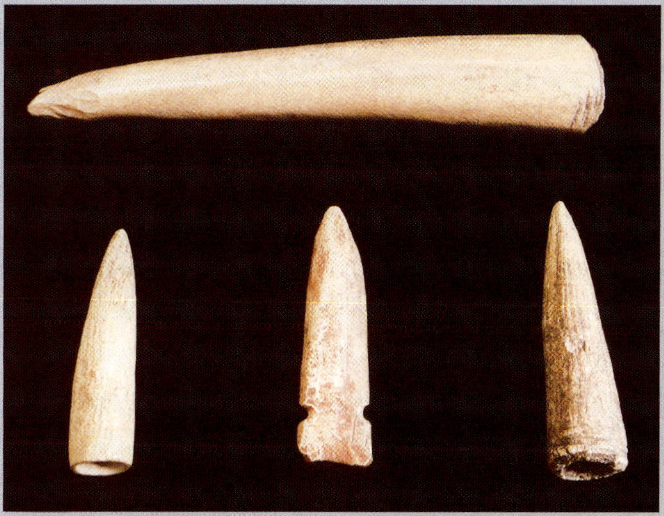

Antler and bone artifacts, large antler spearpoint is 9 cm long, whittled tip, from Alabama. The three projectile points made of antler tines are: a finished point that is carved and polished with basal socket (left); a notched deer bone point with ground tip (center); and, a partially finished antler point with base somewhat smoothed and partially reamed out (right). All of these are from New York. Private collection. Each, **$25.00 – 35.00.**

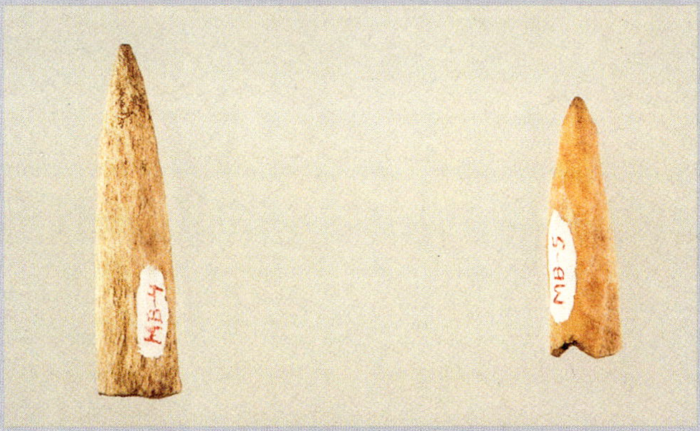

Antler arrowpoints, longest is 1½". Probably shaped with flake knives (judging by small facets), these were found in West Virginia. Doug Hooks collection. Each, **$15.00 – 20.00.**

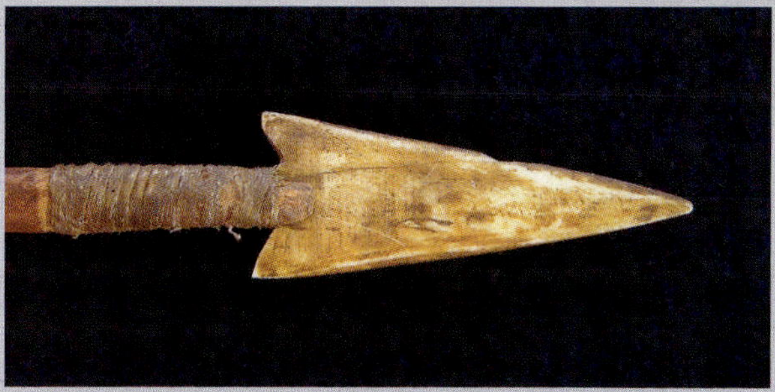

Arrow with bone tip, Plains(?) region, 1¾" long. This is a rare artifact. Victor T. Trujillo collection, Nevada. Museum grade.

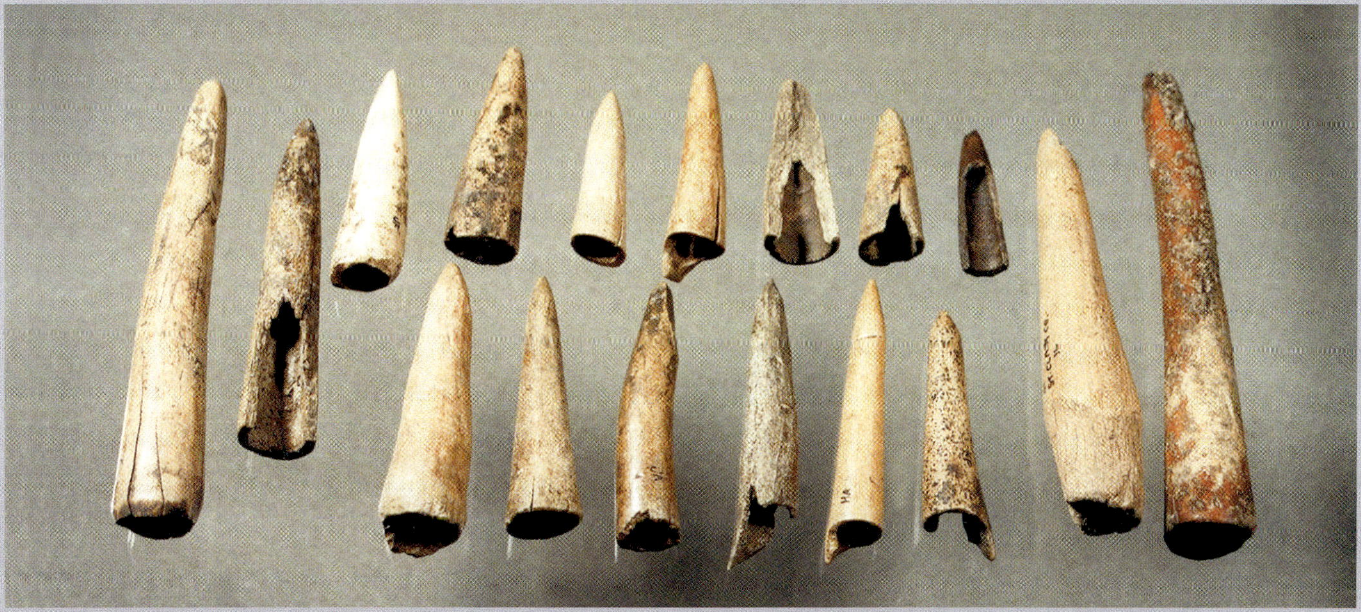

Projectile points, Riverton people of the Late Archaic period, 1 to 3⅝" long. Many of the Riverton sites have produced a few such projectile points and they are far from common. These came from Crawford County, Illinois. John Smith collection, Illinois. Each, **$25.00 – 60.00.**

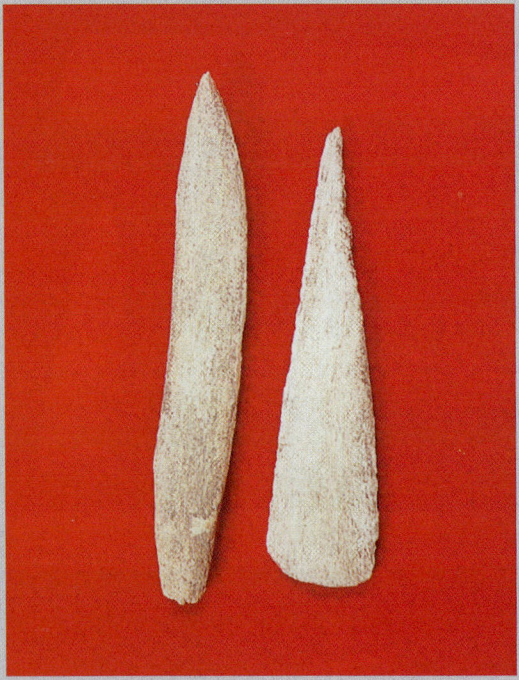

Bone projectile points, left example with base ground to fit socket. Northwest Coast. Pete Timoch collection. Left, 2⅞". **$125.00.** Right, triangular, 2½". **$100.00.**

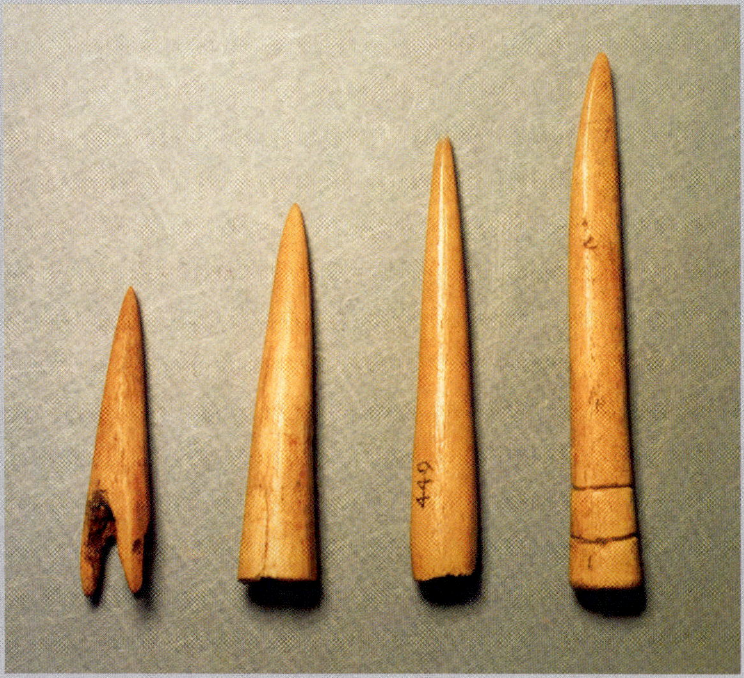

Arrowpoints, historic, ca. AD 1750, the longest is 3¼". These are fine examples. Both the small barbed point on left and the decorated point on right are of special interest. Morton County, North Dakota. Private collection. Each, **$75.00 – 125.00.**

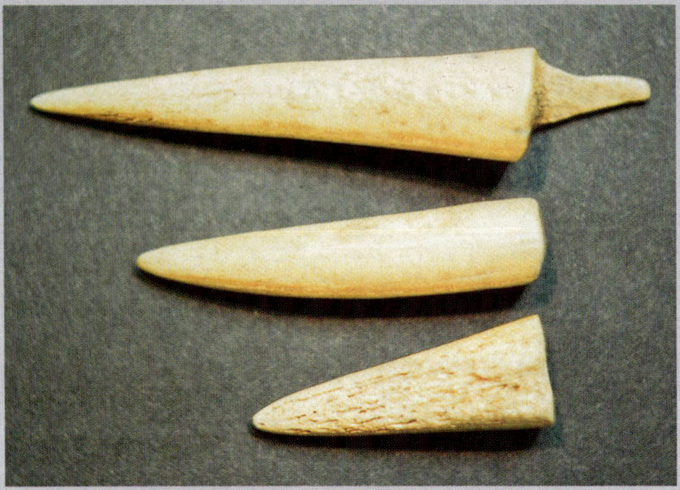

Arrowpoints, antler, longest is 3". These were found in Morton County, North Dakota. Mike Fox collection, Iowa. Each, **$25.00 – 50.00.**

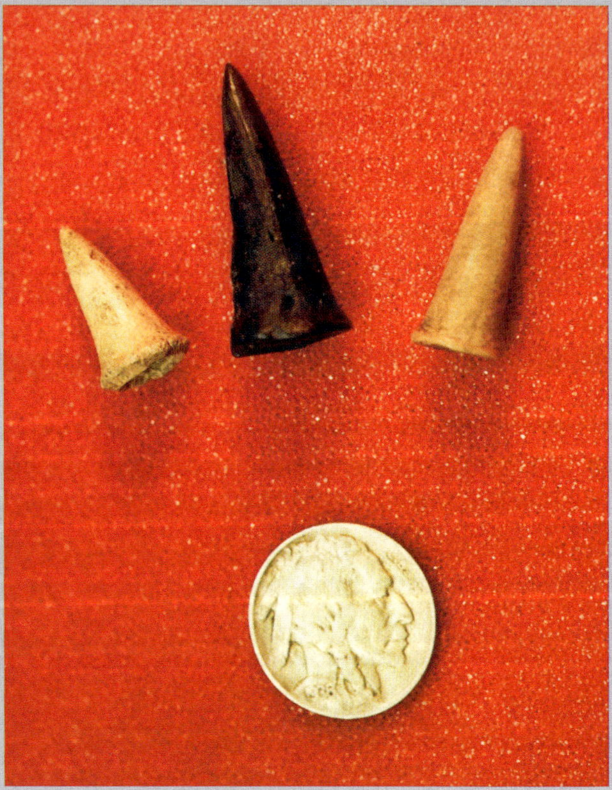

Arrowpoints, deer antler, well-preserved because they were in a trash pit. Fulton County, Illinois. Fred Smith collection, Illinois. Each, **$15.00 – 25.00.**

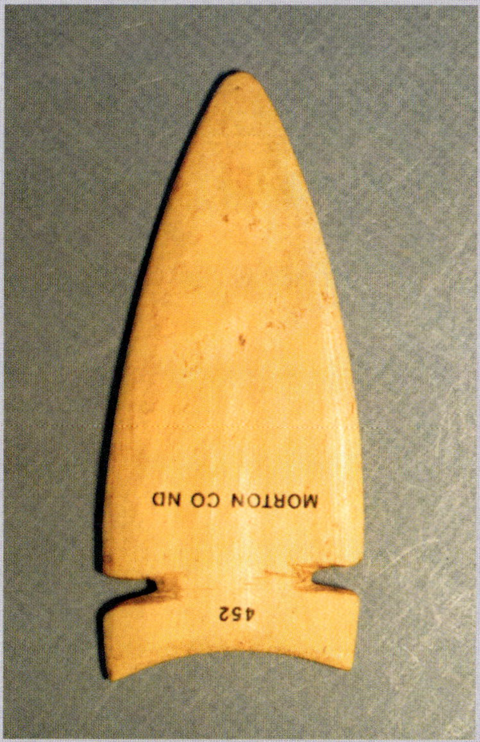

Bone spear point, historic period, ca. AD 1750, 3¼" long. It came from Morton County, North Dakota. Private collection. Museum grade.

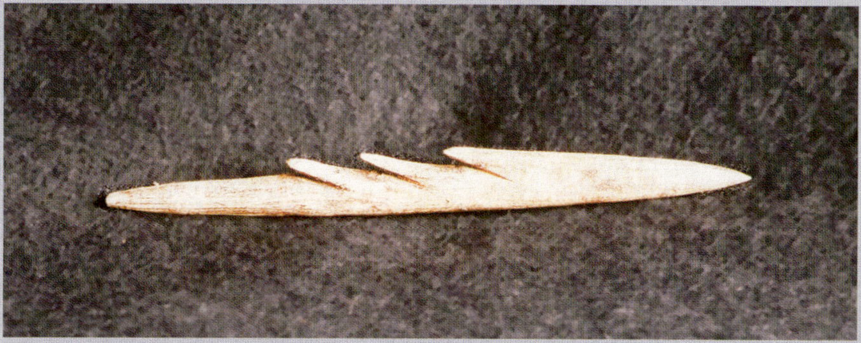

Bone harpoon, three unilateral barbs, 4¼" long. The origin of this fine harpoon is unknown. John F. Wubker collection, Illinois. **$275.00.**

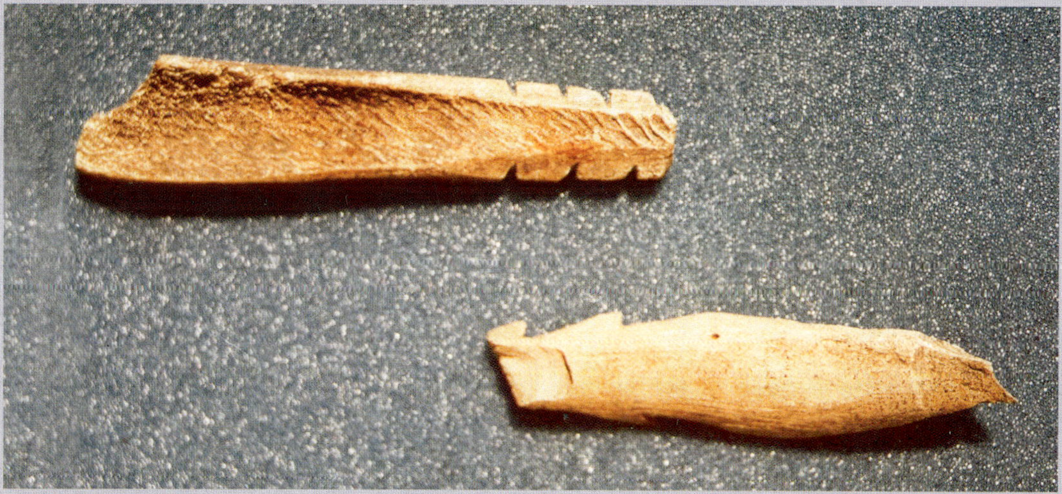

Harpoon sections, made of thick bone, 3½ and 4⅜" long. These are Point Peninsula and Hopewell phases, Middle Woodland period. They were found in Onondaga County, New York. Dave Summers collection, Victor, New York. Each, **$100.00.**

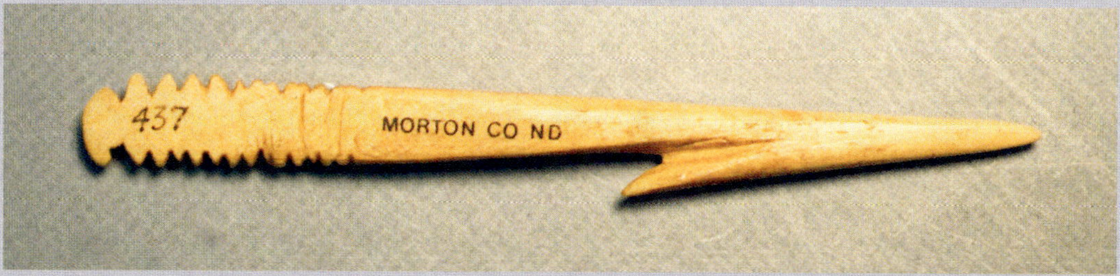

Harpoon, rare, the only example recovered by the finder, C. Hintz. It is 5" long, ca. AD 1750, from Morton County, North Dakota. Private collection. Museum grade.

Fishhooks

It appears that bone fishhooks were made just about anywhere there was fishing water and animals for a supply of bones. Regions with abundant rivers and lakes usually have sites that produce fishhooks from the Archaic, Woodland, and Mississippian periods. Fishhooks, desired by collectors for their graceful beauty, are far from common. Due to the thinness of these artifacts, the survival rate for complete examples is not high and unbroken examples are at a premium.

Most fishhooks were made from deer rib bones; though a few were carved from deer toe bones, the bones of other animals, and shell. Hooks have a U-shape (rounded at the base) or V-shape (angular at the base), and, in outline, resemble modern hooks. In some other respects they are quite different. While a few hook tips are barbed, most are not. Only a very few have the long shaft holed near the end for line attachment, and the majority have the shaft top angled, grooved, or knobbed to help hold the fishing line.

Various manufacturing methods were used, most beginning with a rectangular piece of thin bone. For narrow bones, the center was cut or gouged away, leaving the sides intact. This "frame" was then cut in the appropriate places to produce the hook, and a long bone section could be cut in two places to make two hooks. Another method was to bore a large hole in the bone preform, which then became the inside curve of the fishhook.

The bone was ground to a smooth finish and sometimes polished. In use, the breakage and loss rate must have been very high, a consideration that adds to both the scarcity and desirability of bone fishhooks today. Hooks range in length from about 1 to 3 inches, but examples up to 6 inches have been found. An artifact dealer, Allen Brown of Chicago, once owned the largest known cache of bone fishhooks. There were 95 hooks in the cache, ranging in size from 1½ to 3 inches long. The hooks were found in Kansas.

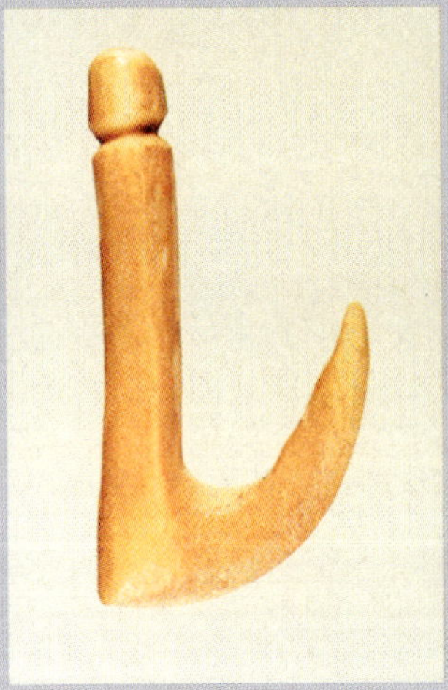

Fishhook, angled tip, 1¾" long. The size and curved hook tip indicate that this piece was made from a deer toe bone. Madison County, Alabama. Robin Fiser collection. **$175.00.**

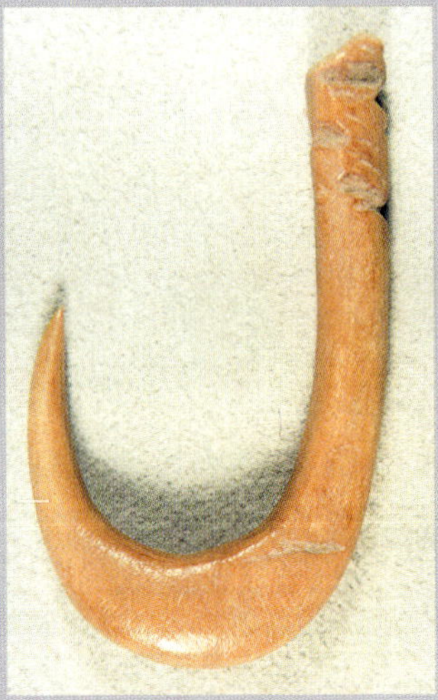

Fishhook, bone, large size at 1-1/10 x 2⁷⁄₁₀". This big hook has attachment grooves on the shaft and has a fine golden patina. Pike County, Illinois. First Mesa, Indiana. **$165.00.**

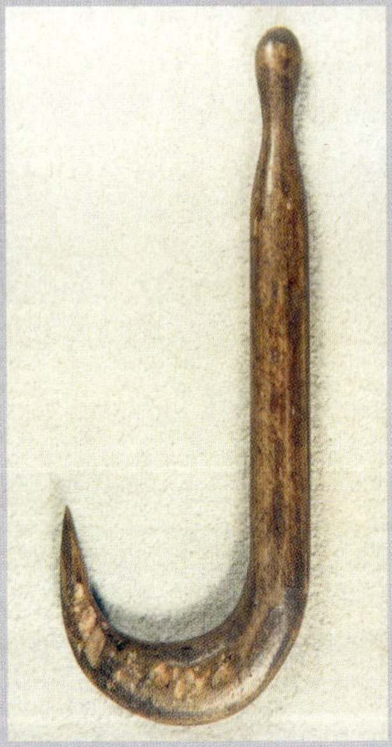

Fishhook, bone, 9/10 x 2½", weathered high polish and mottled brown patina. The shaft top is narrowed for cord attachment. Boone County, Kentucky. First Mesa, Indiana. **$185.00.**

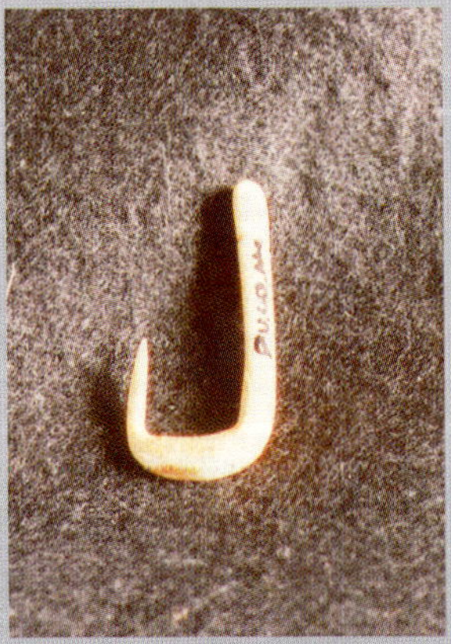

Fishhook, 1³⁄₁₆" long, squared U-shape. The find-site for this hook is not known. John F. Wubker collection, Illinois. **$125.00.**

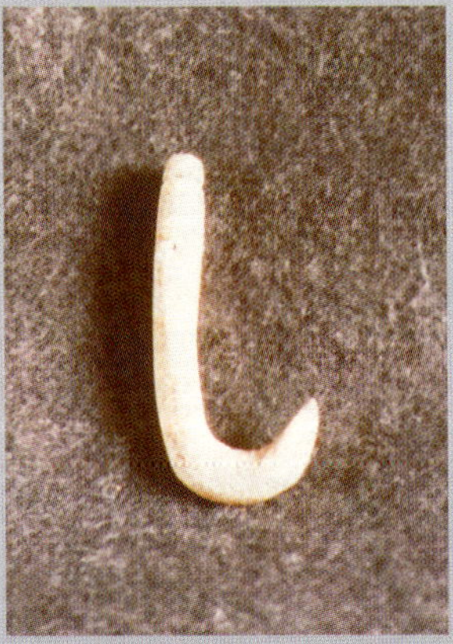

Fishhook, 1⅜" long, bone, grooved shank top. Find-site is unknown for this piece. John F. Wubker collection, Illinois. **$125.00.**

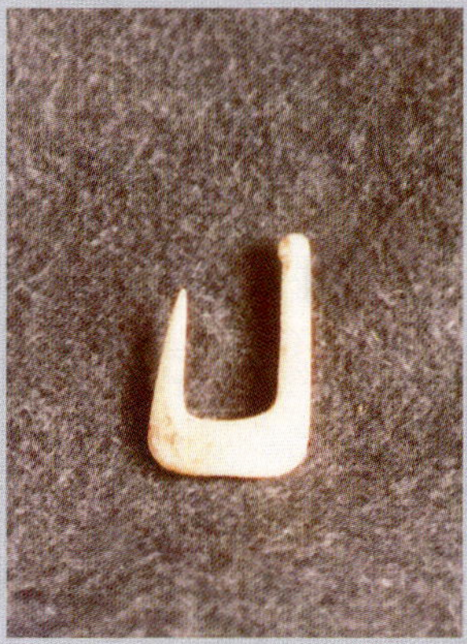

Fishhook, 1⁵⁄₁₆" long, squared configuration. This bone artifact was found in Todd County, Tennessee. John F. Wubker collection, Illinois. **$125.00.**

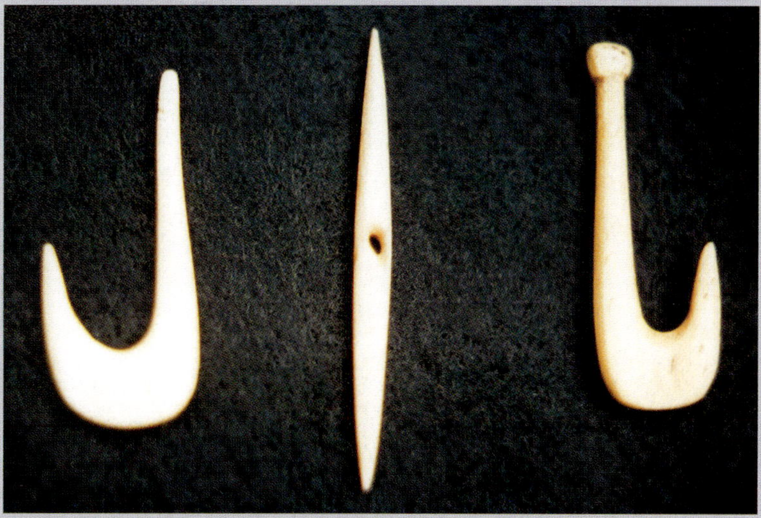

Fishhooks, three different styles including a drilled gorge hook at center, lengths 1¾ to 2⅛". All were found in Kentucky. Bob Hess collection, Indiana. Left, **$125.00;** center, **$150.00;** right, **$175.00.**

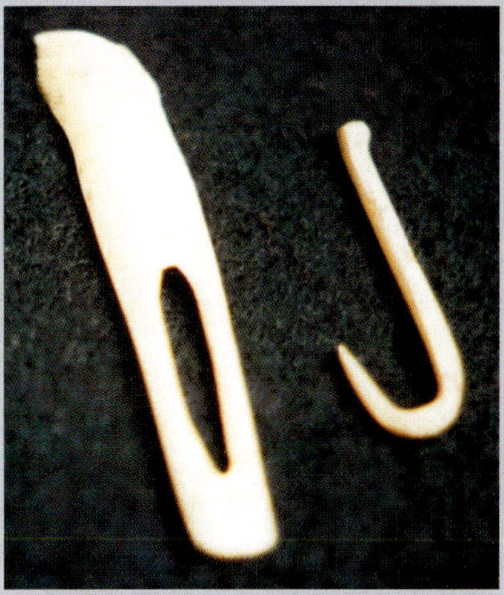

Bone fishhook and fishhook preform, hook is 1¼" long. They were found in Kentucky. Bob Hess collection, Indiana. Preform, **$75.00;** fishhook, **$150.00.**

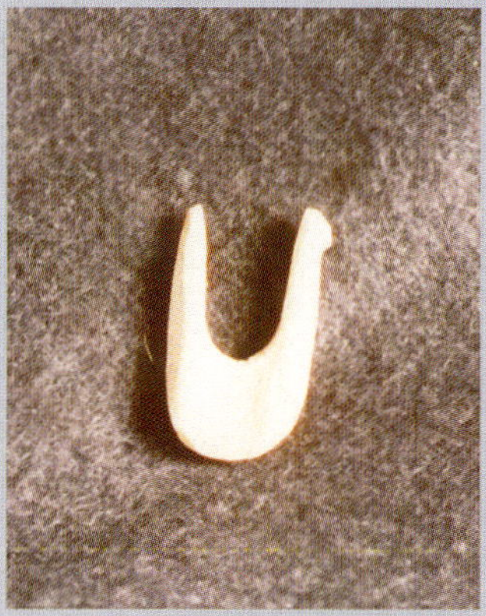

Fishhook, 1⁵⁄₁₆" long, deer bone. U-shaped, the portion between the shank and point is exceptionally thick. Find-site unknown, probably Midwest. John F. Wubker collection, Illinois. **$100.00.**

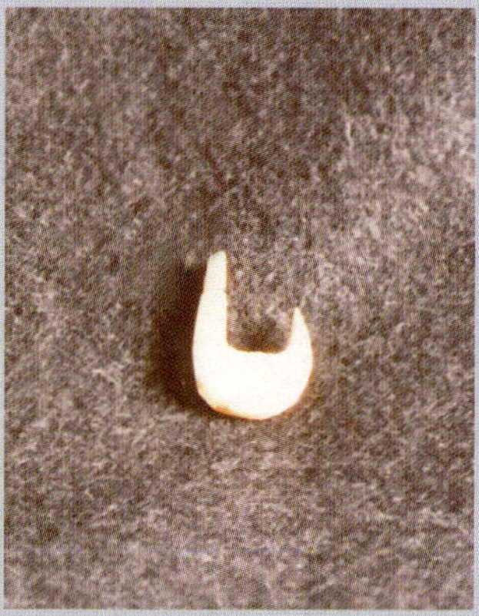

Fishhook, only ½" long, grooved near shank top with thick body. Find-site unknown. John F. Wubker collection, Illinois. **$100.00.**

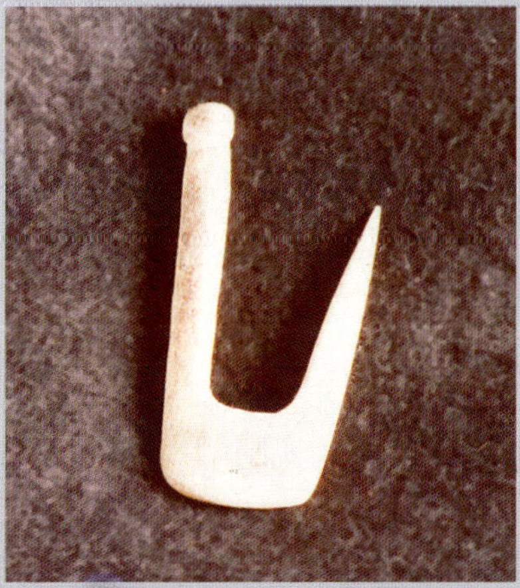

Fishhook, U-shaped and sturdy, shank top grooved. A well-made hook, find-site is unknown. John F. Wubker collection, Illinois. **$150.00.**

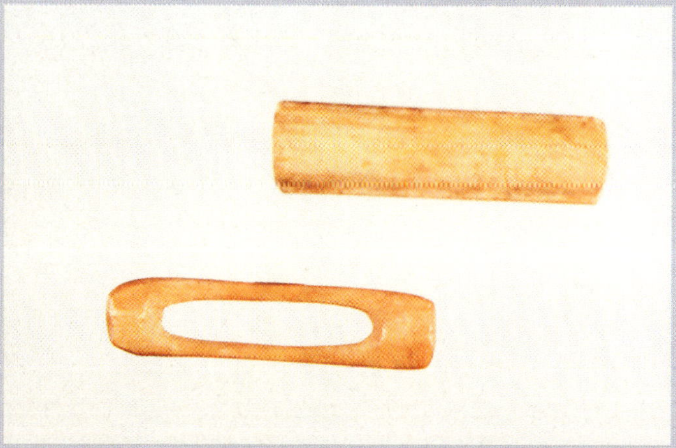

Fishhook forms, top blank is 1½". In the piece at bottom, the center section has been removed. Cut in the proper places, such blanks made two hooks. Scioto County, Ohio. Fred Winegardner collection. Unlisted.

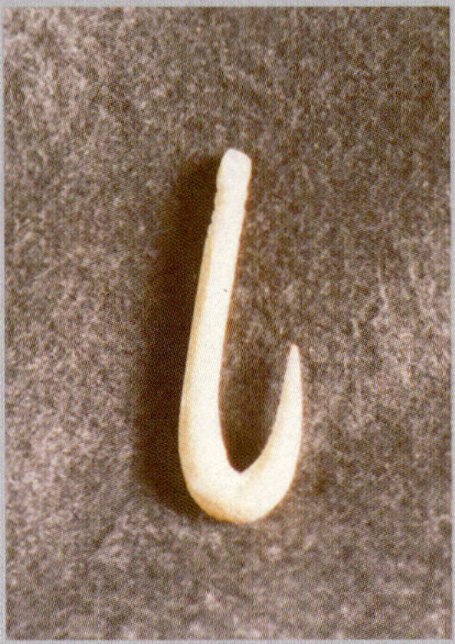

Fishhook, 1¾", ex-collection Reed. This hook is grooved for line attachment and find-site is not known. John F. Wubker collection, Illinois. **$150.00.**

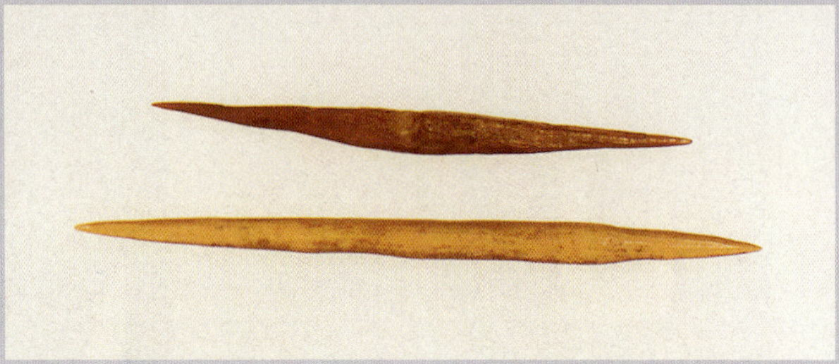

Gorge hooks(?), ivory, double-pointed, both from Alaska. James Timoch collection. Top, very sharp tips, **$60.00.** Bottom, 3⅜", **$100.00.**

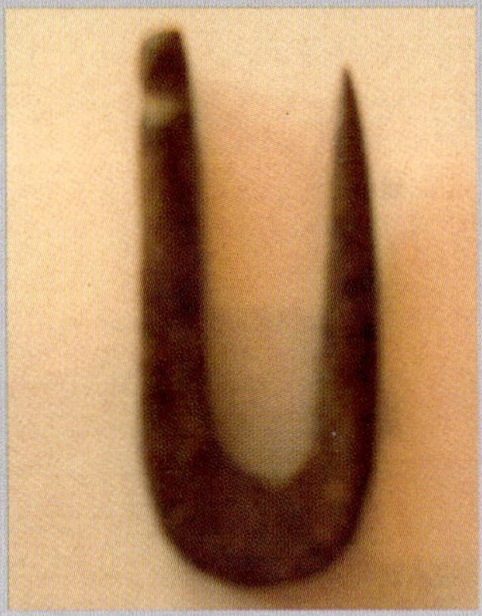

Bone fishhook, Mississippian (late prehistoric), 7/16 x 1". Grooved at the shaft top, it is an Ohio River find. Mason County, West Virginia. Private collection. Rodney Roberts photograph. **$125.00.**

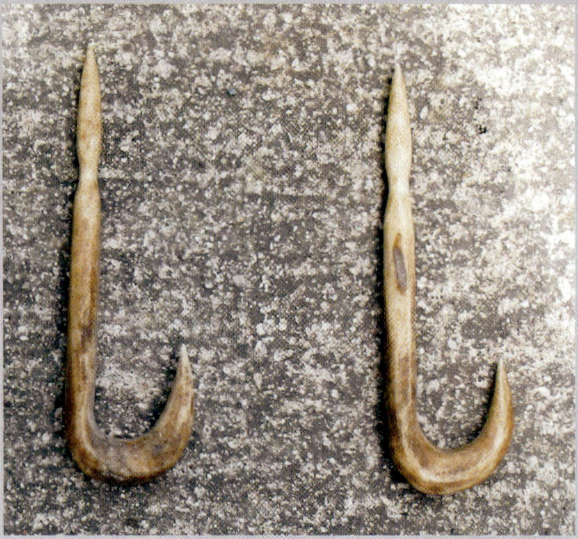

Fishhooks, bone, each 2¼" high, Eskimo. The similarity suggests the same person made them. St. Lawrence Island. John and Susan Mellyn collection, Texas. Each, **$150.00.**

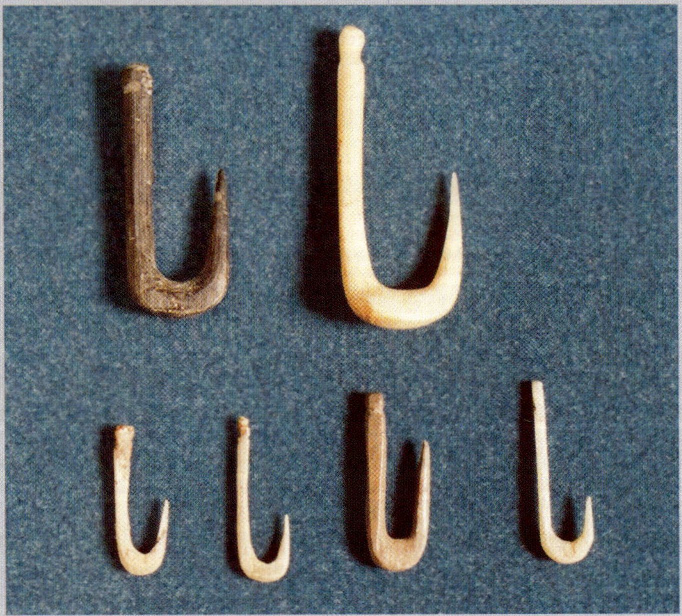

Fishhook collection, all fine and well-made examples. Top, Mississippian period, two large hooks from Meigs County, Tennessee. The white hook is 5 cm long. The other four hooks are Fort Ancient in culture, from Scioto County, Ohio. Private collection. Hooks, each, **$150.00 – 275.00.**

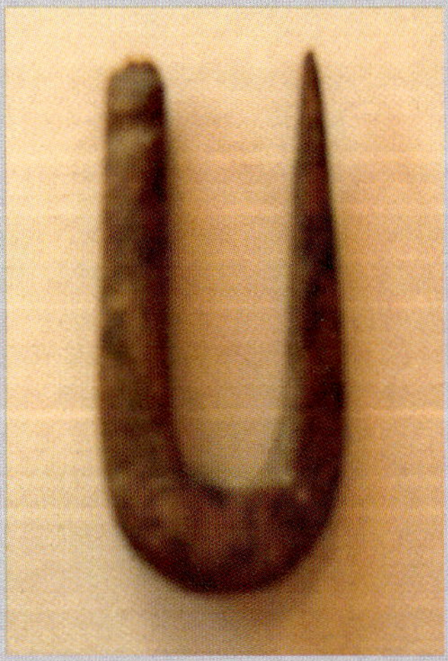

Fishhook, Mississippian period, ½ x 1". Grooved at the top for line attachment, this is one of two fishhooks that were found together. Mason County, West Virginia. Private collection. Rodney Roberts photograph. **$100.00.**

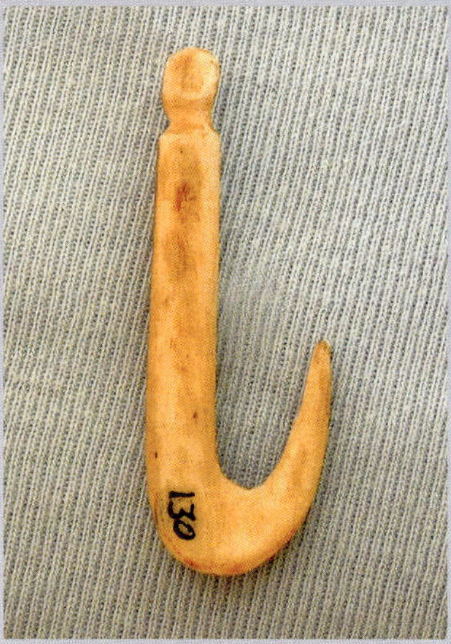

Fishhook, 2¼" high, animal bone. This is a sturdy hook in top condition, grooved for the fishing line. Pettis County, Missouri. Rod Fuller collection, Nebraska. **$200.00.**

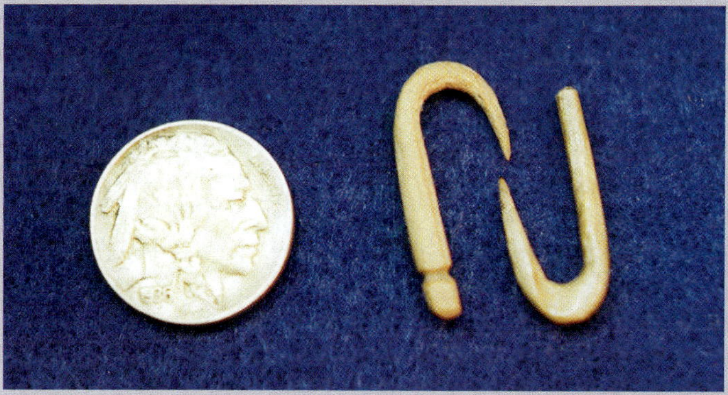

Fishhooks, made from deer toe bones, average length is 1$\frac{1}{16}$", well-shaped and polished. They were found in Fulton County, Illinois. Fred Smith collection, Illinois. Each, **$125.00 – 175.00.**

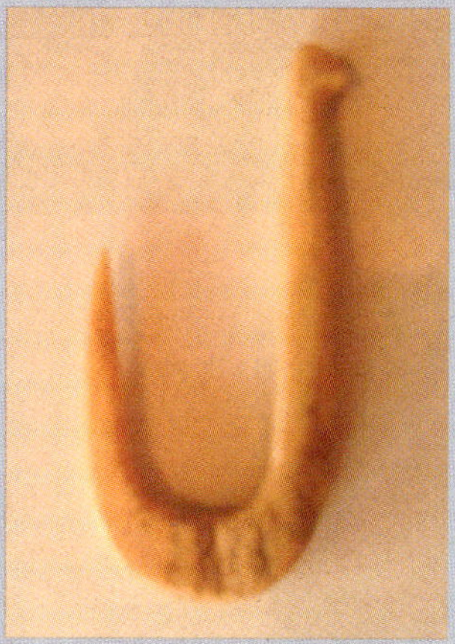

Bone fishhook, Mississippian, $\frac{9}{16}$ x 1$\frac{5}{16}$", with a projecting shaft-top knob. The owner found it in a path leading to the Ohio River. Mason County, West Virginia. Private collection; Rodney Roberts photograph. **$125.00.**

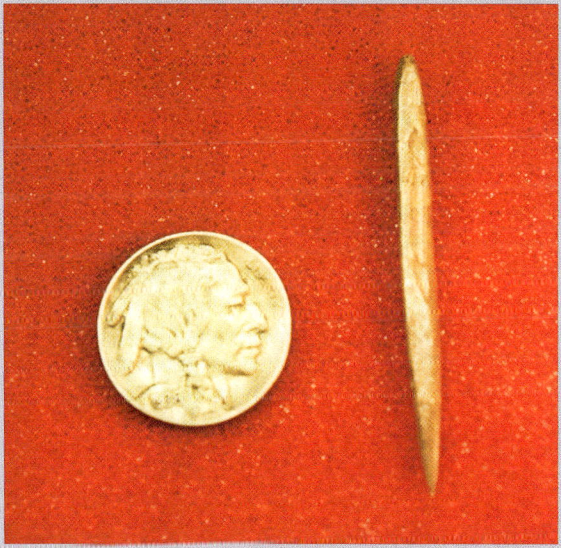

Double-pointed awl or gorge hook, wild turkey bone, 2¼". Such small artifacts could be used for quillwork and other intricate tasks. Fulton County, Illinois. Fred Smith collection, Illinois. **$15.00 – 20.00.**

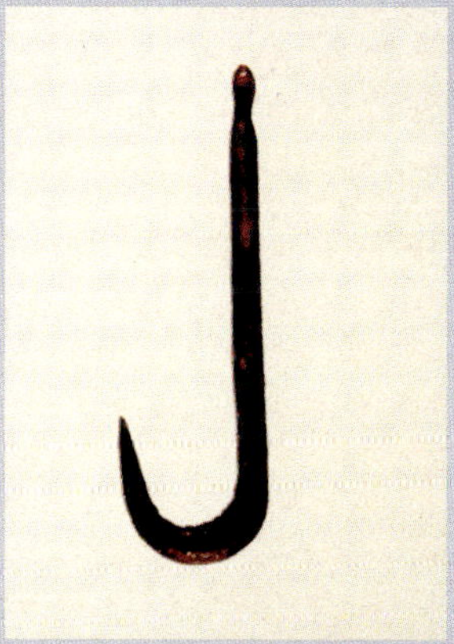

Fishhook, shank top with wide and shallow groove, finely carved. This hook is 1⅜" long and ex-collection Selb. West Virginia. Private collection. **$150.00.**

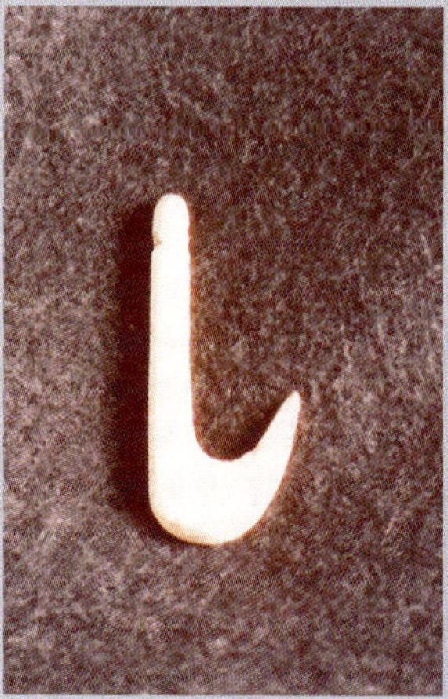

Fishhook, 1⅜" long, deer bone. Grooved at the shaft top, the find-site is not known. John. F. Wubker collection, Illinois. **$125.00.**

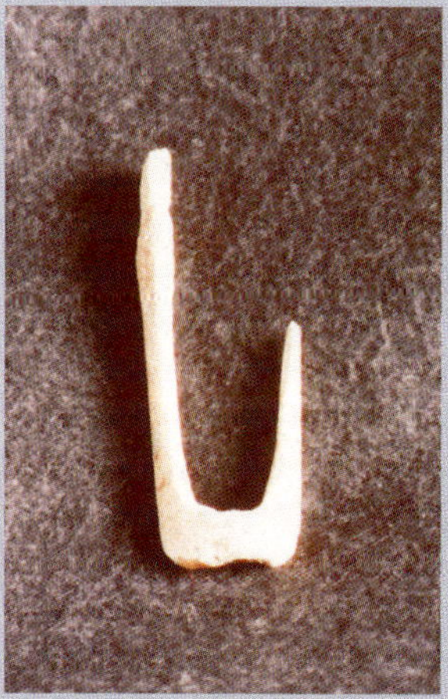

Fishhook, U-shape, deer bone, 1⅝" long. Site-location unknown. John F. Wubker collection, Illinois. **$150.00.**

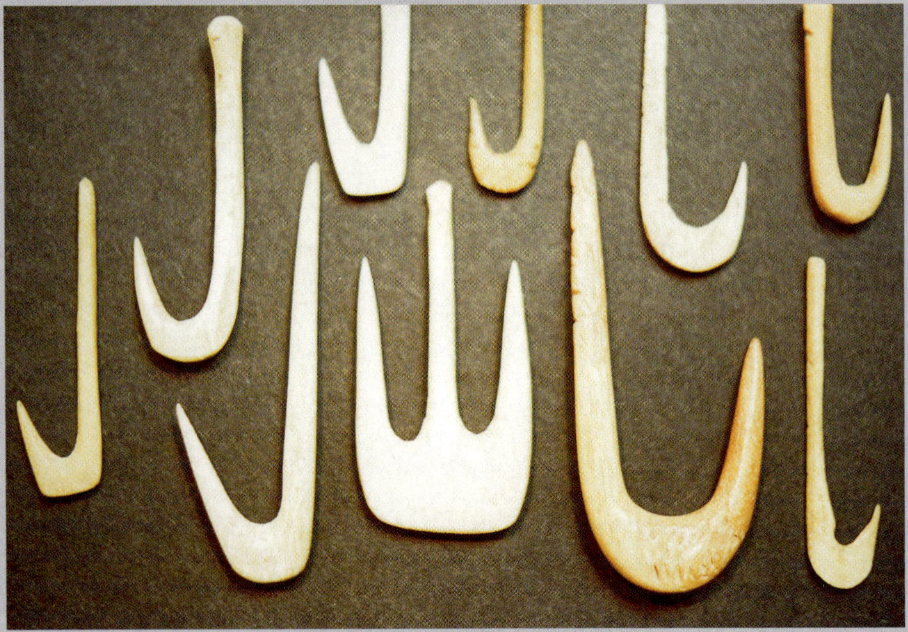

Fishhooks, center double hook is 1¾" long. Historic period, these were picked up near Chamberlain, South Dakota. Mike Fox collection, Iowa. Single hooks, **$75.00 – 150.00;** largest single hook, **$200.00;** double hook, **$250.00.**

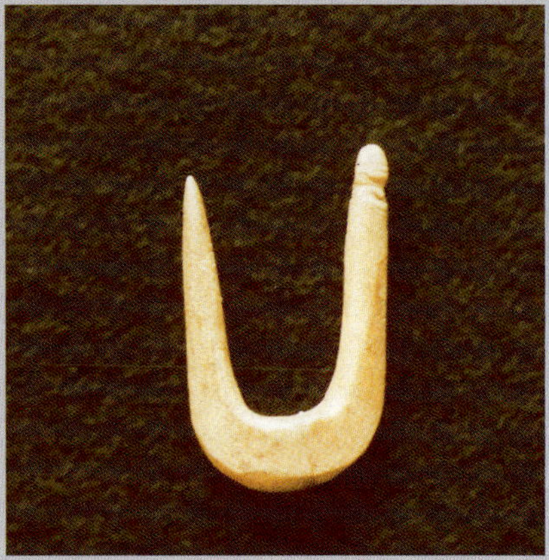

Bone fishhook, 1½" long. It is Mississippian (late prehistoric) and has a grooved shaft top. Polk County, Tennessee. Dave Summers collection, Victor, New York. **$175.00.**

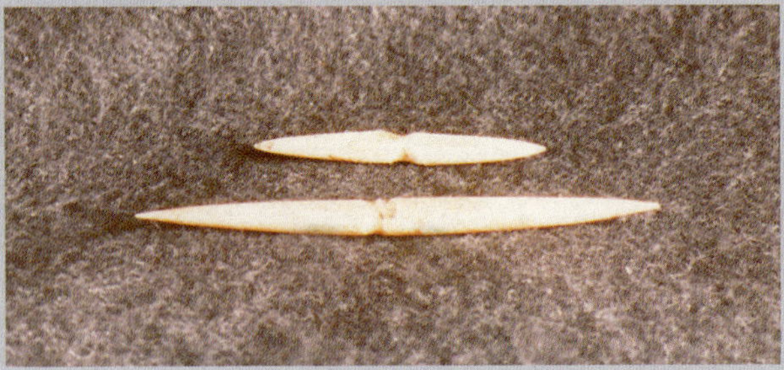

Gorge hooks, line grooves near centers, smaller hook is 1$\frac{5}{16}$" long and larger hook is 2$\frac{7}{16}$" long. These are much scarcer than the typical curved hooks and are ex-collection Quinn. They are from Galatin County, Illinois. John F. Wubker collection, Illinois. Smaller, **$175.00;** larger, **$200.00.**

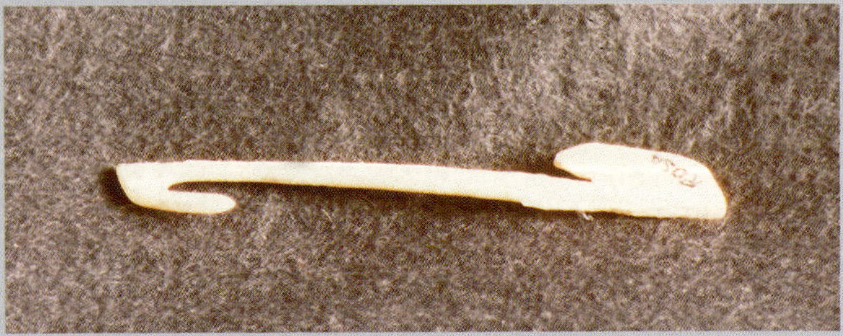

Bone fishhook preform, 3½" long. The work done here suggests this might have been intended to be separated to form two hooks. Rosa site, location unknown. John F. Wubker collection, Illinois. **$175.00.**

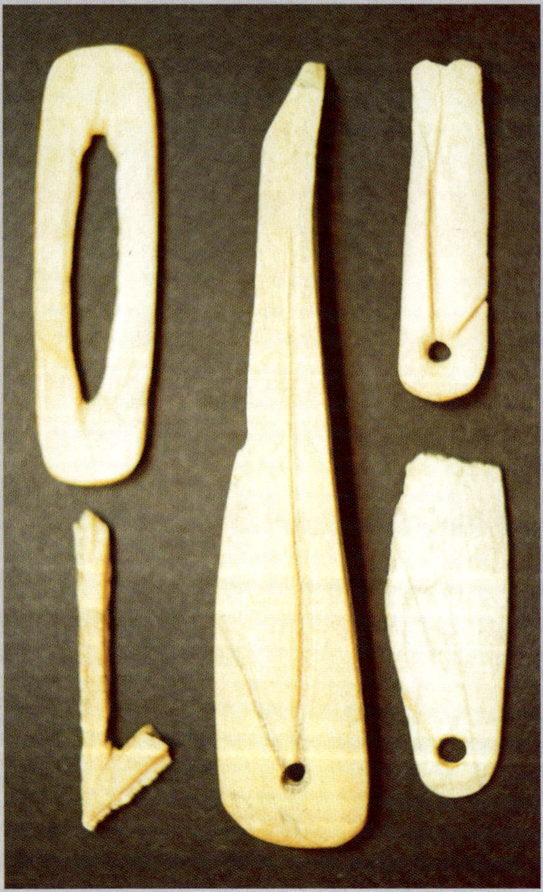

Bone fishhook preforms, illustrating two methods of hook manufacture. Preforms are actually scarcer than the finished hooks. These are historic period and the longest is 4¼". They were found near Mobridge, South Dakota. Mike Fox collection, Iowa. Each, **$50.00 – 150.00.**

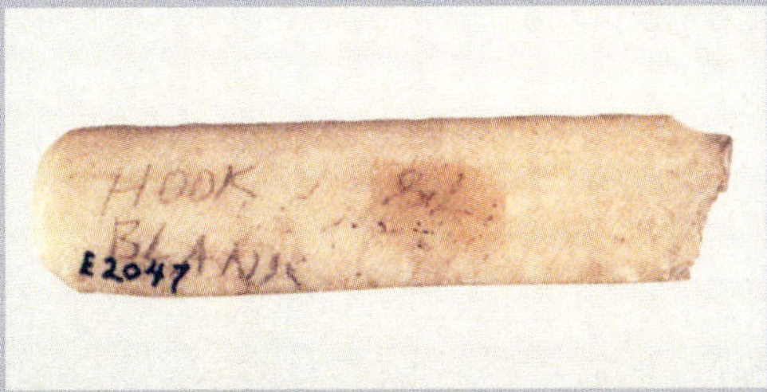

Fishhook blank, highly polished thin bone, 2" long. It was found in 1939 and is ex-collection Copeland. Mississippian in time, it came from southern Ohio. Private collection. **$15.00.**

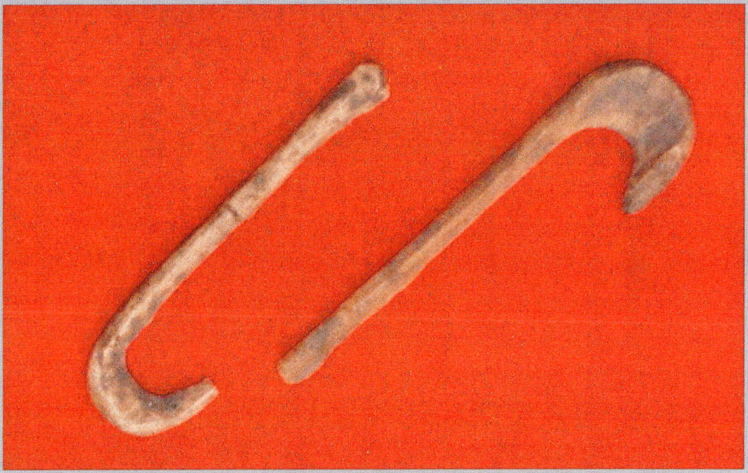

Fishhooks, bone, 5⁄16 x 1⅛", 1⁄16" thick. Prehistoric, the hooks were found at Saginaw, Michigan. Michael F. Slasinski collection, Michigan. Each, **$50.00 $75.00.**

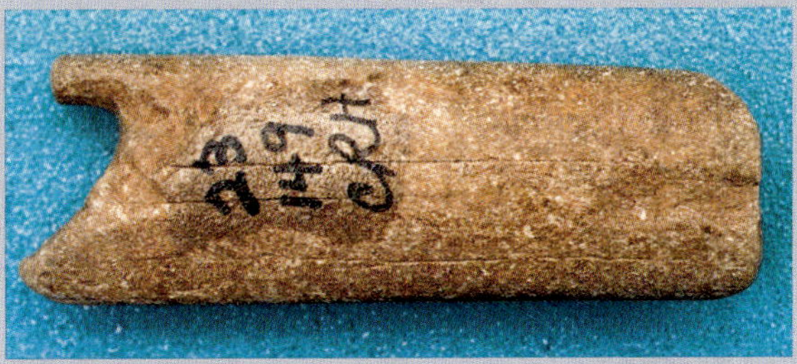

Fishhook preform, Archaic or later, bone, ¾ x 2³⁄16". Harwood found it in 1954. One hook was cut from an end, leaving the two prongs; the curvature between the prongs matches the bend of the hook that was taken off. Limestone County, Alabama. Collection of, and photograph by, Gary Henry, North Carolina. **$50.00.**

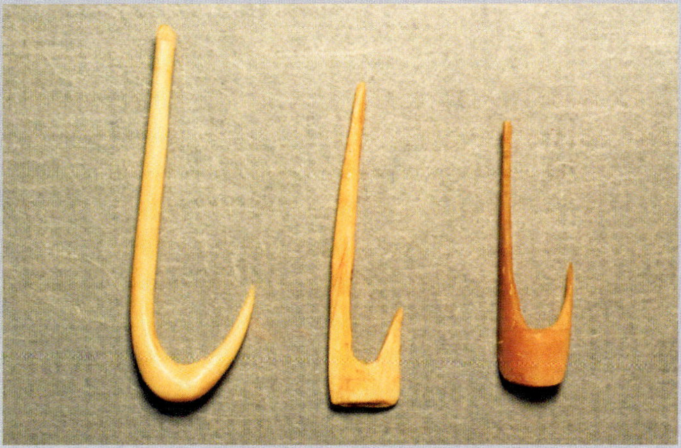

Fishhooks, 1¼ to 1½" long. These historic hooks are ca. AD 1750, from Morton County, North Dakota. Private collection. Each, **$100.00.**

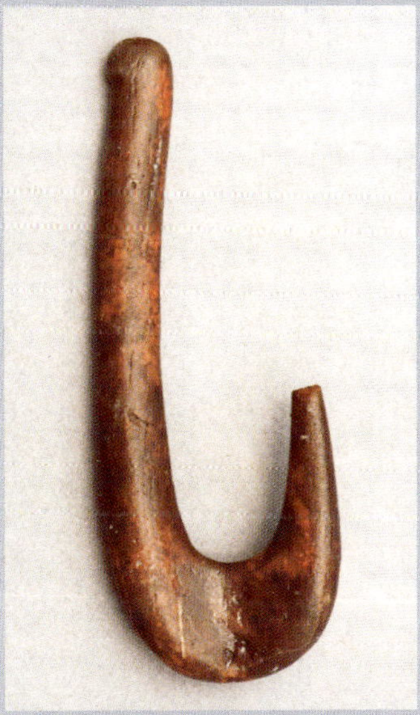

Fishhook, 2⅜" long, prehistoric, from an old collection and thought to be from the Pennsylvania – New York line. Exact site unknown. Elizabeth A. Greene collection, Naples, Florida. **$150.00.**

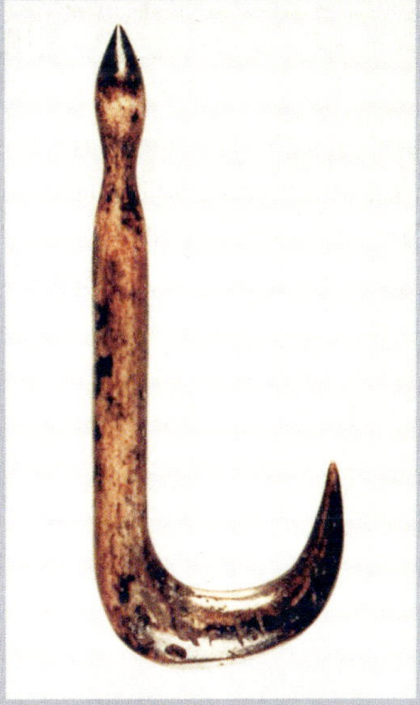

Fishhook, glossy black and brown patina, 2⅜" high. The narrowed shaft top is nicely carved on this piece. Found in Arkansas. Robin Fiser collection. **$175.00.**

Fishhook, indented shaft for cord, 2¼" long. This example was found in Madison County, Alabama. Robin Fiser collection. **$150.00.**

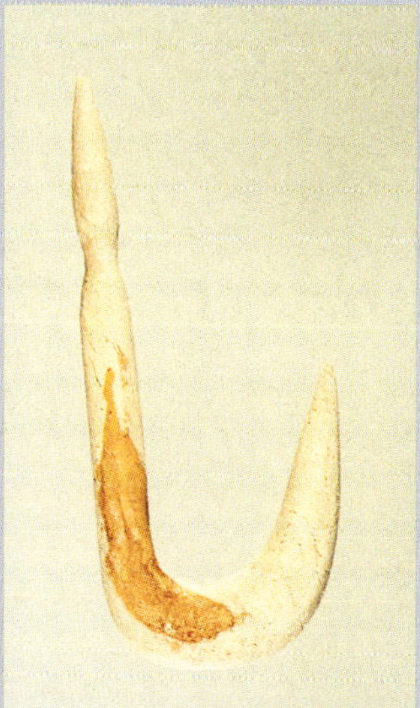

Fishhooks

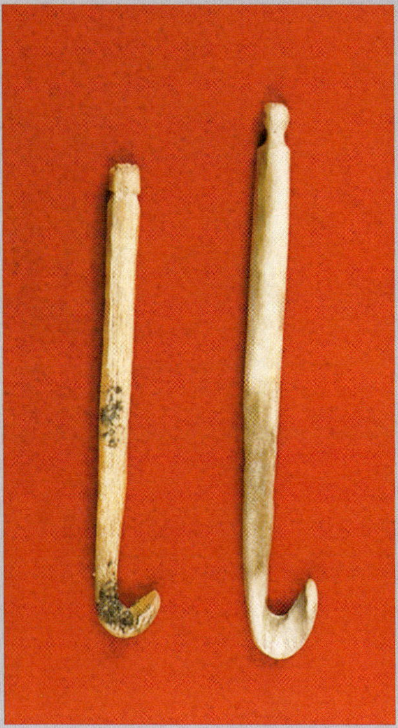

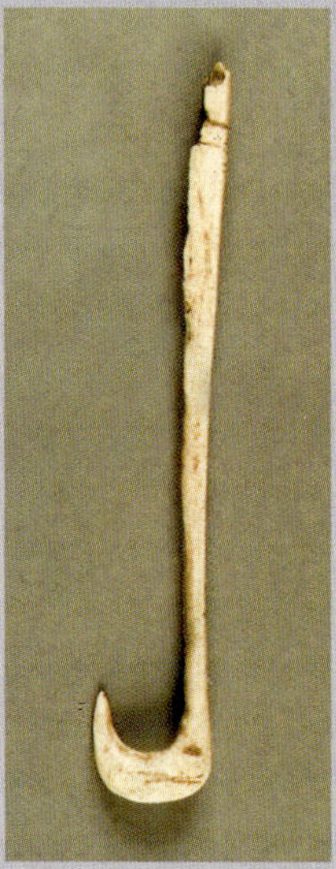

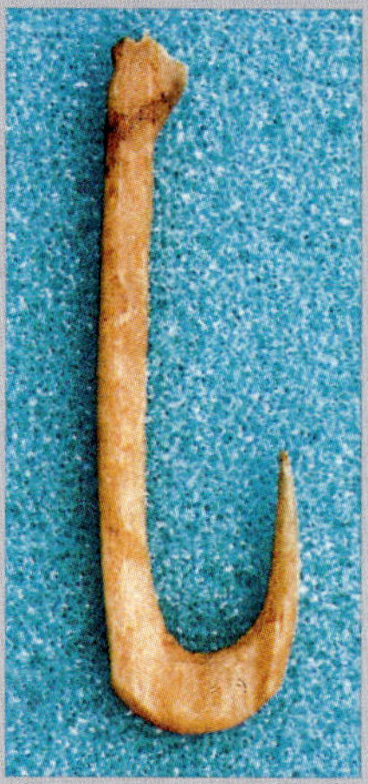

Bone fishhook, ⅜ x 1 3/16" long, Woodland or Mississippian. Unbarbed, it has a knob top and is in excellent condition for a fragile object. Ex-collection Snyder, the hook came from Sullivan County, Tennessee. Collection of, and photograph by, Gary Henry, North Carolina. **$150.00.**

Fishhook, with extra-long shaft, 2¼". The hook is grooved near the top for a fishing line. Northwestern Arkansas. Kenneth Hamilton collection, Arkansas. **$150.00 – 175.00.**

Fishhooks, unusually long shanks with cord knobs, longest hook is 3 3/16". They are ex-collection Vietzen, from southwestern Kentucky. Pete Timoch collection. Long, **$175.00.** Shorter, **$150.00.**

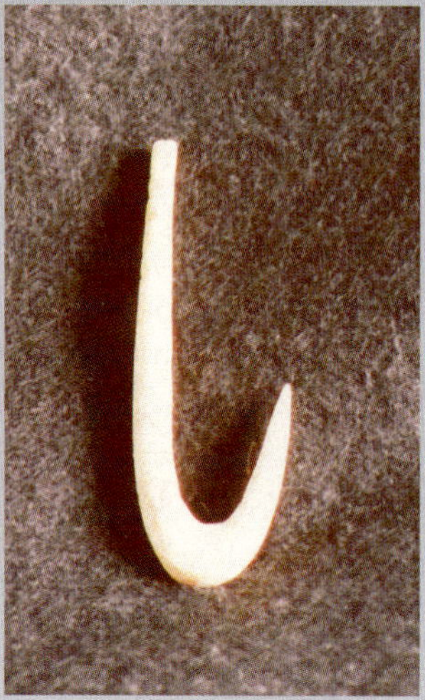

Fishhook, 2 1/16", probably deer bone. Find-site for this piece is unknown. John F. Wubker collection, Illinois. **$150.00.**

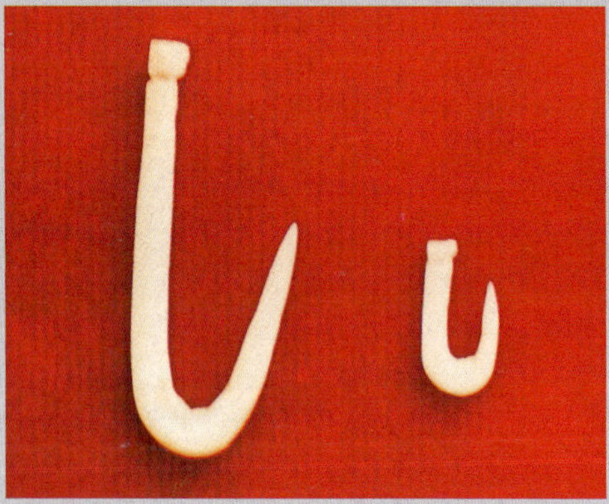

Fishhooks, larger example is 1 1/16" long. The other hook is only ⅜" long and is the smallest complete bone fishhook seen by the author. The two were found in Brown County, Illinois. Tim Liehr collection, Illinois. For both, **$500.00 – 600.00.**

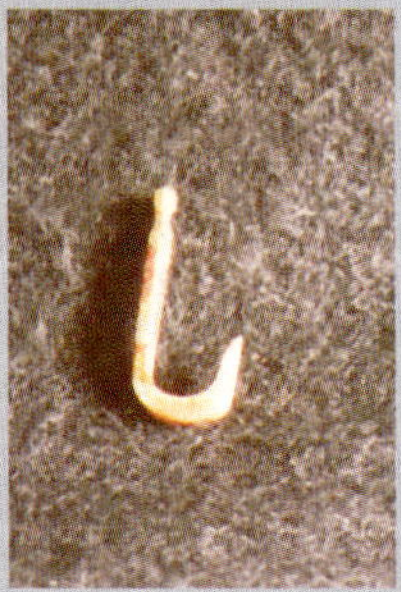

Fishhook, only ⅝" long, ex-collection Ritter. This very small hook is grooved at the shaft top and is probably from the Midwest. John F. Wubker collection, Illinois. **$100.00.**

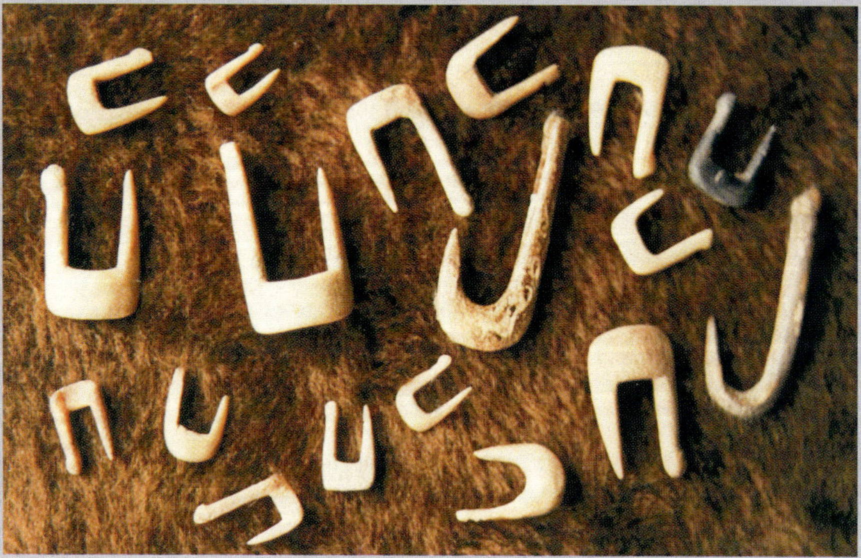

Bone fishhooks, longest example is 1⅝", ex-collection DeLime. The two longest are from Spencer County, Indiana, and the others are from the Clarksville area, Indiana. Dale and Betty Roberts collection, Iowa. Each, **$100.00 – 200.00.**

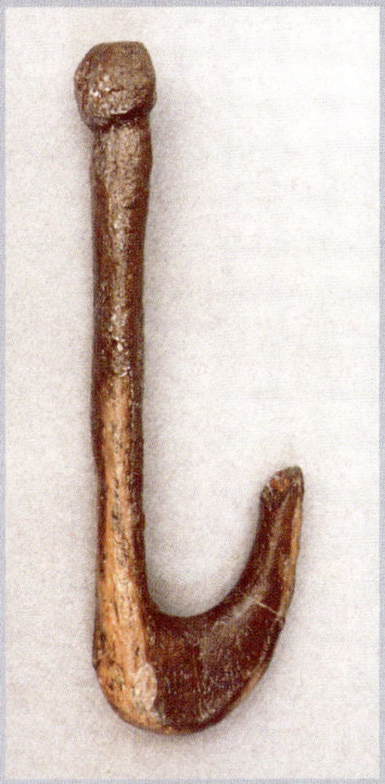

Fishhook, 2½" long, prehistoric. It was in an old collection and believed to be from the Pennsylvania – New York line region. Find-site unknown. Elizabeth A. Greene collection, Naples, Florida. **$150.00.**

Bone fishhooks, each ⅞" long, Iroquois, ca. AD 1540-1560. Once in the Whipple collection, they were acquired in the 1930s. The hooks were found near Richmond Mills, Ontario County, New York. Dave Summers collection, Victor, New York. Each, **$110.00.**

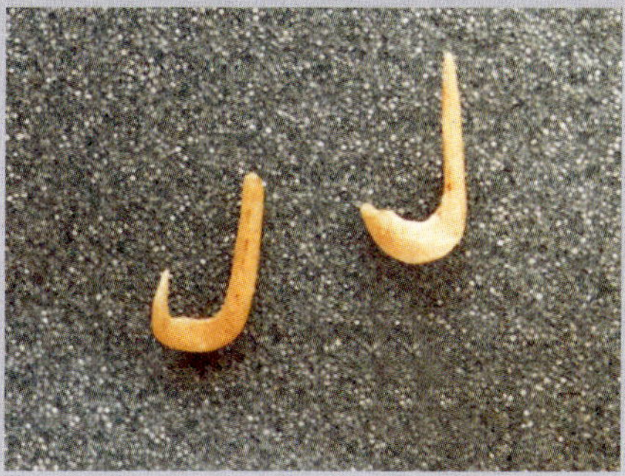

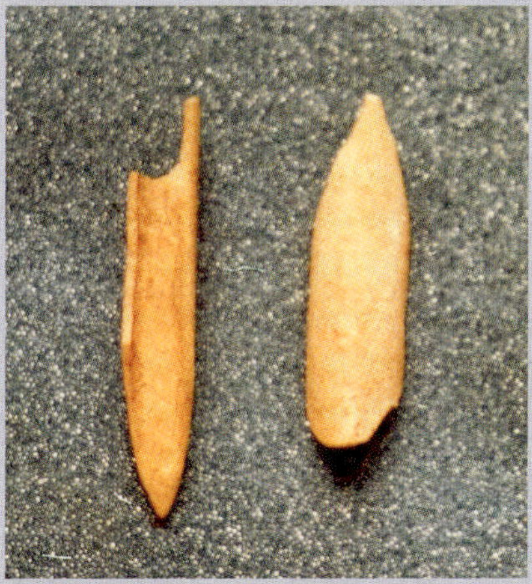

Bone artifacts, fishhook blank (2¼" long) at left and splinter awl (2") at right, Brewerton phase, Late Archaic, ca. 1600 BC. They were found near Brutus, Cayuga County, New York. Dave Summers collection, Victor, New York. Fishhook blank, **$35.00;** awl, **$20.00.**

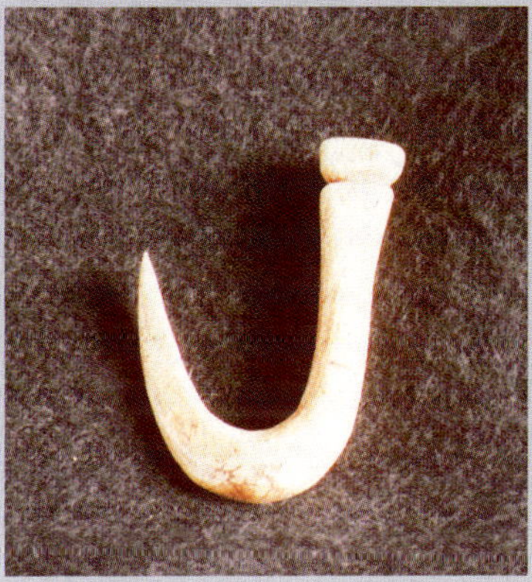

Fishhook, 1⅞" long, deer bone. This is an interesting hook with a narrowed shank and expanded top with a string groove. Find-site unknown. John F. Wubker collection, Illinois. **$175.00.**

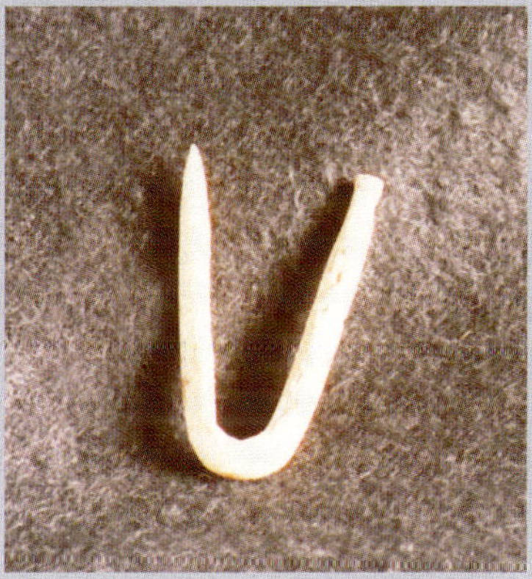

Fishhook, 1$\frac{5}{16}$" long, deer bone. This U-shaped hook has a shallow and wide groove at the shaft top. Find-site unknown, probably Midwest. John F. Wubker collection, Illinois. **$125.00.**

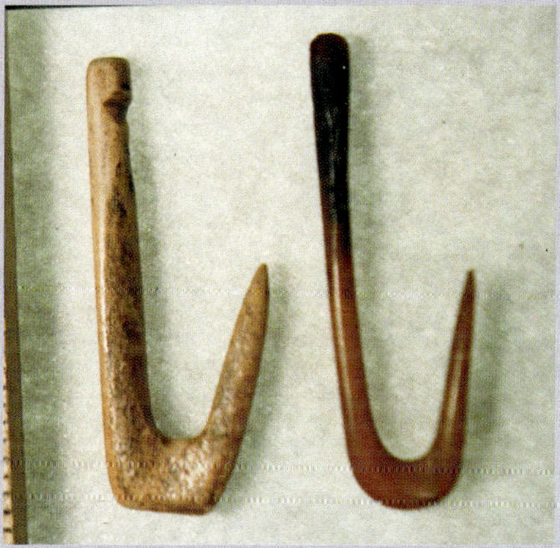

Fishhooks, bone, Fort Ancient of the Mississippian era, finely made. They were found in Bracken County, Kentucky. Back to Earth. Each, **$165.00.**

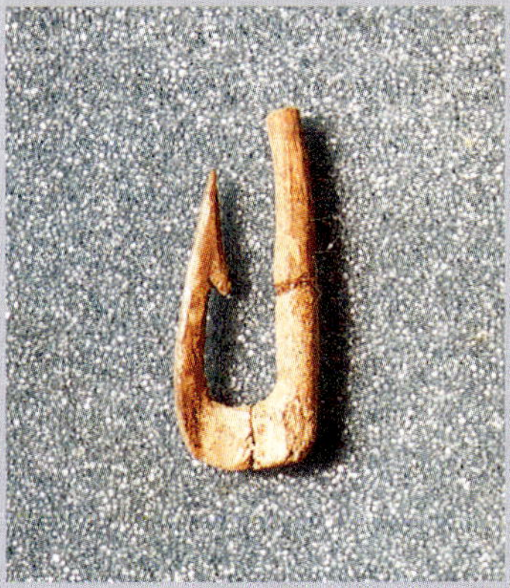

Bone fishhook, barbed, Point Peninsula and Hopewell phases of Middle Woodland times, ca. AD 1 – 1000. Barbed hooks seem to be more prevalent in the East than in the Midwest and perhaps elsewhere in the country. The fishhook is 1⅜" long, from Onondaga County, New York. Dave Summers collection, Victor, New York. **$200.00.**

Bone fishhooks, late prehistoric, left example is 1¼" long. The hook on right resembles a modern fishhook. Bracken County, Kentucky. Back to Earth. Each, **$160.00.**

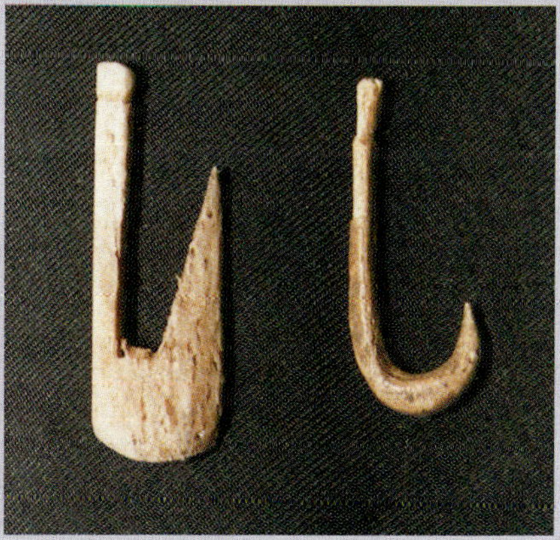

Beads

Understandably, beads near coastal areas are often made of marine shell, while inland areas have beads made of freshwater shell or imported marine shell obtained from prehistoric trade arrangements. In fact, marine shell, due to its greater size and thickness, was certainly a much-desired item, and was widely traded in Middle and Late Archaic times. Adena and Hopewell Indians of Woodland times acquired large numbers of marine shell beads, and their use continued into the Mississippian period. Overall use was for ornamental and ritual purposes.

Beads, whether worn as necklaces and bracelets or used to embellish clothing, were made in many forms. Some were thin and round, and such disc beads might be worn in strands that contained hundreds or even thousands of beads. Bead strands might be in uniform or graduated sizes, or varied in size and shape. Hopewell Indians (Middle Woodland) of the ancient Midwest drilled freshwater pearls for some of their beads, and also made use of mussel shell. In various parts of North America, shell beads might also be rounded or barrel-shaped, oval-shaped, angular, or tubular. In areas where certain animal teeth were in short supply, copies were sometimes made of shell.

Bone beads were often made, and those cut from deer bones were widely used. Necklaces of deer toe bones have been found, as well as bone pendants or necklace elements in various shapes. Bird wing bones (mostly tubular in form) were widely popular, since the bones were lightweight, hollow, and took a high polish. Such beads may be up to four or five inches long, and the ends are typically cut and smoothed.

Mineralized materials were sometimes used when they were available; these include mammoth ivory and walrus teeth. These two were, in a few rare instances, brought into what is now the 48 adjoining United States. Probably the oldest organic bead material, (in terms of pure age and once-living plants) is cannel coal, sometimes called "jet." This black material, formed from the compressed, hardened spores of giant plants of the carboniferous age, polished well and was treasured from Archaic to Mississippian times.

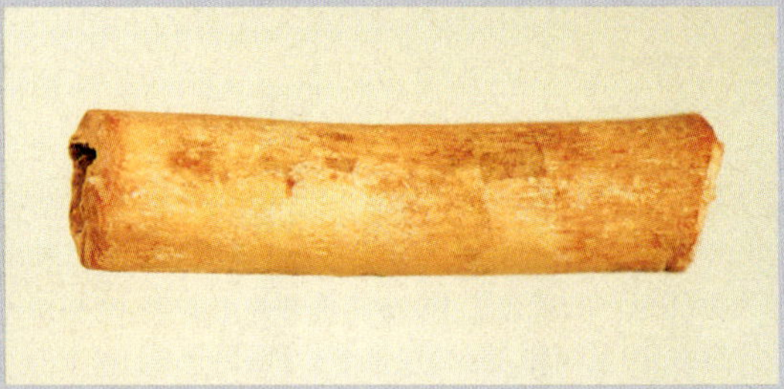

Bead, probably deer bone, cut and rounded ends, 2¼". The bead is hollowed and surface polish is present. Kentucky. Private collection. **$10.00.**

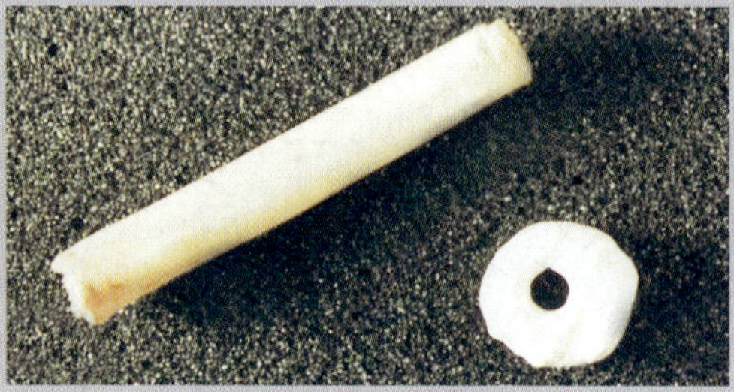

Beads, from the Fort Ancient people, Mississippian period, both from southern Ohio. Private collection. Left, bead made from hollow bird bone, 1$\frac{11}{16}$", **$8.00.** Right, clamshell disc bead. **$2.00.**

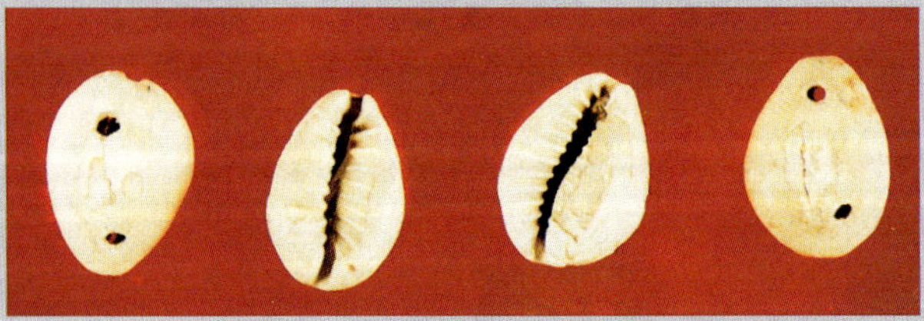

Marine shell beads, Hopewell, average length is ⅝". Each bead is drilled in two places with very small holes. Illinois. Private collection. Each, **$5.00.**

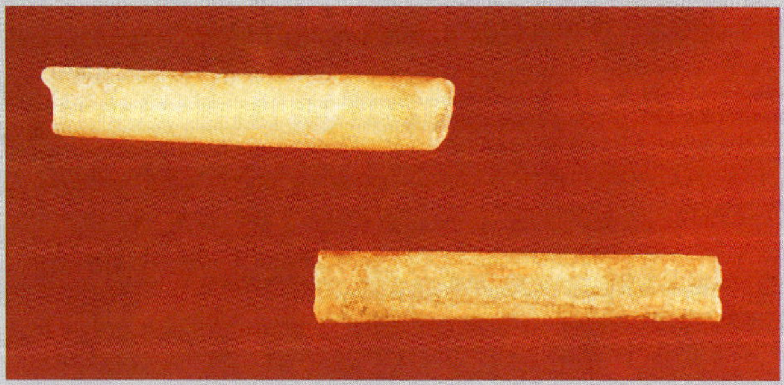

Beads, made of hollow bird bones, longest 1½". The ends were snapped and then lightly ground and flattened. Kentucky. Private collection. Each, **$10.00 – 15.00.**

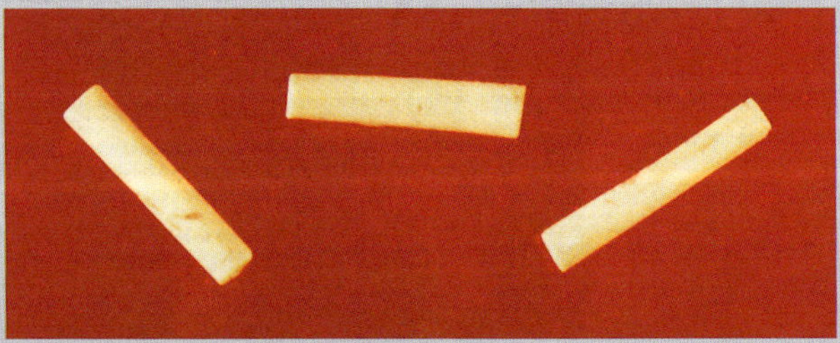

Beads, hollow bird bones, longest is 1$\frac{1}{32}$". The ends were ground flat on these examples from Kentucky. Private collection. Each, **$8.00.**

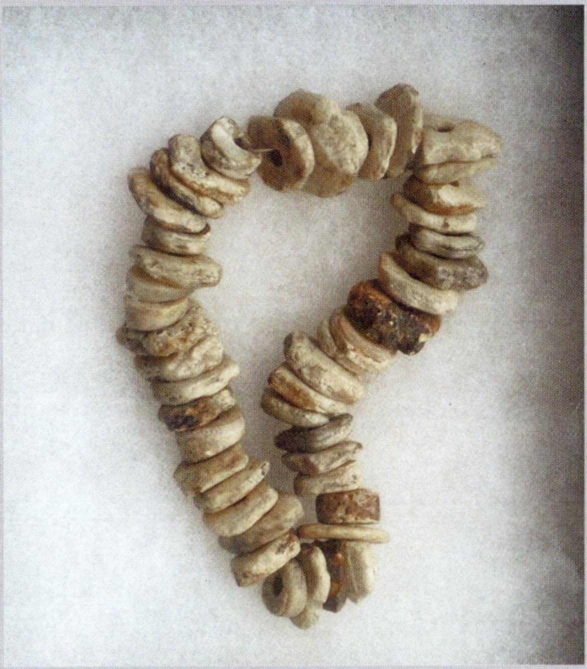

Shell beads, seventeenth and eighteenth centuries, largest is ½" in diameter and ⅛" thick. There are 45 beads in this strand. Ex-collection Levy. They came from Frontier County, Nebraska. Collection of, and photograph by, Gary Henry, North Carolina. **$150.00.**

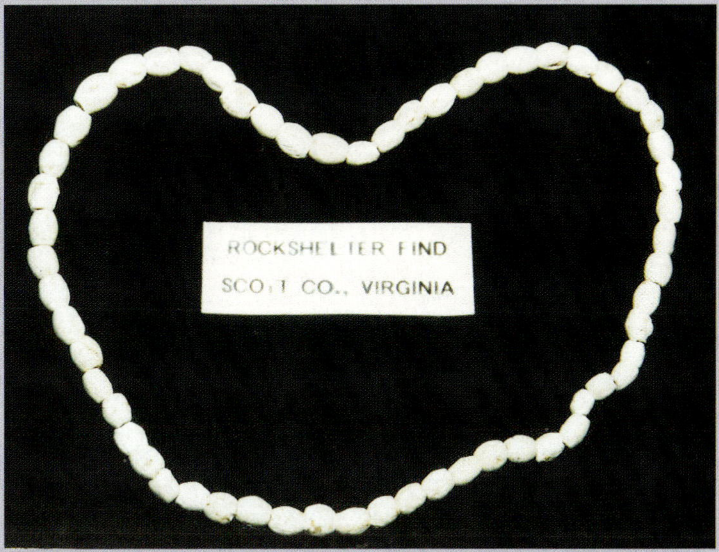

Shell bead strand, oval beads, from a rock shelter. The beads are nicely sized for this ornamental artifact. Back to Earth. Unlisted.

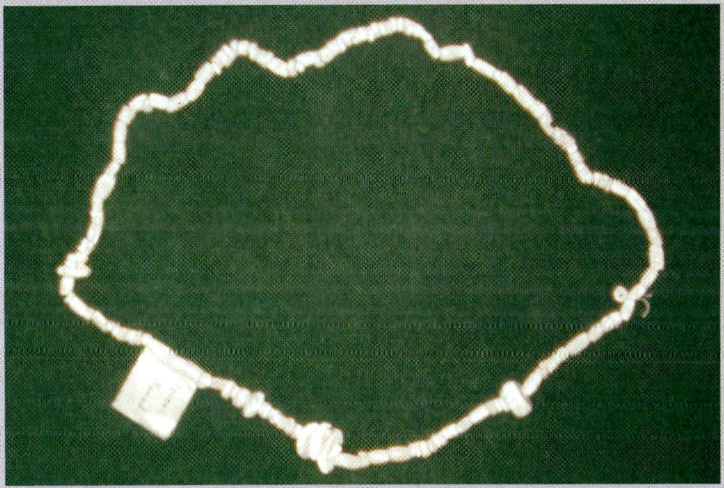

Shell beads, strand is 24" long. Ex-collection Drake, Davis COA. The beads are Mississippian, from Oklahoma. Keith and Rhonda Dodge collection, Michigan. Unlisted.

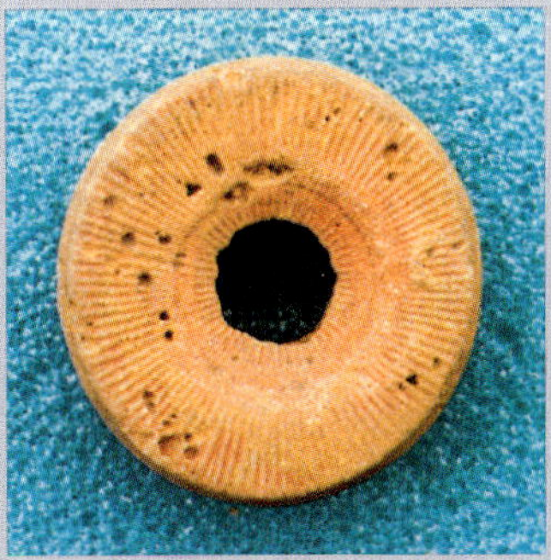

Bead, Woodland or later, ¾" in diameter and 3/16" thick. This is a fossil crinoid, and the artifact is technically from a once-living creature. Harwood found it in 1954. Limestone County, Alabama. Collection of, and photograph by, Gary Henry, North Carolina. **$20.00.**

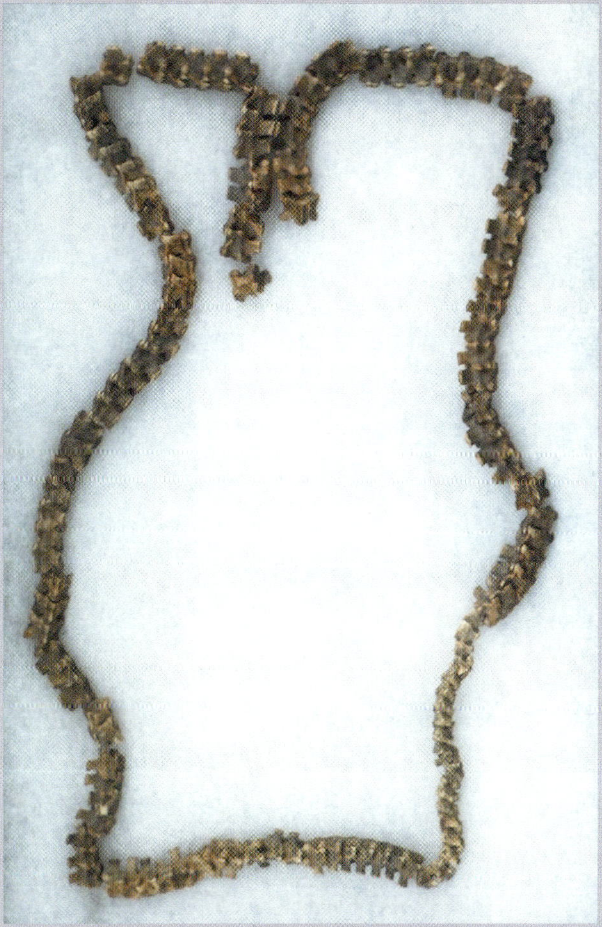

Bead string, prehistoric(?), rattlesnake vertebrae, larger bones are 7/16" in diameter and ⅜" long. These are ex-collection Snyder, from Smyth County, Virginia. Collection of, and photograph by, Gary Henry, North Carolina. **$300.00.**

Beads

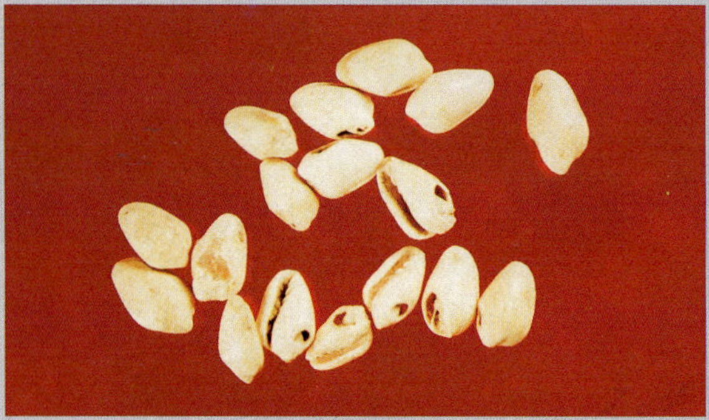

Shell beads, *Marginella*, average length is 3/8". Each bead is holed for suspension. They are Hopewell, from Illinois. Private collection. Each, **$1.00.**

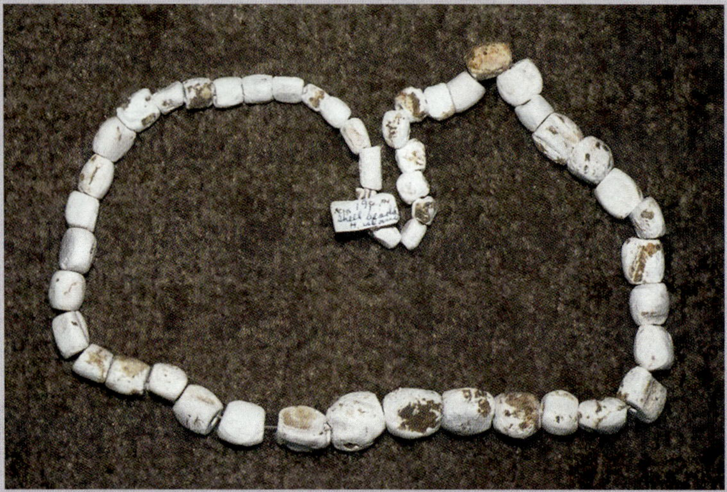

Strand of 49 beads, Woodland or Mississippian, barrel and rounded shell types. Ex-collection Snyder, the largest bead is 1 1/16" long and 5/8" in diameter. Meigs County, Tennessee. Collection of, and photograph by, Gary Henry, North Carolina. **$200.00.**

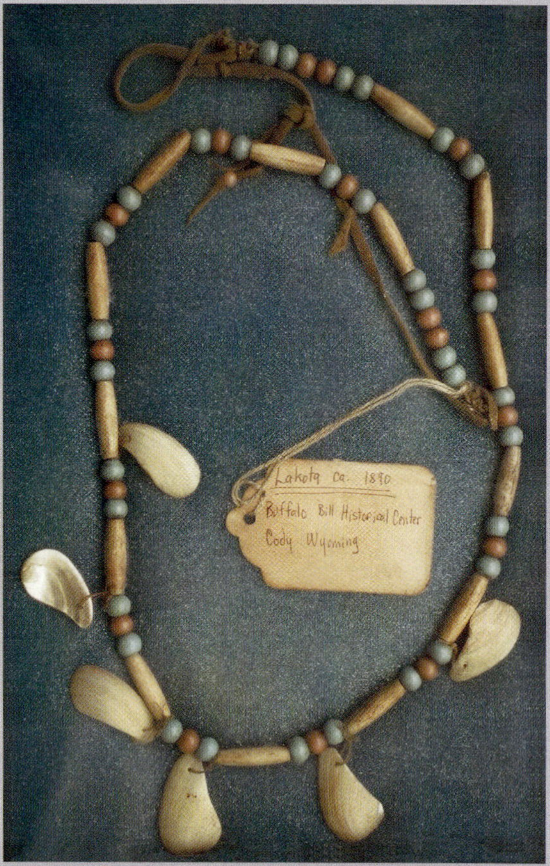

Necklace, 66 beads, ca. 1890. This fine necklace is a mix of 6 clam shell pendants, 14 bone hair-pipe beads and 52 glass trade beads (34 blue, 18 pink). The largest clam shell is 1 3/16 x 1 5/16". Tie-ons are elk sinew and the cord is elk rawhide with brain-tanned tie thongs. The necklace is ex-collection Levy and was once in the Buffalo Bill Historical Center, Cody, Wyoming. Collection of, and photograph by, Gary Henry, North Carolina. Museum grade.

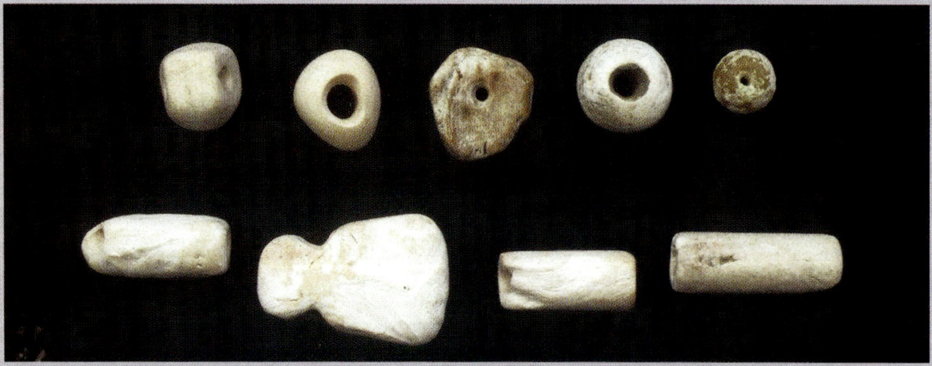

Shell beads, various types, Woodland or Mississippian period. The largest bead is drilled from the side and measures 7/8 x 1 3/8", 1/2" thick. Ex-collection Levy, their origin is unknown. Collection of, and photograph by, Gary Henry, North Carolina. **$50.00.**

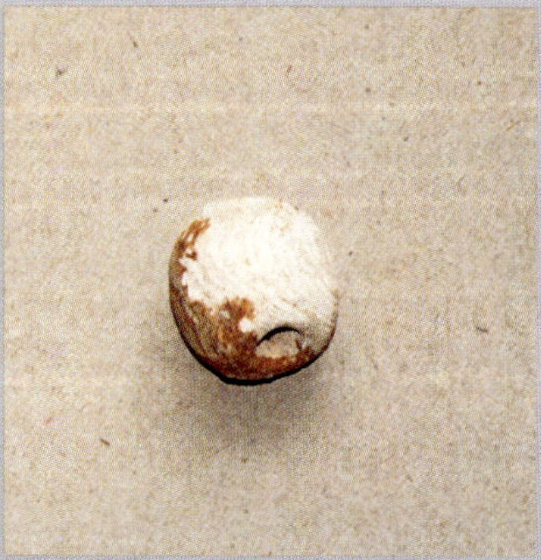

Shell bead, drilled, 3/4 x 1". Probably Mississippian in time, it is from Arkansas. Wilfred Dick collection, Mississippi. **$25.00.**

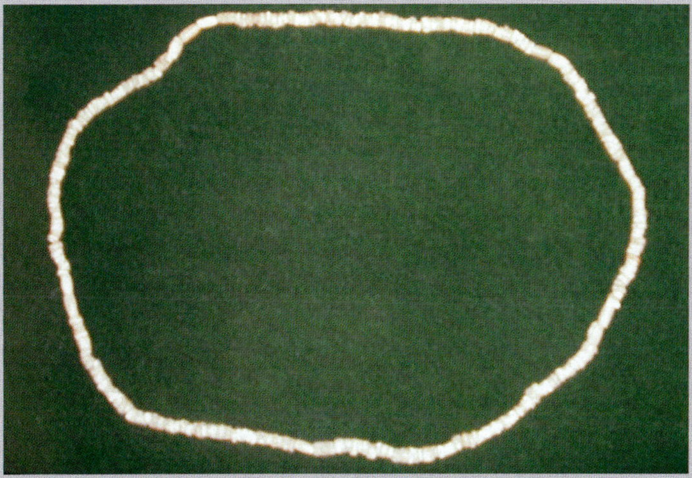

Shell bead strand, 28" long. Ex-collection Drake. The strand has a Davis COA and was found in Oklahoma. Keith and Rhonda Dodge collection, Michigan. Unlisted.

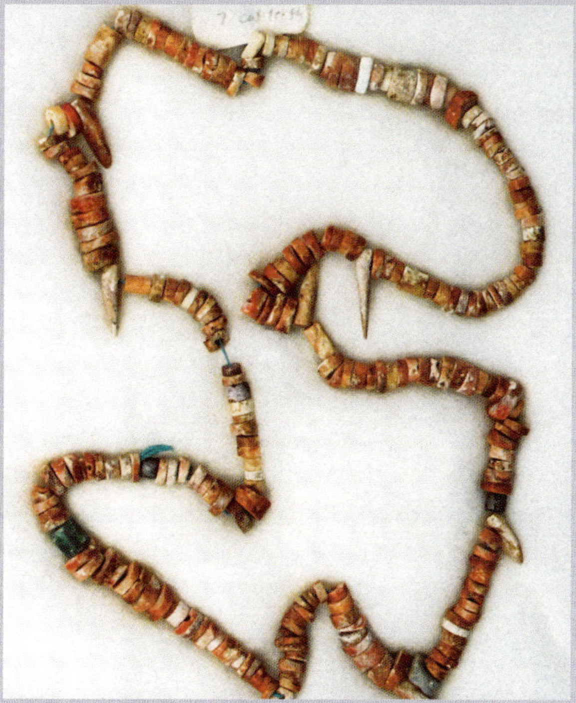

Bead strand, String of 240 beads, 233 made of shell and 7 made from teeth of a large cat (bobcat?). Woodland or later, the largest cat tooth bead is ⅝" in diameter and 3/16" thick. The largest shell bead is ¼" in diameter and ⅛" thick. The beads are ex-collection Snyder, from Meigs County, Tennessee. Collection of, and photograph by, Gary Henry, North Carolina. All, **$300.00.**

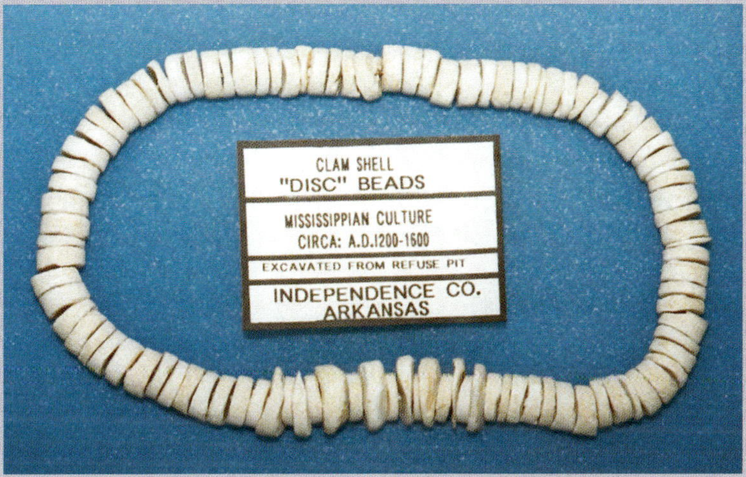

Disc bead strand, freshwater clam or mussel shell, found in a refuse pit or kitchen midden. Independence County, Arkansas. Back to Earth. Unlisted.

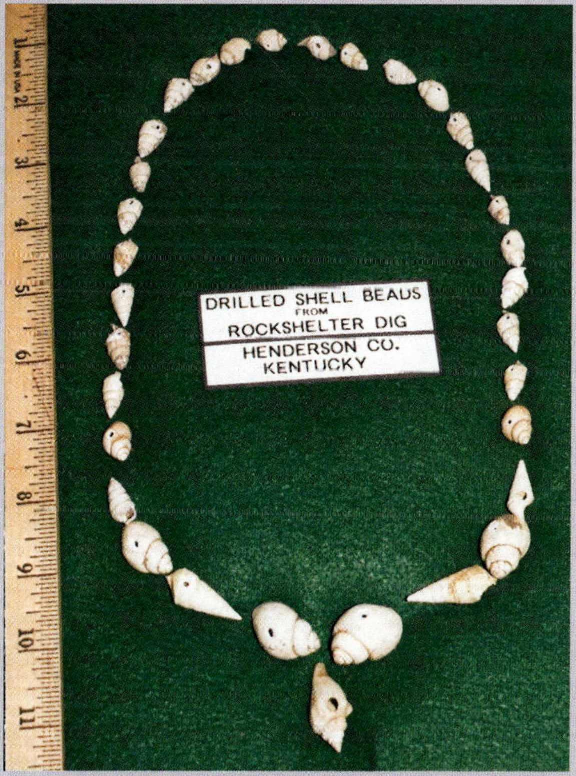

Beads, collection from a rock shelter, frame size is 8 x 12". Made of drilled snail shells, they are from Henderson County, Kentucky. Back to Earth. **$115.00.**

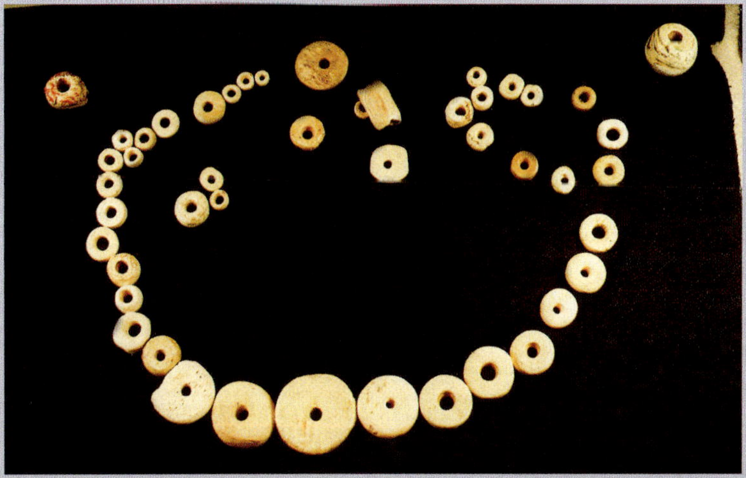

Shell disc beads, most in graduated sizes, largest is 1⅛" in diameter. Top left and right are barrel-type beads, and the left example still has traces of red paint. These were picked up in the Decatur area, Alabama. Robin Fiser collection. All, **$95.00.**

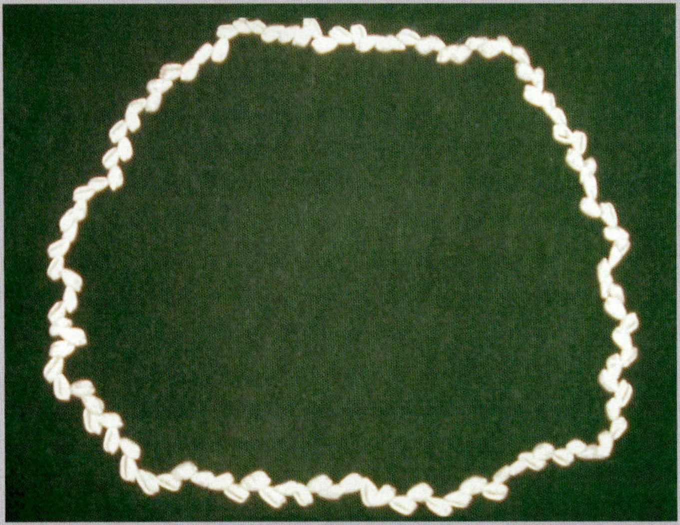

Shell beads, this strand measures 30" long. Davis COA, ex-collection Drake, Oklahoma. Keith and Rhonda Dodge collection, Michigan. Unlisted.

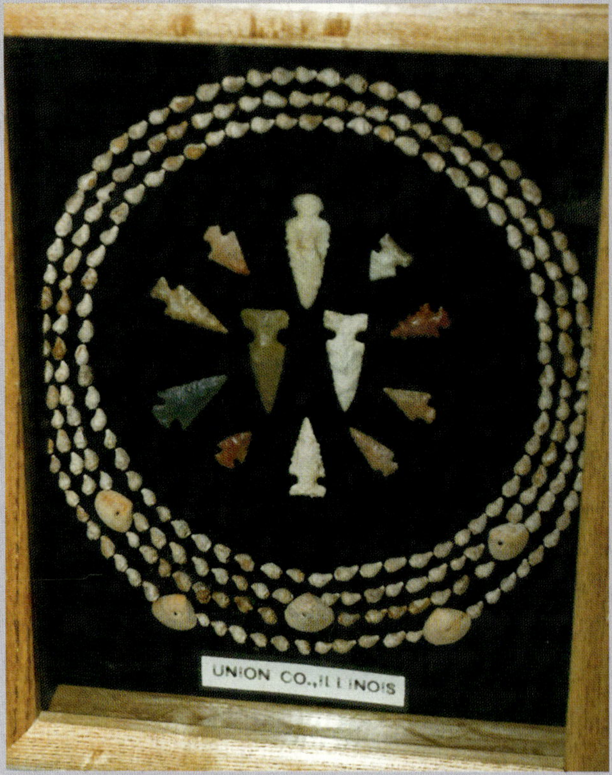

Bead strand, drilled shell necklace with chipped projectile points, bead strand length approximately 60". Frame size, 9 x 11". Union County, Illinois. Back to Earth. **$235.00.**

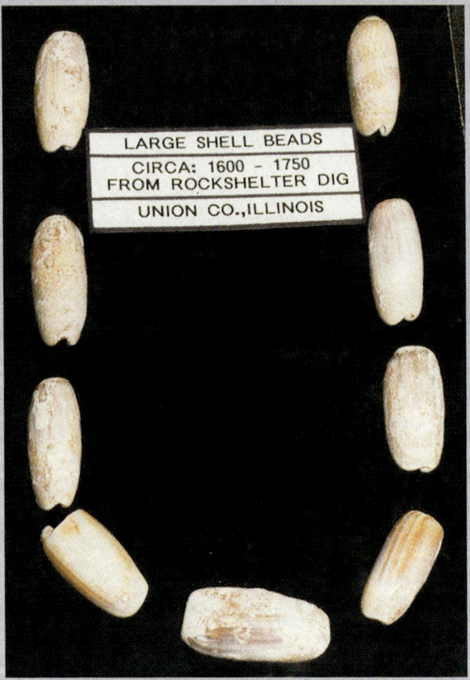

Shell beads, group of nine, early historic period. They were found in a rock shelter. Union County, Illinois. Back to Earth. **$125.00.**

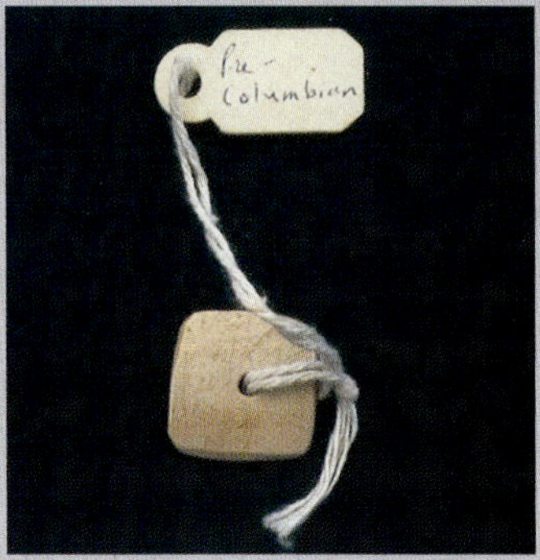

Square shell bead, Woodland or Mississippian, $\frac{5}{8}$ x $\frac{9}{16}$". With atypical shape, the bead is ex-collection Levy and origin is not known. Collection of, and photograph by, Gary Henry, North Carolina. **$10.00.**

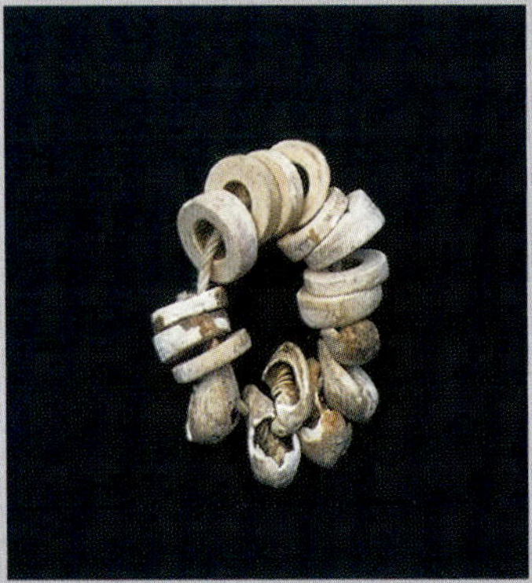

Shell beads, string of 19, ex-collection Levy, Woodland or Mississippian. There are 11 mollusk shell beads and 8 made of snail shell. The shell beads average $\frac{1}{4}$" in diameter. Find-site unknown. Collection of, and photograph by, Gary Henry, North Carolina. **$50.00.**

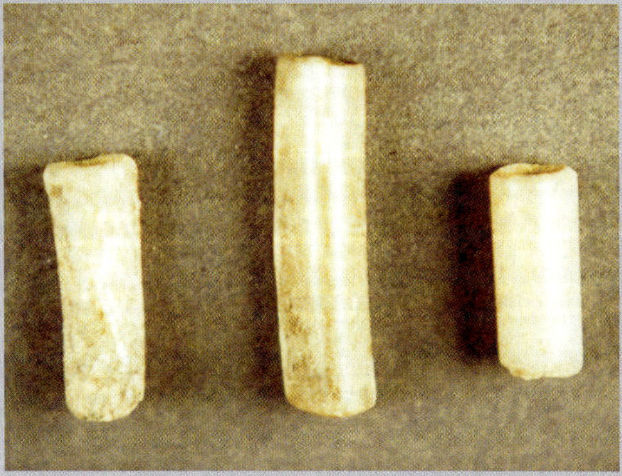

Beads, bird bone, longest 1$\frac{3}{4}$", cut and polished. They were found near Willow Grove, West Virginia. Larry Garvin collection. Each, **$10.00.**

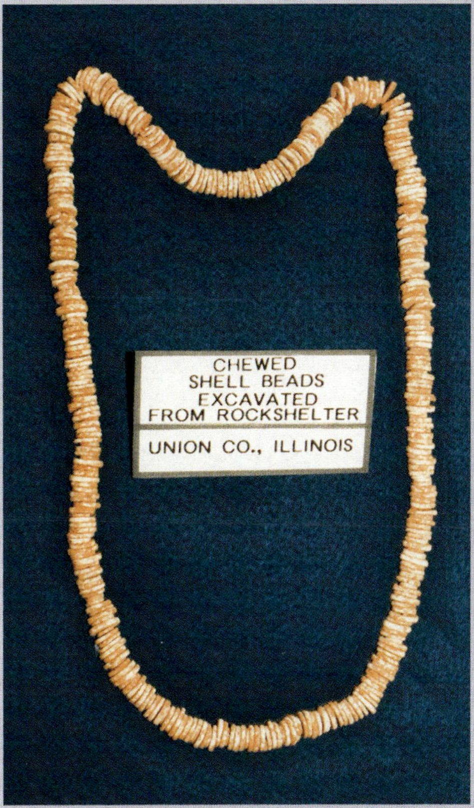
CHEWED
SHELL BEADS
EXCAVATED
FROM ROCKSHELTER
UNION CO., ILLINOIS

Shell bead strand, thin disc form, found in a rock shelter. Union County, Illinois. Back to Earth. Unlisted.

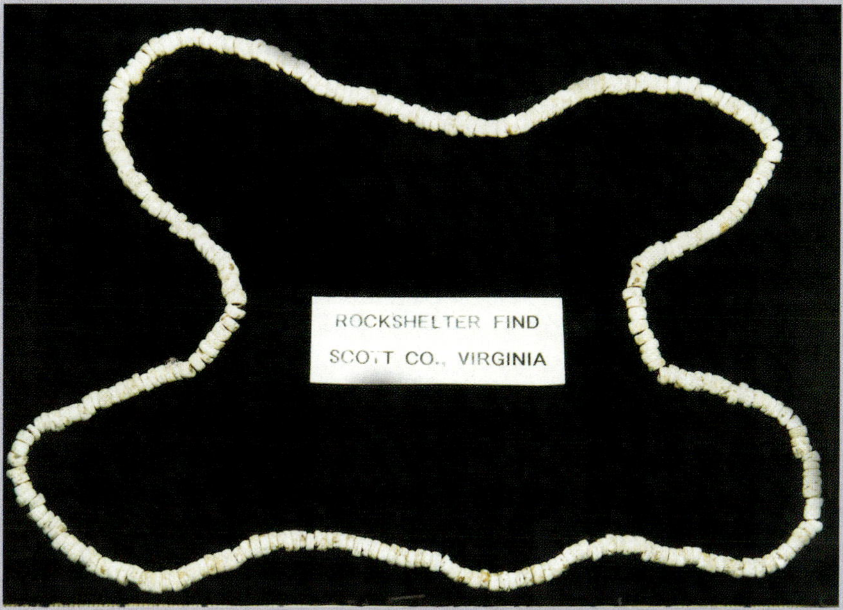
ROCKSHELTER FIND
SCOTT CO., VIRGINIA

Shell bead strand, found in a dry cave or rock shelter. Scott County, Virginia. Back to Earth. Unlisted.

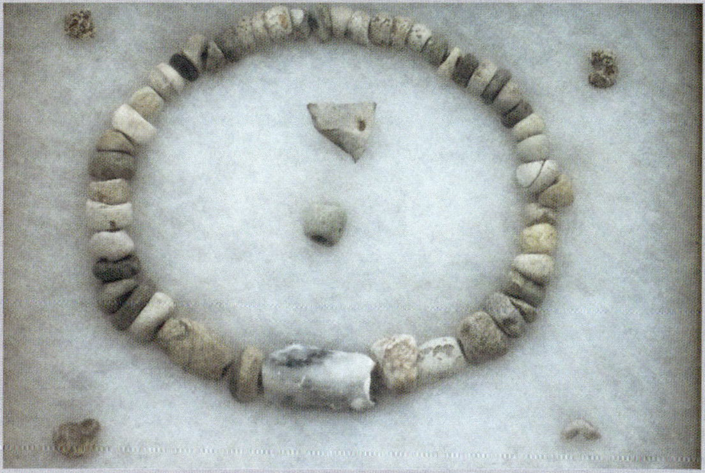

Shell beads and bead pieces, prehistoric(?), largest bead is 1⅝" long and 1" in diameter. The drilled triangular pendant is stone. Found in a rock shelter, these are ex-collection Levy. Blanco County, Texas. Collection of, and photograph by, Gary Henry, North Carolina. **$75.00.**

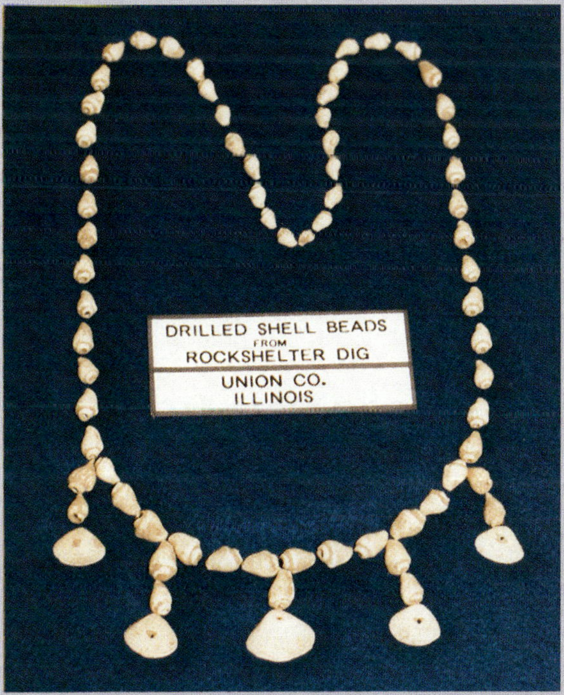

Shell bead strand, with shell drops, rock shelter finds. They came from Union County, Illinois. Back to Earth. Unlisted.

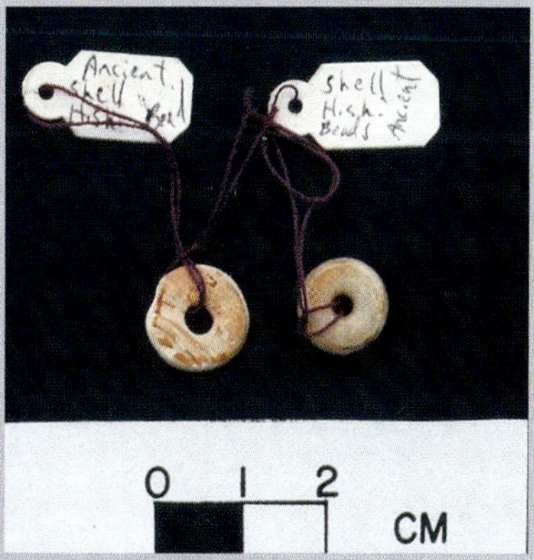

Shell beads, Woodland or Mississippian, right example is ⅜" in diameter and 3/16" thick. They are ex-collection Levy and find-site is unknown. Collection of, and photograph by, Gary Henry, North Carolina. Both, **$10.00.**

Beads

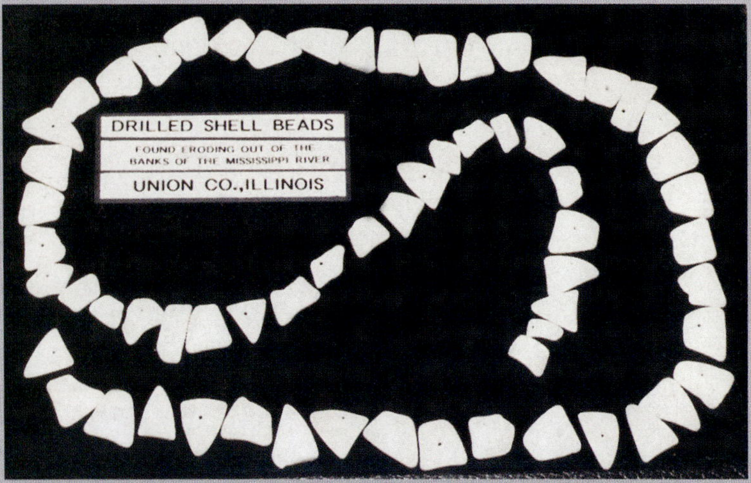

Drilled shell beads, found on the banks of the Mississippi River. Union County, Illinois. Back to Earth. **$155.00.**

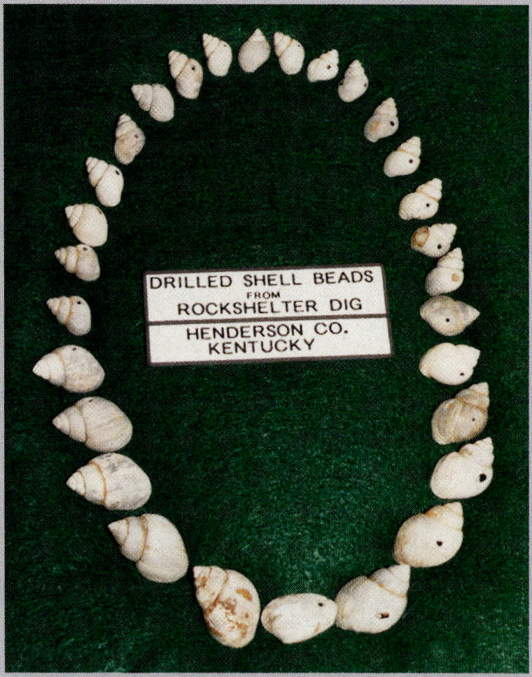

Beads, drilled snail shells, frame size is 8 x 12". Henderson County, Kentucky. Back to Earth. **$115.00.**

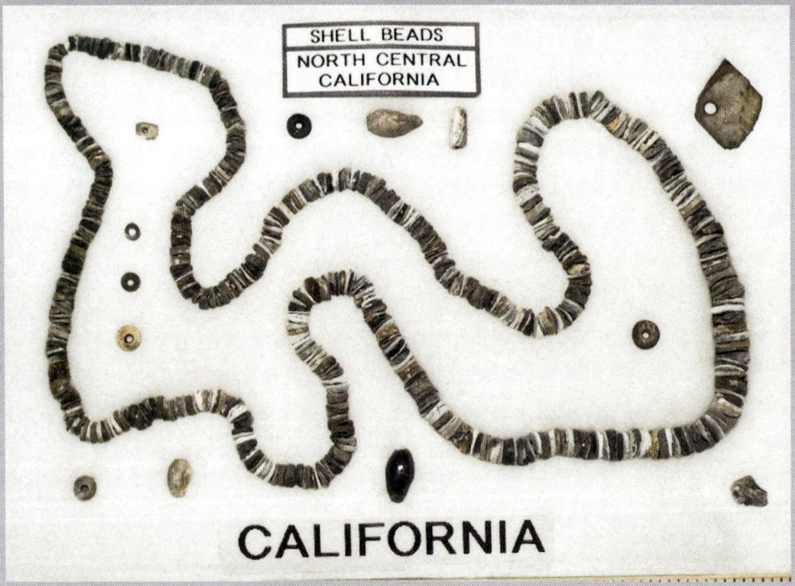

Beads, thin disc type, northcentral California. Coastal areas of the state are noted for fine shell artifacts. Back to Earth. Unlisted.

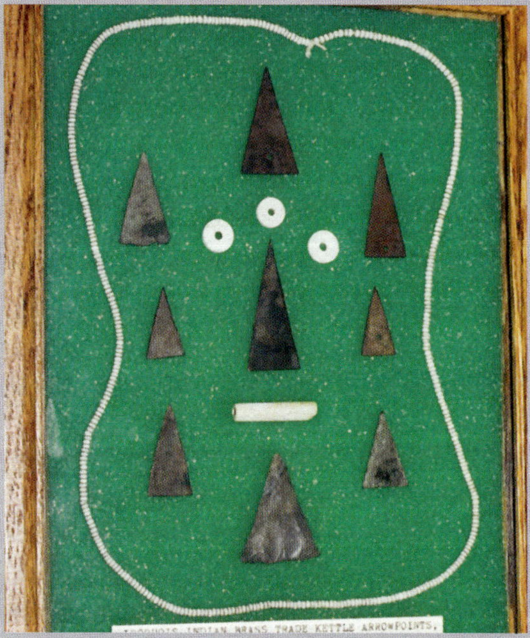

Artifact collection, from an historic village site (ca. AD 1680), including a string of small shell disc beads, a tubular bead, and three disc beads. Eight of the arrowpoints are made of kettle brass. Back to Earth. Unlisted.

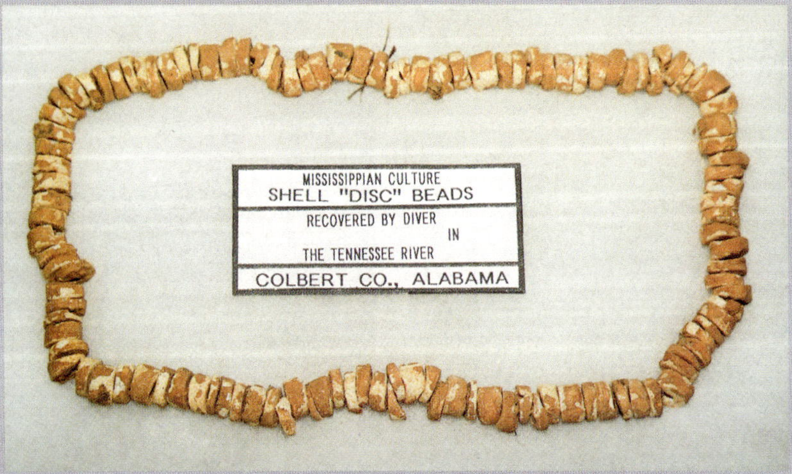

Shell disc beads, Mississippian, found by a diver in the Tennessee River. Colbert County, Alabama. Back to Earth. Unlisted.

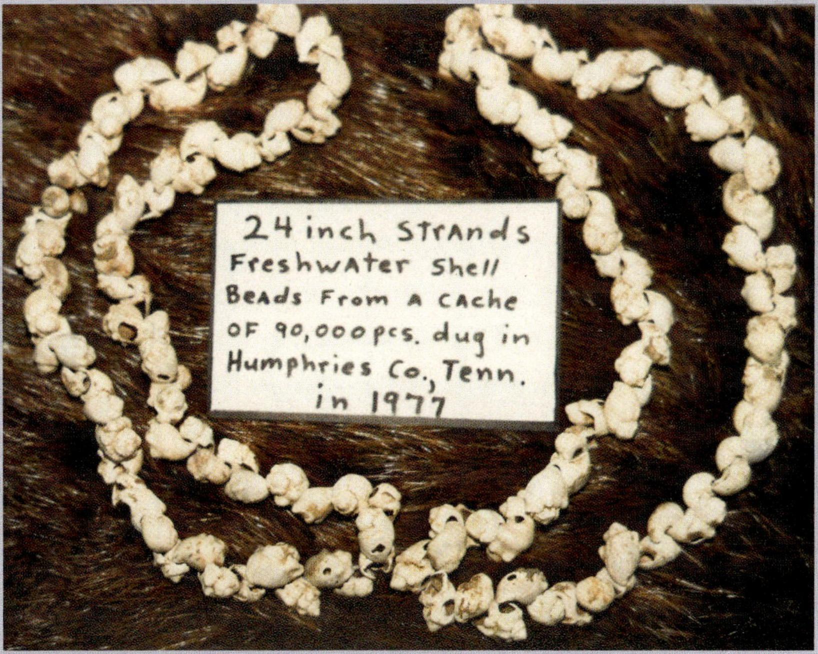
24 inch Strands
Freshwater Shell
Beads From a cache
OF 90,000 pcs. dug in
Humphries Co., Tenn.
in 1977

Shell bead strand, 24" long. It is from a cache of 90,000 beads found in Tennessee. Back to Earth. Strand, **$45.00.**

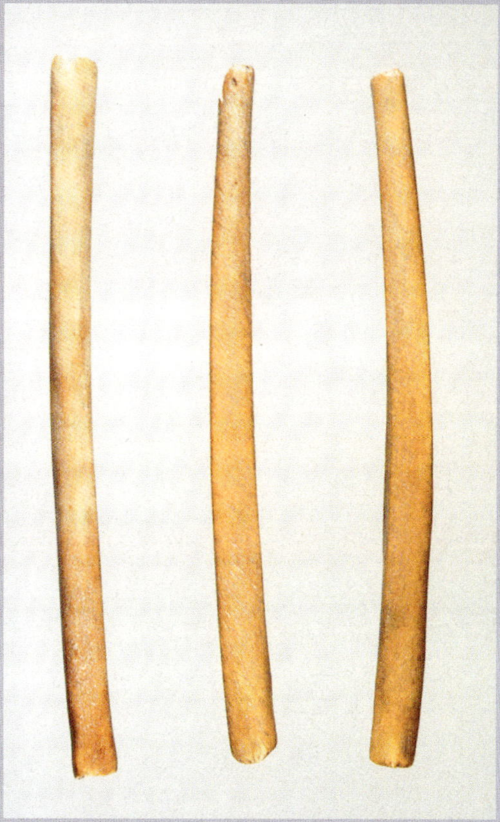

Beads, hollow bird bones, longest example 3⅜". Very long for artifact type, the beads are smoothed at the ends and polished overall. Southern Ohio. Fred Winegardner collection. Each, **$35.00.**

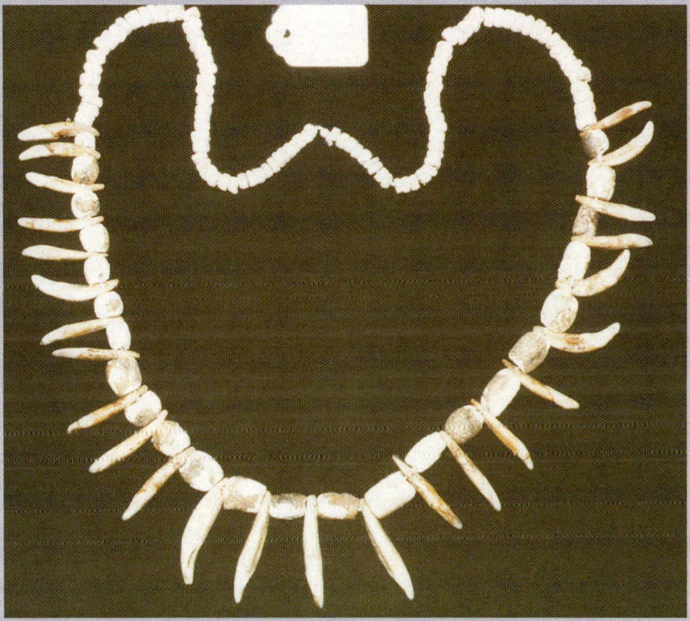

Strand of shell beads and teeth, barrel-shaped spacers, Fort Ancient in time. It was found near Augusta, Kentucky. Back to Earth. Unlisted.

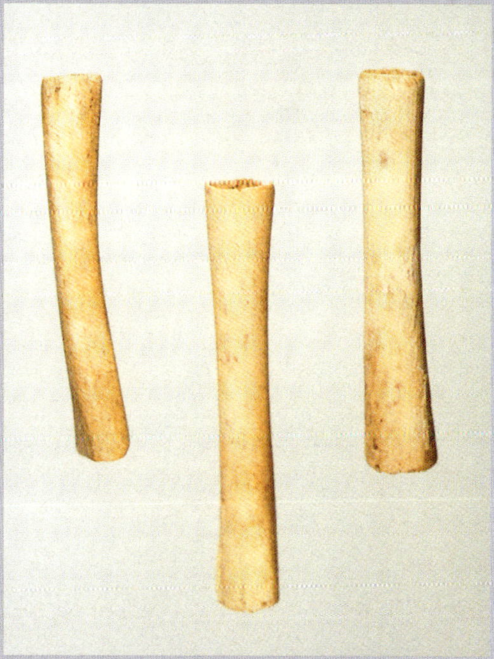

Beads, made of hollow bird bones, longest is 2⅜". The ends are trimmed and smoothed, and shafts are polished. Southern Ohio. Fred Winegardner collection. Each, **$20.00.**

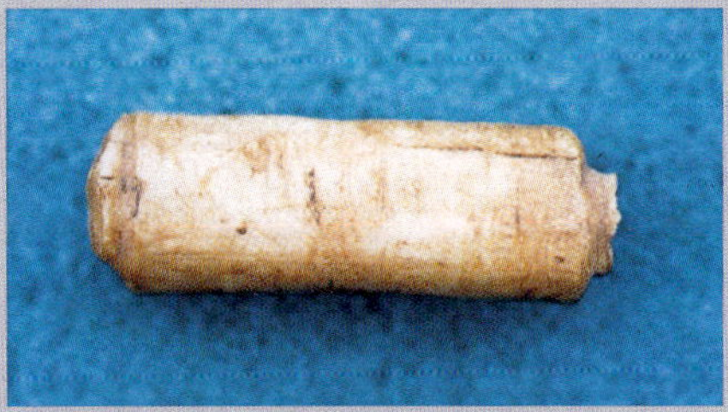

Bone pendant or bead section, ¼ x ⅞", Woodland or later. It is ex-collection Levy, find-location unknown. Collection of, and photograph by, Gary Henry, North Carolina. **$30.00.**

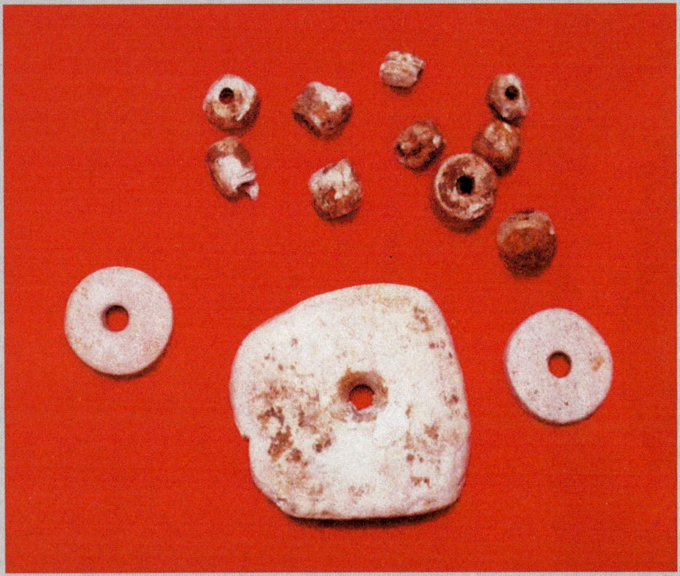

Shell, beads, largest is 1⅛" square and 3⁄32" thick. Small beads average ¼" across. They were found in the Saginaw area, Michigan. Michael F. Slasinski collection, Michigan. All, **$50.00.**

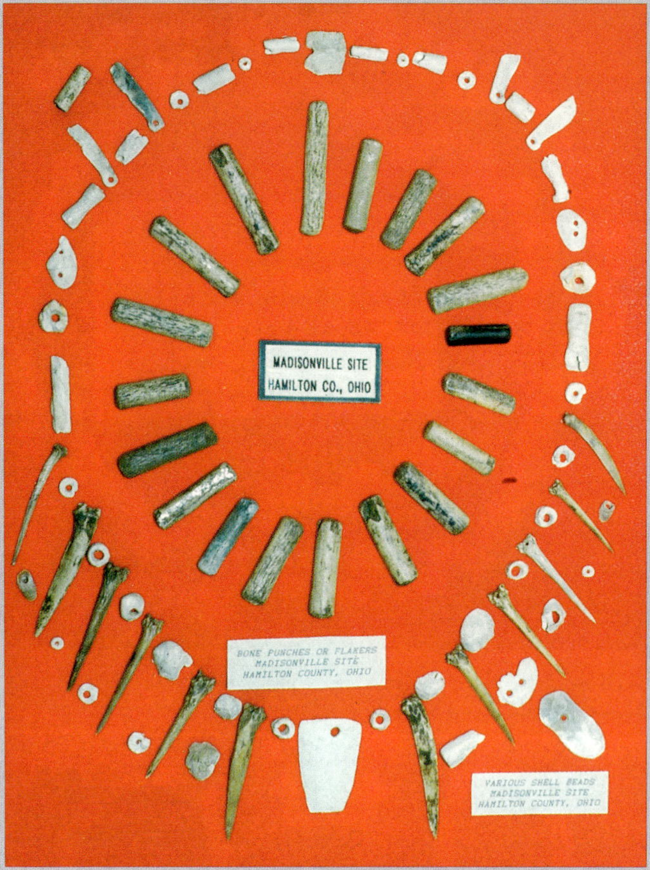

Fort Ancient artifacts, including shell beads, bone flakers, and awls. All are from southern Ohio. Back to Earth. Unlisted.

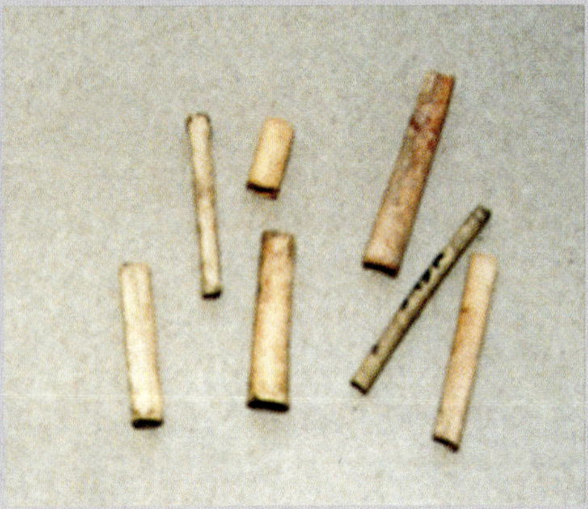

Beads, made of bird bones, all with various degrees of work and polish. They are southeastern United States. Wilfred Dick collection, Mississippi. Each, **$7.00 – 20.00.**

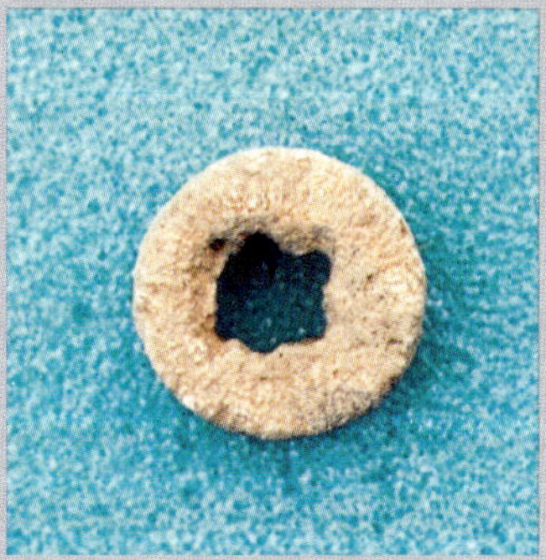

Fossil crinoid bead, Woodland or later, found by Harwood between 1954 and 1982. It is 7⁄16" in diameter and came from Morgan County, Alabama. Collection of, and photograph by, Gary Henry, North Carolina. **$10.00.**

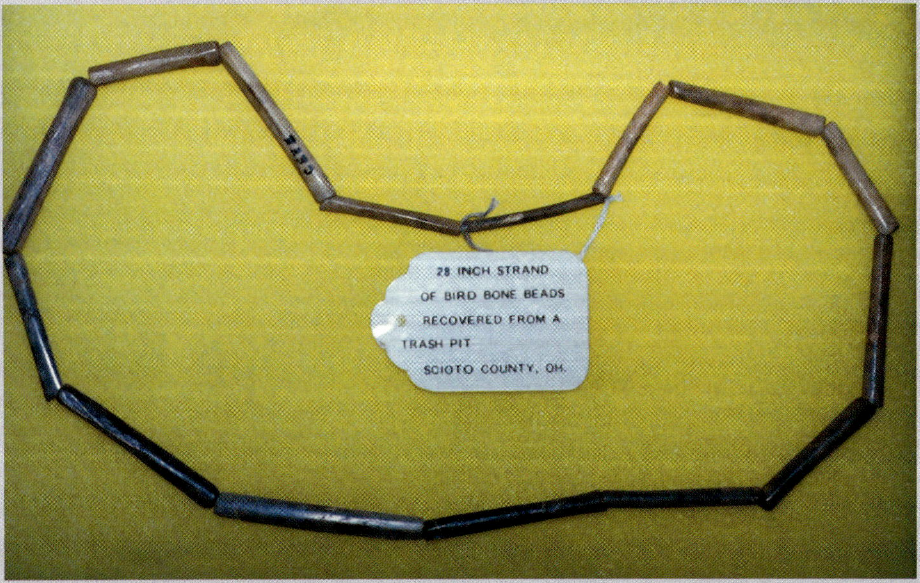

Beads, strand 28" long, polished bird bones, Fort Ancient aspect. These came from a trash pit or midden, Scioto County, Ohio. Back to Earth. Unlisted.

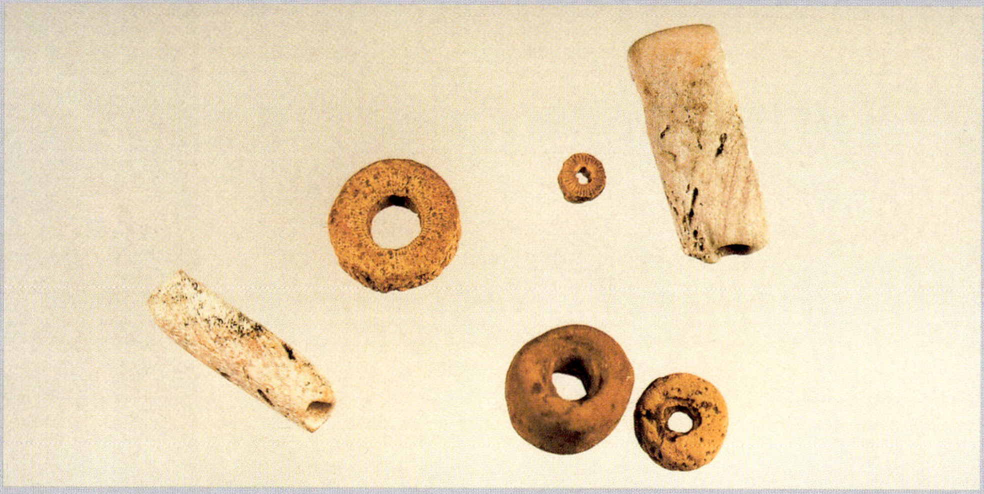

Beads, cylindrical forms made of shell, longest is 1⅛". Of the other four disc beads in different sizes, three are made of pottery and the smallest is a section of fossil crinoid stem. The six came from the Decatur area, Alabama. Robin Fiser collection. All, **$15.00.**

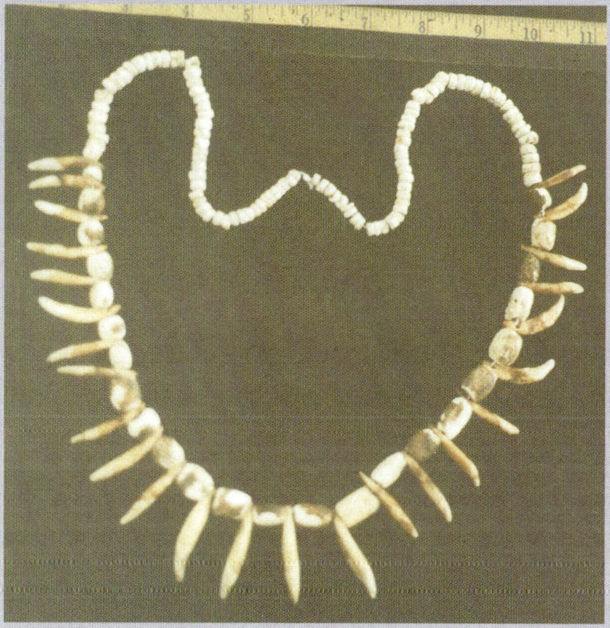

Strand, with 25 drilled canine teeth and spacers made of large beads. The beads and necklace elements are displayed in a custom-built case measuring 15 x 17". Bracken County, Kentucky. Back to Earth. **$750.00.**

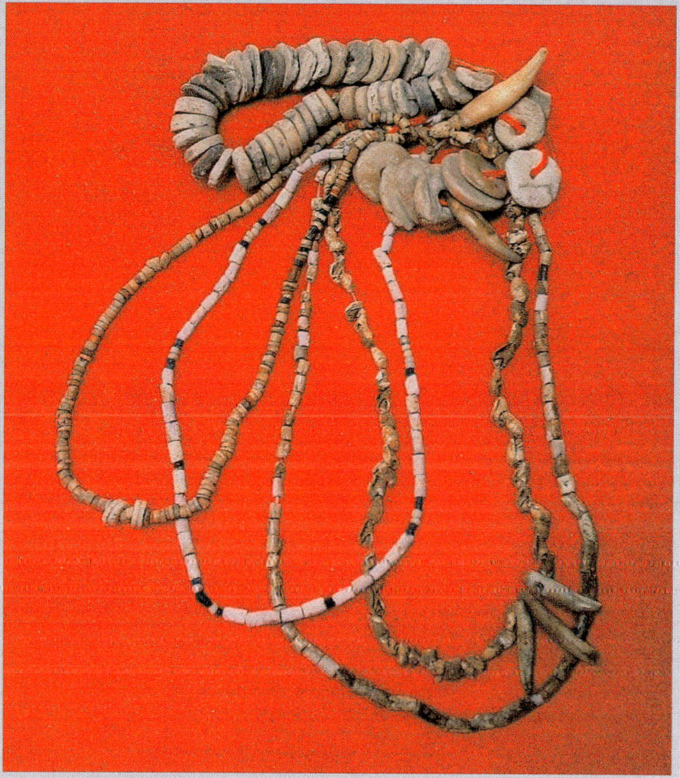

Beads and teeth decorative objects, white and purple wampum beads average ⅛ x 3/16", disc beads are about 3/32 x 9/16", and the shell beads are 3/16 x 5/16". This is a fine regional assemblage of bead types. Michigan. Michael F. Slasinski collection, Michigan. All, **$700.00.**

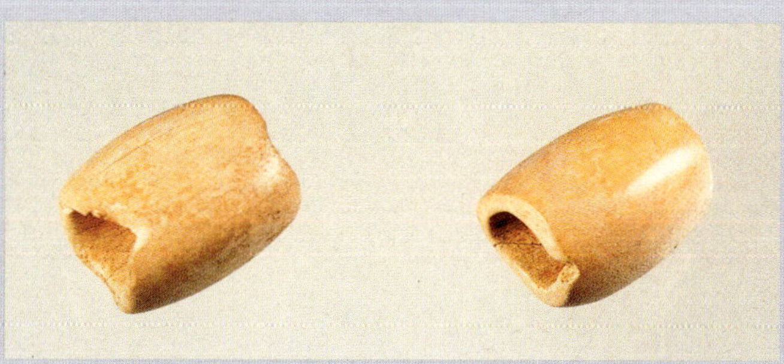

Bone beads, longest is ⅞", both well-shaped and with high polish. Ex-collection Selb, they are from West Virginia. Doug Hooks collection. Each, **$15.00 – 20.00.**

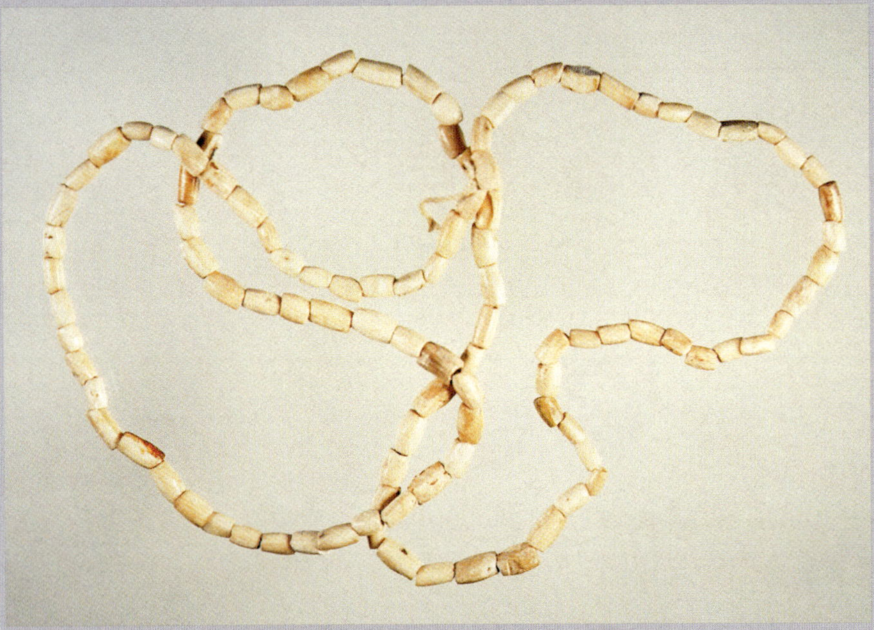

Necklace, barrel-shaped shell beads, average length is ⅜". These were all found in Ross County, Ohio. Fred Winegardner collection. Museum grade.

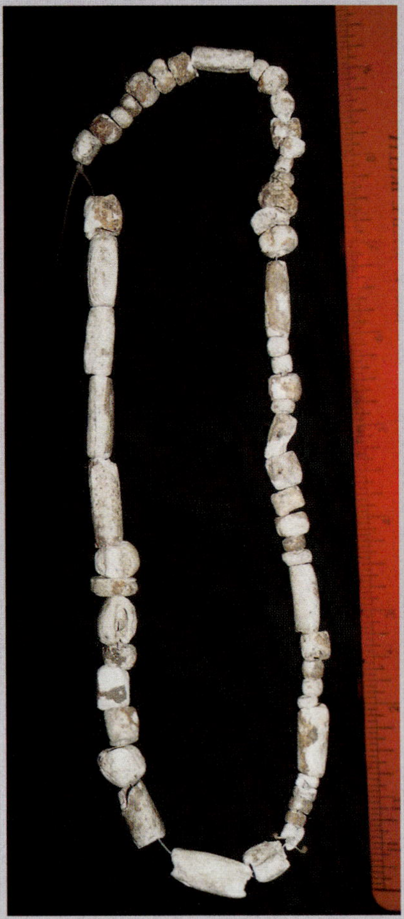

Shell beads, 18" string, longest bead is approximately ¾". These were found in Tennessee. Private collection. Strand, **$150.00 – 200.00.**

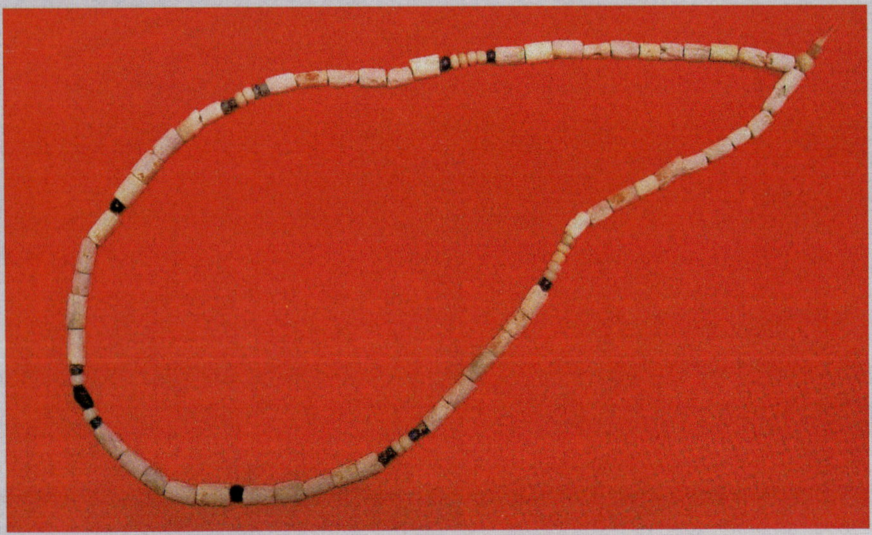

Strand of wampum beads, 13" long, purple and white shell beads with a few glass beads. Shown elsewhere with bead group, this historic example was found in Bay City, Michigan. Michael F. Slasinski collection, Michigan. **$200.00.**

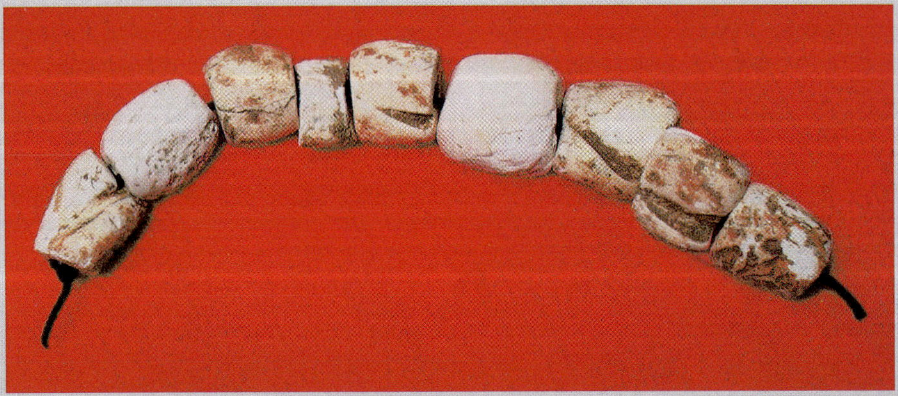

Shell beads, probably Mississippian in origin, average bead diameter is ¾". These were made from large marine mollusks and were found in Tennessee. Michael F. Slasinski collection, Michigan. All, **$125.00.**

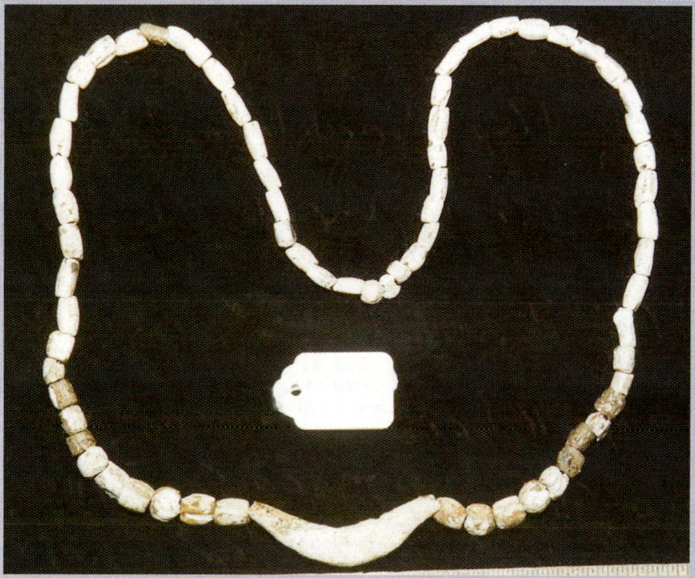

Shell bead strand, unusual and large center bead, strand is 28". The beads were found in Monroe County, Tennessee. Back to Earth. **$185.00.**

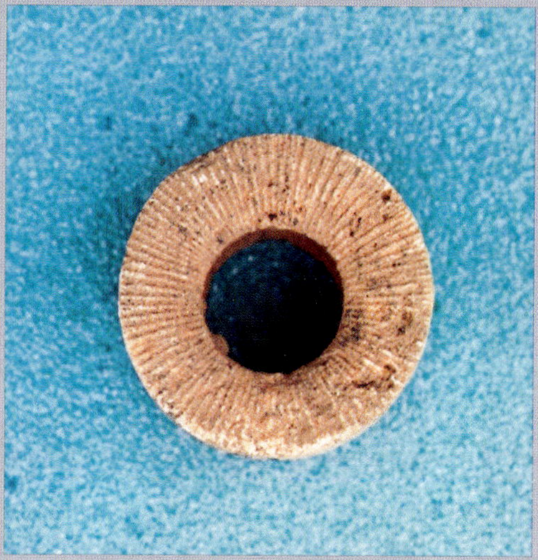

Fossil crinoid bead, Woodland or later, 1¹⁄₁₆" in diameter. This example, found by Harwood in 1954, has been smoothly holed and rounded. Limestone County, Alabama. Collection of, and photograph by, Gary Henry, North Carolina. **$20.00.**

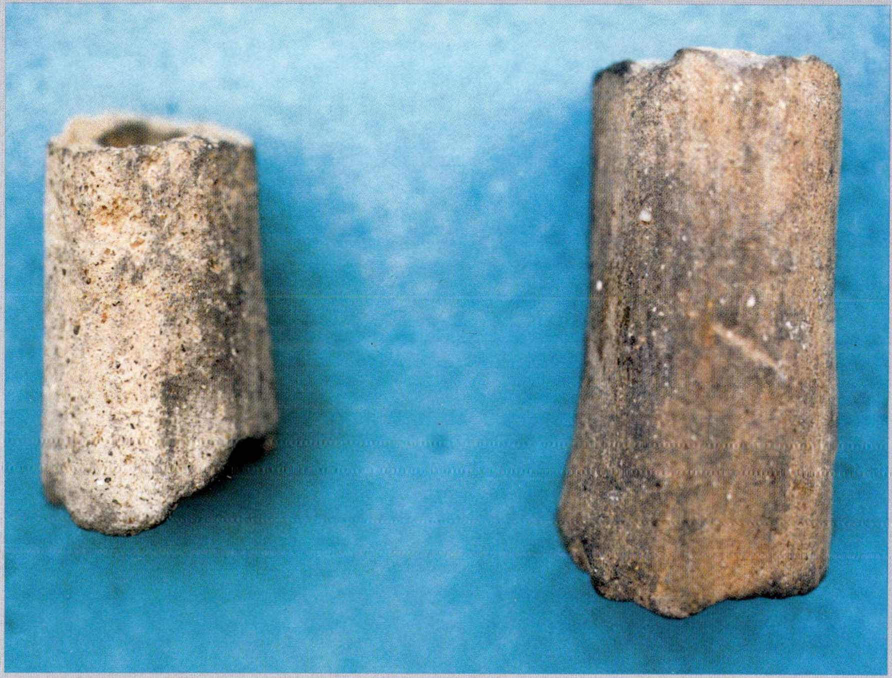

Bone beads, Woodland or later, largest is ¾ x 1½". They are ex-collection Levy, find-location unknown. Collection of, and photograph by, Gary Henry, North Carolina. Each, **$10.00.**

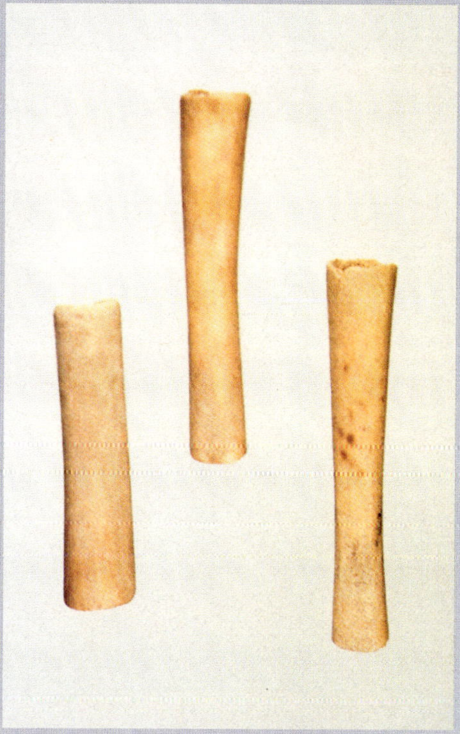

Beads, polished bird bones, longest example is 2¹⁄₃₂". Flared at the ends, the beads came from southern Ohio. Fred Winegardner collection. Each, **$15.00.**

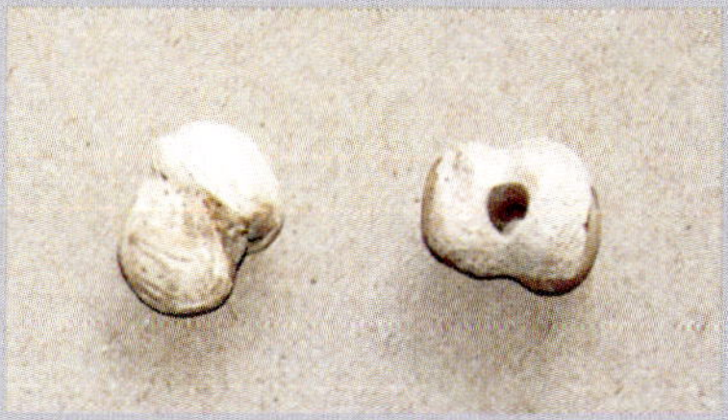

Shell beads, drilled and grooved, beads are ¾" in diameter. Probably Mississippian, they are from Arkansas. Wilfred Dick collection, Mississippi. Each, **$25.00**

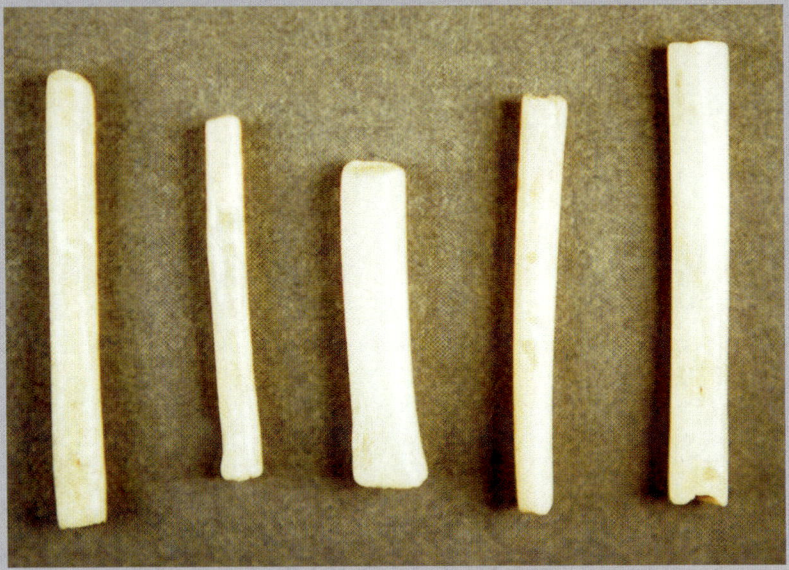

Beads, tubular, bird bone, longest is 2⅜". Such naturally hollow bones, cut to length, were often used for decorative objects. Willow Grove area, West Virginia. Larry Garvin collection. Each, **$15.00.**

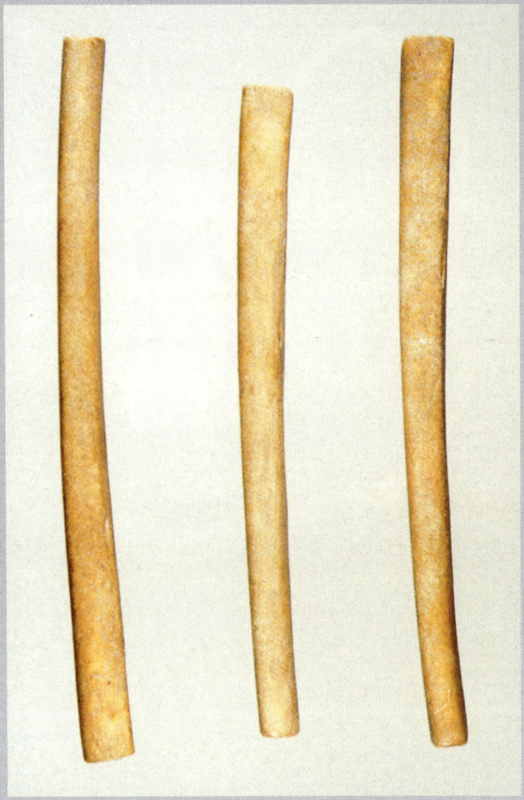

Beads, hollow bird bones, longest bead is 3¹⁵⁄₁₆". These might have been worn as a necklace, ear dangles, or a breastplate. Extra-long in size, they are from southern Ohio. Fred Winegardner collection. Each, **$50.00.**

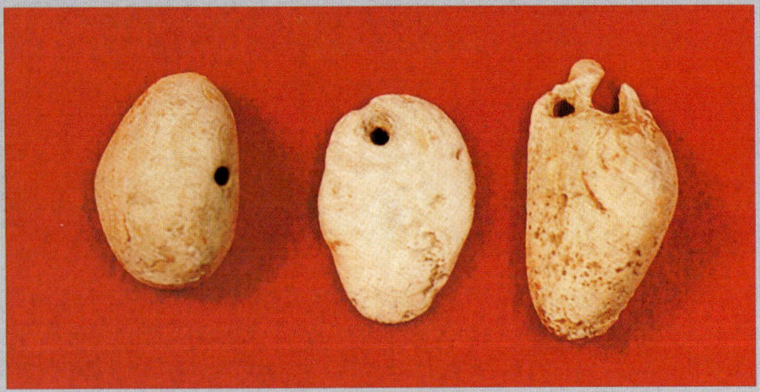

Shell beads, Woodland to Mississippian, longest is 1½", all once in the Vietzen collection. The left example is drilled from the reverse face and the other two are drilled from each face. Southern Ohio. Pete Timoch collection. Each, **$15.00 – 25.00.**

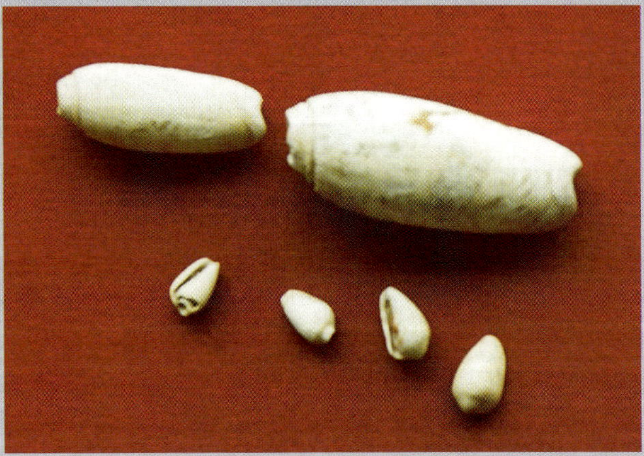

Shell beads, Hopewell olivella shells, 1" and 1¾" long, ca. AD 1 – 300; and four small Seneca marine shell beads, ca. AD 1635 – 1655. All are from Livingston County, New York. Dave Summers collection, Victor, New York. Large shells, **$10.00** and **$20.00;** small shells, four for **$3.00.**

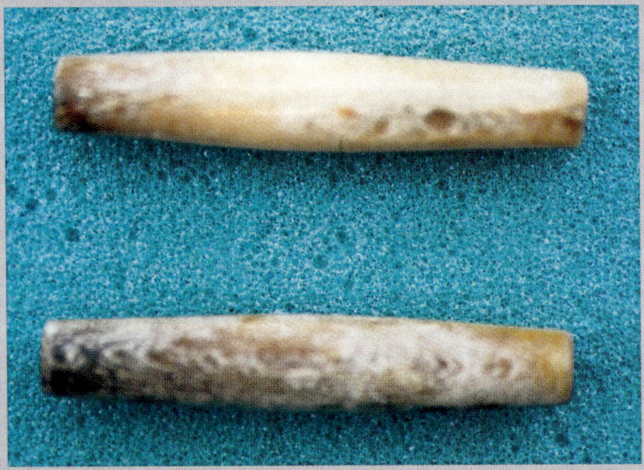

Bone hair-pipe beads, prehistoric(?), each is ¼ x 1½". The beads are ex-collection Levy, origin unknown. Collection of, and photograph by, Gary Henry, North Carolina. Each, **$10.00.**

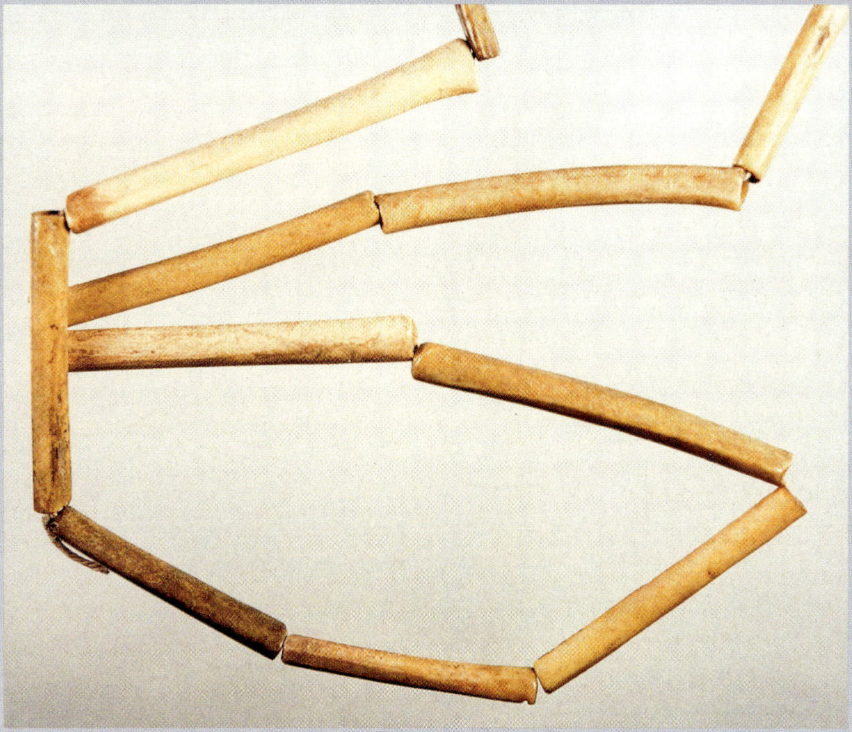

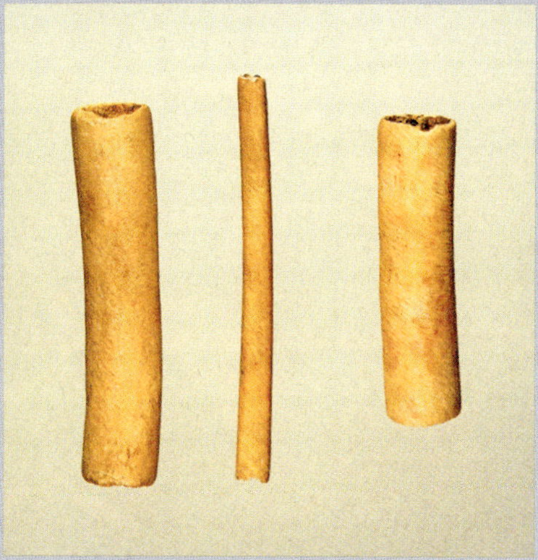

Beads, bird bones, the three showing a width range of such beads. The longest is 2" and all are from southern Ohio. Fred Winegardner collection. Each, **$15.00.**

Necklace, bird bones, longest bead is 2¼". The beads are cut and smoothed on the ends, shafts are polished. Necklace is ex-collections Copeland and Hooks, from southern Ohio. Fred Winegardner collection. Museum grade.

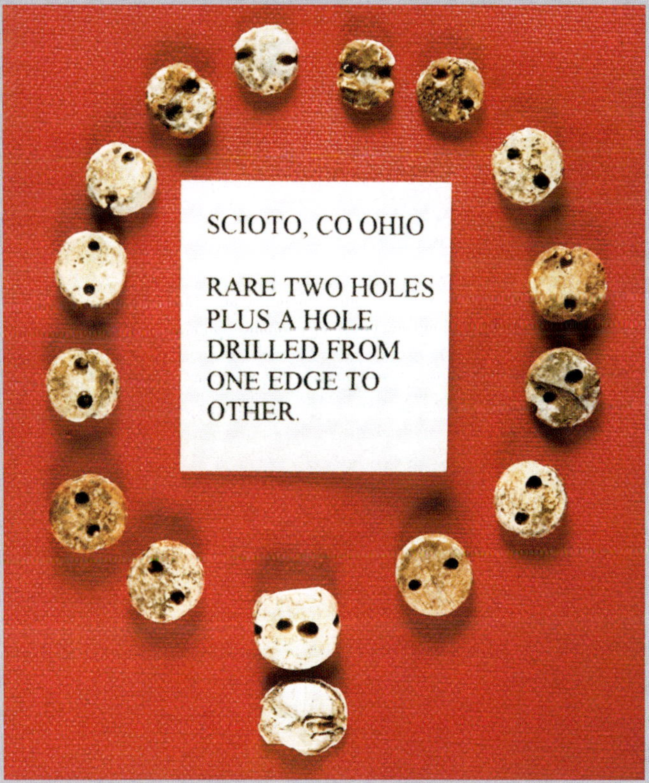

Shell disc beads, each drilled with two small holes, beads are about ½" in diameter. In addition to holes in the two faces, the beads are drilled from side to side. Ex-collection Kientz, they are from Scioto County, Ohio. Don Casto collection. Museum grade.

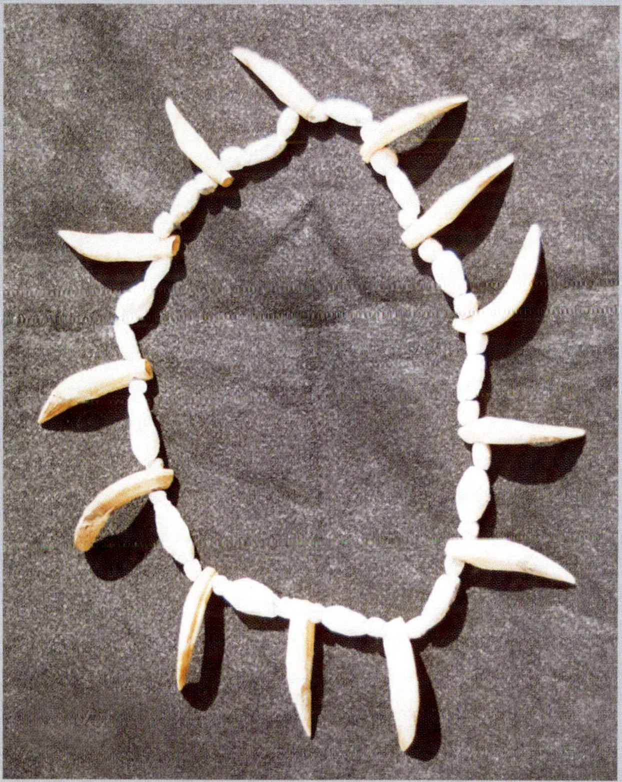

Necklace, shell barrel beads and boar tusks, 27" long, longest tooth is 3⅛". The presence of boar tusks indicates the presence of Europeans and historic times. McDowell County, North Carolina. Jim Maus collection, North Carolina. Unlisted.

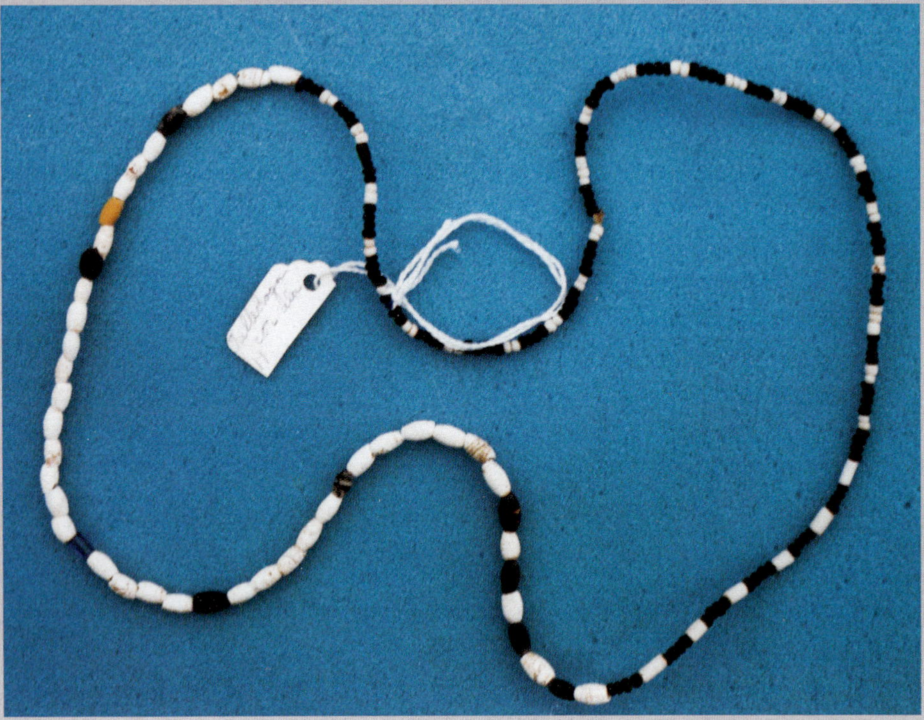

Bead strand, 229 beads with 46 made of shell and 183 black and white glass trade beads, historic period. Glass beads are 1/16 x 1/8". These are ex-collection Snyder, from Talladega County, Alabama. Collection of, and photograph by, Gary Henry, North Carolina. Strand, **$200.00.**

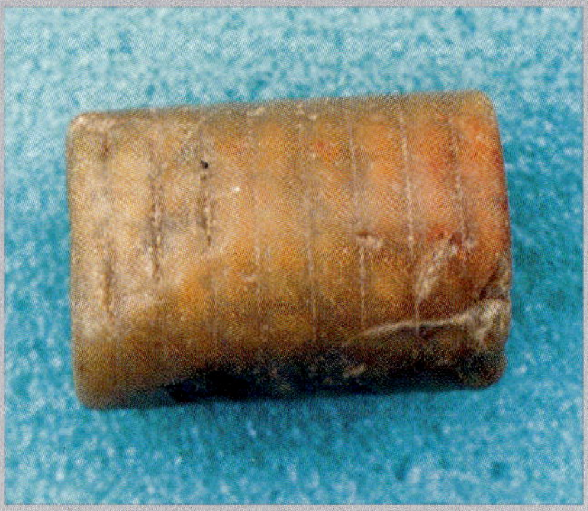

Fossil bead, crinoid, with drilling begun but not completed. Woodland or later, it is 7/8" long and 9/16" across. Found by Harwood between 1954 and 1956, it came from Morgan County, Alabama. Collection of, and photograph by, Gary Henry, North Carolina. **$10.00.**

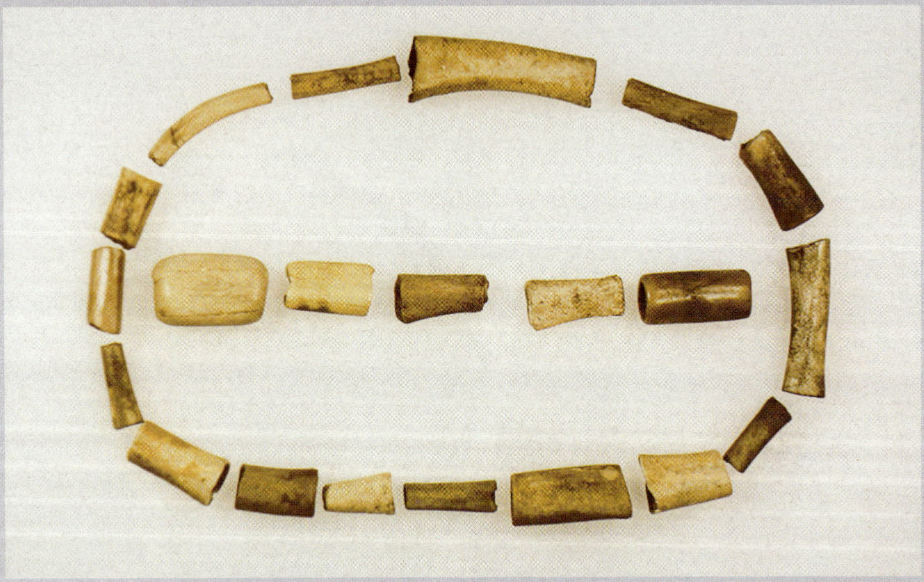

Necklace, Mississippian period, made of bone beads from various sites, longest is 2¾". Note the color variation due to different find-sites. All are ex-collection Vietzen, from Ohio and Kentucky. Pete Timoch collection. Unlisted.

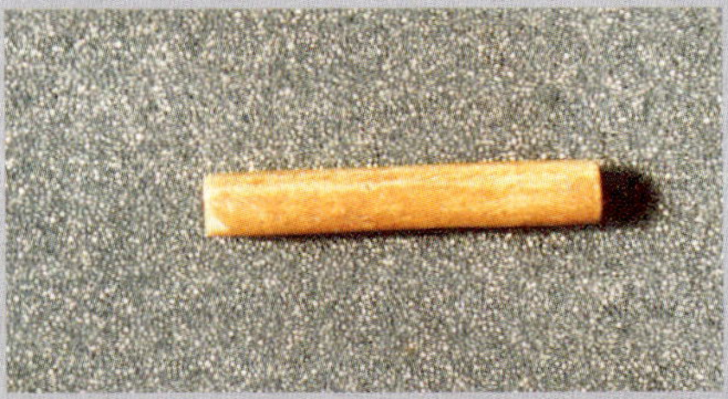

Antler tubular bead, 1¾" long. Antler was not often used for beads in any period. It is historic Iroquois (Seneca), ca. AD 1675 – 1687, and was found near the town of Victor. Ontario County, New York. Dave Summers collection, Victor, New York. **$35.00.**

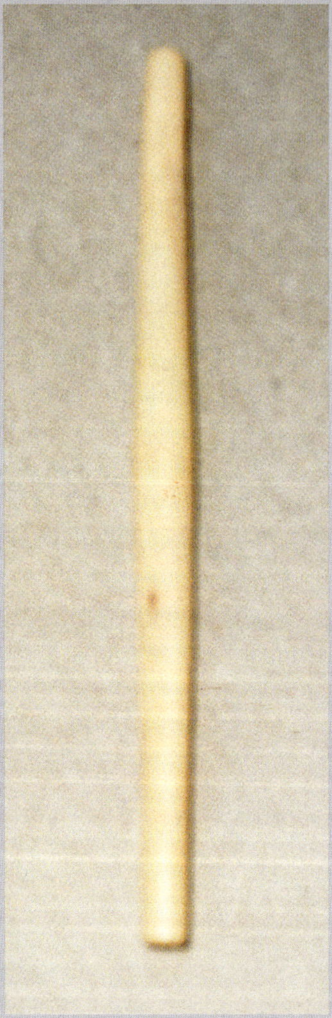

Bead, 4¾" long, nicely shaped and polished. It is from Oklahoma. Wilfred Dick collection, Mississippi. **$175.00.**

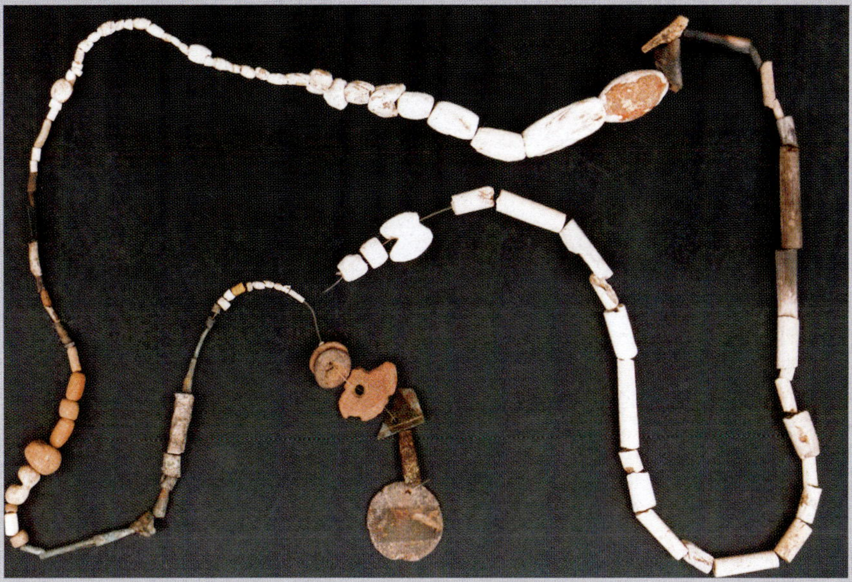

Beads and round metal pendant, prehistoric and historic, beads made of shell, bone, stone, metal, clay, and broken kaolin pipe stems. The longest shell bead is 1⁵⁄₁₆". The owner found these between 1965 and 1968 in Monroe County, Tennessee. Collection of, and photograph by, Gary Henry, North Carolina. All, **$250.00.**

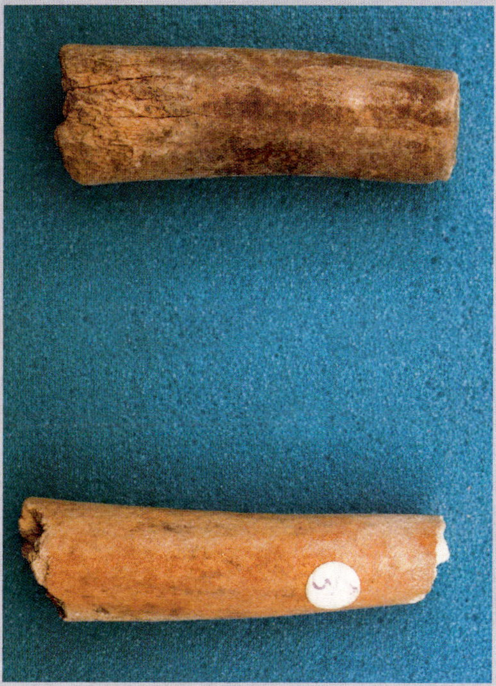

Bone bead preforms, cut but not yet drilled. Woodland or later, the top example is ¾ x 2⁵⁄₁₆". Ex-collection Snyder, they are from Meigs County, Tennessee. Collection of, and photograph by, Gary Henry, North Carolina. Each, **$10.00.**

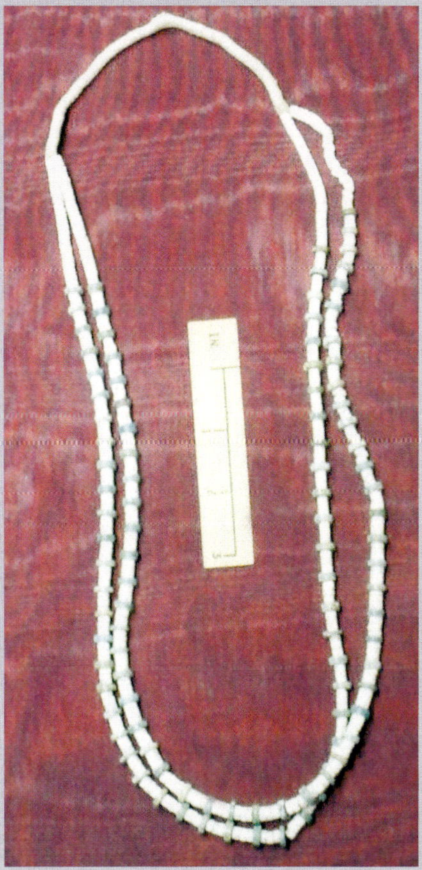

Double-strand bead necklace, made by the Navajo Indians. Ca. 1940, the shell beads are separated with small pieces of turquoise. Southwest. Ben Thompson collection, Missouri. **$450.00.**

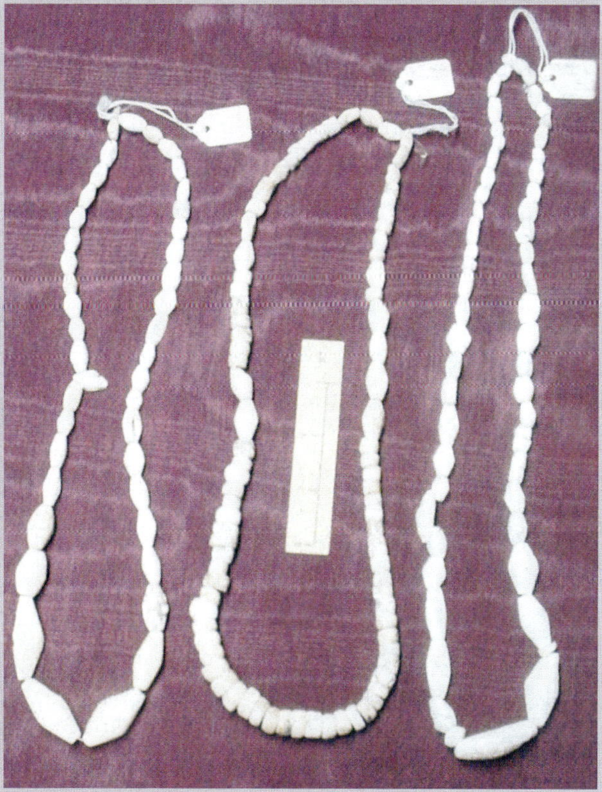

Shell bead necklaces, all beads from Indian campsites in Alabama. These beads are in exceptionally good condition. Ben Thompson collection, Missouri. Each strand, **$400.00 – 650.00.**

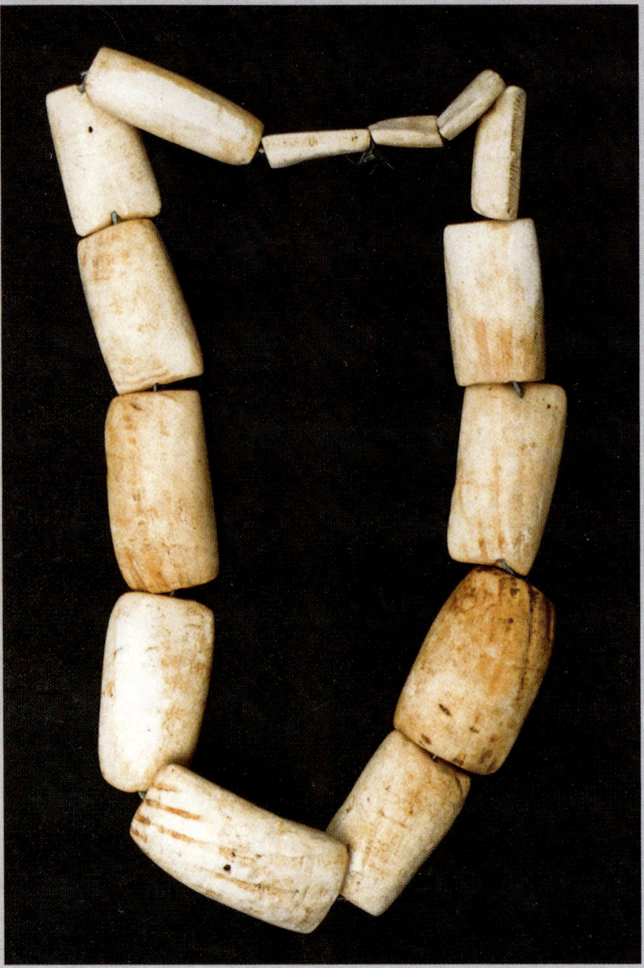

Strand of 14 beads, probably elk antler, Woodland or later. The largest bead is 1½ x 2⅝". These beads are ex-collection Snyder, from Washington County, Virginia. Collection of, and photograph by, Gary Henry, North Carolina. Strand, **$150.00.**

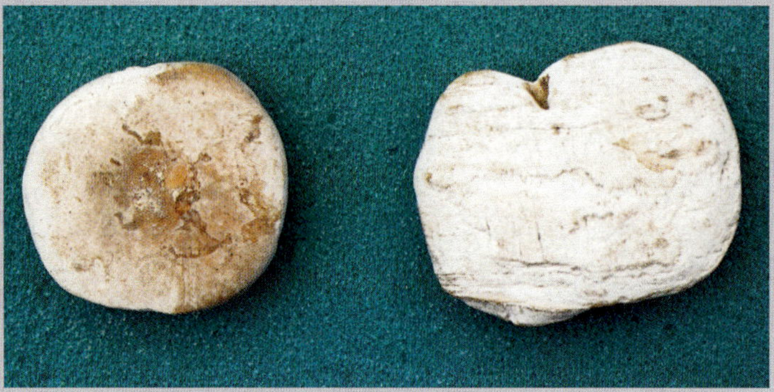

Flattened beads, Woodland or Mississippian, largest is ⅞ x 1⅛", ⅛" thick. Harwood found them in 1957. Clay County, North Carolina. Collection of, and photograph by, Gary Henry, North Carolina. Each, **$10.00.**

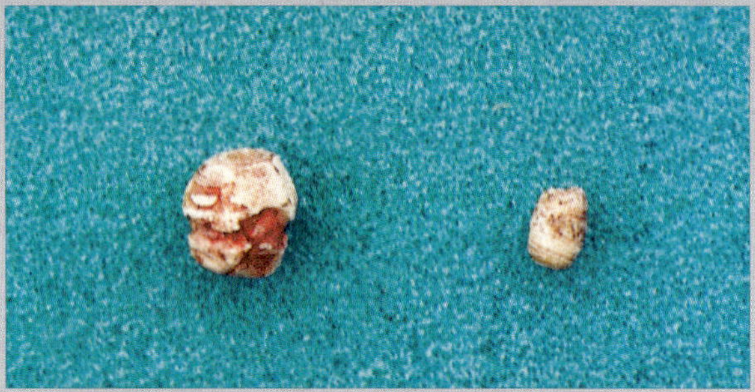

Beads, smaller one is 3⁄16" long and ⅛" in diameter. Found with glass trade beads, these are from the historic period. Harwood found them between 1954 and 1982. Cherokee County, North Carolina. Collection of, and photograph by, Gary Henry, North Carolina. **$10.00.**

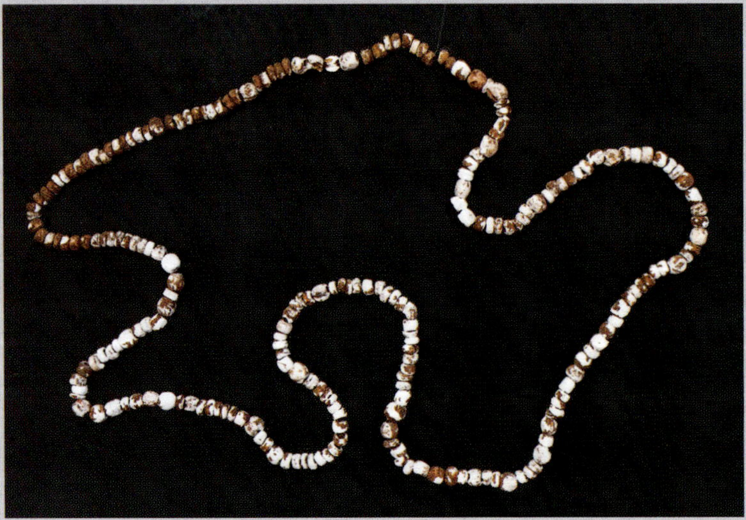

Strand of beads, 227 beads, largest is 5⁄16" both long and thick. These are from the Dallas people, ca. AD 1400 – 1600, very late prehistoric and proto-historic. The owner found them in 1970. Montgomery County, Tennessee. Collection of, and photograph by, Gary Henry, North Carolina. **$200.00.**

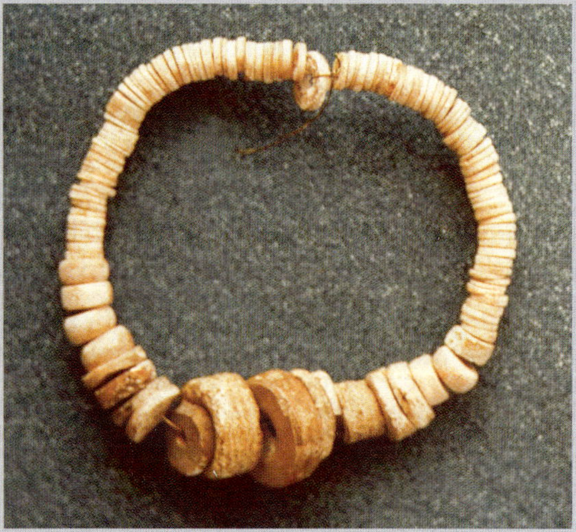

Bead strand, three fish vertebra and 119 marine shell discoidal beads, strand is 9" long. They are Seneca Indian from a site near Livonia dating ca. AD 1565 – 1575. Livingston County, New York. Dave Summers collection, Victor, New York. Strand, **$225.00.**

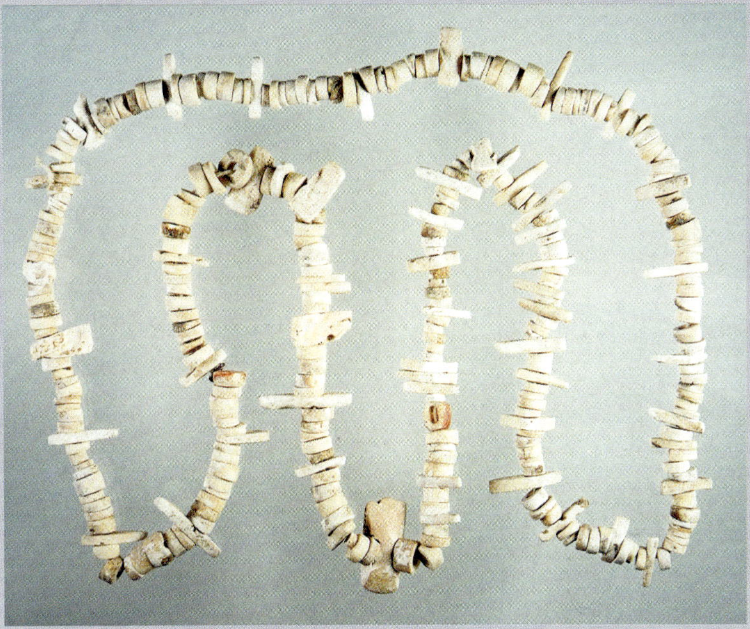

Necklace, disc, barrel, and rectangular beads, bottom pendant is 7/16" long. There are almost 300 beads in the necklace, which came from Ohio or Kentucky. Private collection. Museum grade.

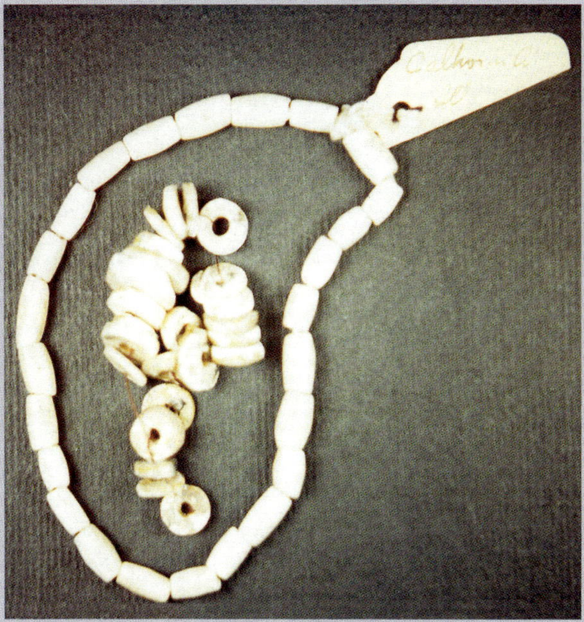

Beads – bone, barrel, and disc types. Found in Calhoun County, Illinois. Lee Hallman collection, Pennsylvania. All, **$225.00.**

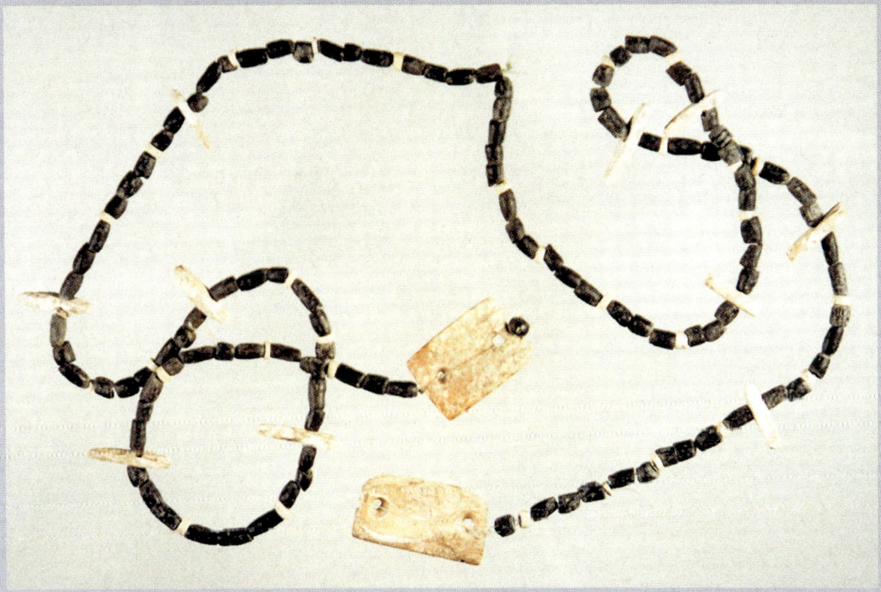

Necklace, shell beads and spacers, longest two pieces at bottom are 1⅛". Probably Mississippian (Fort Ancient), it is from near Marietta, Ohio. Fred Winegardner collection. Museum grade.

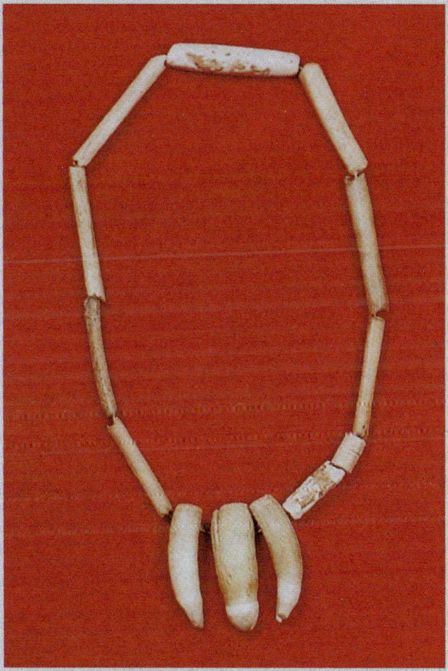

Necklace, bird bones and shells with alligator tooth pendants. Necklace is 16" in circumference. Ex-collection Vietzen, this unusual necklace is from the Gulf Coast region. Pete Timoch collection. **$350.00.**

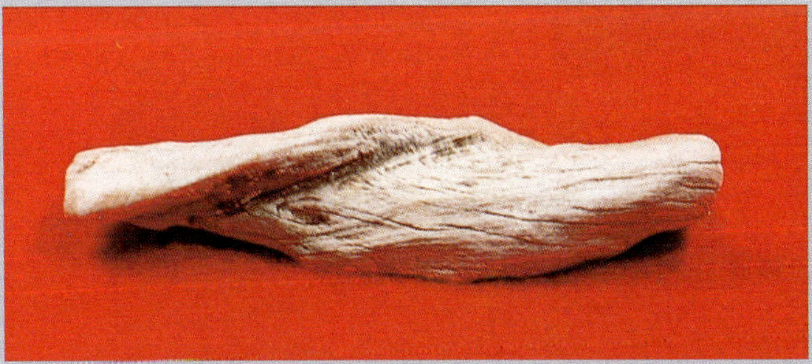

Shell bead, large marine shell column, 3" long. It was once owned by Col. Vietzen and is drilled laterally through the midsection. An old tag indicates it came from Oklahoma. Pete Timoch collection. **$50.00 – 75.00.**

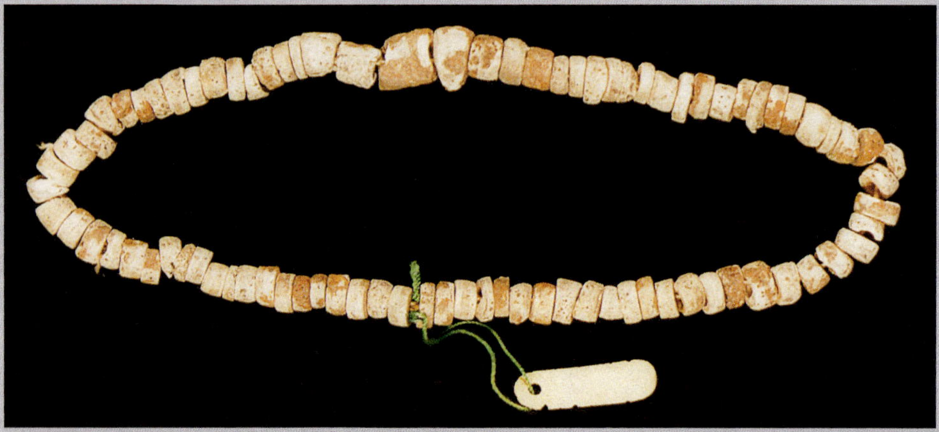

Shell necklace, Mississippian period, circumference of 10½", first collector's string and identification tag present. The strand has a good pedigree, having been found by Peter Bungart in 1918 and later acquired by Col. Vietzen. This particular strand has drawn considerable attention due to its history. It came from Bungart land in the Black River Valley, Lorain County, Ohio. Pete Timoch collection. Museum grade.

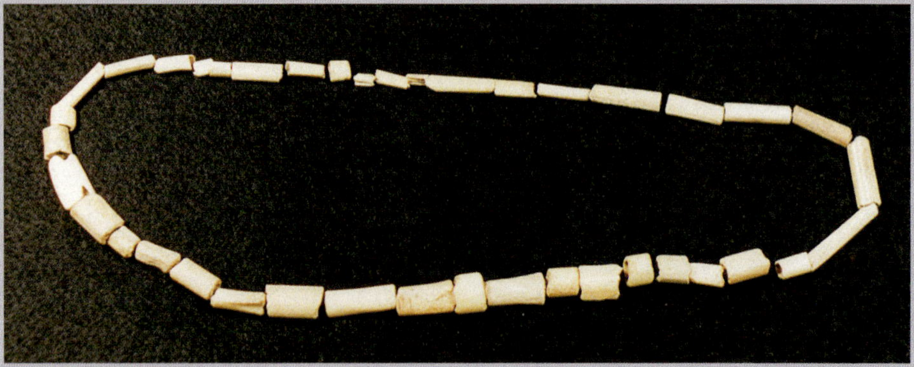

Necklace, polished bird bones, strand is 24" long. These are solid beads, nicely finished, ex-collection Vietzen. Portsmouth area, Ohio. Pete Timoch collection. **$200.00.**

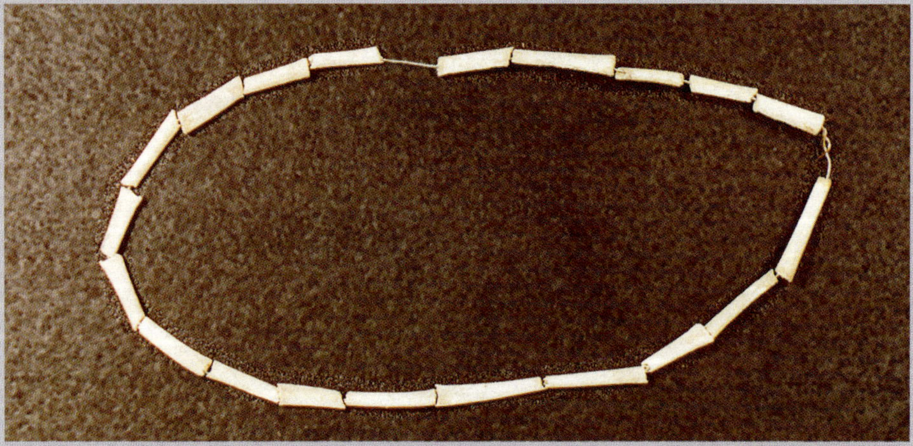

Necklace, Mississippian, small bird bones, 18" total length. Once in the Col. Raymond C. Vietzen collection, the beads are from Ohio or Kentucky. Pete Timoch collection. **$100.00 – 150.00.**

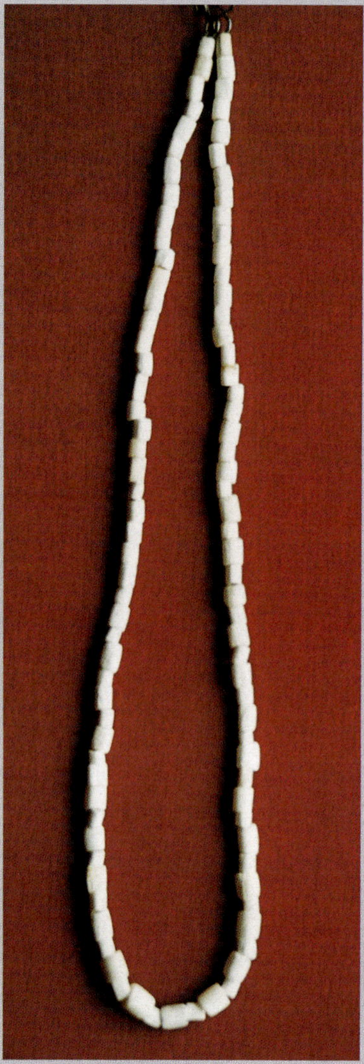

Seneca beads, rare, stone-drilled short tubular beads, marine shell, ca. AD 1560 – 1635. There are 98 beads and the strand is 18" long. Ex-collection Wray, the beads are from West Bloomfield, New York. Dave Summers collection, Victor, New York. **$950.00.**

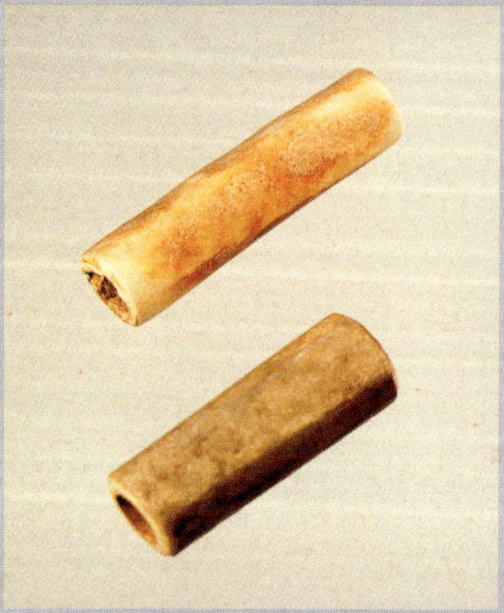

Beads, animal bone, crisply cut and shaped, good polish. The longest bead is 1¾". West Virginia. Doug Hooks collection. Each, **$20.00 – 25.00.**

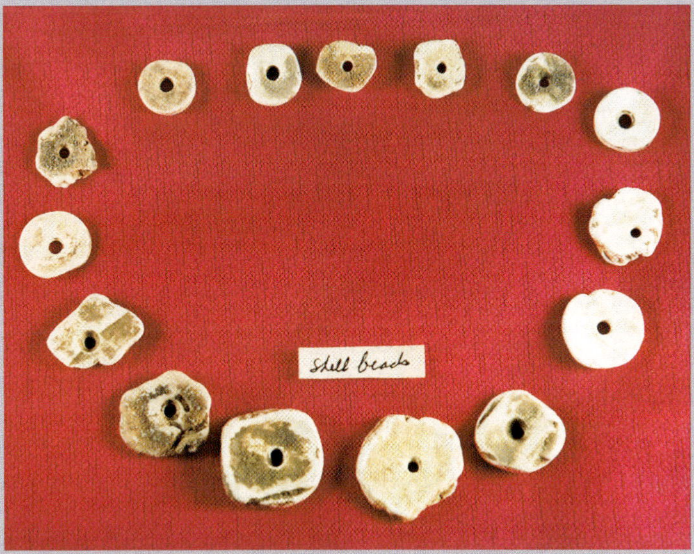

Shell disc beads, drilled for suspension, largest beads are about ¾" in diameter. These are Mississippian in time and ex-collection Kientz. Scioto County, Ohio. Don Casto collection. Museum grade.

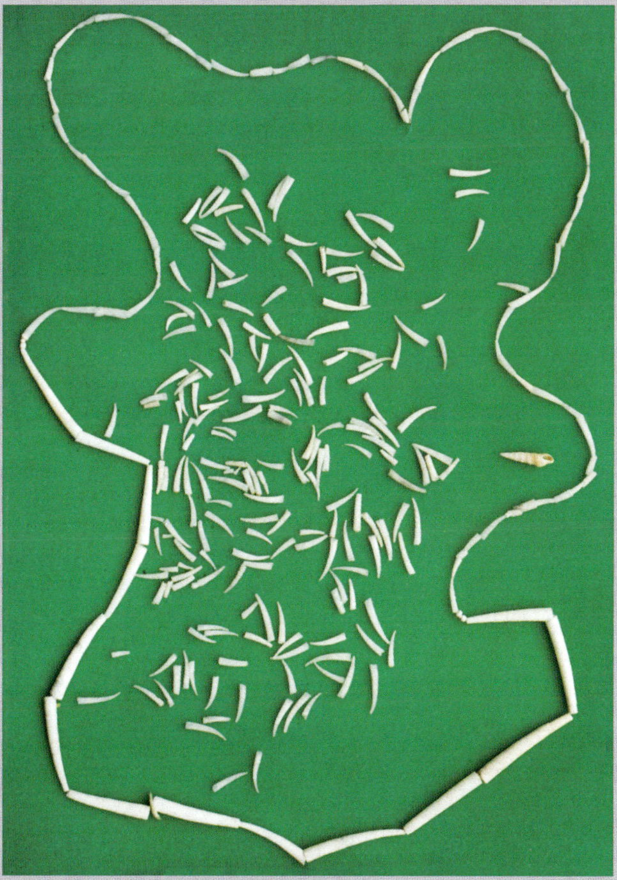

Dentalium shell beads and undrilled examples, prehistoric(?), longest bead is ¼ x 2". These beads were important both for decoration and as a form of money; longer beads were more highly valued. They are from the Pacific Northwest. Collection of, and photograph by, Gary Henry, North Carolina. All, **$200.00.**

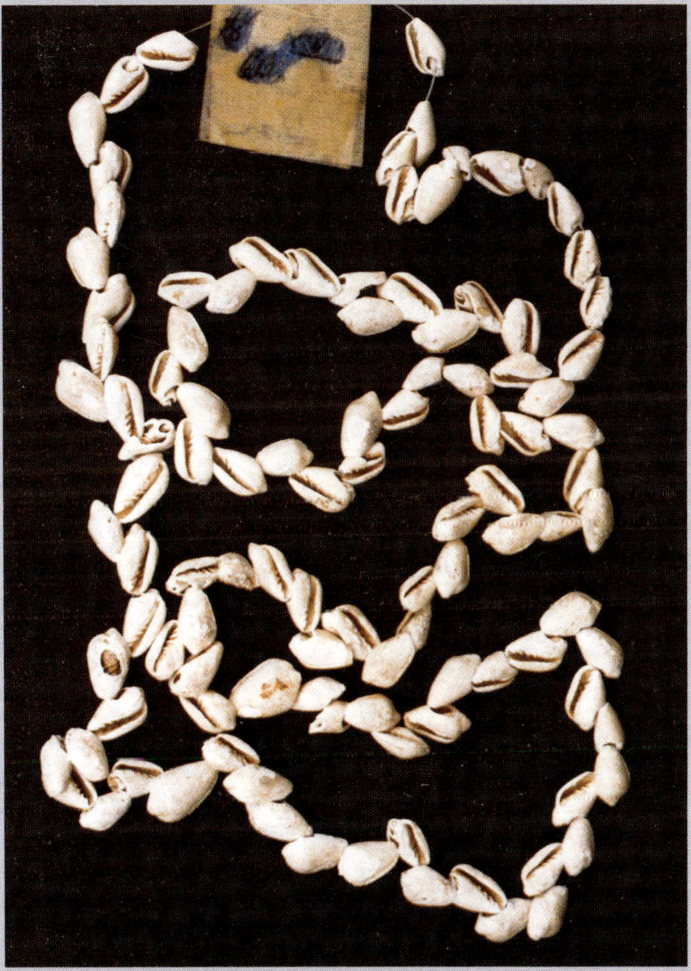

Strand of 109 marginella (snail shell) beads, average size is ½" long and ¼" in diameter. Woodland or Mississippian, they are ex-collection Snyder and were found by him between 1947 and 1958. Polk County, Tennessee. Collection of, and photograph by, Gary Henry, North Carolina. **$100.00.**

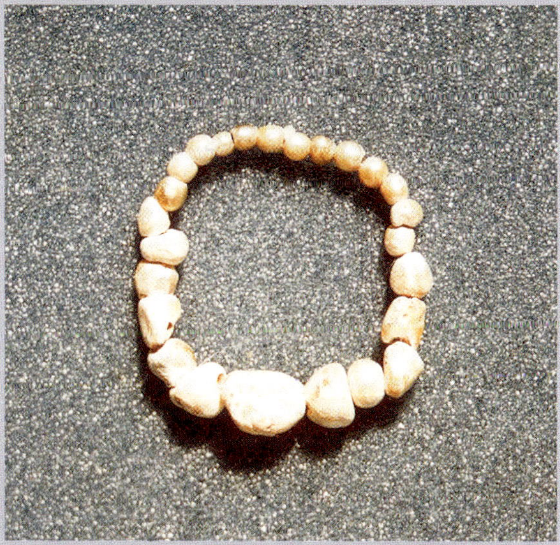

Pearl beads, Hopewell, ca. AD 200, Middle Woodland, strand is 5½" long. Freshwater mussel baroque drilled beads in graduated sizes, they were found near Mt. Morris in Livingston County, New York. Dave Summers collection, Victor, New York. Strand, **$500.00.**

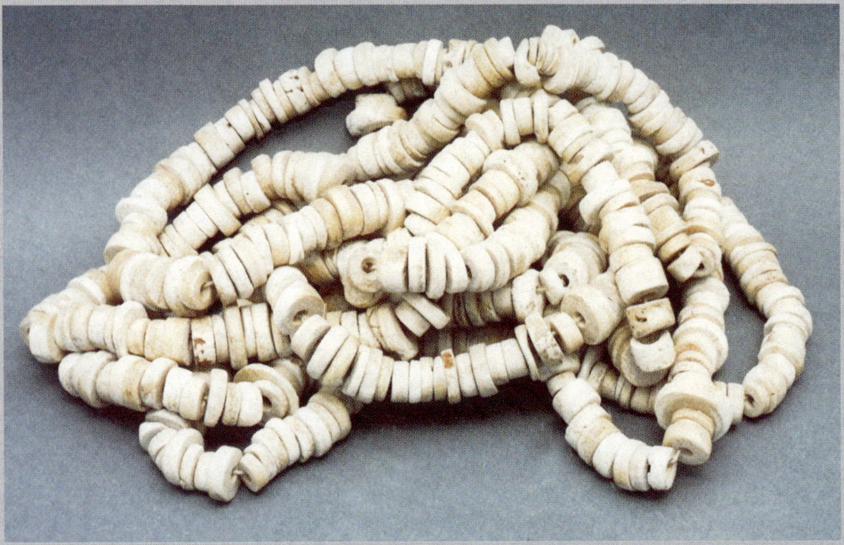

Shell beads, Mississippian period, ca. AD 1200. The individual beads are ½ to ⅝" in diameter and the strand is 8' long. Found during construction activities, it is from a site near Macon, Georgia. H. B. Greene II collection, Naples, Florida. Unlisted.

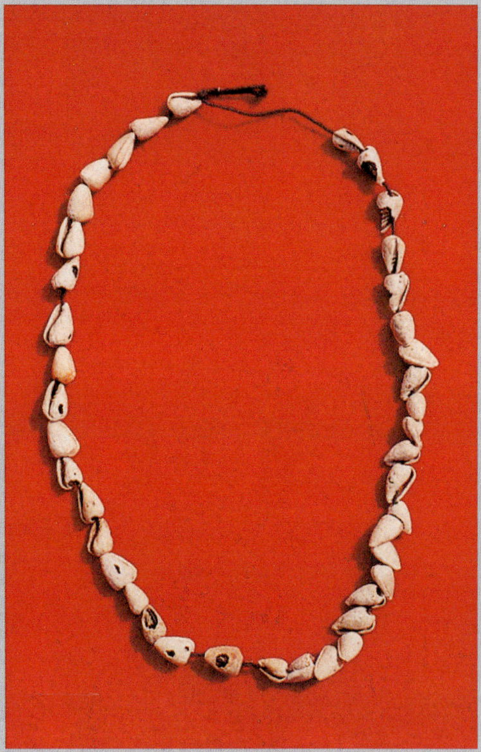

Necklace, probably Woodland in time, strand 16" long. This is ex-collection Vietzen, from Ohio. Pete Timoch collection. **$100.00.**

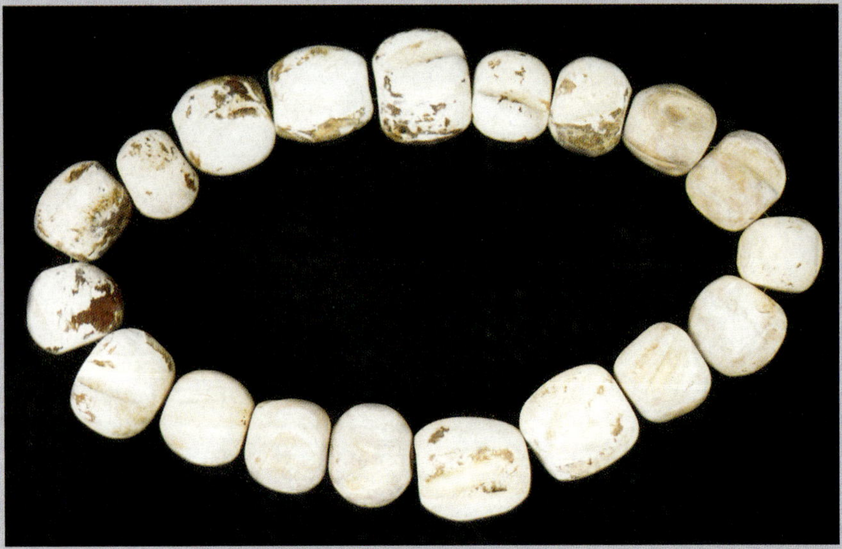

Beads, rounded and barrel shapes, bead size up to 1" long. These were found in Pemiscot County, Missouri. Bob Hess collection, Indiana. Museum grade.

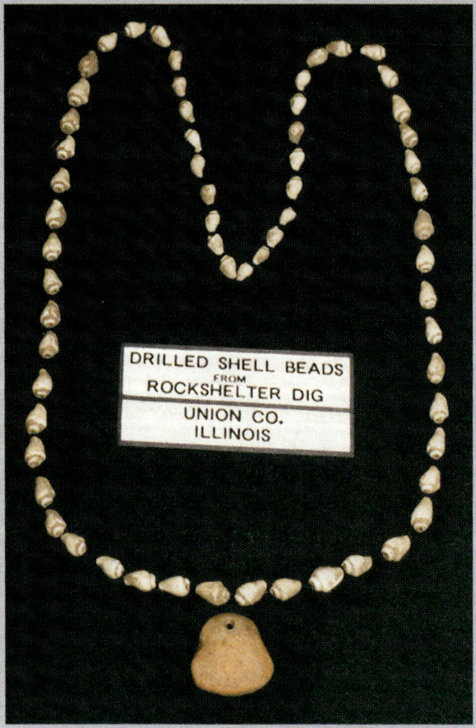

Drilled shell beads, rock shelter find, frame size 8 x 12". The beads are from Union County, Illinois. Back to Earth. Unlisted.

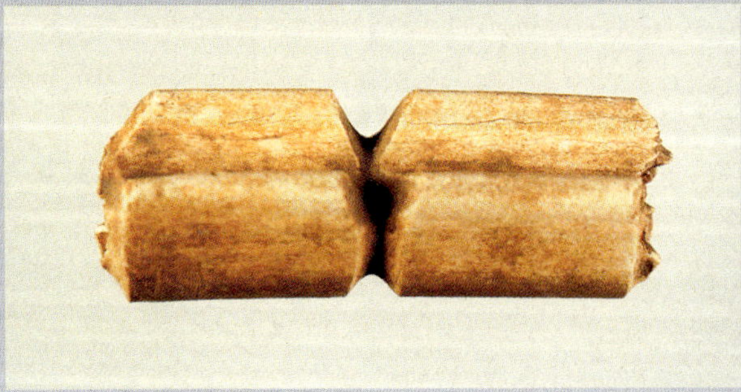

Bead preform, elk bone, sections (two beads) 2¼" long. Bone sections were isolated with V-shaped cuts and broken apart to form the beads. West Virginia. Doug Hooks collection. **$50.00.**

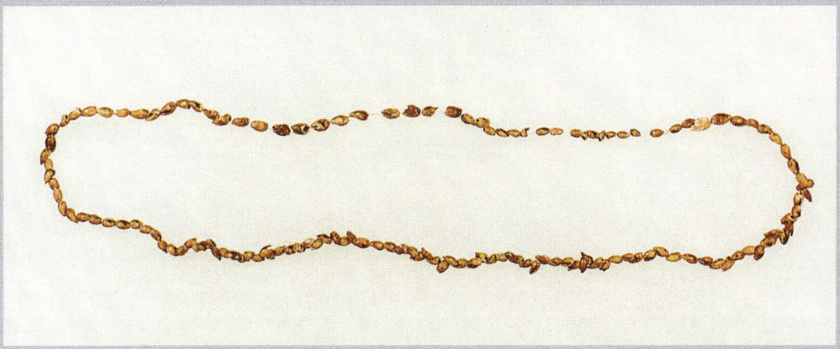

Small shell beads, strand is 26", individual beads are ⅛ to ¼". Mississippian, they are from St. Clair County, Illinois. Pete Timoch collection. Unlisted.

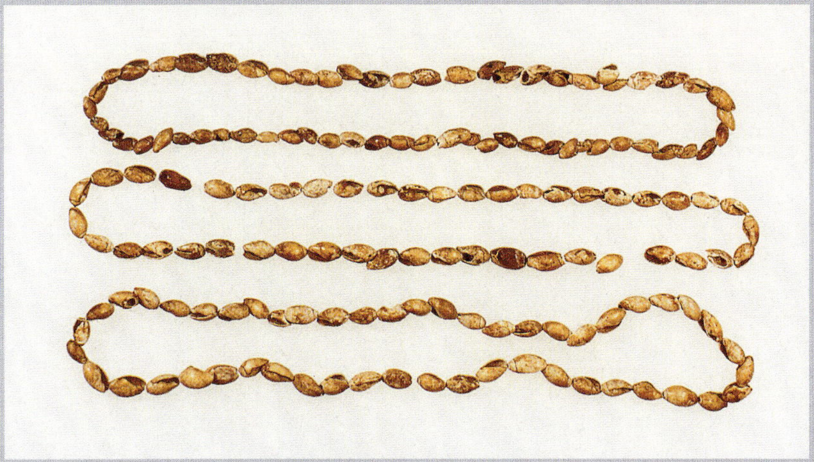

Medium-size beads, shell, three strands 24" long. Individual beads are ½ to 9/16". They are Mississippian, from St. Clair County, Illinois. Pete Timoch collection. Unlisted.

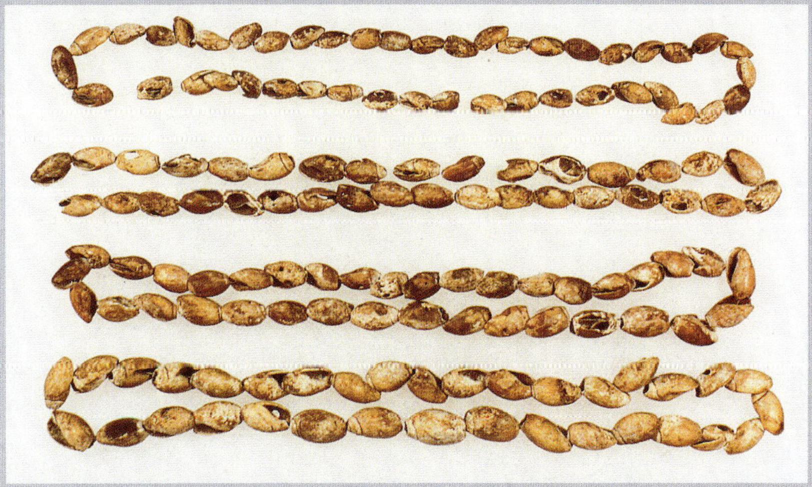

Large shell beads, four strands, longest is 25". These beads measure from ¾ to 1⅛" long. Mississippian period, St. Clair County, Illinois. Pete Timoch collection. Unlisted.

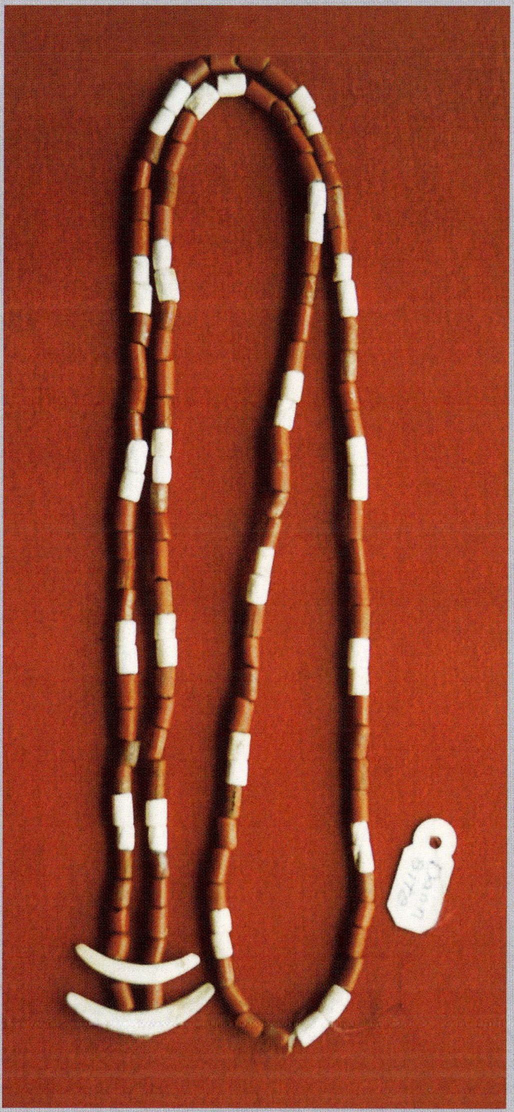

Seneca beads, ca. AD 1655 – 1675, necklace of white Dutch-made shell wampum beads (44, in good condition) with 90 redwood colored glass trade beads and two shell crescents. The necklace is 29" long and is from the Mendon area, Monroe County, New York. Dave Summers collection, Victor, New York. Crescents, **$75.00 – 150.00** each; wampum beads, all, **$100.00.**

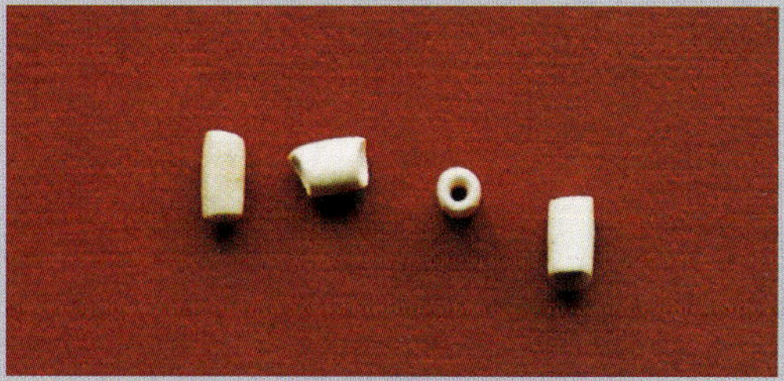

Seneca beads, Indian-made, stone-drilled, thick marine shell beads. The four together are 1½" long, ca. AD 1440 – 1600. Ex-collection Wray, the beads are from Ontario County, New York. Dave Summers collection, Victor, New York. Group, **$60.00.**

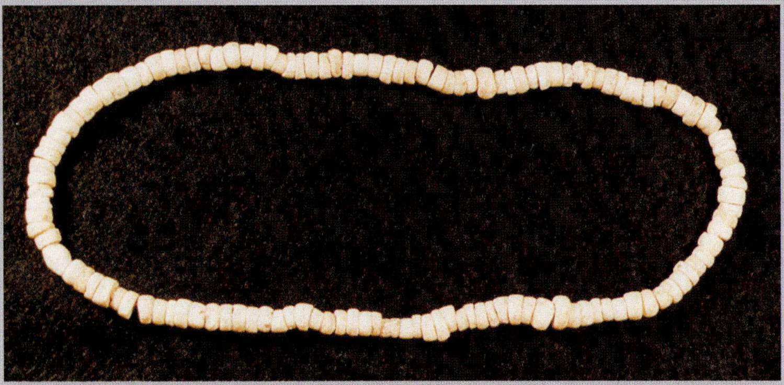

Shell bead necklace, Woodland to Mississippian periods, small discs cut and ground on both faces. The strand totals 16" long and was listed in the Vietzen sale catalog as being from the Pittsburgh, Pennsylvania area. Pete Timoch collection. **$200.00.**

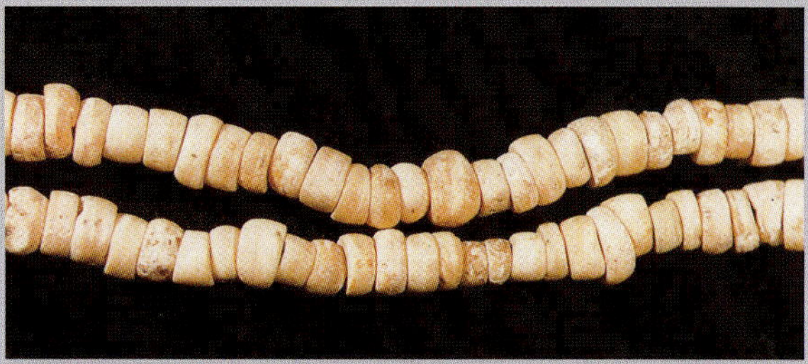

Closeup, of beads in the shell necklace from the Pittsburgh, Pennsylvania area (at left). The beads are quite attractive, being well shaped and polished. They have conical drilling from both faces and the shell retains density and weight. Pete Timoch collection. **$200.00.**

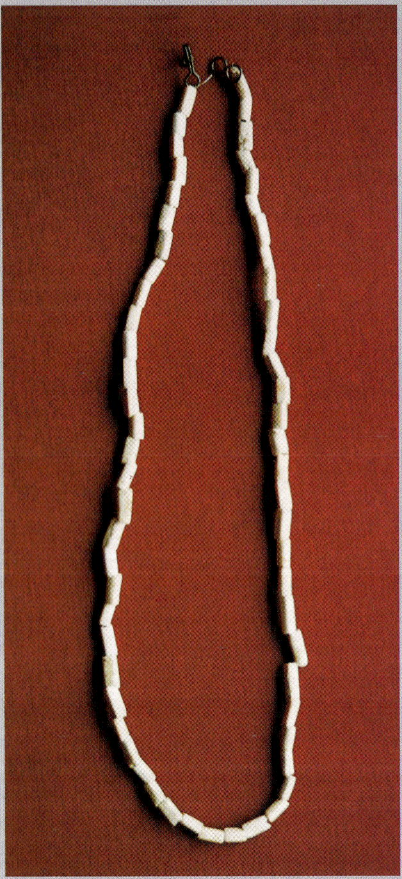

Seneca beads, Indian-made, stone-drilled, square cross-section marine shell, strand is 17" long They are ca. AD 1535 – 1640, ex-collection Wray, from Livingston County, New York. Dave Summers collection, Victor, New York. **$300.00.**

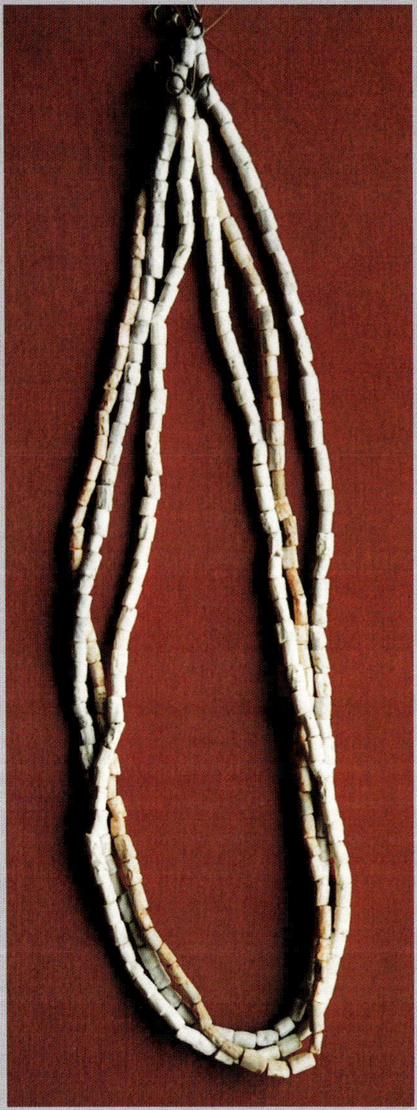

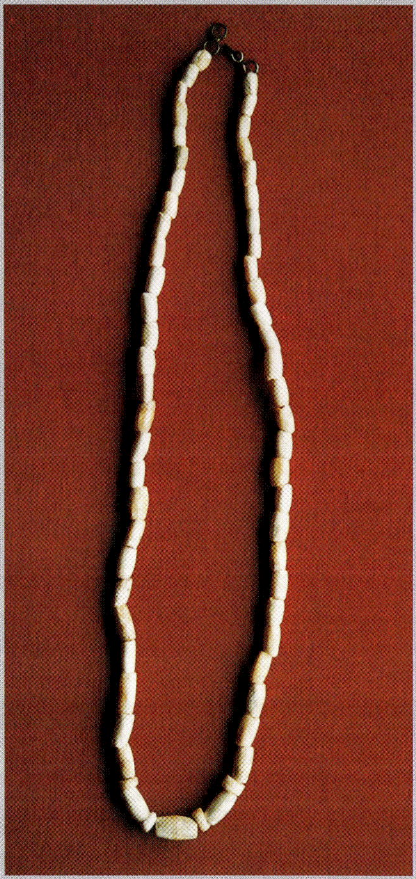

Seneca beads, Indian made, stone-drilled, barrel shape, white marine shell, rare. There are 61 beads and the strand is 17½" long. Ca. AD 1550 – 1590, they are ex-collection Wray. Livingston County, New York. Dave Summers collection, Victor, New York. **$400.00.**

Seneca common beads, lathe-turned, 1650 – 1820, tube-type wampum. There are three strings: 19" purple strand with 95 beads; 18" white strand with 92 beads; and, 18" strand with 85 rare white "War Beads" stained red. These tube beads are thin and short, steel-drilled, and not particularly well made. They are ex-collection Wray, from the Victor area, Ontario County, New York. Dave Summers collection, Victor, New York. Purple beads, **$120.00;** white beads, **$90.00;** red beads, **$250.00.**

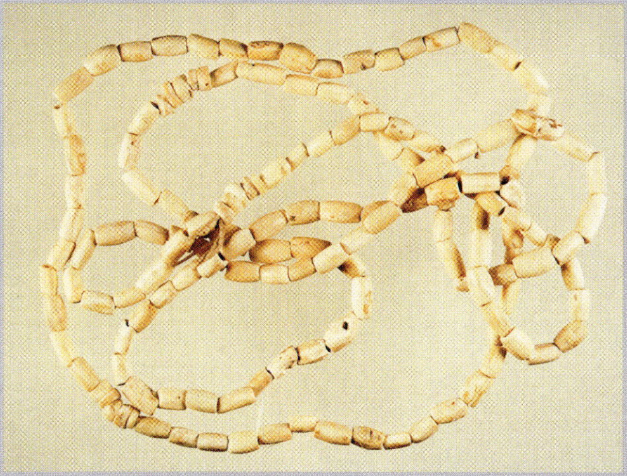

Bead strand, 22½" long, drilled shell. These were found in the Decatur area, Madison County, Alabama. Robin Fiser collection. **$175.00 – 200.00.**

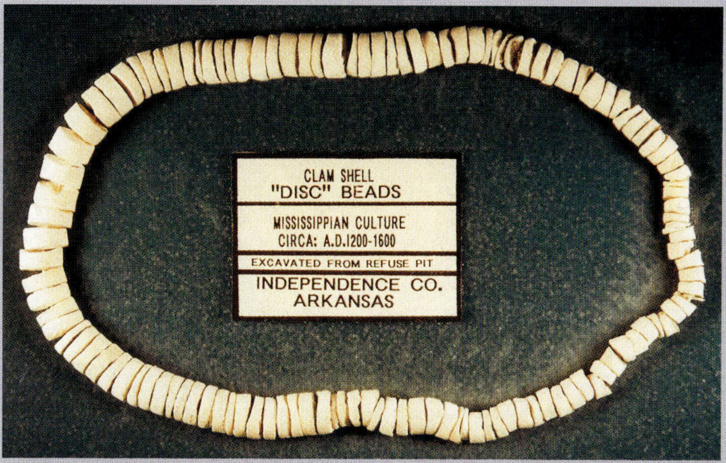

Disc beads, freshwater mussel shell, strand is about 10¼" long. These are Mississippian in time, and the beads are in graduated sizes. Independence County, Arkansas. Robin Fiser collection. Museum grade.

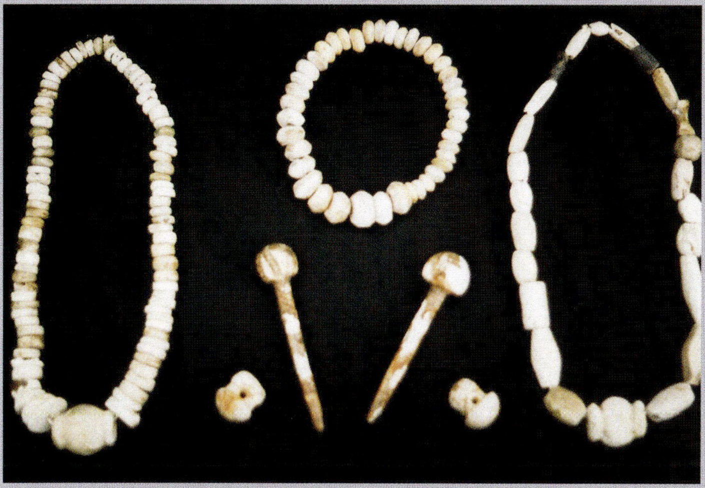

Shell artifacts, left and right strands, Mississippian period and found in Le Flore County, Oklahoma. At lower center are short ear plugs and long ear plugs or hairpins plus unusual rounded disc shell beads at top center. The plugs and beads are from Pemiscot County, Missouri. Bob Hess collection, Indiana. Museum grades.

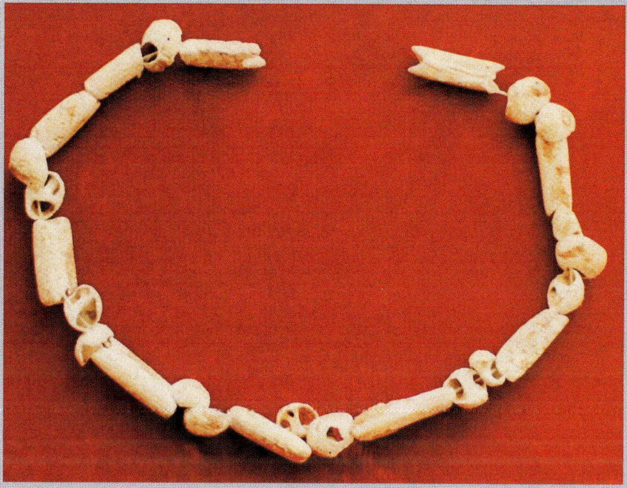

Bracelet, found by A. Scott, mixed bead types. These came from Brown County, Illinois. Tim Liehr collection, Illinois. Unlisted.

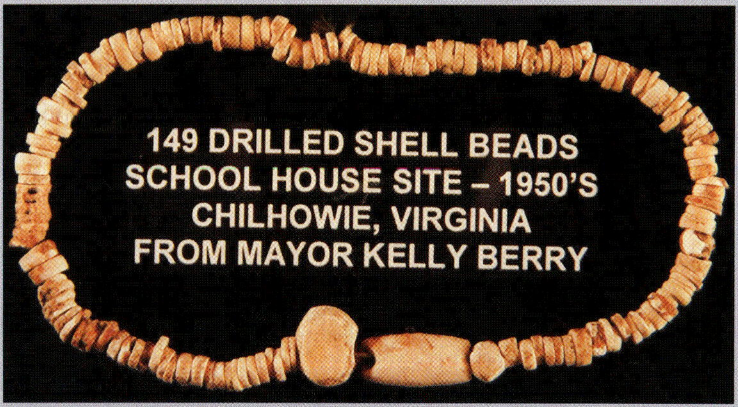

Shell beads, found on a Late Mississippian site in southwestern Virginia. Collection of, and photograph by, Ron Harris, North Carolina. All, **$200.00.**

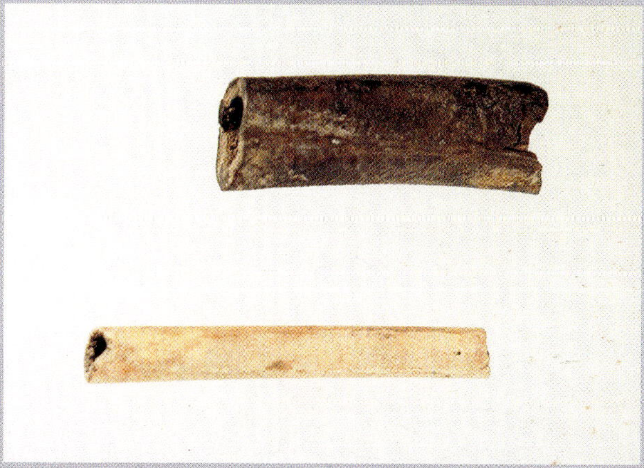

Beads, bird bones, longest is 1⅞". These illustrate the great difference in patina that may be present on bone artifacts. Ex-collection Hall, they are from Wayne County, Kentucky. Private collection. Each, **$4.00 – 6.00.**

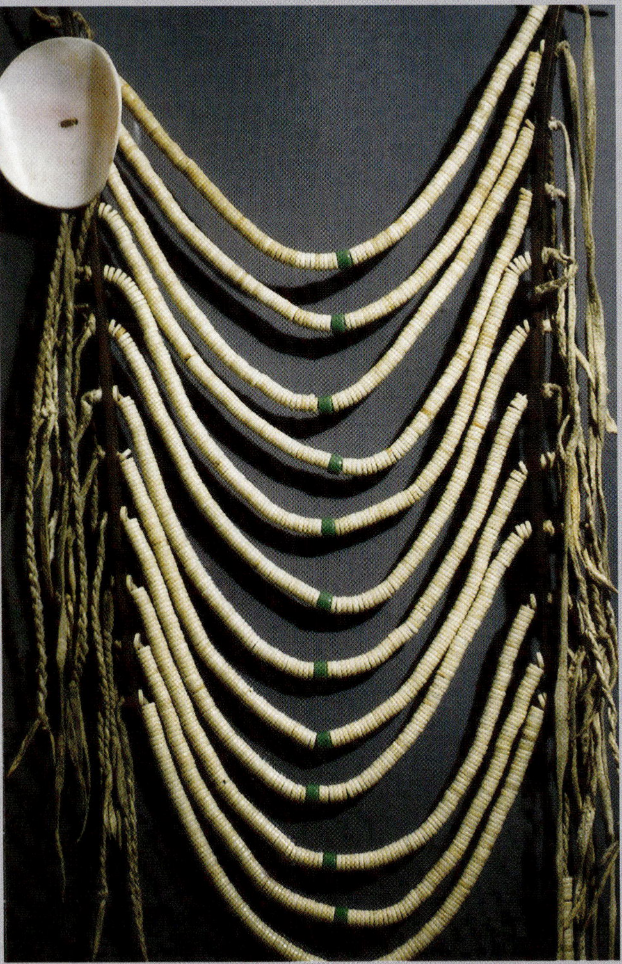

Crow Indian necklace, shell and trade beads strung on hide cords with heavy hide side strips. The bead strands total 143½" long. Made in the 1880s, it was formerly in the B. Van Landingham collection. H. B. Greene II photograph, Naples, Florida. Museum grade.

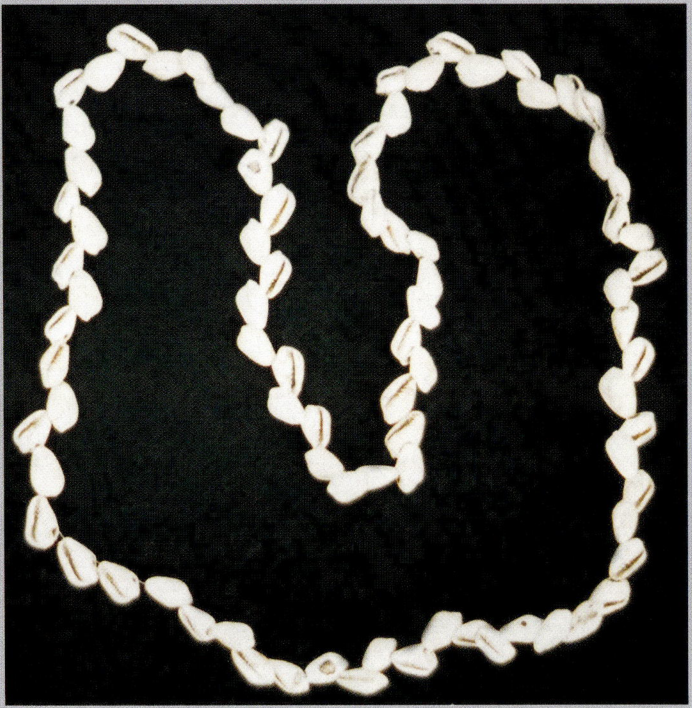

Olivella shell beads, drilled for attachment. All are Mississippian period, from Le Flore County, Oklahoma. Bob Hess collection, Indiana. Unlisted.

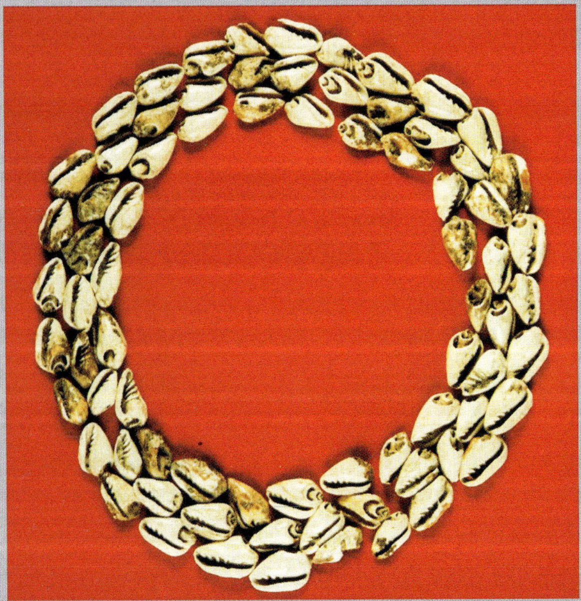

Small beads, grouping is 4" in diameter. These were found in West Virginia. Private collection. **$100.00.**

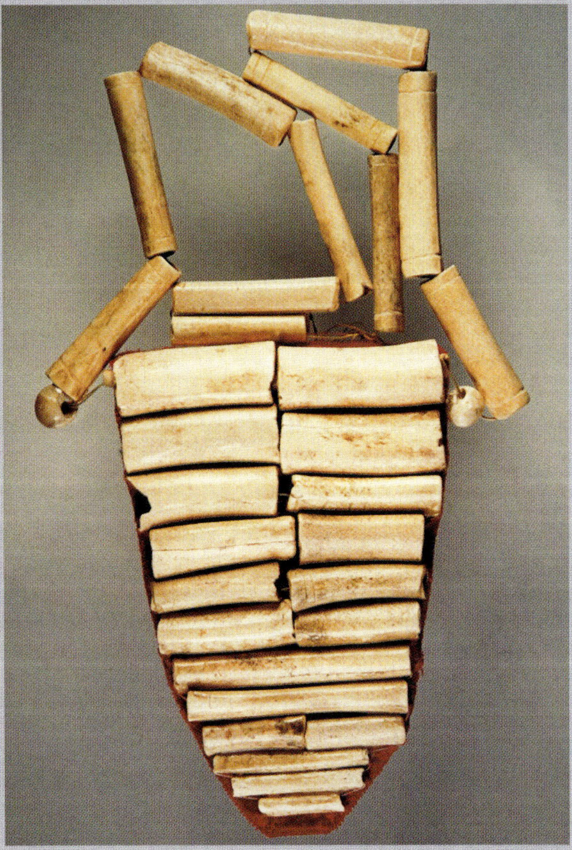

Beads, made from large animal bones, longest bead (sixth from bottom) is 2⅝". These were found by Mr. L. Tolliver, and came from a rock shelter near the Hocking-Perry County line, Ohio. Private collection. Museum grade.

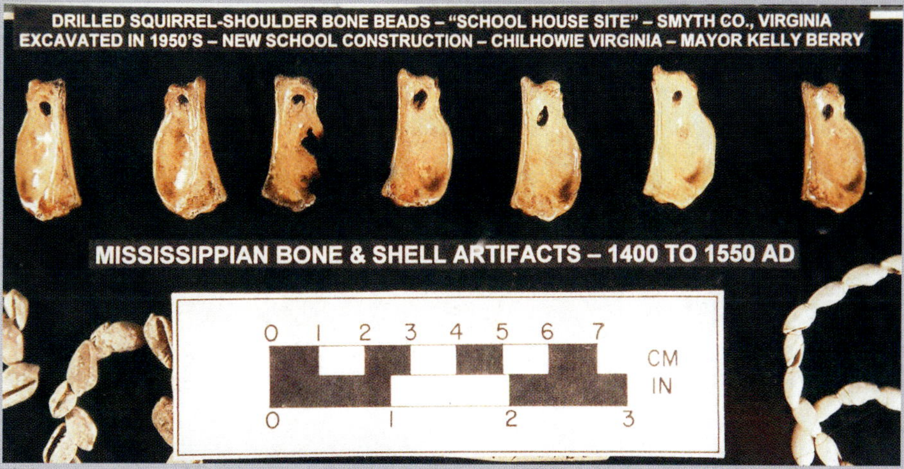

Bone beads or pendants, drilled squirrel shoulder bones, found in the 1950s during construction of a school. The shoulder bones are unusual artifacts, from the Mississippian period. Smythe County, Virginia. Collection of, and photograph by, Ron Harris, North Carolina. Bone beads, all seven, **$125.00.**

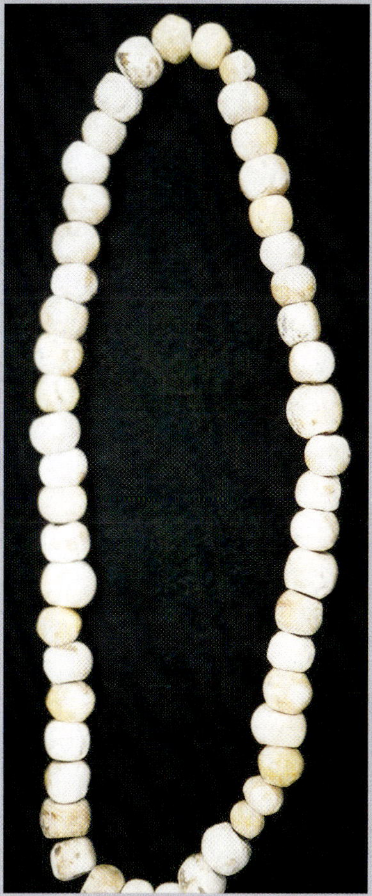

Beads, shell, large strand of rounded beads, good condition. These came from Pemiscot County, Missouri. Bob Hess collection, Indiana. Unlisted.

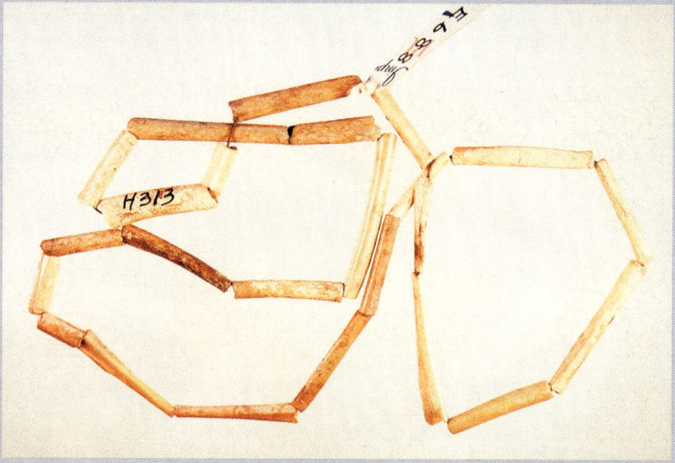

Necklace, bird bones, longest bead is 2". These are ex-collection Copeland, from southern Ohio. Fred Winegardner collection. Museum grade.

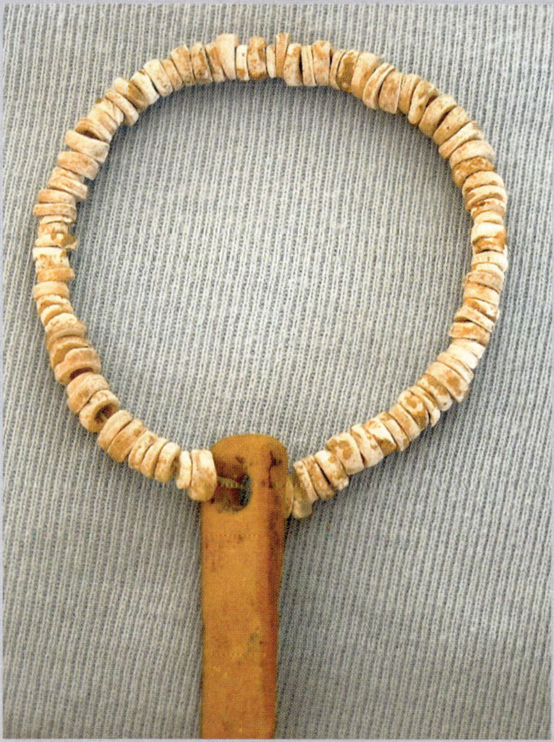

Bracelet, shell beads and stone pendant, strand 3¾" long. This was found near McNeal, Arizona. Rod Fuller collection, Nebraska. Unlisted.

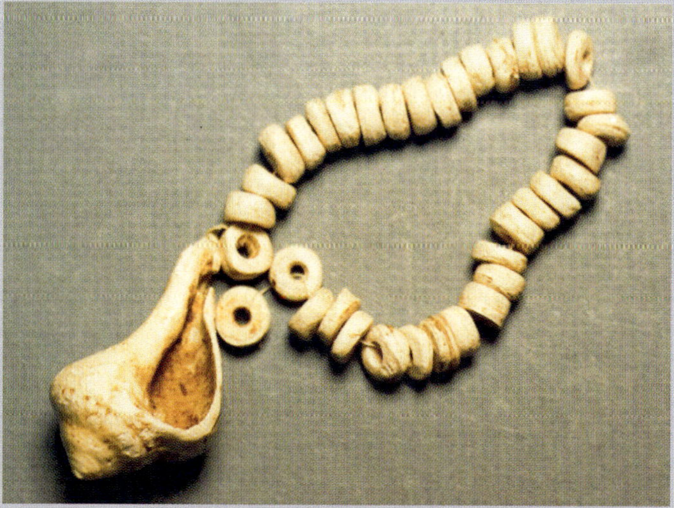

Necklace or bracelet, conch shell and bead, conch only is 1½" long, miniature form. Prehistoric, it has Mississippian Caddo influence, ca. AD 800 – 1350. Arkansas. Private collection. **$350.00.**

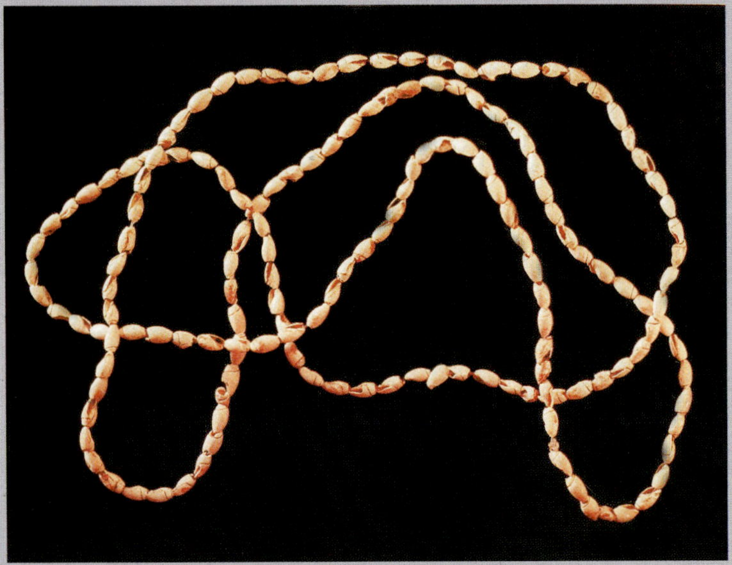

Marginella shell beads, found in the 1970s, ex-collection McCarn. Cabarrus County, North Carolina. Collection of, and photograph by, Ron Harris, North Carolina. **$200.00.**

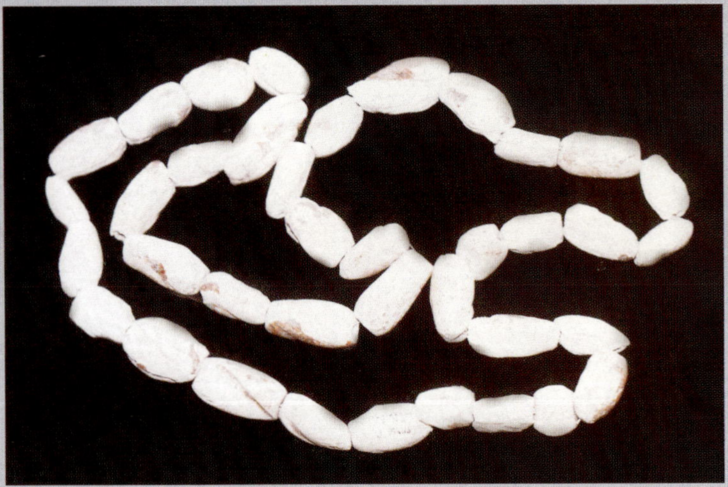

"Knobby" bead necklace, shell, 39" long, all beads drilled for suspension. The beads came from Davidson County, North Carolina. Jim Maus collection, North Carolina. Unlisted.

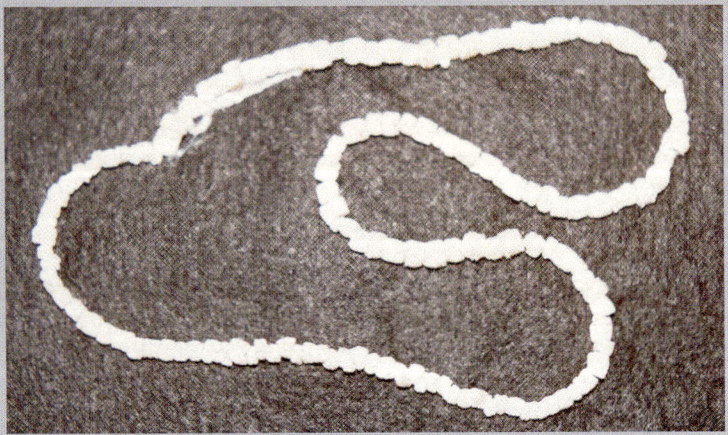

Necklace, fish vertebrate bones, 19" long. This necklace came from Macon County, Alabama. Jim Maus collection, North Carolina. Unlisted.

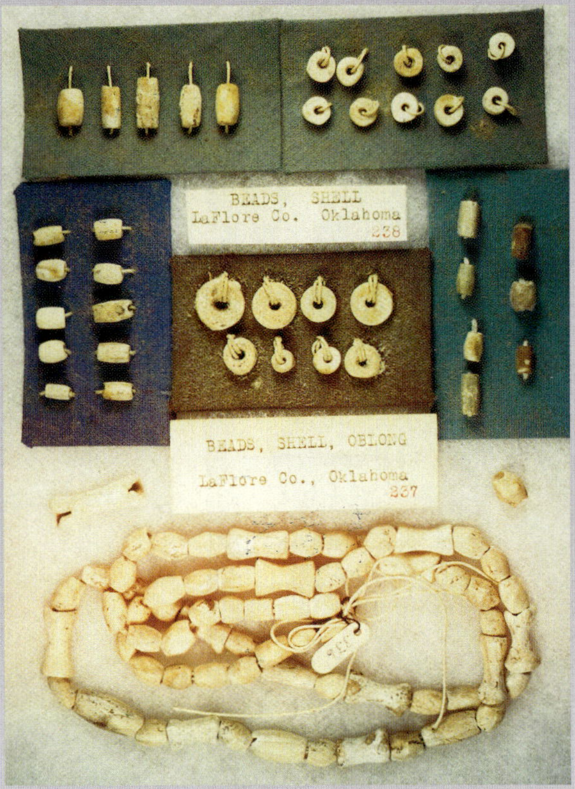

Shell beads, shapes including oblong, tubular, barrel, and disc. All are Mississippian period, from Le Flore County, Oklahoma. Lee Hallman collection, Pennsylvania. Unlisted.

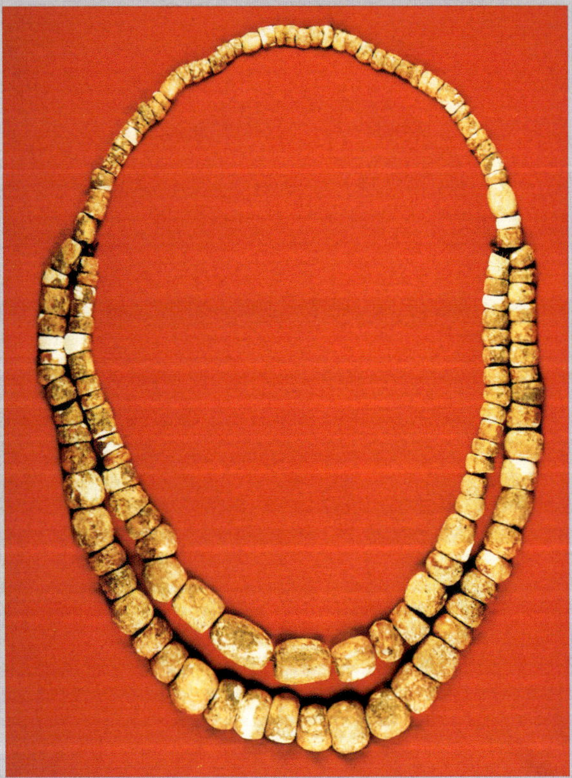

Marine shell beads, strand is 12" high as shown, material probably from the Gulf of Mexico. These were found in West Virginia. Private collection. Museum grade.

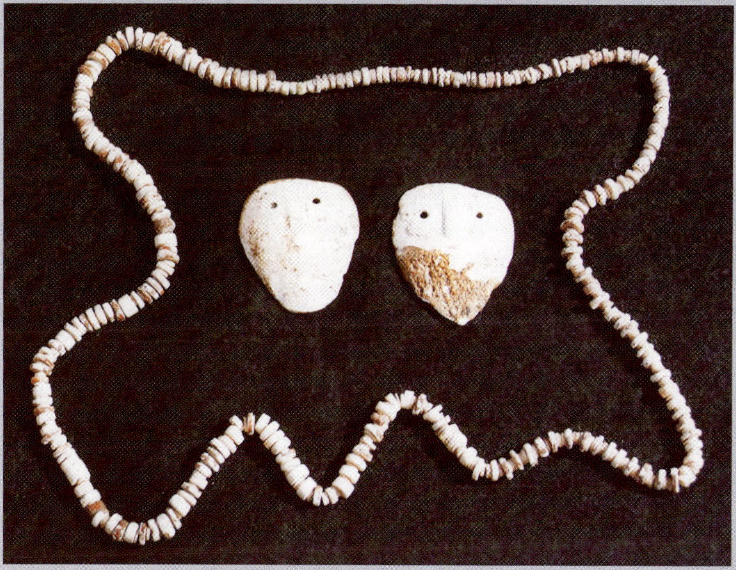

Shell face masks, Chicamauga style, with string of cut shell beads. The left gorget is 2¾6" high and the right gorget is 2⅝6" high. All were found together in Union County, Kentucky. Jim Maus collection, North Carolina. Museum grade.

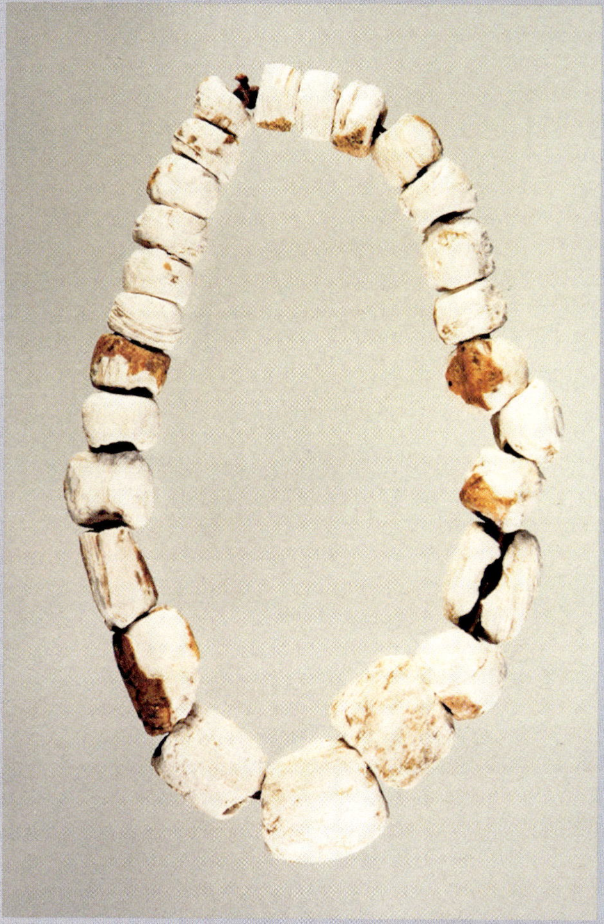

Marine shell beads, strand is 5", longest dimension as shown. These came from a site in West Virginia. Private collection. Unlisted.

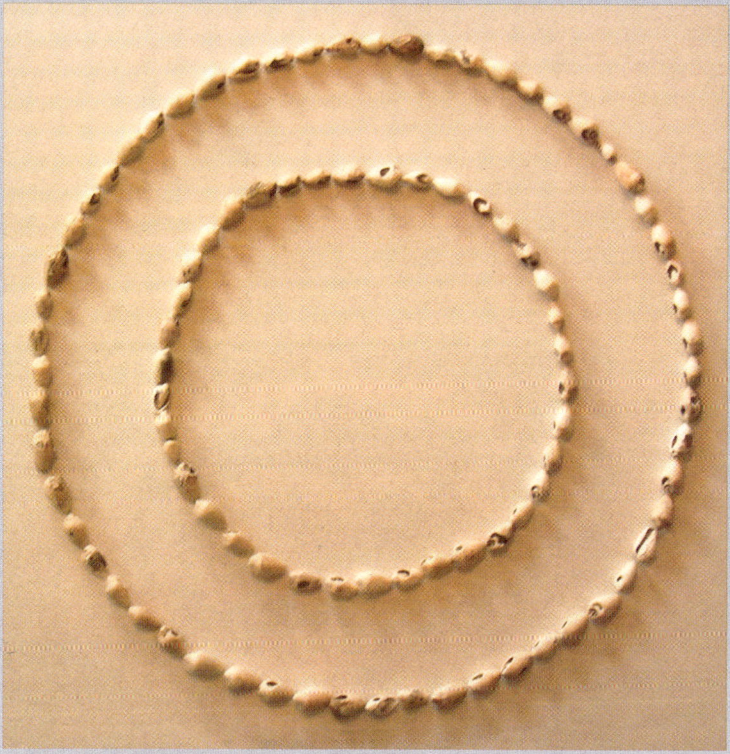

Marginella shell beads, outer strand is 26" long, inner strand is 14" long. Mississippian in time, the beads came from Mason County, West Virginia. Private collection; Rodney Roberts photograph. Shorter strand, **$80.00;** longer strand, **$150.00.**

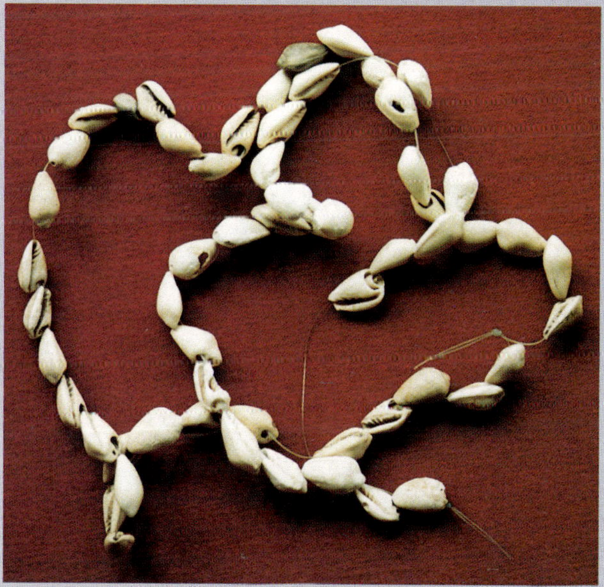

Anculosa shell beads, Point Peninsula, ca. AD 500 – 800. There are 58 shells, ground at the tips to create a small hole for stringing. The strand is 22" long, from Seneca County, New York. Dave Summers collection, Victor, New York. **$100.00.**

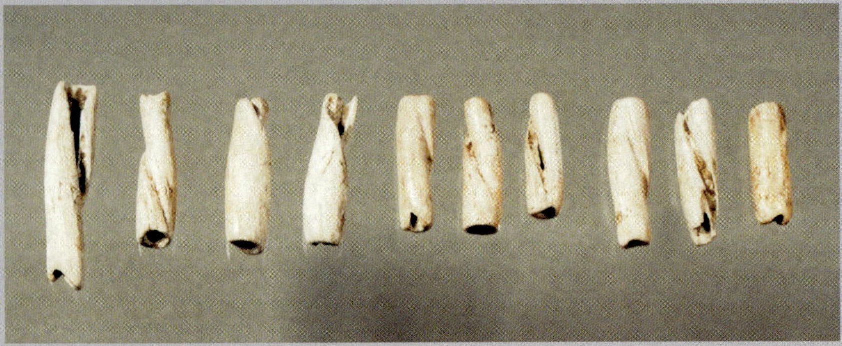

Tubular marine shell beads, sizes range 1 to 1½" long, Mississippian period ca. AD 800 – 1200. Obtained in far-flung trade arrangements, the shells were ground to shape and drilled. These beads are drilled from both ends and were found in a rock shelter in Tennessee. John Smith collection, Illinois. Each, **$10.00.**

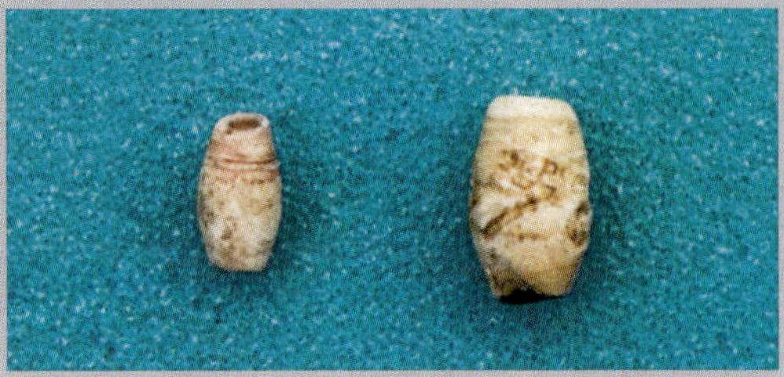

Shell beads, Woodland or later, smaller bead is 5/16" long and 1/8" in diameter. Harwood found these between 1954 and 1982. Origin unknown. Collection of, and photograph by, Gary Henry, North Carolina. Each, **$2.00 – 4.00.**

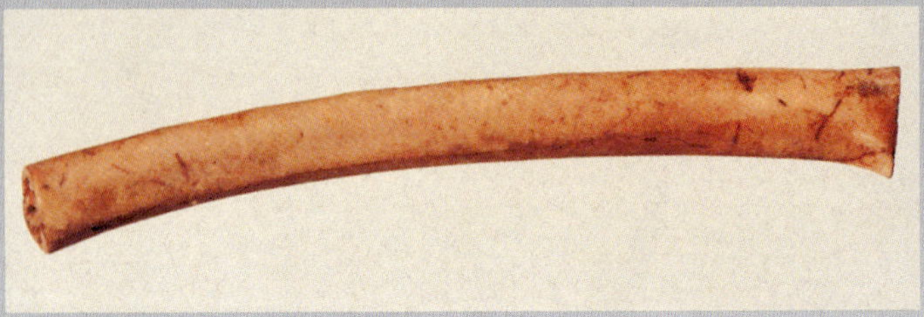

Bead or narrow handle, bird bone, 3¼" long. Both ends were ground off on this piece, found in Wayne County, Kentucky. Private collection. **$20.00 – 25.00.**

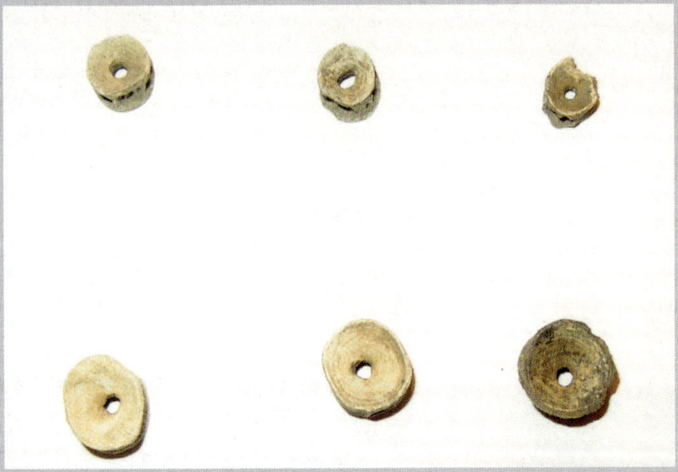

Bone beads, Mississippian period, largest ½" in diameter. They were found in Mason County, West Virginia. Private collection; Rodney Roberts photograph. Each, **$2.00 – 5.00.**

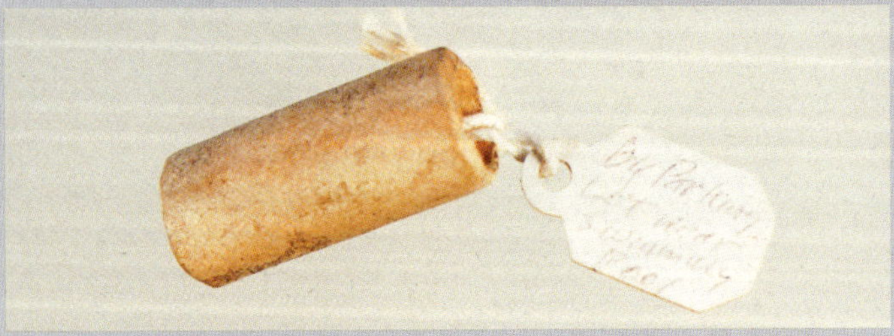

Bead, deer bone, 1¼" long. The tag reads "By parking lot near swimming pool." This is Mississippian, from southern Ohio. Fred Winegardner collection. **$15.00 – 20.00.**

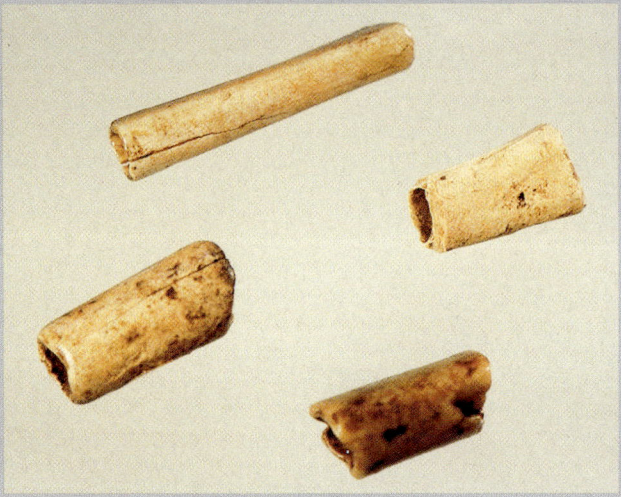

Bone beads, longest example is 1⅝". These were made from a variety of animal bones, and all are from West Virginia. Doug Hooks collection. Each, **$12.00 – 15.00.**

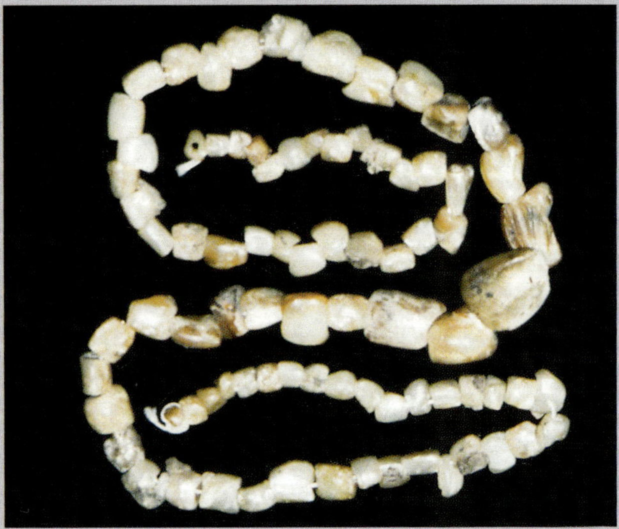

Pearl bead strand, Hopewell and Middle Woodland, graduated sizes. This rare strand is ex-collections Dickson and Fraser, and it has a Berner COA. The beads were found in Fulton County, Illinois. Joseph Sulka collection, Illinois. Museum grade.

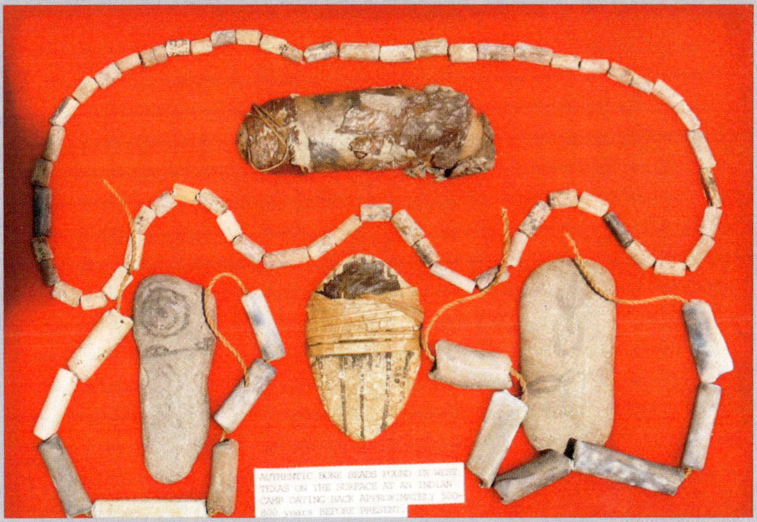

Turkey bone beads, found on a late prehistoric site. These came from western Texas. John and Susan Mellyn collection, Texas. Beads only, **$300.00.**

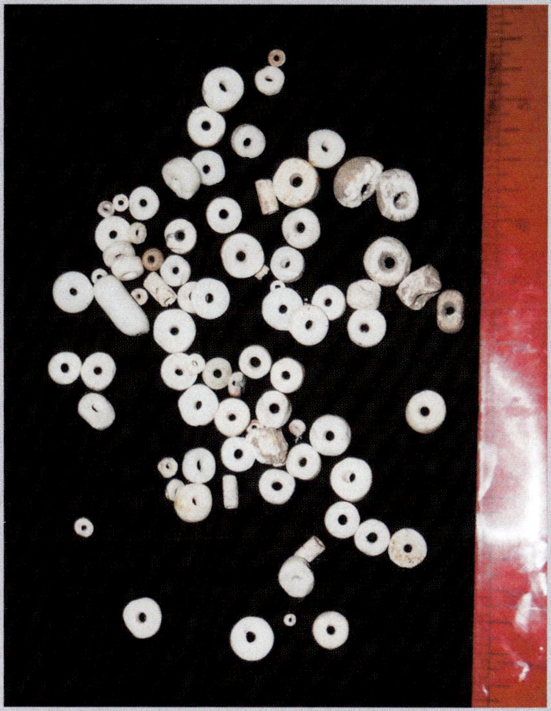

Drilled shell beads, sizes as indicated. All were found in Virginia. Private collection. Each, **$1.00.**

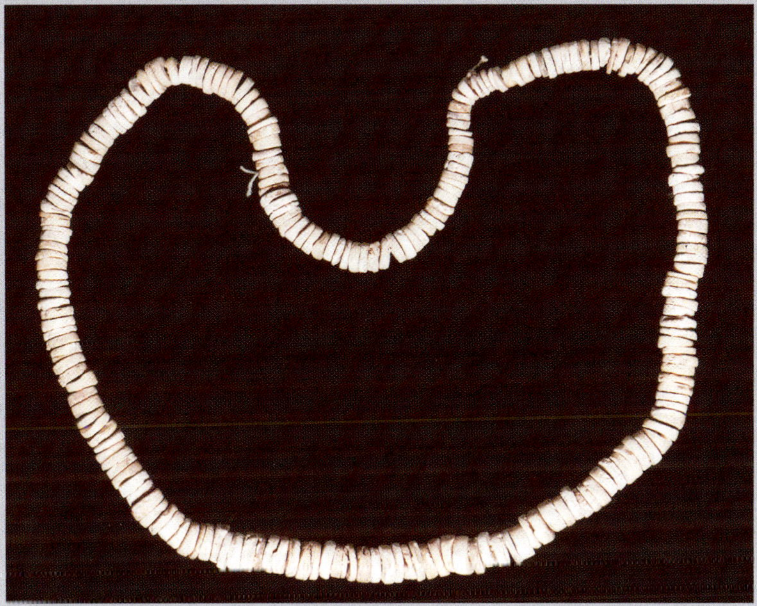

Clamshell bead necklace, 36" long, beads are 7mm to 13mm. in diameter and up to 5mm thick. Drilled, about one-fourth of them have polished edges and the remainder have edges that are weathered dull. Oklahoma. Private collection. Museum grade.

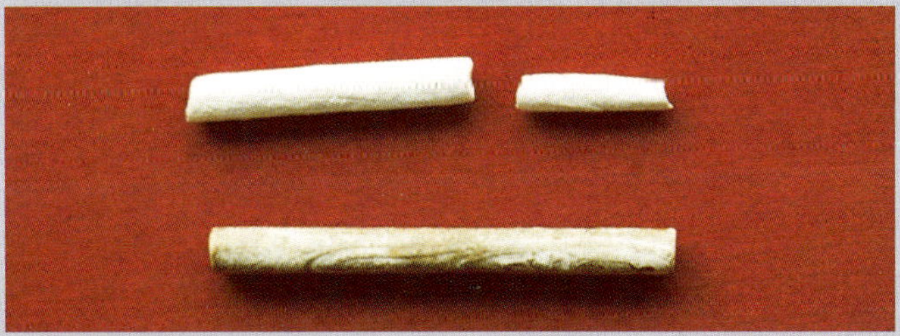

Seneca marine shell "Hair Pipe" beads, mid-sixteenth century, long steel-drilled tubes. These were manufactured commercially by Dutch settlers in Bergen County, New Jersey. Lengths are ⅞", 1½", and 2⅜". Ontario County, New York. Dave Summers collection, Victor, New York. Short, **$2.00;** medium, **$5.00;** long, **$15.00.**

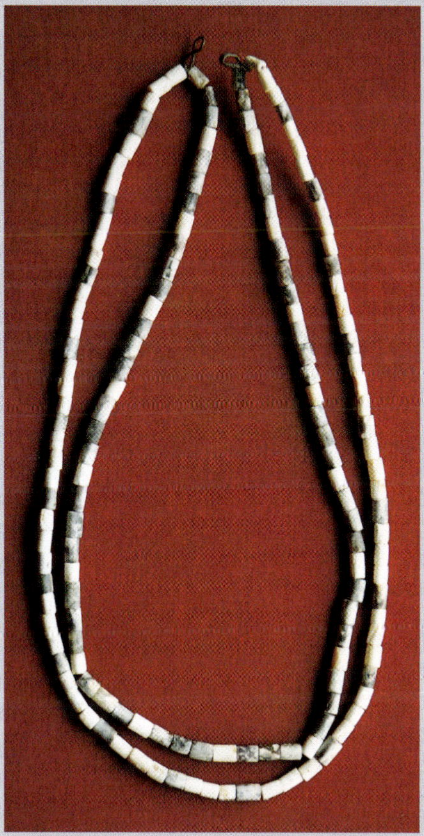

Seneca wampum beads, Dutch-made on Long Island, ca. 1620 – 1730, steel-drilled and polished. True wampum type beads, the two strings have 80 purple and 80 white beads. Each string is 35" long and they are from the Mendon area, Monroe County, New York. Dave Summers collection, Victor, New York. Each, **$400.00.**

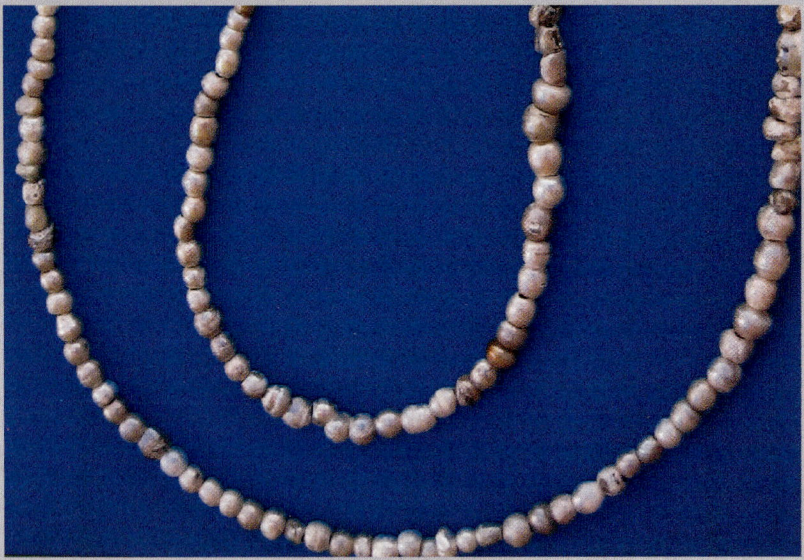

Freshwater pearl beads, strand is 40½" long. The strand has a Perino COA and it contains 255 beads. The beads were found in 1934 and are ex-collections Hathcock, Milsap, Bowen, Stevens and Arbeiter; they were obtained by the owner in 2003. These pearl beads are in fine condition and still retain much of their original lustre. Le Flore County, Oklahoma. William Hamner collection, Alabama. Strand, **$2,000.00.**

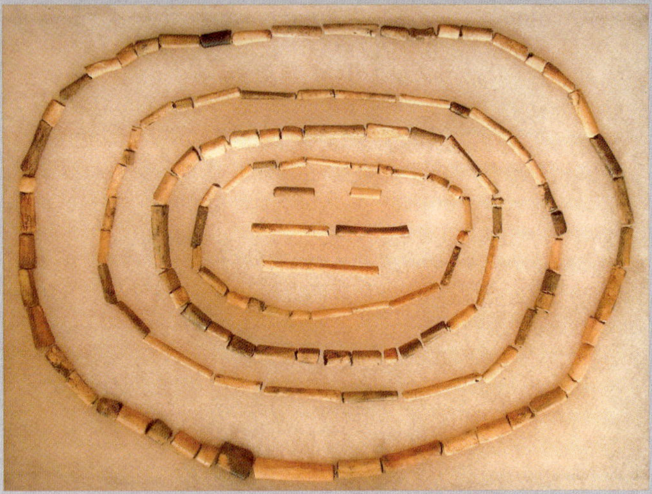

Bone beads, Mississippian period, longest bead is 3⅛". Total length of the beads shown is 128¾". Cabell and Mason Counties, West Virginia. Private collection; Rodney Roberts photograph. Each bead, **$5.00 – 35.00.**

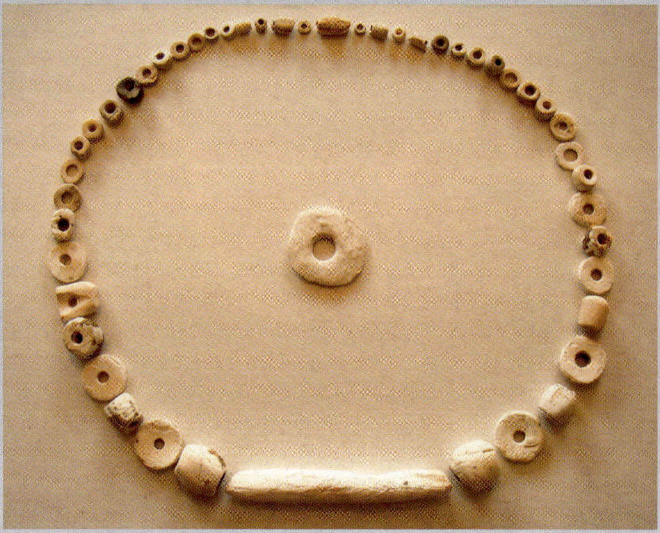

Shell beads, Mississippian period, longest bead (bottom center) is 2⁹⁄₁₆". Total length of all beads is 20", and these consist of shell disc and conch shell forms with disc bead at center measuring 1" across. These were found on Ohio River sites in Cabell and Mason Counties, West Virginia. Private collection. Rodney Roberts photograph. All beads shown, **$175.00.**

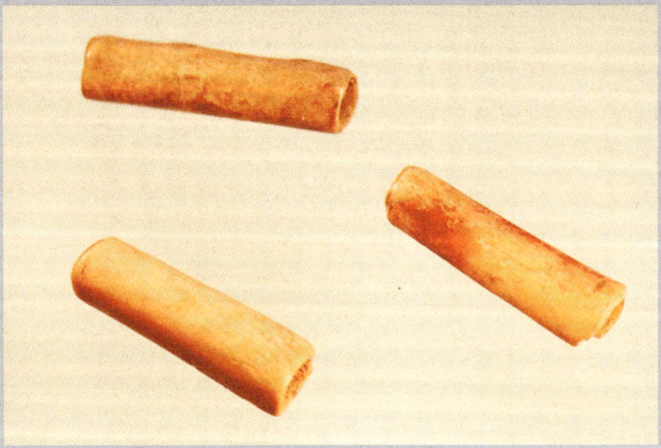

Deer bone beads, hollowed for length, surfaces polished. They average 1³⁄₁₆" in length and were found in southern Ohio. Fred Winegardner collection. Each, **$15.00 – 20.00.**

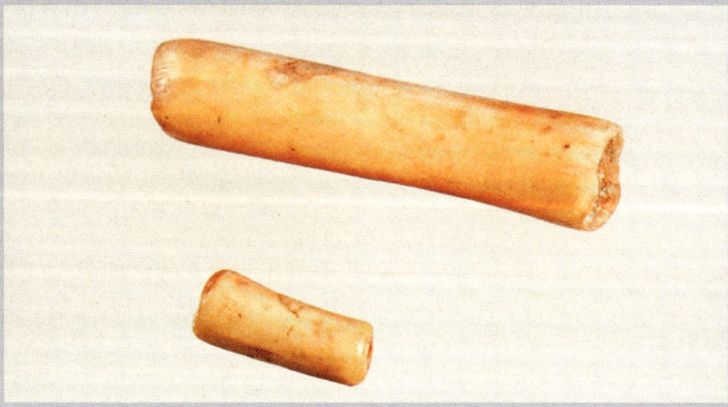

Hollowed deer bone beads, highly polished surfaces. These show the size range usually found, though some are much larger. The longest is 2⅛" and they were collected in 1938. Southern Ohio. Fred Winegardner collection. Large, **$25.00**. Small, **$10.00.**

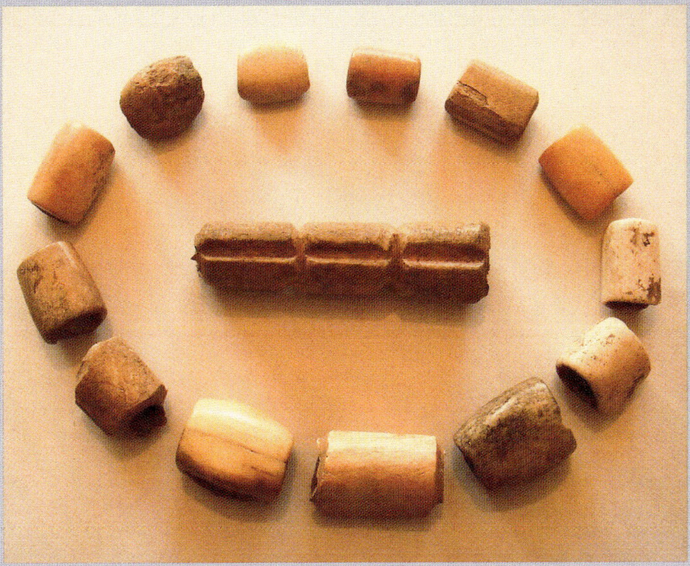

Bone beads, Mississippian, probably deer bone. The beads are ½ to 2⅞" long. At center is a good example of how beads were made by grooving individual beads from a section of bone. Cabell and Mason Counties, West Virginia. Private collection; Rodney Roberts photograph. Beads, each, **$10.00 – 15.00;** bead preform or blank, **$30.00.**

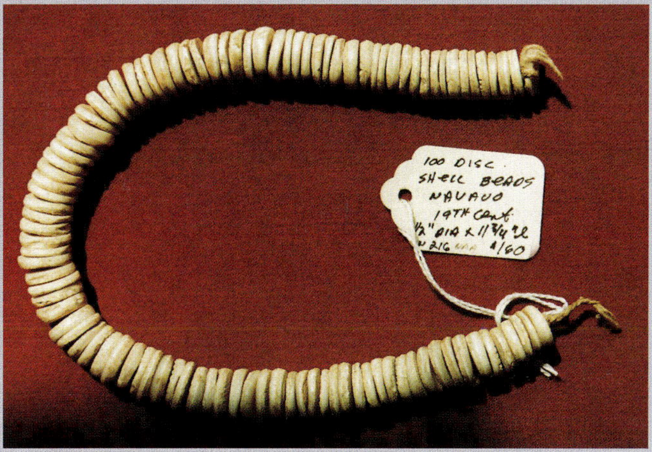

Shell disc beads, Navaho and 1800s, strand is 11¾" long. The 100 beads are thick and ½" in diameter. Origin unknown, but Southwestern. Dave Summers collection, Victor, New York. **$160.00.**

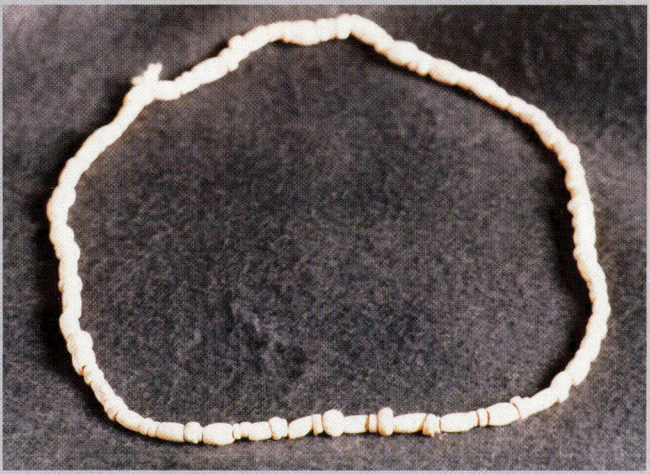

Beads, shell barrel and disc types, find-site unknown but probably Midwestern. John F. Wubker collection, Illinois. **$225.00.**

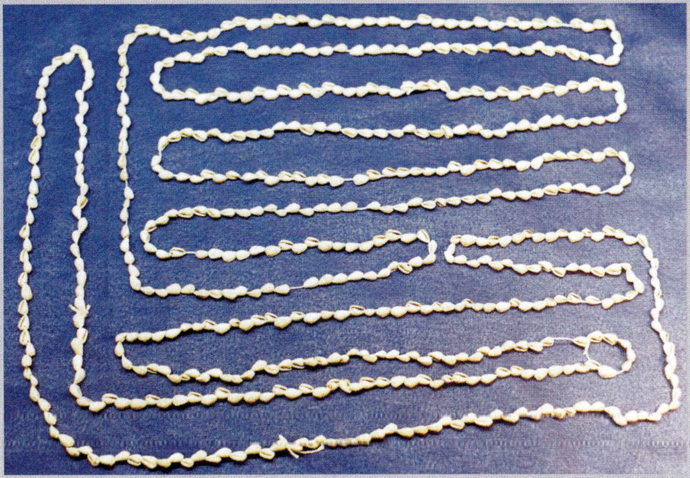

Bead strand, shell, the photograph shows only half of the original find, which measured 19 feet 6" long. The beads came from Peoria County, Illinois. Fred Smith collection, Illinois. Unlisted.

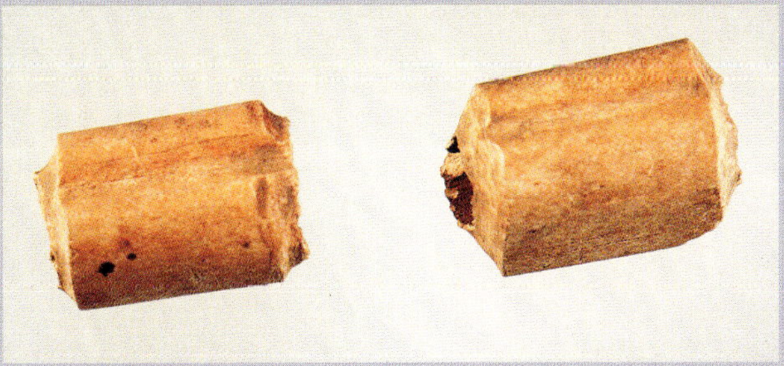

Bone beads, probably elk bone, longest is 1⅜". Cutting bone sections into bead-size pieces made these artifacts. West Virginia. Doug Hooks collection. Each, **$15.00 – 20.00.**

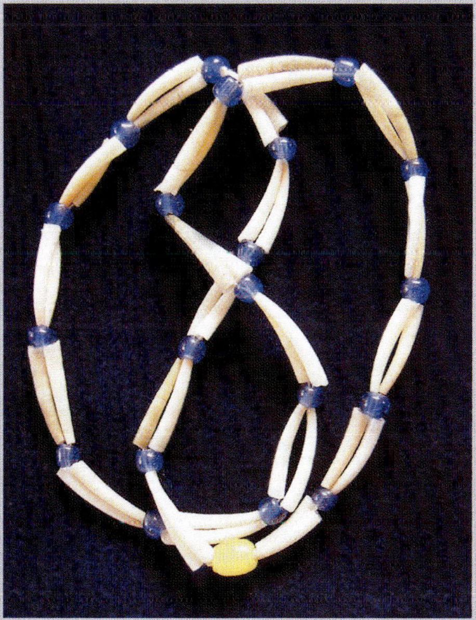

Dentalium shell necklace with Padre beads, historic period. The necklace came from the Great Basin, Nevada. Victor T. Trujillo collection, Nevada. Museum grade.

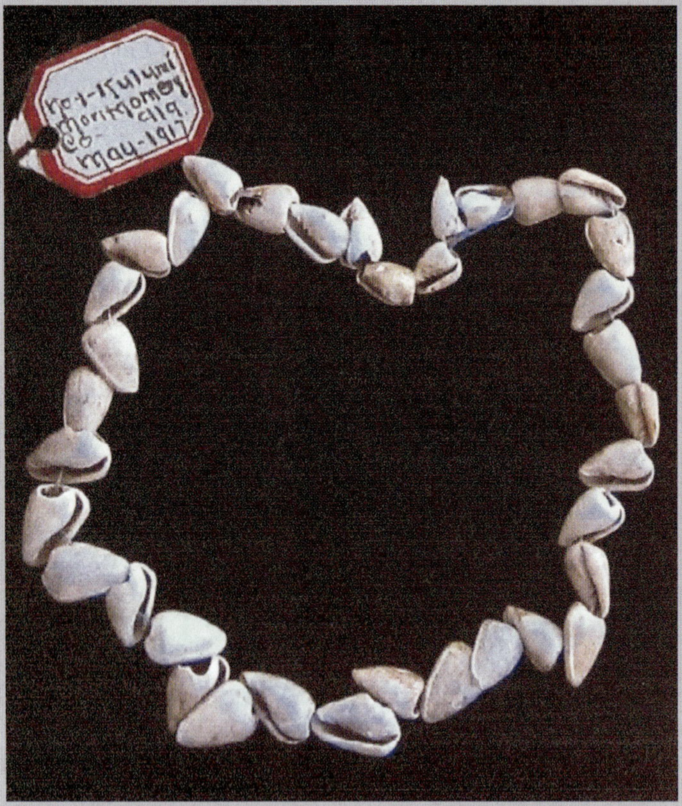

Marginella shell beads, strand is 6" long. Found in May of 1917 by members of the Alabama Anthropological Society. The old tag indicates the beads were found at Kulumi, an Upper Creek town on the Tallapoosa River near old Ware's Ferry. The strand is ex-collection Vietzen and was acquired by the owner in 1998. Montgomery County, Alabama. William Hamner collection, Alabama. Strand, **$80.00.**

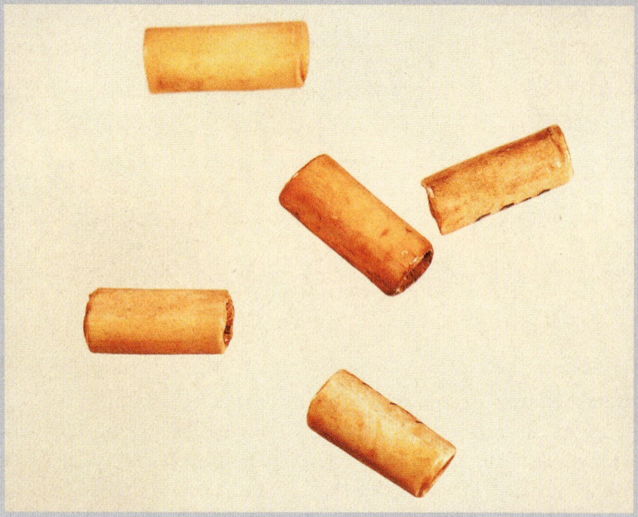

Beads, hollowed deer bones, average length is ⅞". These were found in 1938 at a Fort Ancient site in southern Ohio. Fred Winegardner collection. Each, **$10.00 – 15.00.**

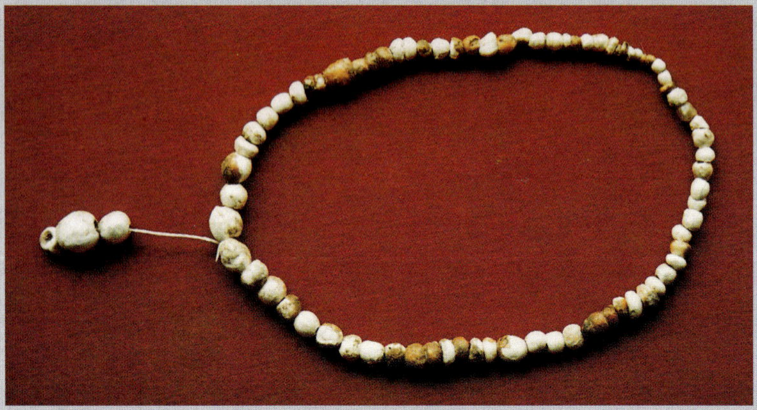

Freshwater mussel pearls, rare, Mississippian period, ca. AD 1000, strand is 12" long. There are 81 drilled beads, found near Elizabethton, Carter County, Tennessee. Dave Summers collection, Victor, New York. **$1,600.00.**

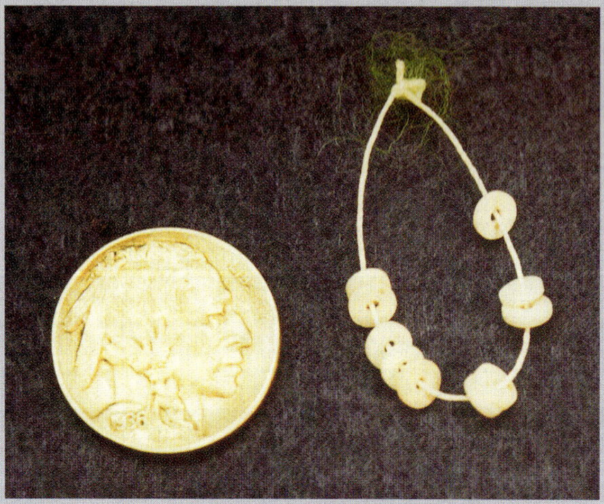

Shell beads, 5/32" in diameter, carefully shaped and polished. They were found about a dozen years ago and were collected from ant hills at village sites. Used for decorating clothing, up to 2500 beads have been found in one ant hill. Mandan, the beads are from South Dakota. Fred Smith collection, Illinois. All, **$20.00.**

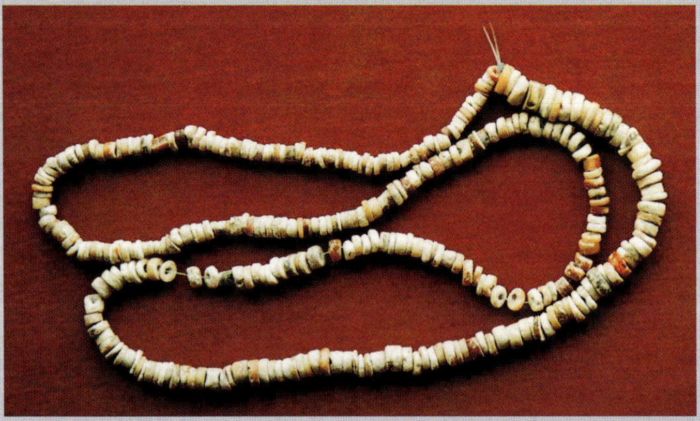

Seneca/Erie disc beads, marine shell and a few made of coral, strand is 20¾" long. They are sixteenth century and the 280-plus beads have traces of copper salts. Western New York. Dave Summers collection, Victor, New York. **$150.00.**

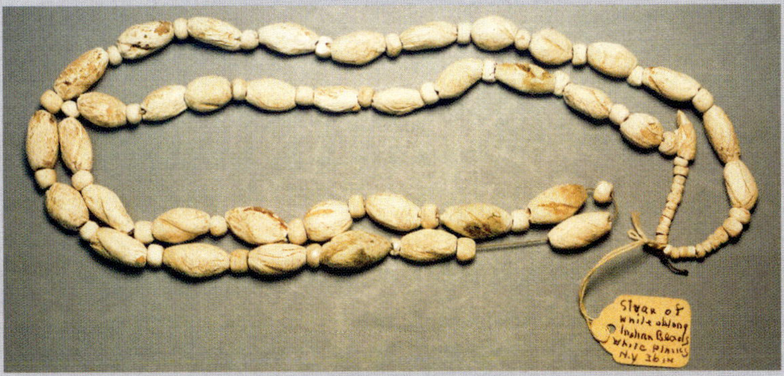

Beads, shell and freshwater pearl, strand is over 36" long, probably Late Woodland period. The beads were found near White Plains, New York. Private collection. **$300.00.**

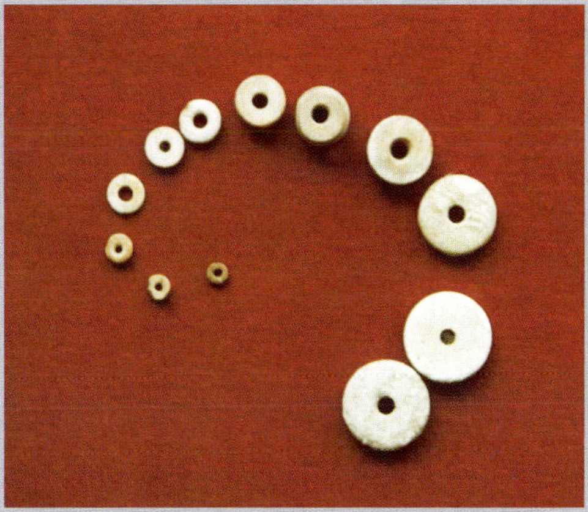

Mixed shell beads, Adena, Hopewell, Owasco, Iroquois (ca. 500 BC – AD 1650). Size range is ⅛ to 9⁄16". Western New York. Dave Summers collection, Victor, New York. Group, **$15.00.**

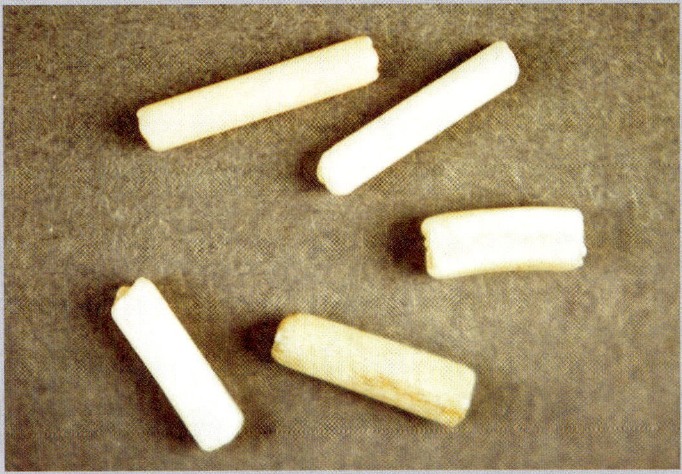

Tubular beads, made of bird bone, longest is 1⅛". With slightly rounded ends, all were found near Willow Grove, West Virginia. Larry Garvin collection. Each, **$10.00.**

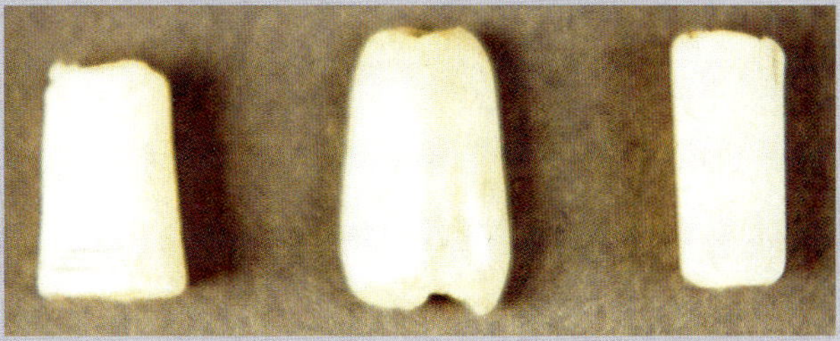

Bone beads, cut and polished, longest is ⅞". These were found near Willow Grove, West Virginia. Larry Garvin collection. Each, **$10.00.**

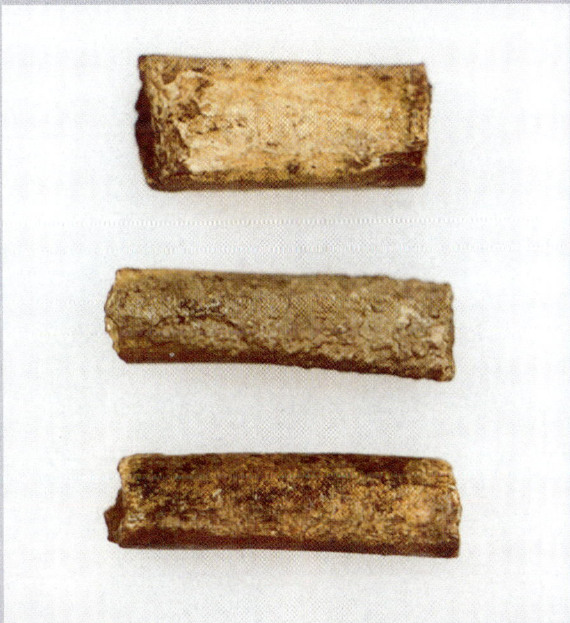

Tool handles, Late Archaic to Woodland, different materials. Top, antler; middle and bottom, bone. Longest is 2⅝". The antler artifact has tapered holes that meet near the center, while the bone handles have end-to-end holes. Ex-collection Vietzen, Christian County, Kentucky. Pete Timoch collection. Each, **$75.00 – 100.00.**

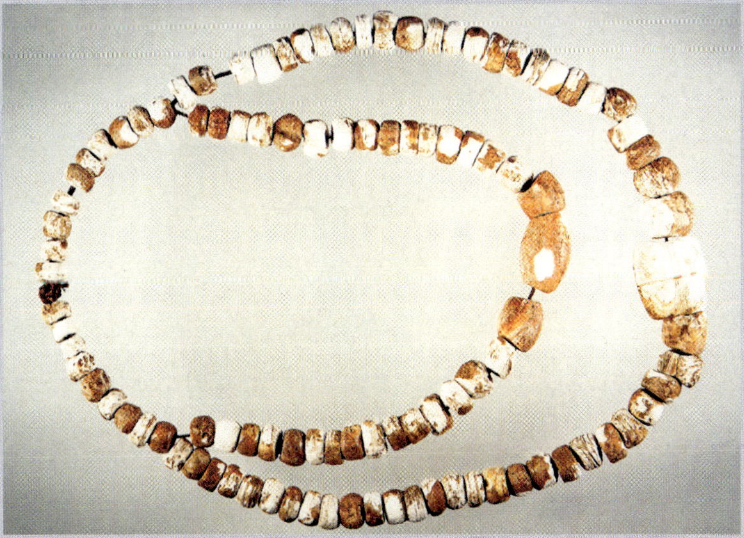

Marine shell beads, strand (as shown) is about 12" long. The large beads were found in West Virginia. Private collection. Museum grade.

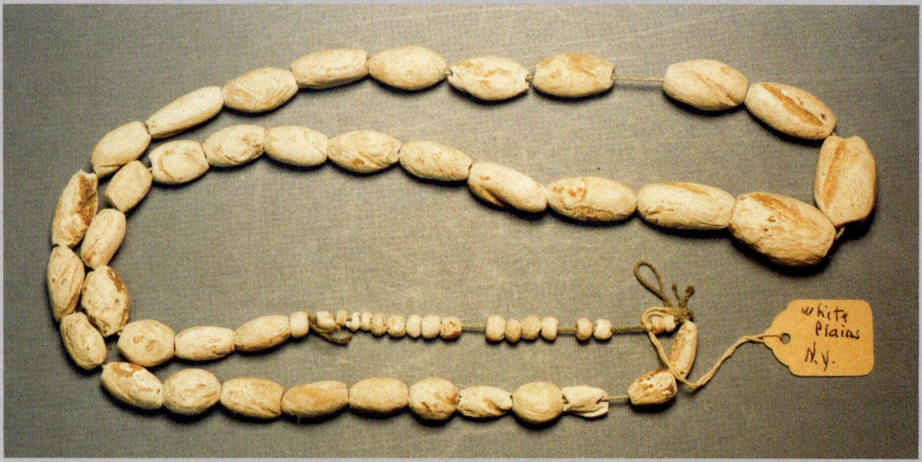

Beads, graduated sizes, strand is over 34" long. Probably Late Woodland, it was found near White Plains, New York. Private collection. **$250.00.**

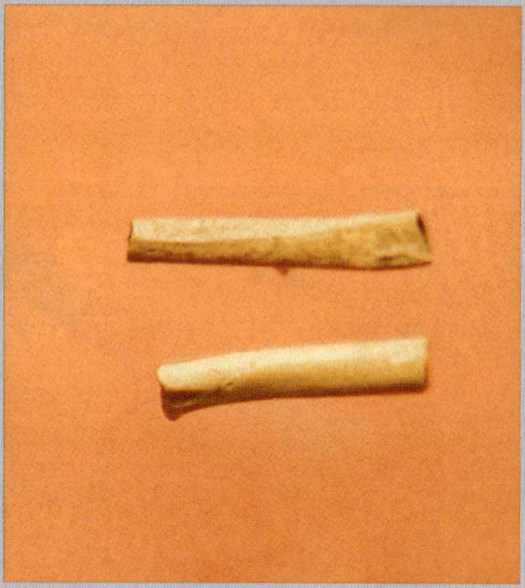

Tubular beads, bird bones, average length is 1¼" long. They are Lamoka phase, Middle Archaic, and were found in Schuyler County, New York. Dave Summers collection, Victor, New York. Each, **$50.00.**

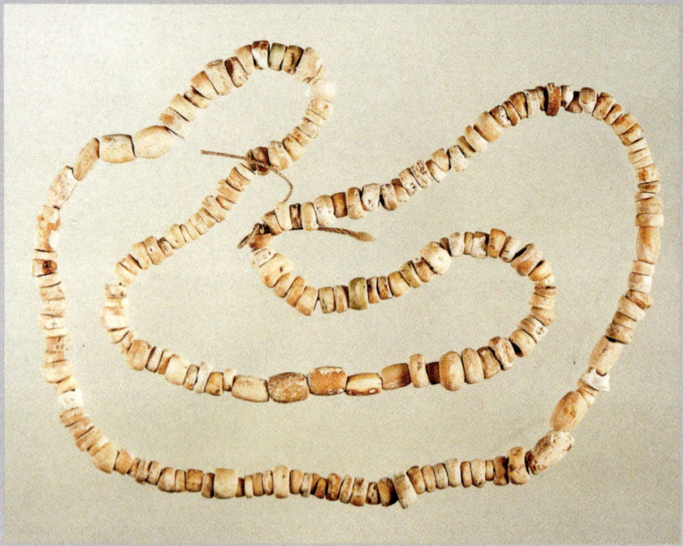

Freshwater mussel shell beads, strand is 23" long, barrel-type. The disc and beads came from the Ohio Valley in southern Indiana. Private collection. **$125.00.**

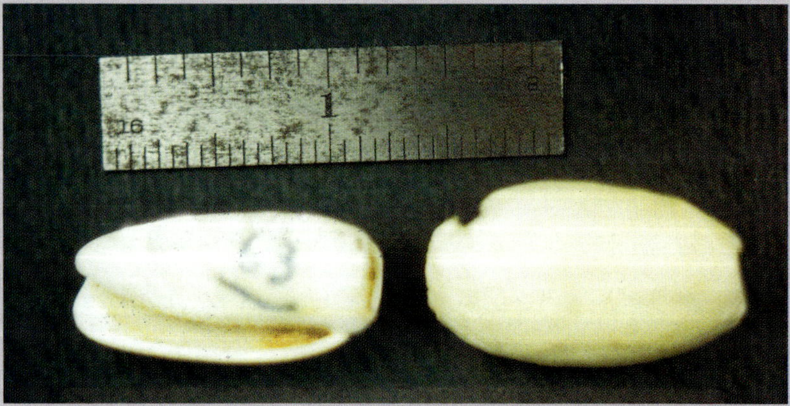

Olivella shell beads, fine condition. Lee Hallman collection, Pennsylvania. Unlisted.

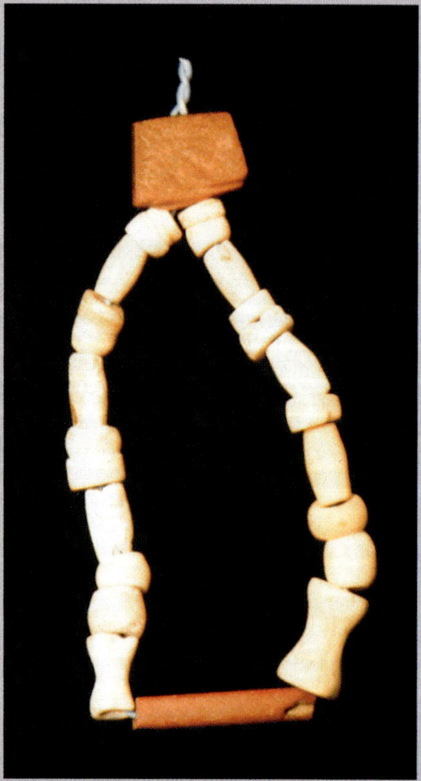

Beads, various shapes including disc, barrel, and hourglass, strand is 5" long. In fine condition, they were found in New York state. Tom Sekula collection, Pennsylvania. Strand, **$100.00.**

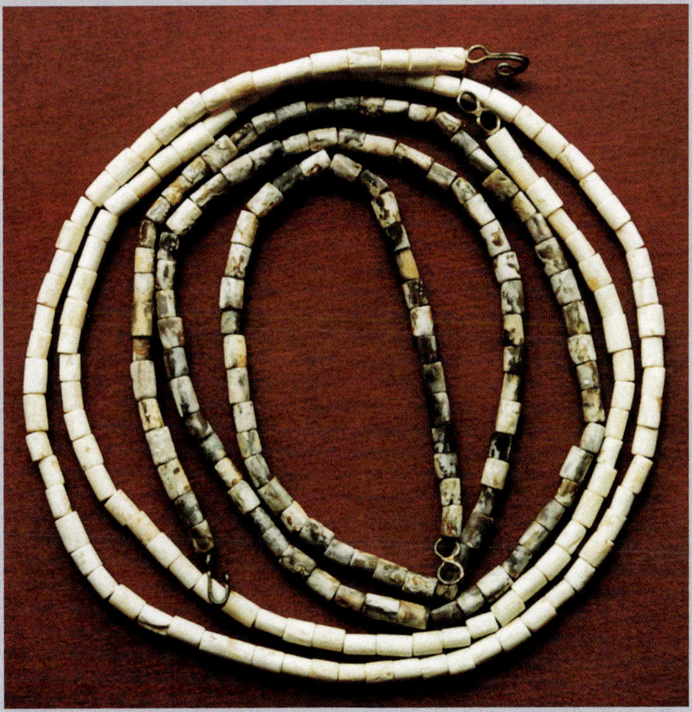

Seneca wampum beads, Dutch-made on Long Island, ca. 1620 – 1730. These are thick and long steel-drilled tube beads, well made and polished. These are the true wampum type, used to make wampum belts. The two strings are 57" long; one has 111 purple beads and one has 128 white beads. Ex-collection Wray, they are from the Mendon area, Monroe County, New York. Dave Summers collection, Victor, New York. Each, **$600.00.**

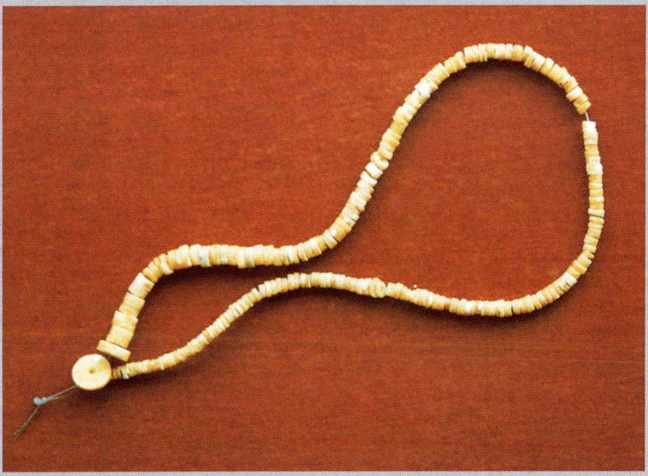

Seneca/Erie disc beads, thin marine shell, sixteenth century, stained orange. The 200-plus beads are 1/16 to 1/4" in diameter and the strand is 9½" long. Western New York. Dave Summers collection, Victor, New York. **$100.00.**

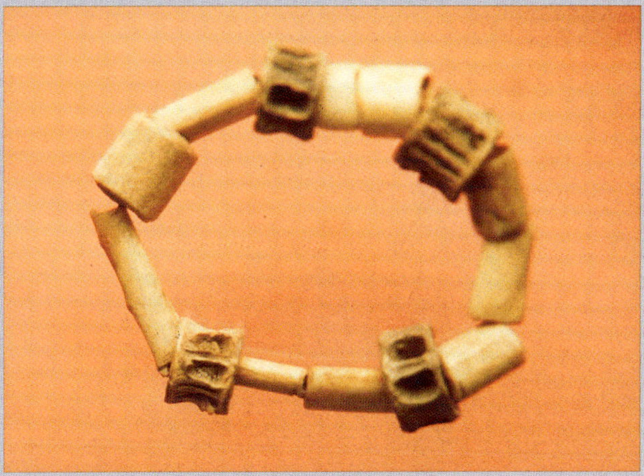

Beads, Lamoka phase of the Middle Archaic, strand is 6" long. The smooth beads are made of bird bone; the others are fish vertebra beads. They were found in Schuyler County, New York. Dave Summers collection, Victor, New York. Strand, **$100.00.**

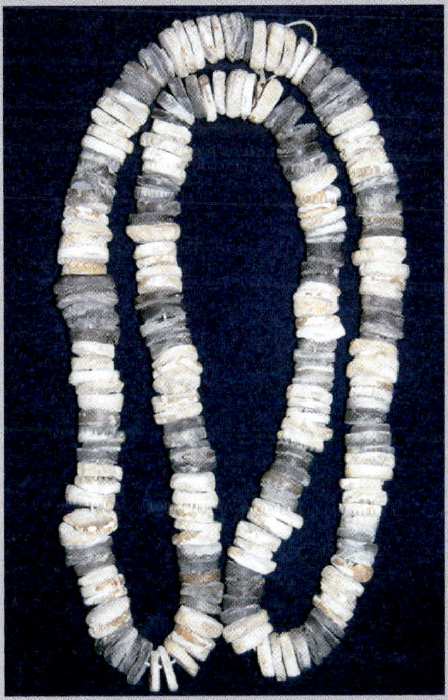

Disc beads, clamshell, strand 32" long. The beads, in two colors, are from California. Victor T. Trujillo collection, Nevada. **$300.00.**

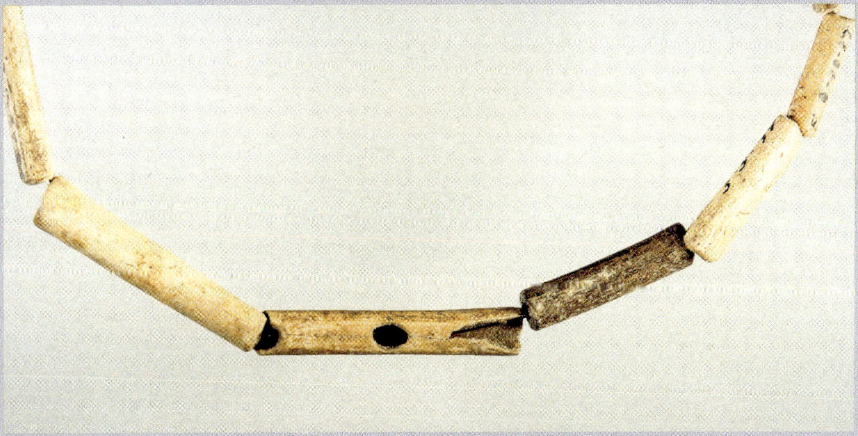

Necklace section, Fort Ancient period, bottom bead is 1¾" long. While the other beads made of bird bone are typical, the bottom example was salvaged from a flageolet and still retains one-and-a-half finger holes. Southern Ohio. Private collection. Museum grade.

Musical Instruments

Prehistoric Indians used many different kinds of musical instruments, and there were undoubtedly great numbers of instruments that did not outlast the years. Bone was the preferred material almost everywhere. Flageolets (commonly called flutes) were made in late prehistoric times from the radii of birds – hawk and wild turkey bones were frequently used for this purpose. Two to seven or more drilled, in-line holes on the topside of the bone changed the tones when the instrument was played.

Shorter bones from the same birds were sometimes drilled with one hole only, and these artifacts are termed whistles. Capable of producing only one pitch, it is thought that while the instruments might have made music, they also might have served as game calls or for giving signals in long-distance communication. Bone whistles up to ten inches long have been found in Manitoba, Canada. Other bone whistles used by historic Indians in the U. S. West are referred to as war-whistles.

Deer rib bones were sometimes notched or grooved for most of the length, and it is likely that they were rubbed with a wood or bone wand to serve as rasps or rhythm sticks. Rattles were made, and these were often box tortoise tops and bottoms containing pebbles. Historic Iroquois made similar rattles from the shells of snapping turtles. Deer hooves were used as rattlers or tinklers, sometimes bunched at the end of a handle and sometimes fastened to clothing.

Almost nonexistent in private collections (or museums for that matter) is a rare musical instrument, known as a panpipe, made by the Hopewell Indians in the Middle Woodland times. To make this instrument a row of short, hollow tubes made of reed or bone was held together by thin sheet copper. The tubes had one end closed, and apparently were played by blowing across the open ends. Instruments something like them are played in the Andes Mountains today, and they produce a breathy, haunting music. Probably fewer than two dozen of these Hopewell musical instruments have been found, mainly in the Midwest.

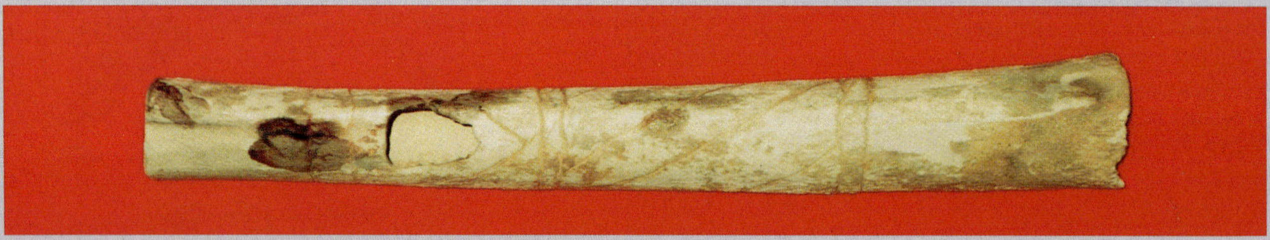

Bone whistle, with incised decorations, historic Arikara, ca. AD 1700, 6¼" long. The whistle is from the Missouri River area, South Dakota. Richard Krueger collection, Iowa. Sandra Krueger photograph. **$350.00 – 400.00.**

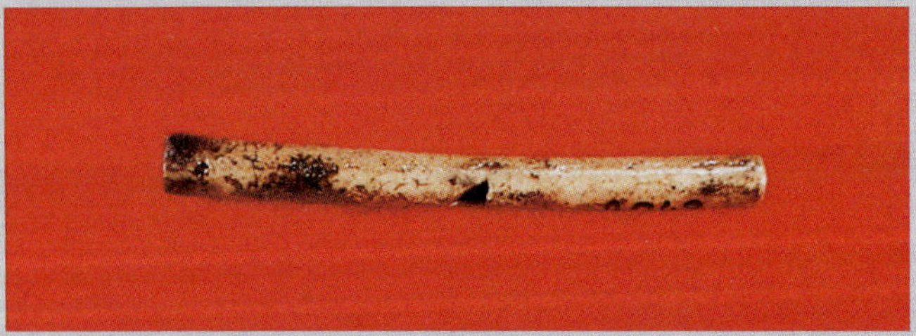

Bone whistle, from a large bird, 3⅛" long. Formerly in the Hovan collection, the whistle has very high polish and is from a Fort Ancient site in southern Ohio. Pete Timoch collection. **$100.00.**

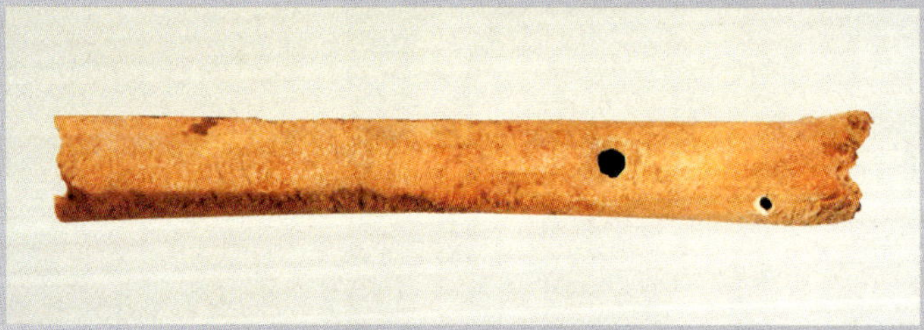

Flageolet section, probably Mississippian period, 3¼" long. Made from a bird bone, it is ex-collection Selb. West Virginia. Doug Hooks collection. Unlisted.

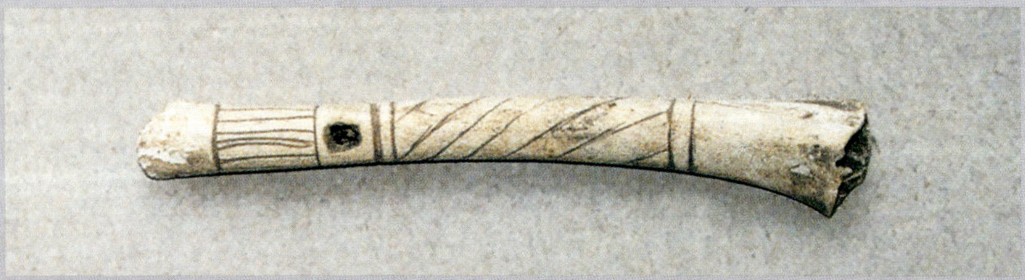

Bone whistle, bird bone with much exterior incising, 4⅜" long. Most whistles are not decorated to this extent. Find-location unknown. Wilfred Dick collection, Mississippi. **$350.00.**

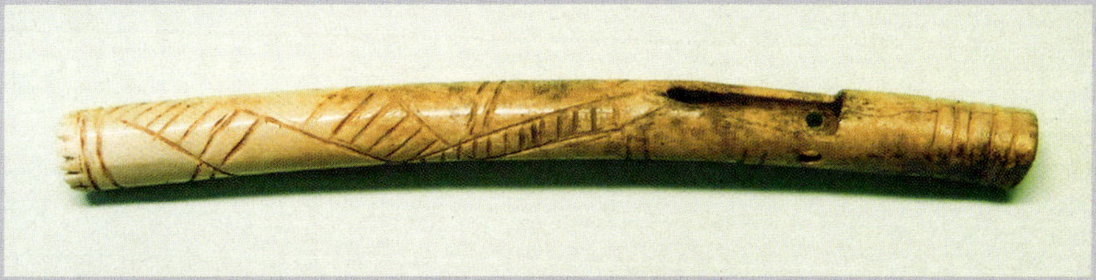

Whistle, hollow bird bone, ⅜ x 4¼". It is fully incised, serrated/tallied at one end, and has a cut vent hole and two drilled side holes. In fine condition, the whistle came from Weber County, northern Utah. Dann Russell collection, Utah. $350.00.

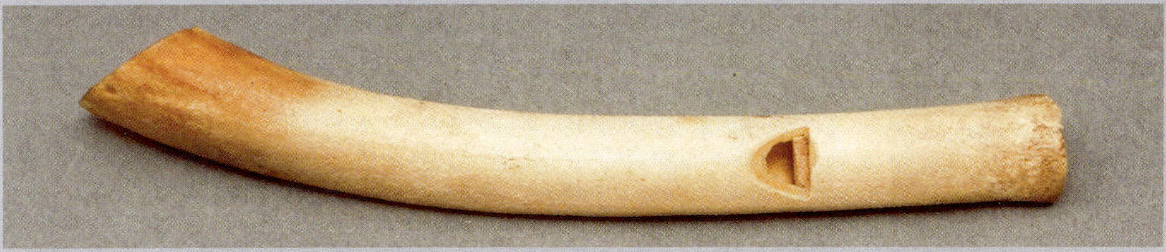

Whistle, bird wing bone, 5⅛" long. Made about 1950, this whistle (used for ceremonies) was given to the owner by a Hopi friend. H. B. Greene II collection, Naples, Florida. Unlisted.

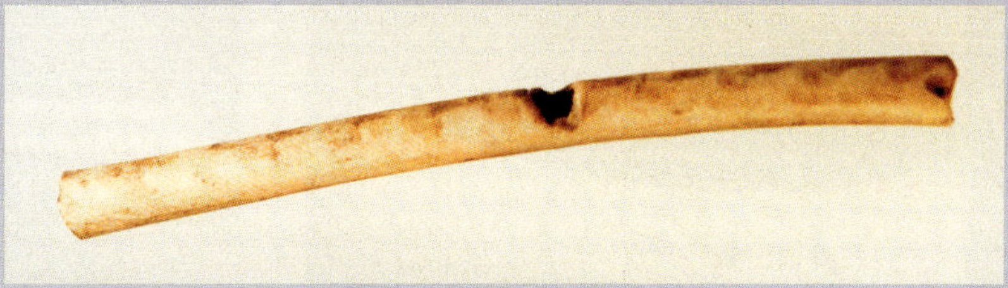

Whistle or game call, wild turkey bone, 3¾". This musical instrument is from the Midwest. Don Casto collection. **$75.00.**

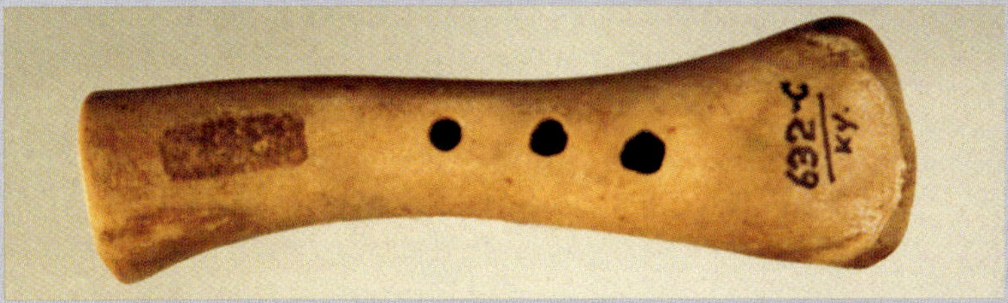

Musical bone, possibly bear bone, 3½" long. It was picked up in 1943. Kentucky. Robin Fiser collection. Museum grade.

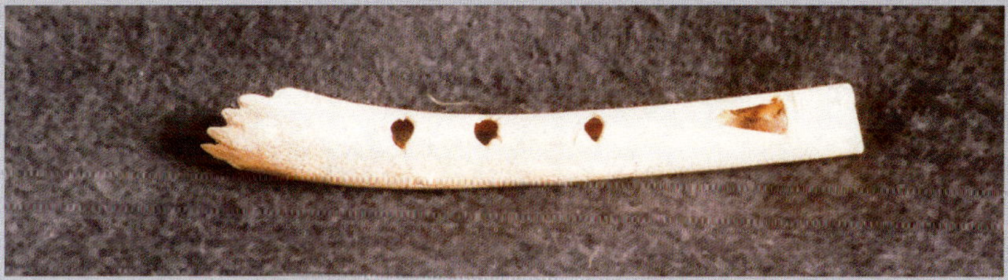

Flageolet, three holes and fringed end, 3⅞" long. This is an especially ornate example compared to others of the type. Find site unknown, but probably Midwestern. John F. Wubker collection, Illinois. **$400.00.**

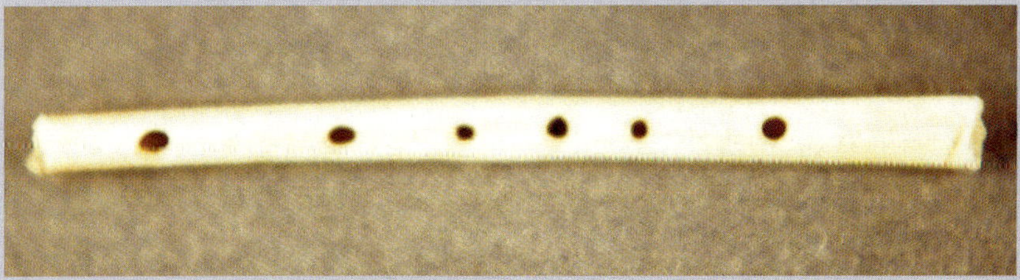

Flageolet, hollow bird bone, six holes. Found in 1945, it is 3⅞" long and came from a site in West Virginia. Larry Garvin collection. Museum grade.

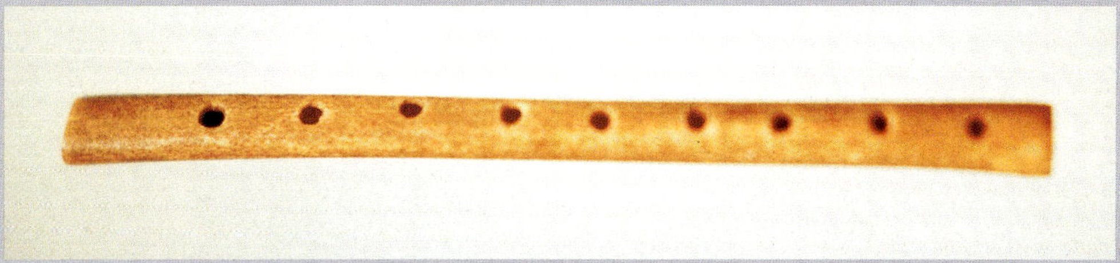

Bone flageolet, nine drilled holes, 4¾", made from the wing bone of a wild turkey. It was found in the 1940s and is ex-collection Shipley. Scioto County, Ohio. Larry Garvin collection. Museum grade.

Musical Instruments

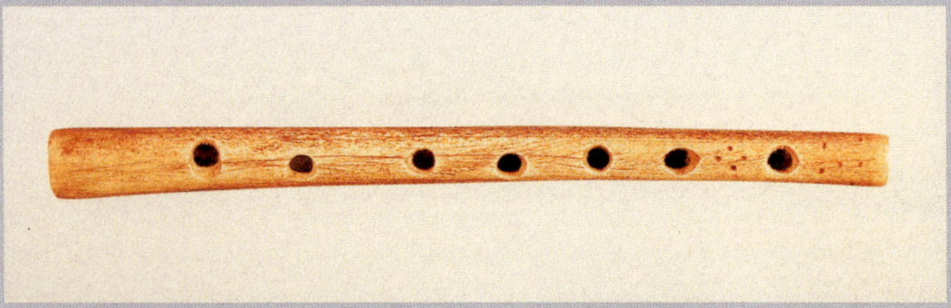

Flageolet, seven holes, exactly 3½" long. This is an exceptional musical instrument due to fine condition and the presence of pinhead patterned dots at one end. Ex-collection Copeland, the artifact came from southern Ohio. Fred Winegardner collection. **$300.00.**

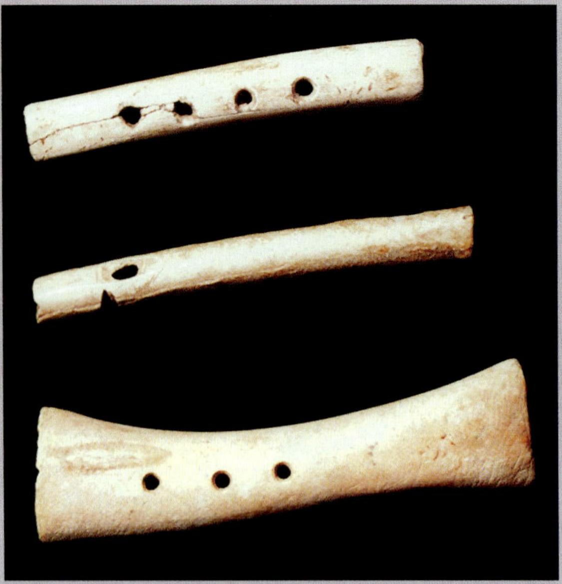

Flutes or flageolets, largest bone is 9 cm long, unknown animal, from Kentucky. The other two are made of turkey bones; top example has four holes and the center piece (broken at one end) has two holes showing but it also has a third hole. Private collection. Top, **$225.00;** center, **$125.00;** bottom, **$225.00 – 250.00.**

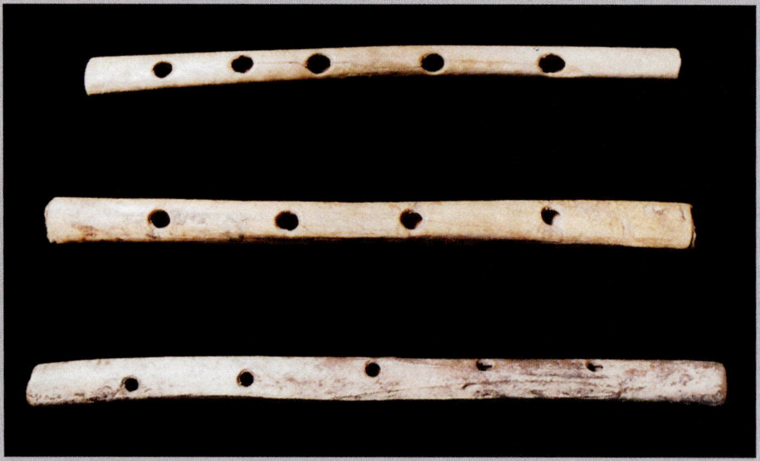

Flutes or flageolets, bird bones, four and five finger holes. The bottom example is of special interest in that the holes spiral around the hollow bone. At 10 cm long, the middle example is from Kentucky. The owner suggests that these musical instruments may once have had reed mouthpieces. Private collection. Each, **$250.00 – 325.00.**

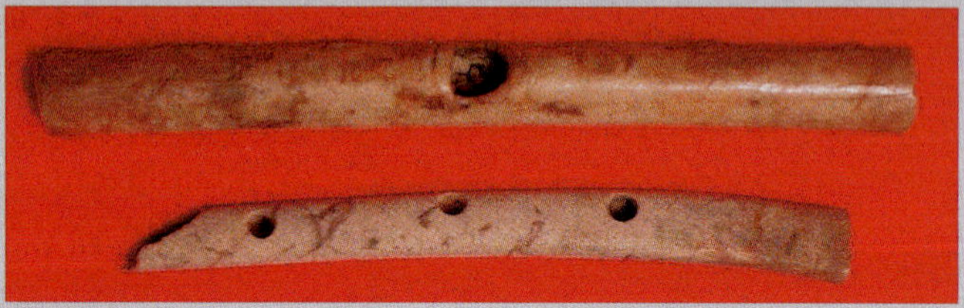

Bone musical instruments, late prehistoric or early historic, longer whistle is ⅜ x 3½". Canada. Michael F. Slasinski collection, Michigan. Whistle, **$150.00;** flageolet section, **$100.00.**

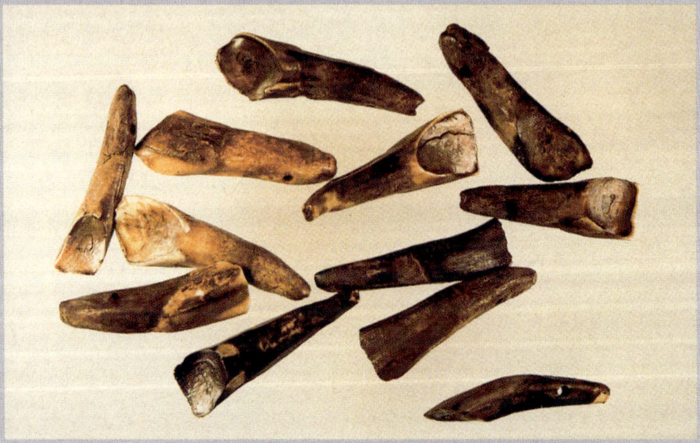

Bison Teeth, found near a "buffalo jump," average tooth length is 1¾." While not in an established musical artifact category, teeth like these were often joined with other objects like deer dew claws to create rattles and noise-makers. These, darkened with age and exposure, came from near Winslow, Arizona. Robin Fiser collection. Each, **$5.00.**

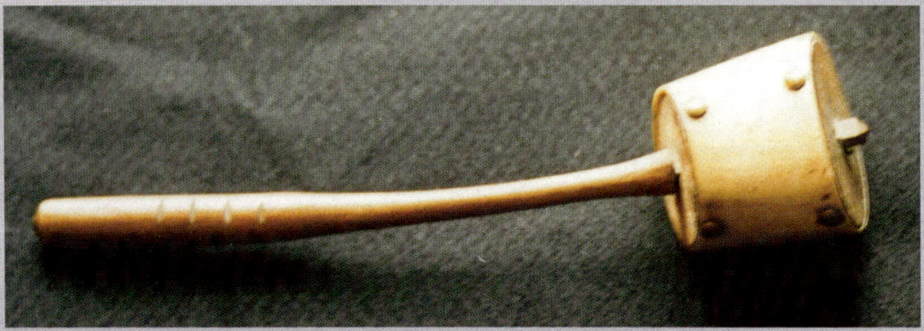

Rattle, cow horn body and wooden handle, late historic Seneca Indian, ca. 1880, 10½" long. It came from the Tonawanda Reservation, Niagara County, New York. Dave Summers collection, Victor, New York. **$200.00.**

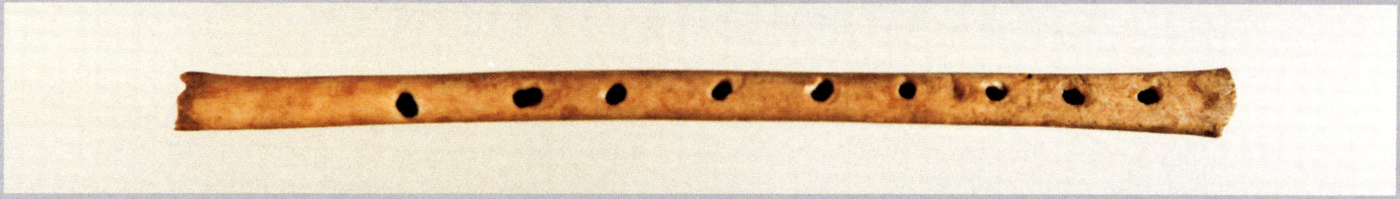

Flageolet, bird bone, 4¾" long. There are nine holes in this musical instrument, which was found in the midwest. Don Casto collection. **$200.00.**

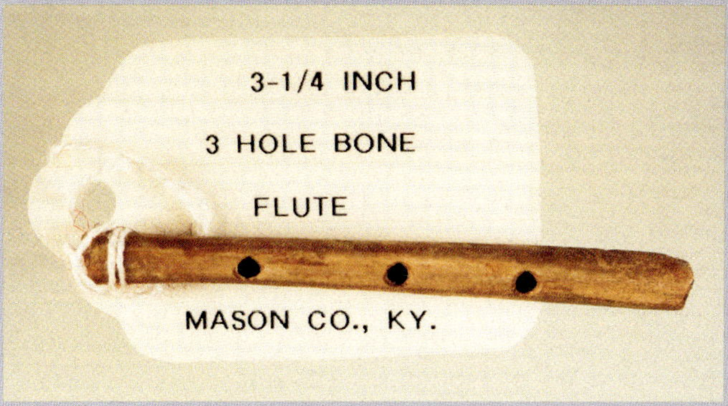

Flageolet, three-holed, 3¼" long. It is Mississippian and in good condition with a brown patina. Mason County, Kentucky. Robin Fiser collection. **$225.00 – 250.00.**

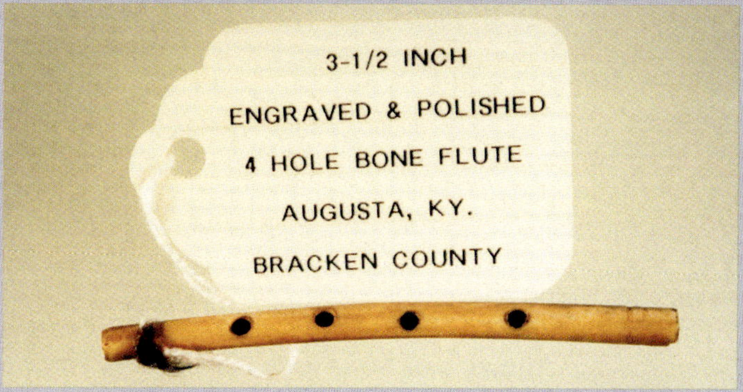

Flageolet, four-holed, 3½" long. This is a fine example made of bird bone and it has incised lines. Bracken County, Kentucky. Robin Fiser collection. **$300.00.**

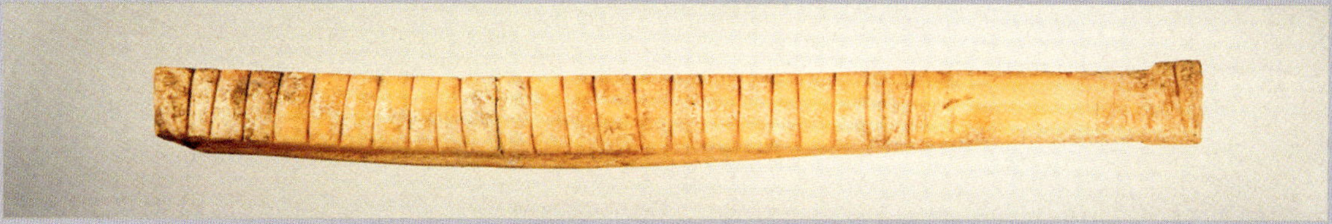

Rasp or rhythm stick, deer rib bone, 7⅜" long. These were "played" with a piece of wood or bone. Ex-collection Selb, it is from West Virginia. Doug Hooks collection. **$225.00 – 275.00.**

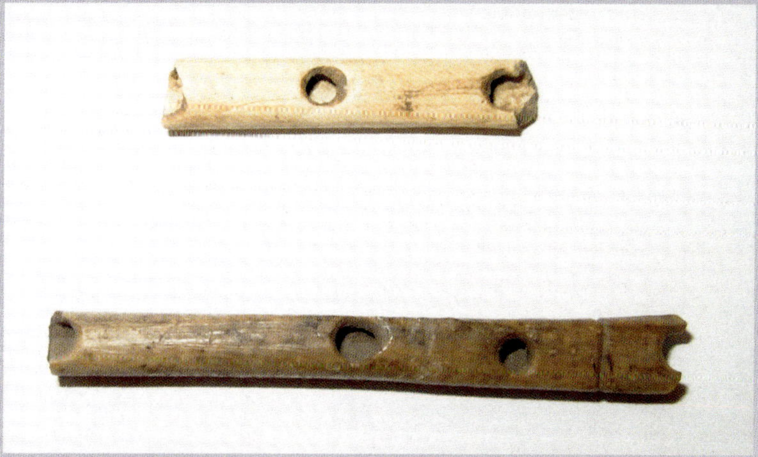

Bone flageolet fragments, the longer one has an incised groove. Sometimes pieces like this were salvaged to make tubular beads. They are Mississippian in time, from Mason County, West Virginia. Private collection. Rodney Roberts photograph. Each, **$15.00 – 30.00.**

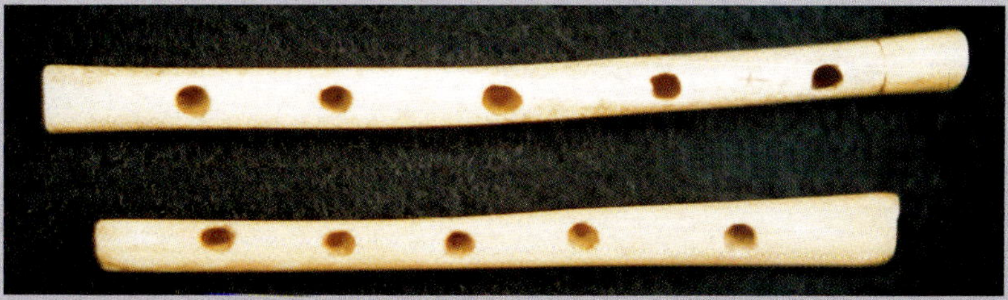

Flageolets, Mississippian period, 3¼ and 3¾" long, respectively. They were found in Kentucky. Bob Hess collection, Indiana. Each, **$200.00 – 275.00.**

Ornamental Artifacts

While bone was regularly and widely used for ornamental and decorative purposes, shell was also used when it was available. Most shell was a convenient size, naturally attractive, and easily worked with traditional methods. A thriving prehistoric trade brought West Coast shell into the Southwest, and Gulf Coast shell into the Midwest. Similar exchanges took place elsewhere in North America. Only a fraction of the shell artifacts once made have been found, and the original exchange quantities must have been enormous. Bone was also used in many regions.

Shell beads ranged from small freshwater snails and clamshells to objects cut from large conch and abalone shells. Necklaces were often all shell in some form, or shell interspersed with animal teeth or claws. Stone or cannel coal beads were sometimes used with shell, providing a pleasing contrast of color and texture. Shell earpins, often in matching sets, were carved from thick marine shell, and the Southeast is particularly rich in such artifacts.

Intricate shellwork was done in California, where shell was cut and drilled to make an almost endless variety of pendants and small decorative objects of many uses. Even a few finger rings were made in the Southwest, plus bracelets carved so that the outer rim of certain shells made the ornament. In this region, prehistoric workers learned to inset shell with bits of jet or turquoise, and even etched designs on shell using an acid derived from cactus.

In the eastern U. S., fine pendants were made of large shell sections which were often incised with geometric designs or figures of snakes, spiders, birds, or humans. Rounded to oblong, such pendants (usually referred to as gorgets) often have two suspension holes at the top. Some Mississippian people made large marine shell engravings; these are among the finest depictions of prehistoric ritual activities.

Many groups used bone for specialized ornamental purposes, such as the figural combs of the Iroquois and pre-Iroquois of the Northeast. The Hopewell in the Midwest also used carved bone, perhaps for clothing enhancement, and cut tortoise and turtle shell into graceful forms.

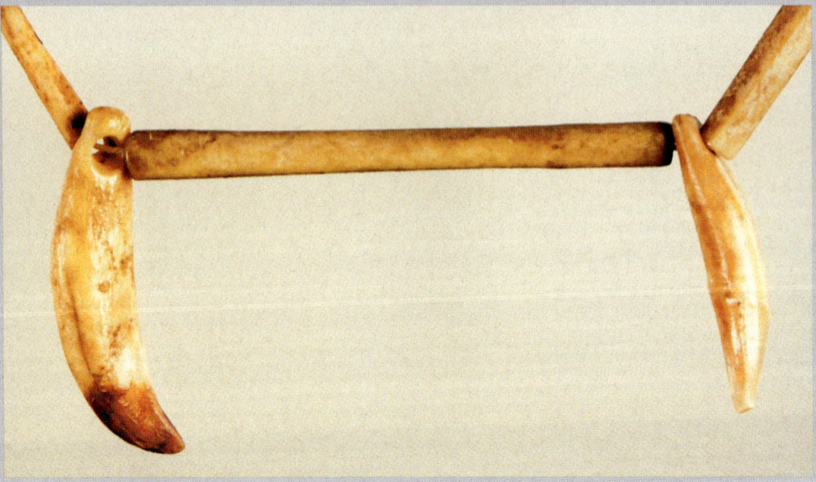

Necklace elements, drilled animal teeth and bird bones. The longest bead in the strand (shown at center) is 3 1/16". Ex-collections Copeland and Hooks, it is from Ohio. Fred Winegardner collection. Museum grade.

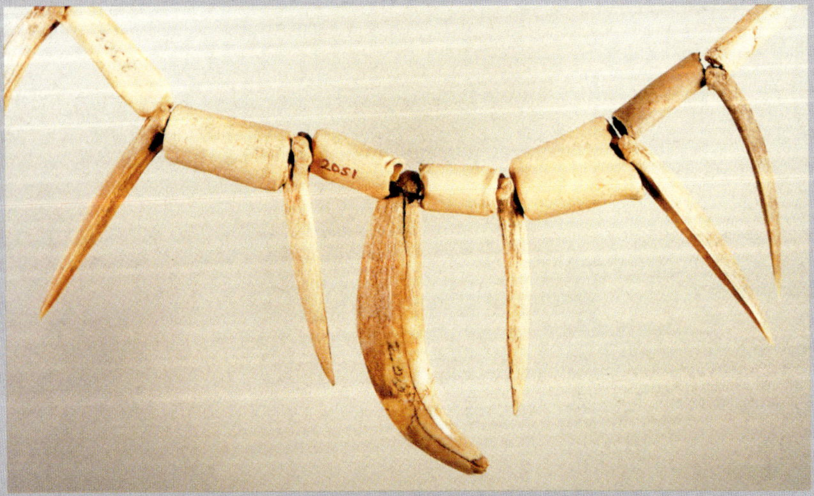

Necklace elements, bear tooth (canine), fish spines, and deer bone beads. Bear tooth is 2 3/16" long. Mississippian period, northern Ohio. Fred Winegardner collection. Museum grade.

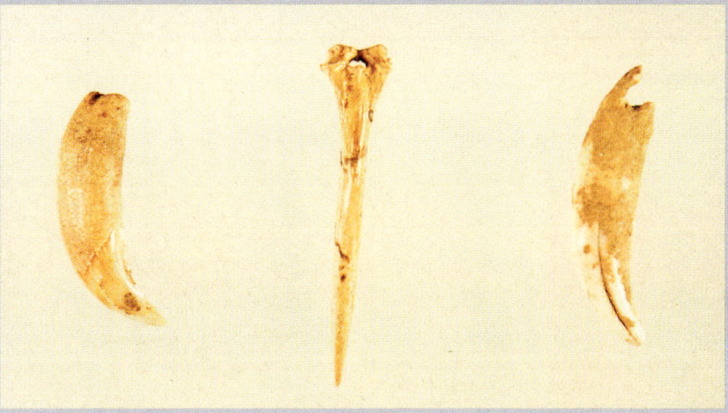

Necklace elements, animal tooth (left); drilled fish spine (center), 1¼". Drilled dog(?) tooth (right). All from southern Ohio and private collection. Group, **$20.00.**

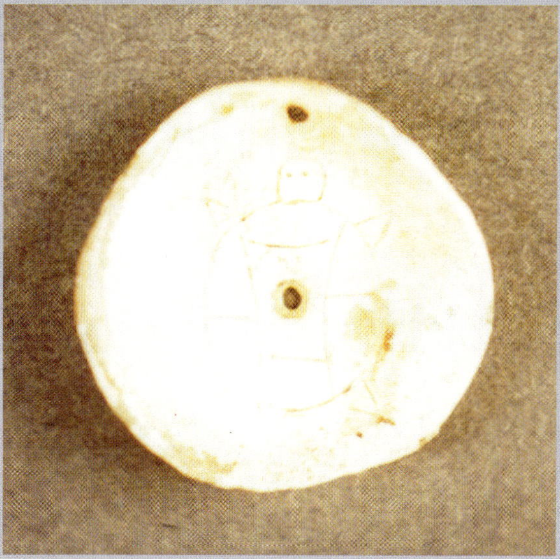

Shell pendant or gorget, with central suspension hole. This example is 1⅞" in diameter and has an incised turtle design on the concave (facing) surface. Southeastern United States. Larry Garvin collection. Museum grade.

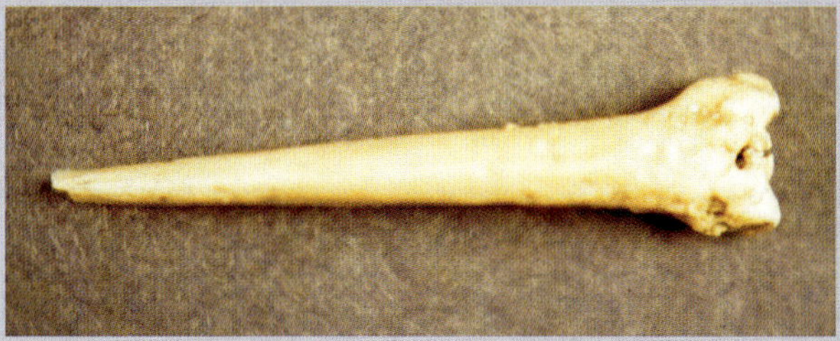

Pendant, fish bone, suspension hole drilled in larger end, 2⅜" long. Mississippi County, Arkansas. Back to Earth. **$10.00.**

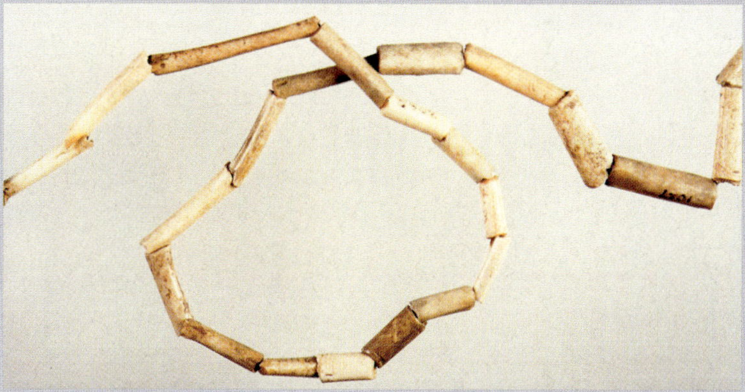

Necklace, bird bone beads, average length is ¾". The polished beads are from northern Ohio. Fred Winegardner collection. Museum grade.

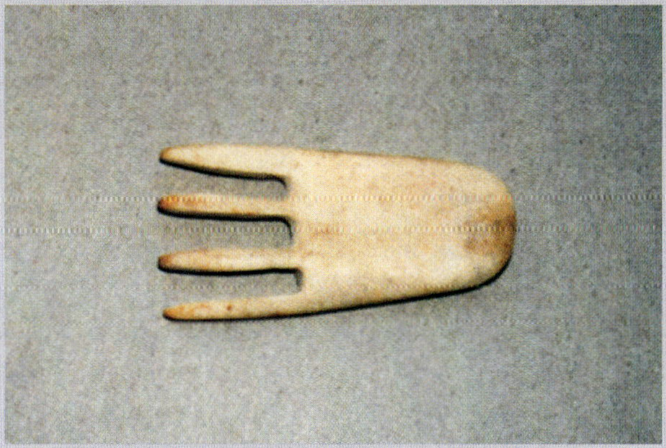

Hair comb or adornment, 2 x 3", well-shaped and polished. It was found on a site in Illinois. Wilfred Dick collection, Mississippi. **$300.00.**

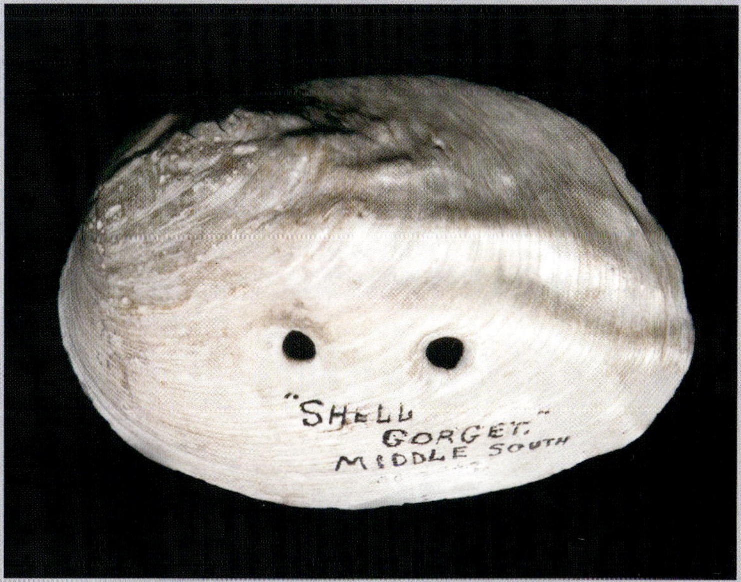

Shell gorget, two-hole, 5⅝" long. It is Mississippian period, ca. AD 1200 – 1600. A good, solid example of a scarce artifact type, the gorget was found in Tennessee. Back to Earth. **$125.00 – 160.00.**

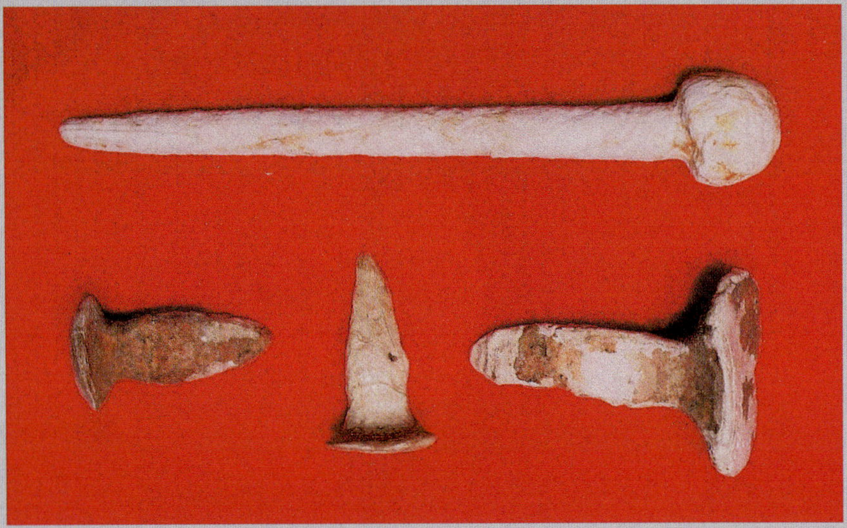

Shell ear plugs and hairpin(?), plugs are 1½ to 1¹⁵⁄₁₆" long, hairpin is 5⅛" long. These are probably Mississippian in time and were found in Ohio. Michael F. Slasinski collection, Michigan. Unlisted.

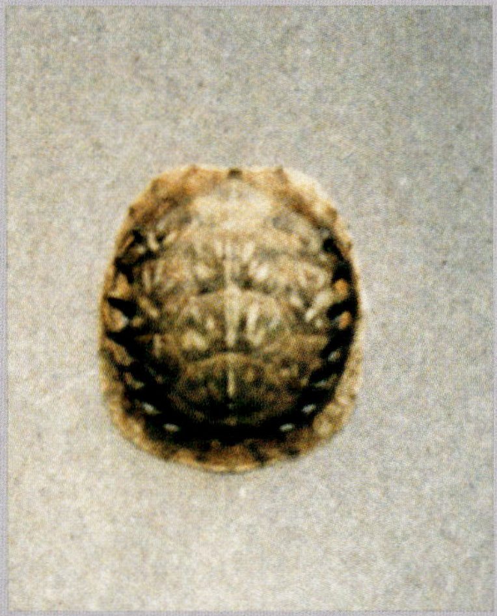

Turtle shell with edge carving, shell size is 1½ x 2". This piece was found on a camp site in Mississippi. Wilfred Dick collection, Mississippi. **$40.00.**

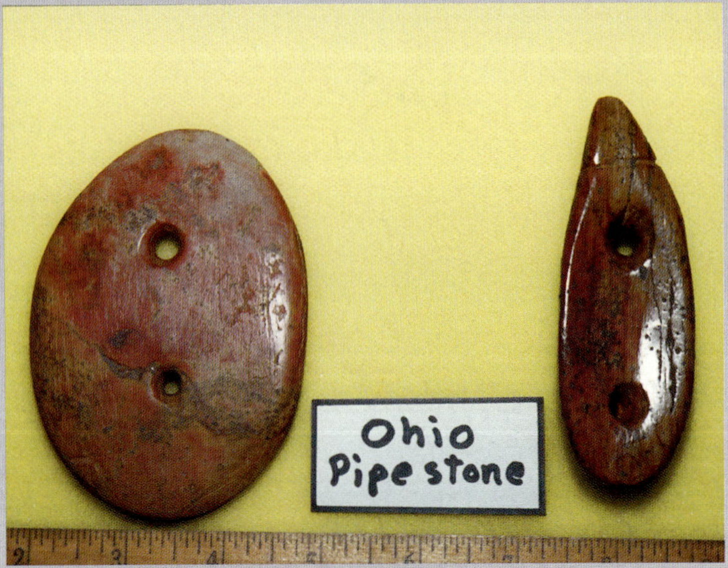

Pipestone artifacts, gorgets on left and pendant on right. It is probably a tooth effigy and is both drilled and grooved at the top. Back to Earth. Unlisted.

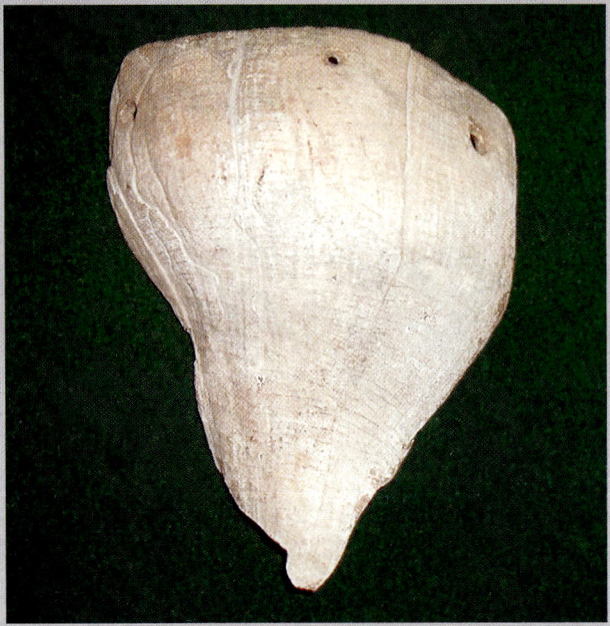

Shell mask, 5 x 5", large marine shell. It was found in the Logan area, Tennessee. Keith and Rhonda Dodge collection, Michigan. Unlisted.

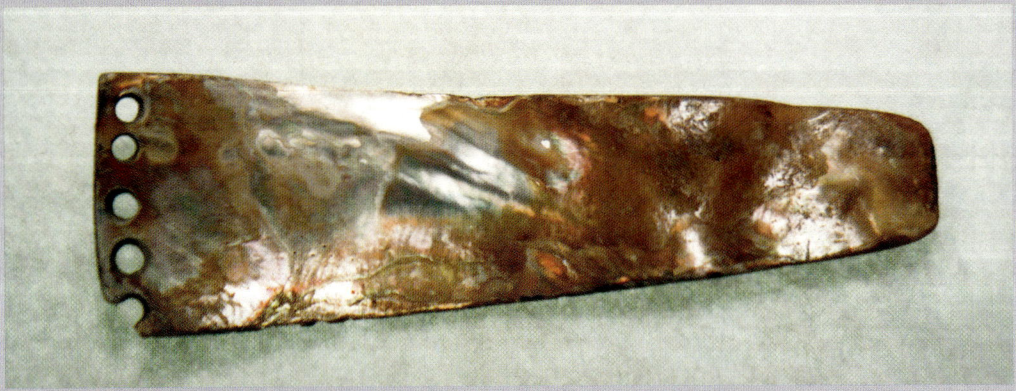

Abalone shell pendant, iridescent surface, 5⅛". It was found at Rio Oso, Yuba County, California. Back to Earth. **$225.00.**

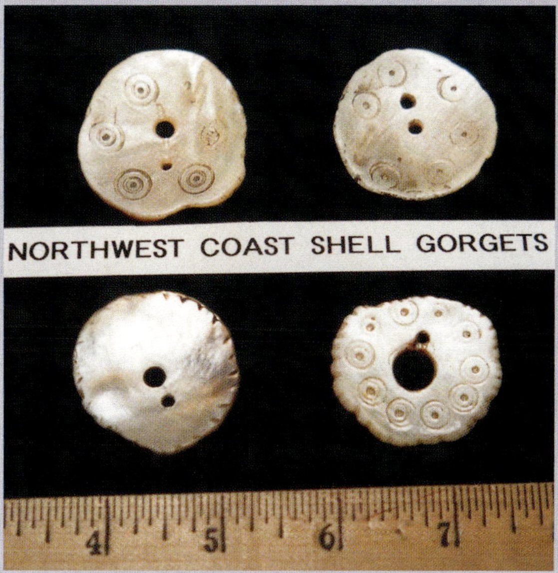

Shell gorgets, incised decorations and central hole, all from the Northwest Coast. Back to Earth. Unlisted.

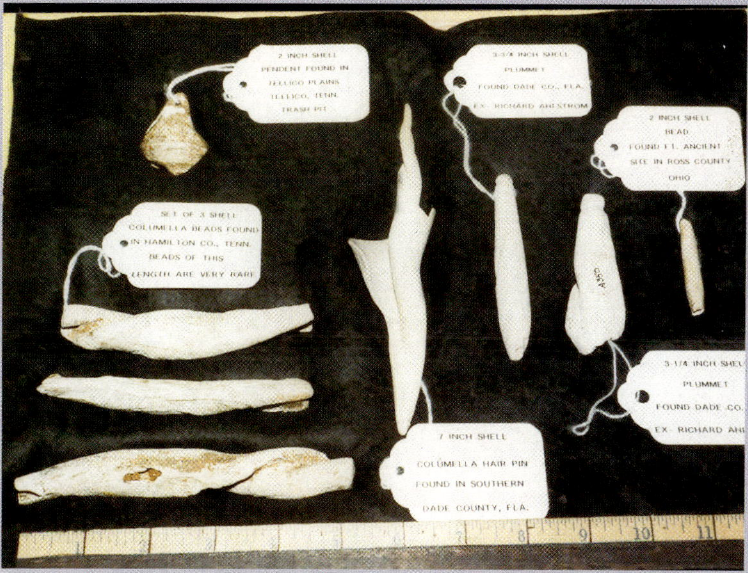

Shell artifacts, plummets, beads, and a pendant. These are from the states of Ohio, Tennessee, and Florida. Back to Earth. Unlisted.

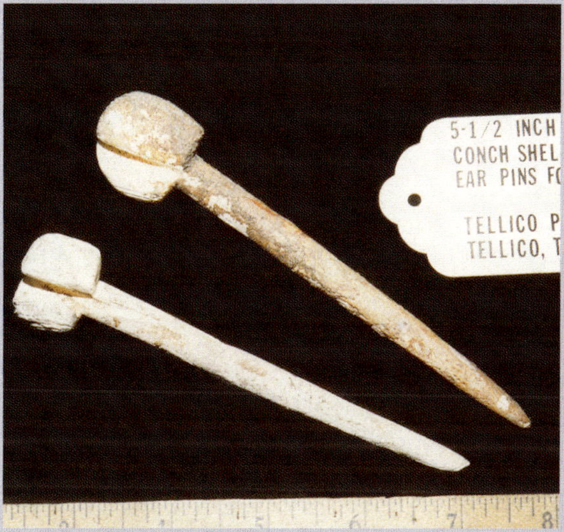

Conch shell ear pins, 5½" long. These Mississippian artifacts were found in Tennessee. Back to Earth. Museum grade.

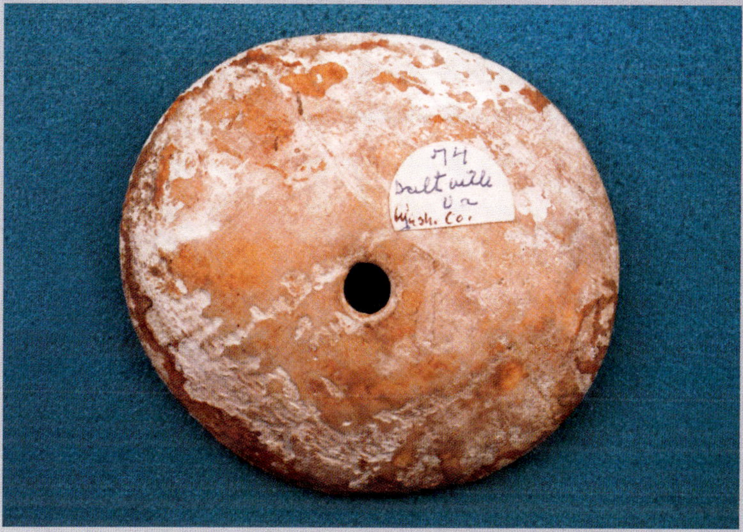

Shell gorget, probably Archaic, 2¹⁵⁄₁₆" in diameter. Ex-collection Snyder, it is from Washington County, Virginia. Collection of, and photograph by, Gary Henry, North Carolina. **$250.00.**

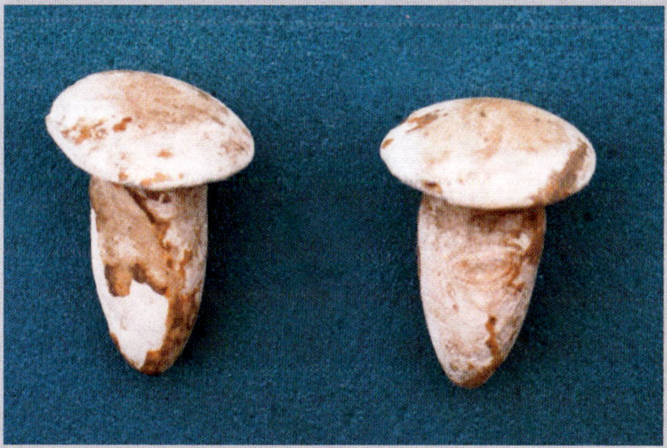

Shell earplugs, Mississippian period, each ⅞ x 1¼". They are ex-collection Snyder, from Monroe County, Tennessee. Collection of, and photograph by, Gary Henry, North Carolina. Pair, **$150.00.**

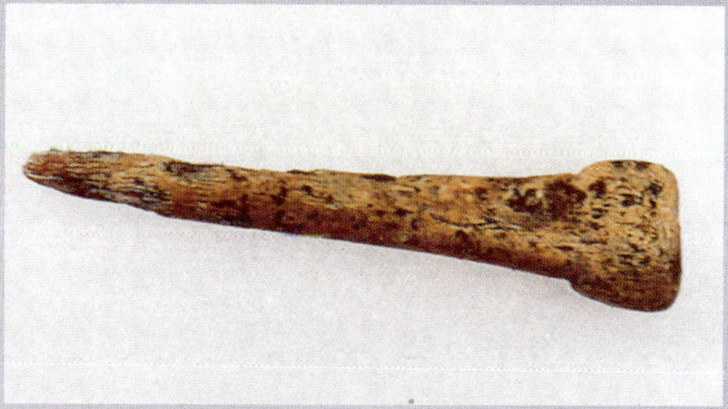

Hairpin or earplug, Woodland to Mississippian period, knobbed top, 2⅝" long. It has a black and brown patina and is ex-collection Vietzen. Ohio-Kentucky region. Pete Timoch collection. **$100.00 – 150.00.**

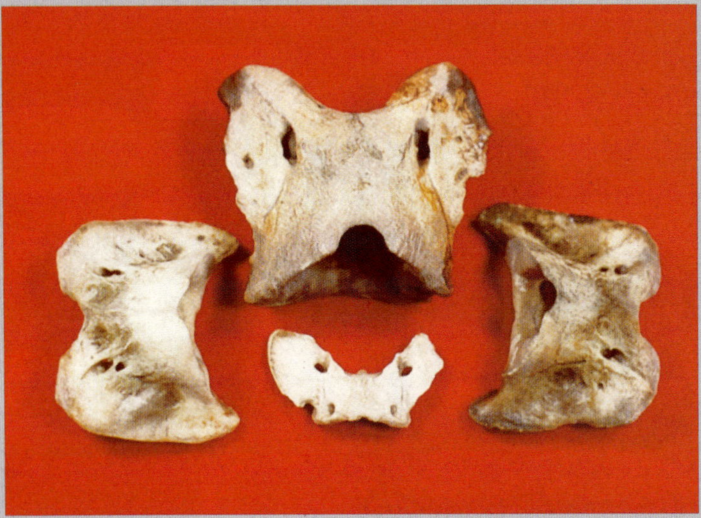

Elk vertebras beads or pendants, Late Archaic to Woodland. Ex-collection Vietzen, the largest is 3⅜ x 4". Polish and wear indicate these were worn in some fashion. Christian County, Kentucky. Pete Timoch collection. Each, **$40.00 – 70.00.**

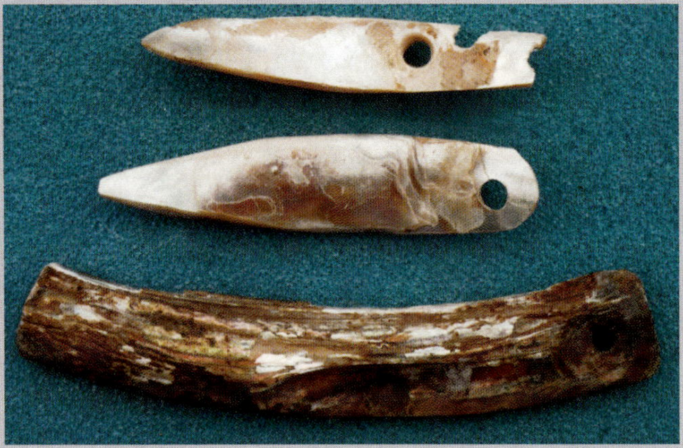

Abalone shell pendants, prehistoric(?), longest (bottom) ½ x 2¹³⁄₁₆", ¹⁄₁₆" thick. They are ex-collection Levy and were probably found in California. Collection of, and photograph by, Gary Henry, North Carolina. Each, **$50.00 – 100.00.**

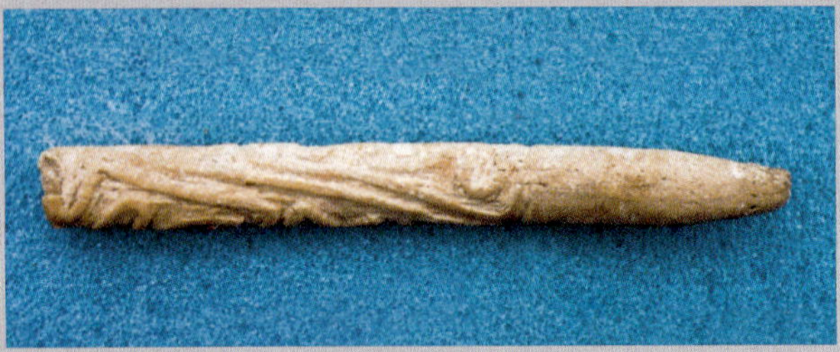

Engraved pin, bone, Woodland period or later, ¼ x 2¼", ⅛" thick. This artistic example is ex-collection Levy, origin unknown. Collection of, and photograph by, Gary Henry, North Carolina. **$50.00.**

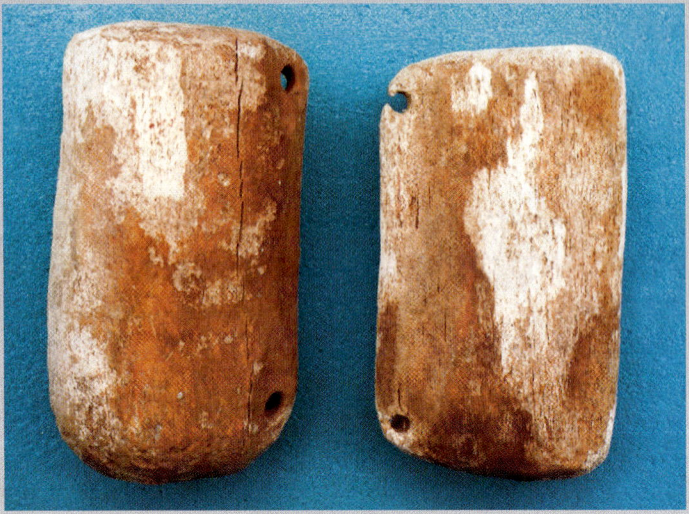

Elk bone gorgets, Woodland or later. Each gorget is 2¹⁄₁₆ x 3⅝" and thickness is 1⅝ and 1¹⁄₁₆". The matching artifacts are from the Levy collection, find-site unknown. Collection of, and photograph by, Gary Henry, North Carolina. Each, **$100.00.**

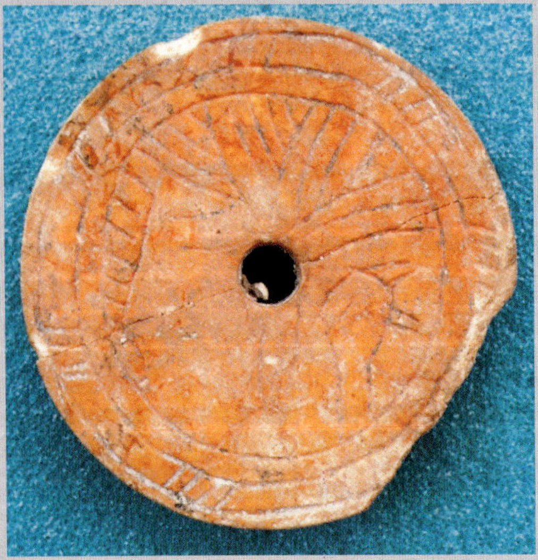

Shell gorget or earspool, incised turkey motif. Mississippian in origin, it is 1⅝" in diameter and ³⁄₁₆" thick. Ex-collection Levy, the find-location is unknown. Collection of, and photograph by, Gary Henry, North Carolina. **$175.00.**

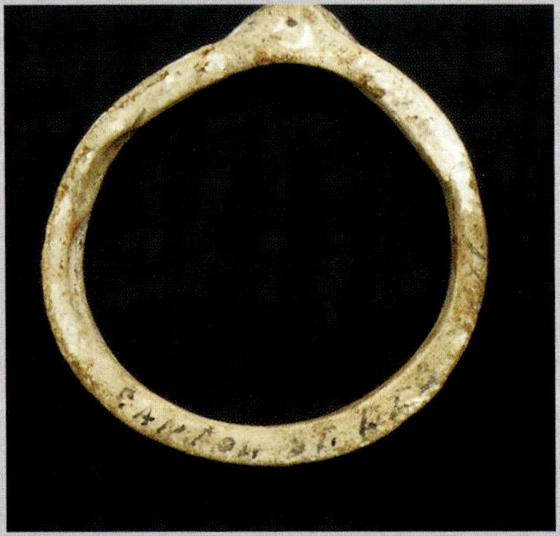

Shell bracelet, prehistoric(?), 2⅛ x 2¼", ³⁄₁₆" thick. The example is ex-collection Levy and probably from the American Southwest. Collection of, and photograph by, Gary Henry, North Carolina. **$150.00.**

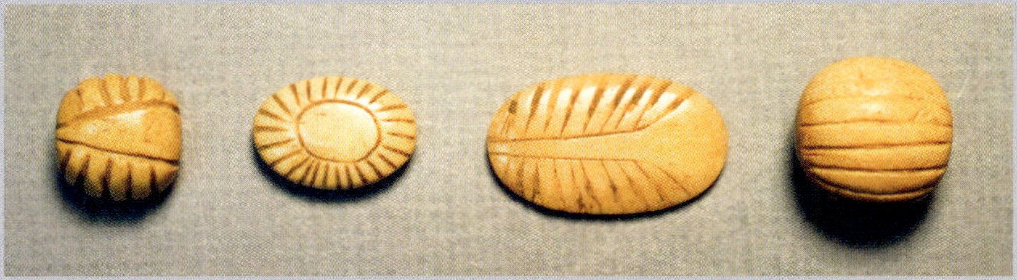

Gaming pieces, polished bone, all with incised line designs. They are about 1" in diameter, ca. AD 1750. Morton County, North Dakota. Private collection. Each, **$75.00.**

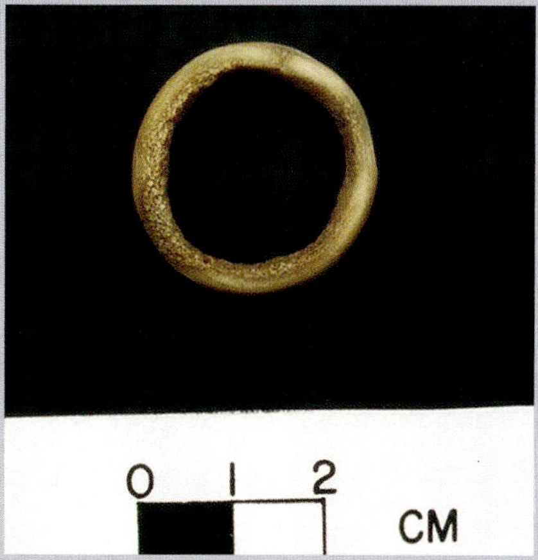

Bone ring, prehistoric(?), 1" in diameter and 1/4" thick, ex-collection Levy. This example is probably from California. Collection of, and photograph by, Gary Henry, North Carolina. **$50.00.**

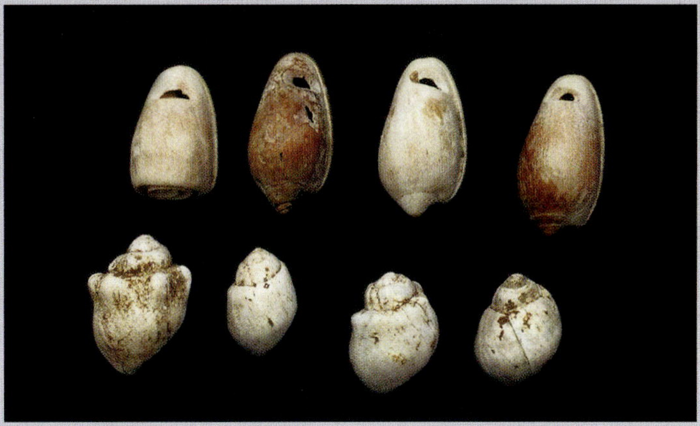

Snail shell beads, Woodland and later, largest is 9/16 x 1". Ex-collection Levy, origin is unknown. Collection of, and photograph by, Gary Henry, North Carolina. Each, **$2.00.**

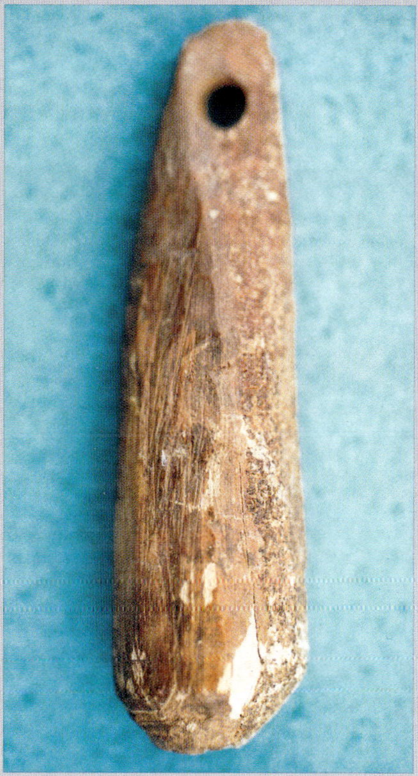

Bone pendant, Woodland or later, 1 5/16 x 2 3/8" long. It is ex-collection Levy, origin unknown. Collection of, and photograph by, Gary Henry, North Carolina. **$20.00.**

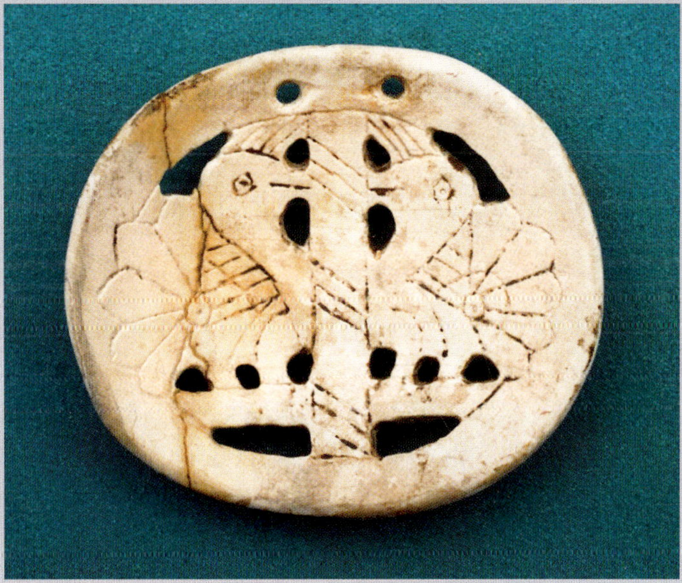

Shell gorget, cutaway turkey motif, Mississippian period, 2 3/4 x 3 1/8". Washington County, Tennessee. Collection of, and photograph by, Gary Henry, North Carolina. **$750.00.**

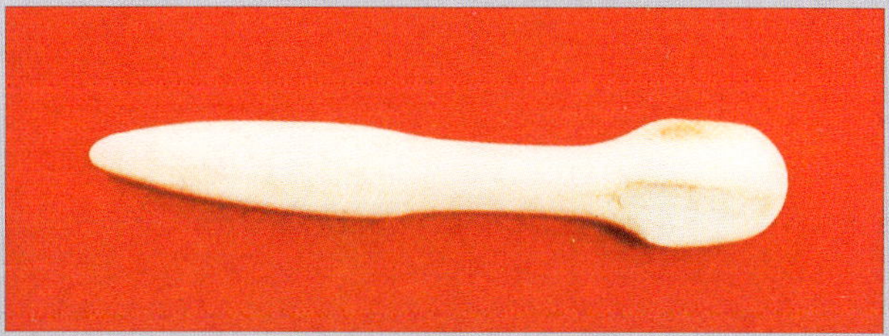

Bone hairpin or ornament, 2 11/16". This has an unusual shape, being expanded both near the base and tip. It is highly polished, ex-collection Vietzen, Ohio-Kentucky region. Pete Timoch collection. **$100.00 – 150.00.**

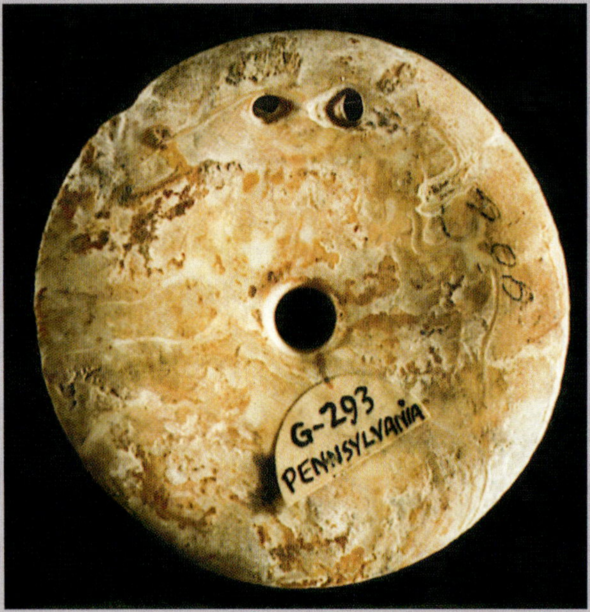

Shell gorget, probably marine mollusk, Glacial Kame people of the Late Archaic period. It has two small suspension holes and a large central hole. Once in the B. W. Stephens collection, it originally came from Pennsylvania. Jon Boyes collection, Illinois. **$950.00.**

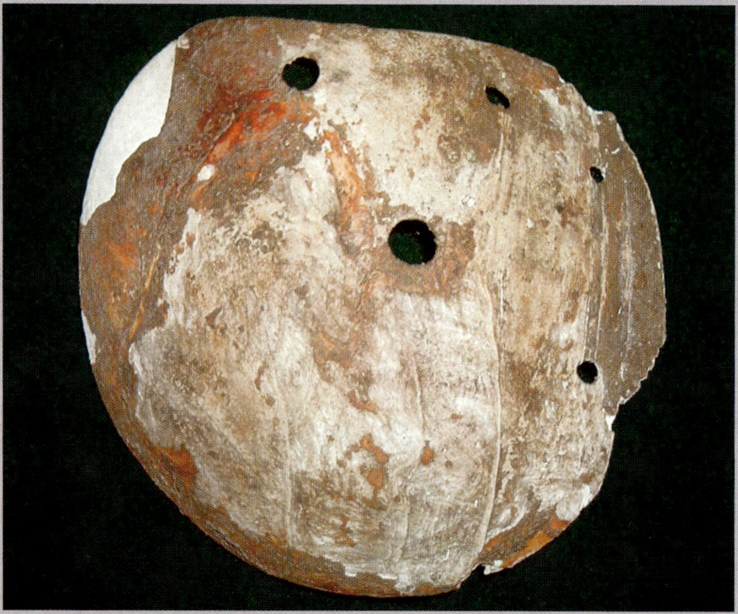

Shell mask, with perforations, ex-collection Noel, 4¼ x 4¾". It was found in Casey County, Kentucky. Keith and Rhonda Dodge collection, Michigan. Unlisted.

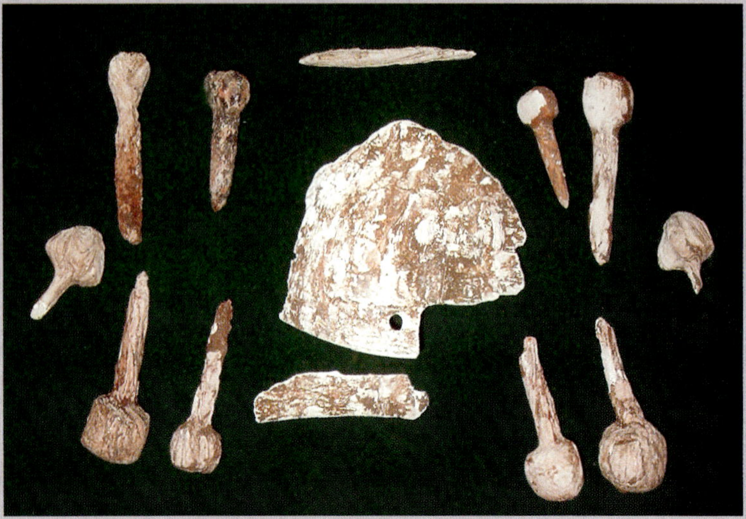

Artifacts, bone or shell, Davis COA, lengths range from 1½ to 3". All were found in Polk County, Tennessee. Keith and Rhonda Dodge collection, Michigan. Unlisted.

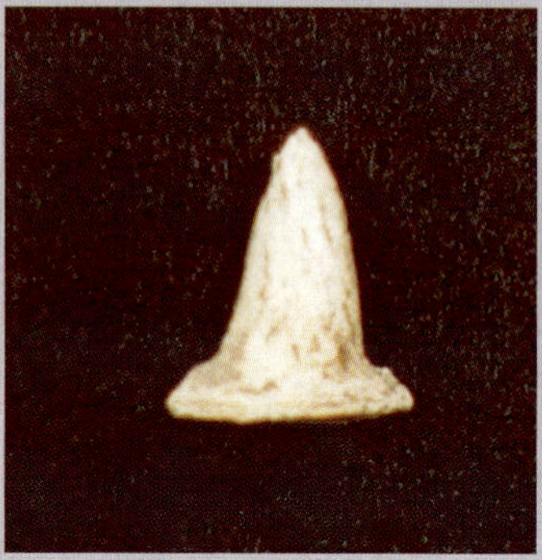

Decoration or charm, cut and ground wild turkey leg spur, Mississippian period, ca. AD 800 – 1500, 1⁵⁄₁₆" long. Ex-collection Vietzen, southern Ohio. Pete Timoch collection. **$50.00.**

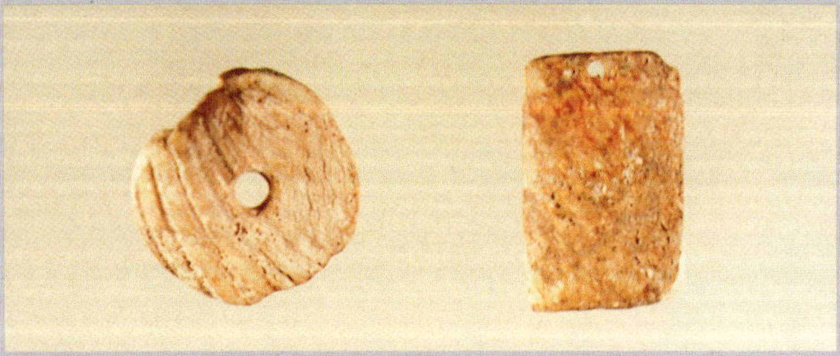

Necklace elements, drilled shell pieces, largest is 1¼" across. These were found in Florida. Robin Fiser collection. Unlisted.

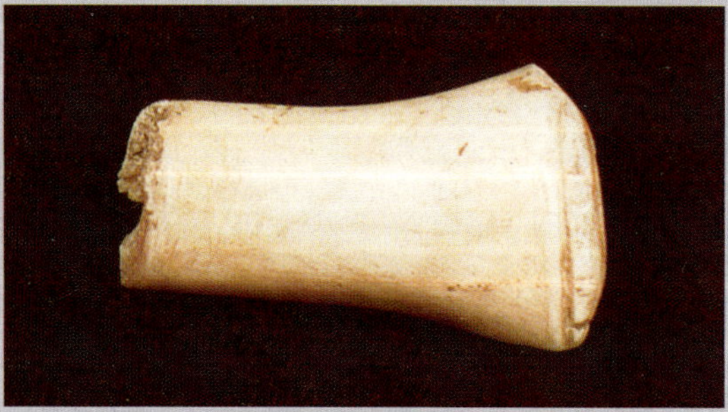

Hair ornament, Late Archaic to Woodland, interior whorl of conch shell, which was brought from the Gulf of Mexico. It is 2¼" long, ex-collection Vietzen. The ornament is pictured in Col. Vietzen's book *The Saga of Glover's Cave* on three different pages. Christian County, Kentucky. Pete Timoch collection. **$150.00.**

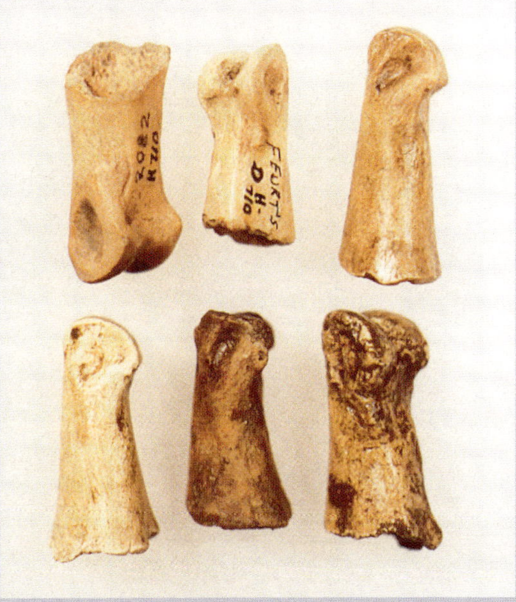

Pendants, deer toe bones (astragalus), longest is 1⅝". These have been hollowed from the thicker end and are drilled at the smaller end. All are ex-collection Vietzen, and came from various Mississippian sites in Ohio. Pete Timoch collection. Each, **$40.00 – 50.00.**

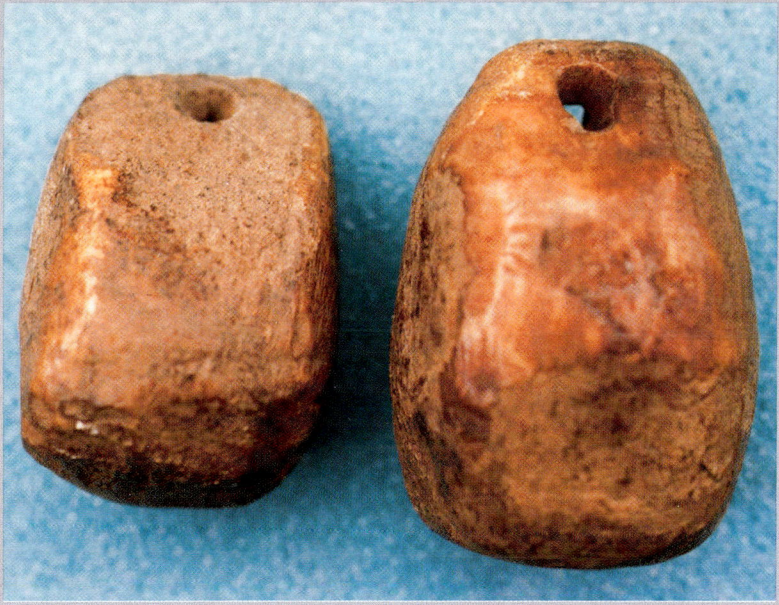

Pendants, drilled at top, elk antler, Woodland or later, larger one is 1$\frac{1}{16}$ x 1$\frac{9}{16}$", smaller one is 1$\frac{5}{16}$ x 1⅜". They are ex-collection Levy, origin unknown. Collection of, and photograph by, Gary Henry, North Carolina. Each, **$40.00.**

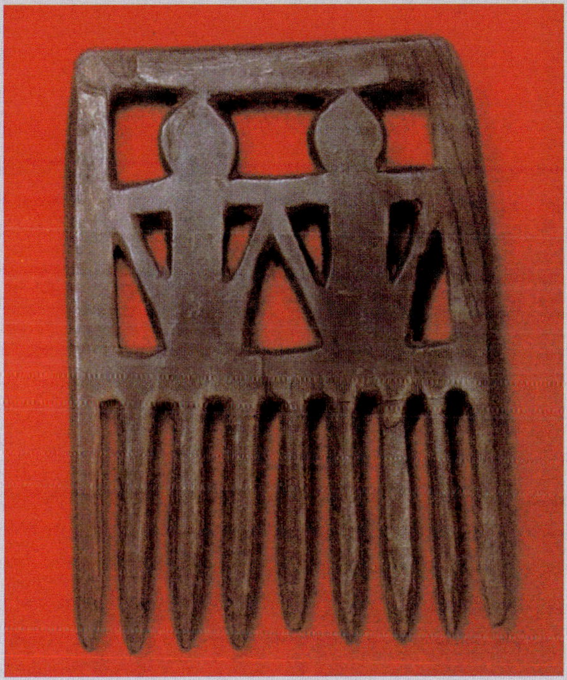

Antler comb, 2⅛ x 3", ¼" thick. It is historic Iroquois, from Ontario, Canada. Michael F. Slasinski collection, Michigan. **$350.00.**

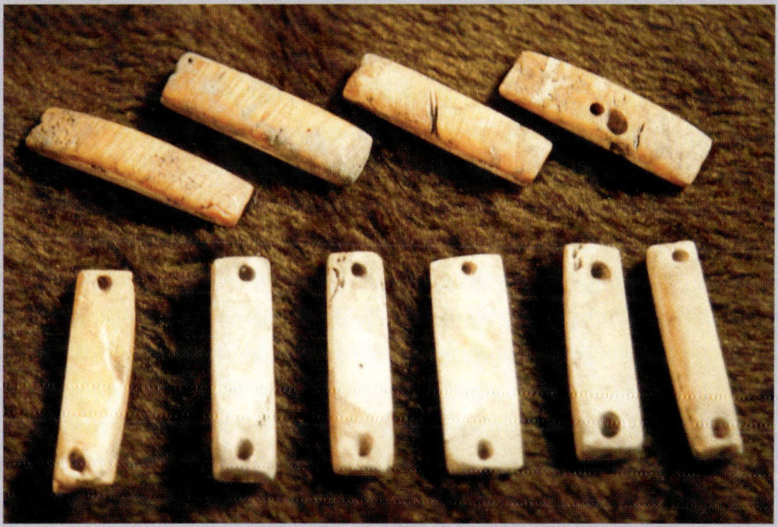

Shell beads, rectangular and with L-shaped holes drilled at each end, average length is 1¾". This is an exceptional ten-piece set, ex-collections Jenkins, Daily, and Adam. The beads came from Davidson County, Tennessee. Dale and Betty Roberts collection, Iowa. Museum grade.

Shell earpin, 2" long, Mississippian period. It came from the Arkansas – Tennessee line. Wilfred Dick collection, Mississippi. **$40.00.**

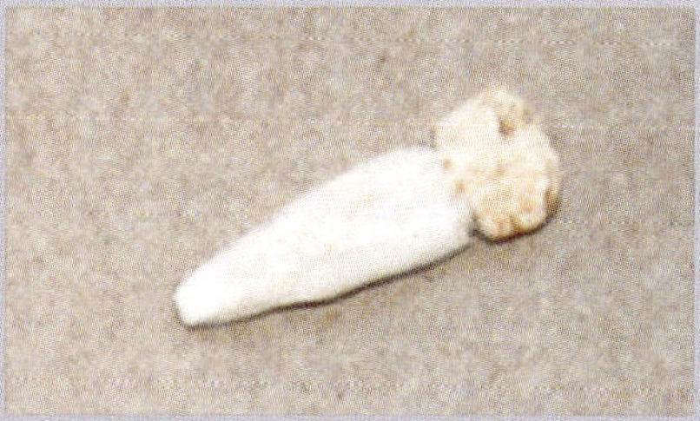

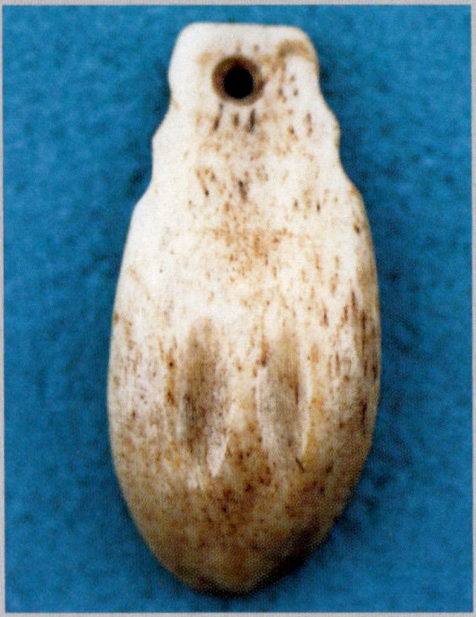

Bone pendant, shaped and drilled, prehistoric, 1 1/16 x 1½". The artifact is ex-collection Levy, origin unknown, and may be a copy of an elk canine tooth. Collection of, and photograph by, Gary Henry, North Carolina. **$50.00.**

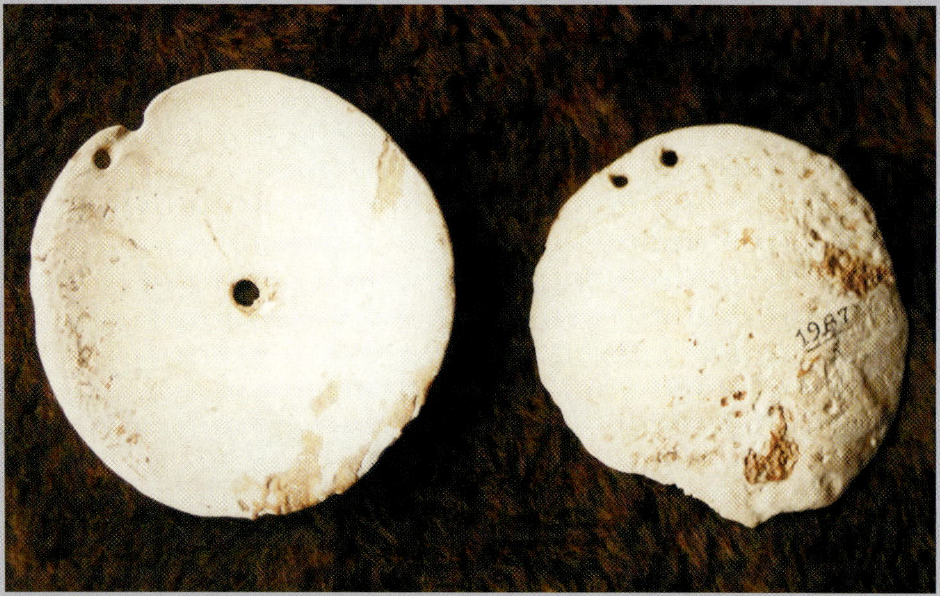

Shell gorgets, 2¾" in diameter, one with central drill-hole. These are ex-collection Meuser and are pictured in *The Meuser Collection*, page 143. Butler County, Ohio. Dale and Betty Roberts collection, Iowa. Each, **$225.00 – 275.00.**

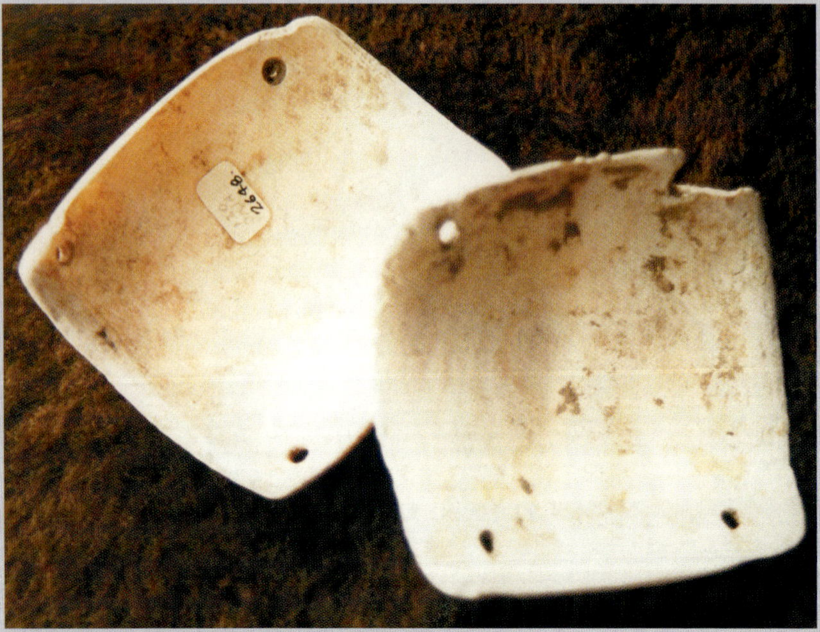

Square shell gorgets, pair, 2⅞" square, curved marine shell. These are ex-collection Thompson and were found at a Mississippian site in Oklahoma. Dale and Betty Roberts collection, Iowa. Pair, **$450.00.**

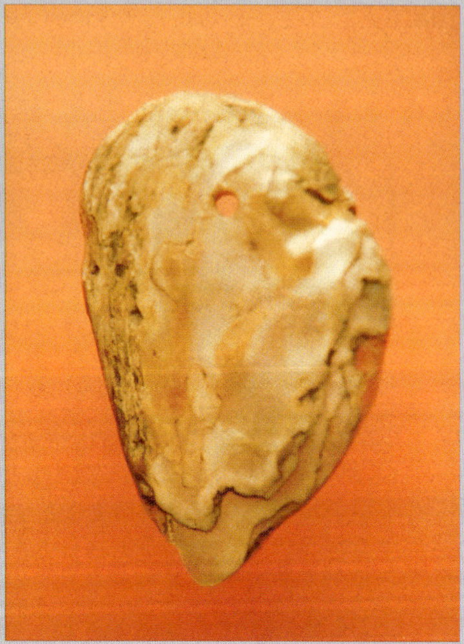

Oyster shell pendant, 2¾" long, drilled for suspension. Late Archaic, this Frontenac phase piece is ca. 2000 BC. Cayuga County, New York. Dave Summers collection, Victor, New York. **$100.00.**

Gaming pieces, ground and smoothed mammal bone, left example is ½ x 2", 3/32" thick. The left piece has incised lines at one end and in the middle. The elongated piece is from Weber County, northern Utah, and the circular example is from Box Elder County, Utah. Dann Russell collection, Utah. Elongated piece, **$20.00;** circular piece, **$15.00.**

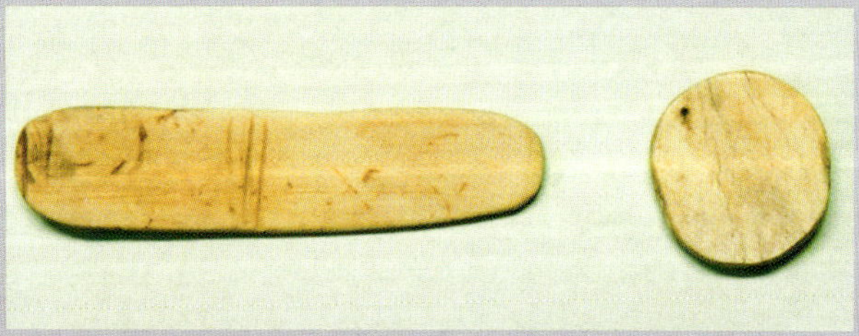

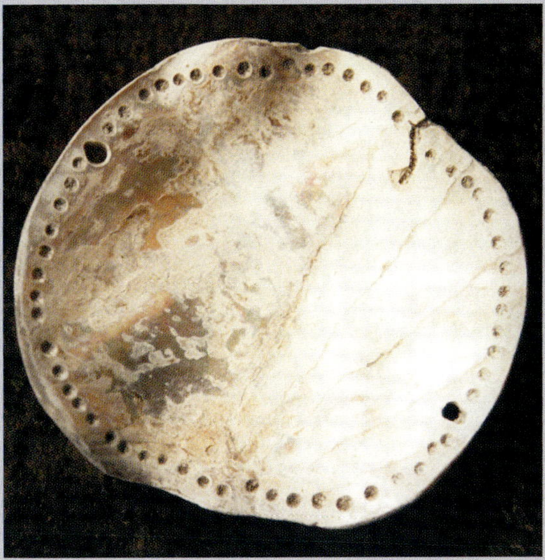

Abalone gorget, 2¾" in diameter. This is a finely decorated piece with drilled holes and spaced rim indentations. Ex-collection Petrie, the gorget is from California. Dale and Betty Roberts collection, Iowa. **$200.00.**

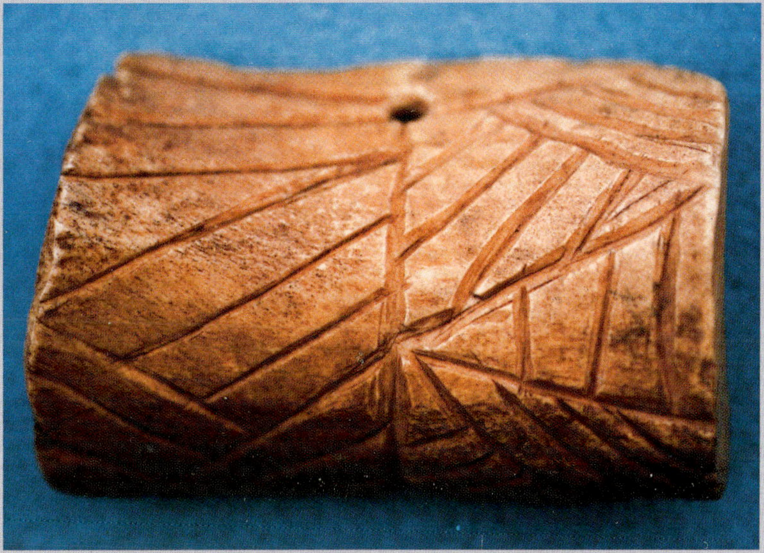

Engraved pendant, elk antler, ex-collection Levy. The artifact is 1¹⁵⁄16 x 2⁵⁄16" and Woodland or later in time. Find-location unknown. Collection of, and photograph by, Gary Henry, North Carolina. Museum grade.

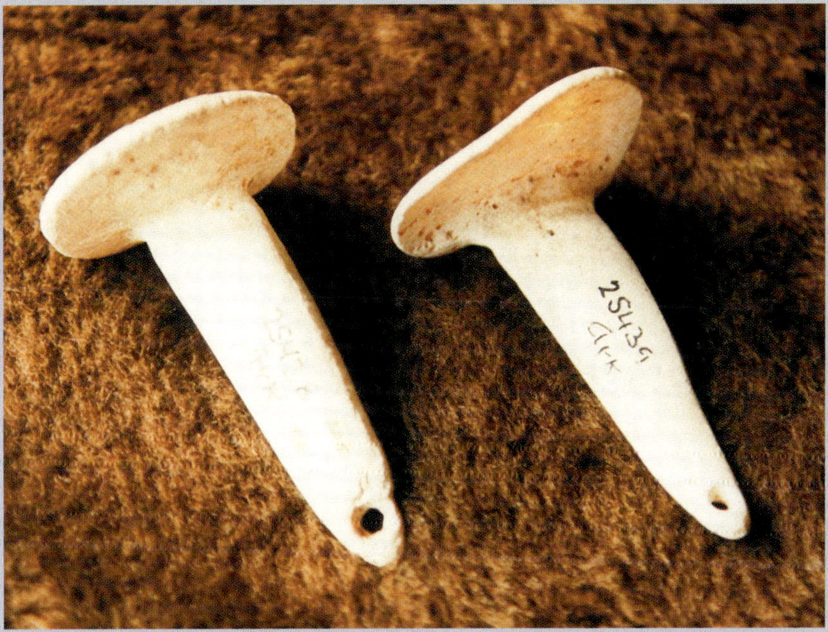

Earplugs or pendants, each 2⅝" long. These are finely made from marine shell and ex-collections Guthrie and Jenkins. Arkansas. Dale and Betty Roberts collection, Iowa. Unlisted.

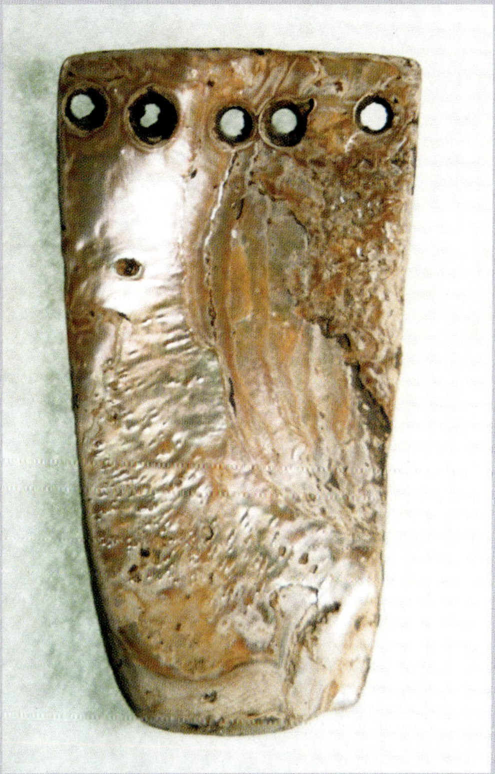

Abalone shell pendant, 3⅝" long. It was found before 1940 in Yuba County, California. Back to Earth. **$275.00.**

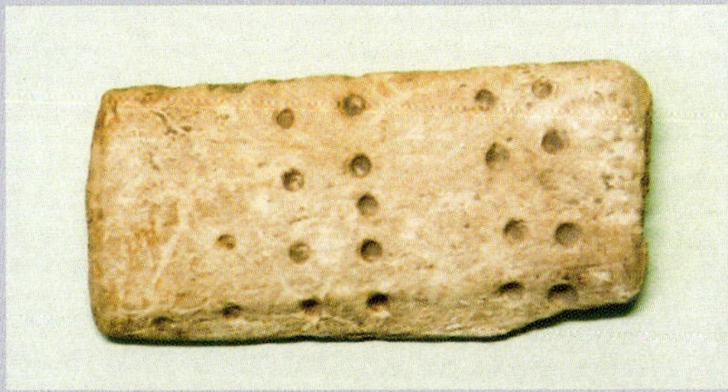

Tally bone or gaming piece, 1 x 2⅛", split bone from a large mammal. The edges have been ground smooth and it has dot decoration. Weber County, northern Utah. Dann Russell collection, Utah. **$25.00.**

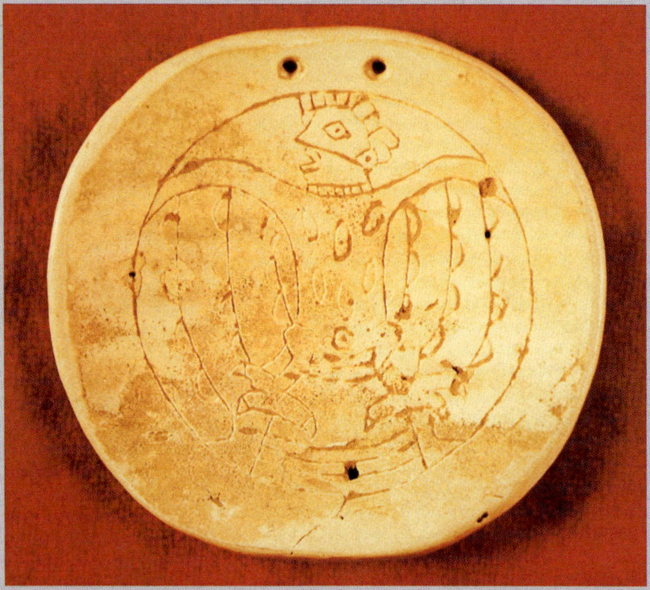

Shell gorget, Eagle Dancer motif, gorget is 2¾" high. Mississippian in time, it is from Tennessee. Robin Fiser collection. Museum grade.

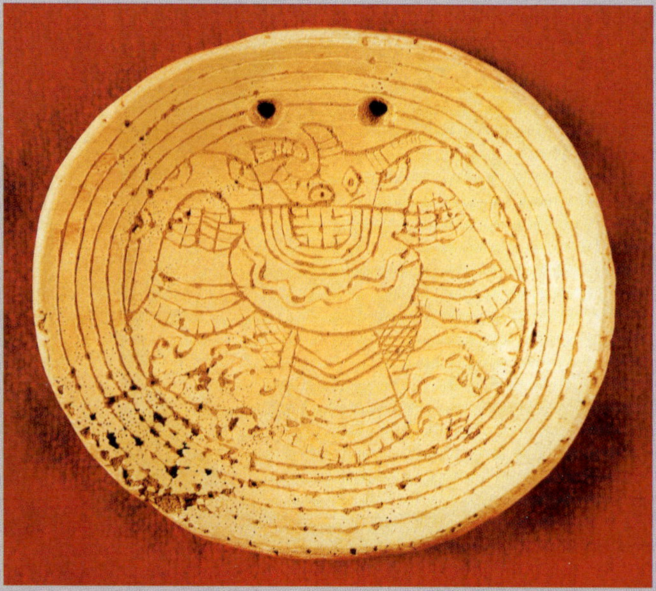

Shell gorget, Mississippian period, 2⅝" high. The incised figure is a stylized bird. This piece came from Tennessee. Robin Fiser collection. Museum grade.

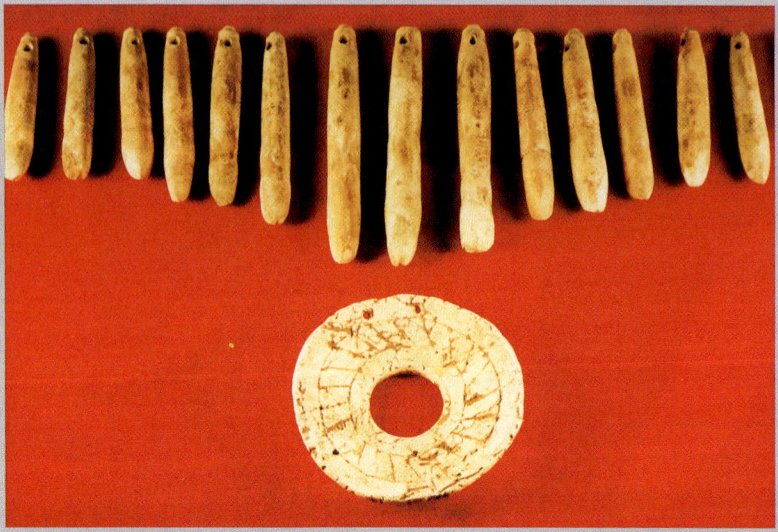

Shell beads and gorget, longest bead is 3⅞" and gorget diameter is 3¹⁄₁₆". These are Mississippian in time, location unlisted. Robin Fiser collection. Museum grade.

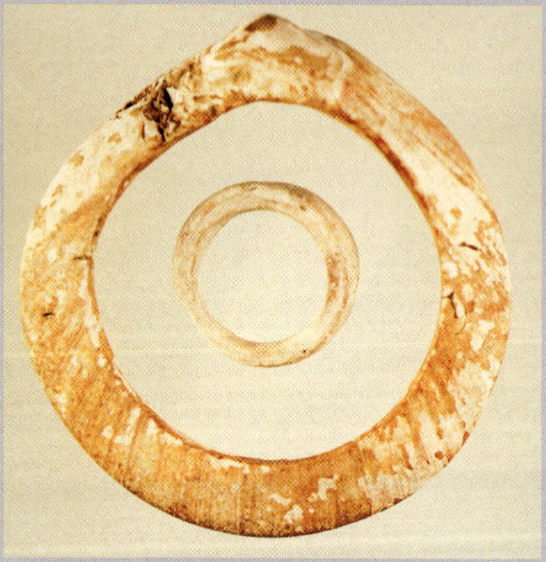

Bracelet and finger ring, both carved from marine shell, bracelet is 2⅞" in diameter. The two came from the American Southwest. Robin Fiser collection. Unlisted.

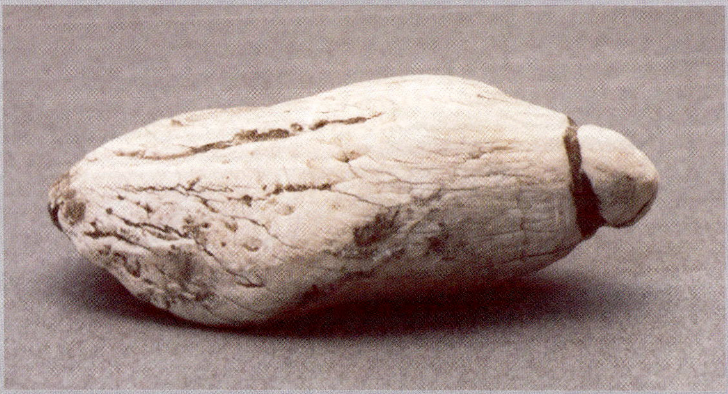

Shell pendant or plummet, 2" long, Calusa culture, AD 1450 or earlier. Found on the south end of Key Marco, now Marco Island, it is from Collier County, Florida. H. B. Greene II collection, Naples, Florida. **$75.00.**

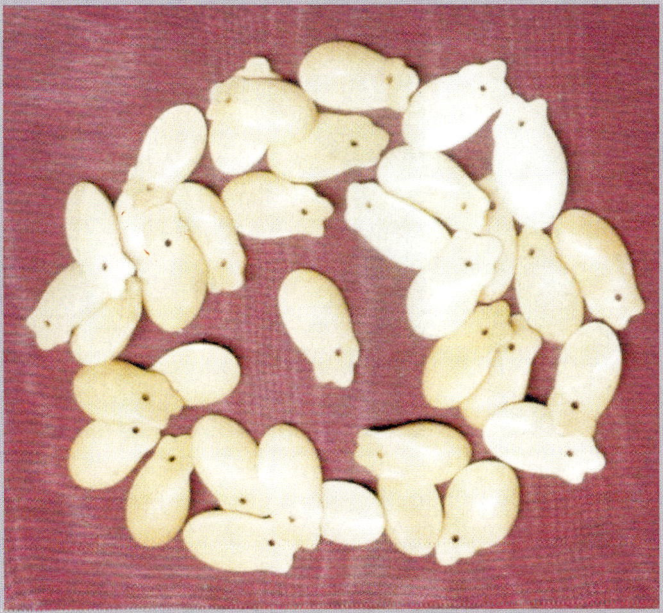

Beads, made of bone which represent the tusks of male elk. These elk had only two of the teeth, and copying the teeth in bone increased the supply. The beads could be used as jewelry or fastened to clothing as decorations. Ben Thompson collection, Missouri. Each, **$25.00.**

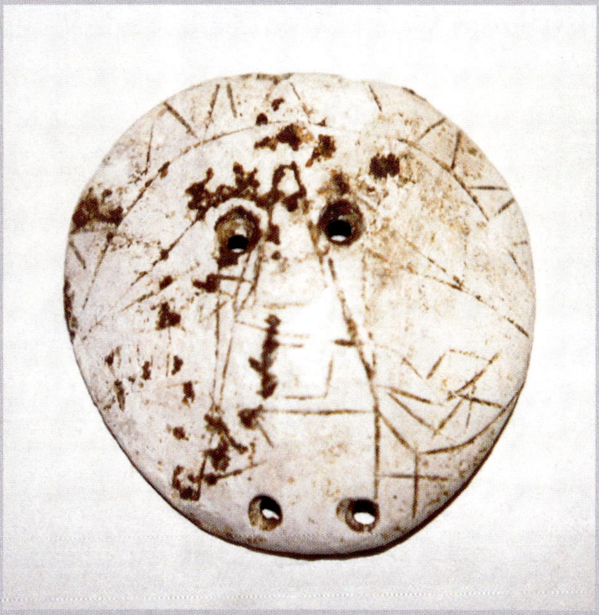

Shell face mask gorget, Buffalo style, 2¼ x 2½". It has rare secondary engraving of a human and two extra suspension holes at the bottom. St. Francis County, Arkansas. Jim Maus collection, North Carolina. Unlisted.

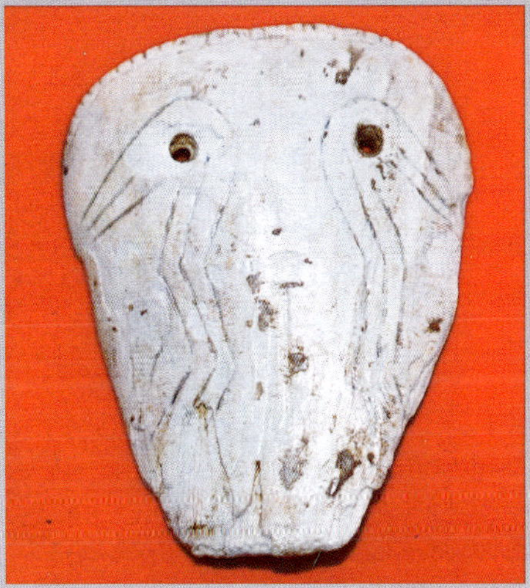

Shell face mask gorget, Buffalo style, 2³⁄₁₆ x 2¾". It has the classic Weeping Eye incising of the Mississippian period and was found in Russell County, Virginia. Jim Maus collection, North Carolina. Unlisted.

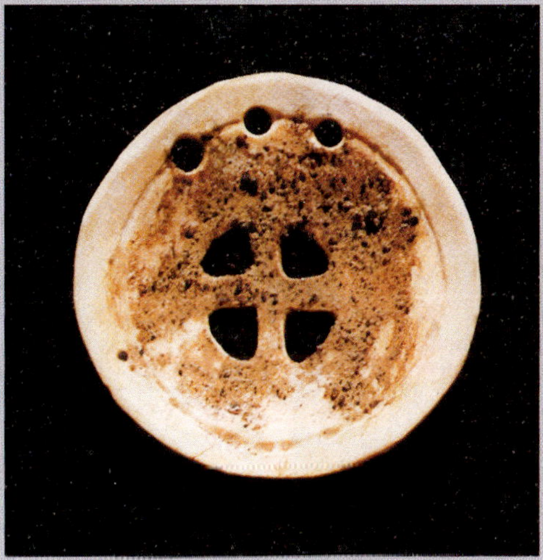

Shell gorget, cruciform, Pine Island style, 2⅜" across, Mississippian period. It is drilled with three suspension holes and was found in Burke County, North Carolina. Jim Maus collection, North Carolina. Unlisted.

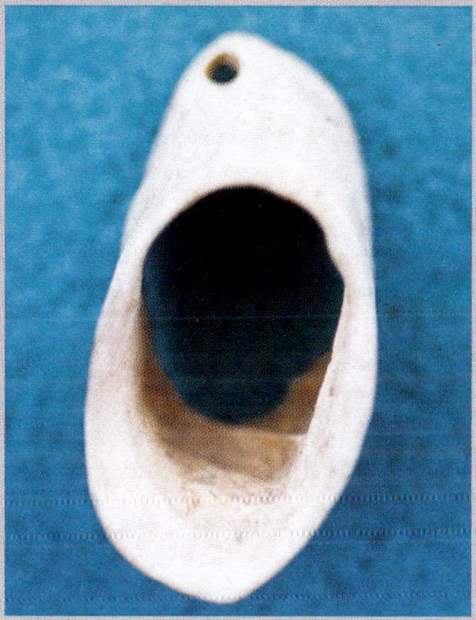

Bone pendant, Woodland or later, ex-collection Levy. The pendant is ⅝ x 1¼", find-location unknown. Collection of, and photograph by, Gary Henry, North Carolina. **$20.00.**

Shell earpin, Mississippian period, 1³⁄₁₆ x 5¼". Though weathered, this is an excellent example with an expanded head. Found by Snyder between 1947 and 1958, it is from Polk County, Tennessee. Collection of, and photograph by, Gary Henry, North Carolina. **$150.00.**

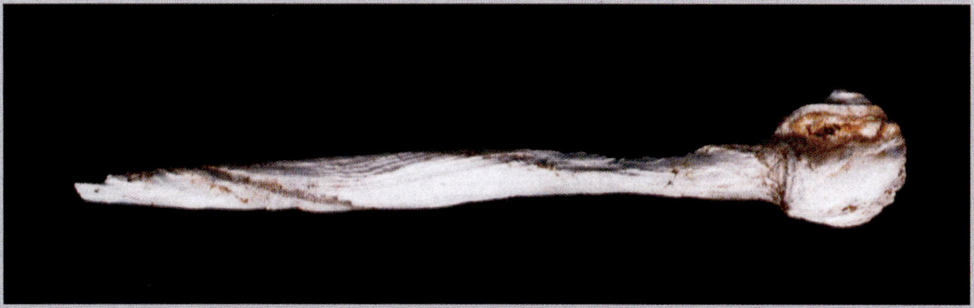

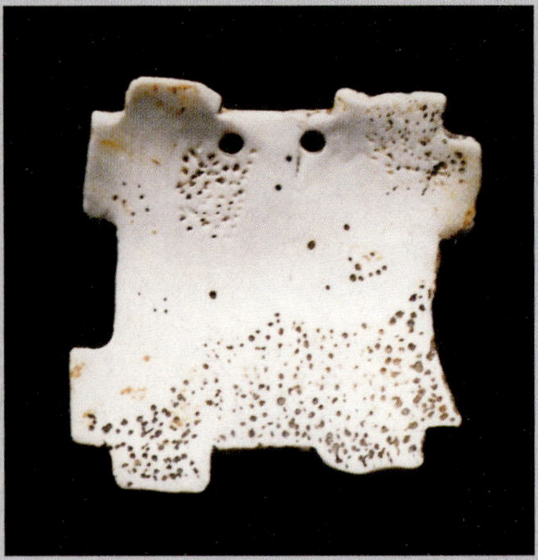

Shell gorget, Square Cross form, 1 15/16" high and 1 7/8" wide, Mississippian. It came from Davie County, North Carolina. Jim Maus collection, North Carolina. Unlisted.

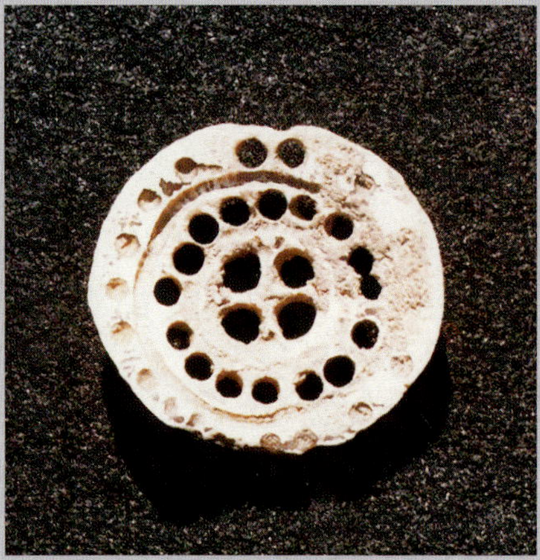

Shell gorget, Geometric style, Mississippian, 1 5/8" in diameter. It was found in Stokes County, North Carolina. Jim Maus collection, North Carolina. Unlisted.

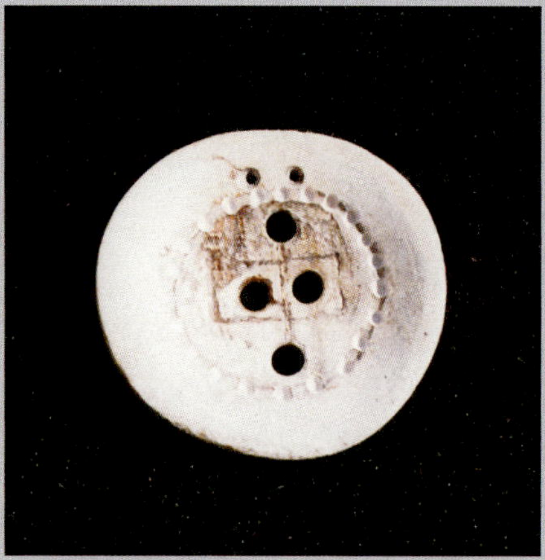

Shell gorget, Mississippian, Cruciform style, 1 9/16" in diameter. It was found in Monroe County, Tennessee. Jim Maus collection, North Carolina. Unlisted.

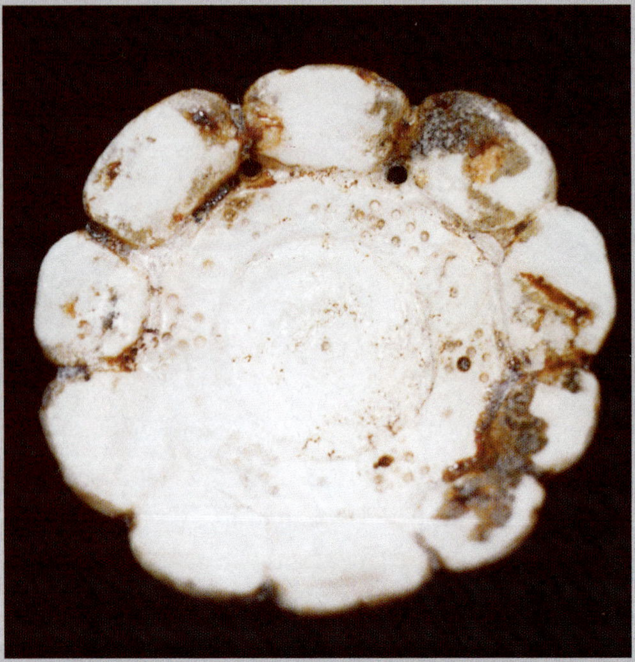

Shell gorget, Triskele, Nashville II style, 3 5/8" in diameter. Boldly engraved, this piece is Mississippian (Fort Ancient) and was found in Kentucky. Jim Maus collection, North Carolina. Unlisted.

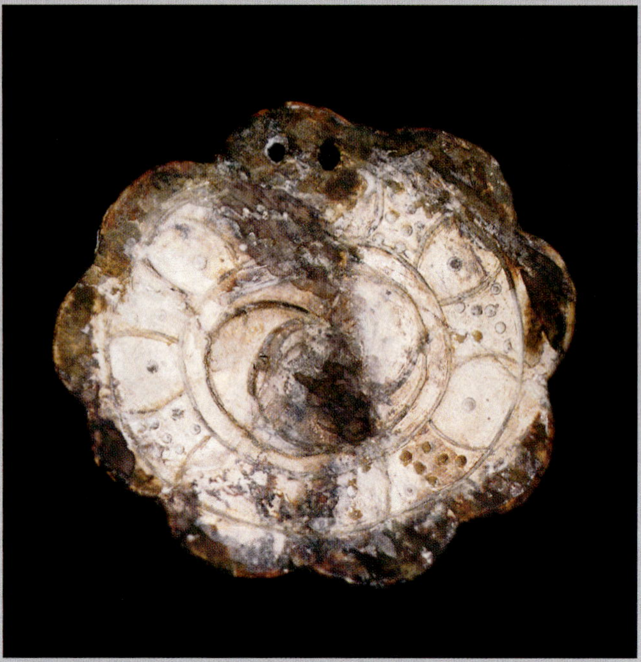

Shell gorget, Triskele, Nashville II style, 3 1/2" in diameter. It has two suspension holes, scalloped rim, and came from Meigs County, Tennessee. Jim Maus collection, North Carolina. Unlisted.

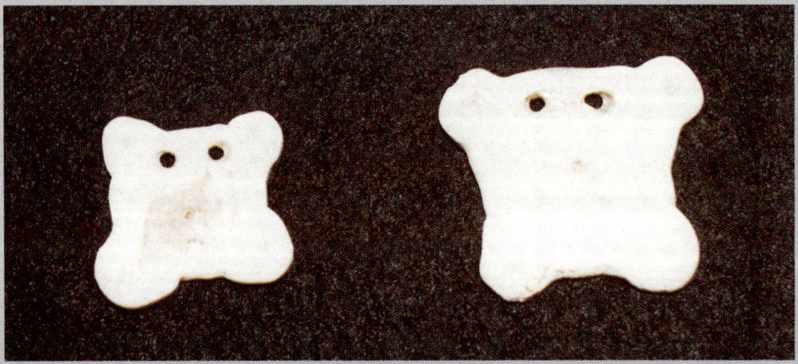

Shell gorgets, Warren Wilson style, left example is 1 1/16 x 1 1/8", right example is 1 5/16 x 1 1/2". Also known as "Mickey Mouse" gorgets, they came from the Chattanooga area, Tennessee. Jim Maus collection, North Carolina. Unlisted.

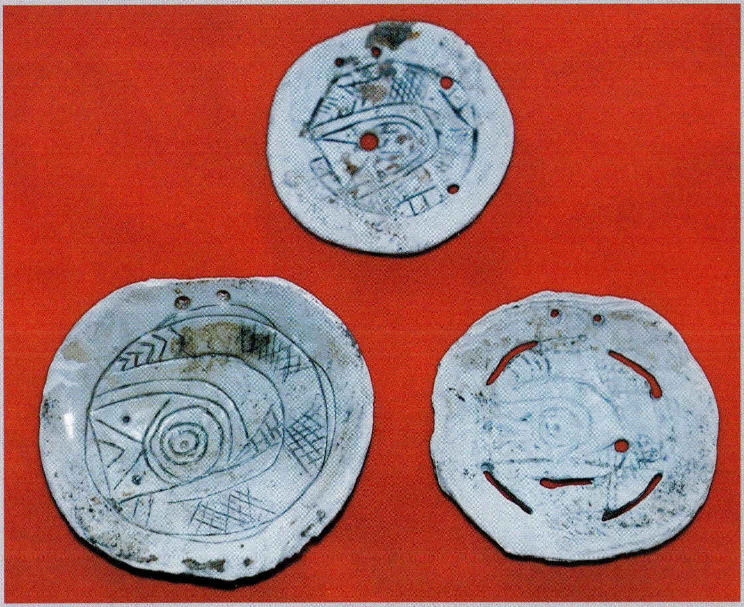

Shell gorget, Rattlesnake designs, Mississippian period. Top, Saltville style, 2½" in diameter. Left, Saltville style, 3¼" in diameter. Right, Lick Creek style, 2⅞" in diameter. All were found on the same site in Stokes County, North Carolina. Jim Maus collection, North Carolina. Unlisted.

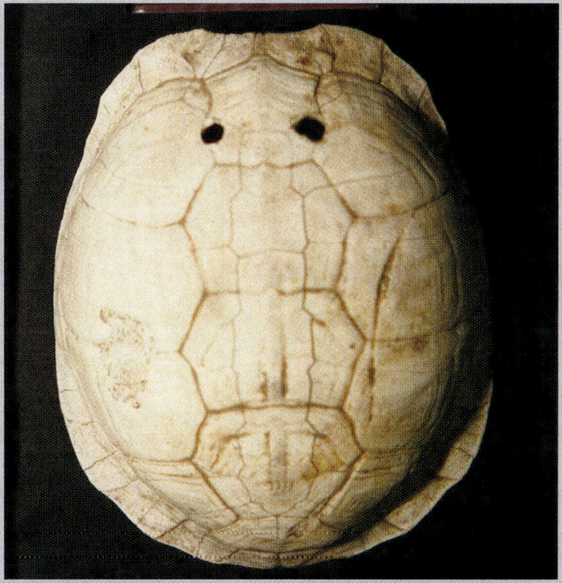

Tortoise shell pendant or gorget, Anasazi, Southwestern United States. Back to Earth. Unlisted.

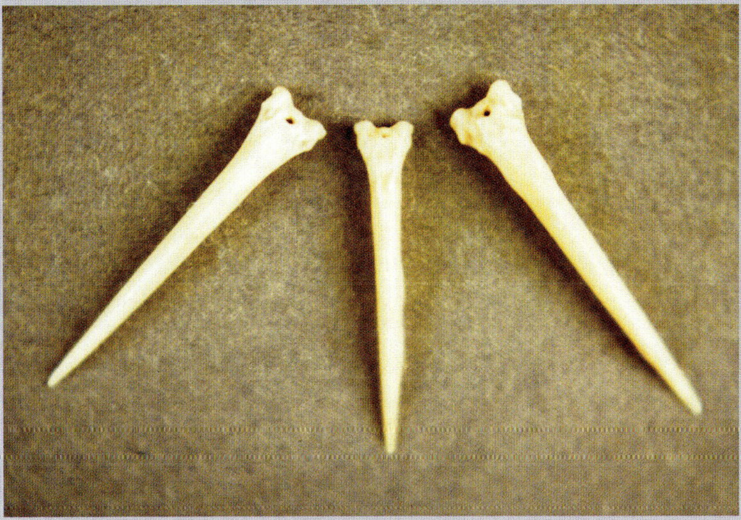

Fish bone necklace elements, longest is 1⅞". Each of the artifacts is drilled at the thick end with a small hole, and all came from near Willow Grove, West Virginia. Larry Garvin collection. Each, **$15.00.**

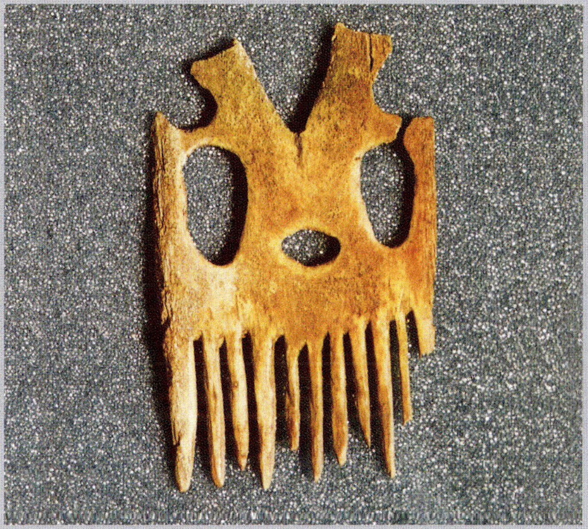

Antler comb, two bears climbing trees, 3" long. Stained with deep green copper salts, it is historic Iroquois (Seneca) and ca. AD 1650 – 1675. These combs may have been used to decorate hair or scalp locks and not for combing. The effigy comb was found near Honeoye Falls, Monroe County, New York. Dave Summers collection, Victor, New York. **$1800.00.**

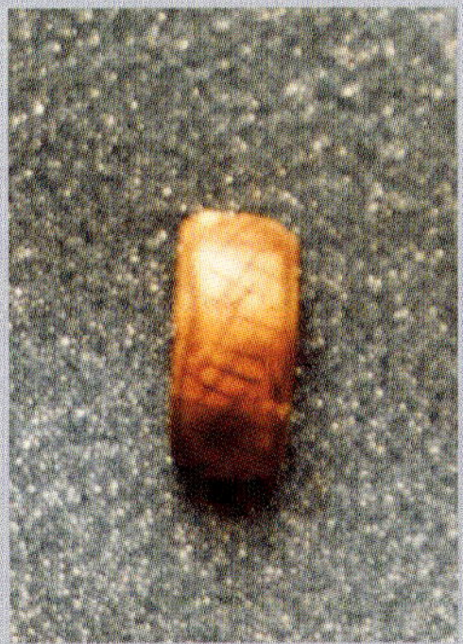

Finger ring, incised bone, ¾" in diameter. The ring is Late Archaic, Brewerton phase, ca. 1600 BC. Onondaga County, New York. Dave Summers collection, Victor, New York. **$125.00.**

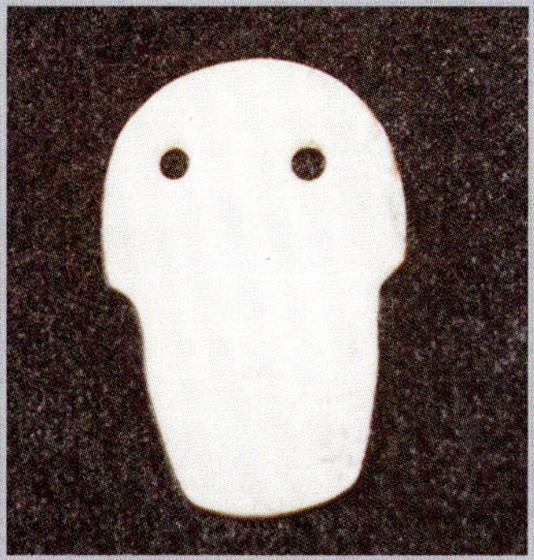

Shell face mask gorget, miniature, McBee style, 1⅛ x 1⁹⁄₁₆". It was found in Hamilton County, Tennessee. Jim Maus collection, North Carolina. Unlisted.

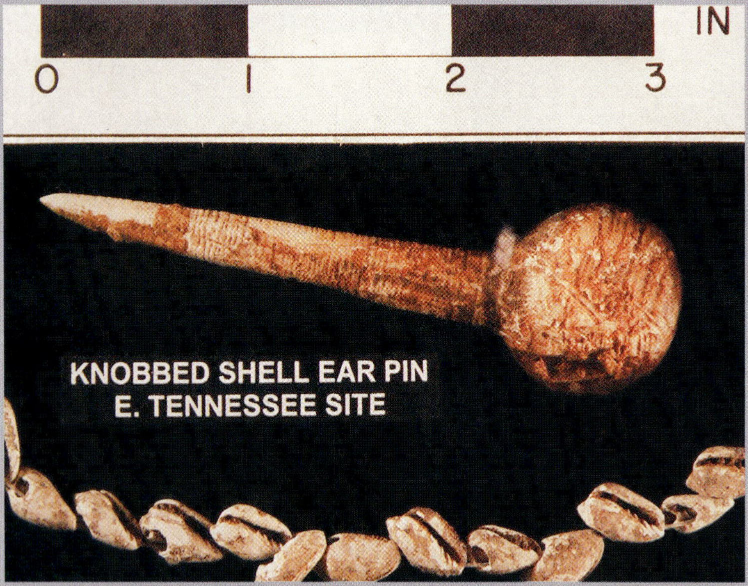
IN
0 1 2 3
KNOBBED SHELL EAR PIN
E. TENNESSEE SITE

Hair or ear pin, shell with marginella shell beads. The carefully shaped pin came from an eastern Tennessee site, while the beads are from Cabarrus County, North Carolina. Collection of, and photograph by, Ron Harris, North Carolina. Beads, unlisted; pin, **$200.00.**

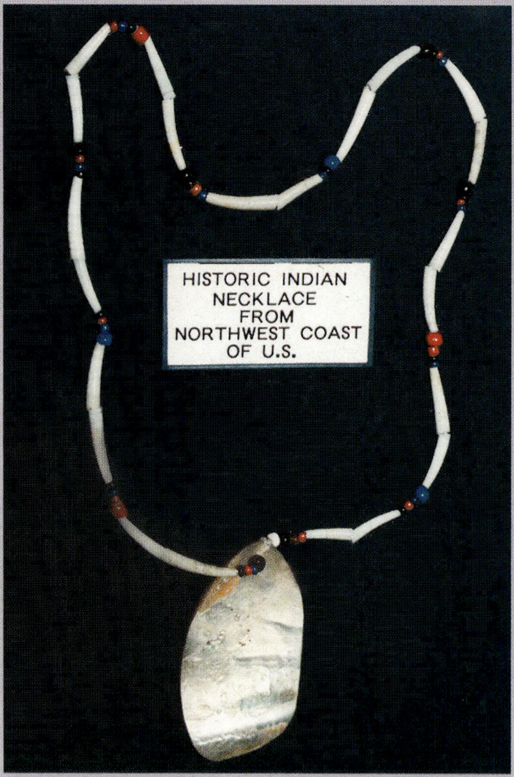
HISTORIC INDIAN
NECKLACE
FROM
NORTHWEST COAST
OF U.S.

Necklace, with dentalium and glass beads with a large shell pendant. Dentalium shells came mainly from the Vancouver Island area and were either obtained from the seafloor or found on the beach. Northwest Coastal region. Back to Earth. Unlisted.

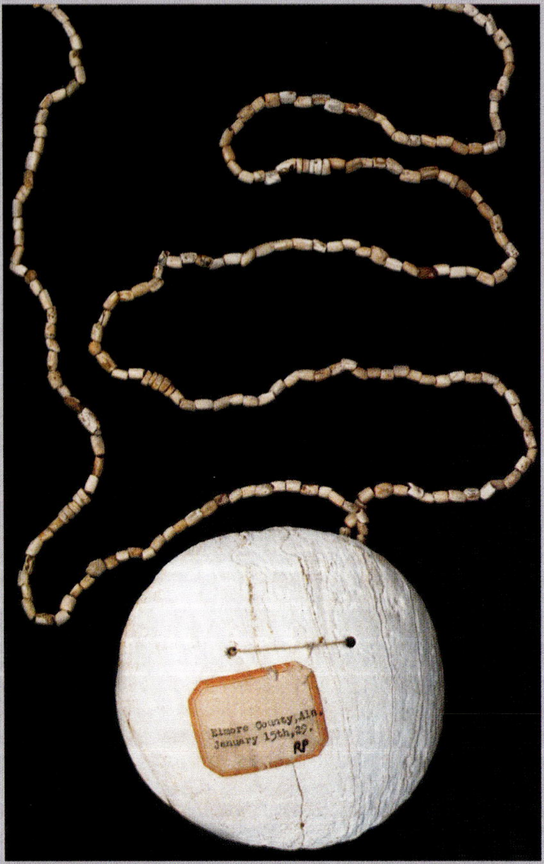

Shell gorget, with 274 shell beads. The gorget is 4½" across and the average bead is ¼" long and ⅛" in diameter. Mississippian in time, this is ex-collection Snyder. Elmore County, Alabama. Collection of, and photograph by, Gary Henry, North Carolina. Museum grade.

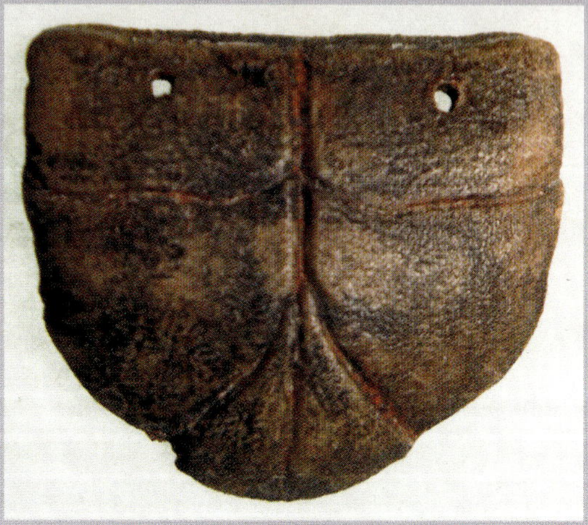

Shell pendant, land tortoise, fully intact. It was found in a rock shelter in Union County, Illinois. Back to Earth. **$275.00.**

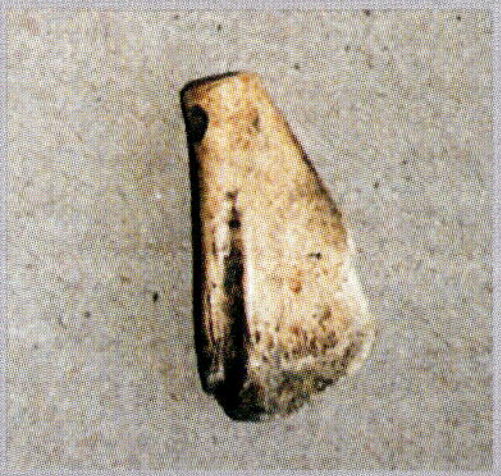

Bone pendant, with drilled hole and two side grooves, pendant size is ½ x 1". It was found in Arkansas. Wilfred Dick collection, Mississippi. **$60.00.**

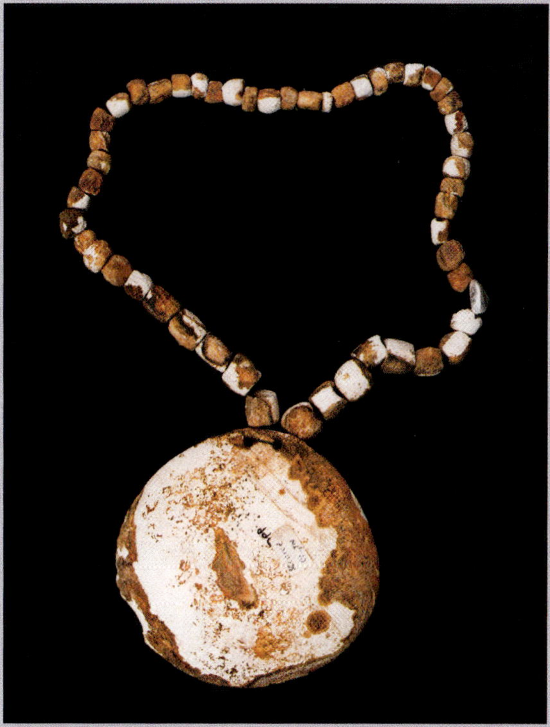

Shell gorget and pendant with beads, (with one freshwater pearl bead), Mississippian period. The gorget is 4" in diameter and the largest bead is 9/16" both long and wide. This piece is ex-collection Snyder, from Monroe County, Tennessee. Collection of, and photograph by, Gary Henry, North Carolina. Museum grade.

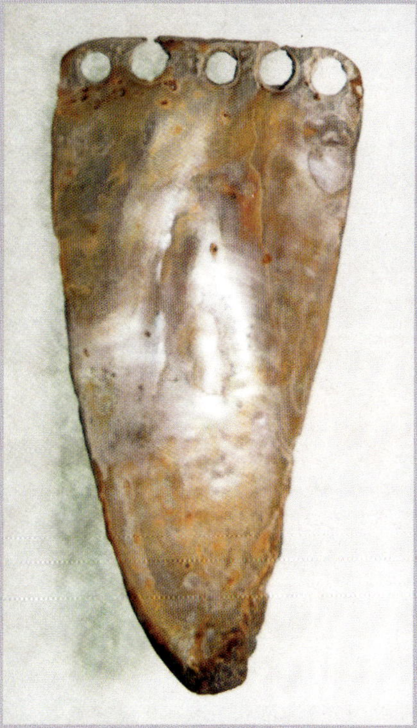

Abalone shell pendant, 3½" long, possible claw effigy. The pendant was found before 1940 in Yuba County, California. Back to Earth. **$215.00.**

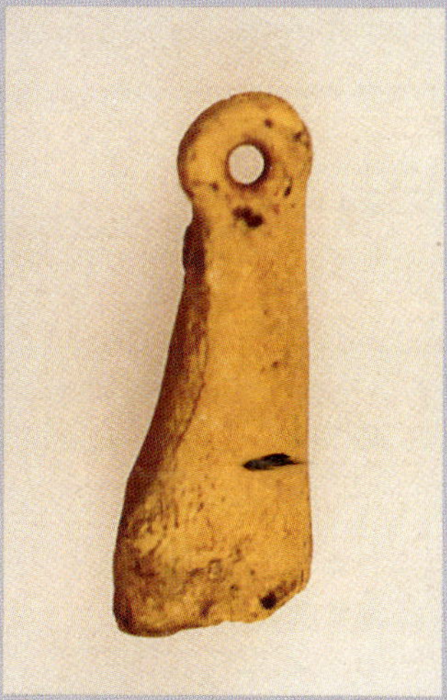

Pendant, deer toe bone, 2¼" long. Precisely drilled at the top, the bone itself is solid and has not been hollowed. Such bones were sometimes used for arrowpoints and fishhooks, but this example was made into an ornament. Ex-collection Vietzen, Ohio River Valley. Pete Timoch collection. **$50.00 – 75.00.**

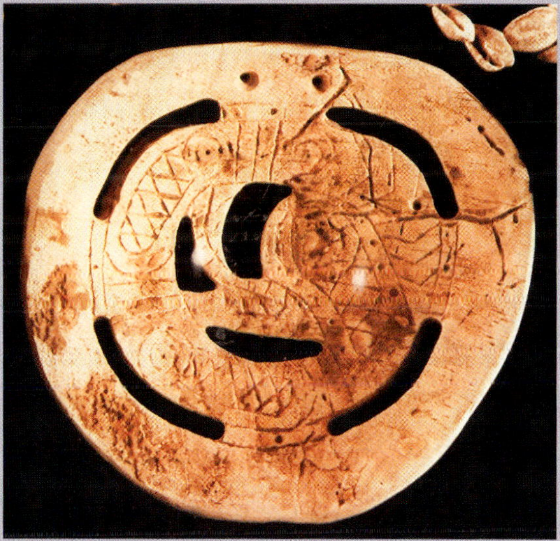

Shell gorget, Brakebill style Fenestrated (windowed) design, 3½" across at widest point. Mississippian, it was found at a site in southwestern Virginia. Collection of, and photograph by, Ron Harris, North Carolina. Museum grade.

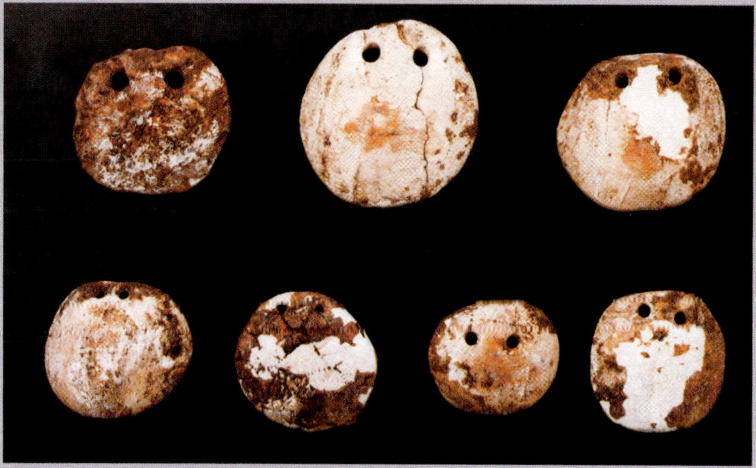

Shell gorget, Woodland or Mississippian, largest is 1⅝ x 1 15/16". Drilled with two suspension holes, these are plain but artistic pieces. Ex-collection Snyder, they are from Blount County, Alabama. Collection of, and photograph by, Gary Henry, North Carolina. Each, **$75.00 – 125.00.**

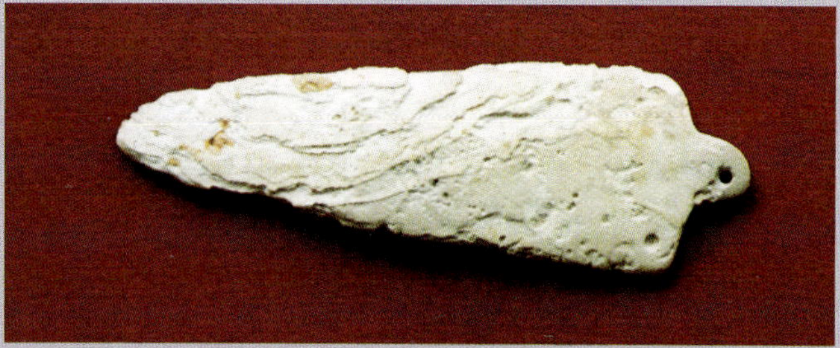

Arrowhead pendant, shell, Iroquois ca. AD 1650, perforated for suspension. It is 4⅜" long, from central New York. Dave Summers collection, Victor, New York. **$350.00.**

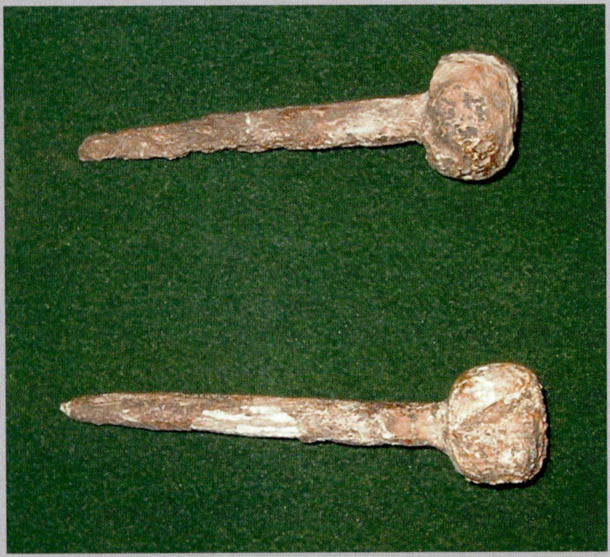

Earpins, bone or shell, 4½ and 4" long, Davis COA. The pins came from Polk County, Tennessee. Keith and Rhonda Dodge collection, Michigan. Unlisted.

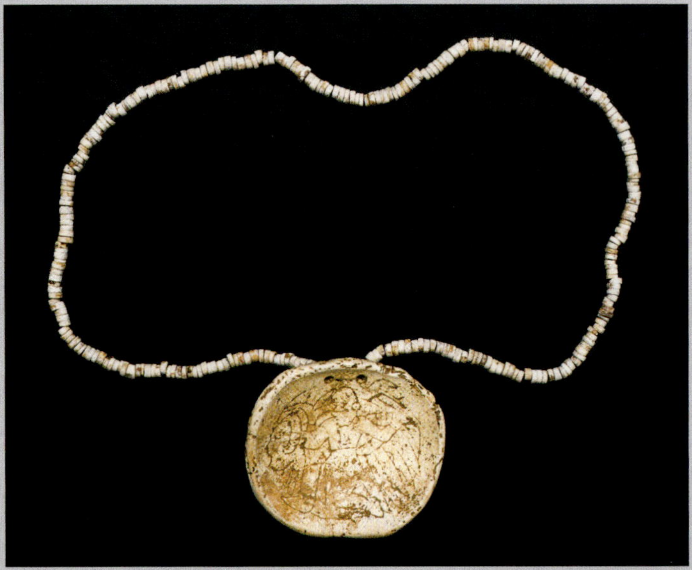

Shell gorget, with incised feathered dancer, Mississippian period, strand with 276 beads, 2⅝ x 2$^{15}/_{16}$". This fine example is ex-collection Snyder. Meigs County, Tennessee. Collection of, and photograph by, Gary Henry, North Carolina. **$1,000.00.**

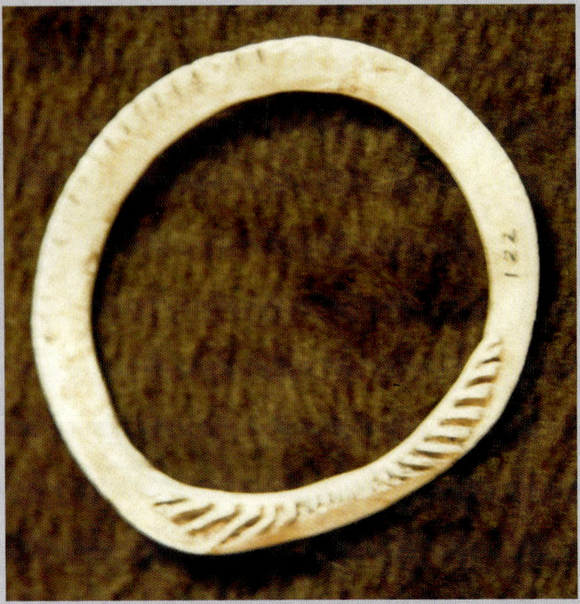

Engraved shell bracelet, 3" in diameter, ex-collection Petrie. This carved and decorated bracelet was found in Arizona. Dale and Betty Roberts collection, Iowa. **$250.00.**

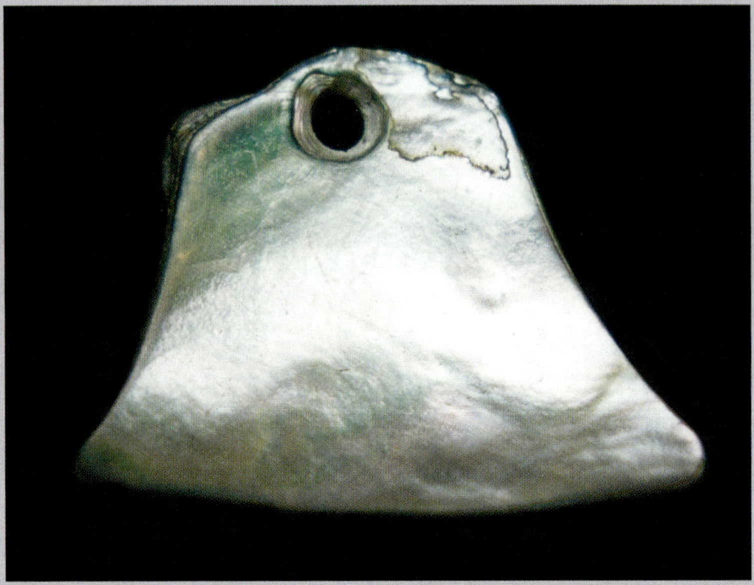

Drilled abalone shell pendant, 1¾ x 2⅛". This ornament was found in Erie County, Ohio. Garvin collection. Unlisted.

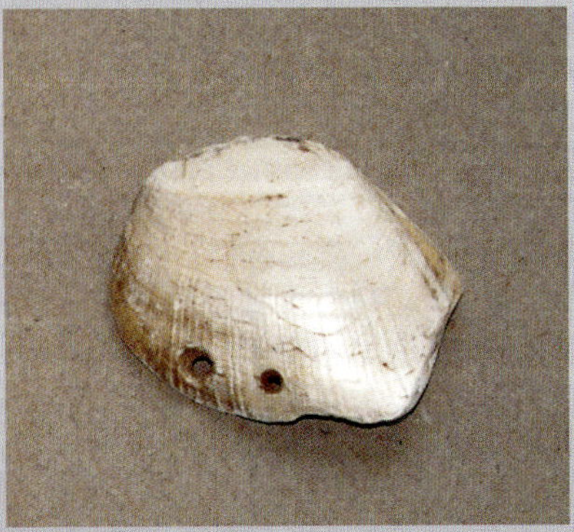

Shell pendant, 1¾ x 2½", two drilled holes. This example, probably Mississippian, was found near the Tennessee River. Wilfred Dick collection, Mississippi. **$65.00.**

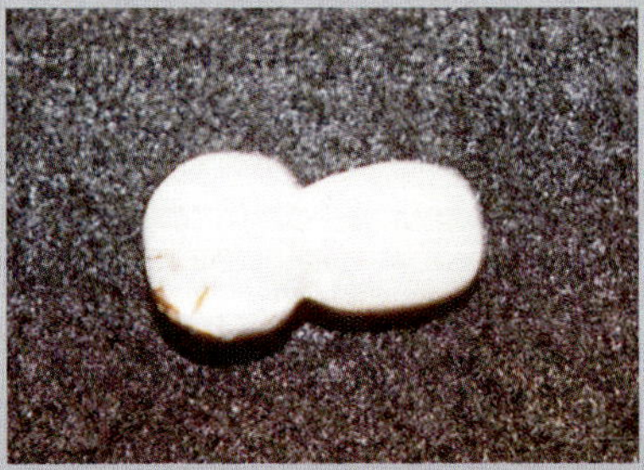

Marine shell nose plug, 1$^{3}/_{16}$". It was found at Tick Island, Florida. Jim Maus collection, North Carolina. Unlisted.

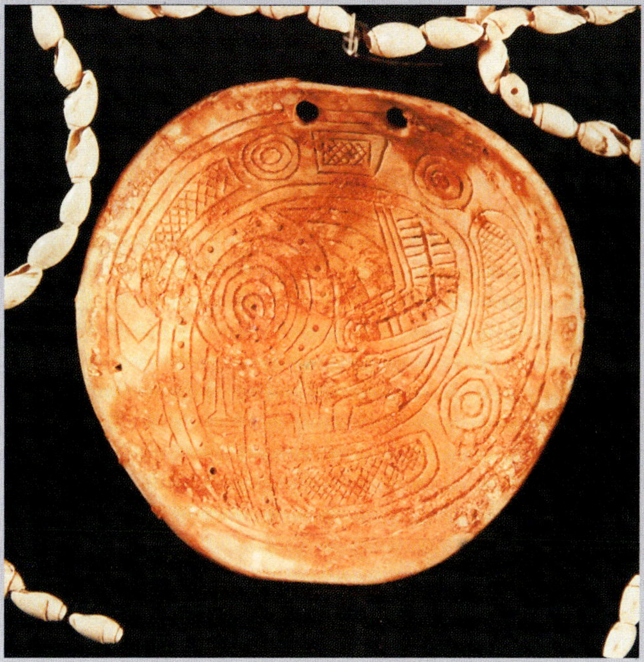

Shell gorget, outer whorl of conch shell, Mississippian, 3" across at widest. Drilled at the top, this is a Citico style Rattlesnake gorget with marginella shell beads. The gorget is from a site in eastern Tennessee, while the beads are from Cabarrus County, North Carolina. Collection of, and photograph by, Ron Harris, North Carolina. Museum grade.

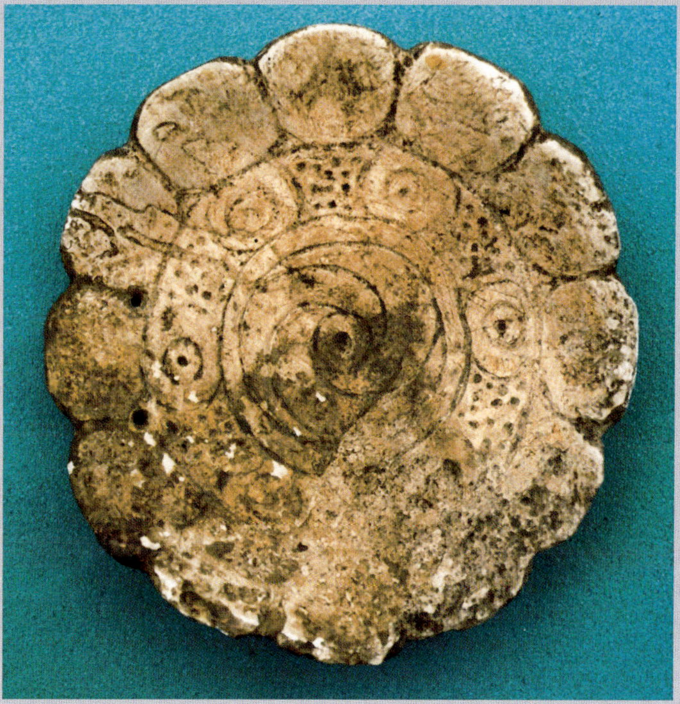

Scalloped shell gorget, with sun circles and triskele center, 3 13/16" across. It is pictured in *Who's Who in Indian Relics* No. 8, and is ex-collection Snyder. Mississippian, it was found in Rhea County, Tennessee. Collection of, and photograph by, Gary Henry, North Carolina. **$1,250.00.**

Pendant, unusually thick conch shell, ca. AD 1650-1675, Seneca's Huron captives. Grooved for suspension, it is 4 3/4" long and from East Bloomfield, New York. Dave Summers collection, Victor, New York. **$325.00.**

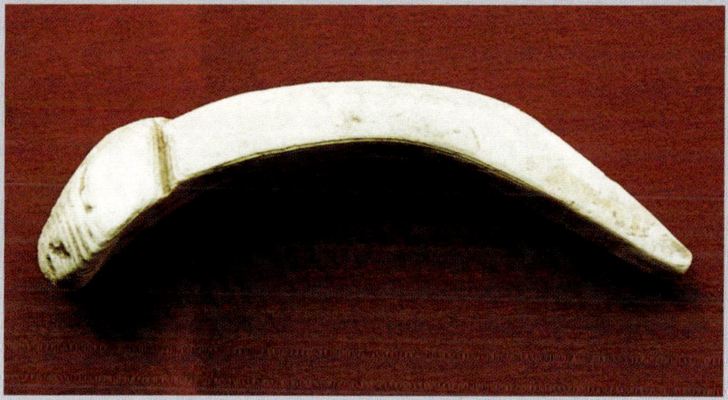

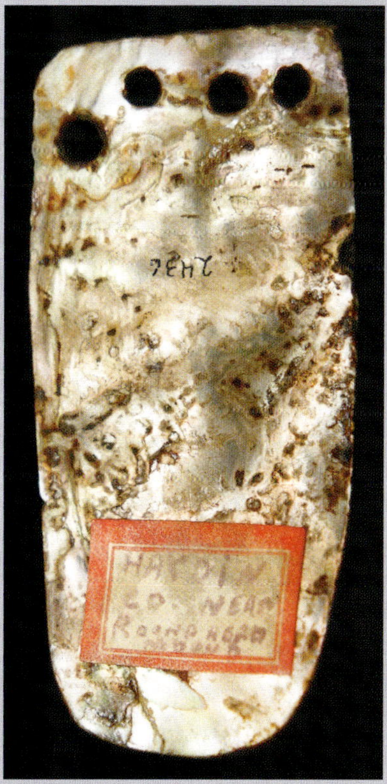

Pendant, 1 5/8 x 3 1/4", drilled suspension holes. It is made of abalone shell, imported from the West Coast. The find-location suggests this piece might be Glacial Kame and Late Archaic. Roundhead Township, Hardin County, Ohio. Garvin collection. **$250.00.**

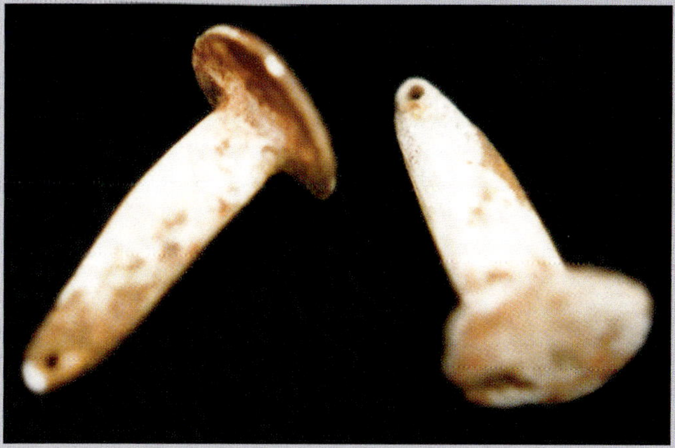

Shell earplugs, marine shell, 1 5/16" and 2 1/2" long, respectively. These were found in Pemiscot County, Missouri. Bob Hess collection, Indiana. Unlisted.

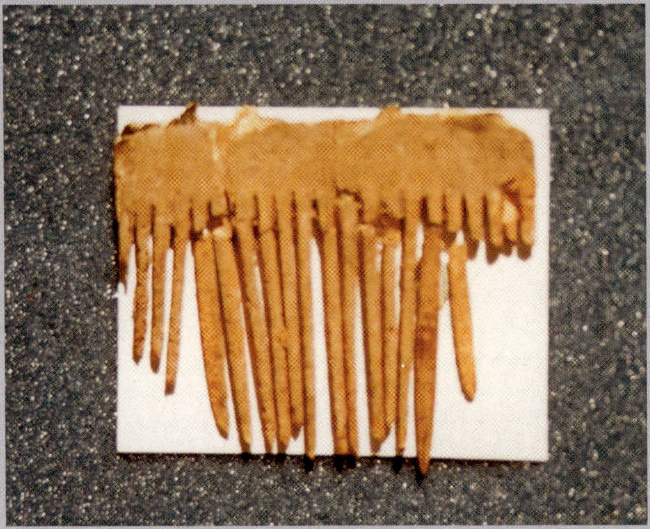

Bone "cootie comb," European-made, ex-collection Schroff (ca. 1930), 2 x 2½". It is historic Iroquois (Seneca) and dates to AD 1675 – 1687. The comb was found near Victor, Ontario County, New York. Dave Summers collection, Victor, New York. **$150.00.**

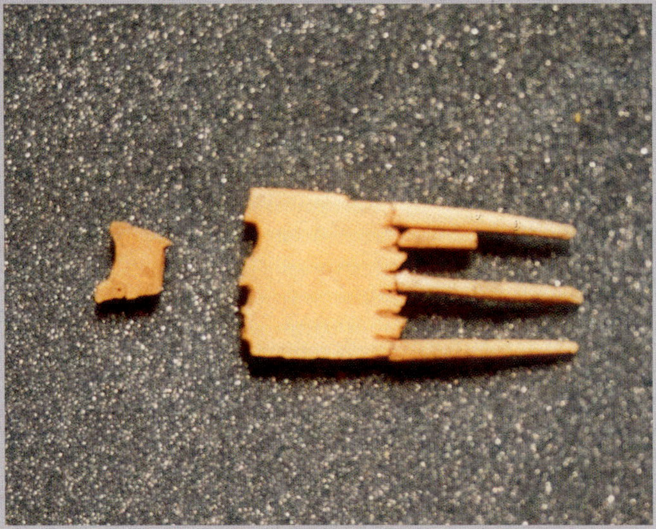

Broken bone effigy comb, 3" as shown. It is historic Iroquois (Seneca) and ca. AD 1670 – 1687. The comb was found near Victor, Ontario County, New York. Dave Summers collection, Victor, New York. **$300.00.**

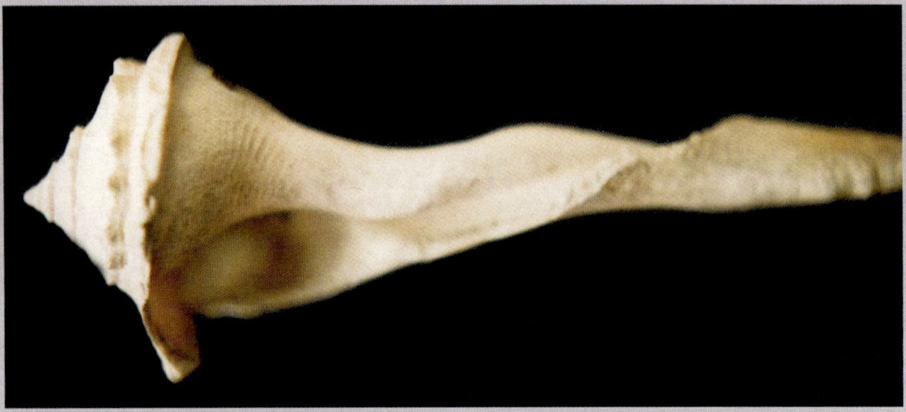

Central whorl, conch shell, worked to shape, 6½" long. It is ex-collection Dr. Gish and was found in a shell midden. Florida. Bob Hess collection, Indiana. **$75.00.**

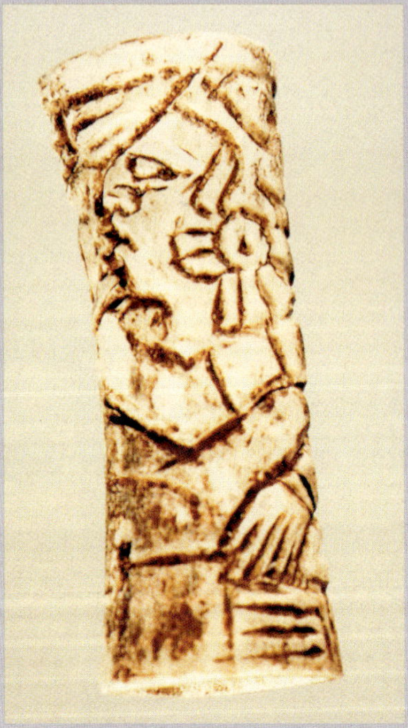

Handle, hollowed bone, 2⅞" long. The smaller end has two drilled holes, and the effigy figure is deeply incised. While the figure appears to be Mayan, the artifact was supposedly found along the Tennessee River in Alabama. Robin Fiser collection. Unlisted.

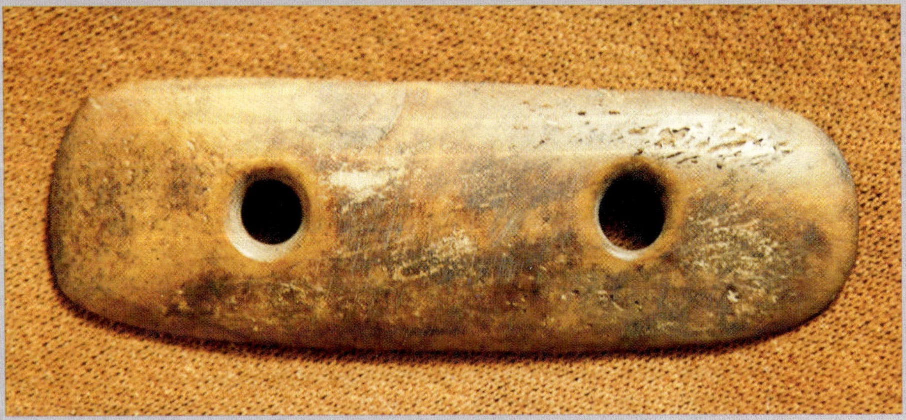

Bone gorget, Archaic or Woodland period, 4⅛" long. It is well-shaped and polished, with large holes. Ex-collection Fryer, the gorget is from northwestern Arkansas. Dale and Betty Roberts collection, Iowa. **$375.00.**

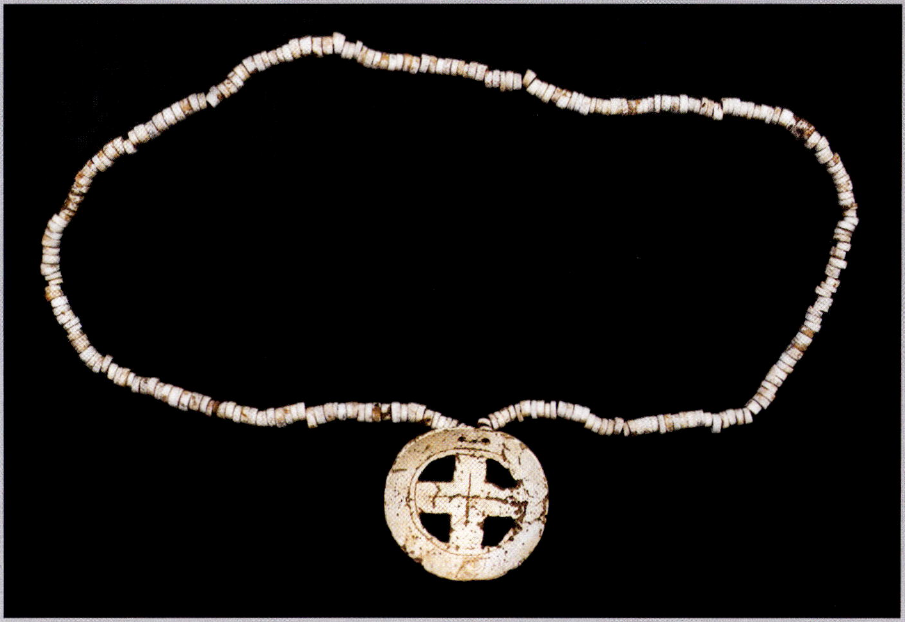

Shell "cross-and-circle" gorget, with 253 beads, Mississippian period, gorget is 1¾ x 1$^{15}/_{16}$". The beads average ¼" in diameter and ⅛" thick. This piece is ex-collection Snyder, from Meigs County, Tennessee. Collection of, and photograph by, Gary Henry, North Carolina. **$600.00.**

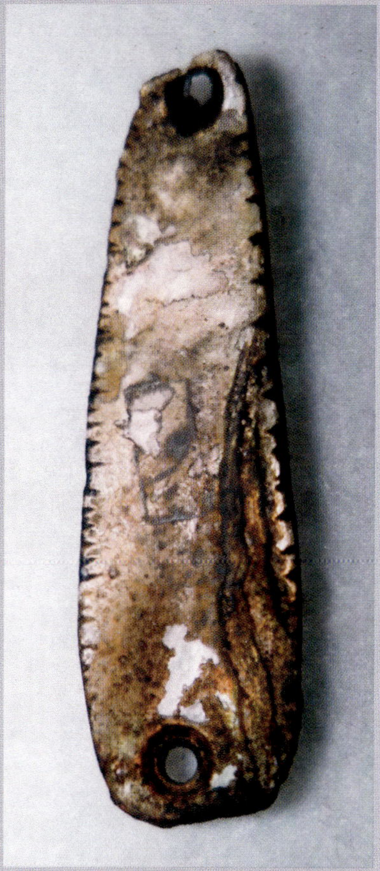

Abalone shell pendant, 2¼" long. This drilled ornament has tally marks and came from Bartow County, Georgia. Garvin collection. **$75.00 – 100.00.**

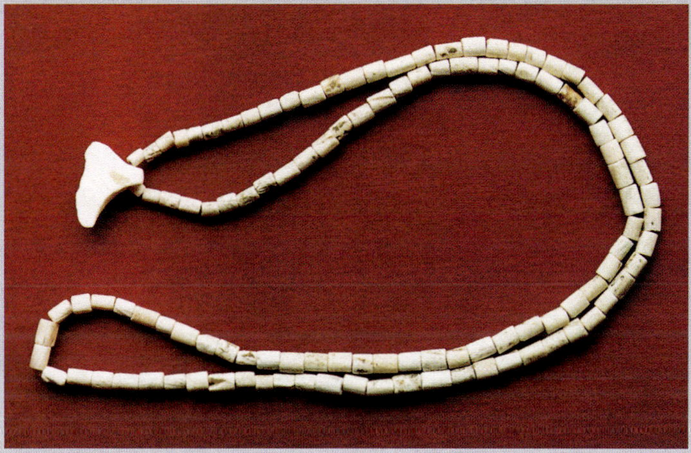

Seneca beads, ca. AD 1655 – 1675, 116 white Dutch-made shell wampum beads in good condition with a claw-shaped pendant. The necklace is 24" long. These ornamental objects are from the Mendon area, Monroe County, New York. Dave Summers collection, Victor, New York. **$300.00.**

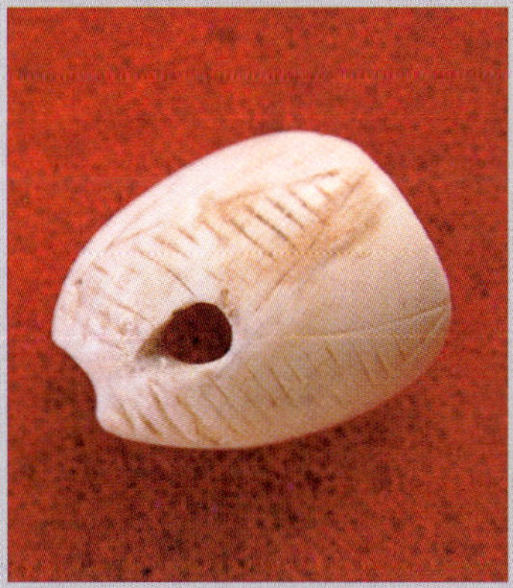

Carved olivella shell bead, 1¼". This example was found in the Great Basin, Nevada. Victor T. Trujillo collection, Nevada. **$30.00.**

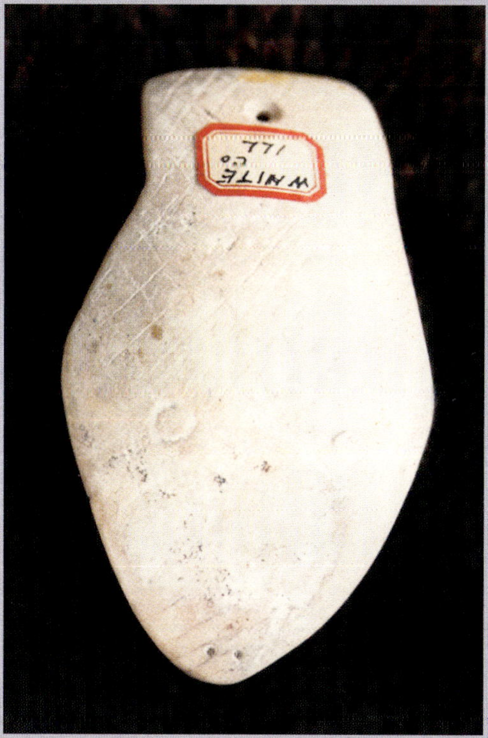

Shell pendant, snake head effigy, engraved eyes, drilled nostrils and cross-hatched head top. It is 3½" long, ex-collection Cheeseboro. White County, Illinois. Dale and Betty Roberts collection, Iowa. Museum grade.

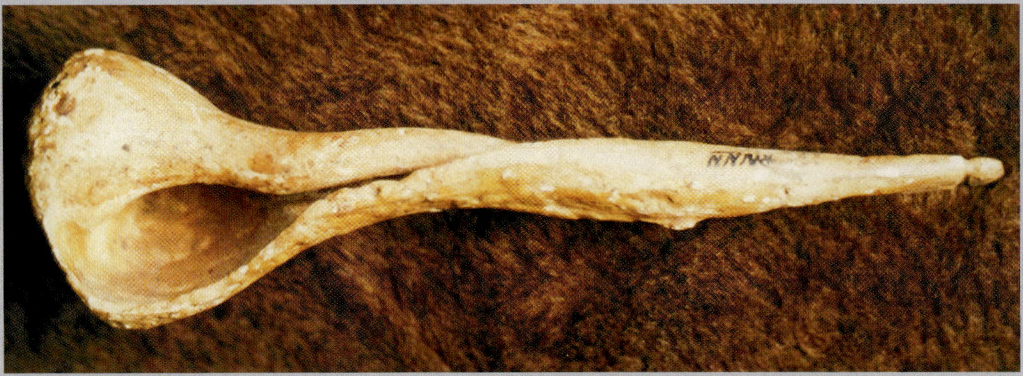

Conch shell pendant, 8½" long, central section with grooved tip. Ex-collection Stroud, this very long ornamental piece is from Mason County, Kentucky. Dale and Betty Roberts collection, Iowa. **$375.00.**

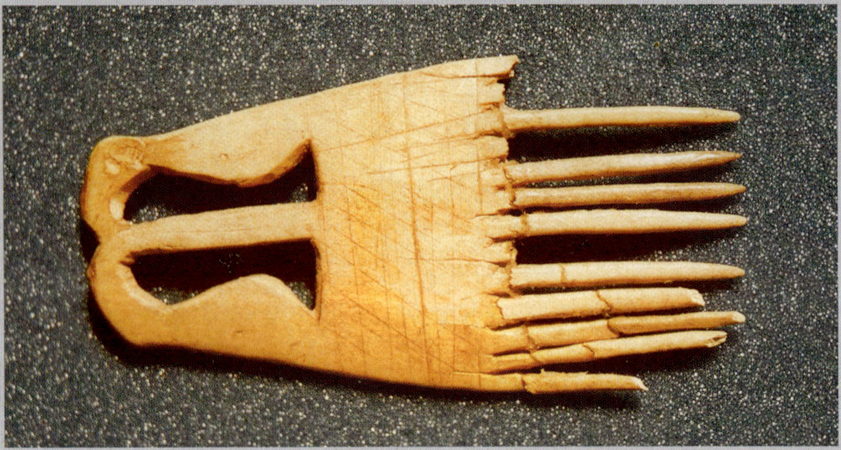

Effigy comb, moose antler, Bird Clan totem engraved with spirit lines, 4½" long. Effigy combs are very scarce to rare on New York sites. It is ex-collections Quinlin (ca. 1935) and Casterline. Historic Iroquois (Seneca), it came from near East Bloomfield and is dated AD 1630 – 1650. Ontario County, New York. Dave Summers collection, Victor, New York. **$2,800.00.**

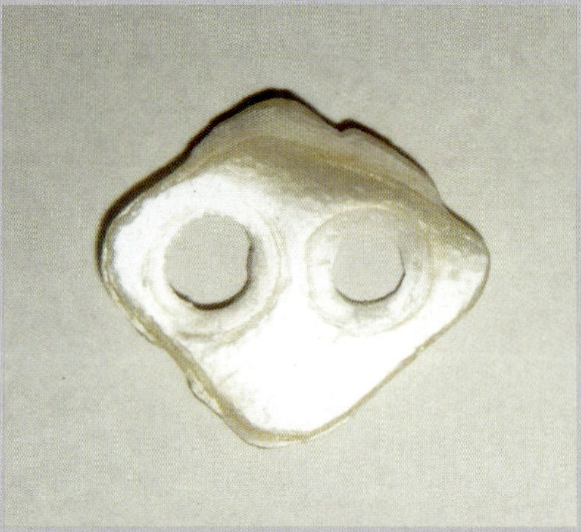

Shell gorget, Mississippian period, 1 3/16 x ¾". It has incised lines around the eye-holes and was found in the Ohio River by the owner's wife. Mason County, West Virginia. Private collection. Rodney Roberts photograph. **$100.00.**

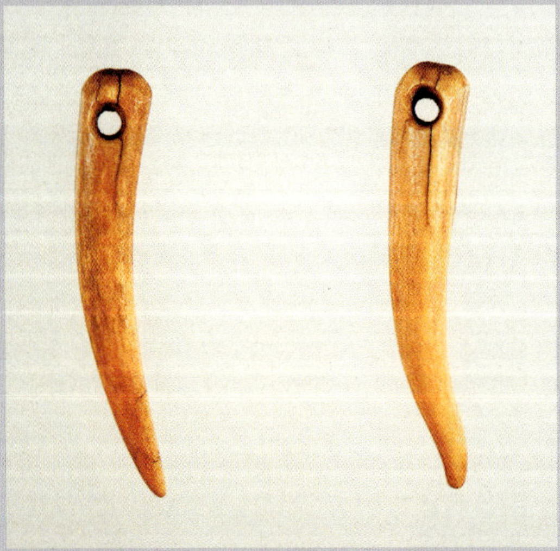

Pendants, deer antler tines, longest is 2⅝". Probably also necklace elements, they may be Hopewell (200 BC – AD 500) in time. Ross County, Ohio. Fred Winegardner collection. Museum grade.

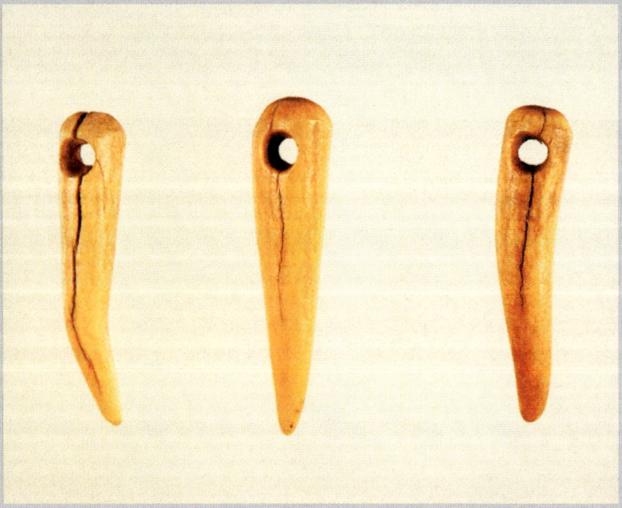

Pendants or necklace elements, polished deer antler, longest is 1⅞". Possibly Hopewell (Middle Woodland), they came from Ross County, Ohio. Fred Winegardner collection. Museum grade.

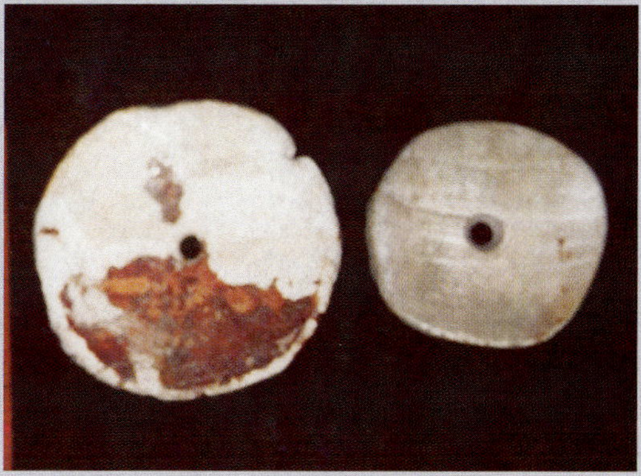

Shell ornaments, diameter of largest (at left) is 1⅝". The center holes were for cord suspension or for use as beads. Provenance unlisted. Private collection. Small, $30.00. Large, **$75.00.**

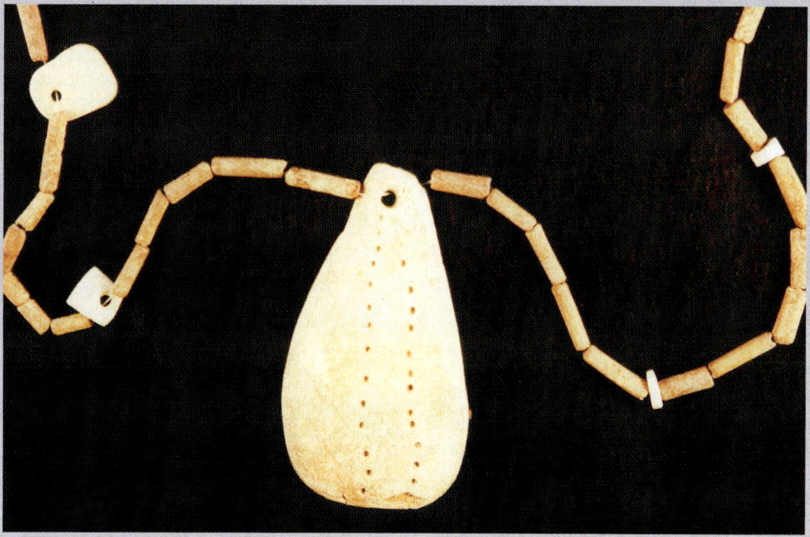

Pendant, with necklace beads. The pendant, 2½" high, is an exceptional piece with incised markings. These include two rows of dots, two sets of zigzag lines, and ladder or railroad track lines. A fine piece, it is Mississippian period, from northern Ohio. Fred Winegardner collection. Museum grade.

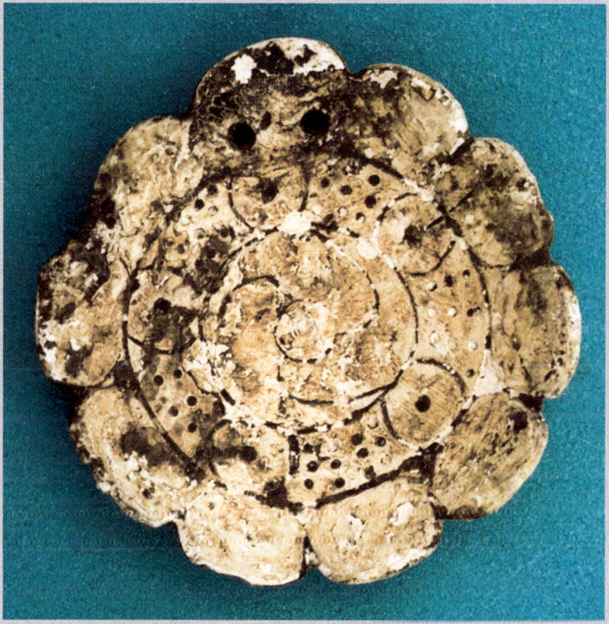

Scalloped shell gorget, with sun circles and triskele center, pictured in *Who's Who in Indian Relics* No. 8, size 3³⁄₁₆" across. Deeply incised, this is an exceptional Mississippian piece. Ex-collection Snyder, it is from Meigs County, Tennessee. Collection of, and photograph by, Gary Henry, North Carolina. **$1,000.00.**

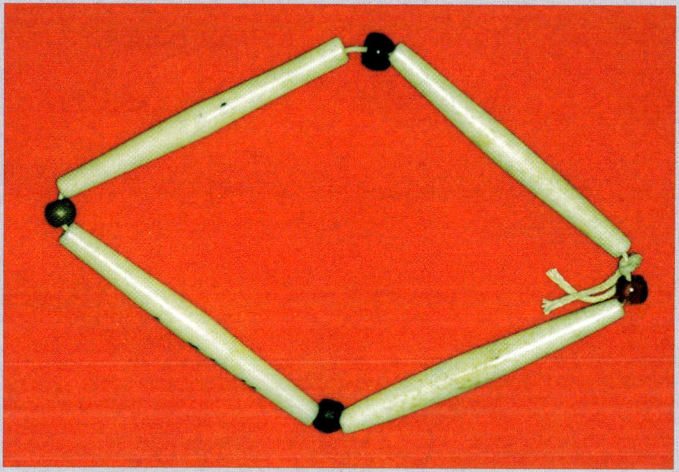

Bone hairpipes and glass trade beads, historic Lakota, beads 3" long. These came from western South Dakota. Richard Krueger collection, Iowa; Sandra Krueger photograph. Unlisted.

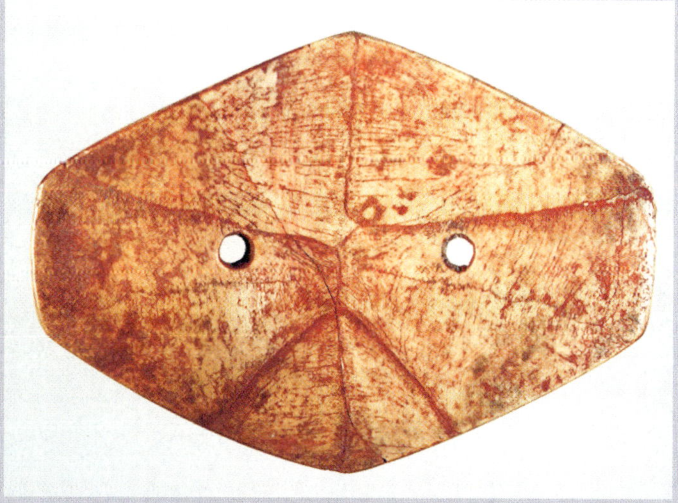

Tortoise shell gorget, 3³⁄₁₆" long, made from a land tortoise plastron. Quite rare, it is ex-collection Tolliver. Hocking County, Ohio. Private collection. Museum grade.

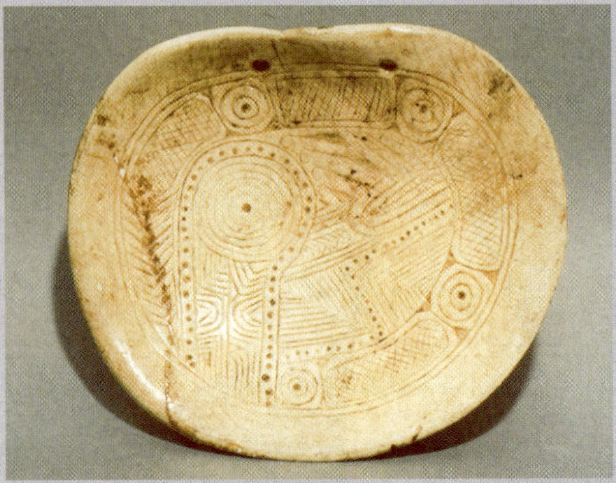

Marine shell gorget or pendant, with engraved designs, 4⅜ x 5¼". It is Mississippian period, probably from the southeast United States H. B. Greene II collection, Naples, Florida. Museum grade.

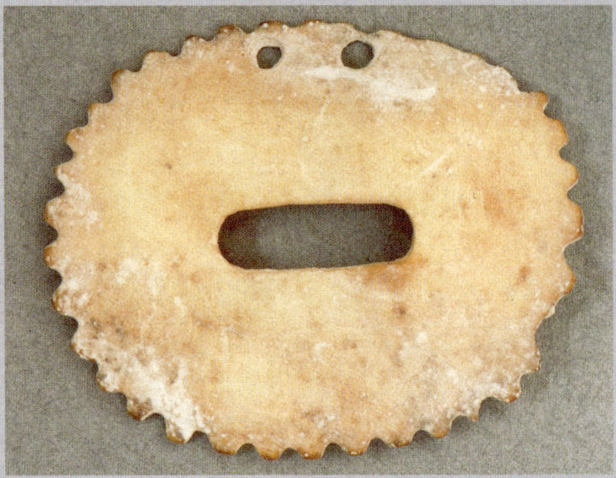

Shell pendant, two suspension holes, 1 x 1⅞", serrated edge. Thin and nicely shaped, the age of this piece is unknown. West Coast, Florida. H. B. Greene II collection, Naples, Florida. **$100.00.**

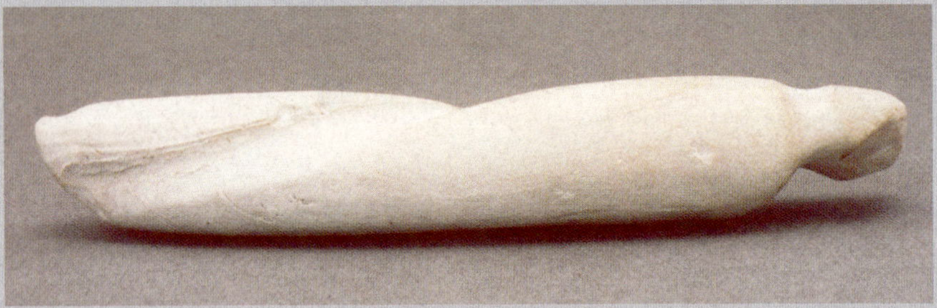

Columella shell pendant, Calusa culture, (AD 1450 or earlier), 4⅜" long. It was found on the south end of Key Marco, Collier County, Florida. H. B. Greene II collection, Naples, Florida. **$75.00.**

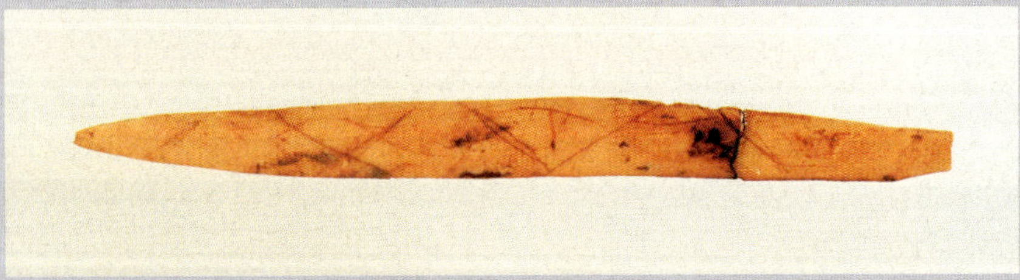

Bracelet section, thin, probably split deer rib, incised decorative lines, 4⅝" long. This is a scarce and fragile piece, and artifacts like this are not often found. It is from Indiana. Don Casto collection. Museum grade.

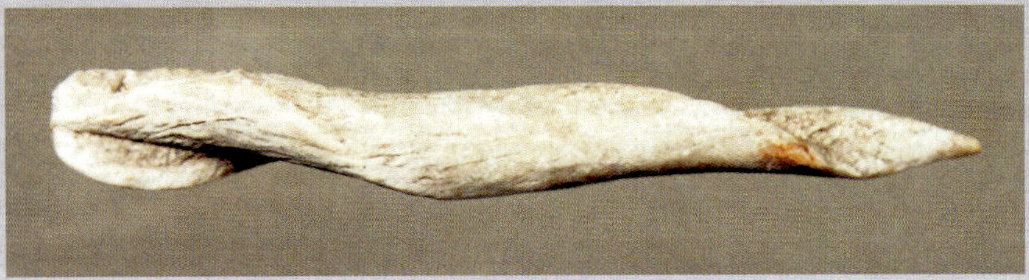

Pendant, conch shell, Middle Woodland period. The artifact has been worked and shaped but not drilled. Fulton County, Illinois. John Smith collection, Illinois. **$20.00.**

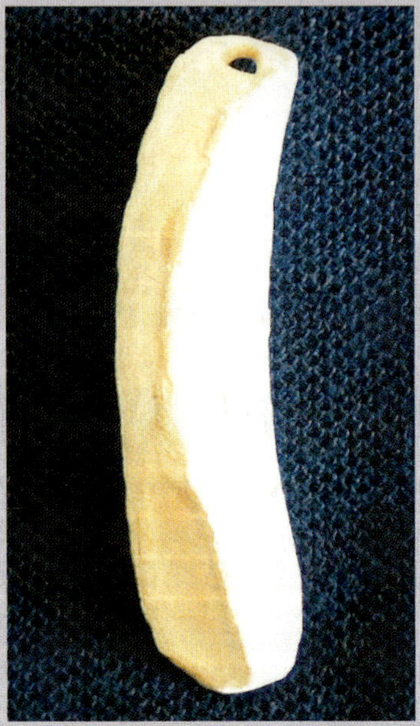

Abalone shell pendant, 2½" long. An early trade item, the pendant is from North Platte, Nebraska. Rod Fuller collection, Nebraska. **$75.00.**

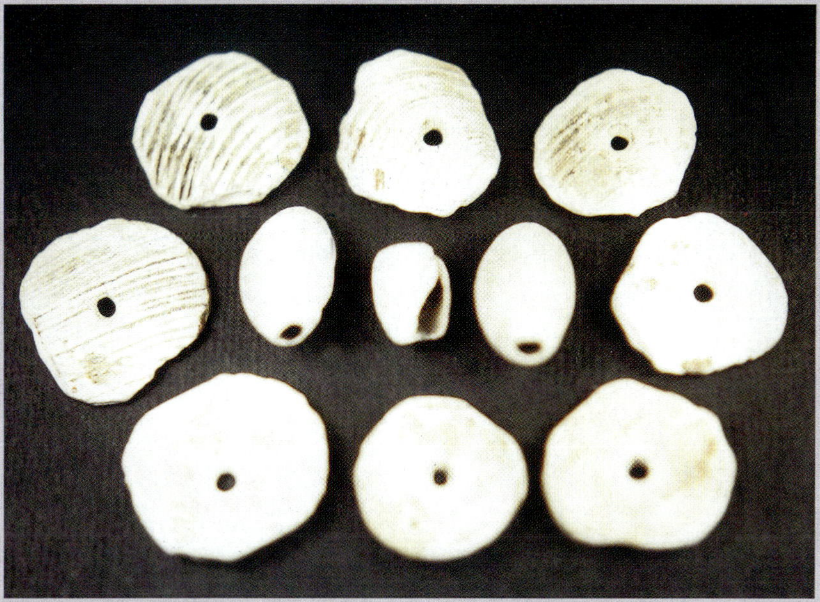

Shell drilled ornaments, found in Lycoming County, Pennsylvania. Lee Hallman collection, Pennsylvania. All, **$90.00.**

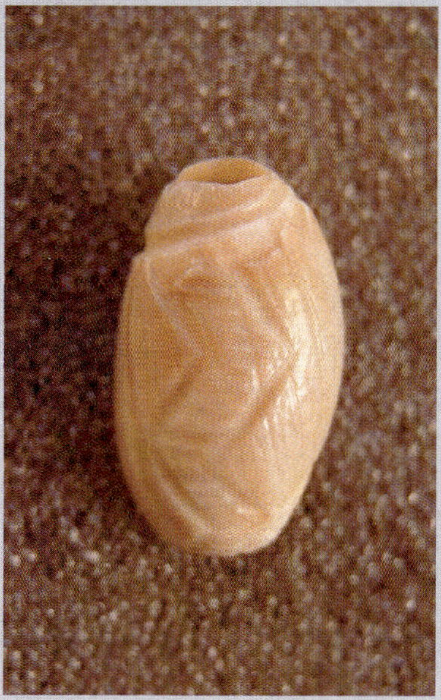

Olivella shell bead, carved design, 1½" long. This unusual bead was found in the Great Basin, Nevada. Victor T. Trujillo collection, Nevada. **$35.00.**

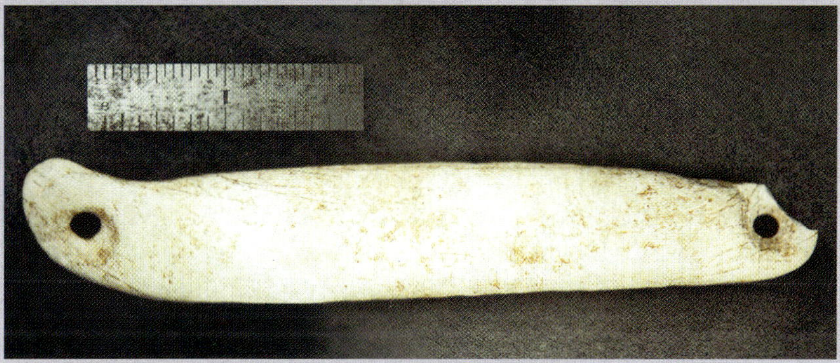

Gorget or decorative object, made of heavy bone, possibly that of extinct elephant-like creatures. This rare piece was found at a yard sale in 1968 and was obtained for $4.00. Monroe County, Pennsylvania. Lee Hallman collection, Pennsylvania. Museum grade.

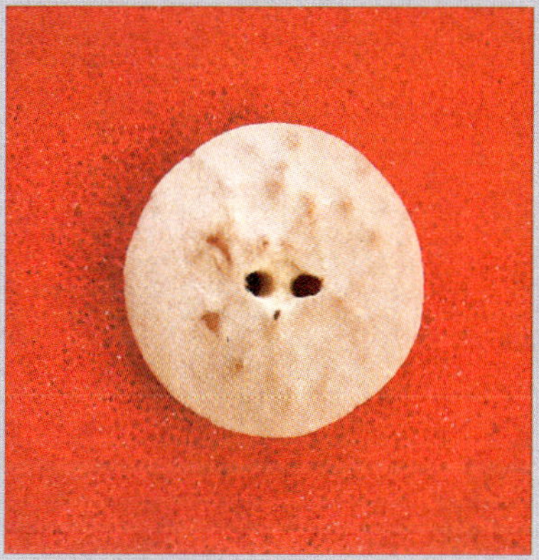

Antler button, two fastening holes, 1" in diameter. This button came from the Great Basin, Nevada. Victor T. Trujillo collection, Nevada. **$12.00 – 15.00.**

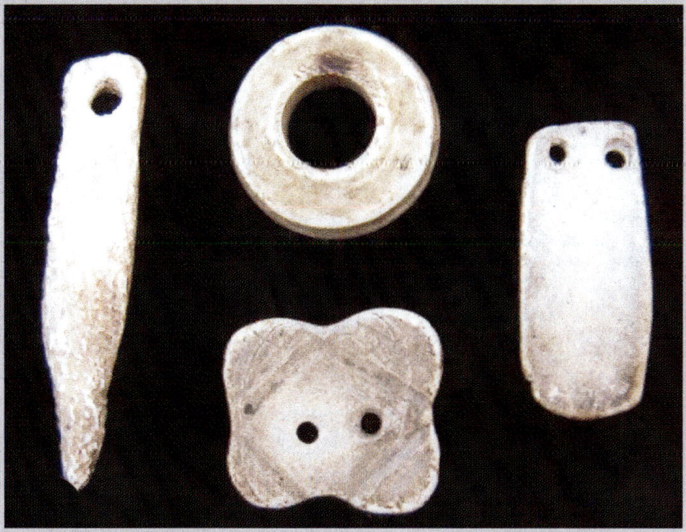

Shell artifacts, top center, ½" in diameter, fish vertebral centrum fashioned into an ornament, faint cross-hatch lines, found in the late 1940s. Ex-collection Phillips, it was acquired by the owner in 1999. Bottom center, "Mickey Mouse" type gorget bead, engraved Passementerie bead with lines and small dots; the word Passementerie refers to any fancy spangle thought to have been sewn to a garment. Ex-collection Phillips, it was obtained by the owner in 1999. Left, whelk spiral pendant, 1½". Right, two-hole shell pendant, 1" long. All came from near Miami, Ottawa County, Oklahoma. William Hamner collection, Alabama. Each, **$25.00.**

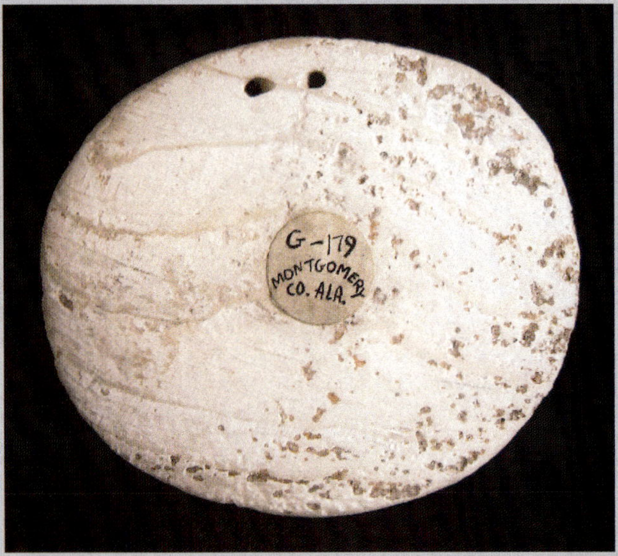

Gorget, whelk shell, reverse view, 3¼" across. It still retains the B. W. Stephens catalog number, G-179. Montgomery County, Alabama. William Hamner collection, Alabama. **$500.00.**

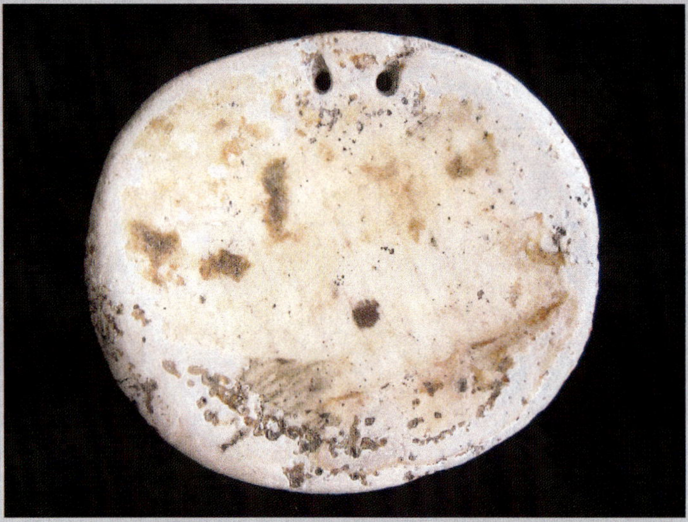

Gorget, whelk shell obverse view, 3¼" across. It was probably found with marginella beads in 1917 at Kulumi, an Upper Creek site on the Tallapoosa River. Ex-collections Stephens and Vietzen, it is also pictured in Onken's *Legends of Prehistoric Art* page 47, and was featured on two pages in *Who's Who in Indians Relics* No. 1. Montgomery County, Alabama. William Hamner collection, Alabama. **$500.00.**

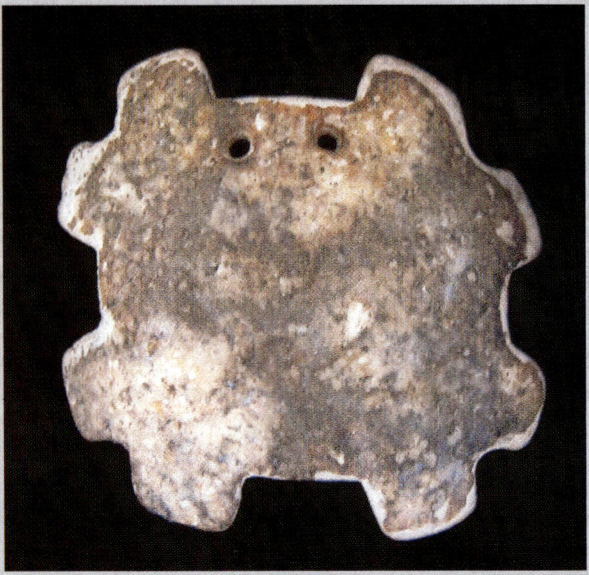

Shell gorget, reverse view, 2½" wide. Mississippian, this is sometimes called a "litter" gorget in reference to a litter for carrying a person of some importance. Davidson County, Tennessee. William Hamner collection, Alabama. **$1,000.00.**

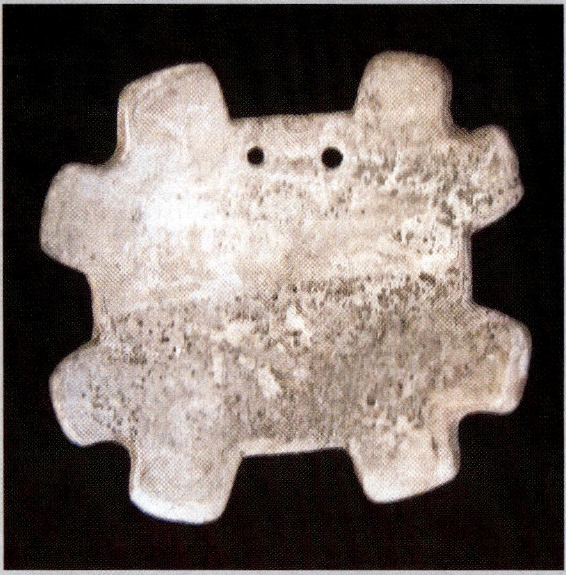

Shell gorget, a rare Double Cross motif, obverse view. It is 2½" wide and was found in the 1950s by Col. Vietzen near Nashville. It is pictured Vietzen's *The Saga of Glover's Cave,* page 238. Davidson County, Tennessee. William Hamner collection, Alabama. **$1,000.00.**

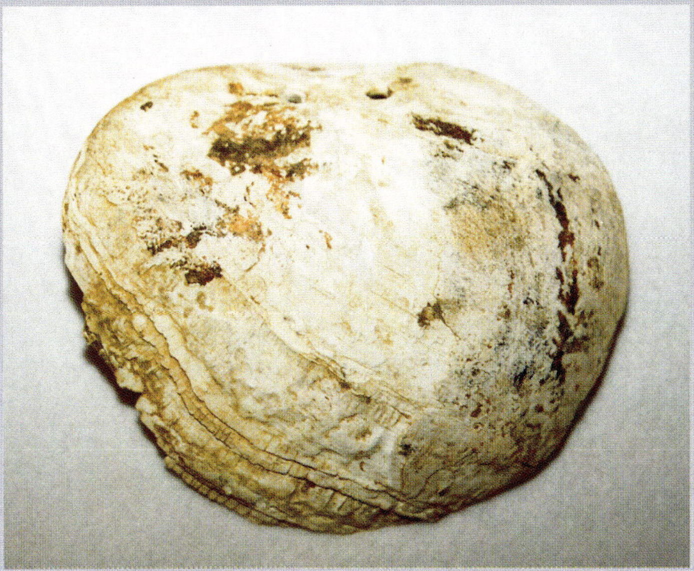

Conch shell gorget, Mississippian period, 5 x 6". The owner found it on the Ohio River bank in Mason County, West Virginia. Private collection. Rodney Roberts photograph. **$125.00.**

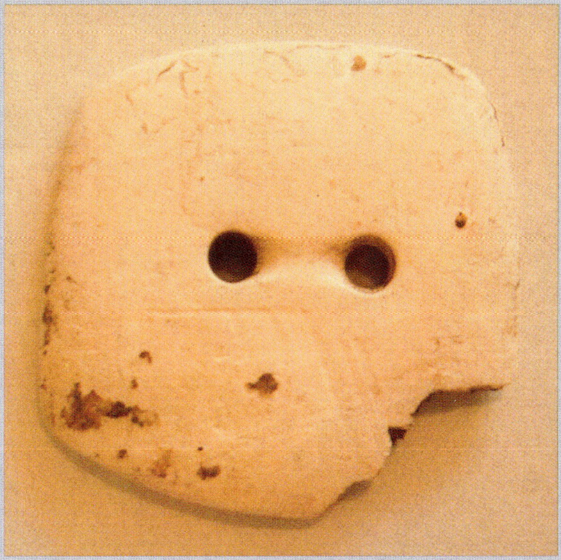

Shell gorget, corner damage, 1¼ x 1⁵⁄₁₆". Mississippian, the owner found it in May of 2002. Mason County, West Virginia. Private collection. Rodney Roberts photograph. **$30.00.**

Choker, with bone tubular beads and elk tooth pendant, 20" long. This ornamental piece came from Douglas County, Nebraska. Rod Fuller collection, Nebraska. Museum grade.

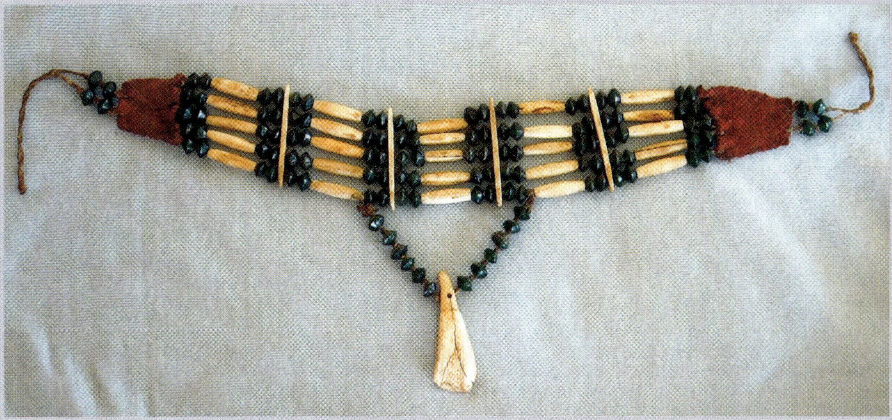

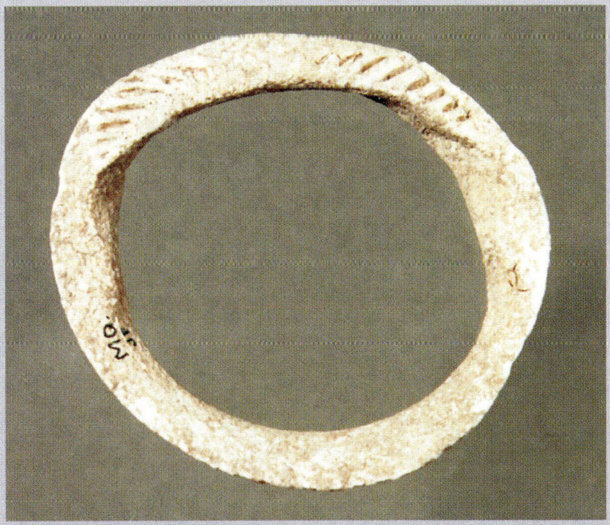

Bracelet, freshwater clam shell, 2½" in diameter and without incising. Mississippian period, ca. AD 800 – 1200, the example was found in Missouri. John Smith collection, Illinois. **$50.00.**

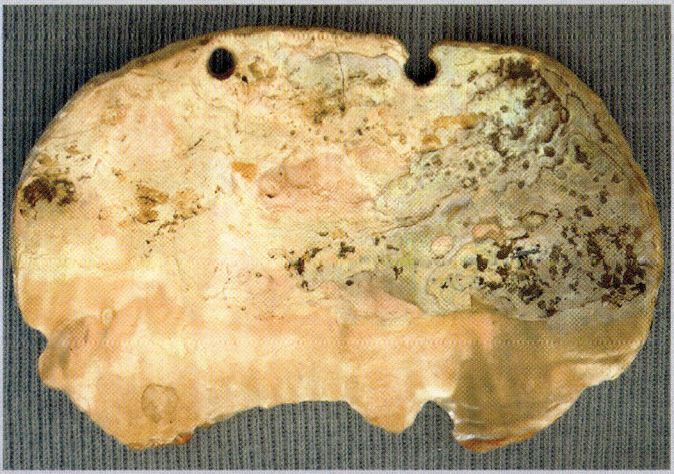

Abalone shell gorget, 3" across. Probably Fort Ancient (Mississippian period), the material would have come from the Pacific Coast by trade. Mayfield area, Kentucky. Rod Fuller collection, Nebraska. **$125.00.**

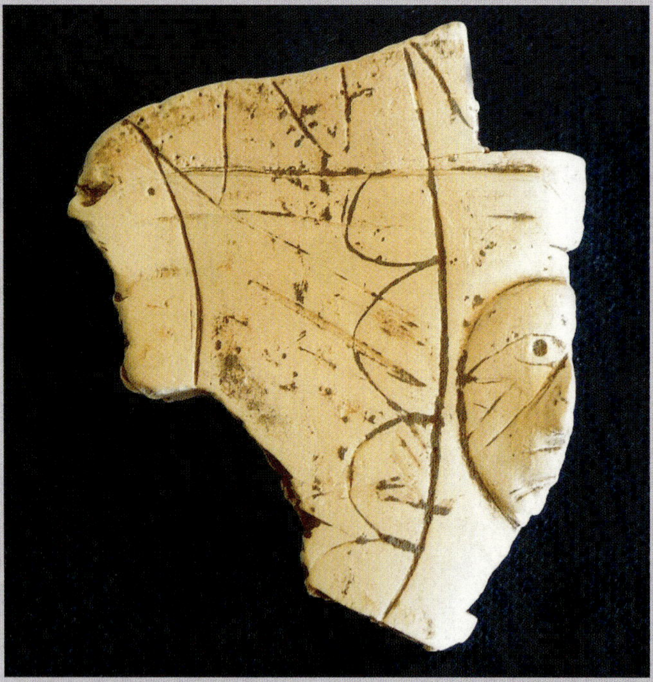

Shell section, engraved with lines and portion of human face, 3¼" across. This piece was found near North Platte, Nebraska. Rod Fuller collection, Nebraska. Unlisted.

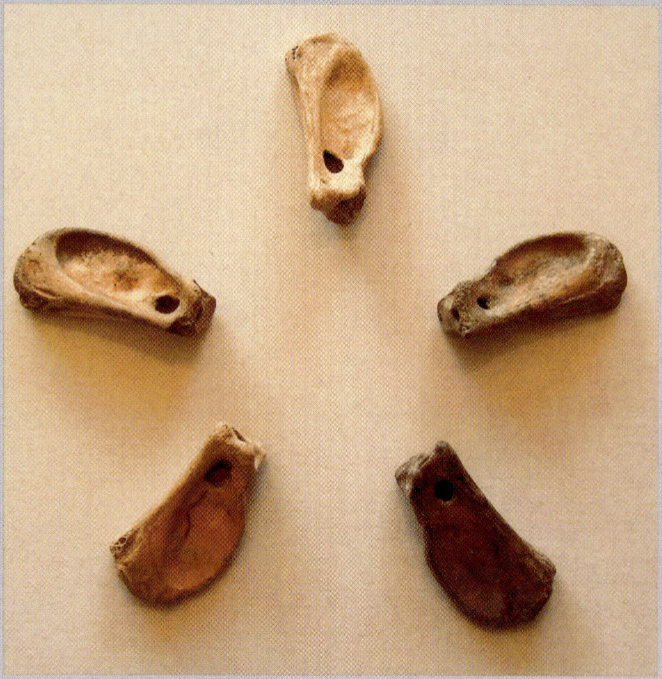

Bone beads, turtle bone, Mississippian period, longest is 1⅛". Drilled, these came from Ohio River Valley sites in Cabell and Mason Counties, West Virginia. Private collection. Rodney Roberts photograph. Each, **$15.00.**

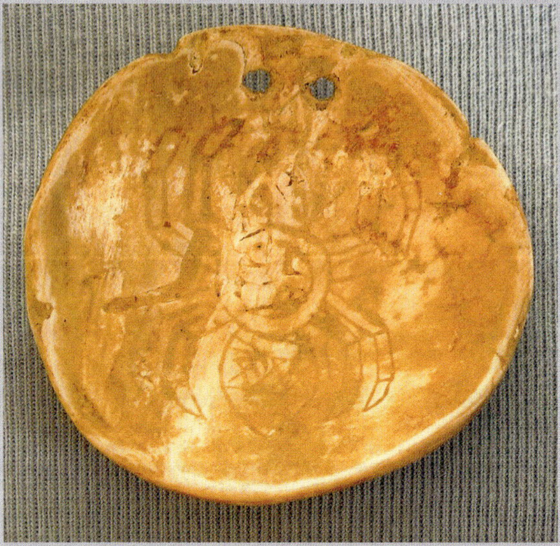

Conch shell gorget, Mississippian period. It is 2½" in diameter and has an engraved spider. Faxon area, Tennessee. Rod Fuller collection, Nebraska. Unlisted.

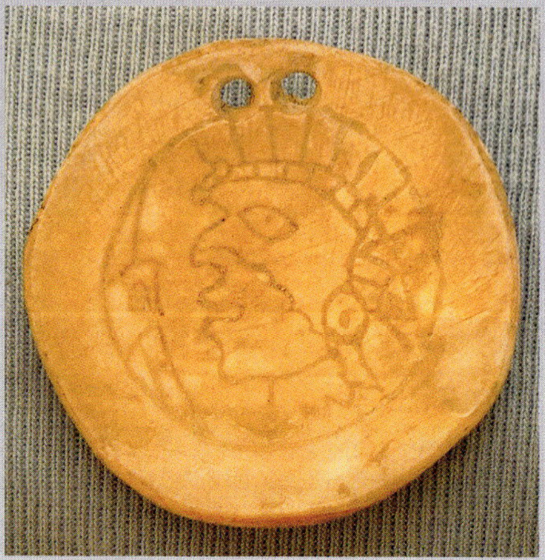

Conch shell gorget, 1¾" in diameter. This example is engraved with a warrior's head and was found near Hurley, Tennessee. Rod Fuller collection, Nebraska. Unlisted.

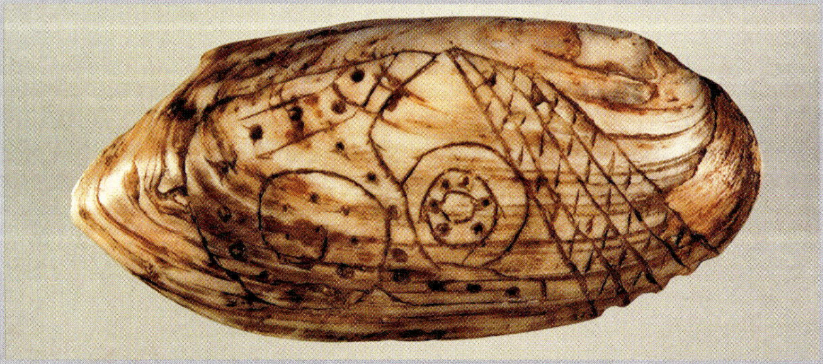

Spoon or dipper, freshwater clamshell, Mississippian period, engraved designs. This specimen is 3⅞" long. Ex-collection Tolliver, Hocking County, Ohio. Museum grade.

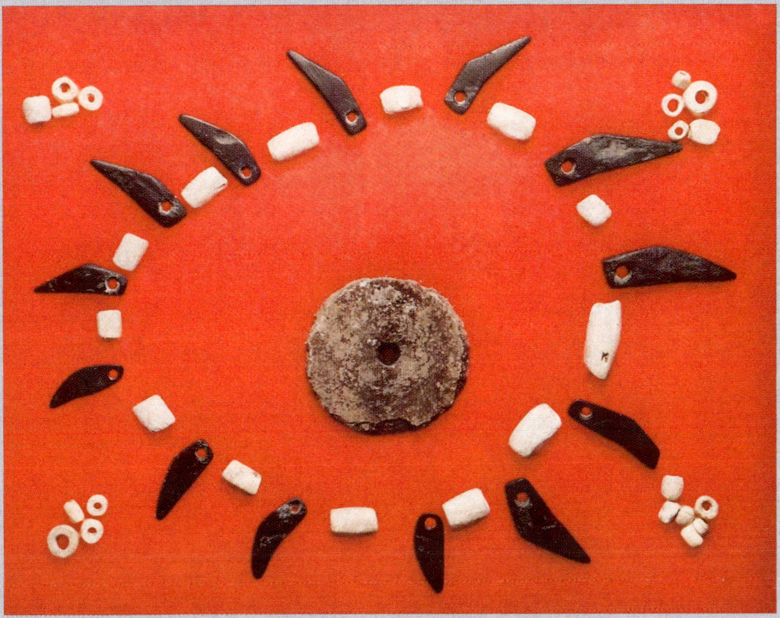

Beads and pendants or necklace pieces, Cannel coal and shell, all found in Greenup County, Kentucky. There are 13 cannel coal tooth effigies, all drilled, longest is 35mm. The shell beads are disc and barrel in shape, and all are drilled. The center pendant or gorget is made of pottery and the edge has been modified to make it round. Private collection. Museum grade.

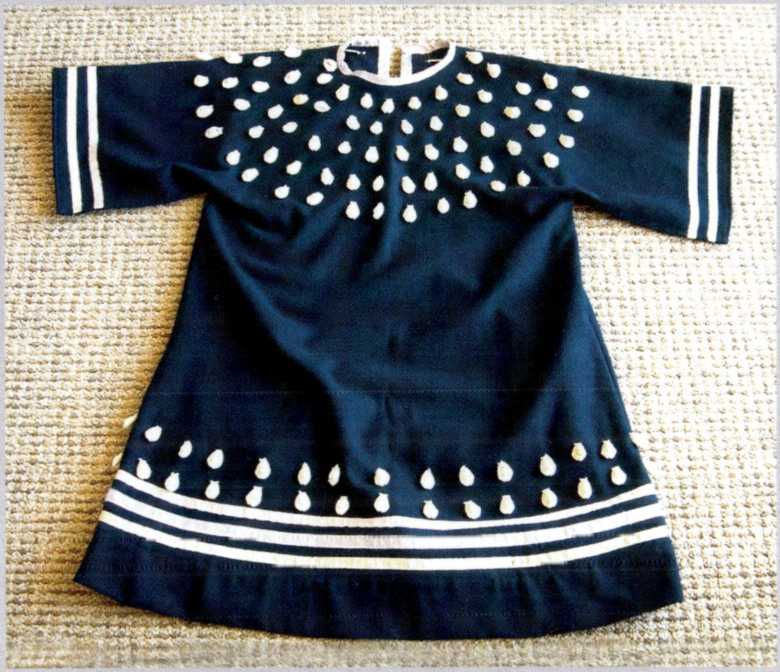

Child-size dress with shell decorations, 33" long. In very fine condition, it is from the Billings area, Montana. Rod Fuller collection, Nebraska. Museum grade.

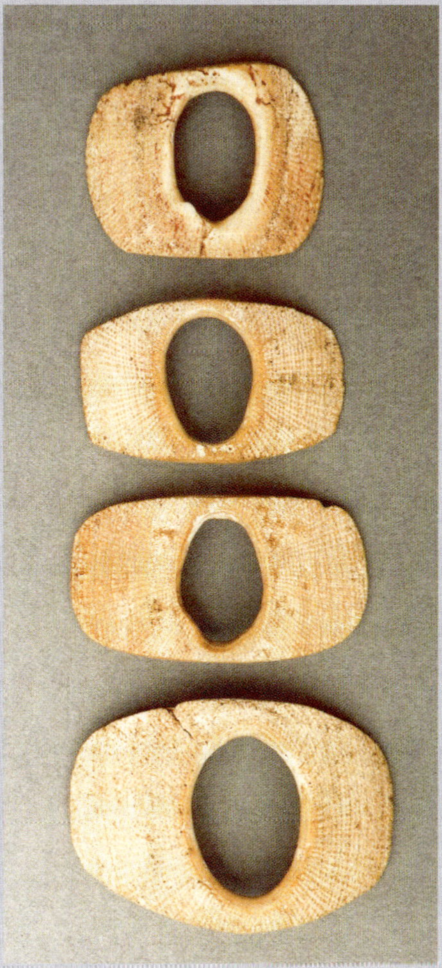

Limpet shell artifacts, 1 to 1½" long. They have been shaped and polished on both ends and faces. Probably too small for composite Atl-atl weights, their purpose may be decorative. Southwestern Florida. H. B. Greene II collection, Naples, Florida. Unlisted.

Decorated ivory piece, Eskimo, 2" long. While exact use is unknown, this is an appealing small artwork. Eek, Alaska. Rod Fuller collection, Nebraska. **$100.00 – 125.00.**

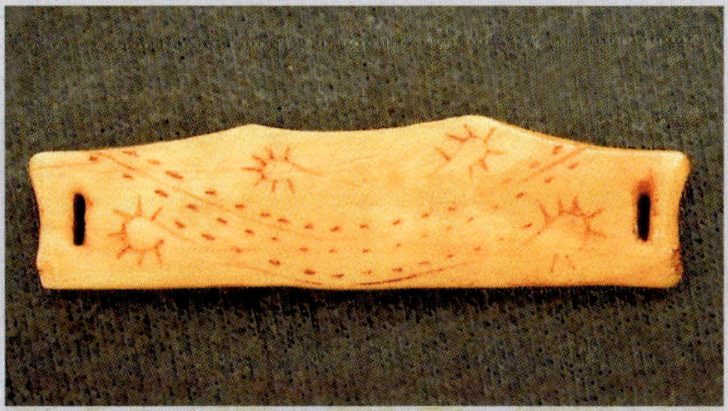

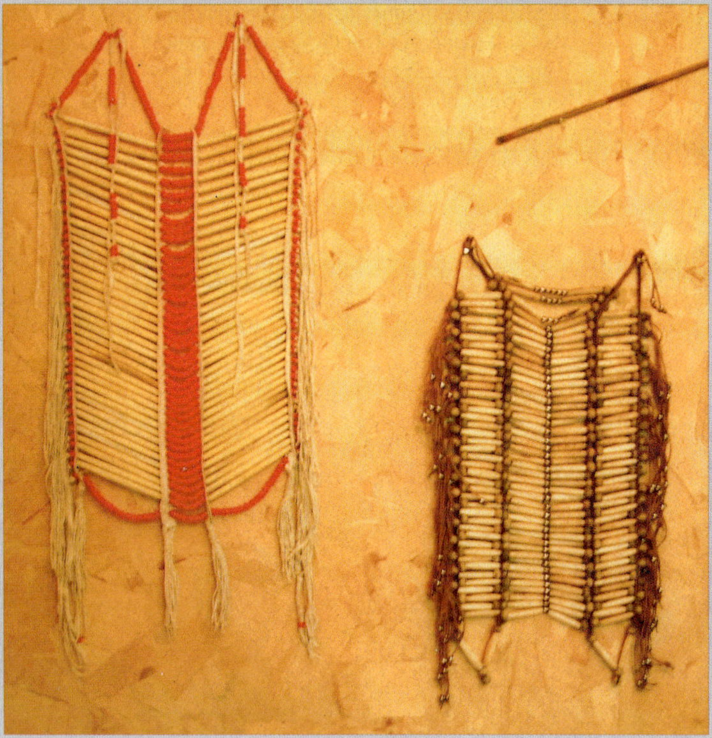

Breast plates, child size and man size, 19" and 26" long, respectively. These historic artworks have long tubular bone beads. Ogalala, South Dakota. Rod Fuller collection, Nebraska. Each, museum grade.

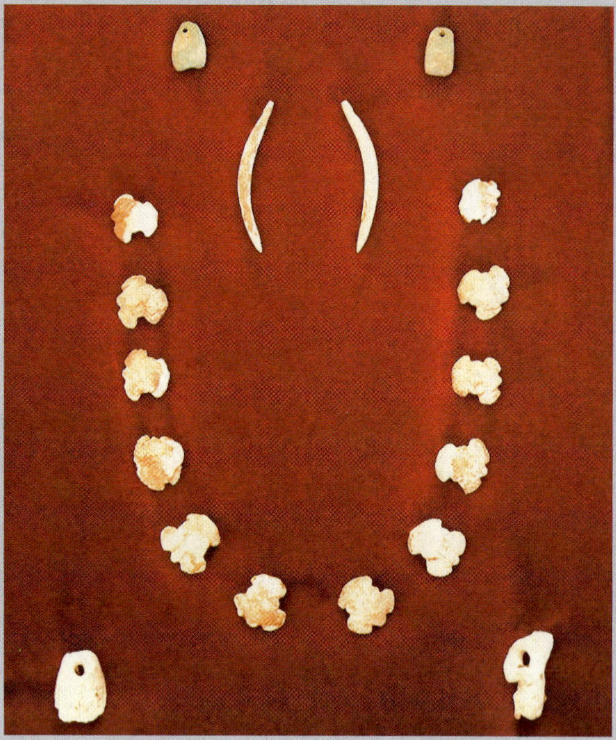

Shell beads, bone pendants and turquoise ear decorations (drilled, at top) all child size, frame is 6½ x 8½". These artifacts came from Gila County, Arizona. Rod Fuller collection, Nebraska. Unlisted.

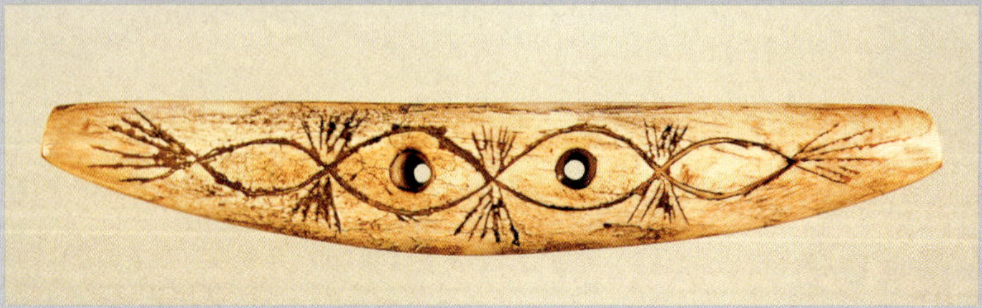

Gorget, ivory-like polished bone, 4¼" long. This incised artifact is ex-collection Tolliver, possibly from Hocking County, Ohio. Private collection. Museum grade.

Effigy handle(?), obverse, bear bone, image in the form of a wolf. This very rare piece is 5½" long and was found in Hocking County, Ohio. Private collection. Museum grade.

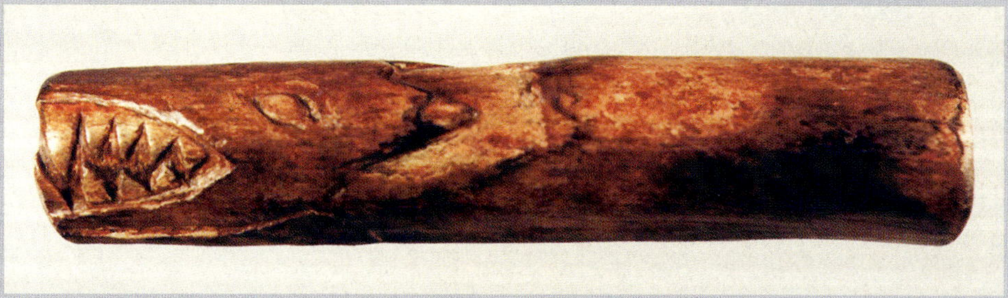

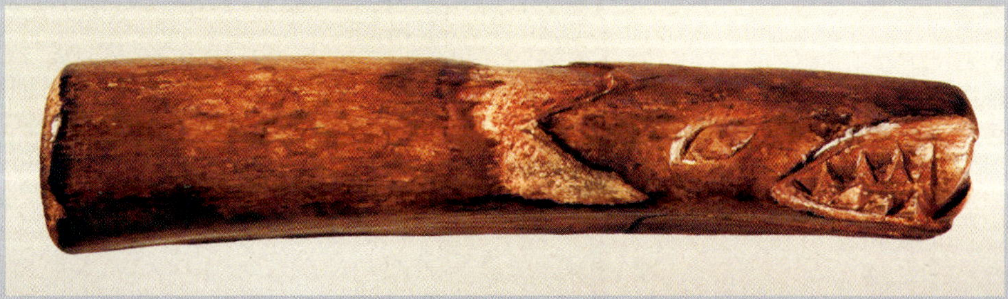

Effigy handle, reverse, bear bone, wolf effigy. The bone has a rich brown patina and the handle(?) is 5½" long. The time-period for this piece is unknown. Ex-collection Tolliver, Hocking County, Ohio. Private collection. Museum grade.

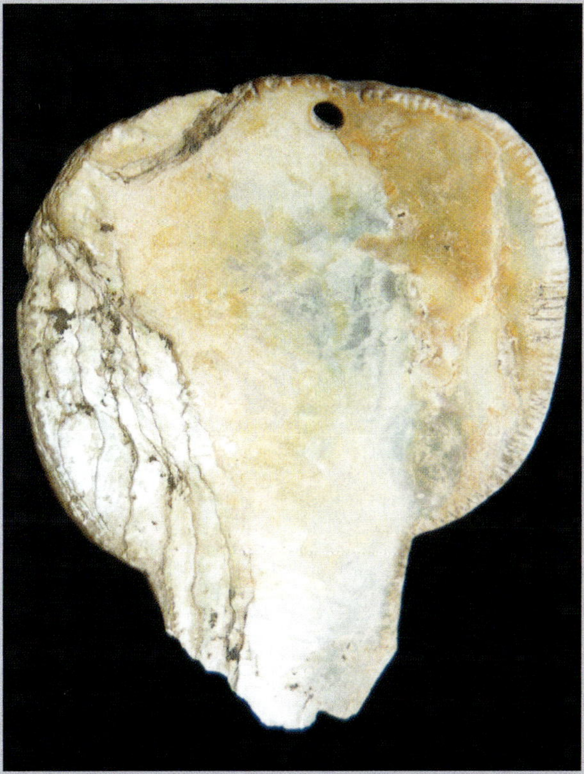

Shell pendant, drilled, 2½" wide and 3" long, exterior edge with many narrow tally marks. It was found in Bartow County, Georgia. Garvin collection. **$75.00 – 100.00.**

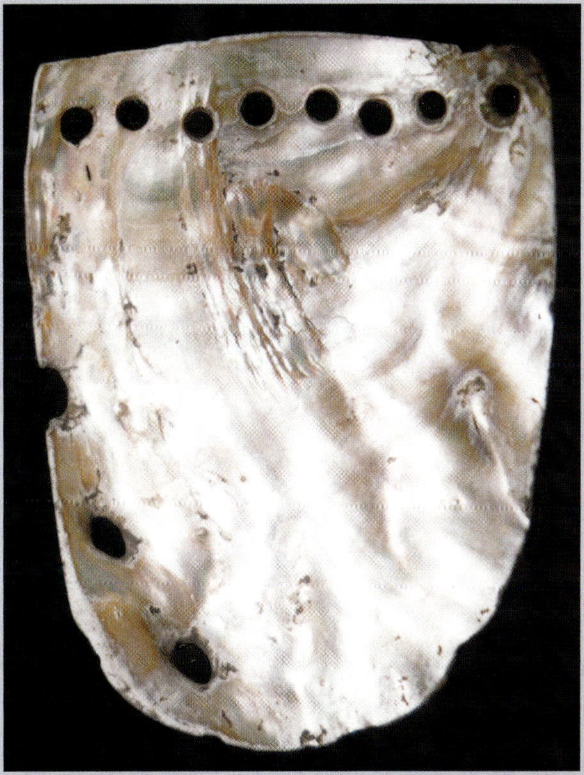

Abalone shell pendant, 2¾ x 3¾", multiple drilled holes, abalone shell. Found by Herbert Enochs in 1939, it was picked up at Rio Oso, Yuba County, California. Garvin collection. **$350.00.**

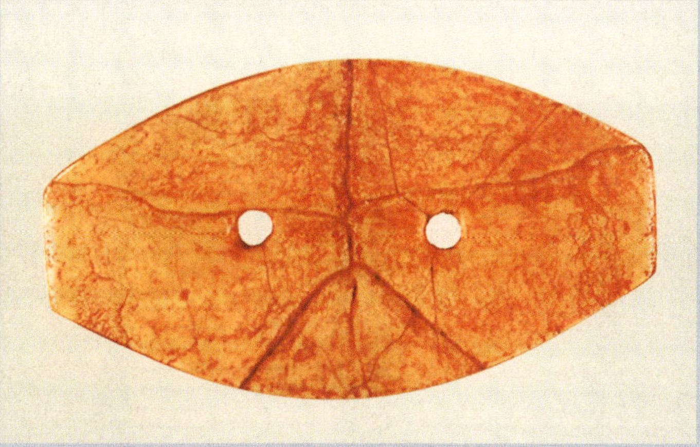

Tortoise shell gorget, 3" long. It is made from the plastron or ventral surface of a land tortoise. This rare artifact is ex-collection Tolliver, from Hocking County, Ohio. Private collection. Museum grade.

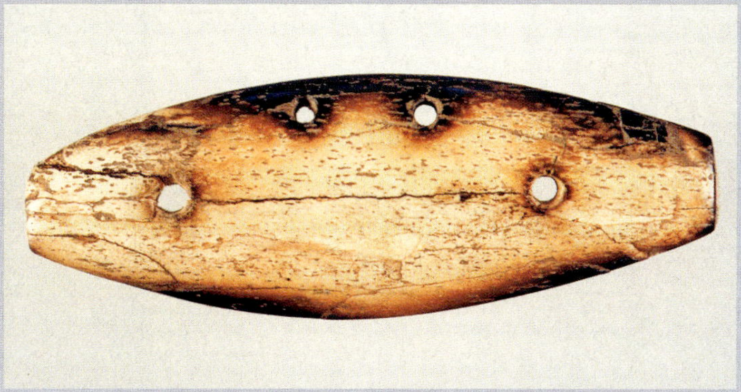

Gorget, polished bone, about 3¼" long. The two smaller holes are in unusual positions. Ex-collection Tolliver, Hocking County, Ohio. Private collection. Museum grade.

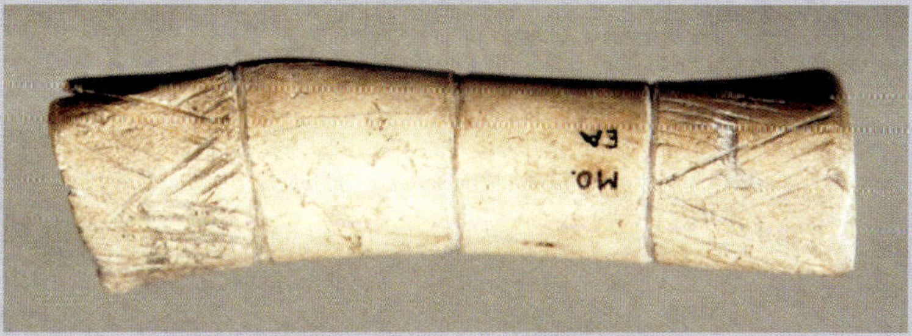

Engraved bone tube, probably Woodland period, and likely used as a handle for a tool. It is 3⅝" long and came from a rock shelter in Missouri. John Smith collection, Illinois. **$75.00.**

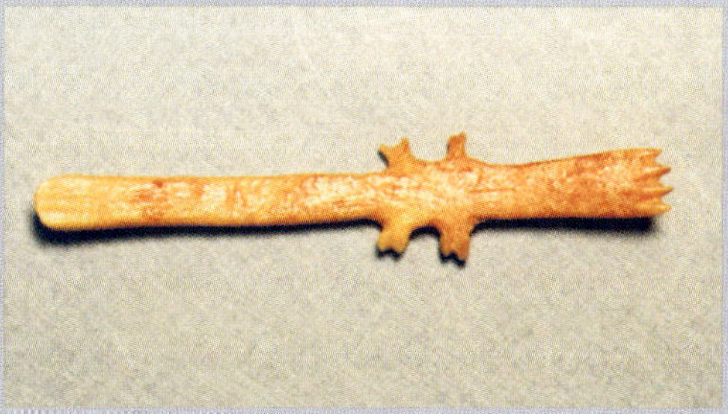

Scarifier(?), perhaps used to prepare the skin for tattoos, quite unusual. It is 2" long, ca. AD 1750, Morton County, North Dakota. Private collection. Museum grade.

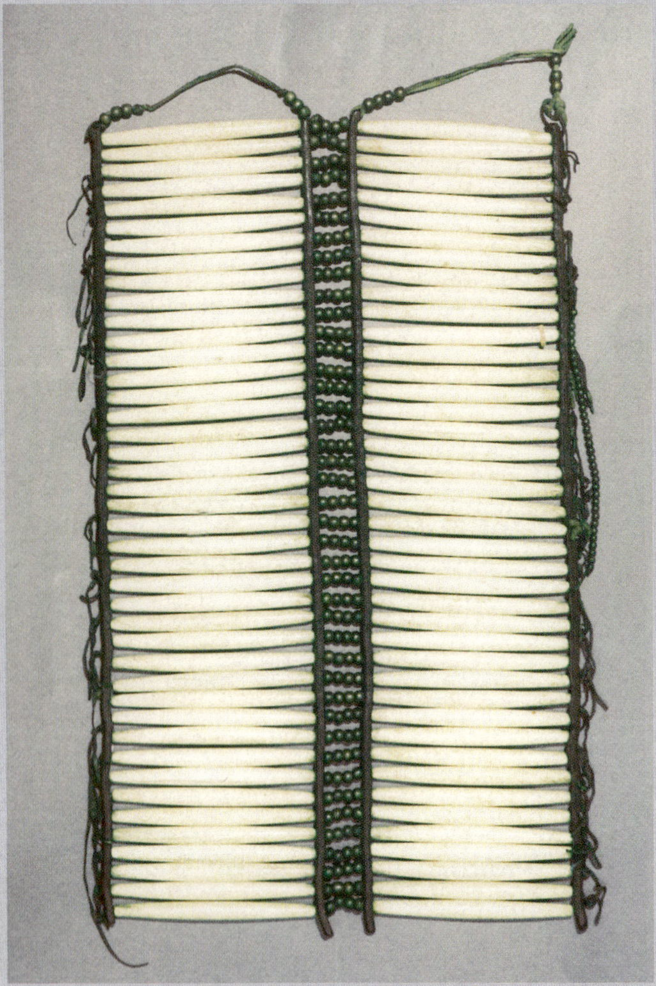

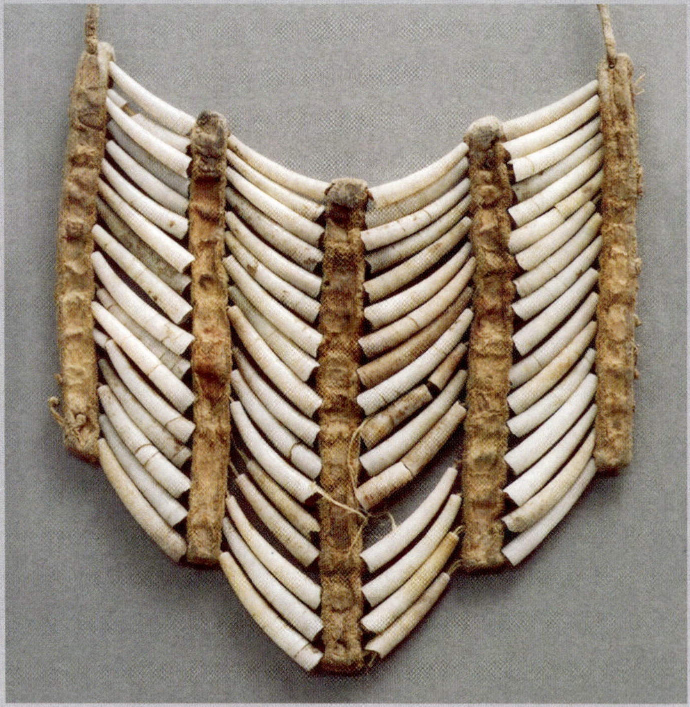

Child's breastplate, tusk shell, 5½ x 5½", hide and string. This fine piece is ca. AD 1870s and pre-reservation. The breastplate is western U. S. and shells are from the Puget Sound area. H. B. Greene II collection, Naples, Florida. Museum grade.

Bone breastplate, with metal beads, man size, 10⅝ x 17½". This historic piece, (ca. AD 1870s) with 42 bone pipes on each side, is fastened together with harness leather. Northern Plains region. H. B. Greene II collection, Naples, Florida. Museum grade.

Marine shell pendant, Mississippian period, 1½" long. This example, likely obtained in trade, is grooved at the top. Such examples were attached to necklaces or clothing. The pendant came from a rock shelter in Tennessee. John Smith collection, Illinois. **$40.00.**

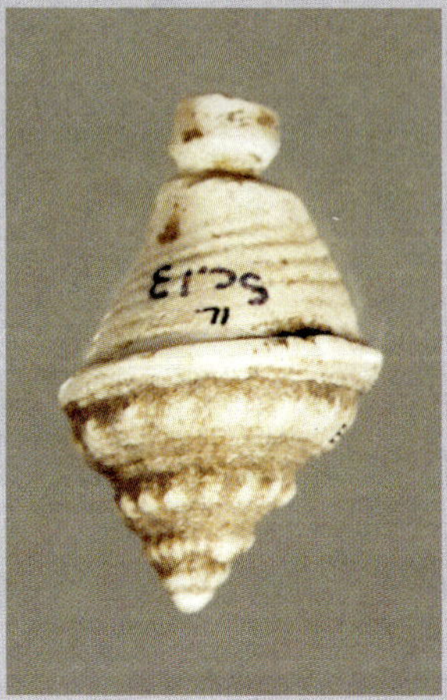

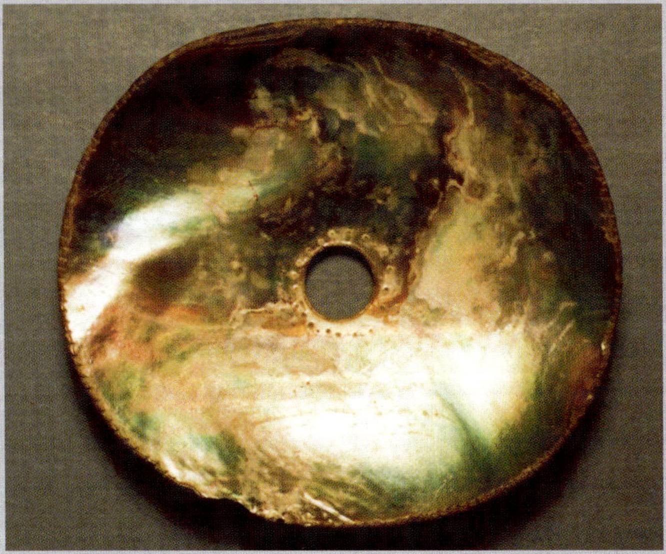

Abalone shell pendant, dots around central hole and tally marks around circumference, 3" in diameter. It is ex-collection Lighthauser and was acquired in the early 1970s. Nevada. Private collection.

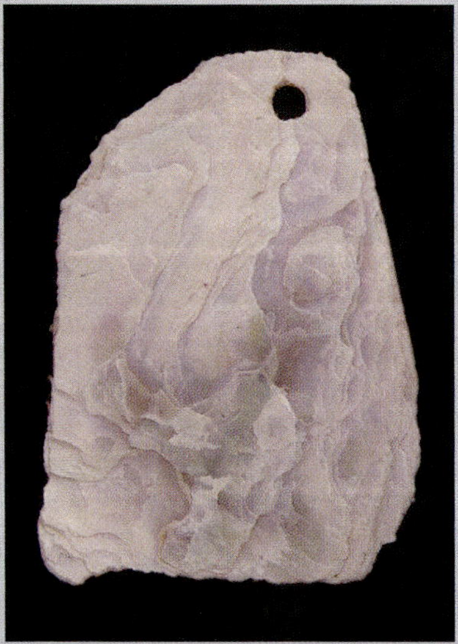

Abalone shell pendant, 2¼" high, with suspension hole. This ornament is from the Great Basin area, Nevada. Victor T. Trujillo collection, Nevada. **$75.00.**

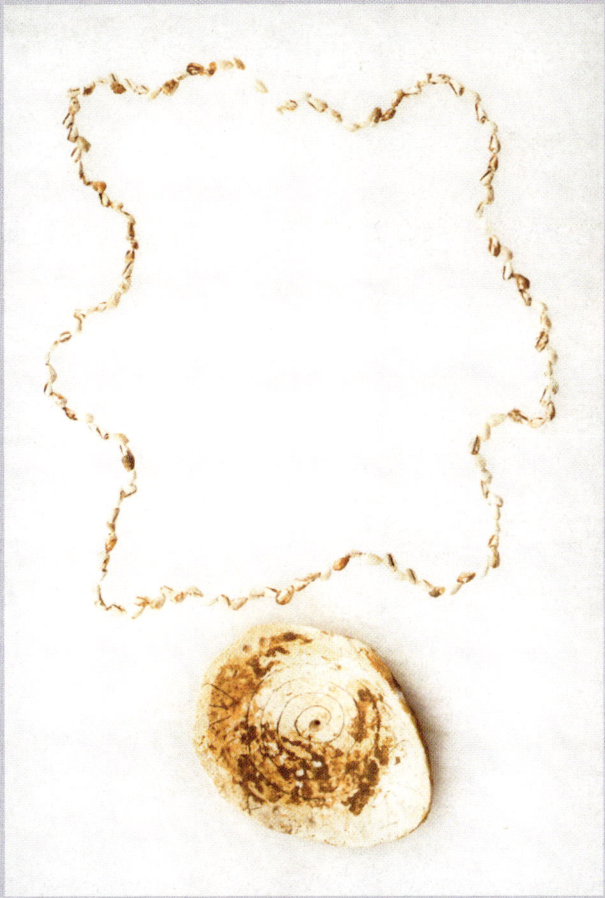

Necklace, shell beads with whelk shell gorget, Dallas phase (Temple Mound II) of the Middle Mississippian period. The gorget is 4¼" across and the necklace is 43½" long. An engraved spiral design is on the gorget reverse and it has a drilled center hole. These artifacts are ex-collection Fergerson (Piffard, New York) and came from the Hiawassee River area, Polk County, Tennessee. Dave Summers collection, Victor, New York. **$800.00.**

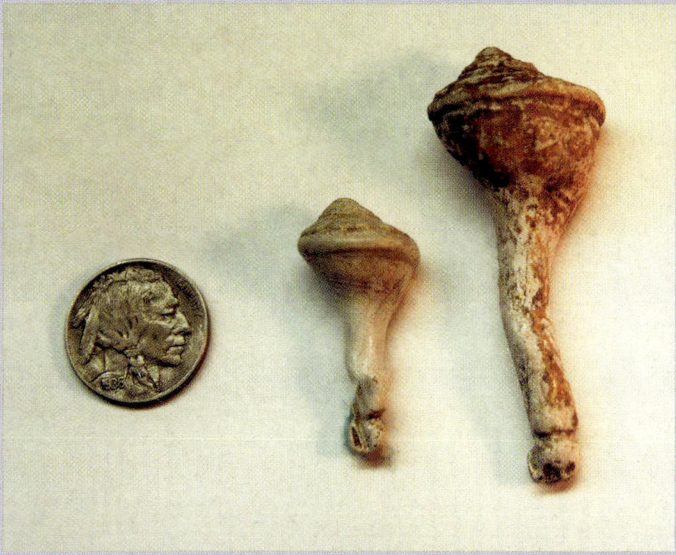

Shell whorl pendants, Gulf of Mexico, each cut, polished, and grooved on the small end. Decorations or ornaments, the longest is 2⅜". Fulton County, Illinois. Fred Smith collection, Illinois. Each, **$75.00 – 100.00.**

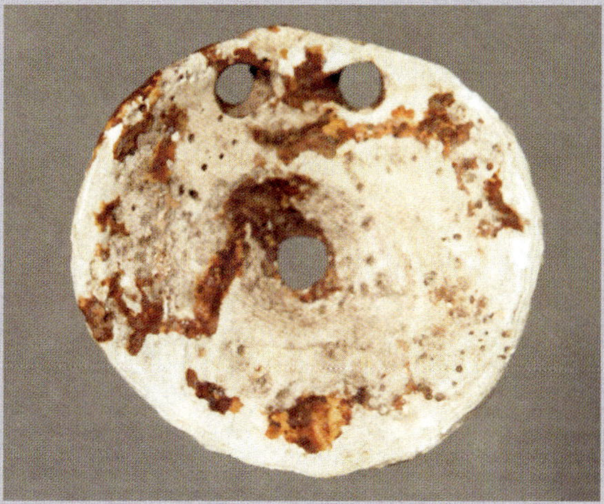

Three-hole gorget, one of the most desired ornaments from the Mississippian culture, 2" in diameter. This form is called an Annular gorget because of the central hole. Ex-collection Marion Dickson, it is from Fulton County, Illinois. John Smith collection, Illinois. **$125.00.**

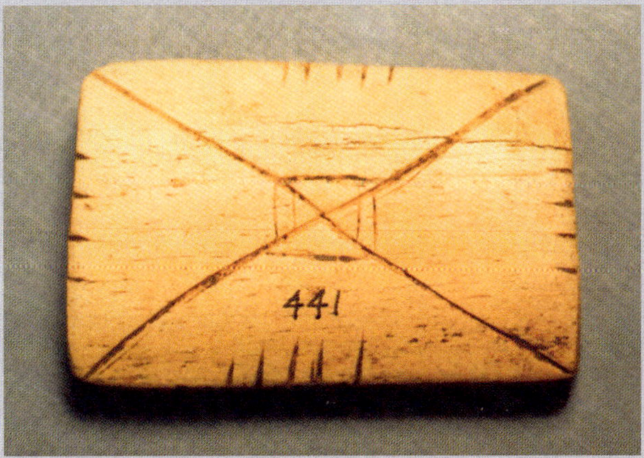

Bone gaming piece, incised line decorations, 2¾" long. It is ca. AD 1750 and was found in Morton County, North Dakota. Private collection. **$150.00.**

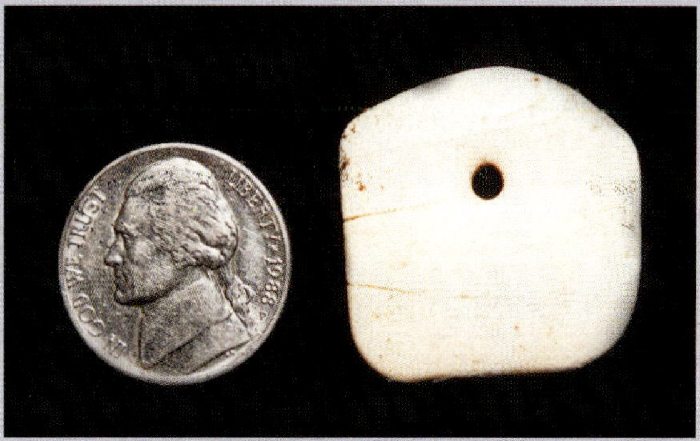

Shell bead or pendant, size as indicated, drilled for suspension. It was found in northwestern Arkansas. Kenneth Hamilton collection, Arkansas. **$15.00 – 25.00.**

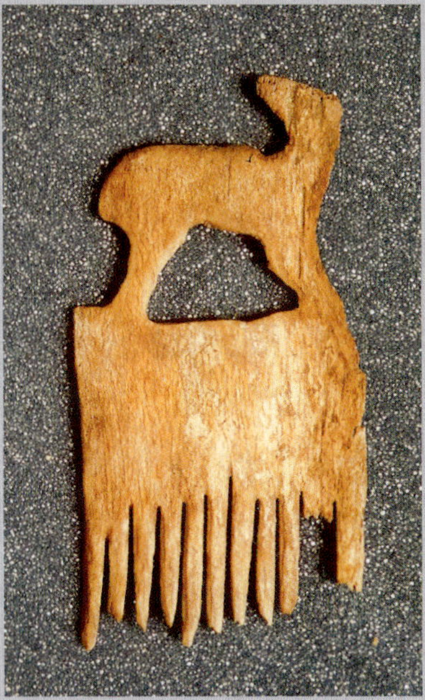

Deer effigy comb, bone, 3⅛" long. This piece is historic Iroquois (Seneca), ca. AD 1650 – 1675. Animal forms are usually clan totems. As to rarity, the owner remarked that only some 251 Seneca combs are known to exist. The example is from near Honeoye Falls, Monroe County, New York. Dave Summers collection, Victor, New York. **$1,600.00.**

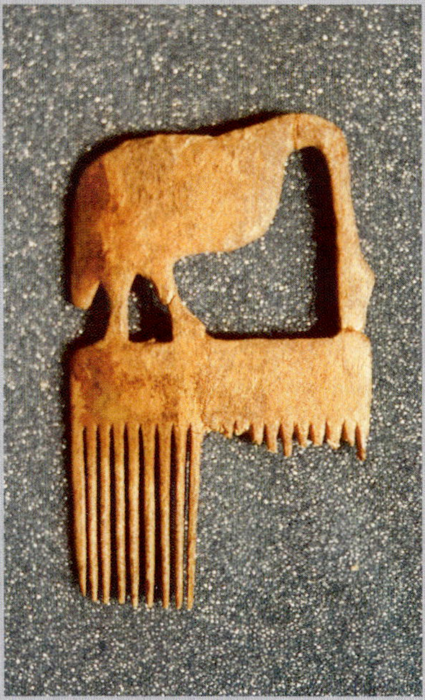

"Feeding Goose" comb, antler, ex-collections Schroff (ca. 1940), Casterline and Hesse. It is 3" long and historic Iroquois (Seneca), ca. AD 1675 – 1687. The comb was found near Mendon, Monroe County, New York. Dave Summers collection, Victor, New York. **$2,000.00.**

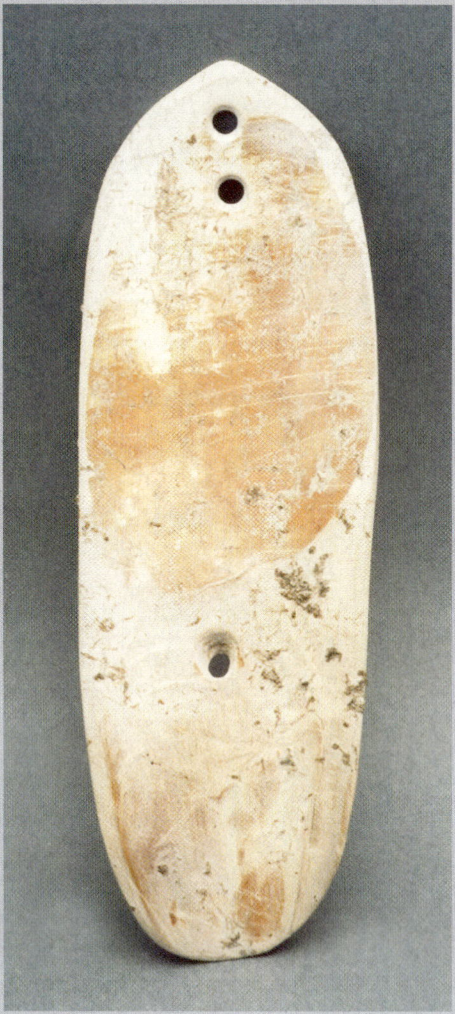

Shell pendant, elongated form with three suspension holes, 1⅞ x 5⅜". It was found in a creek by Bill Piper around 1938. Pre-1400, this pendant or gorget form is similar to shell forms from the Late Archaic Glacial Kame people (1500 BC) of the eastern Midwest. There the form is known as the sandal-sole gorget and it, too, has three in-line holes. This example is from northern Collier County, Florida. H. B. Greene II collection, Naples, Florida. Unlisted.

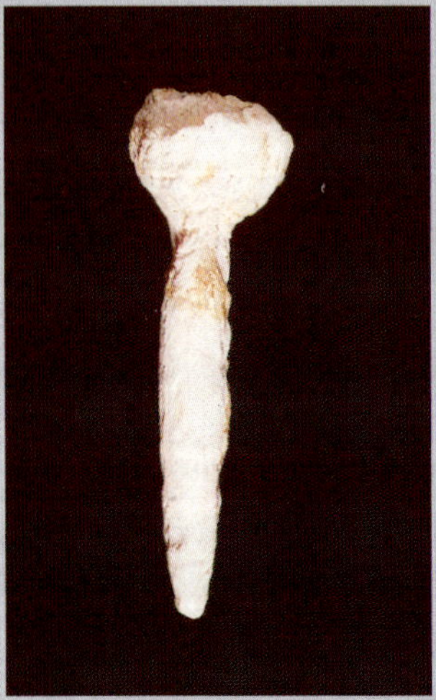

Ear plug, Mississippian period, weathered shell. It is 45mm long and was found in Alabama. Private collection. Unlisted.

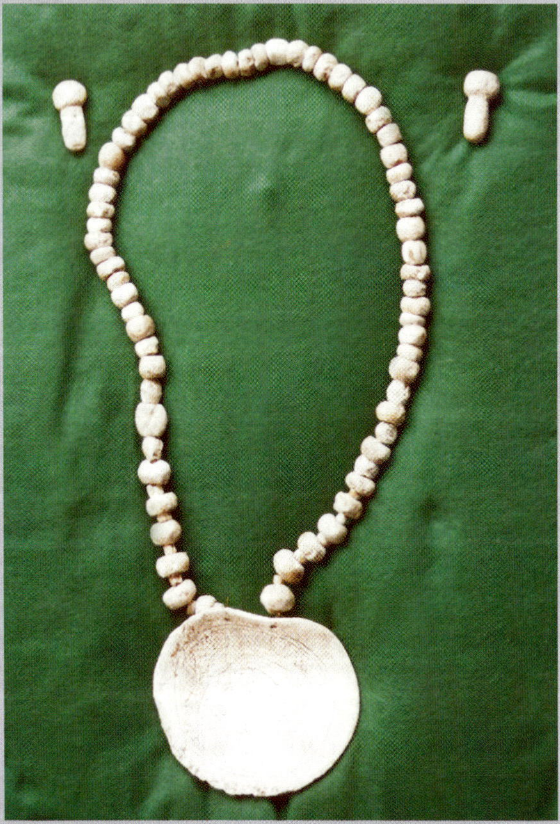

Necklace, shell beads with whelk shell gorget, Dallas phase (Temple Mound II) of the Middle Mississippian, ca. AD 1200. This gorget has a stylized rattlesnake motif, and the necklace consists of 81 large drilled conch shell beads. The gorget is 4 x 4¾", the necklace is 18" long, and the two shell ear pins are each 1½" long. Ex-collection Fergerson (Piffard, New York), these artifacts are from the Hiawassee River area, Polk County, Tennessee. Dave Summers collection, Victor, New York. All, **$1,850.00.**

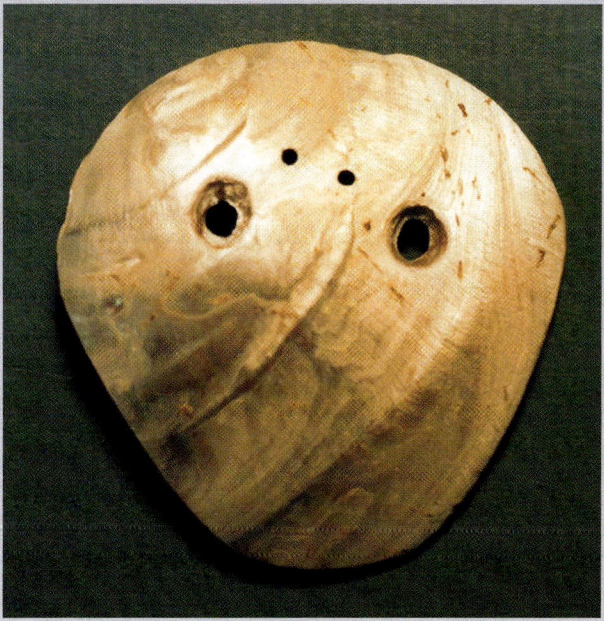

Mask gorget, shell, just over 2" in diameter. This piece is historic, ca. AD 1500 – 1750. Mobridge area, South Dakota. Private collection. **$350.00.**

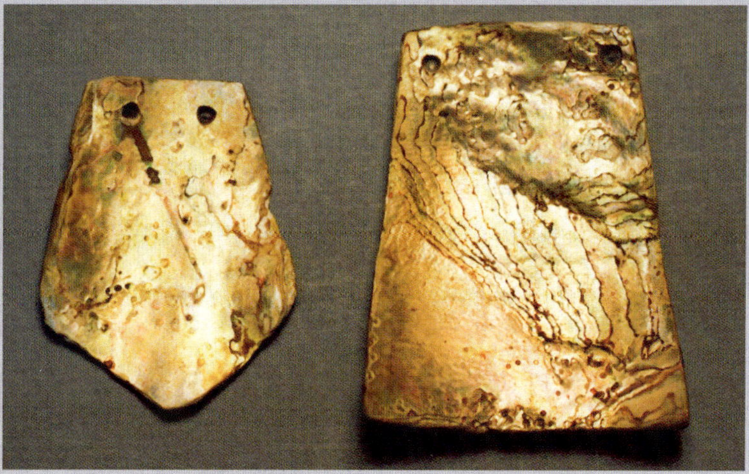

Abalone shell gorgets or pendants, largest is 3" long, ca. AD 500 – 1500. These were found by Ben Woodworth about 1940. California. Private collection. The two, **$250.00.**

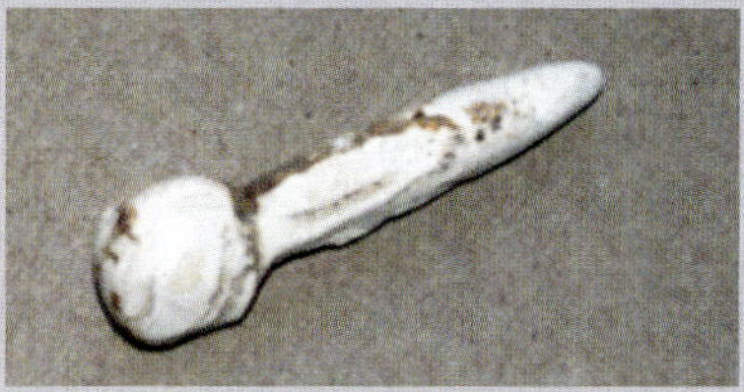

Shell earpin, probably Mississippian, 1½" long. It was found in Arkansas. Wilfred Dick collection, Mississippi. **$40.00.**

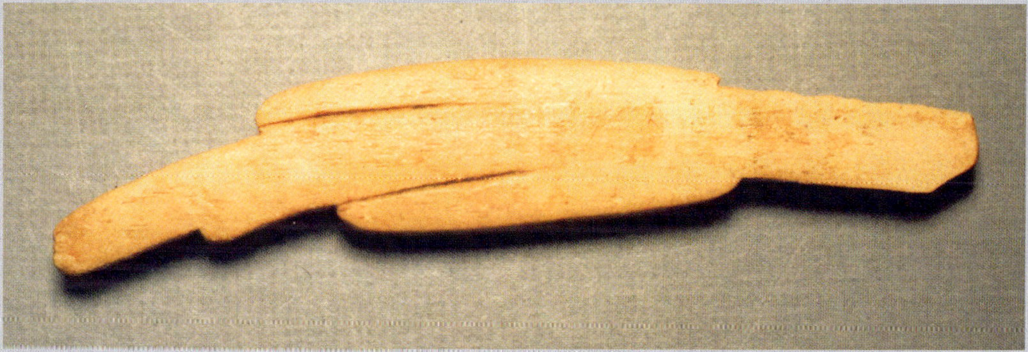

Bone knife handle, in effigy of a flying bird, 5" long. A stone knife blade was inserted into a slot cut in the edge of the handle. Historic, (ca. AD 1750), it came from west of Gettysburg, South Dakota. Private collection. **$125.00.**

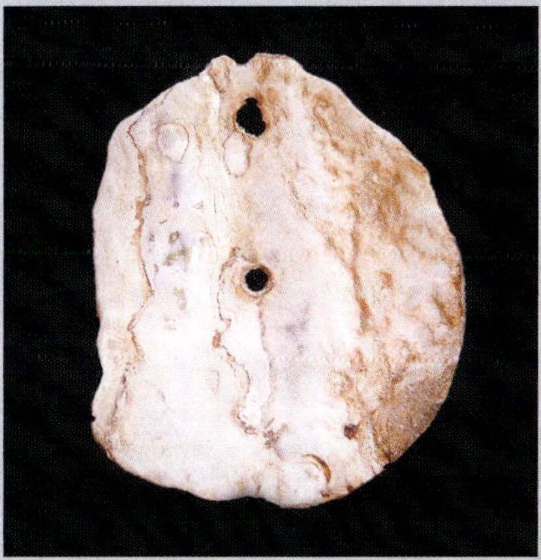

Abalone shell ornament, 1¾" high, with two in-line holes. This artifact is from the Great Basin, Nevada. Victor T. Trujillo collection, Nevada. **$50.00.**

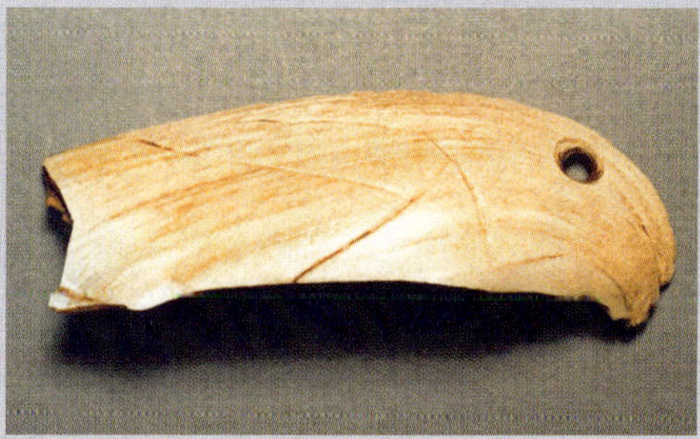

Abalone shell thunderbird effigy, one wing missing, 1½" long. The chest area is incised on this example, ca. AD 1500 – 1750. Found in the 1950s, it came from west of Gettysburg, South Dakota. Private collection. **$250.00.**

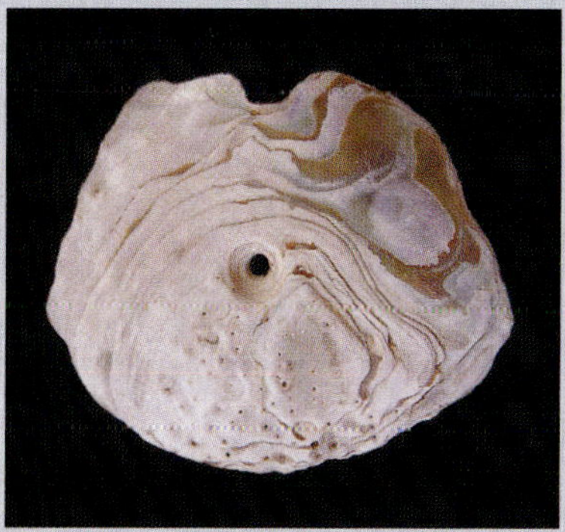

Abalone shell ornament, 1½" long, with central drilled hole. The ornament came from the Great Basin, Nevada. Victor T. Trujillo collection, Nevada. **$65.00.**

Ornamental Artifacts

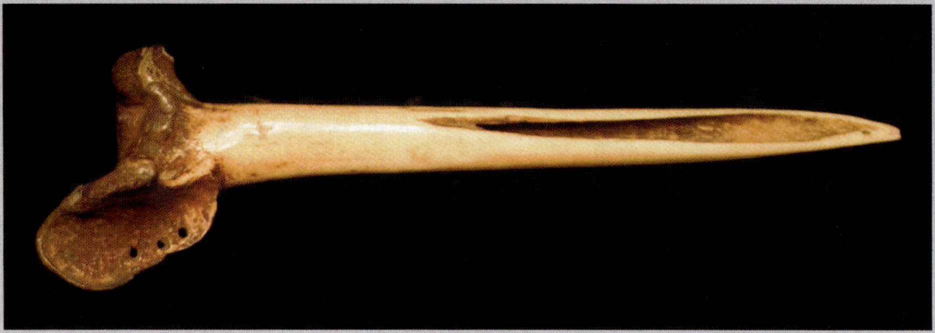

Awl or ornamental artifact, the head portion has red ochre and polish, while the shaft is polished to a gloss. An incised line is around the artifact and the head has three small holes. Possibly an elk leg bone, it is 15" long. Ex-collection Bush. Western United States, Tom Sekula collection, Pennsylvania. **$550.00.**

Bone whistle, 4⅜" long. This is a highly refined example, decorated with incised lines and dots. Ex-collection Liehr, it is probably Midwestern. John F. Wubker collection, Illinois. Museum grade.

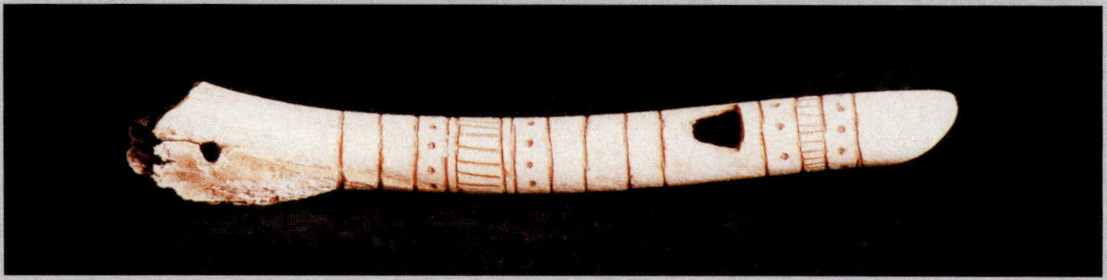

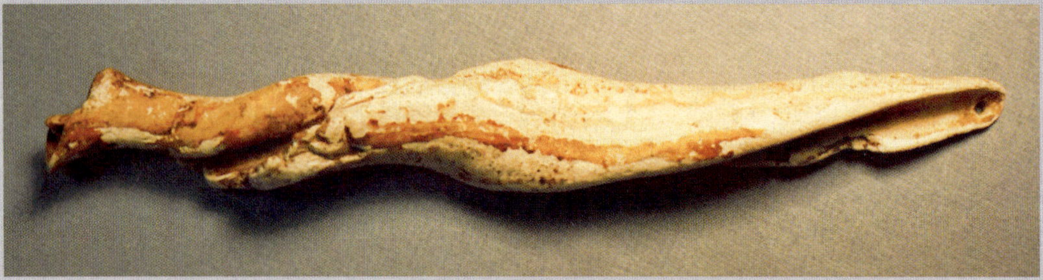

Busycon conch gorget, drilled at small end, historic period, ca. AD 1750. It is over 7" long and was found in the 1950s near Chamberlain, South Dakota. Private collection. **$350.00.**

Bone arm band, drilled with holes at each end for cord ties, diameter is 5". It is historic (ca. AD 1750) and came from Morton County, North Dakota. Private collection. **$200.00.**

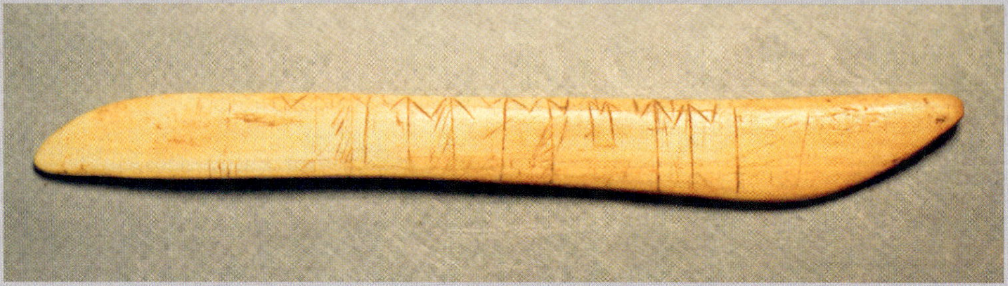

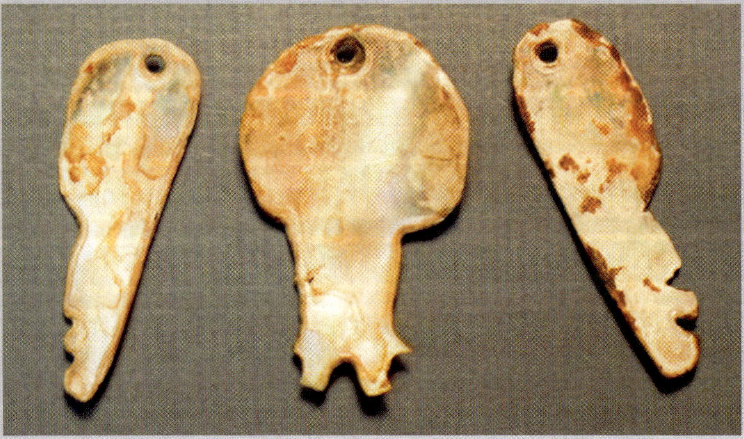

Abalone shell ornaments, known as key shapes due to outlines, 2 to 2¼" long. Ca. AD 500 – 1500, they were found by Ben Woodworth around 1940. Central California. Private collection. Group, **$200.00.**

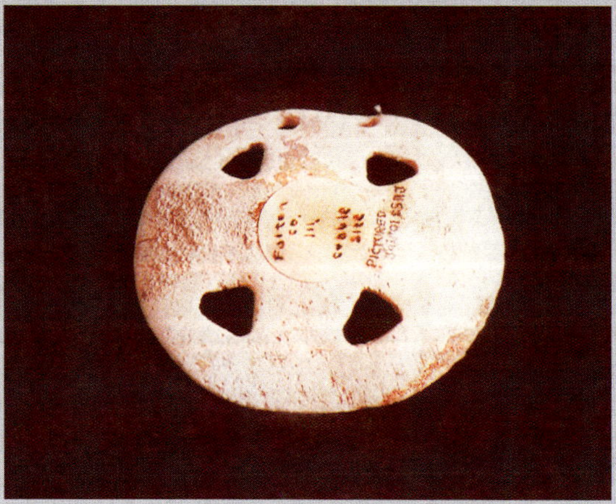

Shell gorget, two suspension holes and cross design, 1$^{13}/_{16}$" high and 2$^{1}/_{16}$" wide. It was found in Fulton County, Illinois. John F. Wubker collection, Illinois. **$275.00.**

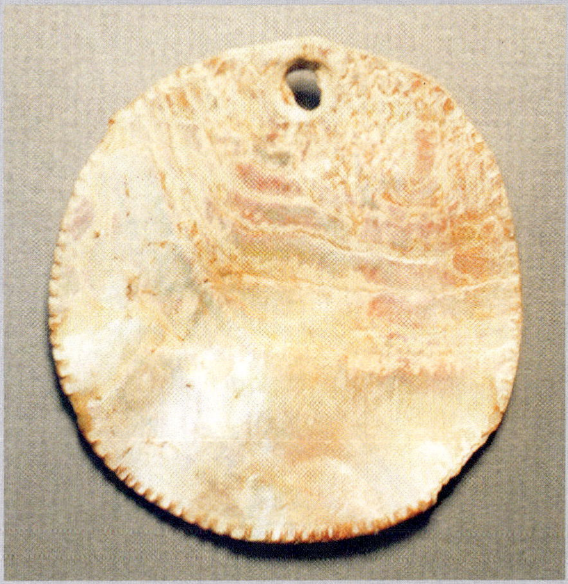

Abalone shell pendant, 2½" in diameter. The shell has tally marks around the outer edge and is drilled for suspension. It is ca. AD 500 – 1500 and was found by Ben Woodworth about 1940. Central California. Private collection. **$200.00.**

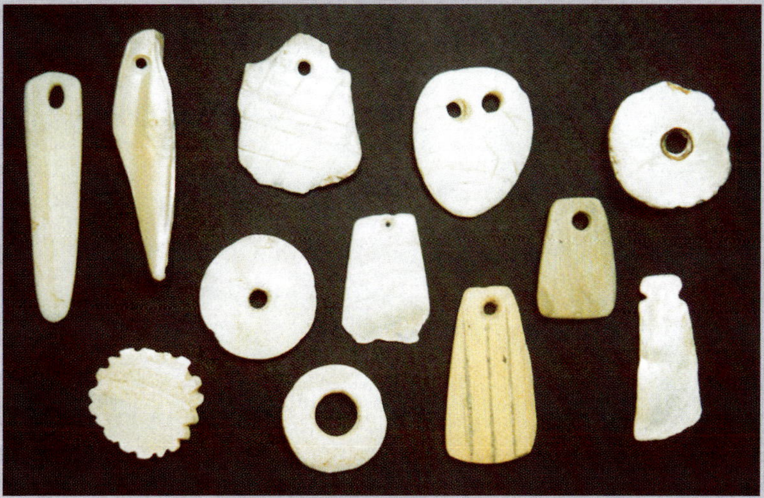

Pendants, drilled or holed (one notched), longest shell pendant is 1⅝". Of the two bone pendants, the longest (with incised lines) is 1⅛." These are probably all historic period and were found near Chamberlain, South Dakota. Mike Fox collection, Iowa. Shell pendants, each, **$35.00 – 60.00;** bone pendants, **$65.00 – 85.00.**

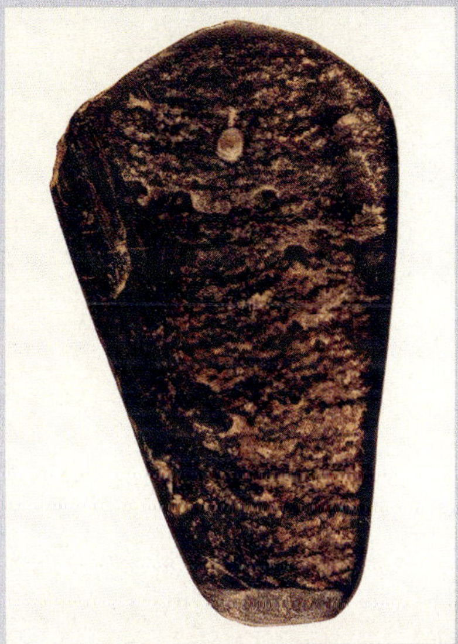

Pendant or necklace element, drill-hole just started, 2⅝" high. It is made of cannel coal, fossilized plant pollen. This piece is from West Virginia. Doug Hooks collection. Unlisted.

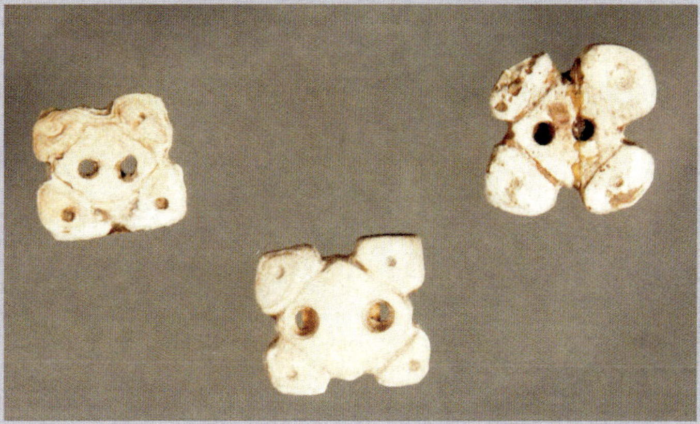

Ornamental shell buttons, perforated and engraved, largest is ¾ x 1". This type of small button or gorget is known only from the southern United States. Mississippian period, ca. AD 800 – 1200, they are from Alabama. John Smith collection, Illinois. Each, **$25.00 – 35.00.**

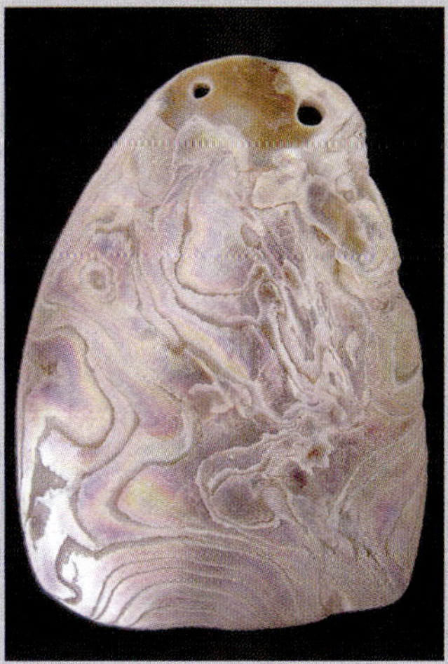

Abalone shell pendant, two suspension holes, 2½" high. It was found in the Great Basin, Nevada. Victor T. Trujillo collection, Nevada. **$85.00.**

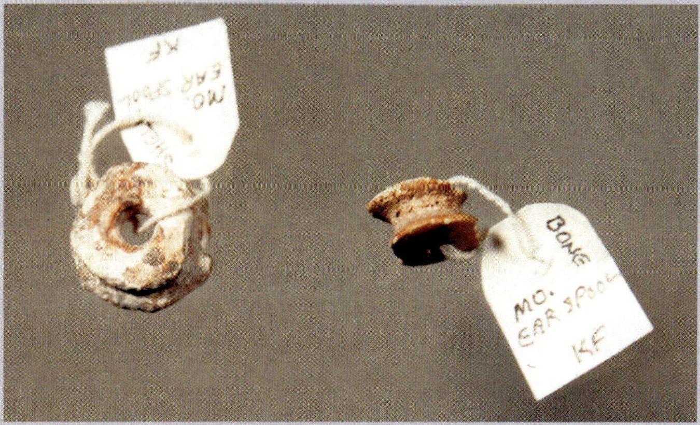

Earspools, left example is made of shell and the right is made of bone. These are scarce specimens from the Mississippian culture, and they were rock shelter finds in northern Missouri. John Smith collection, Illinois. Each, **$25.00 – 35.00.**

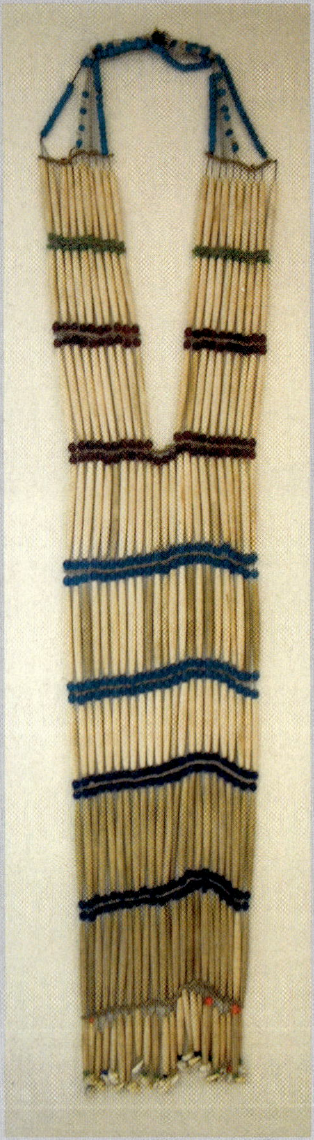

Breast decoration, bone and glass beads, 50" long. This historic piece came from near Chadron, Nebraska. Rod Fuller collection, Nebraska. Museum grade.

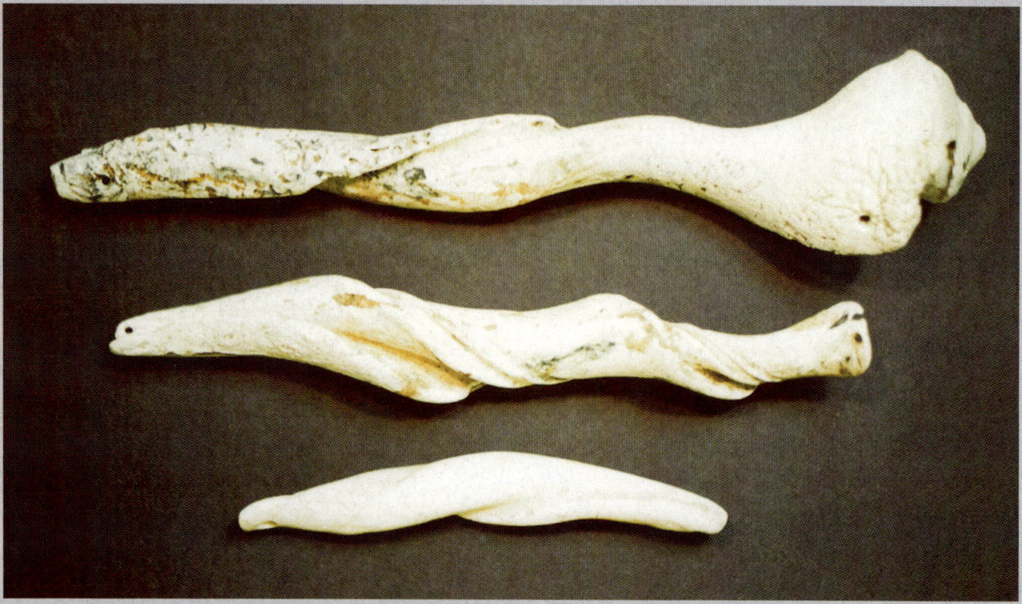

Columella pendants or gorgets, conch shell, lengths range from 5½ to 8½ inches. These marine shell artifacts are historic period and were found near Chamberlain, South Dakota. Mike Fox collection, Iowa. Each, **$150.00 – 350.00.**

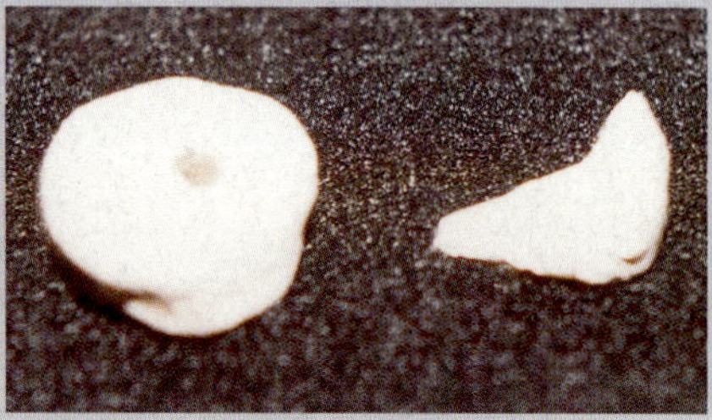

Shell cloak fasteners, perforated button with pin, button is ⅝" in diameter and pin is 9/16" long. They are proto-historic Creek, from Macon County, Alabama. Jim Maus collection, North Carolina. Unlisted.

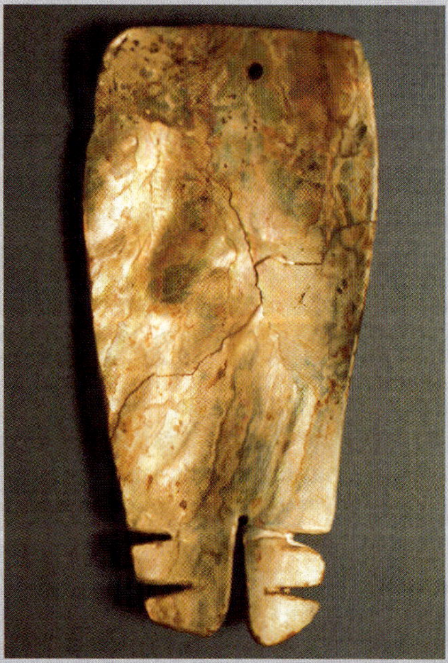

Banjo shape ornament, abalone shell, found about 1940 by Ben Woodworth. This prehistoric pendant is ca. AD 500 – 1500, from central California. Private collection. -

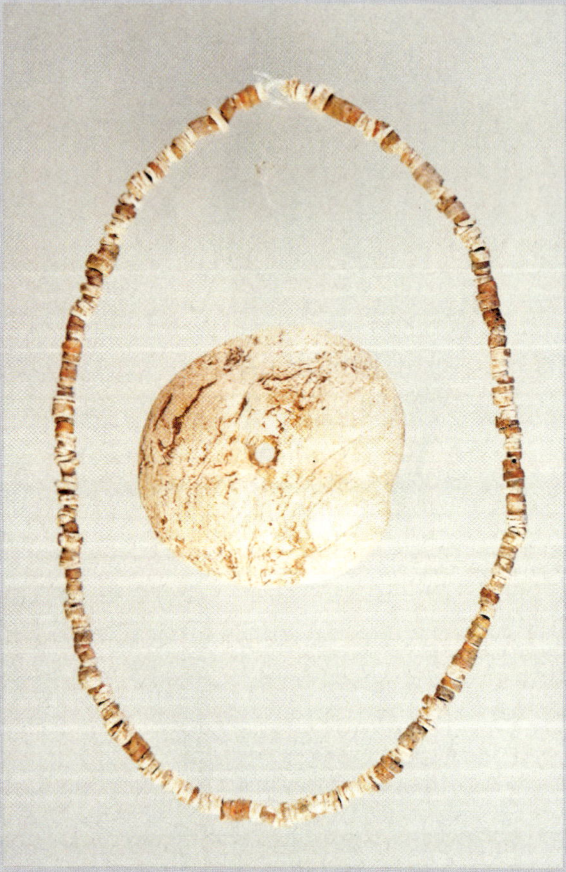

Shell gorget and string of tiny beads, gorget is 1¾" across. Probably Fort Ancient (AD 800 – 1500), they were found in Franklin County, Ohio. Fred Winegardner collection. Museum grade.

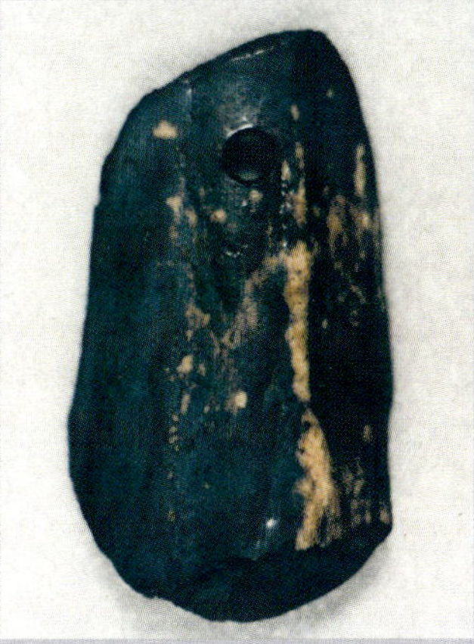

Fossil ivory pendant, mammoth or mastodon ivory, 1½" long. This unique piece was found in Posey County, Indiana. First Mesa, Indiana. **$165.00.**

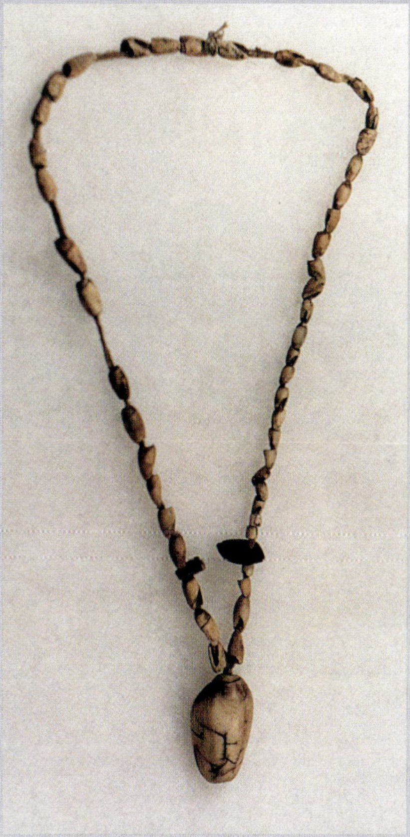

Necklace, shell beads and pendant, Mississippian, strand is 24" around and pendant is 1⅛" long. The beads were not indigenous to the area where they were found. Ex-collection Vietzen, St. Clair County, Illinois. Pete Timoch collection. **$200.00 – 250.00.**

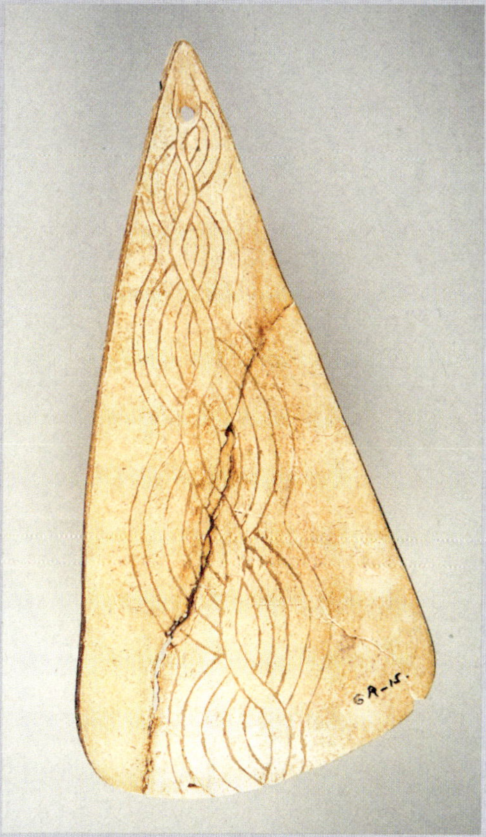

Pendant, animal shoulder bone, incised decoration, 8⅓₂" high. This is a very rare decorative/ornamental object with line designs that may represent a snake. It is ex-collection Tolliver, from Hocking County, Ohio. Private collection. Museum grade.

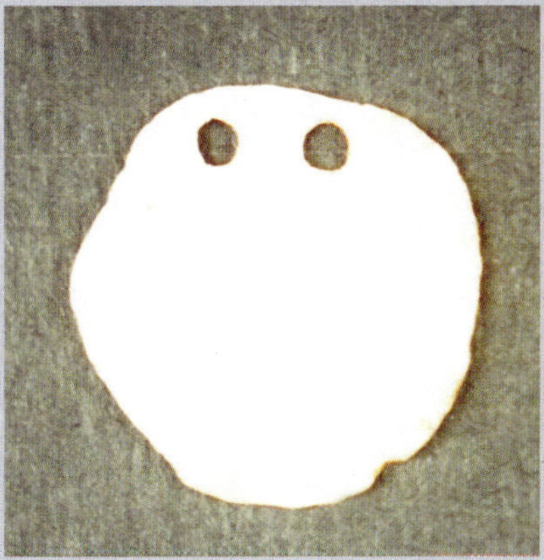

Shell pendant, two suspension holes. It came from the Emmaus area, Lehigh County, Pennsylvania. Lee Hallman collection, Pennsylvania. **$35.00.**

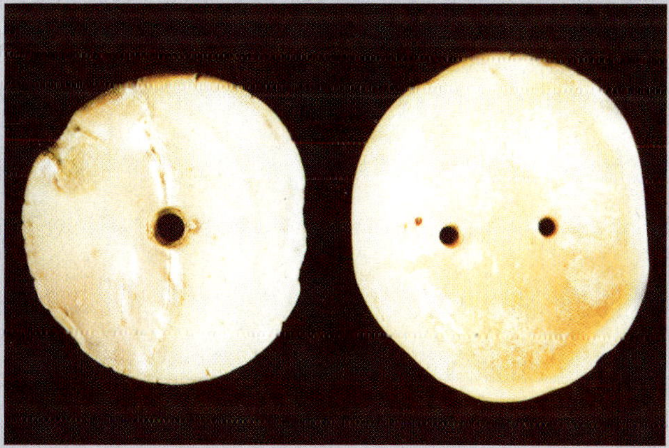

Shell ornaments, pendant with edge tally marks (left) is 1¼" in diameter, shell gorget (right) is 1⅝" in diameter. These are historic period, found near Mobridge, South Dakota. Mike Fox collection, Iowa. Pendant, **$100.00;** gorget, **$150.00.**

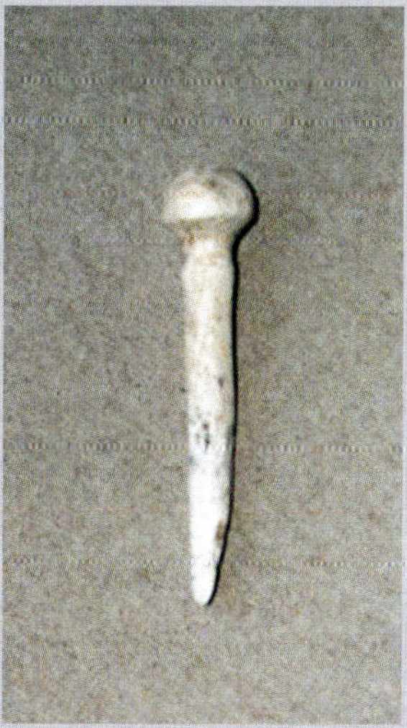

Shell earpin, Mississippian period, 2" long. It was found near the Arkansas – Tennessee line. Wilfred Dick collection, Mississippi. **$70.00.**

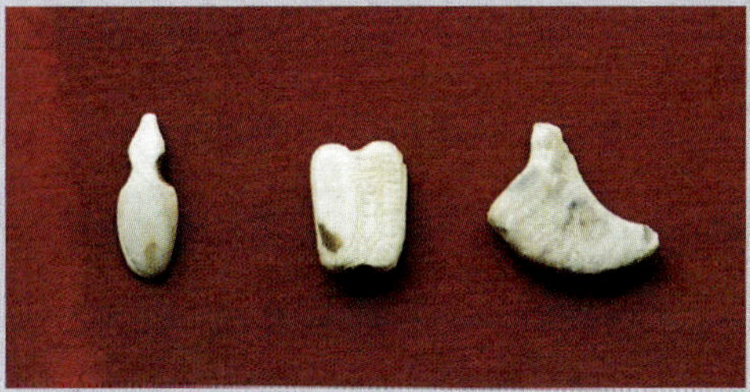

Drilled marine shell pendants, Seneca, duck effigy (left), rectangular runtee (center) with hole through the longest dimension, and claw (right). The runtee is ¾" long, the duck is 1", and the claw is 1⅛". All are from sites in Ontario County, New York. Dave Summers collection, Victor, New York. Runtee, **$60.00;** claw, **$140.00;** duck, **$150.00.**

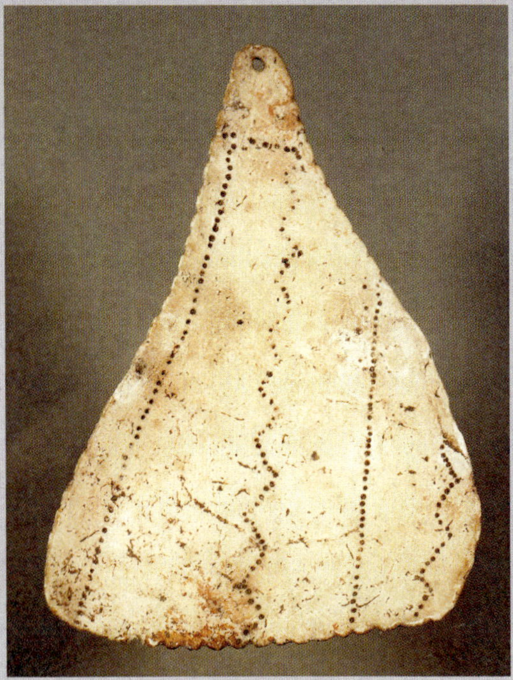

Marine shell pendant, with punctated design and scalloped edges. A rare piece, it is Late Archaic and was found in Texas. Private collection. **$2,000.00.**

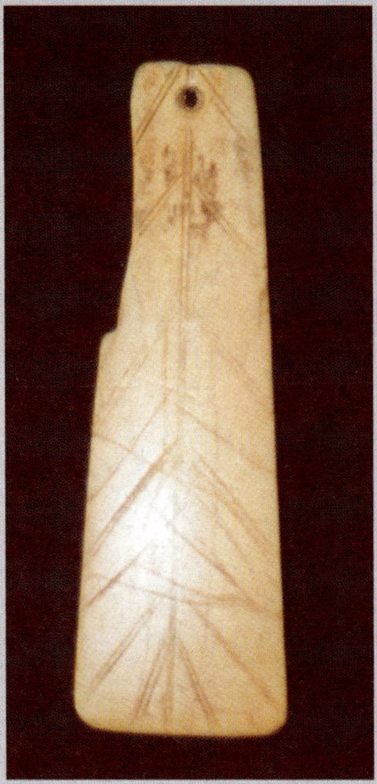

Bone pendant, engraved line design, 1¼ x 3½". This unusual piece has an unlisted provenance. Private collection. Museum grade.

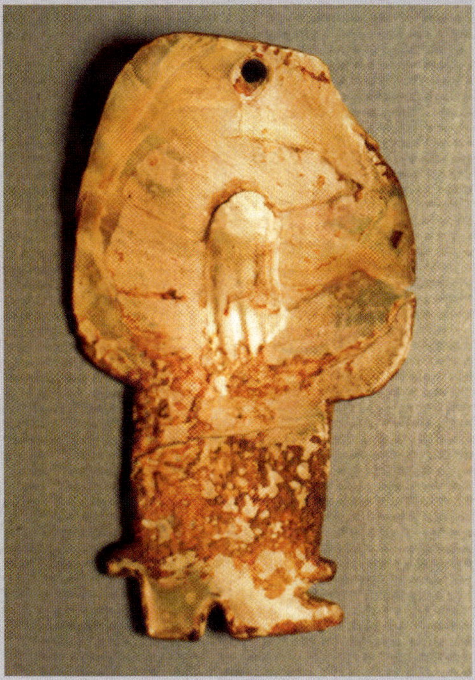

Abalone shell ornament, called a banjo shape, it is prehistoric (ca. AD 500 – 1500), 3" long. It was found by Ben Woodworth in about 1940. From central California, private collection. **$250.00.**

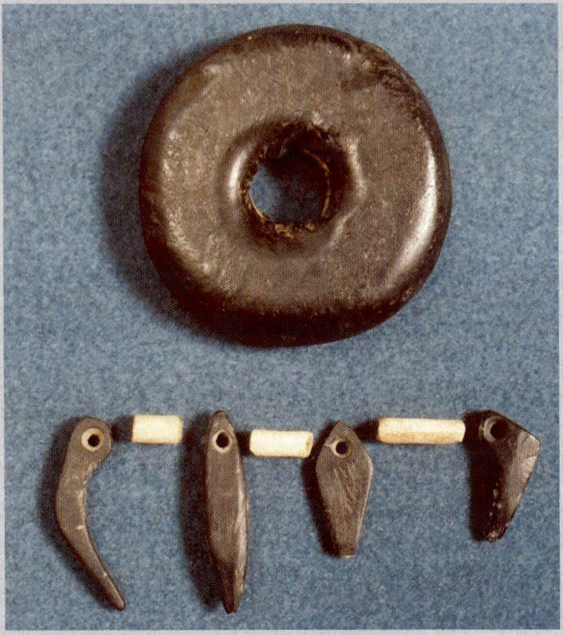

Discoidal, cannel coal Fort Ancient discoidal, top, four cannel coal necklace elements (talon effigy, tooth effigy, coffin-shaped and icicle shaped. The discoidal, Mississippian period, is 2½" in diameter. All of these artifacts, including the three bird bone beads, are from Ohio. Private collection. Discoidal, **$350.00 – 450.00;** necklace elements, each **$35.00 – 100.00;** beads, **$5.00 – 10.00.**

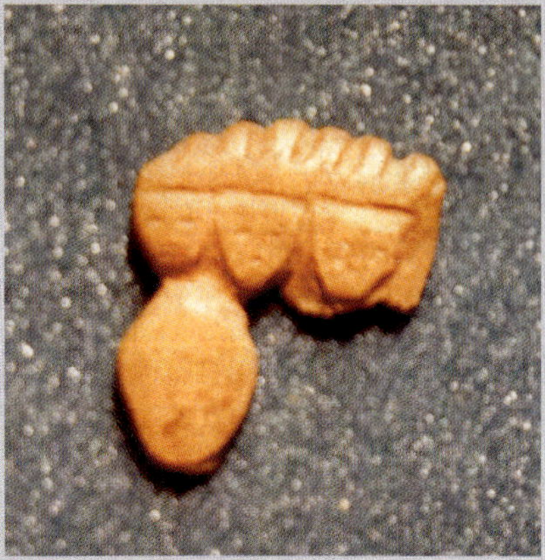

"Four Faces" comb section with teeth missing, ex-collections Schroff (ca. 1935) and Casterline. It measures 1½ x 1½" and is historic Iroquois (Seneca). Many of such combs were made from the wide section of elk or moose antler or from bone. The effigy comb section was found near Victor, Ontario County, New York. Dave Summers collection, Victor, New York. **$800.00.**

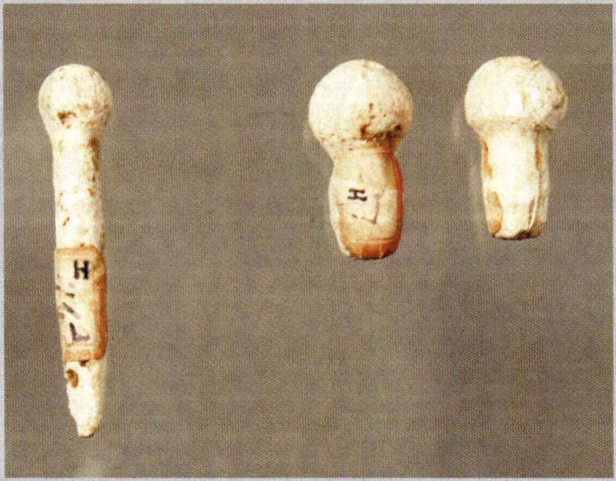

Knobbed ear pins, shell, Mississippian period ca. AD 800 – 1200. They are probably from the southern U. S. John Smith collection, Illinois. Each, **$20.00** and more if paired.

Hafted Tools

Most of the prehistoric artifacts found in North America are only part of the original, complete, and as-used tool. Most arrowpoints had wooden shafts, and axes had handles. This is also true for some organic material artifacts. Beads were held together with cord to form necklaces and bracelets, and most flint knives had handles of wood, bone, or antler. While that part of the original artifact made of durable matter (like knife blades) in most cases survived, usually the handle, string, or shaft did not.

Only a comparatively few complete artifacts have been found. Split-bone awls, those ubiquitous Indian tools, are usually recovered without a haft or handle, even though a great many seem designed to have one. It is probable that some awls were used with a leather wrap, and this would have disappeared in a relatively short time on the average site.

Some awls have been recovered with the handle intact, and these are often made of bone or antler. It is interesting to speculate about this. Since so many bone awls have been found, it is a puzzle why there are so few bone awls found in handles made of the same material. It is possible that awls were quickly replaced as they wore out or were damaged. Handles and the various awls that might fit them could have been stored separately and the awls fitted into them and used as required. In short, the awl and awl handle might have been only a temporary pairing for work around the prehistoric campfire. Many bone and antler handles have a small hole in one end, which suggests they might have been handles for awls.

Knives and handles found together are sometimes of the typical and expected combination, which is handle at one end and blade at the other, like most of the knives today. Many prehistoric hafted knives, however, have the blade set in and projecting from the side of the handle. It is, in fact, likely that many blades that are fairly small and asymmetrical and have resharpening mainly on one edge were mounted in this fashion.

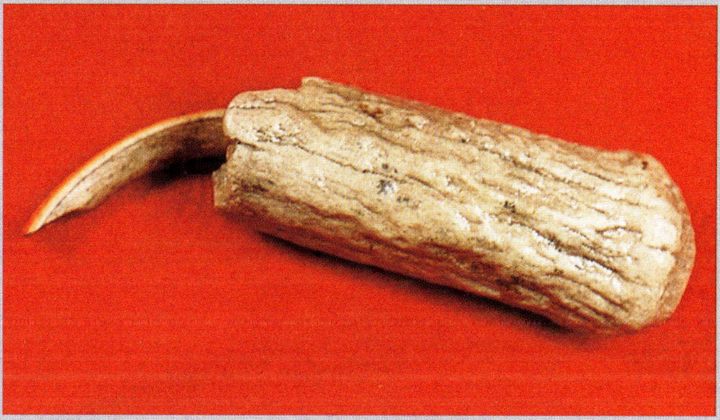

Graver/gouge set, rodent tooth and antler handle, handle is 3⅛" long. The oval hole, 2¼" deep, measures ⅜" x ⅝". This configuration wedges and seats the tooth, making a solid connection. The two were placed together for the photograph, and both are ex-collection Vietzen. Christian County, Kentucky. Pete Timoch collection. Set, **$250.00.**

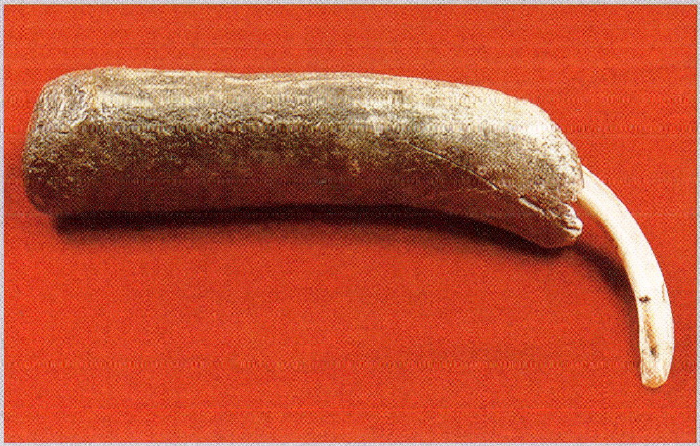

Tool handle (antler) and beaver tooth, both found at the same site and placed together for the photograph. The handle is 3½" long and the set could be used for graving or gouging. Shaped for a good grip, the handle is balanced and polished. Ex-collection Vietzen, Christian County, Kentucky. Pete Timoch collection. Set, **$250.00 - $300.00.**

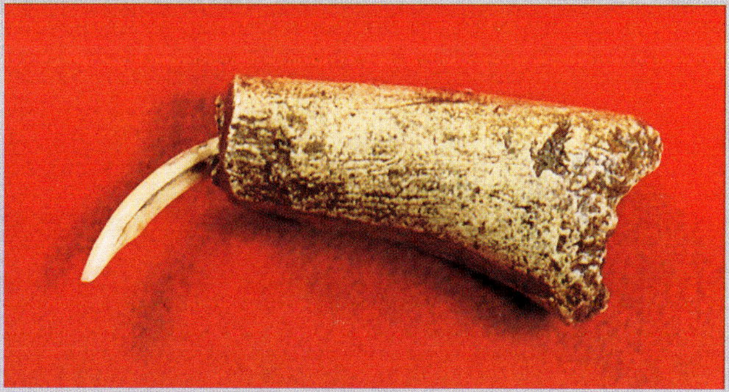

Tool, antler handle and rodent (groundhog) tooth, handle is 2 5/16". Col. Vietzen found the two (not together as shown) while exploring a large rock shelter. The handle is fully drilled, so the curved tooth wedges tightly in the hole. Christian County, Kentucky. Pete Timoch collection. Set, **$200.00.**

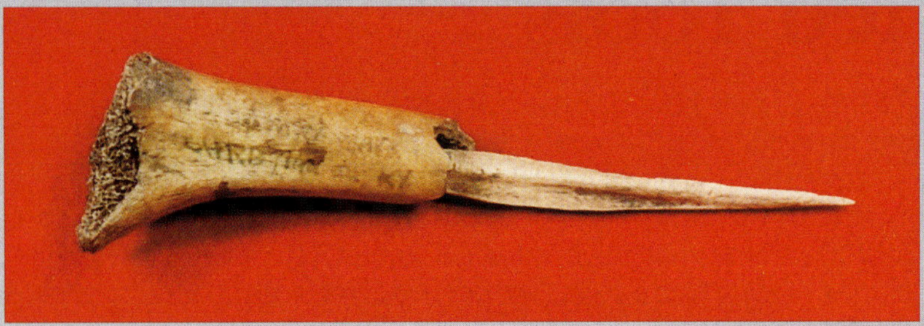

Bone handle, with split bone awl, Woodland period, handle $3\frac{1}{4}$" long. The natural bone hole was bored out and a $\frac{1}{2}$" hole was drilled from the larger end. Not found as a set, the artifacts were assembled for the photograph. They are ex-collection Vietzen and were found in Christian County, Kentucky. Pete Timoch collection. Set, **$250.00.**

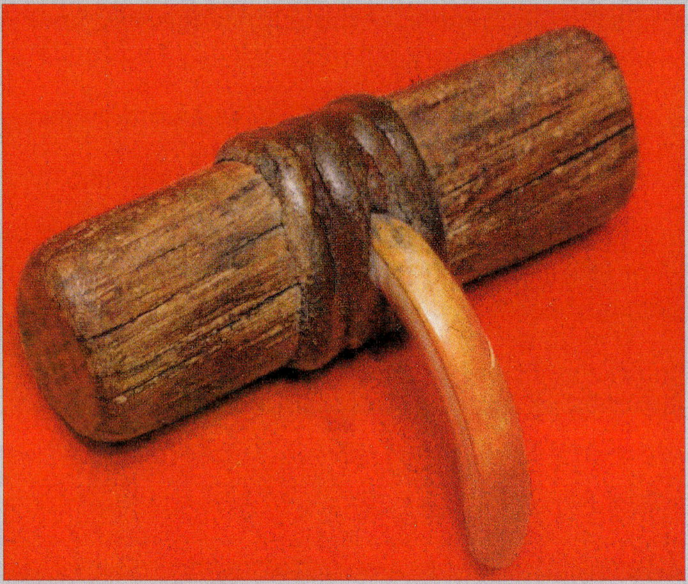

Gouge, beaver tooth, wood handle and leather wrap, 1 x $3\frac{5}{16}$". Of recent origin, the owner saw this being used by an elderly Iroquois to carve a wooden bowl. Canada. Michael F. Slasinski collection, Michigan. **$175.00.**

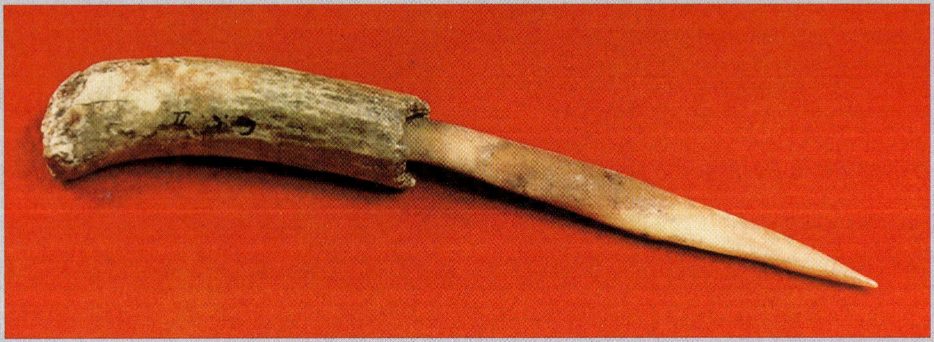

Handle (antler) and split bone awl, Late Archaic to Woodland, handle length is $2\frac{15}{16}$". The round handle hole is $\frac{3}{8}$" across and 1" deep. The handle has almost a modern look, and both pieces were found in the same large rock shelter and were fitted together for the photograph. Ex-collection Vietzen, Christian County, Kentucky. Pete Timoch collection. Set, **$250.00 - $300.00.**

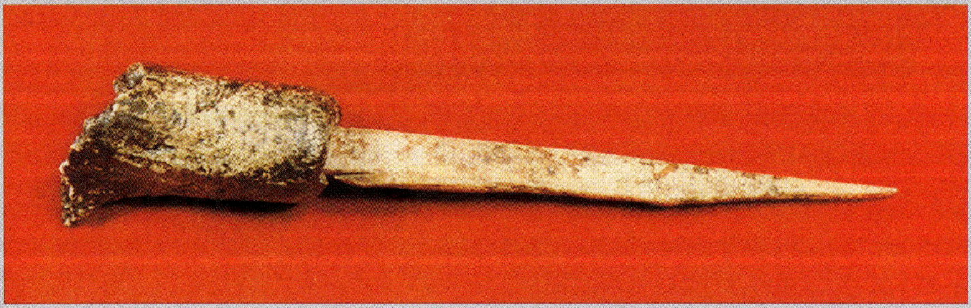

Handle and awl, found in the same rock shelter but placed together for the photograph, handle is $2\frac{1}{4}$" long. An oval hole runs the length of the handle and is larger at the awl end. The awl could have been wedged or glued in position. These artifacts were in the Vietzen collection and were found in Christian County, Kentucky. Pete Timoch collection. Set, **$250.00.**

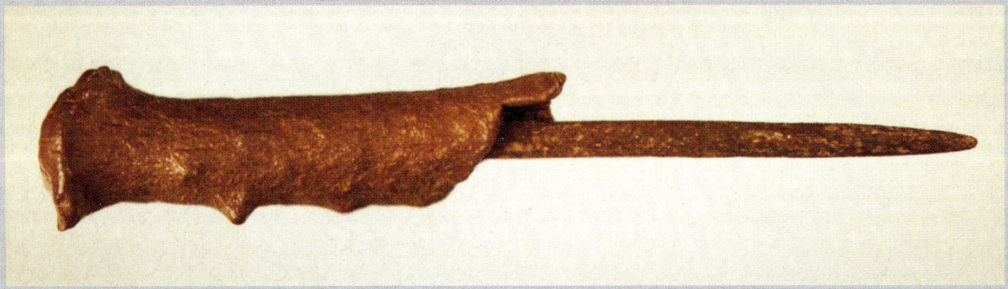

Perforator or awl, antler handle with bone blade in place, both mineralized to the same degree. This very scarce set is $5\frac{15}{16}$" long and was found in the Midwest. Larry Garvin collection. Museum grade.

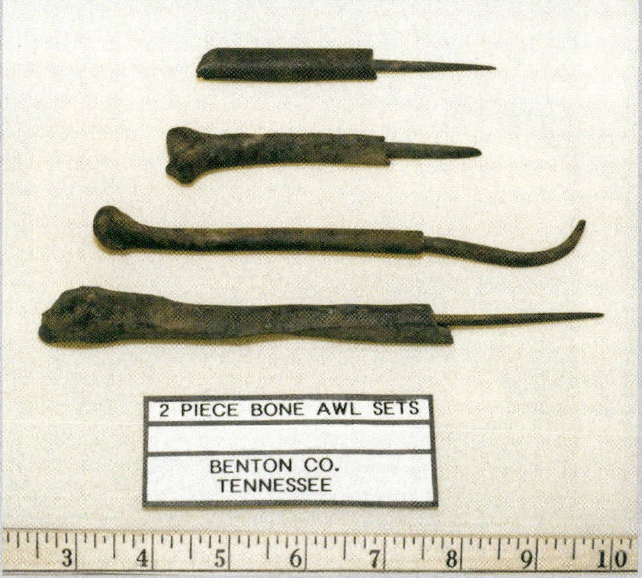

Awl or perforator sets, hollowed bone handles and bone awls, sizes as indicated. Now mineralized and stained dark, these were river finds in Benton County, Tennessee. Back to Earth. Unlisted.

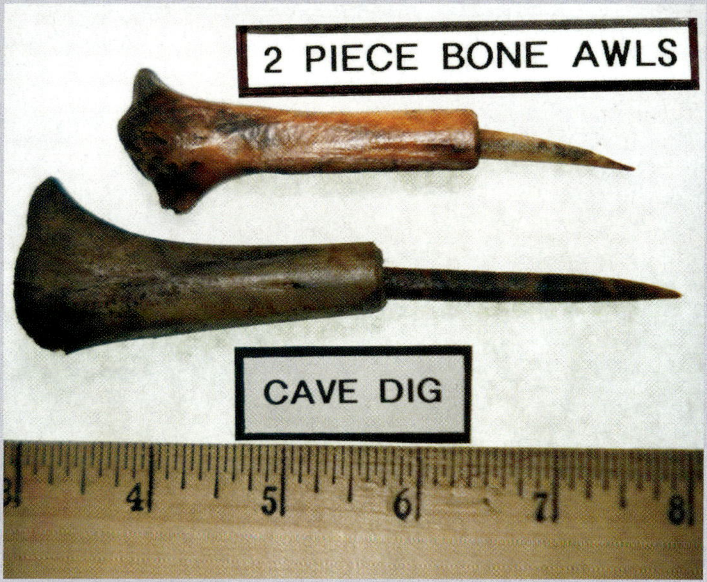

Awls set in bone handles, bone, two-piece sets, deeply patinated. These scarce examples were found in Robertson County, Tennessee. Back to Earth. Each, **$150.00.**

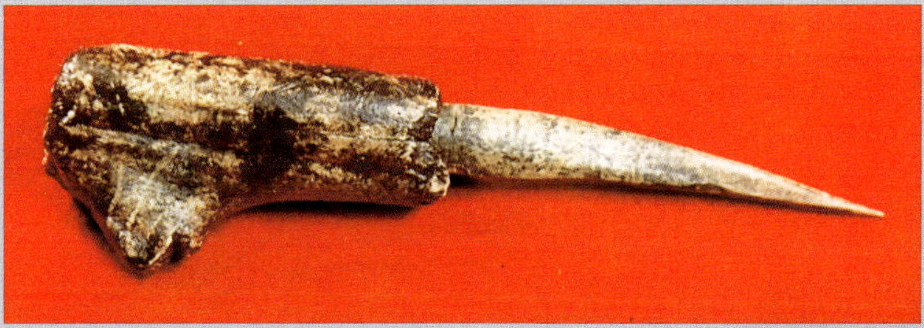

Antler handle and bone awl, handle, with full-length hole that tapers from 7/16" at the awl end to 3/16" at the hilt, handle is 2⅞" long. Both were found, but not together, at the same site. Formerly in the Vietzen collection, the artifacts are from Christian County, Kentucky. Pete Timoch collection. Set, **$250.00.**

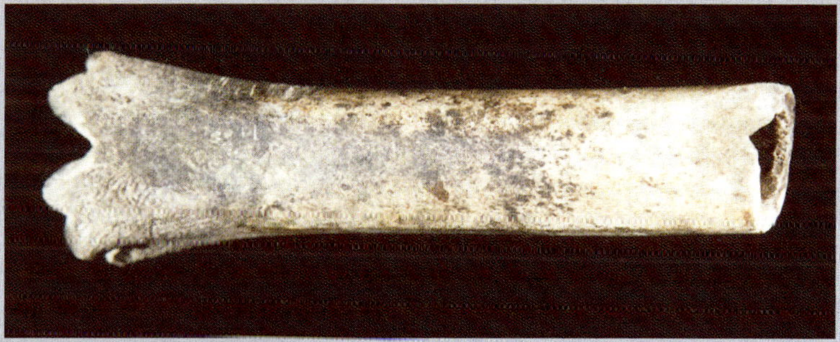

Deer bone handle, 4⅜" long. This artifact was pictured in *Indian Artifacts of the Midwest*-V, and was found in a creek. It is from Lee County, Iowa. Pat Clark collection, Iowa. John Gorham photograph. **$200.00.**

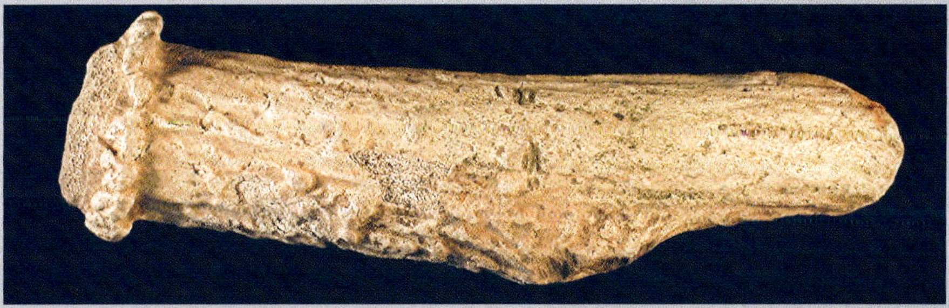

Deer antler handle, 6¼" long. This piece was found in the same creek that also produced the deer bone handle, and they were found two years apart. Lee County, Iowa. Pat Clark collection, Iowa; John Gorham photograph. **$200.00.**

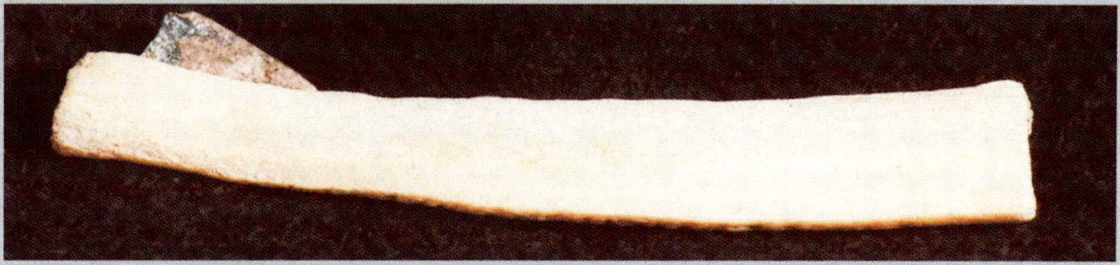

Knife, bone handle with thin copper blade, overall length is 5 7/16". From the historic period, the knife was found in Morton County, North Dakota. John F. Wubker collection, Illinois. **$375.00.**

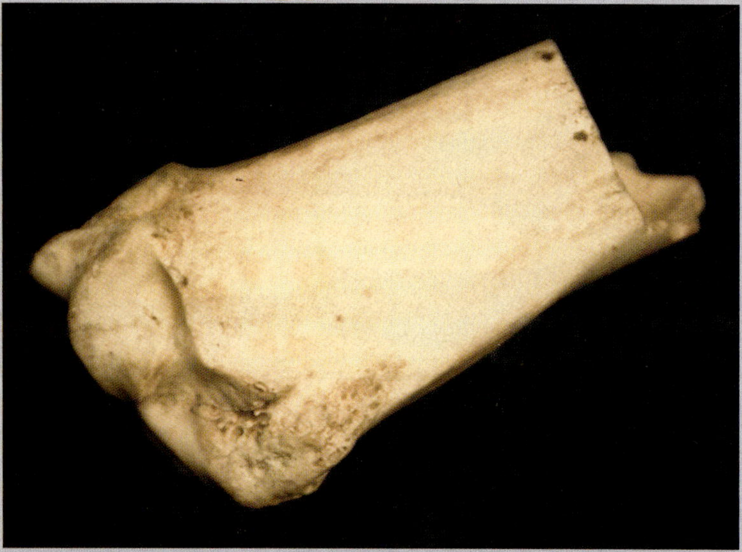

Bone handle, found by the owner in a field, 2½" long. Such handles were used for awls, knives, and Atl-atls. Erie County, Pennsylvania. Tom Sekula collection, Pennsylvania. **$25.00.**

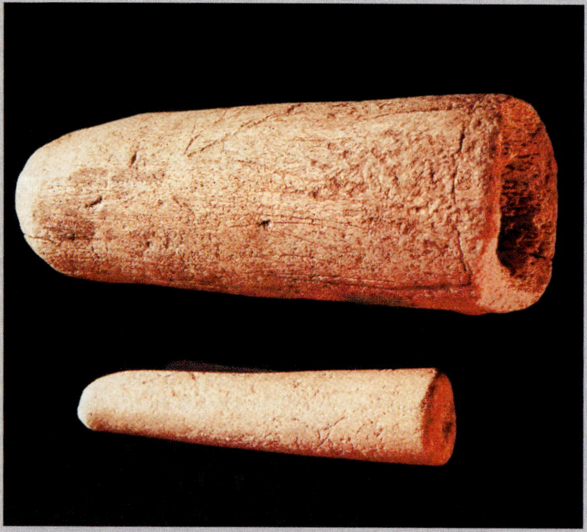

Bone artifacts, socketed handle with tapered bone insert, use unknown. The tool combination is 3⅛" long when assembled, and they came from a site dated ca. AD 1450 – 1600 on the east side of Yadkin River. Davidson County, North Carolina. Collection of, and photograph by, Ron Harris, North Carolina. Both, **$150.00.**

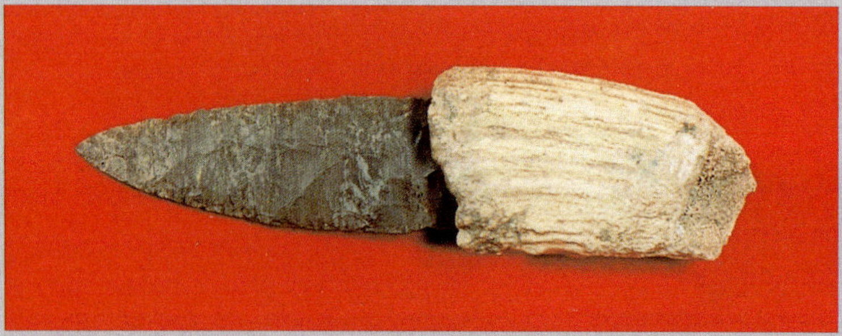

Handle (antler) and flint blade, Late Archaic to Woodland, handle is 3¼". Ex-collection Vietzen, the knife blade is from the same time period and the two were placed together for the photograph. The handle came from Christian County, Kentucky. Pete Timoch collection. Handle only, **$300.00 – 400.00.**

Bone tool or knife handle, 2⅝" long, cutmarks on side. The accompanying river-stained awl was not found with the handle, but the photo illustrates how they might have been paired. Florida. Dwight Wolfe collection. Handle, **$75.00.** Awl, **$25.00.**

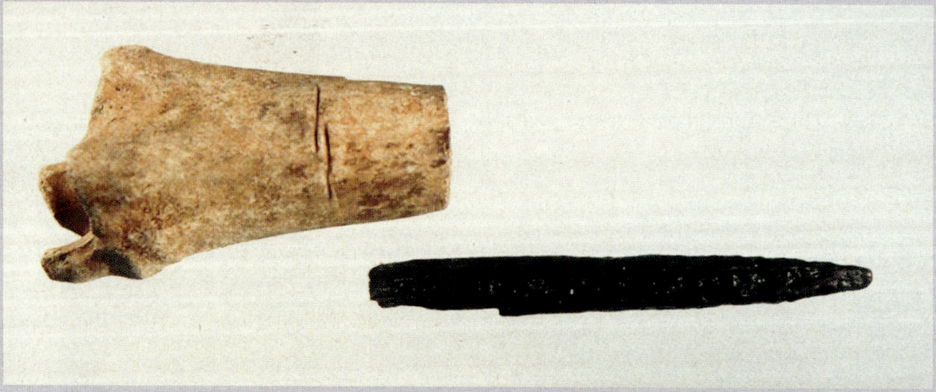

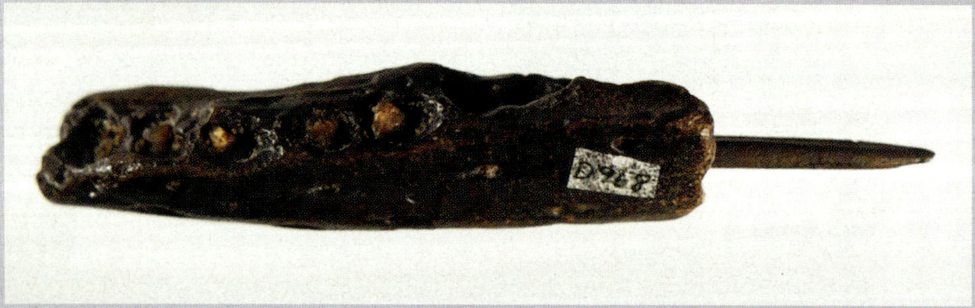

Tool set (handle with punch or awl), handle 4" long. The handle is made of scarce material, an alligator jawbone with some tooth stubs remaining. This dark stained tool combination was found in the Suwannee River, Florida. Dwight Wolfe collection. Museum grade.

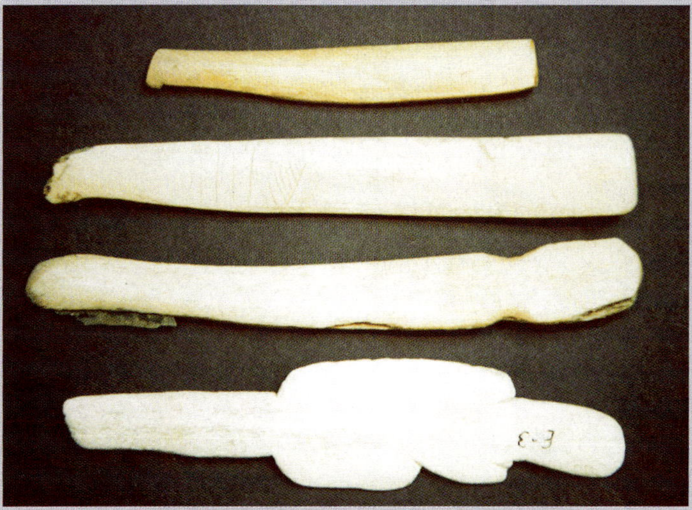

Bone knife handles, bottom example an unusual form. The longest handle (second from bottom) is 6½" and it still retains some of the copper blade. The handles came from Morton County, North Dakota. Mike Fox collection, Iowa. Each, **$100.00 - $200.00;** handle with blade remnant, **$350.00.**

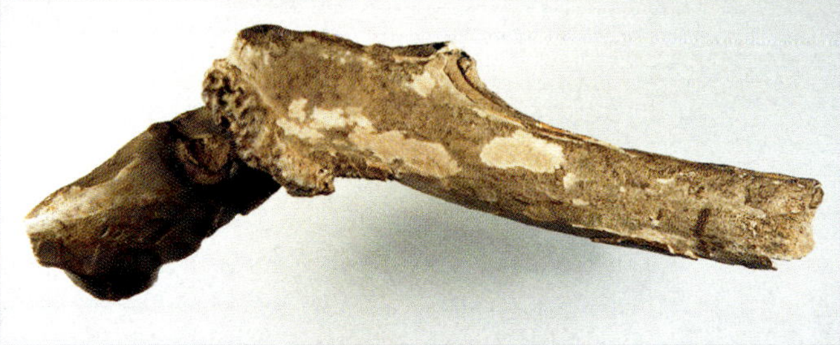

Celt and original antler handle, not North American Indian but included here to show the widespread use of such combinations. The broken handle and extended flint celt are 9⅜" long. Interestingly, the polished flint celt is wedged into the antler base with small wooden shims. France. Dwight Wolfe collection. Museum grade.

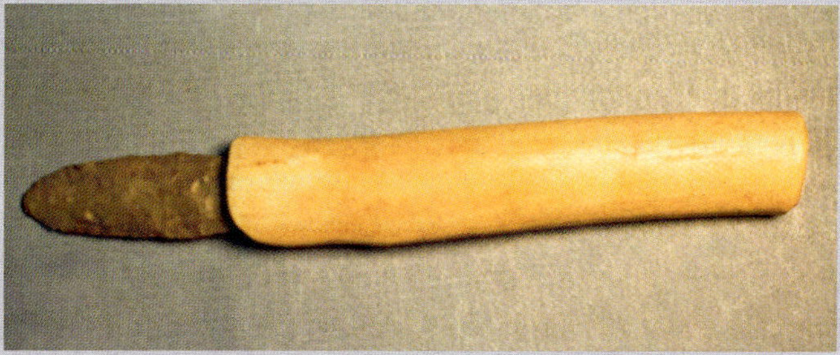

Knife, bison rib handle and flint blade, overall length is 5½". Ca. AD 1750, it is from Morton County, North Dakota. Private collection. Museum grade.

Knife, copper blade inset into bison rib handle, 6¼" long. Despite the cleaver-like appearance, knives like this were probably used for slicing meat and roots into thin strips. It is 6¼" long, ca. AD 1750. Morton County, North Dakota. Private collection. **$350.00.**

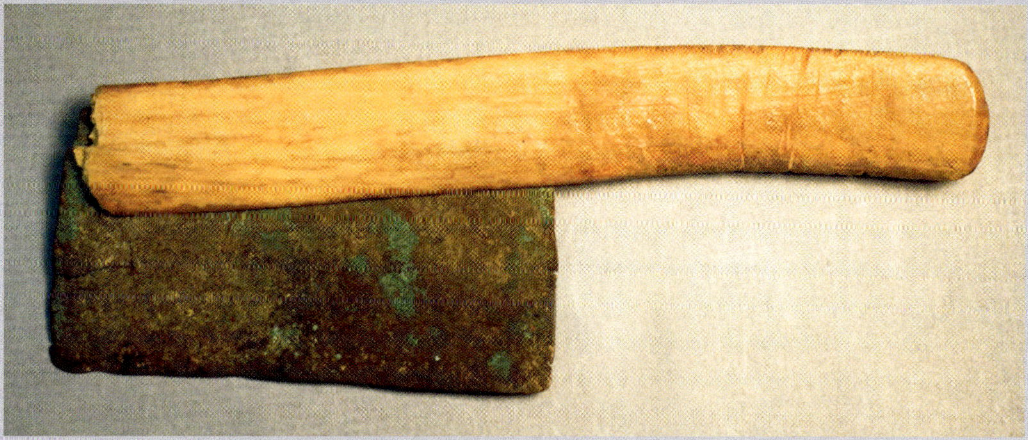

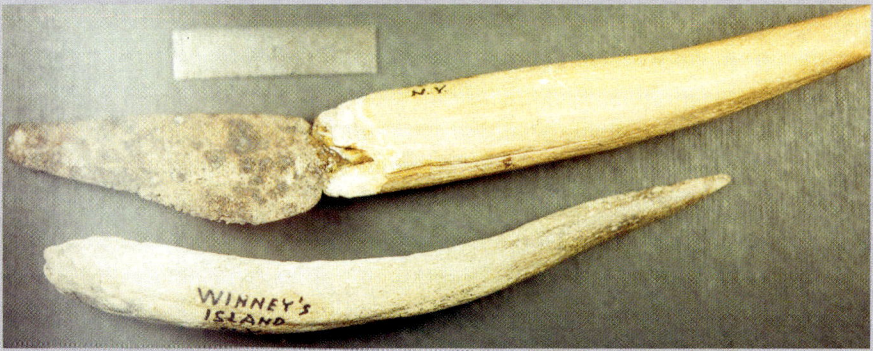

Artifacts, antler. Upper, long knife handle with inset metal blade. Lower, antler awl or punch. Both came from Winney's Island, New York. Lee Hallman collection, Pennsylvania. Knife, Museum grade; awl or punch, **$25.00.**

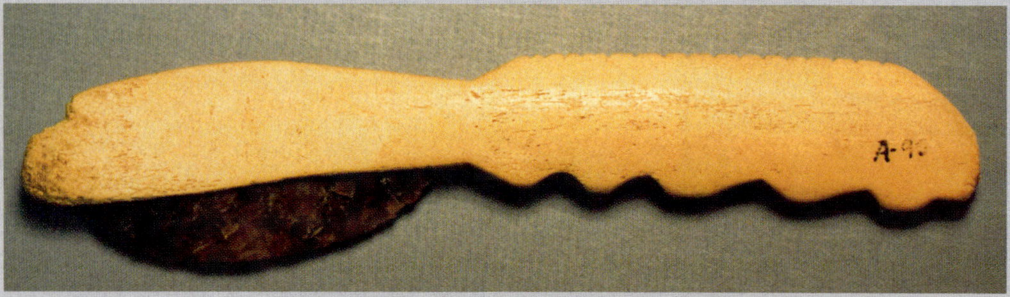

Knife, complete with Knife River flint blade, overall length is 8" long. The handle edge of this artistic piece has many tally marks. The knife is historic, ca. AD 1750, and was found near Chamberlain, South Dakota. Private collection. **$400.00.**

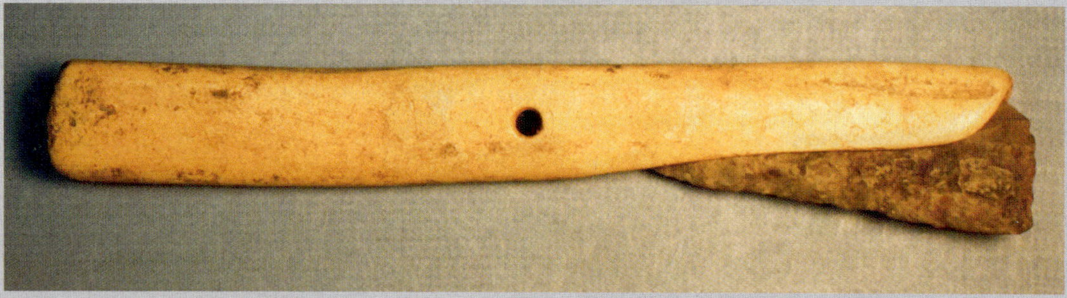

Knife, flint blade inset into bison bone rib. Historic period, the knife is 7½" long and has a suspension hole near the handle center. Morton County, North Dakota. Private collection. **$300.00.**

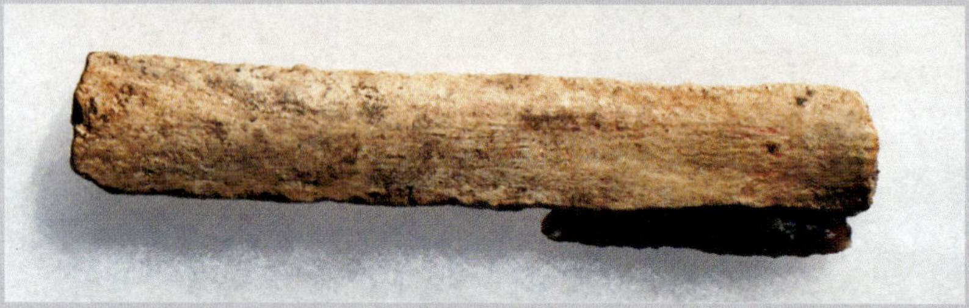

Knife, bone handle, 6⅜" long, inset blade with straight edge made of Knife River flint. Ex-collection Gregory Perino, it has a Perino COA. A rare piece, the complete knife was found near Bismarck, North Dakota. Earthworks Artifacts. Museum grade.

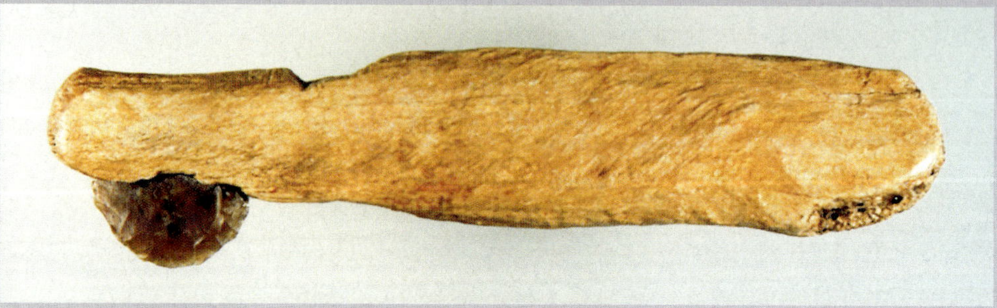

Knife with bison bone handle, small inset side blade made of Knife River flint. The handle is 7⅞" long and the handle and blade were found as pictured. Fort Bennett area, South Dakota. Dwight Wolfe collection. Museum grade.

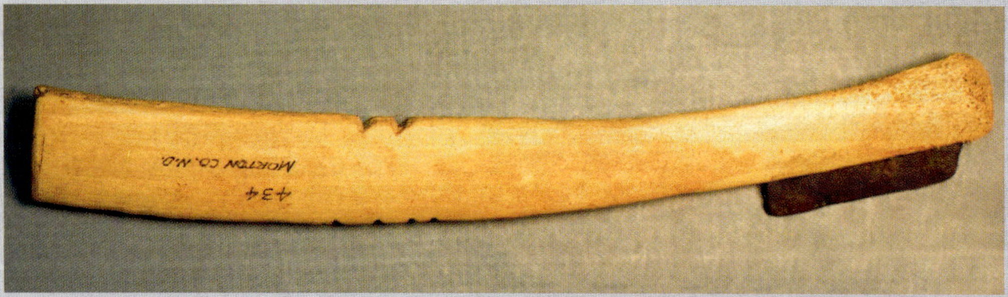

Knife, copper blade inset into side and end of bison rib, 6½" long. It has several tally marks on the handle and is ca. AD 1750. Morton County, North Dakota. Private collection. **$350.00.**

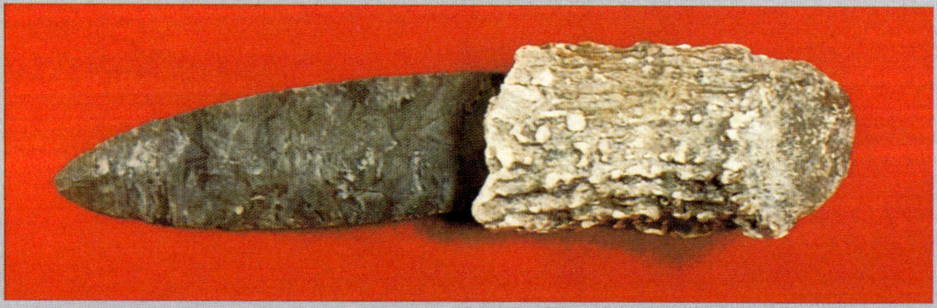

Handle (antler) and flint blade, handle is 4 inches long. From the Vietzen collection, the handle only is pictured in his book *The Saga of Glover's Cave*, page 219. The knife blade is from the same period (Late Archaic to Woodland) and the handle hole is rectangular and tapered, 1⅝" deep. Christian County, Kentucky. Pete Timoch collection. Handle only, **$300.00 – 400.00.**

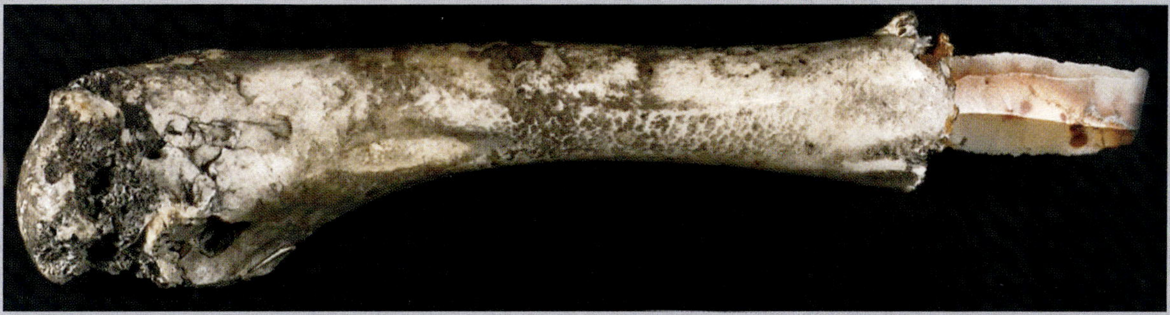

Hopewell knife, bone-hafted bladelet made of Flint Ridge translucent core flint in pink and tan, overall knife length is 5¾". One of the most important artifacts pictured in this book, this knife indicates how at least some of the gem quality Hopewell (Middle Woodland) bladelets were hafted. (It also suggests an exchange distance, since the flint came from Licking County, Ohio.) The blade fits a loose slot in the bone end, and the bladelet and handle were certainly a tool unit. The knife was found in a rock shelter in Daviess County, Indiana. Tracy Spradlin collection, Illinois. Tony Clinton photograph. Museum grade.

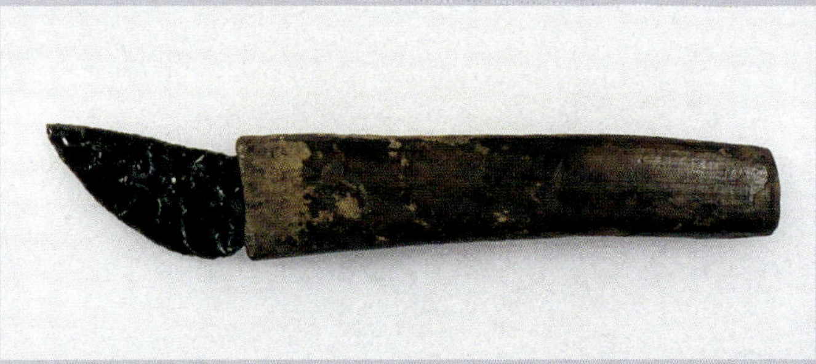

Antler knife handle, shown with a modern blade placed in the centered haft receptacle, handle is 5¾" long. A helpful feature is a slotted hole on one narrow side of the handle, either for a wedge or so that a broken blade could be punched out. Alaska. Pete Timoch collection. **$150.00 – 200.00.**

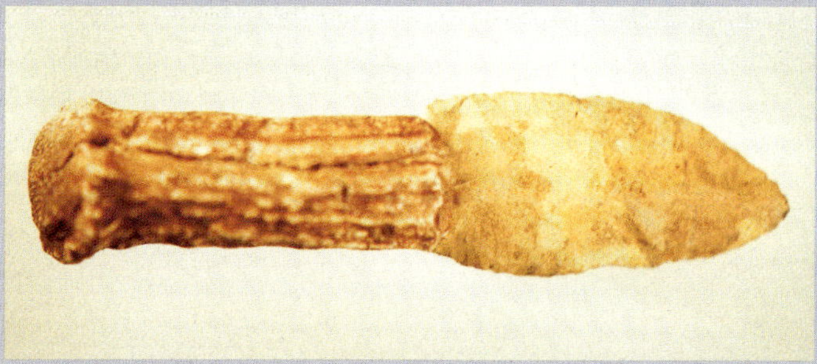

Knife, chert blade with original antler handle, 6⅜" long. An as-used knife and handle set is extremely scarce. This came from Hardin County, Tennessee. Larry Garvin collection. Museum grade.

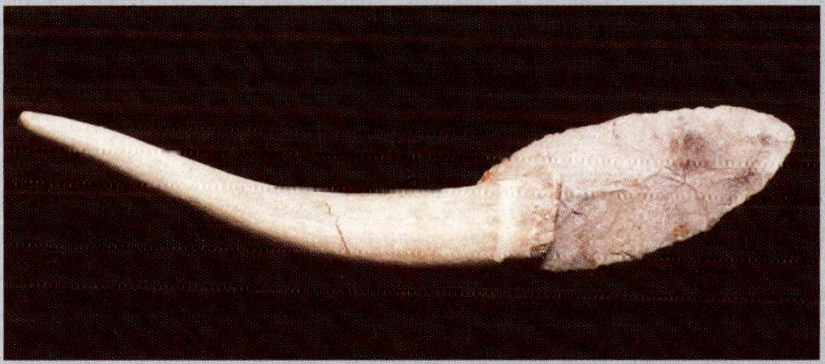

Complete knife – tine handle possibly from elk antler, 6½" long. The inset flint blade is 4½" long. This rare tool was found in a dry cave excavation in New York state. Private collection. Museum grade.

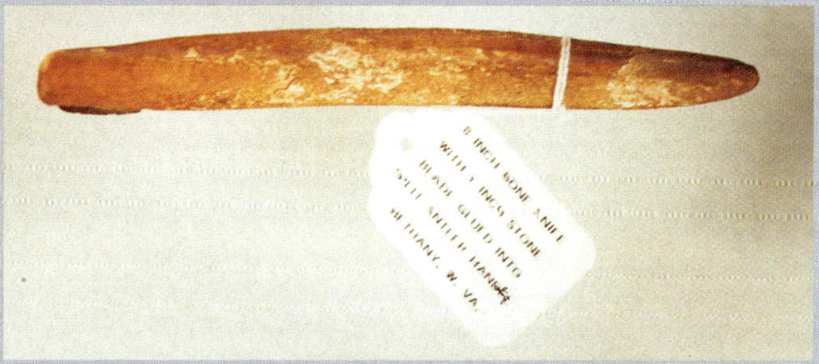

Bone knife, with inset short stone knife blade on the side at one end, 8" long. A rare artifact, it was found near Bethany, West Virginia. Larry Garvin collection. Museum grade.

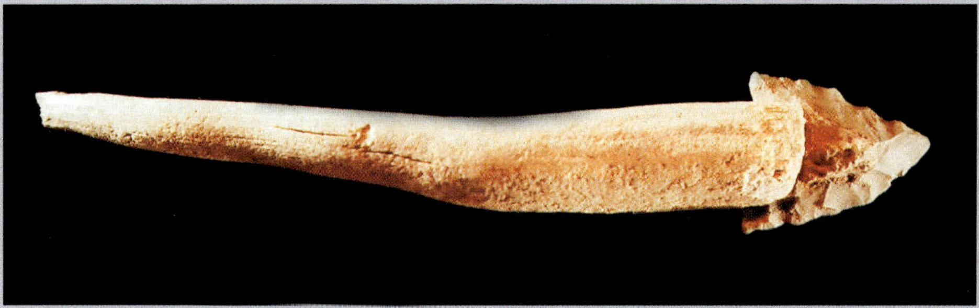

Complete knife, antler handle and flint blade, entire artifact is 5½" long. The blade is set firmly in the handle and is further secured by asphaltum (tar) on both sides. This is an exceptional find for the area (site dates ca. AD 1450 – 1600) considering the acidic soil. Davidson County, North Carolina. Collection of, and photograph by, Ron Harris, North Carolina. Museum grade.

Hairpins

Even though they seem to look much like what we think hairpins should be, no one really knows what this particular class of artifacts was really used for. The word persists, however, even though many examples may have been clothing toggles, fasteners for bundles, or game pieces. We know so little about prehistoric hairstyles that we cannot be certain hairpins were even widely used.

This said, hairpins are known to have been made from Late Archaic times into Contact times (ca. AD 1500), and they exist in plain and decorated forms. A classic hairpin is rounded, long and narrow, pointed at one end, and expanded, flattened, knobbed, or blunt at the other end. Lengths vary from 3 or 4 inches to 10 inches or more. Most are made of large animal bones. Plain examples are like giant needles, and a few may even have a drilled hole in the end opposite the tip. Ornamental hairpins may have incised markings, and some Late Archaic examples are elaborately carved with geometric designs. In the Northeast, hairpins have been found with traces of red paint.

The difference between long, slender, well-made awls and some hairpins is difficult to determine; some examples, indeed, might have served interchangeable purposes. Today, one collector might call a particular object an awl while another might consider it a hairpin. However, if an artifact has about the same diameter for much of the length, is seemingly too long for comfortable or practical awl use, is finely finished, and shows no signs of heavy use-wear, it might be a hairpin, toggle, or fastener.

Whatever the descriptive word and actual prehistoric use, hairpins are admired for their beauty and the skill it took to make them. No antler, bone, or shell collection is truly complete without some examples of this artifact class.

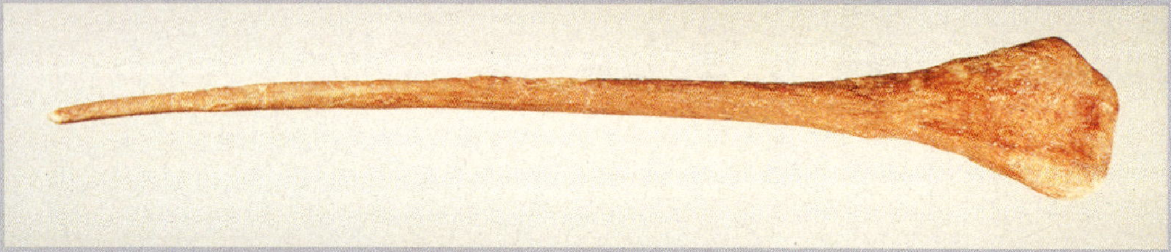

Hairpin, chemically stabilized animal bone, 7⁹⁄₁₆" long. It has a knobbed head and the small end was retipped (cream color) recently. The pin is from Kentucky or Tennessee. Private collection. **$60.00.**

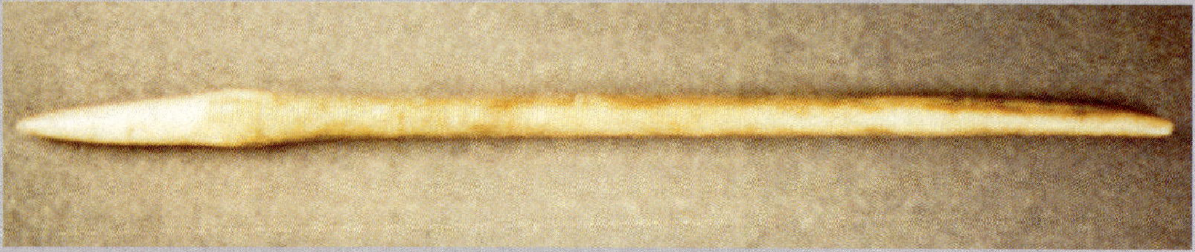

Bone hairpin, polished and ivory-like, 7" long. This pin was found near Willow Grove, West Virginia. Larry Garvin collection. **$250.00.**

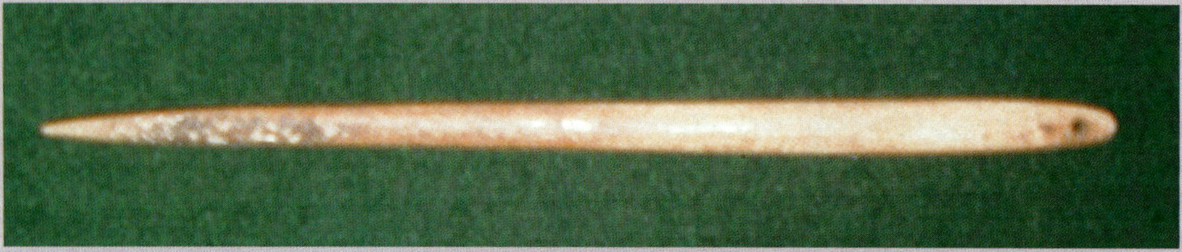

Bone needle or hairpin, drilled, ex-collection Noel. Nicely shaped, this example is from Kentucky. Keith and Rhonda Dodge collection, Michigan. **$225.00.**

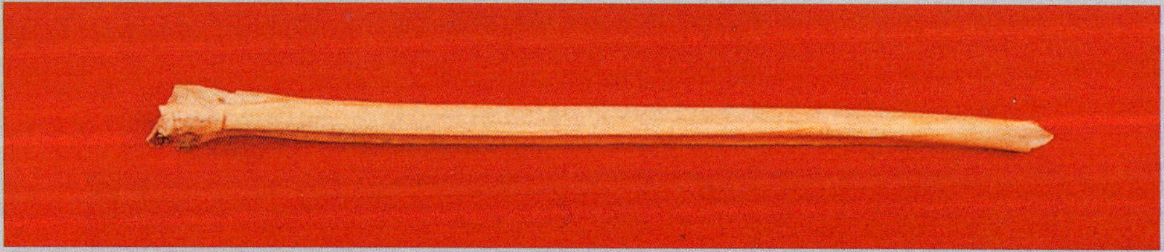

Hairpin, Late Archaic to Woodland, 9". This long, lightweight artifact may be made of trumpeter swan bone. Col. Vietzen found it in a large rock shelter. Christian County, Kentucky. Pete Timoch collection. Museum grade.

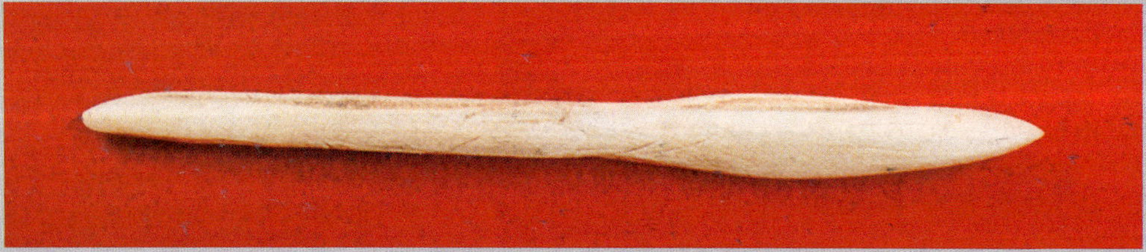

Hairpin, expanded near the more pointed tip, smooth bone, highly polished. Ex-collection Vietzen, it is 3¹⁵⁄₁₆" and from the Ohio-Kentucky region. Pete Timoch collection. **$100.00 – 150.00.**

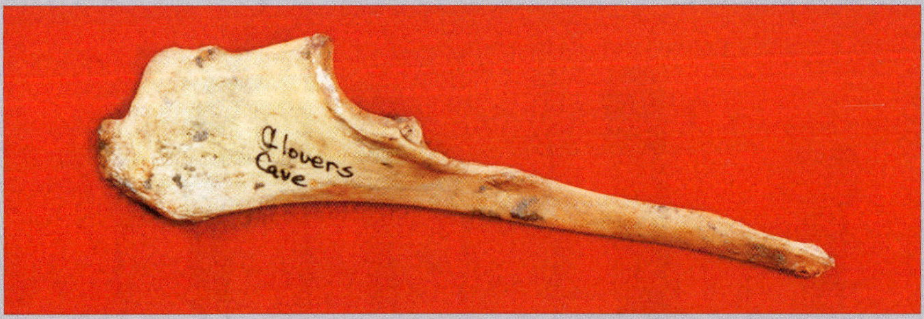

Hairpin(?), worked bone, Late Archaic to Woodland times, 6" long. It is ex-collection Vietzen, from Christian County, Kentucky. Pete Timoch collection. Unlisted.

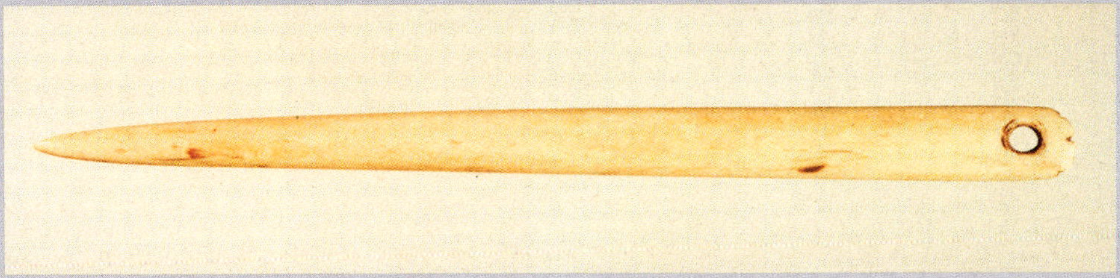

Hairpin, highly polished overall, bird bone with very thin walls. It is 4½" long and has a worn basal hole that might have held a tassle or other decoration. There are three tally marks or narrow notches at the wide end. Hocking County, Ohio. Lar Hothem collection. **$150.00.**

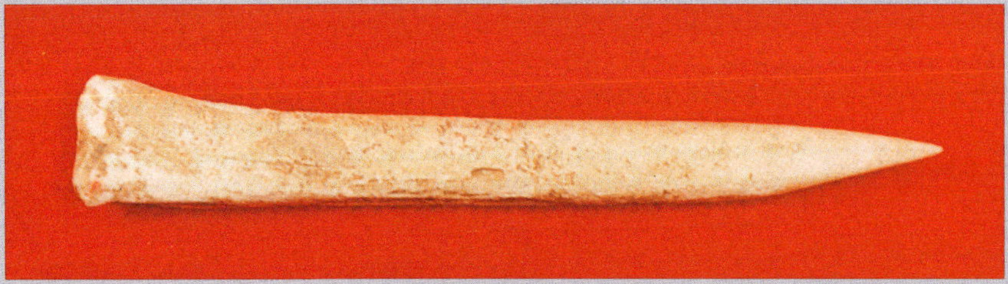

Hairpin, split animal leg bone, 4¹¹⁄₁₆". Woodland period, the bone has become chalky with age. It was ground flat on the sides and is so well-worked it is probably not just an awl. Ex-collection Vietzen, it was found in Ohio. Pete Timoch collection. **$100.00.**

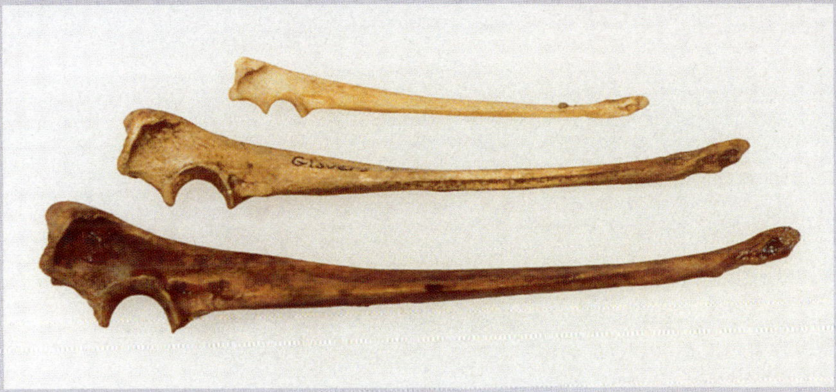

Hairpins, Late Archaic to Woodland, longest is 7¾". All are ulna bones, probably from deer, with the original animals' different ages and sizes. The left or largest portion of the ulna was often made into trigger awls. Once collected by Col. Vietzen, they are from Christian County, Kentucky. Pete Timoch collection. Unlisted.

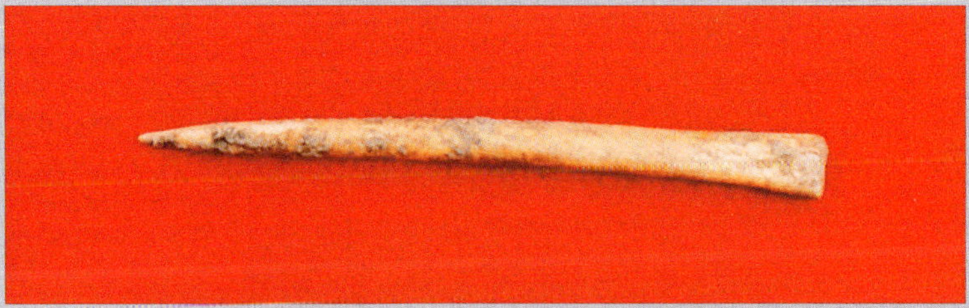

Bone hairpin, Woodland or Mississippian, 3⅛". Tapered full-length and slightly curved, it is from the well-known Vietzen collection. Ohio-Kentucky region. Pete Timoch collection. **$100.00 – 150.00.**

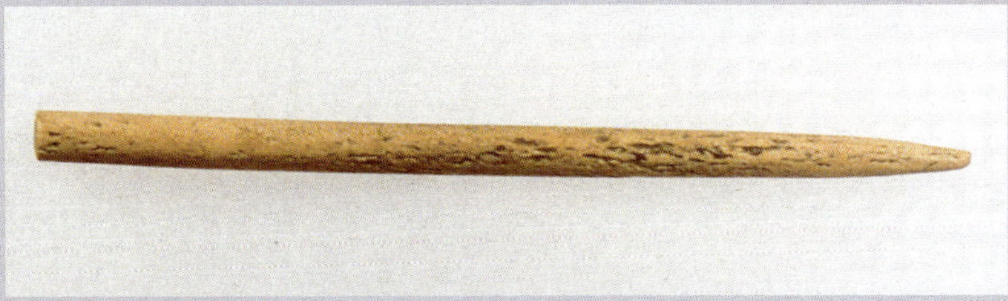

Bone hairpin, pencil-like profile, 3½" long. Well-shaped and finished, Col. Vietzen owned it. Ohio-Kentucky region. Pete Timoch collection. **$100.00 – 150.00.**

Hairpins

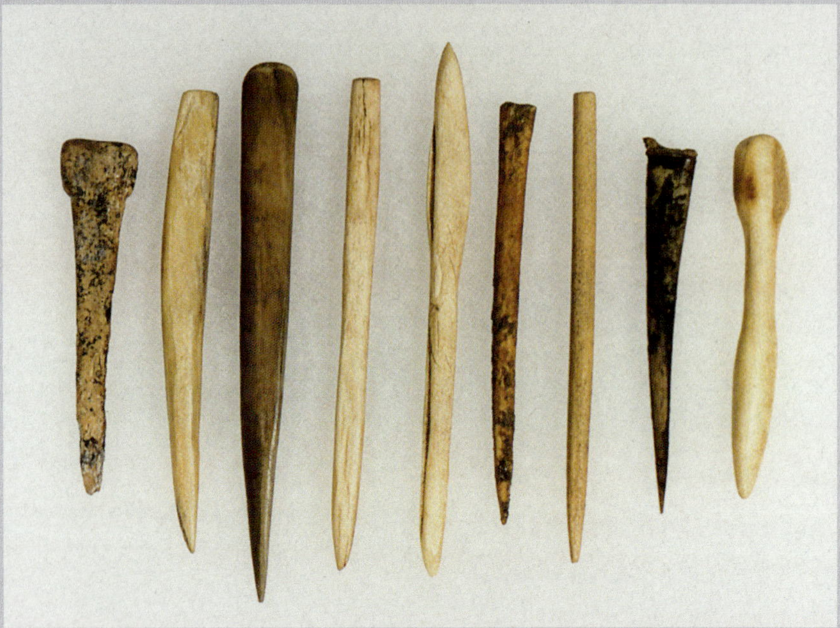

Bone hairpin group, longest is 4", individual specimens are shown elsewhere in this book. All are ex-collection Vietzen, from sites in Ohio and Kentucky. Pete Timoch collection.

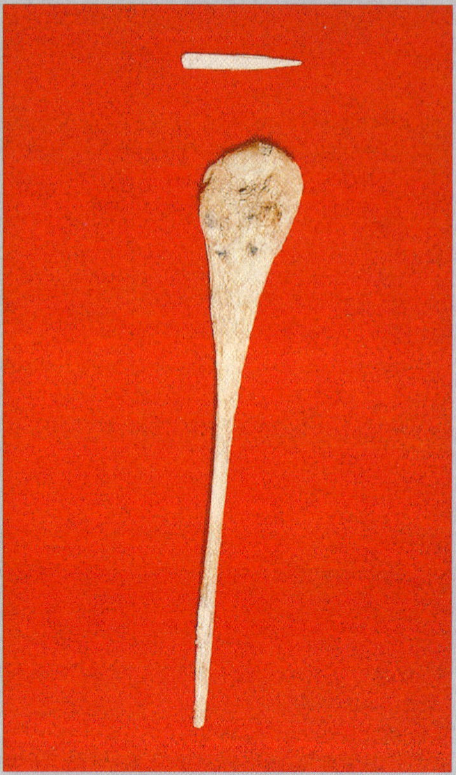

Bone hairpin and awl, Mississippian period, ca. AD 1200 – 1550. The awl is 1¼" long and the hairpin is 6½" long. Southwestern Iowa. Richard Krueger collection, Iowa. Sandra Krueger photograph. Awl, **$10.00;** hairpin, **$125.00.**

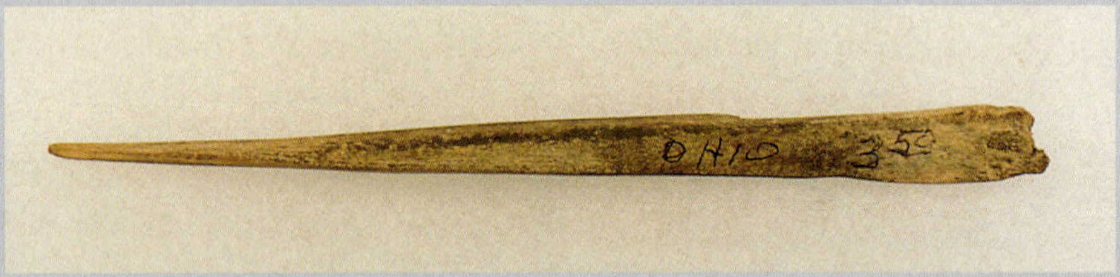

Hairpin or large needle awl, 5¾", split animal bone, Woodland period. The head is flattened while the remainder is triangular in cross-section. From the Vietzen collection, it was found in Ohio. Pete Timoch collection. **$75.00.**

Awl, bird bone, 5⅞" long. This fragile piece has survived undamaged, and was found in Lawrence County, Ohio. Fred Winegardner collection. **$45.00.**

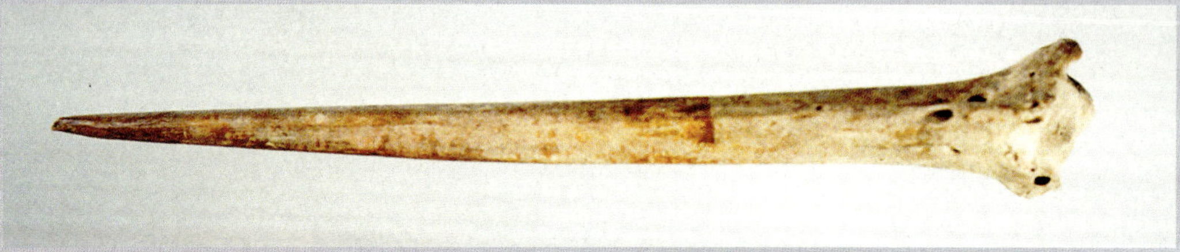

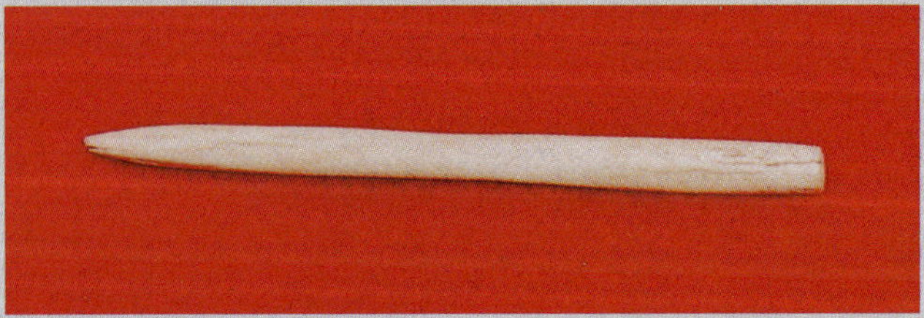

Bone hairpin, Woodland to Mississippian in time, slender shape and slightly constricted near the middle, 3⅝". Highly smoothed and polished, the example has an ivory-like finish. Once in the Vietzen collection, it is from the Ohio-Kentucky region. Pete Timoch collection. **$100.00 – 150.00**.

Awl or hairpin, polished bone, 4⁵⁄₁₆", well-shaped and nicely finished. It was found in the Midwest. Don Casto collection. **$50.00.**

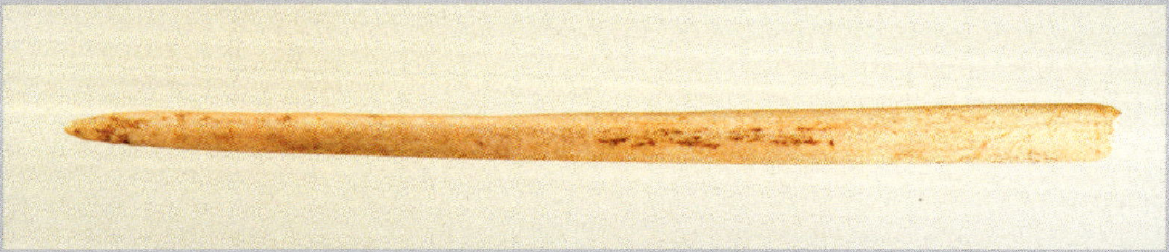

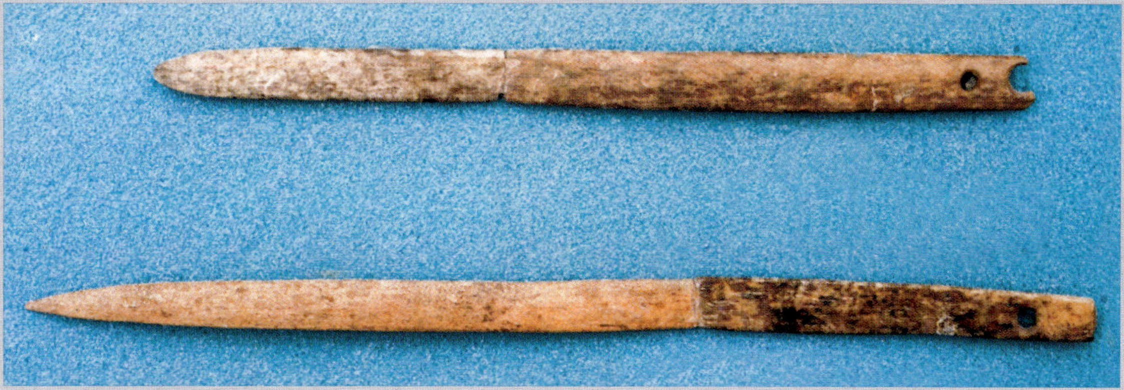

Needles or hairpins, drilled eyes, smaller example broken and glued. Made of animal bone, these Woodland or Mississippian pieces are ex-collection Snyder. The top needle is 5/16 x 5⅜" and the bottom needle is 5/16 x 6⅛". Both are only 1/16" thick. Snyder found them between 1947 and 1958 in Polk County, Tennessee. Collection of, and photograph by, Gary Henry, North Carolina. Small, **$100.00;** large, **$150.00.**

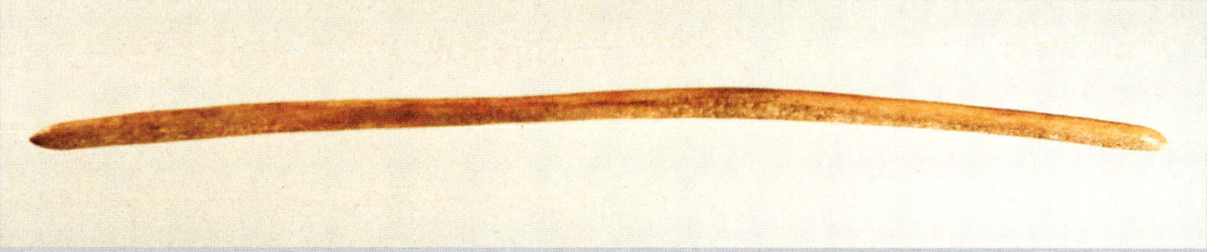

Hairpin, double-tipped, 6¾" long. Polished bone, this is a delicate but durable piece that luckily survived in fine condition. Midwestern. Don Casto collection. **$75.00.**

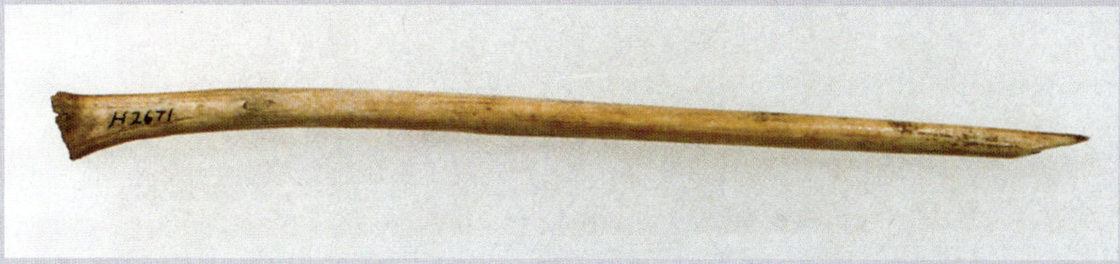

Hairpin, Mississippian period, deer lower leg bone, 7⅜" long. Well-made, this piece also has narrow incised lines from the base to the tip. Ex-collection Hovan, the hairpin was found at a Fort Ancient site. Southern Ohio. Private collection. **$200.00.**

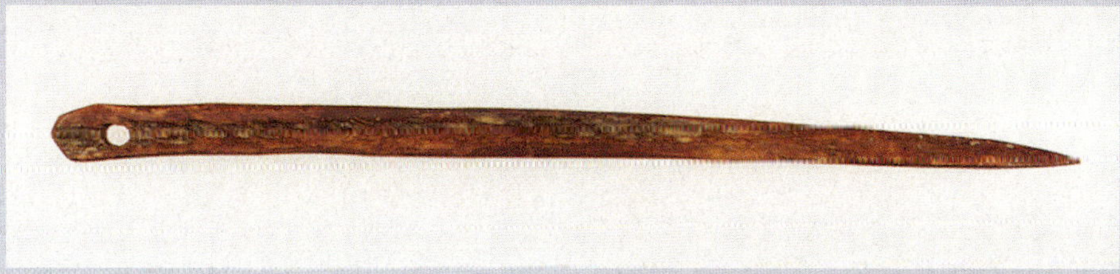

Needle or hairpin, probably split deer bone, Woodland period, 6½" long. The artifact is from eastern Tennessee. Pete Timoch collection. **$150.00.**

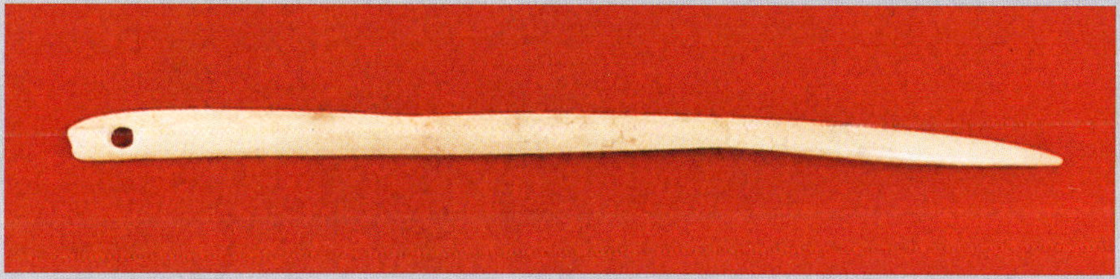

Needle, Woodland period, 4⅞", polished split bird bone. It is quite thin and has a glossy surface sheen. Hocking County, Ohio. Private collection. **$75.00.**

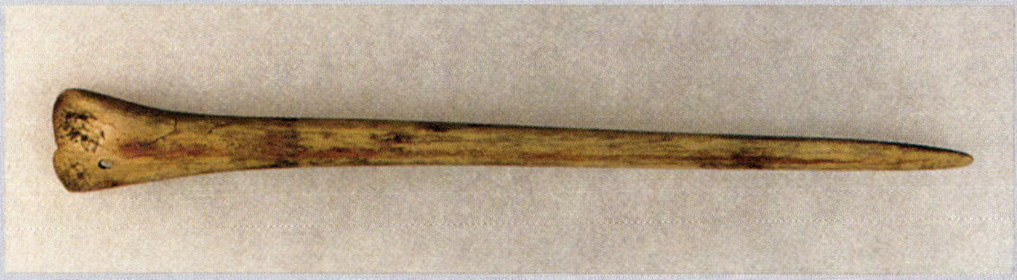

Hairpin, Late Woodland, 6⅞". Probably made from a deer leg bone, the small hole is natural to the bone and the wide end has been ground into a wedge shape. Well-polished overall, this is an outstanding piece. Eastern Tennessee – North Carolina region. Pete Timoch collection. Museum grade.

Hairpins

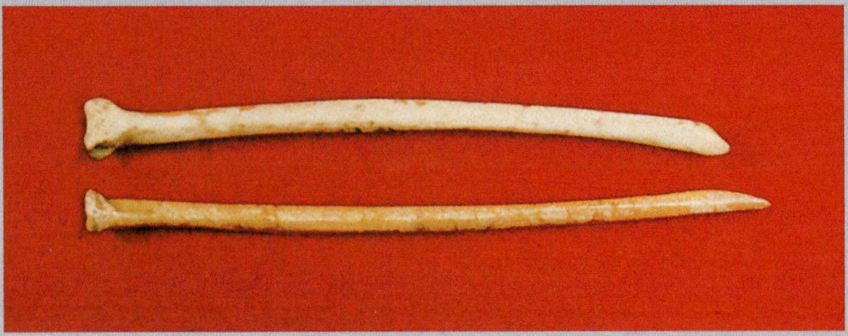

Awls or hairpins, bird bones, Late Archaic to Woodland, bottom example is 5" long. These are made from large birds, possibly the swan or wild turkey. They are from the Vietzen collection, and the shorter example is pictured in the 1956 book, *The Saga of Glover's Cave*, page 230. Christian County, Kentucky. Pete Timoch collection. Each, **$100.00.**

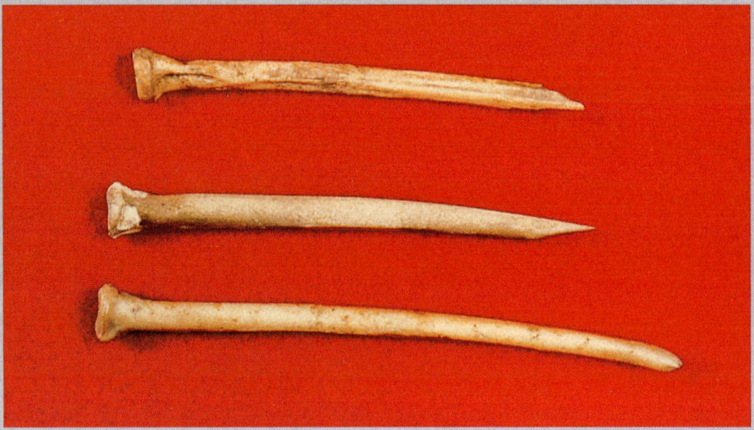

Awls or hairpins, bird bones, Late Archaic to Woodland. The bottom example is 4³⁄₁₆" long. Such thin-walled and dense bones, as here, often have high polish. Ex-collection Vietzen, the top and bottom specimens are pictured in his 1956 book, *The Saga of Glover's Cave*, page 230. Christian County, Kentucky. Pete Timoch collection. Each, **$50.00 – 100.00.**

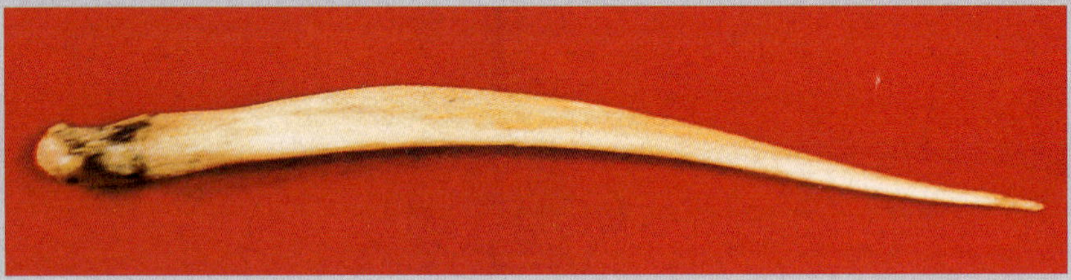

Hairpin, Late Woodland, 7¼". Made from the penis bone of a large animal, probably a bear, it is ex-collection Vietzen. He wrote that the use of such bone was common enough in the area where found, though the majority of hairpins were made from deer leg bones. Eastern Tennessee – North Carolina region. Pete Timoch collection. Museum grade.

Awl, historic Oto-Missouri, bone, 6⅛" long. The shaft is polished on this large awl which was found in eastern Nebraska. Richard Krueger collection, Iowa. Sandra Krueger photograph. **$150.00 – 175.00.**

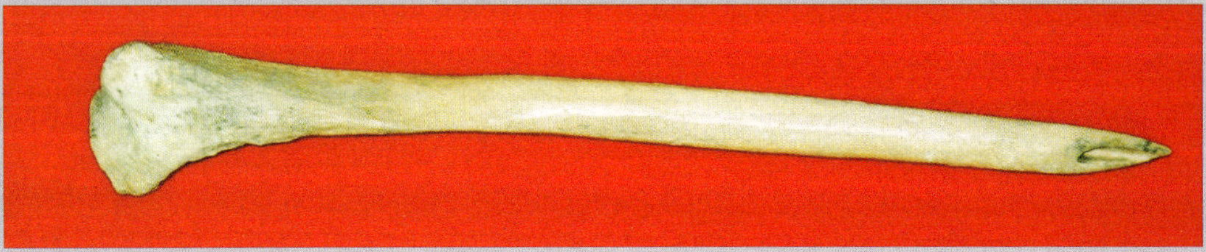

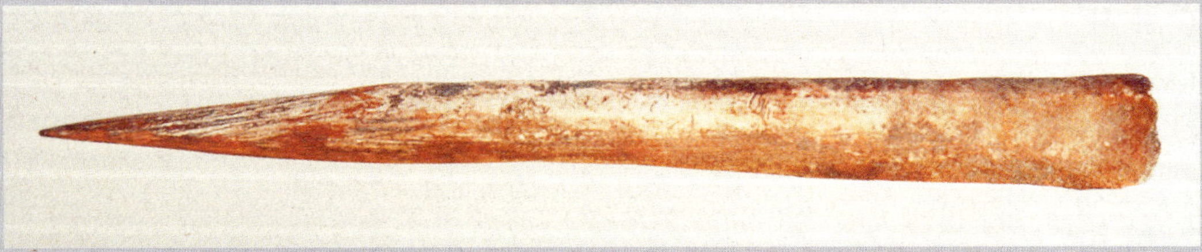

Hairpin or awl, bird bone, 5¼". The artifact, with very thin walls, was found in the eastern Midwest. Fred Winegardner collection. **$45.00.**

Hairpin or awl, polished bone splinter, 4⅝". This has a graceful simplicity of form that would be difficult to match. Eastern Midwest. Fred Winegardner collection. **$65.00.**

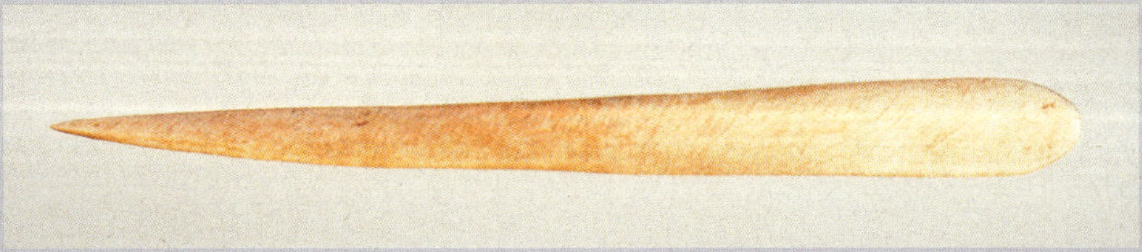

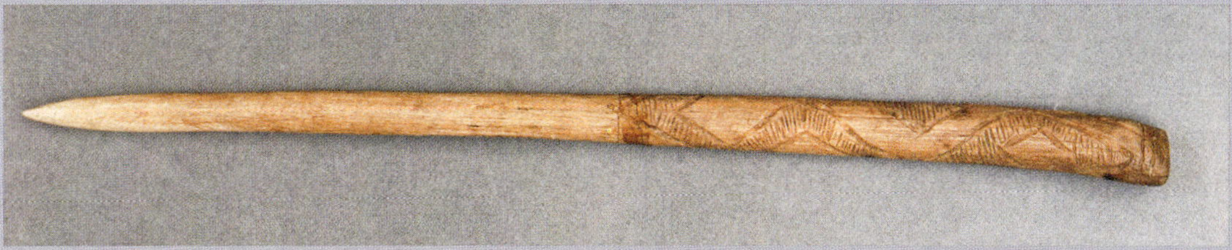

Hairpin, incised design, 6⅛" long. Late Archaic, ca. 1550 BC, it was found at Stallings Island, Georgia. H. B. Greene II collection, Naples, Florida. Museum grade.

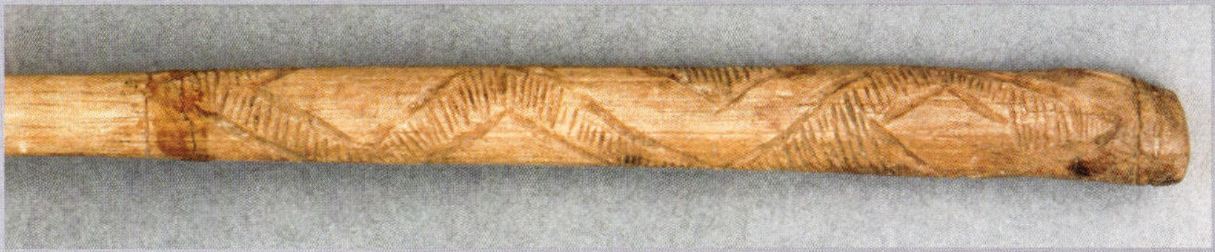

Hairpin, closeup of incised artwork, overall length is 6⅛". The design is similar to that on some ceramics of the period. Stallings Island, Georgia. H. B. Greene II collection, Naples, Florida. Museum grade.

Hairpin, polished bone, "railroad spike" type, 7⅞" long. Well-carved and in fine condition, it is ex-collection Perino. Location unlisted. Earthworks Artifacts. **$1,000.00.**

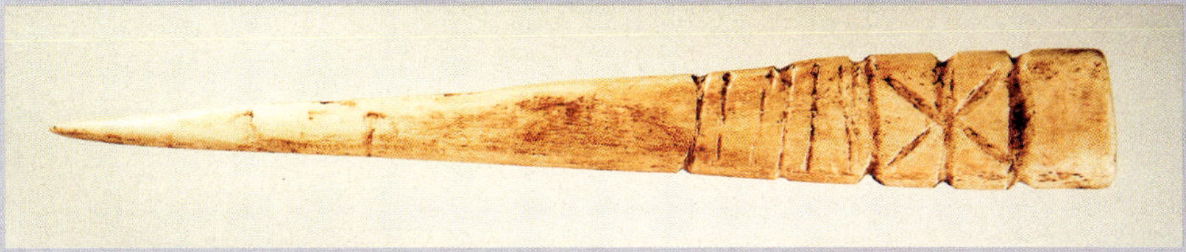

Decorative hairpin, carved line designs, 8⅜" long. It is made from a rib bone and came from Alaska. Robin Fiser collection. **$100.00.**

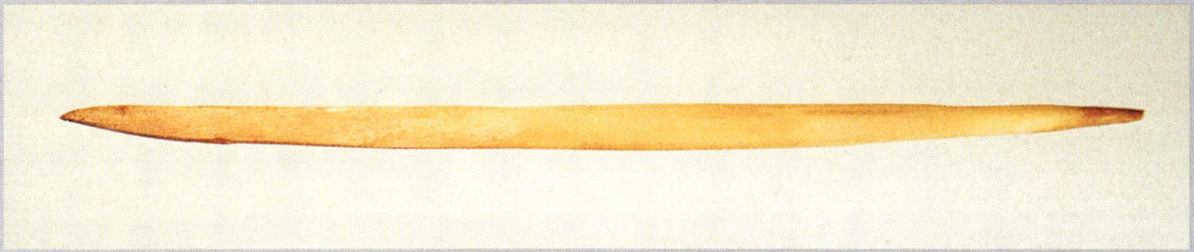

Double-tipped awl or pin, animal bone, 6½" long. This artifact came from Limestone County, Alabama. Robin Fiser collection. **$55.00.**

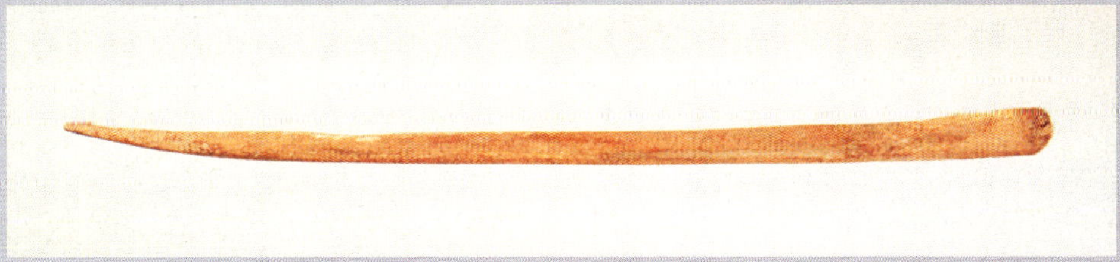

Awl or hairpin, 6¹⁄₃₂" long, slender animal bone. It was found in Limestone County, Alabama. Robin Fiser collection. **$60.00.**

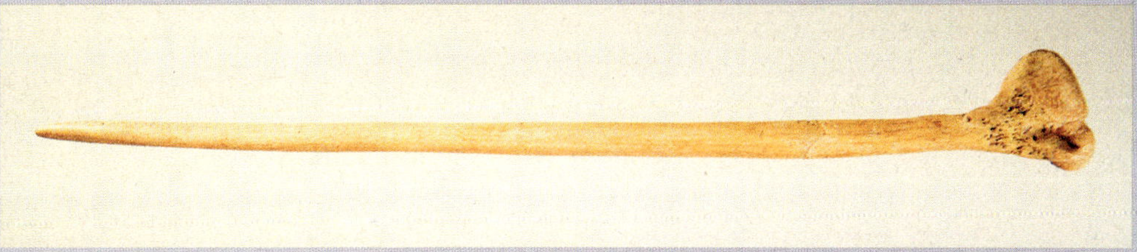

Hairpin, narrow tapered shaft, large animal bone. It is 7½" long and was found in Hamilton County, Ohio. Robin Fiser collection. **$125.00.**

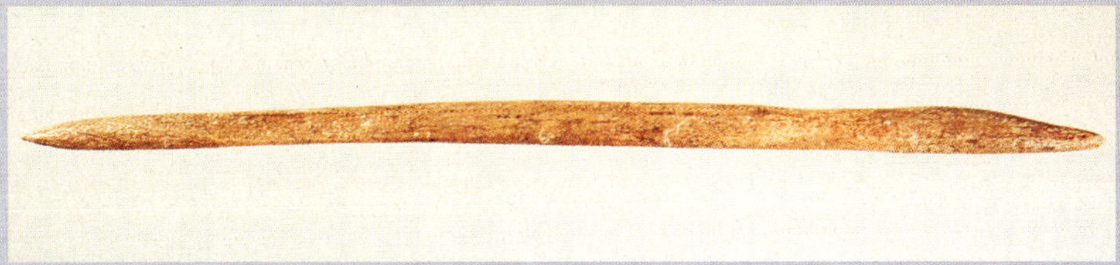

Bone pin, bipointed, brown patina. This example is 5½" long and was found near Augusta, Kentucky. Robin Fiser collection. **$45.00.**

Hairpins

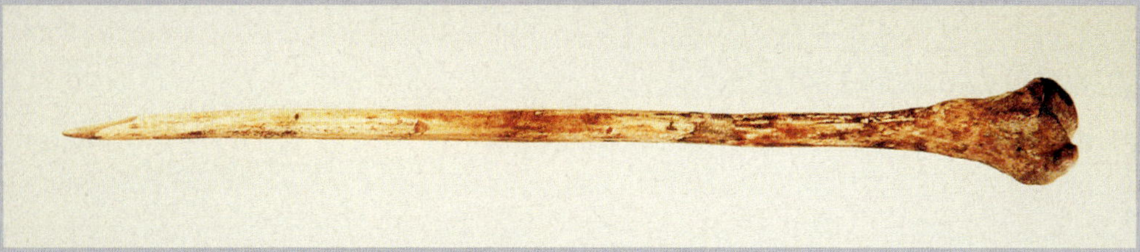

Hairpin, probably Mississippian, polished and patinated shaft. This pin is 8" long and came from Mason County, Kentucky. Robin Fiser collection. **$85.00.**

Hairpin, red ochre coating, bird bone. This long (8") example came from Union County, Kentucky. Robin Fiser collection. **$90.00.**

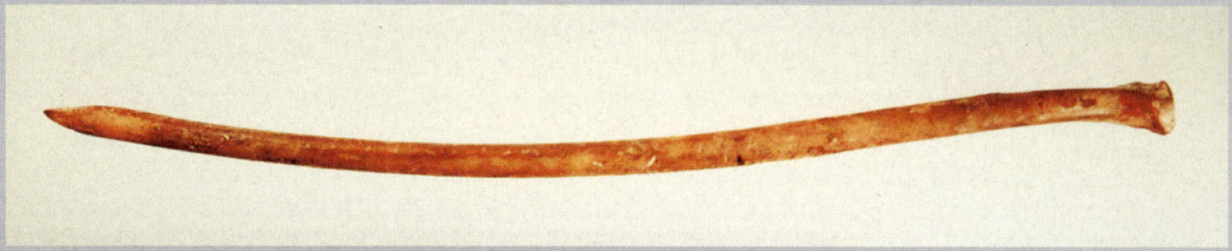

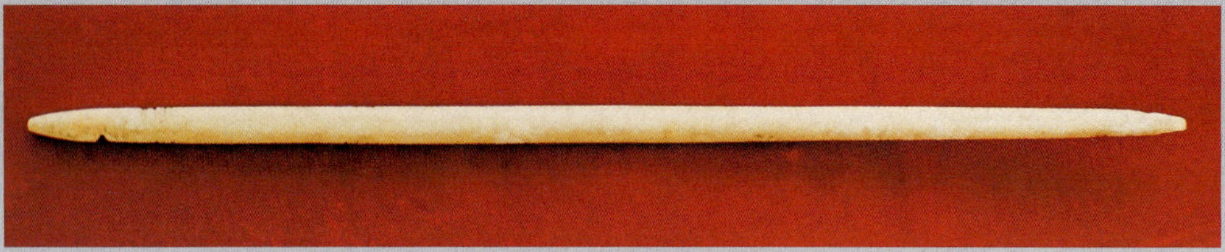

Hairpin, found with seven bone needles or pins, hairpin is 7¼" long. This is a fine example, from Brown County, Illinois. Tim Liehr collection, Illinois. **$300.00.**

Needle, 3½" long, polished, very thin, Mississippian period. One of the finest examples to come from the state, it was found in southern Ohio. Fred Winegardner collection. **$150.00.**

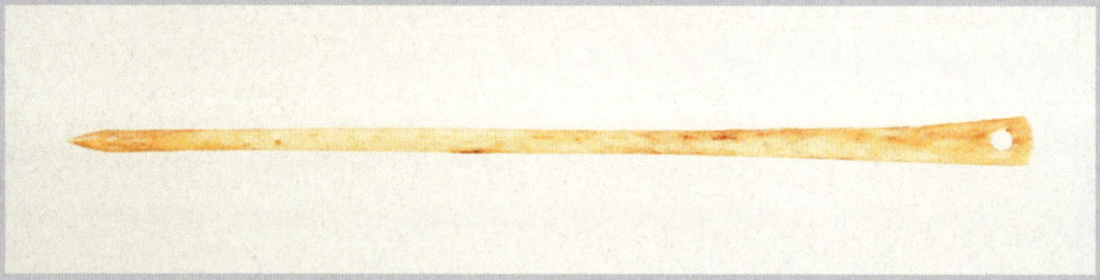

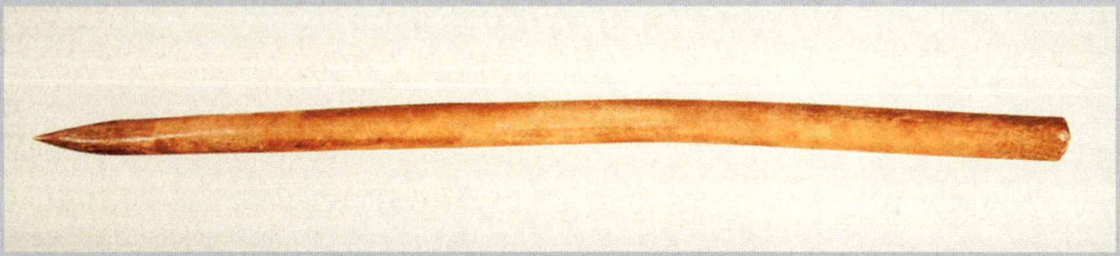

Hairpin, Mississippian (Fort Ancient), 6⅛" long. Polished full-length, it is 6⅛" long and came from southern Ohio. Fred Winegardner collection. **$150.00.**

Hairpin, Mississippian period, 5⅝" long. This decorated pin has seven incised lines that encircle the shaft. Scioto County, Ohio. Fred Winegardner collection. **$200.00.**

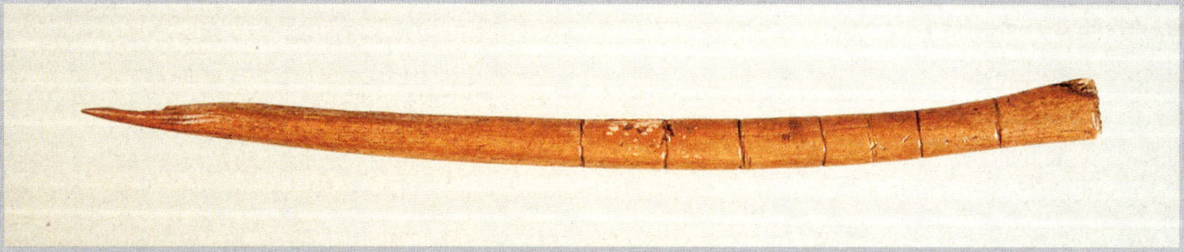

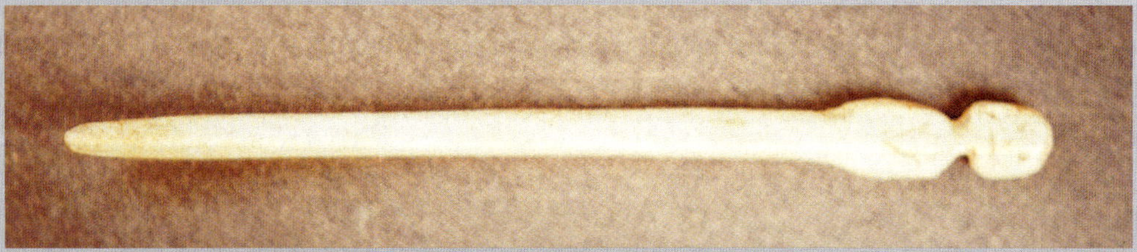

Bone hairpin, human effigy form, 6¼" long. The pin, found in 1980, is from Marion County, Tennessee. Back to Earth. **$375.00.**

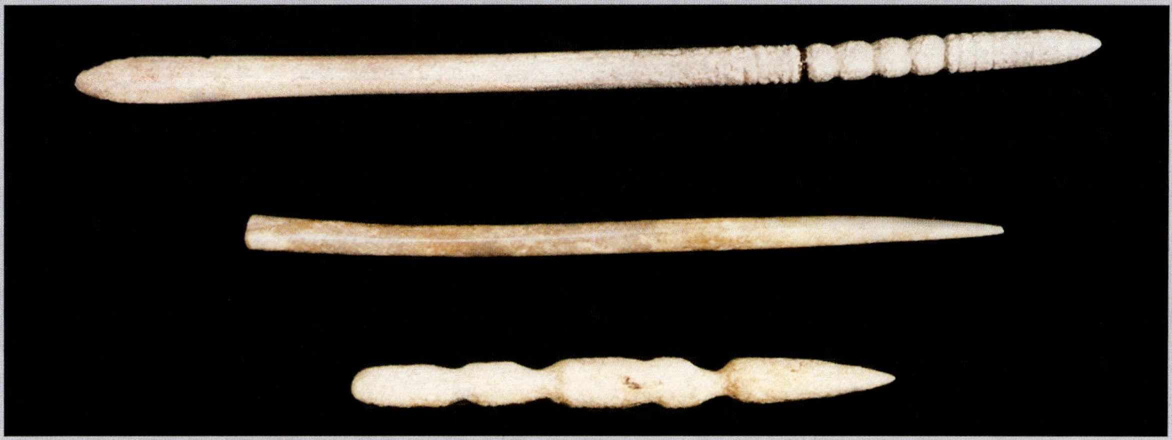

Artifacts, bone and antler, top example broken and glued, concentric carving and etching. It is made from a deer fibula, is 22 cm long, and probably came from Ohio. Center, hairpin or awl, made from a deer fibula. Bottom, antler awl, with finger grips carved into the shaft. It was found in Ontario, Canada. Private collection. Top, **$300.00;** center, **$125.00;** bottom, **$150.00.**

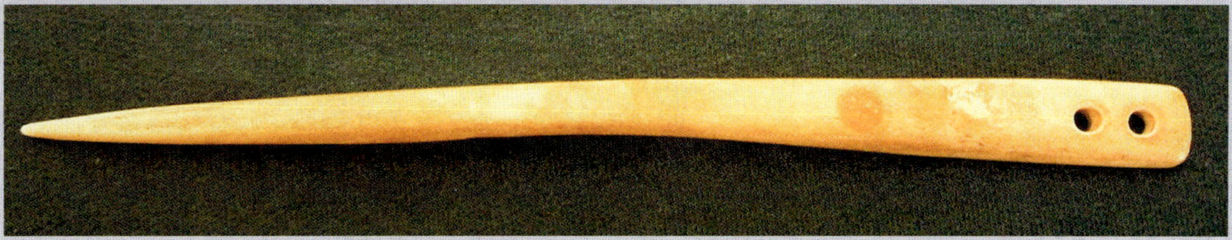

Hairpin or large awl with eyes, heavy animal bone splinter, 6⅝" long. This fine piece came from Osage County, Missouri. Rod Fuller collection, Nebraska. **$200.00.**

Hairpin or very ornate awl, carved and incised with tally marks, fire-darkened in places and highly polished, 4³⁄₁₆" long. Ex-collection Tolliver, Hocking County, Ohio. Private collection. Museum grade.

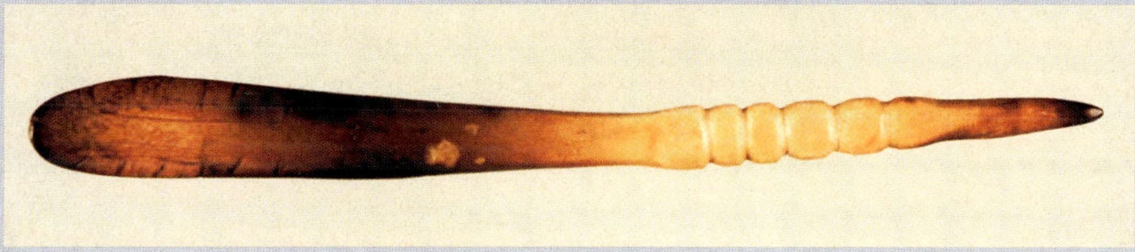

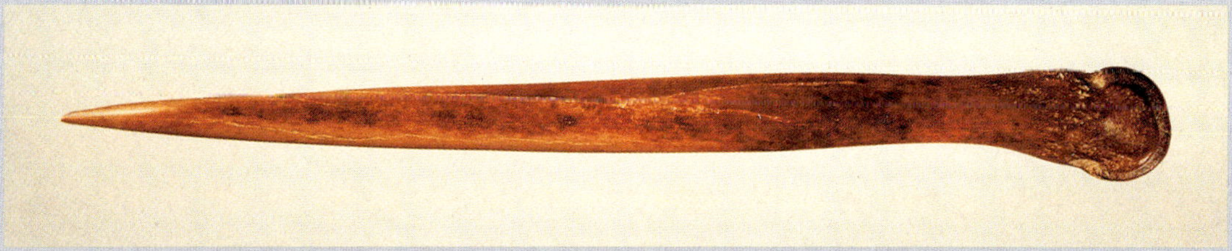

Narrow dagger or wide hairpin, patinated and highly polished animal bone, 7⅜" long. It is flat on the reverse face and is overall a very fine artifact. Ex-collection Tolliver, Hocking County, Ohio. Private collection. **$450.00.**

Hairpin, thin bone, 7⅛" long, polished near tip. This pin is quite delicate and well-made. Ex-collection Selb, West Virginia. Doug Hooks collection. **$350.00.**

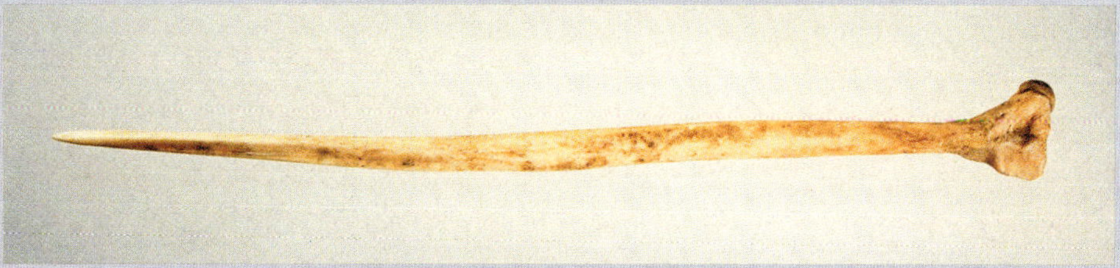

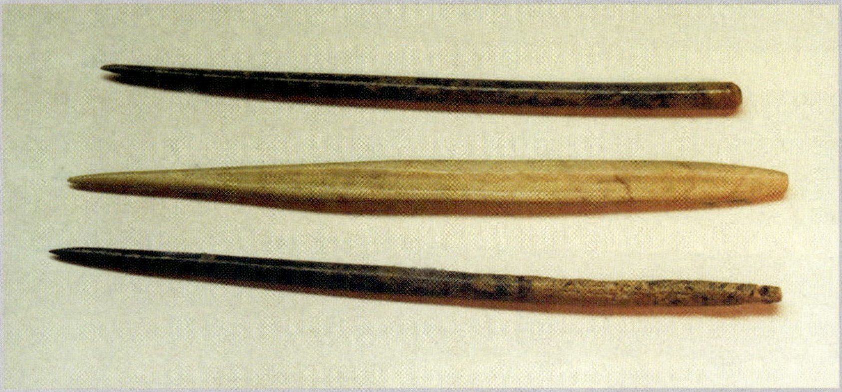

Bone hairpins, longest is 6". One has a grooved end and all are delicate and well-shaped. Fulton County, Illinois. Fred Smith collection, Illinois. Each, **$100.00 – 150.00.**

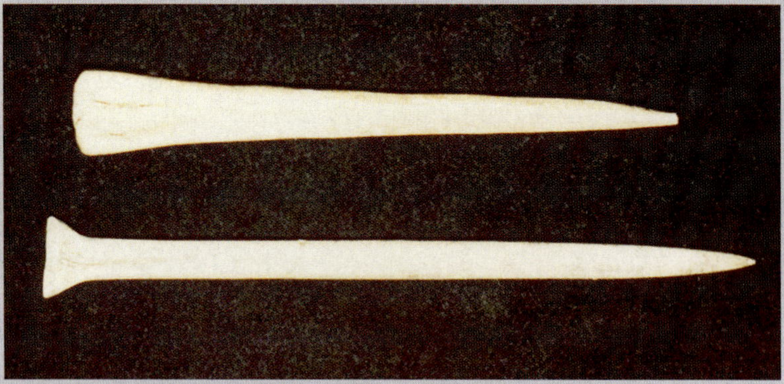

Hairpins, top example 6¼" and bottom example with flared head 8½" long. These are well-made and in fine condition. Northwestern Arkansas. Kenneth Hamilton collection, Arkansas. Top, **$150.00;** bottom, **$300.00.**

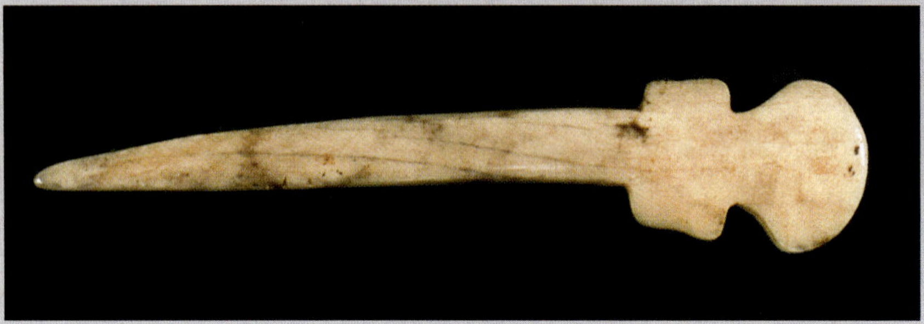

Hairpin, Woodland period, deer leg bone, ¾" wide at base and nearly 4" long. Well-designed and highly polished, the shaft is slightly curved. This piece was pictured in *Central States Archaeological Journal*, Vol. 7 No. 2, April 1960, p 75. St. Clair County, Illinois. Tracy Spradlin collection, Illinois. Tony Clinton photograph. Museum grade.

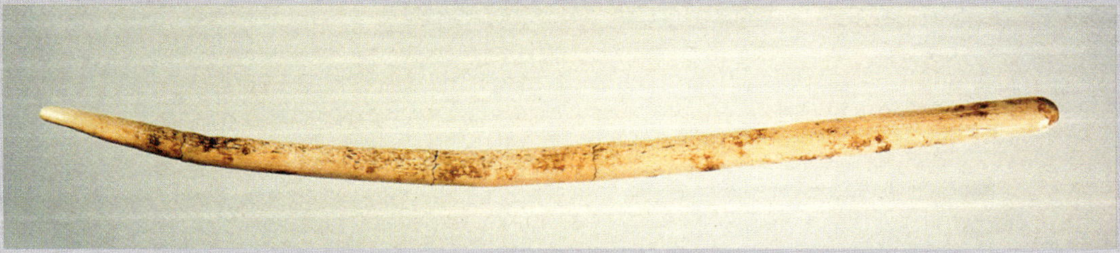

Hairpin, broken in three places and glued, 8⅛" long. Made of animal bone, this is an exceptional specimen in both size and workmanship. West Virginia. Doug Hooks collection. Unlisted.

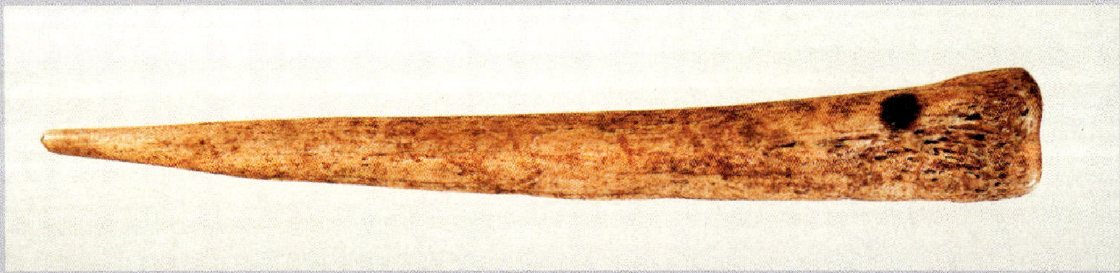

Bone awl or hairpin, polished overall, 4" long. The small black spot is a fire mark. The artifact was found in a rock shelter. Southern Tennessee. Private collection. **$25.00.**

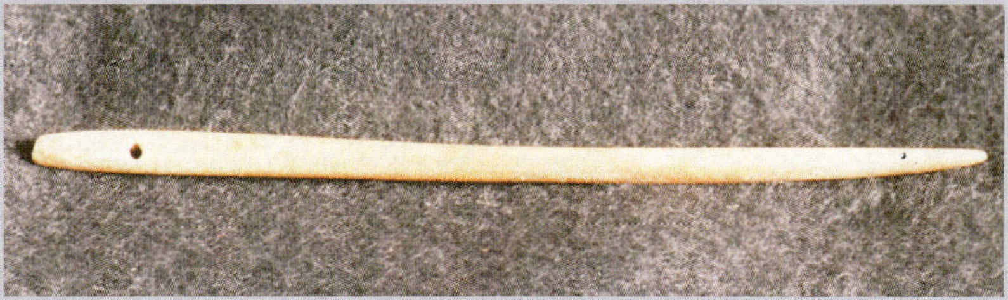

Bone needle or hairpin, $5\frac{1}{16}$" long, ex-collection Liehr. It has high overall polish and was found in Spencer County, Indiana. John F. Wubker collection, Illinois. **$200.00.**

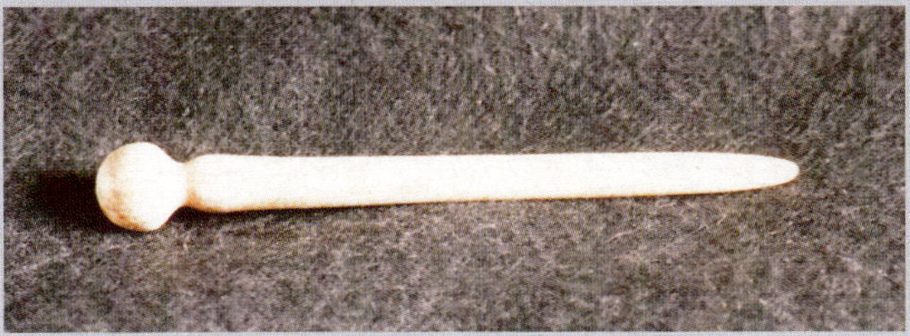

Shell hairpin, finely shaped and finished, $3\frac{5}{16}$" long. It has a knobbed head-like end and tapered shaft. Find-site unknown. John F. Wubker collection, Illinois. **$275.00.**

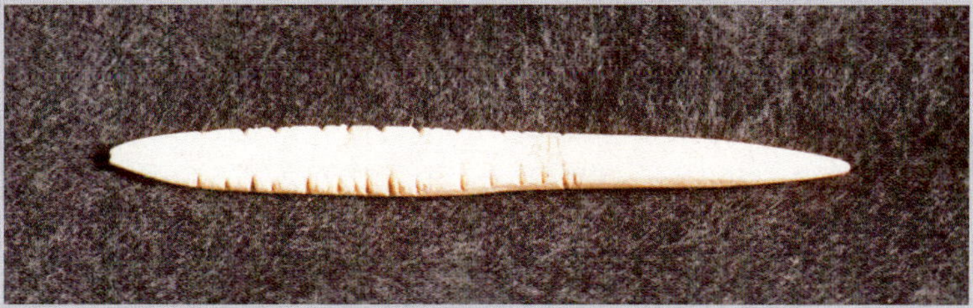

Bone hairpin, with tally marks on both sides, $3\frac{15}{16}$" long. This is an unusual artifact, decorated and polished. Brown County, Illinois. John F. Wubker collection, Illinois. **$275.00.**

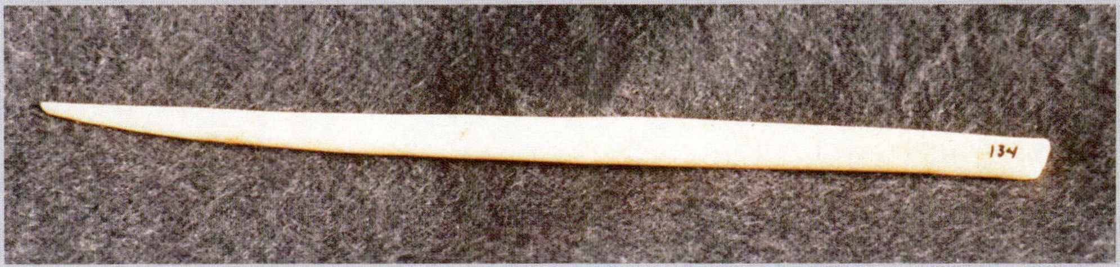

Hairpin, good polish, nicely tapered, $5\frac{3}{4}$" long. This pin is likely from the Midwest. John F. Wubker collection, Illinois. **$100.00.**

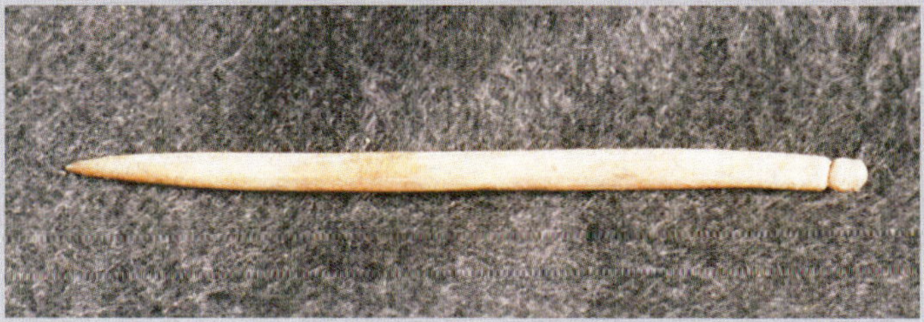

Hairpin or needle, $3\frac{1}{2}$" long, narrow groove at the thick end. It has good overall polish and is probably Midwestern. John F. Wubker collection, Illinois. **$75.00.**

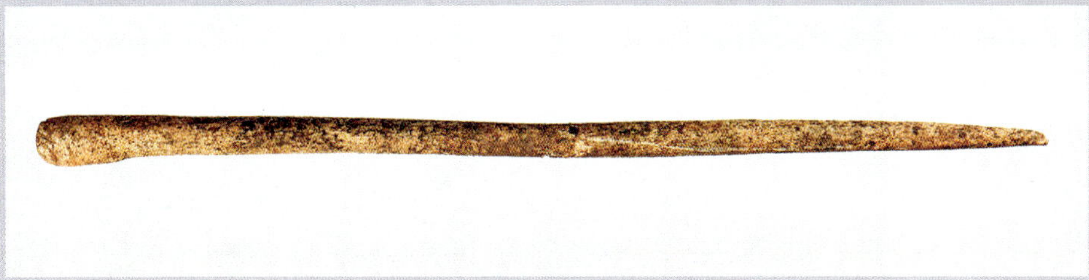

Hairpin, broken and glued, thin and delicate. It is $5\frac{1}{2}$" long, well-worked and polished. Unbroken, it would be in the **$150.00** range. Southern Tennessee. Private collection. **$30.00 – 40.00.**

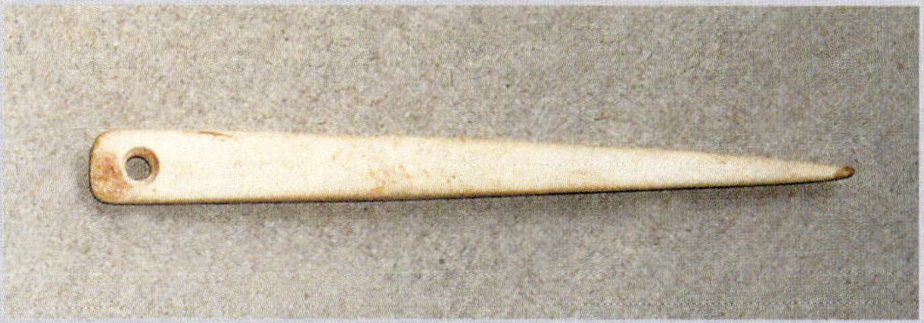

Bone hairpin or well-made needle, 5" long, highly polished. Found in Union County, Illinois. Wilfred Dick collection, Mississippi. **$200.00.**

Effigies

Many small figures (figurines) were made that represent either the entire form or body parts of humans, animals, and birds. While materials were often stone and slate, some effigies were also made with organic materials. Sometimes the figures were naturalistic and sometimes they were so stylized it is difficult to be certain what they represent. Most effigies of any kind seem to belong mainly to the Woodland and Mississippian periods, ca. 1000 BC – AD 1500.

Effigies in antler, bone, and shell can be placed in two groups. One is effigy-only, meaning the figurine is simply a small representation of a living thing and it exists by itself and is complete. Examples in bone from the Northeast often portray men or women or human heads. The other group combines an effigy with an artifact; the effigy portion is part of the whole. A good example would be the pre-Iroquois combs already mentioned, which have effigy handles. These often depict animals and birds, but humans are represented as well.

Shell was also used for effigies, and representations of fish were sometimes made. The effigy gorgets of the southern U. S. are well known, and almost any living thing might be incised on, or carved in, the shell. These of course would be in the second effigy group, and are part of the artifact.

There has long been speculation about the purpose of effigies. Suggestions include their use in magic, decoration, religion, storytelling, and more. As with many artifacts from prehistoric America, they seem to be part of a greater mystery that may never be solved.

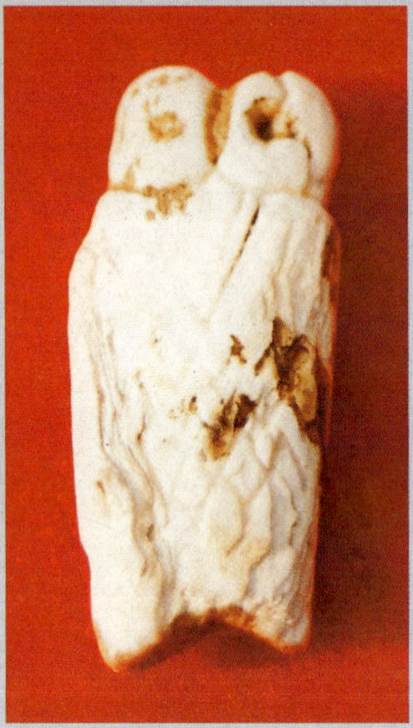

Owl effigy pendant, ⅝ x 1½", conch shell spine. Ex-collection Barron, this bird effigy was made by the Fort Ancient (Mississippian) people of late prehistoric times. Northern Kentucky. Douglas E. McIlwain collection. **$650.00.**

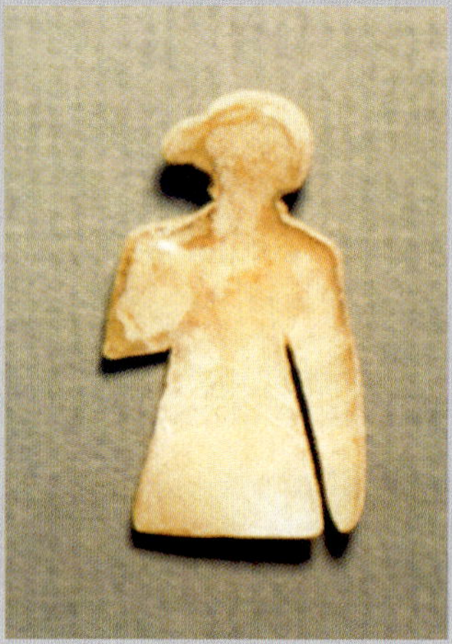

Thunderbird shell effigy, one wing missing, 1½" long. The chest area is incised on this example, ca. AD 1500 – 1750. Found in the 1950s, it came from west of Gettysburg, South Dakota. Private collection. **$250.00.**

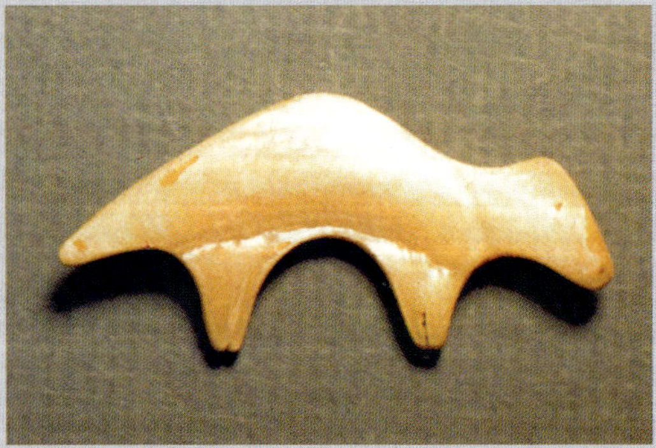

Bison or bear effigy, shell, perfect condition with incising that outlines the legs, nose and eyes. The effigy is 2" long, ca. AD 1500 – 1750. It was picked up near Chamberlain, South Dakota. Private collection. **$350.00.**

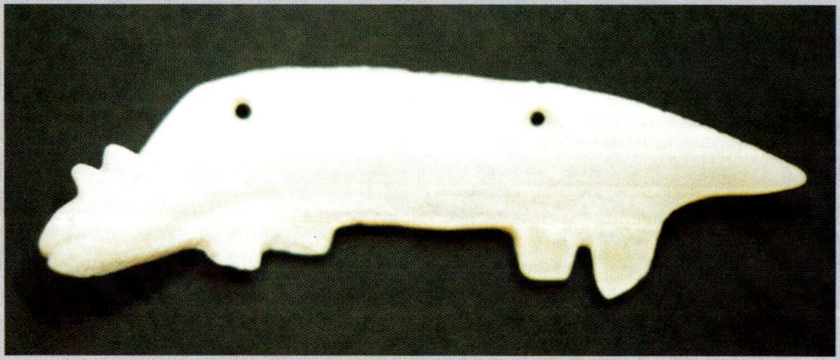

Bear effigy gorget, shell, 3¼" long. Nicely made and with small suspension holes, this historic piece came from near Chamberlain, South Dakota. Mike Fox collection, Iowa. **$550.00.**

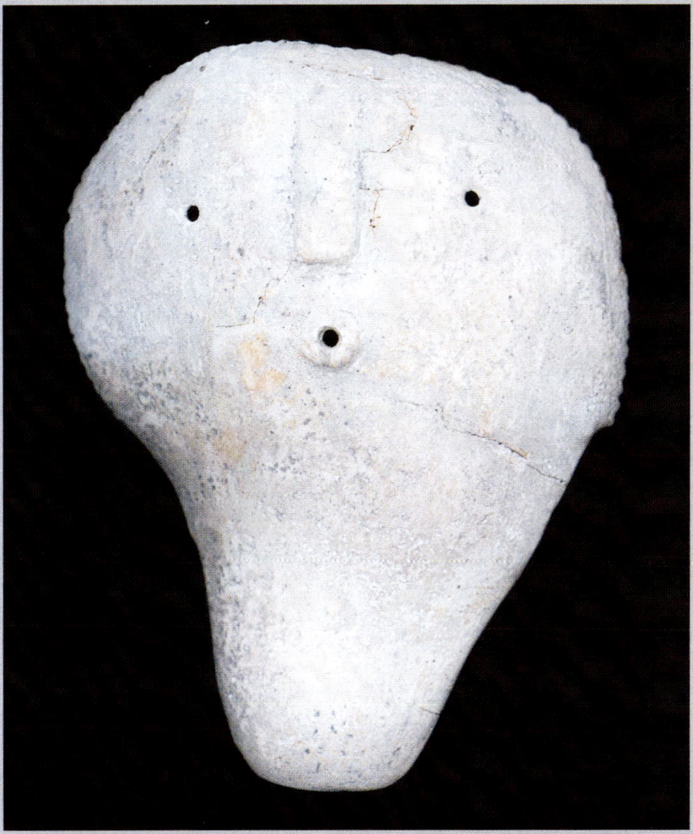

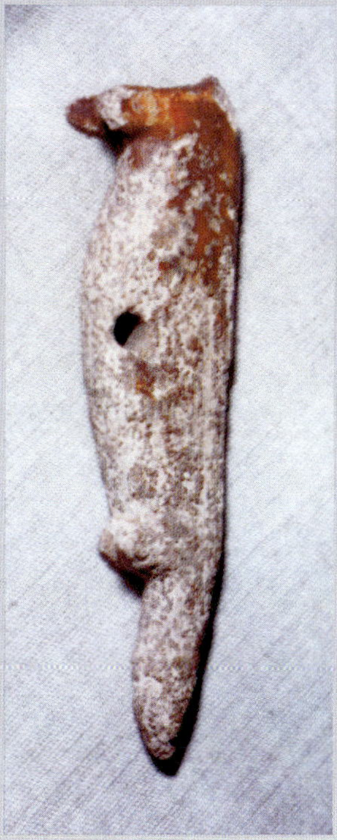

Bear effigy figure, Eskimo, a shaman's tool for curing. This piece is from the Dorset culture of northeastern Canada. The effigy is 4" long and was purchased in a Taos, New Mexico shop in 1989. J. Steve and Anita Shearer collection, California. **$1,000.00.**

Chicamauga style face mask gorget, 5 9/16 x 7 1/16". This large marine shell gorget came from an island in the Tennessee River. Marion County, Tennessee. Jim Maus collection, North Carolina. Museum grade.

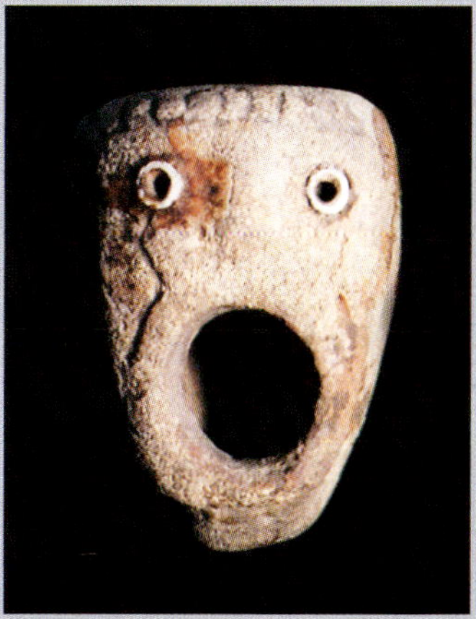

Weeping eye pipe, Fort Ancient (Mississipian), made of sandstone, 3 cm high. The eye inserts are made of drilled shell and are still in position, the nose is in bas relief, and hair and ears are detailed. It is probably Ohio River Valley. Private collection. Museum grade.

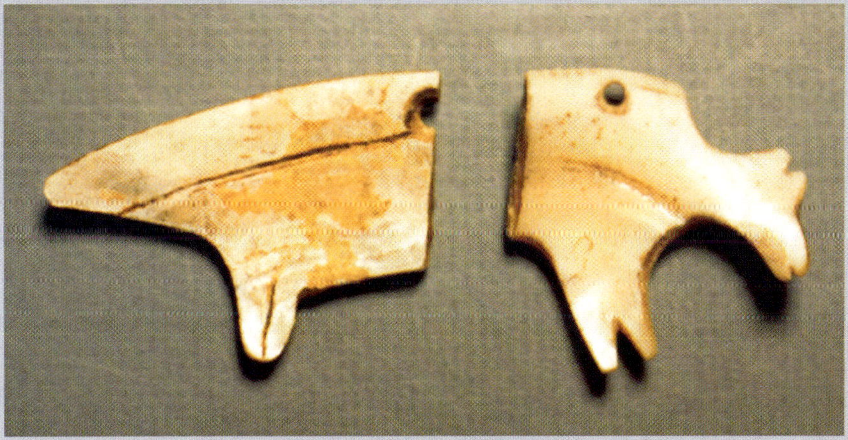

Animal effigy halves, each about 1¾" long. Made of shell, the front represents a bison with cut out and detailed ears, hoofs, and mouth. The other is the back end of an animal with incising at legs and tail. They are ca. AD 1500 – 1750, from the Chamberlain area, South Dakota. Private collection. Each, **$125.00.**

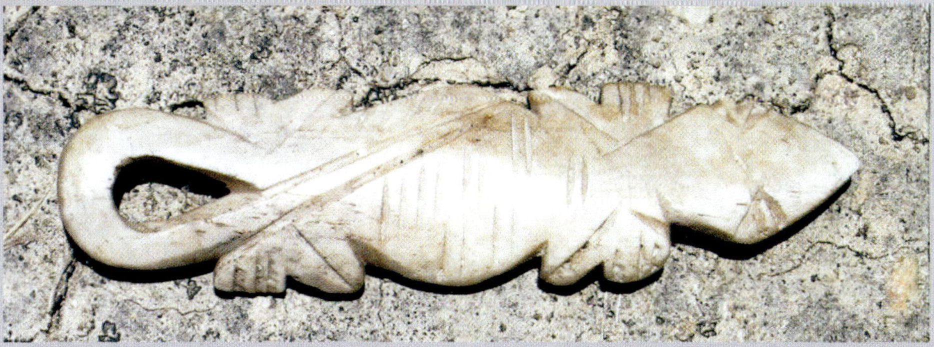

Bone effigy form, 2½" long. This interesting and well-done piece is from Alaska. John and Susan Mellyn collection, Texas. Museum grade.

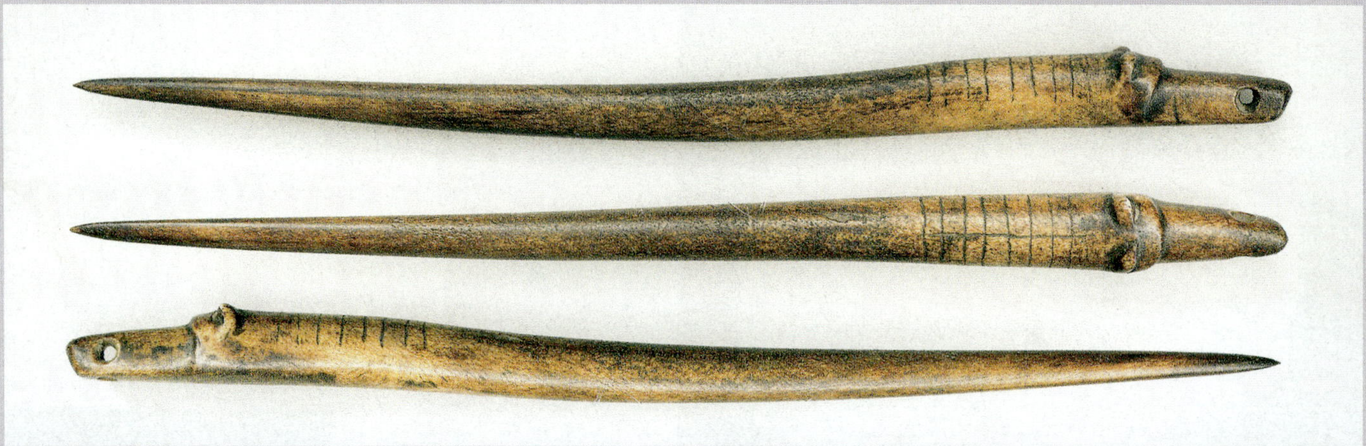

Effigy awl or hairpin – right side view, top view, left side view, bone, 7½" long. This is an exceptional piece in size, workmanship, and condition. It may be an Iroquois piece, from the AD 1700s, and the animal depicted may be a bear or wolf. Found in New York state. Ex-collection Channing. Kirk Spurr collection. Museum grade.

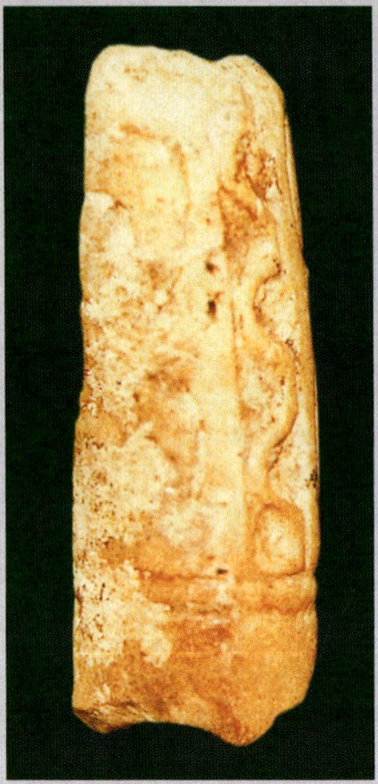

Carved bone with snake effigy on one side, part broken. Unusual, the artifact was found in northwestern Arkansas. Kenneth Hamilton collection, Arkansas. Unlisted.

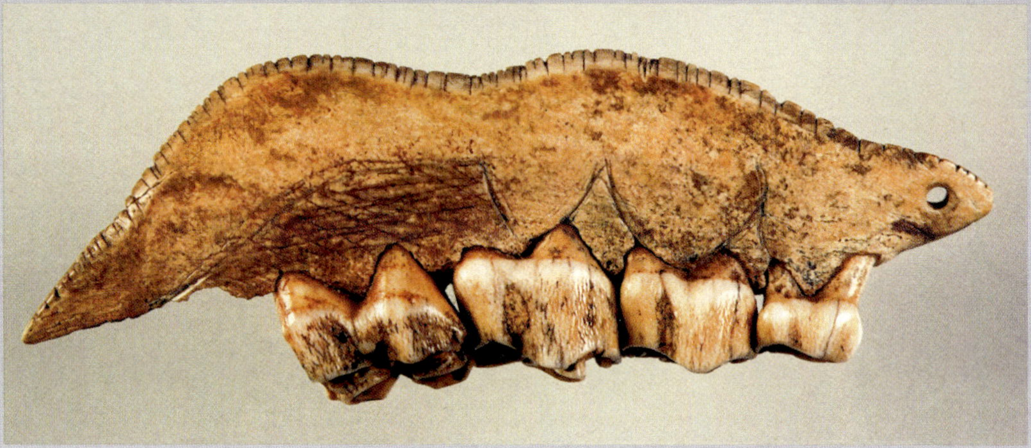

Otter(?) effigy, deer mandible, artifact is 5¹⁄₃₂" long. It is incised and tally-marked, and there is an eye/suspension hole at the right end. This piece is ex-collection Tolliver, from Hocking County, Ohio. Private collection. Museum grade.

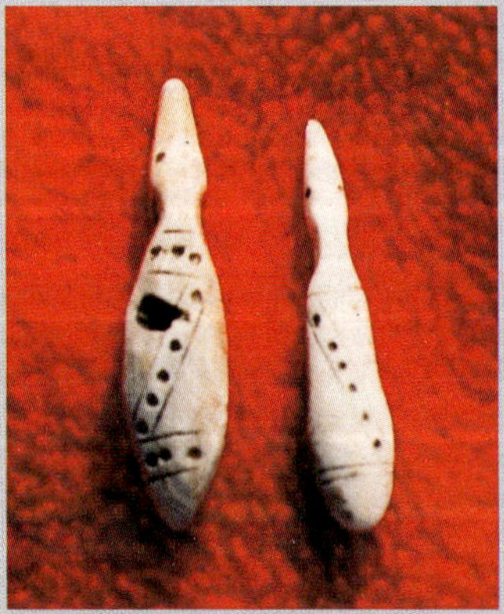

Duck effigies, shell, each about 1" long. They are ex-collections Cameron and Fogelman, and came from a Seneca-Iroquois site that dated ca. AD 1650 – 1670. Brandon Trivette collection, North Carolina. Museum grade.

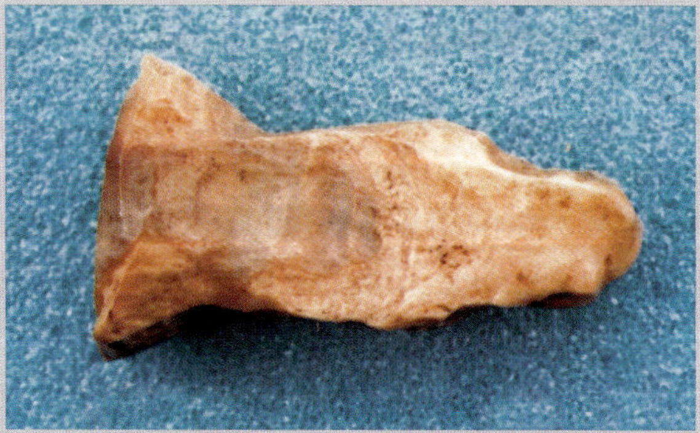

Carved effigy figure, prehistoric(?), ivory, ⅞ x 2³⁄₁₆". Formerly in the Cantrell collection, it is from Alaska. Collection of, and photograph by, Gary Henry, North Carolina. **$15.00.**

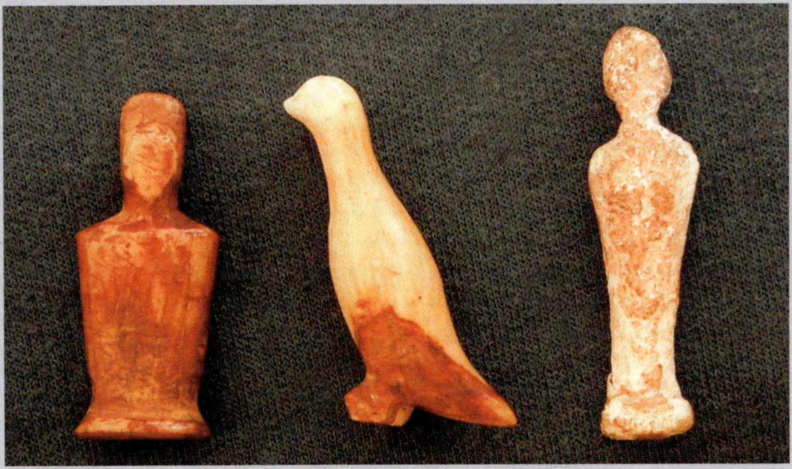

Fetishes or effigies, Eskimo, average heights is 1½". Left to right: Human, fossilized ivory; bird, fossilized ivory; human, bone. These came from Eek, Alaska. Rod Fuller collection, Nebraska. Each, **$75.00 – 125.00.**

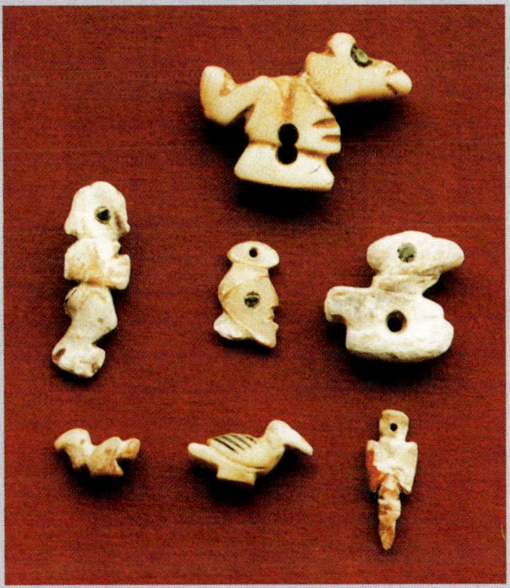

Chavin culture anthropomorphic fetish beads, mother-of-pearl material obtained by trade from coastal Ecuador, ca. 1200 – 500 BC. These are rare pieces of art from the Andean highlands and size range is ½ to 1½" long. The top example and all pieces in the center row have turquoise eyes. Peru. Dave Summers collection, Victor, New York. All, **$800.00 – 1,000.00.**

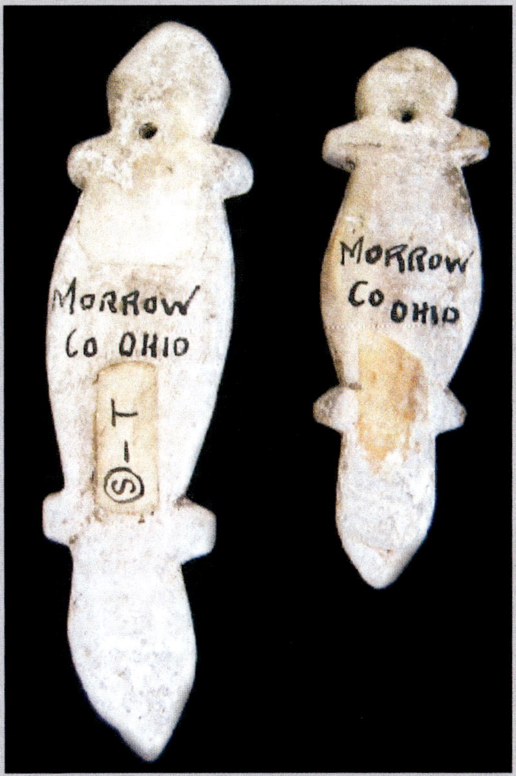

Beaver effigies, shell, probably Woodland period, 3¼" long and 2⅜" long, respectively. The owner obtained the larger effigy at the Vietzen auction in 1998. The smaller effigy is ex-collection Mike Barron, and the two were reunited in 2002. Both were pictured in Vietzen's *Prehistoric Americans* page 100, and Mr. Vietzen termed them "Rare finds." The pair was also illustrated in *Who's Who in Indian Relics* No. 1, and were in the B. W. Stephens collection at that time. Morrow County, Ohio. William Hamner collection, Alabama. Pair, **$1,000.00.**

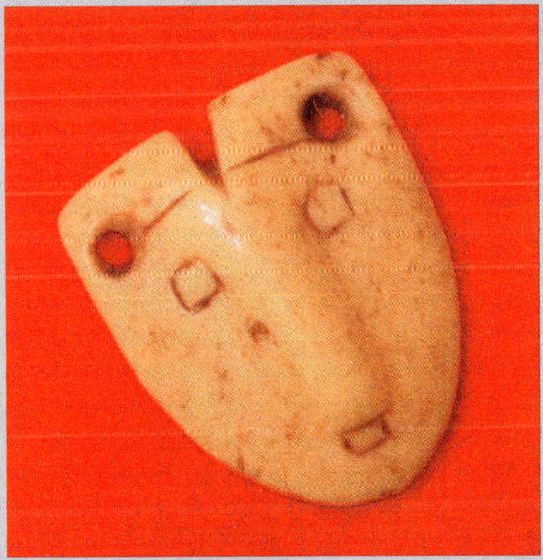

Maskette, human face effigy in bone, ¾ x $1\frac{5}{16}$", $\frac{3}{16}$" thick. Nicely carved and with fastening or suspension holes, it is probably early historic. From New York state. Michael F. Slasinski collection, Michigan. Museum grade.

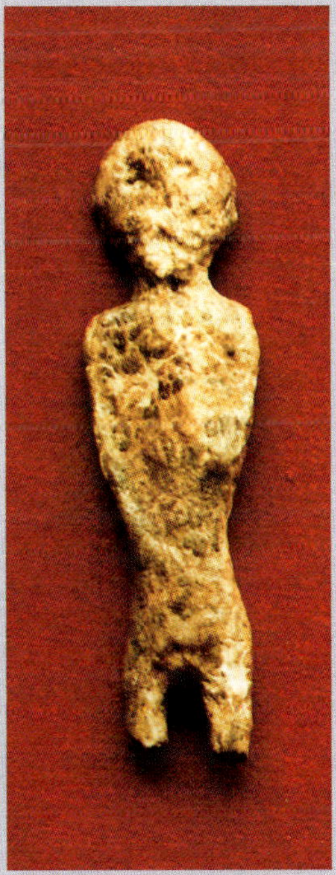

Rare "September Morn" figurine, 3¼" high, antler. It is Susquehannock, ca. AD 1550 – 1575. These received the name from the nude figure in Paul Chabas' famous painting. This example was found with a broken Shultz style pottery jar, and it came from Queen Esters Flats, Pennsylvania. Dave Summers collection, Victor, New York. **$1,200.00.**

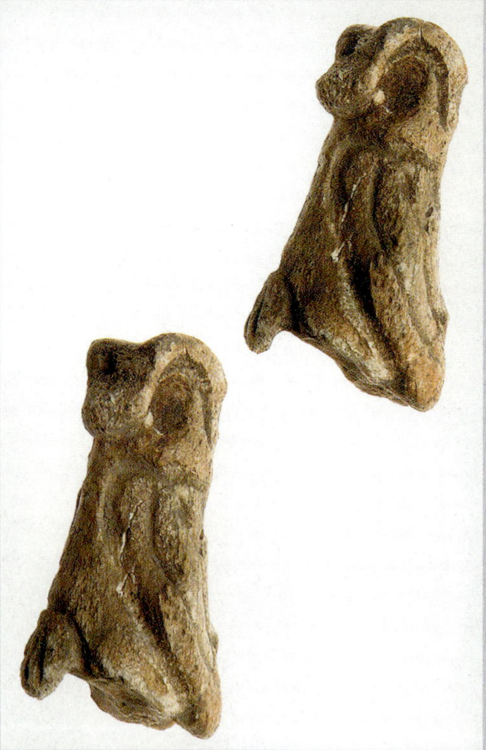

Owl effigy, two views, artifact made from a deer toe bone. It is 1½" high and was found in Pemiscot County, Missouri. Bob Hess collection, Indiana. Art Gerber photograph. Museum grade.

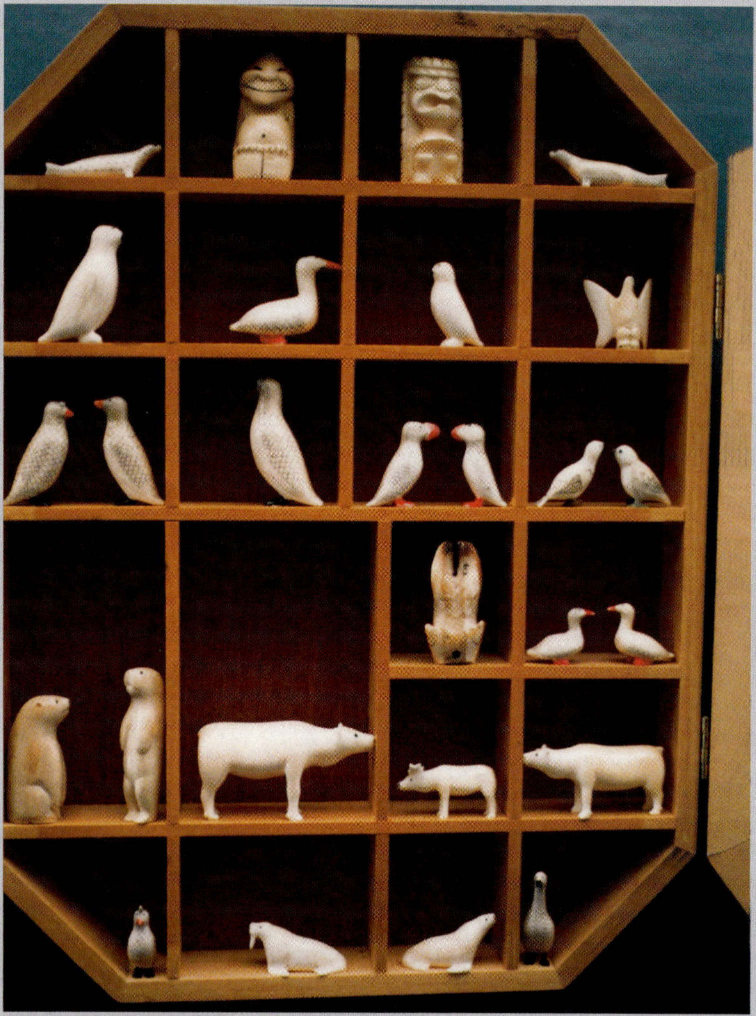

Ivory figurines, birds and animals, caribou 1½ x 2¾", ¾" thick. These images are recent to contemporary and are Eskimo, from Alaska. Collection of, and photograph by, Gary Henry, North Carolina. All, **$500.00.**

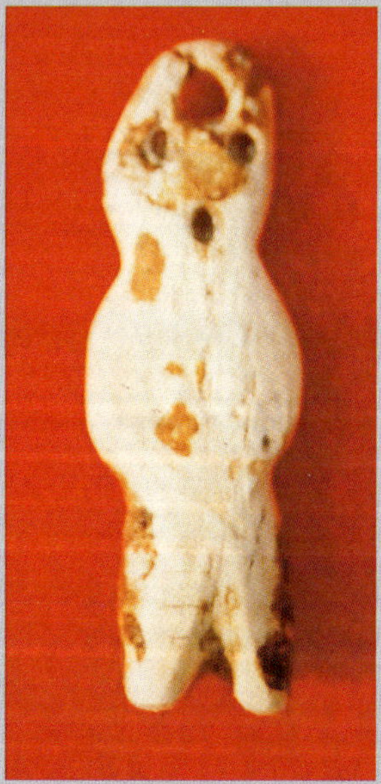

Human effigy figure pendant, with engraving and weeping eye motif, ⅝ x 1⅞", ex-collection Barron. This Mississippian-era piece was made from a conch shell spine and is drilled for suspension. Human effigies from any prehistoric North American period are rare. Northern Kentucky. Douglas E. McIlwain collection. **$650.00.**

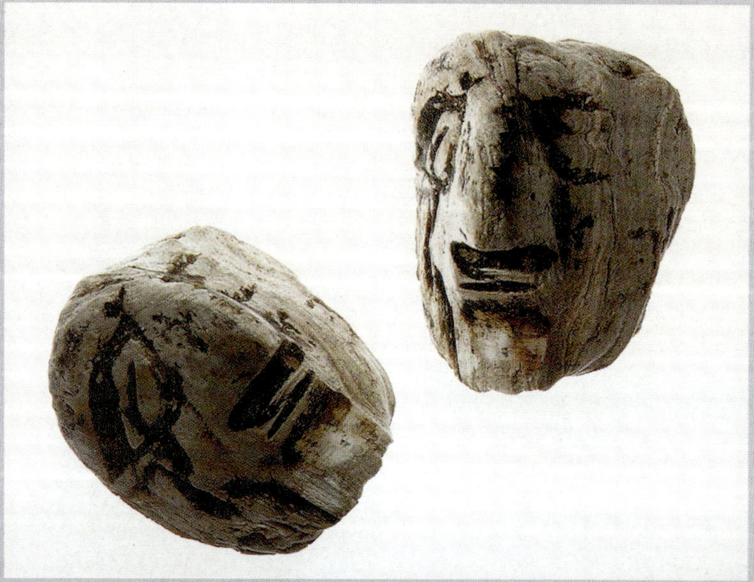

Human face effigy, shell, 1 x 1¼" high. This rare piece was found in Pemiscot County, Missouri. Bob Hess collection, Indiana. Art Gerber photograph. Museum grade.

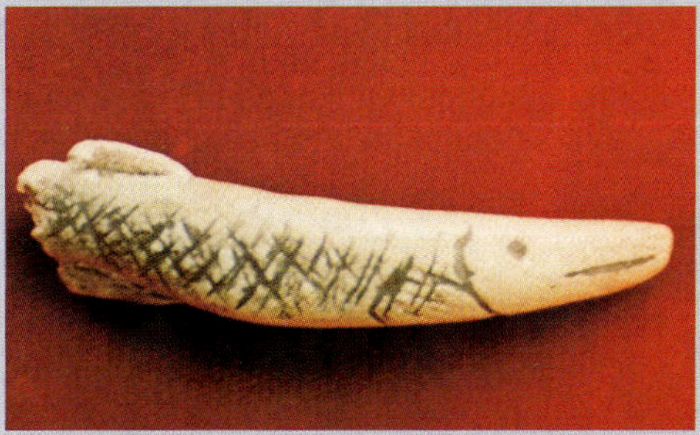

Fish effigy, bone, 2" long. ex-collection Ritter. Find-location unknown. Tim Liehr collection, Illinois. Museum grade.

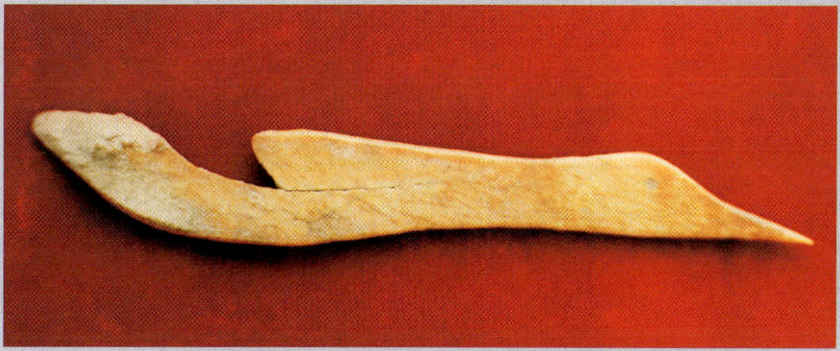

Flying bird effigy, bone, 3⅞" long. Ex-collection Ritter, this is a highly stylized image. Origin unknown. Tim Liehr collection, Illinois. Museum grade.

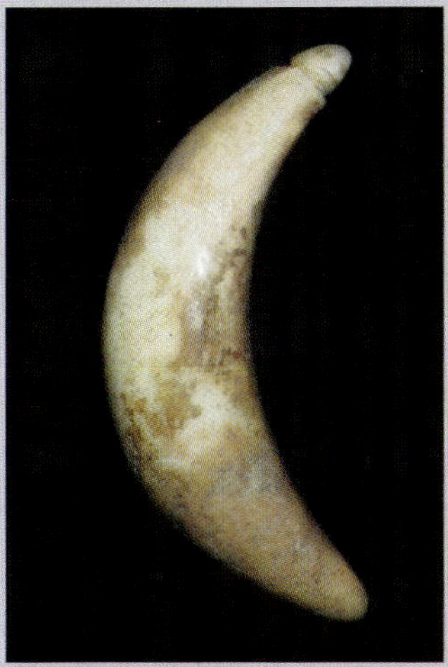

Effigy claw, antler, 1⅞". The tip on this example is grooved, and overall it is well-shaped and polished. Provenance unlisted. Private collection. Museum grade.

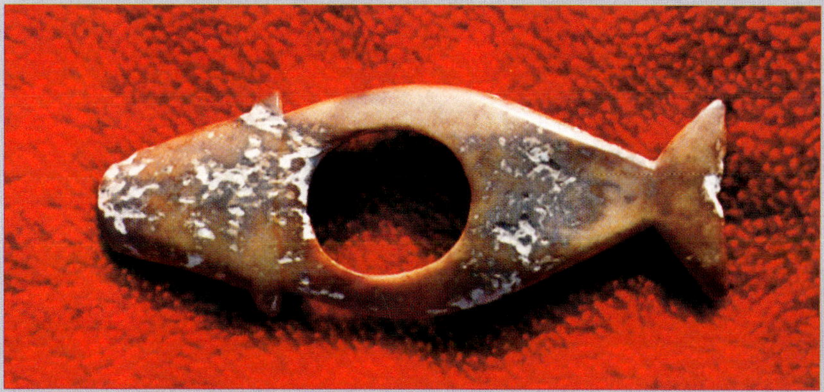

Whale effigy toggle, probably Punik culture, 1.25 x 3.81" long, bone or ivory. This Alaskan piece, once housed in an historical museum, is nicely carved and finished. Brandon Trivette collection, North Carolina. **$250.00.**

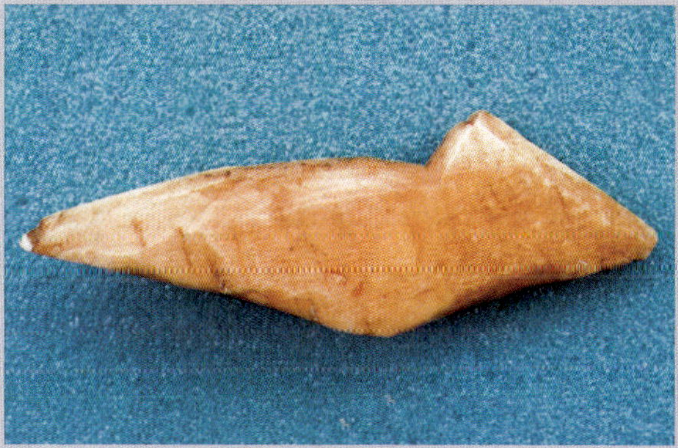

Ivory effigy, prehistoric(?), unknown figure, ⅞ x 2³⁄₁₆". It is ex-collection Cantrell. Alaska. Collection of, and photograph by, Gary Henry, North Carolina. **$25.00.**

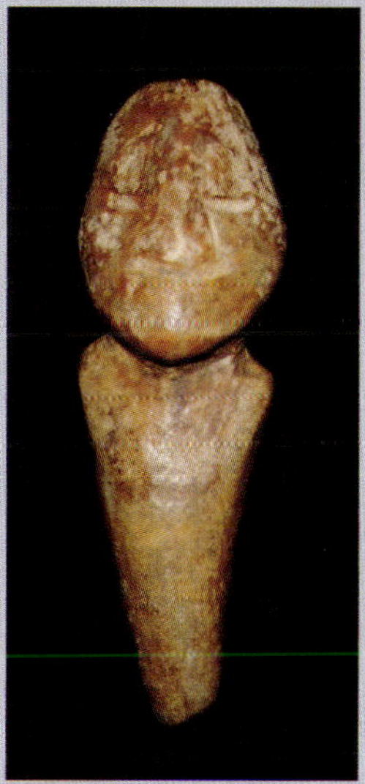

Human figure effigy, made of antler, 3¹⁄₁₆" high. Well-carved and polished, it was found in southcentral Pennsylvania. Private collection. Museum grade.

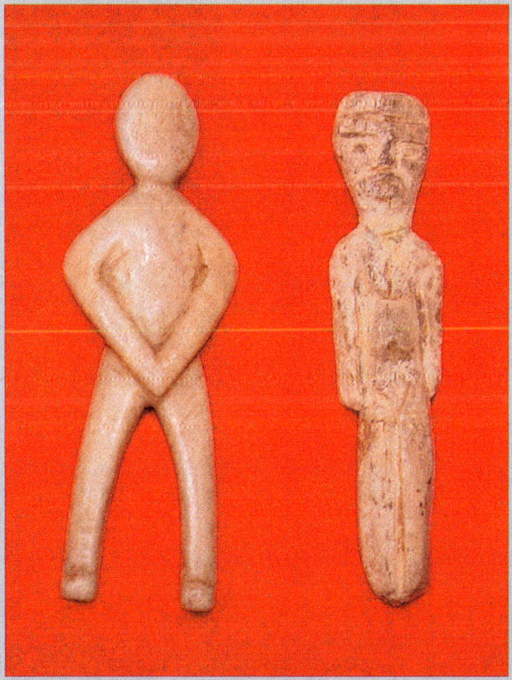

Bone figurines, so-called Virginity dolls or September Morn effigies. They average ³⁄₁₆" thick and 2⅝" long and are probably early historic. Iroquois, they are from Upstate New York. Michael F. Slasinski collection, Michigan. Both, Museum grade.

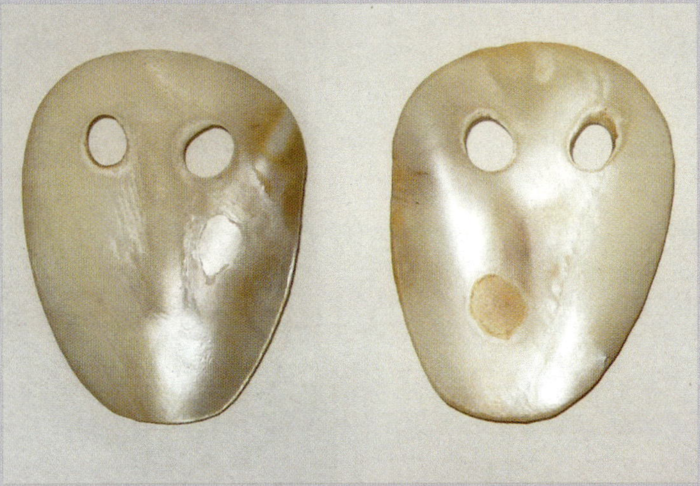

Shell mask gorget, Mississippian period, front and back views. The mask pendant has two eyes and the obverse has a nose. Picked up in July of 1995, it was found in the Ohio River. Mason County, West Virginia. Private collection. Rodney Roberts photograph. Unlisted.

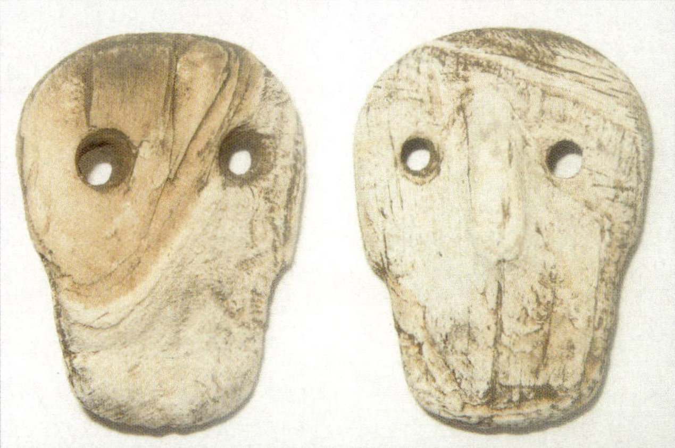

Shell mask gorget, front and back views, Mississippian period. The eyes are drilled and the obverse has a nose. This is the third shell mask gorget found by the owner, two with noses and one without. It came from a plowed field in May of 2003. Mason County, West Virginia. Private collection. Rodney Roberts photograph. Museum grade.

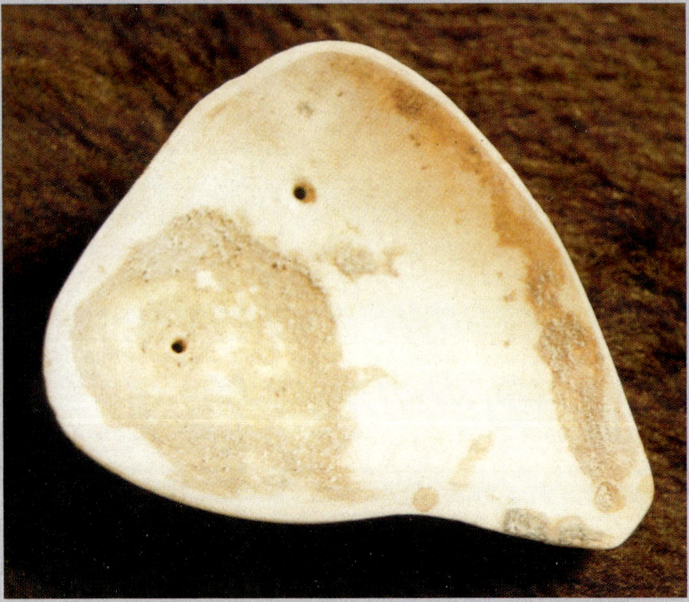

Mask pendant or gorget, 3¼" high, drilled marine shell. The specimen is Mississippian in time, ex-collection Parker. Smythe County, Virginia. Dale and Betty Roberts collection, Iowa. Unlisted.

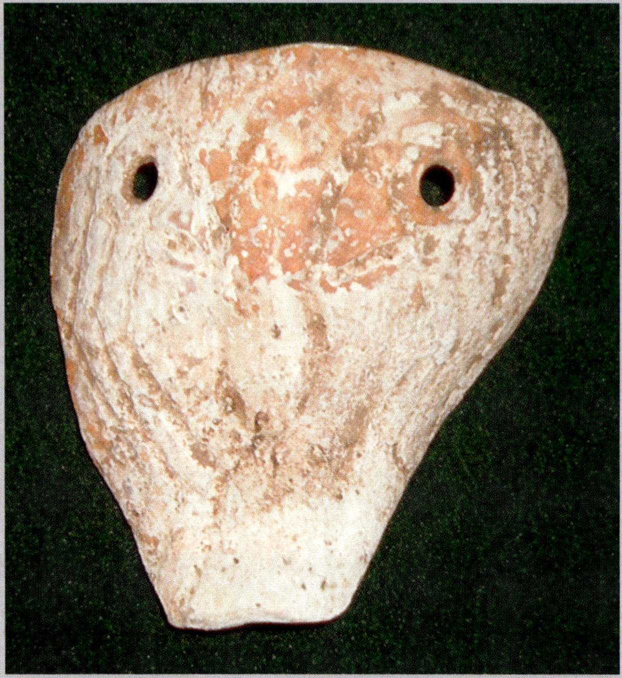

Shell mask pendant, two suspension/eye holes, 3 x 3". The pendant has a Davis COA and it was found in the Batesville area, Arkansas. Keith and Rhonda Dodge collection, Michigan. Unlisted.

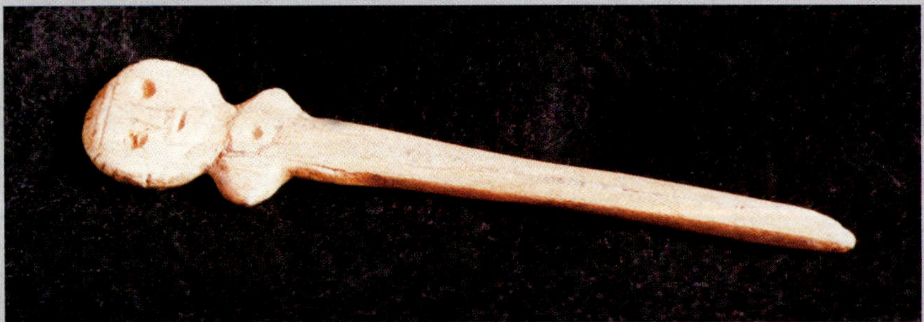

Effigy hairpin, human face and shoulders, 4½" long. It was found in a rock shelter along the Tennessee River near Scottsboro, Alabama. John F. Wubker collection, Illinois. Museum grade.

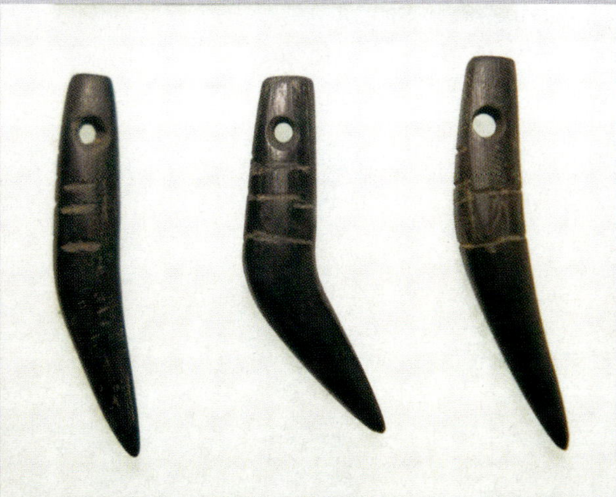

Effigies of talons or claws, cannel coal, each about 2" long. Ex-collections Hardin and Hooks, they are from Mason County, Kentucky. Back to Earth. Each, **$125.00.**

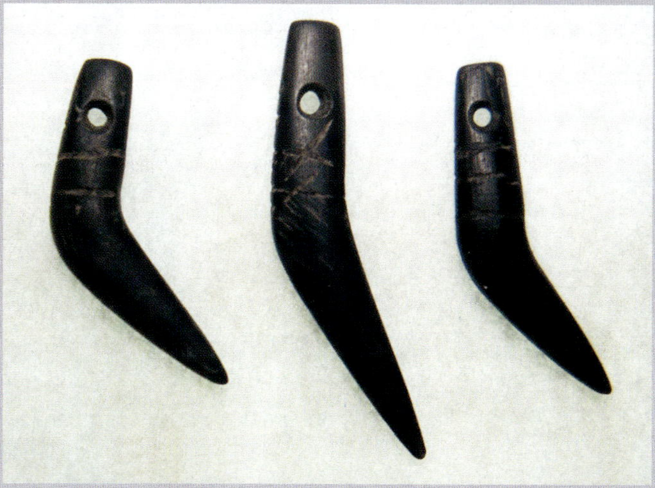

Effigy claws or talons, Fort Ancient aspect of the Mississippian period, incised markings. The cannel coal artifacts were found in Mason County, Kentucky. Back to Earth. Each, **$125.00.**

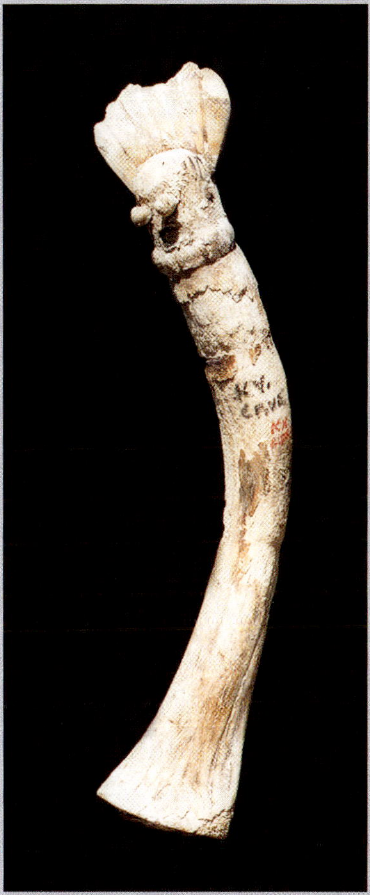

Effigy artifact, probably Woodland, carved antler, 14" long. This mysterious object is possibly a headdress component or ritual wand; it is one-of-a-kind and had an uncertain purpose. From the Col. Raymond Vietzen collection, it was found in Christian County, Kentucky. Pete Timoch collection. Museum grade.

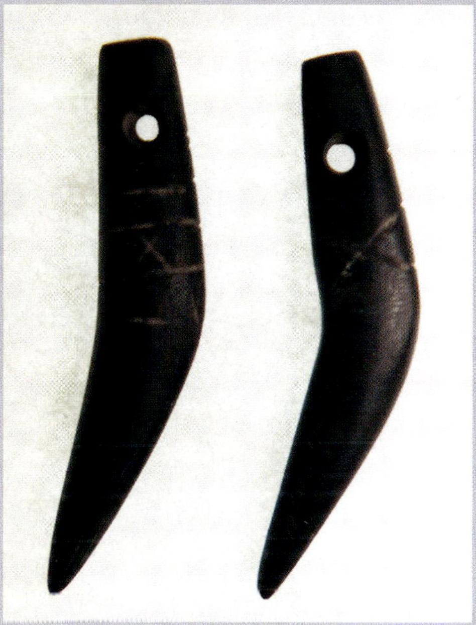

Effigy claws or talons, made of cannel coal, each about 2" long. They have line incising between the drilled hole and the bend. Mason County, Kentucky. Back to Earth. Each, **$125.00.**

Ivory fetish necklace, small animal effigies. The pendant is a bear; nine other birds or animals are represented by the smaller figures. The bear measures $1\frac{1}{16}$ x $2\frac{3}{16}$", and the necklace is recent or contemporary. Alaska. Collection of, and photograph by, Gary Henry, North Carolina. Necklace, **$300.00.**

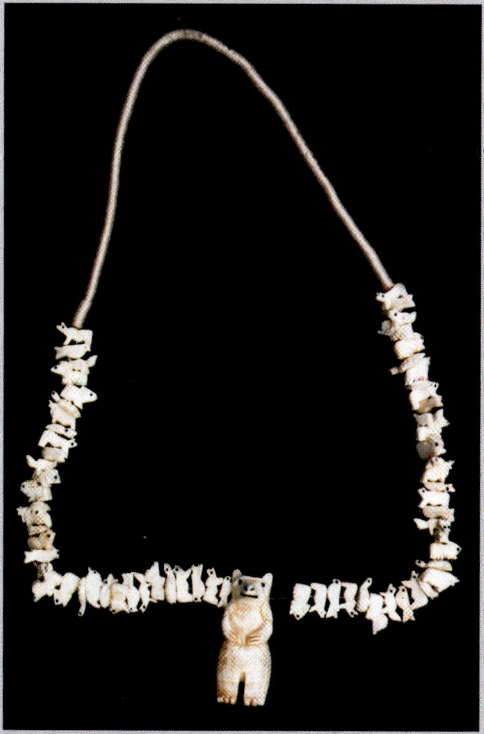

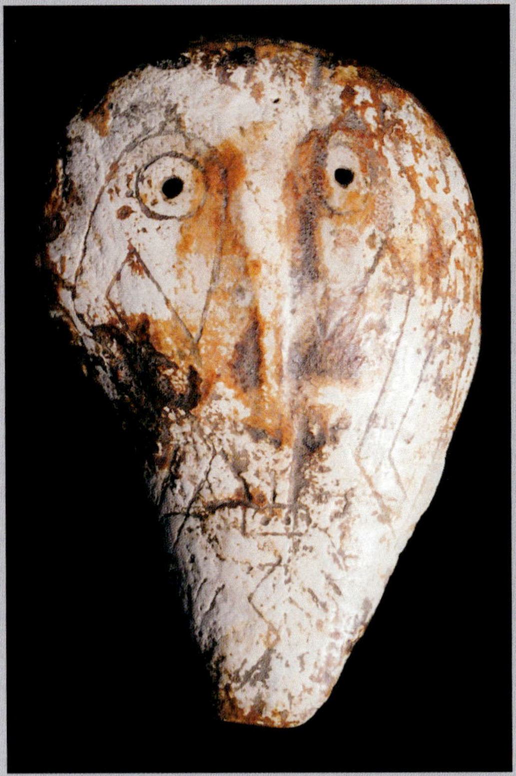

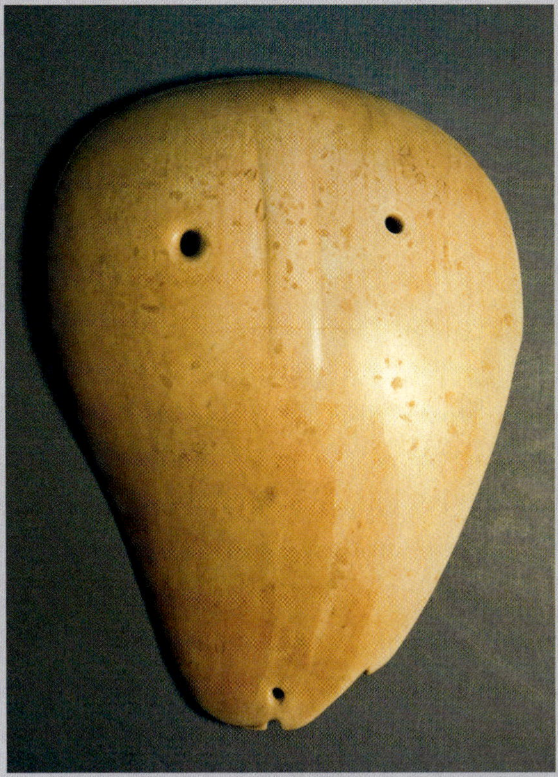

Shell face mask gorget, Buffalo style, 2¼ x 2½". It has rare secondary engraving of a human and two extra suspension holes at the bottom. St. Francis County, Arkansas. Jim Maus collection, North Carolina. Unlisted.

Weeping Eye gorget, 11 cm high. It has a square mouth with two dots and a zigzag line from mouth to chin. The material is tan whelk shell and the hairline is etched. This is a fine artifact from Mississippian times, and the eye tear-drop lines may also represent the long necks of cranes, herons, or storks while the suspension holes represent eyes. Eastern Tennessee. Museum grade.

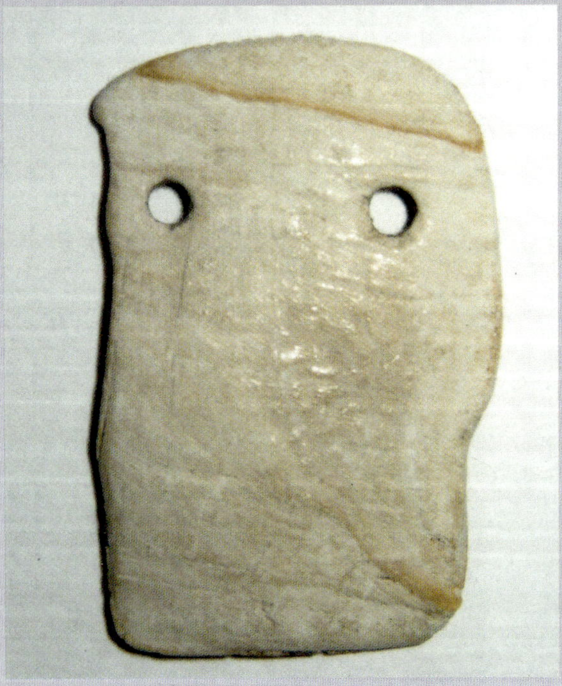

Shell mask gorget, Mississippian, some damage to left side of face, 1⁵⁄₁₆ x 1⁵⁄₁₆". West Virginia. Private collection. Rodney Roberts photograph. Unlisted.

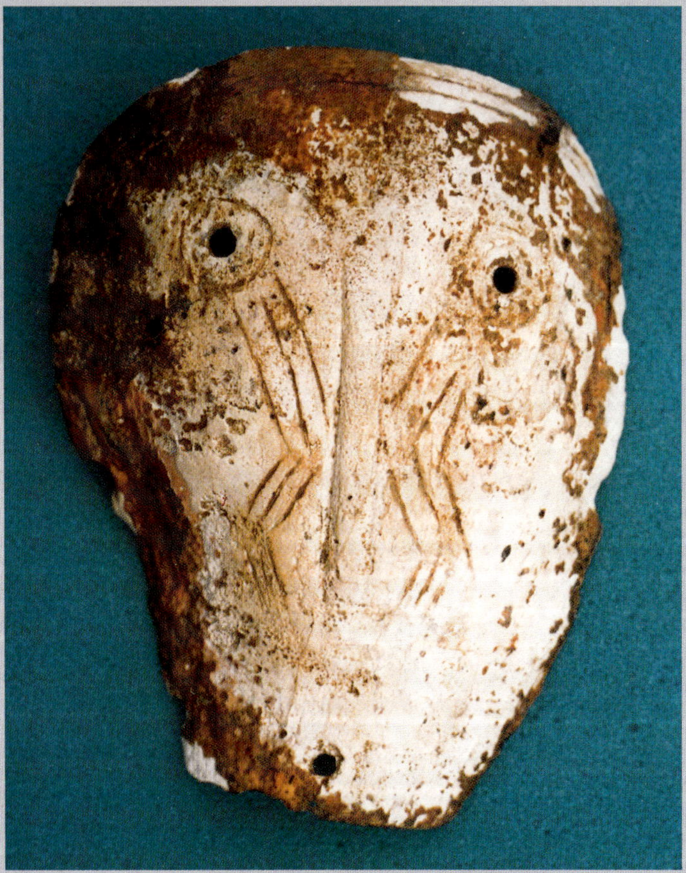

Weeping Eye shell mask gorget, Mississippian period, 3½ x 4½". Pictured in *Who's Who in Indian Relics* No. 8, this example is ex-collection Snyder and was found in Meigs County, Tennessee. Collection of, and photograph by, Gary Henry, North Carolina. **$1,250.00.**

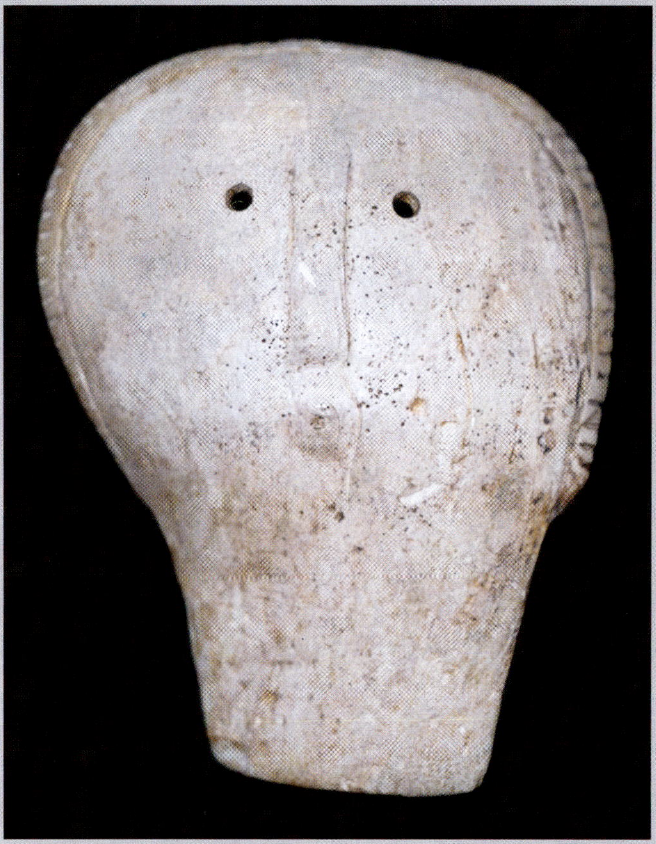

Shell face mask gorget, Chicamauga style, 5½ x 6 15/16". With suspension-hole eyes, nose, mouth, and tally-marked upper edge, it is a superb Mississippian artifact. Talledega County, Alabama. Jim Maus collection, North Carolina. Museum grade.

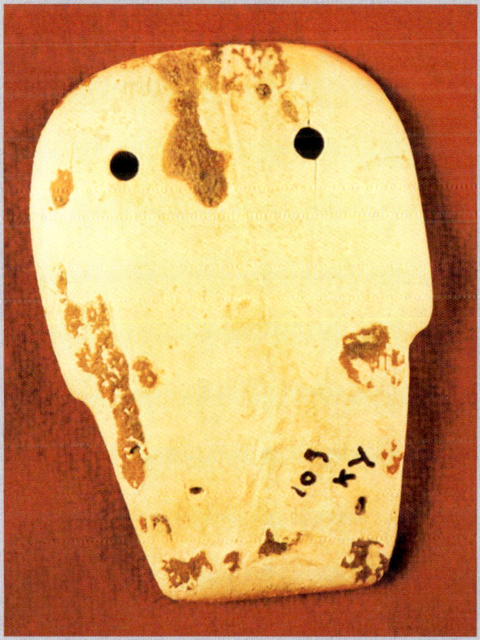

Shell mask gorget, 2⅝" high, drilled eyes/suspension holes. This mask, Mississippian, came from Kentucky. Robin Fiser collection. Museum grade.

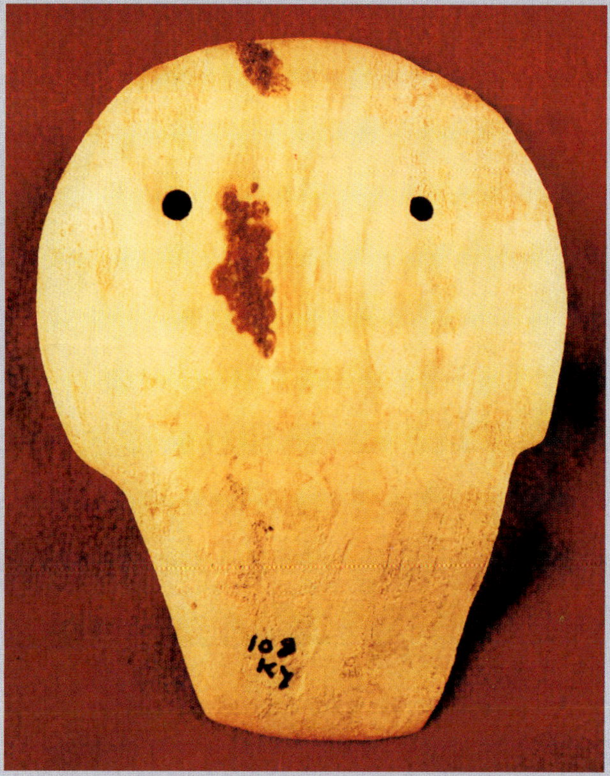

Shell mask gorget, Mississippian period, 3⅜" high. This example was found in Kentucky. Robin Fiser collection. Museum grade.

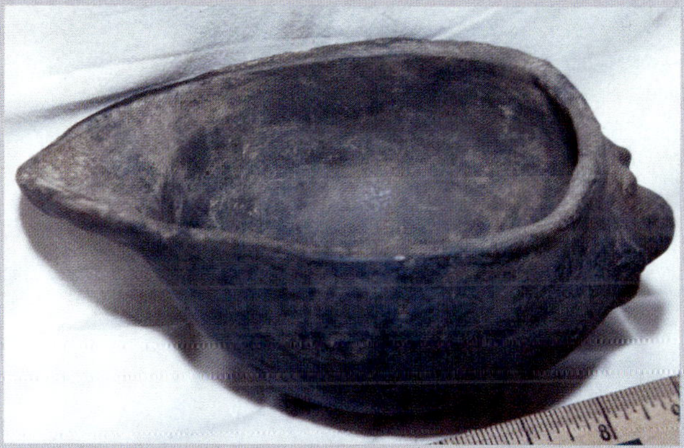

Effigy ceramic pot, marine conch shell, Mississippian era. Pottery pieces like this example are quite rare. Southern United States. Back to Earth. Unlisted.

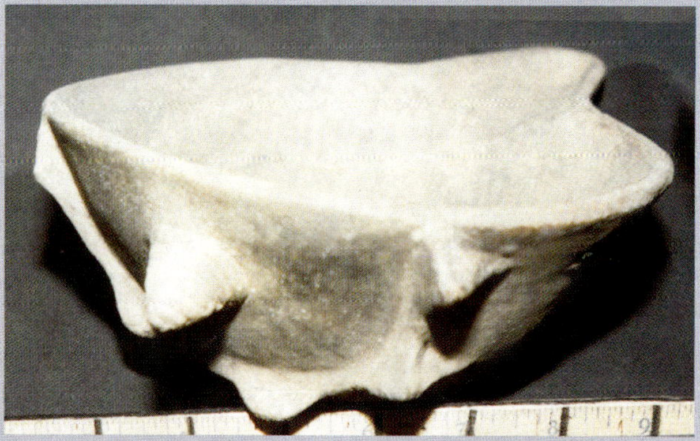

Effigy pottery, in the form of a conch shell, Mississippian people. Back to Earth. Unlisted.

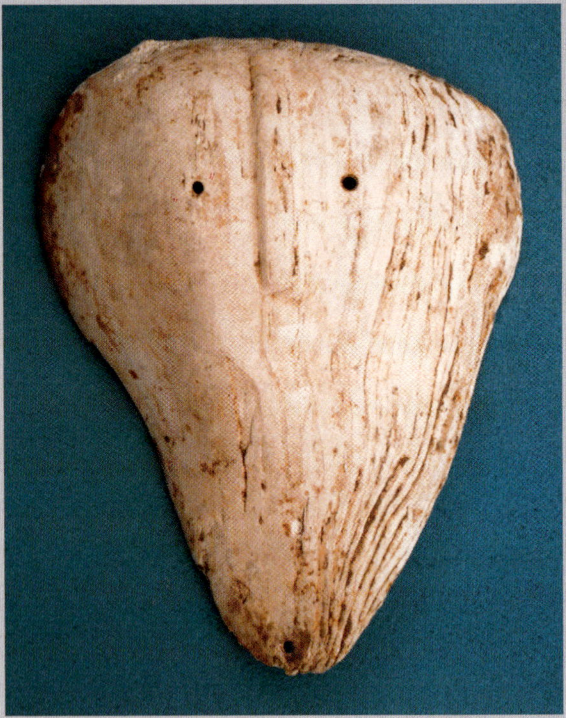

Shell mask gorget, Mississippian period, it measures 5 x 6". Well-made and in fine condition. Snyder found the mask between 1947 and 1958 in Polk County, Tennessee. Collection of, and photograph by, Gary Henry, North Carolina. **$1,000.00.**

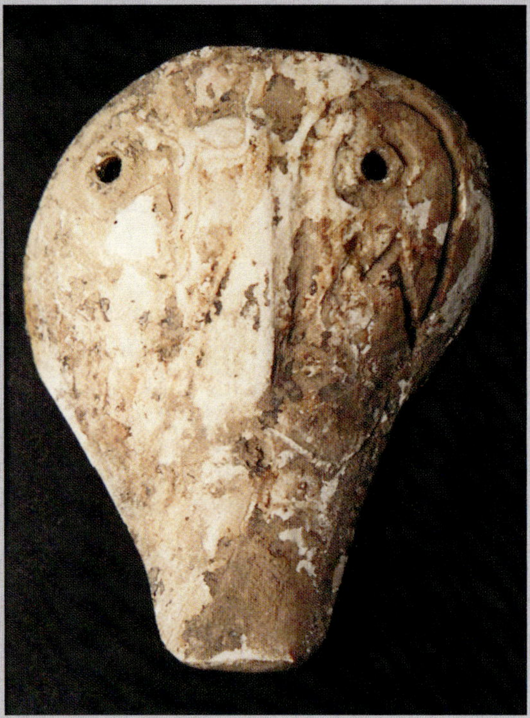

Mask, shell, ex-collection Col. Vietzen, Mississippian period, 3⅜" high. It was found in Lorain County, Ohio. Back to Earth. Museum grade.

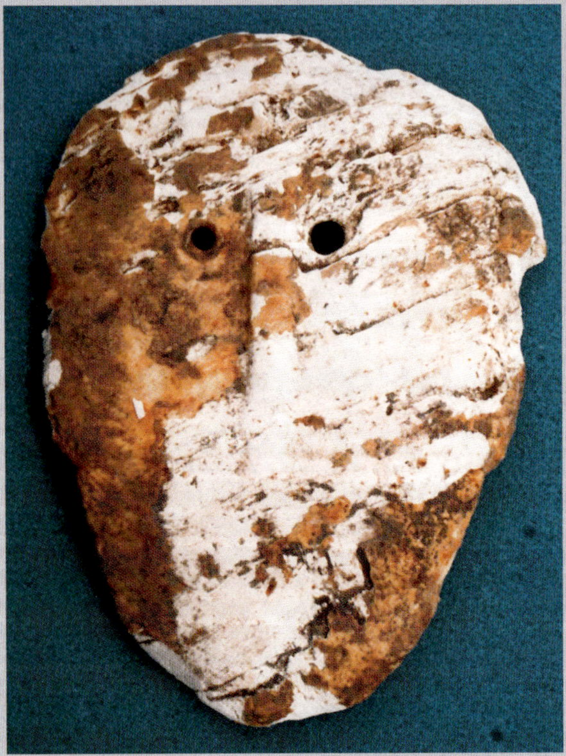

Shell mask gorget, Mississippian period, 2½ x 3¼". Ex-collection Snyder, it has an elongated nose below the eyes, which also served as suspension holes. Monroe County, Tennessee. Collection of, and photograph by, Gary Henry, North Carolina. **$800.00.**

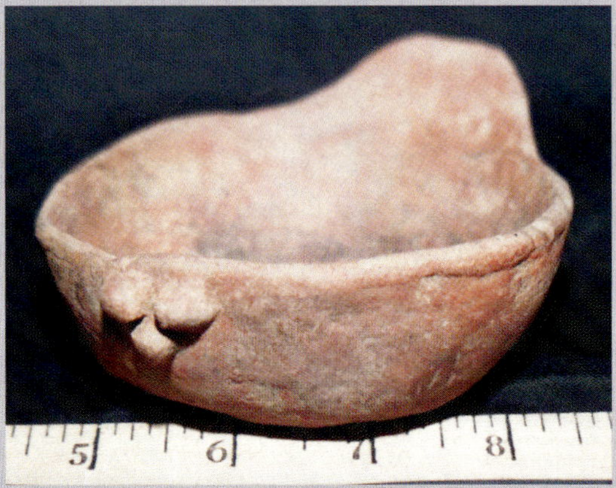

Effigy pottery, conch shell painted red, Mississippian period. Painted effigy pottery is a minority form. Back to Earth. Unlisted.

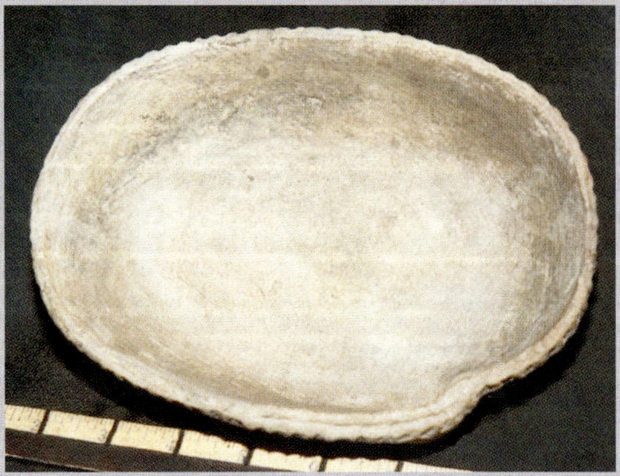

Effigy ceramic pot, mussel shell form, Mississippian people. The actual large shells were used for bowls and dippers. Back to Earth. Unlisted.

Teeth and Ivory

These materials were highly sought-after in prehistoric North America because of their pleasing shapes, color, and durability. There may also have been an emotional or ritual association with the animal that provided teeth and ivory. The teeth of many different animals were used, some for tools (groundhog, porcupine, and beaver) and some for decoration (deer, elk, bison, wolf, cougar, dog, bear, and more.) Large single teeth, like those of black and grizzly bears, were sometimes used individually as pendants; smaller teeth were more often used to make necklaces, anklets, and bracelets.

Teeth would be drilled, grooved, or knobbed so that they could be secured with sinew, leather, or fiber cords. Teeth were almost always worked at the root end, because, there, the material was less hard. Also, when suspended from the root end, the teeth gravity-positioned so that the uniform light color always displayed to best effect. The hardness of teeth provided a natural polish that basically lasted as long as did the teeth.

Ivory is generally considered to be the tusks of large animals, like mammoth and mastodon ("fossil" ivory), and, as relates to North America, the tusks of walrus. The single long "unicorn" tusk of the narwhal is by far the rarest ivory used for artifacts, and little of it went beyond Eskimo (Inuit) lands and waters. Technically, ivory means teeth of any kind, especially the hard yellowish-white dentine portions.

Teeth and ivory were so desired in prehistoric times that it appears that shortages arose now and again. Then, facsimile teeth might be made, usually carved in shell (sometimes bone) which looked much like the material being replaced. In general, the teeth of carnivores (meat eaters) were used most often, but herbivores (vegetation eaters) were employed as well. Wapiti (elk) teeth were favored where that animal was available.

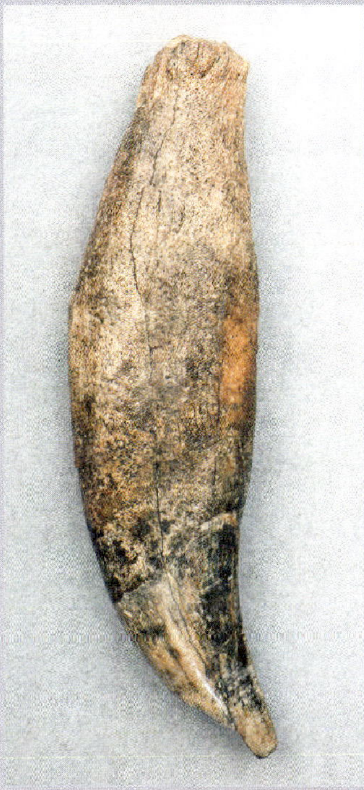

Bear tooth, 2⅜" long, prehistoric. The find-site of this mineralized tooth is unknown. H. B. Greene II collection, Naples, Florida. **$40.00.**

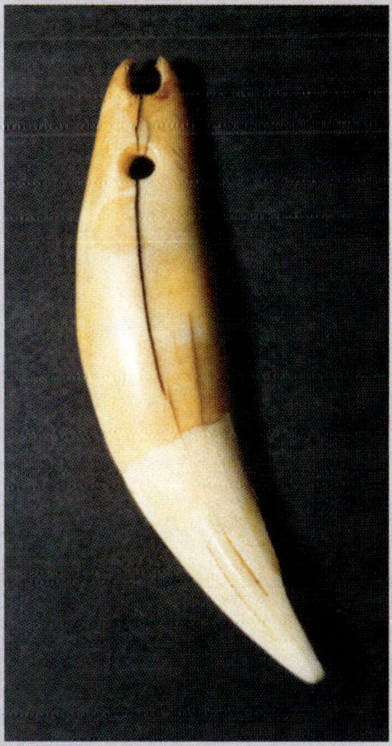

Bear tooth, highly polished, 2⅞" long. This tooth has experienced much use as a pendant; the original drill-hole has worn through and a second was drilled further wear. Found at a Fort Ancient site in Augusta County, Kentucky. Back to Earth. **$275.00.**

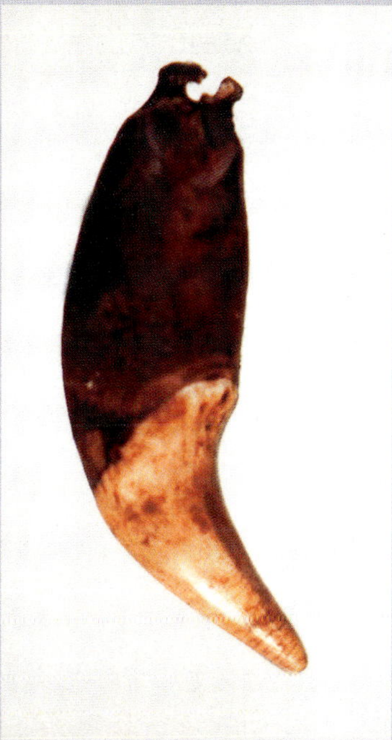

Grizzly bear tooth, suspension hole worn or broken through, 2½". It is from Kotzebue, Alaska. Larry Garvin collection. **$185.00.**

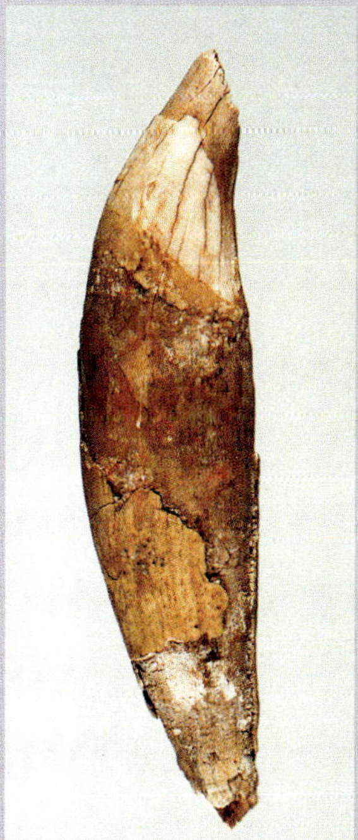

Bear tooth, weathered and partly decomposed, 2¾" long. This example was recovered from a rock shelter. Because the tooth is not drilled or grooved, and in poor condition, value is not high. Southern Tennessee. Private collection. **$10.00.**

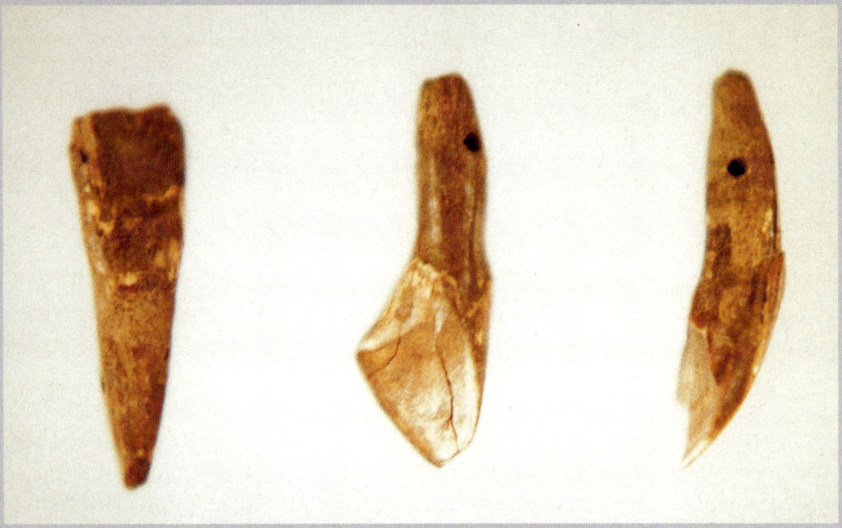

Bison teeth, darkened with age and soil content, longest is 1¾". With narrow drill-holes, the teeth are from Arizona. Back to Earth. Each, **$10.00.**

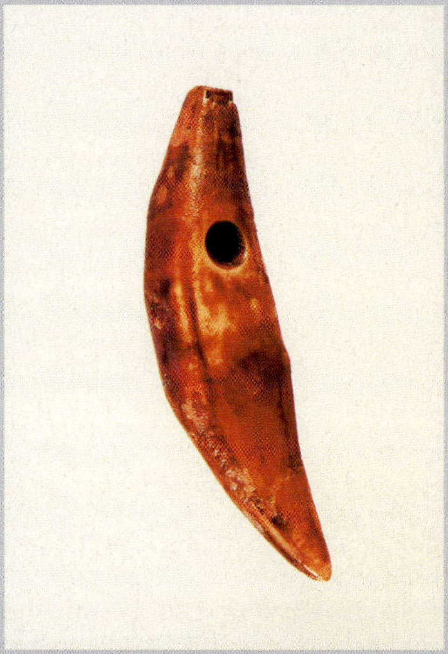

Cougar tooth, shellac coating, 2¼" long. This piece was drilled on the obverse with one hole, on the reverse with two holes, and was also drilled with a small hole from the base into the tooth. Cougar teeth are shorter, more slender, and straighter than bear teeth. Southern Ohio. Fred Winegardner collection. **$125.00.**

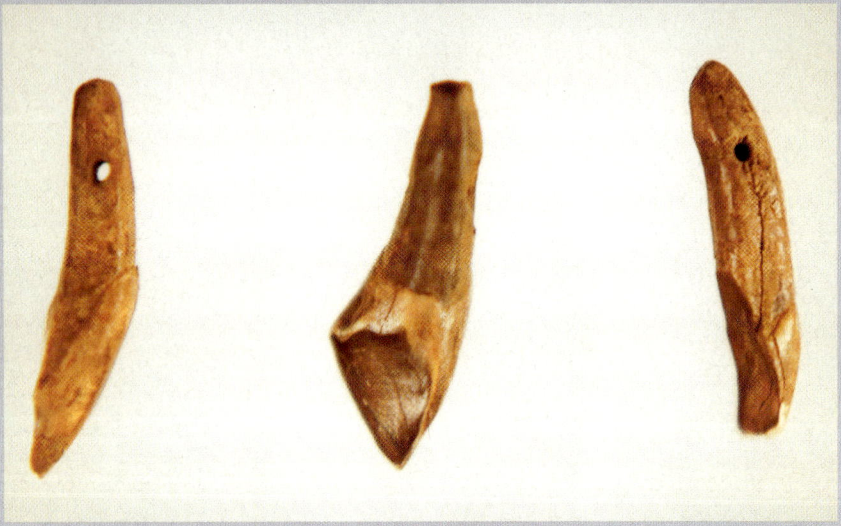

Bison teeth, drilled for suspension, longest 1⅞". Made as pendants or necklace elements, they are from Arizona. Back to Earth. Each, **$10.00.**

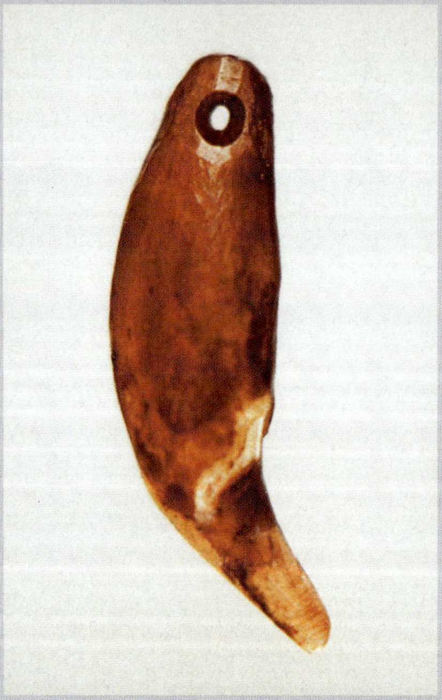

Grizzly bear tooth, drilled at top, 2⅝" long, mineralized. It came from the Kotzebue area, Alaska. Larry Garvin collection. **$250.00.**

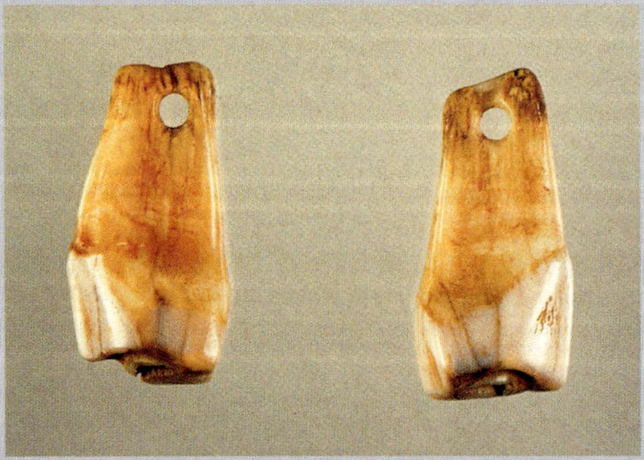

Elk teeth, drilled for suspension as necklace elements or pendants, longest is 1⅜". Ex-collection Tolliver, they are probably from a rock shelter. Hocking County, Ohio. Private collection. Each, **$25.00 – 35.00.**

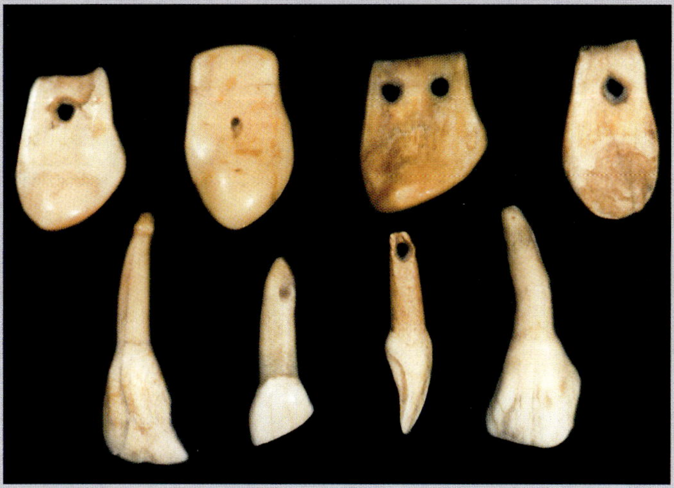

Pendants or pieces for necklaces, elk teeth (top) 1 to 1⅛" long, and buffalo teeth (bottom). They were all found in Greene County, Indiana. First Mesa, Indiana. Elk teeth, each **$85.00 – 125.00;** buffalo teeth, each **$35.00 – 65.00.**

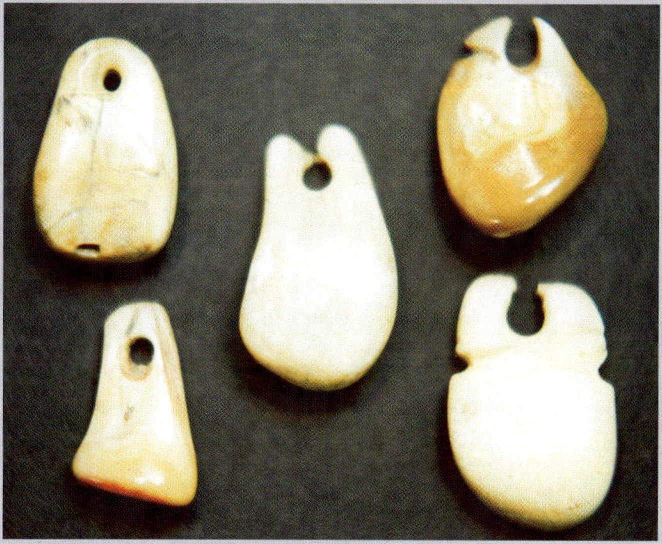

Elk incisors, drilled, and three examples are also grooved. The longest is 1" and all were found near Chamberlain, South Dakota. Mike Fox collection, Iowa. Each, **$35.00 – 65.00.**

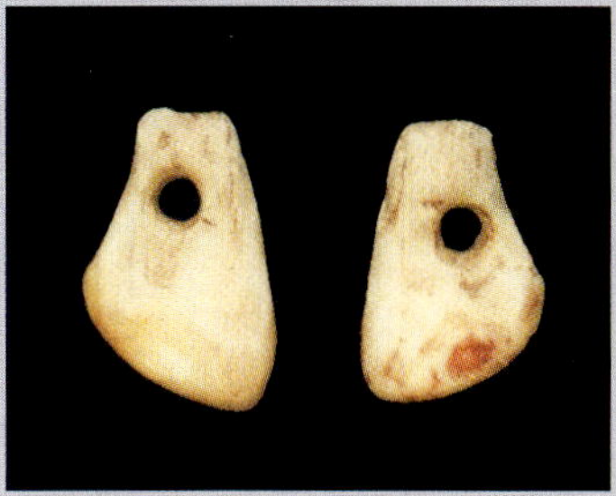

Pendants, Woodland period, mammal premolar teeth, largest is ⅝ x 1⁵⁄₁₆", ⁵⁄₁₆" thick. These drilled examples are ex-collection Levy, origin unknown. Collection of, and photograph by, Gary Henry, North Carolina. Each, **$25.00.**

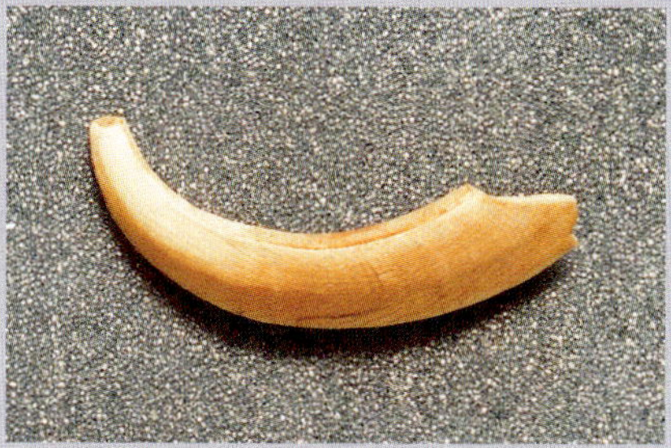

Beaver incisor, with one side ground flat and used as a shaver or knife, from an historic Iroquois (Onondaga) site dated AD 1600 – 1620. It is 2⅛" long and was found near Pompey. Beaver teeth were often used for tools beginning in Late Archaic times. Onondaga County, New York. Dave Summers collection, Victor, New York. **$40.00.**

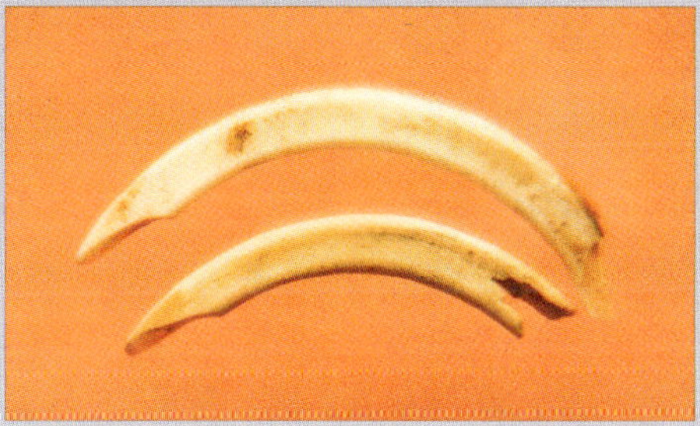

Cutting tools, beaver incisors, 1⅝" and 1⅞" long. They are Lamoka phase, Middle Archaic (ca. 3000 – 2500 BC), and came from Schuyler County, New York. Dave Summers collection, Victor, New York. Each, **$5.00.**

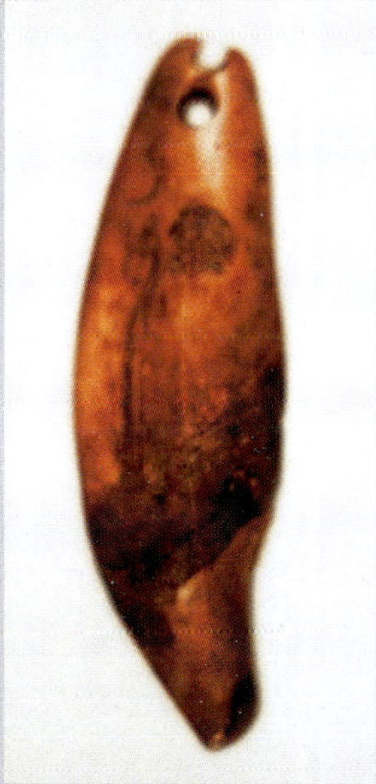

Grizzly bear tooth, mineralized, drilled, and polished, 2⅝" long. When the original suspension hole wore through, a second was made just below the first. Kotzebue, Alaska. Larry Garvin collection. **$250.00.**

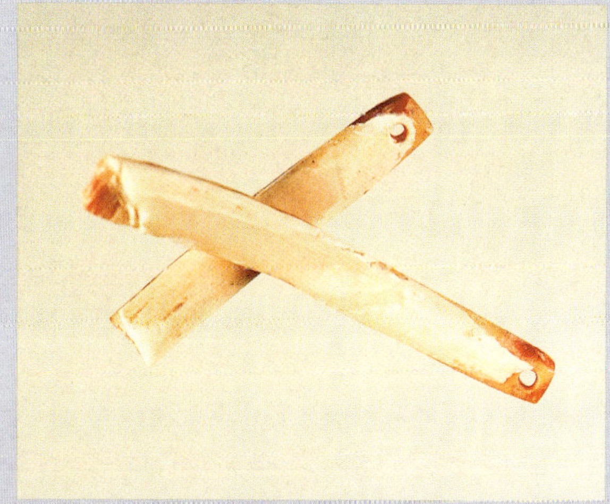

Beaver incisors, drilled for suspension, longest is 2¼". Highly unusual, these are from Ross County, Ohio. Robin Fiser collection. Each, **$25.00 – 35.00.**

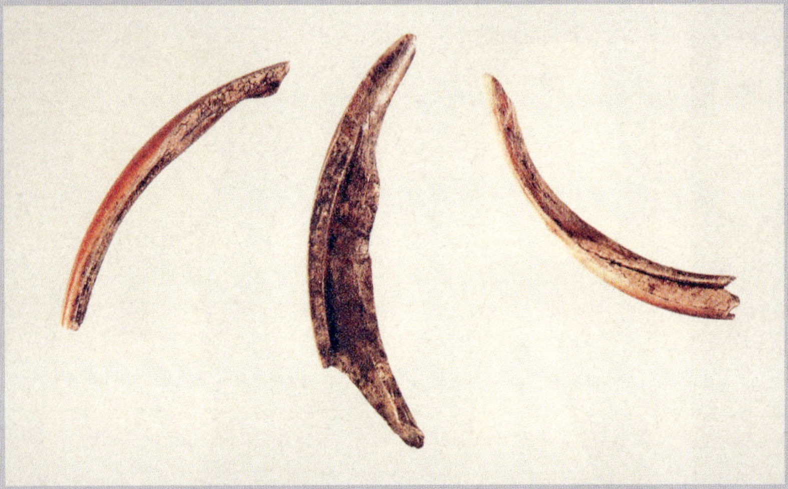

Beaver teeth, probably tool parts, center example split longitudinally, 2⅜". The three came from a Fort Ancient site where collections (among others) were made in 1937 and 1977. Southern Ohio. Private collection. Each, **$2.00 – 4.00.**

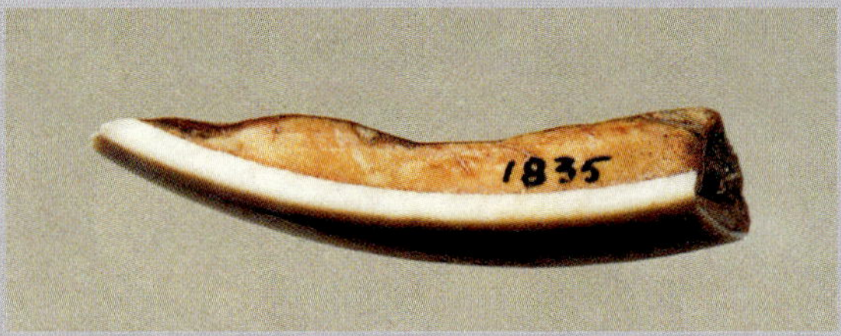

Chisel, beaver incisor, Riverton people of the Late Archaic period. Ca. 1550 BC and later, this cultural manifestation (living sites were often deep mussel-shell middens) is defined by a micro-tool industry. This included wood-carving tools like this chisel, which is polished at both ends from usage. Crawford County, Illinois. John Smith collection, Illinois. **$25.00.**

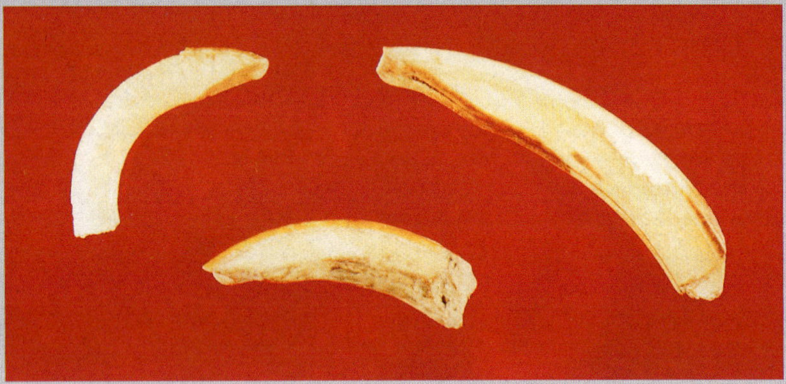

Rodent teeth, prehistoric. Longitudinally split groundhog tooth (left), 1¼"; broken beaver tooth (center); beaver tooth (right), 2" long. Found in Kentucky. Private collection. **$1.00, $5.00,** and **$7.00,** respectively.

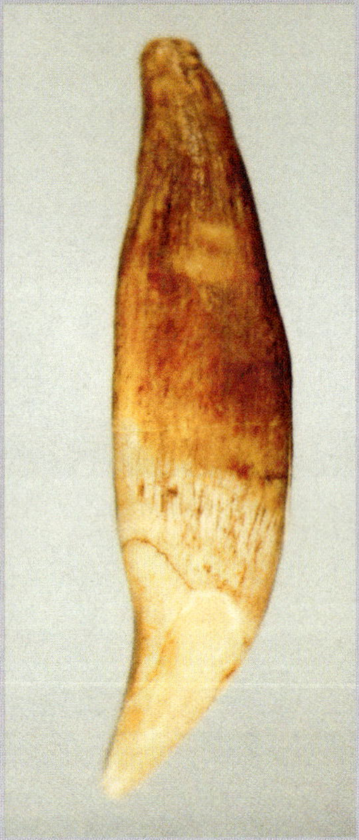

Bear tooth, undrilled, 3½" long. This large tooth was found in a rock shelter in Tennessee. Larry Garvin collection. **$85.00.**

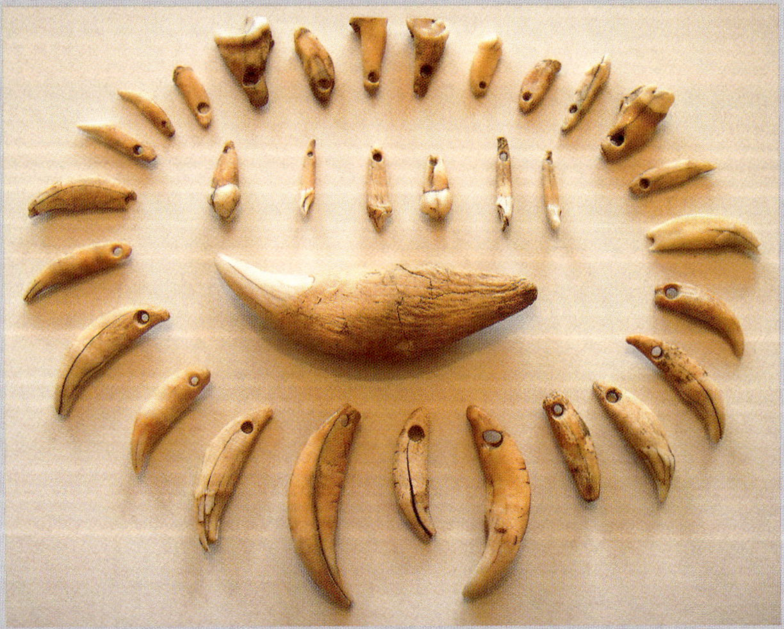

Drilled pendants, made of animal teeth, large bear tooth is 3¼" long. The two larger teeth at bottom are also tally-marked. Mississippian (Fort Ancient), they are from Mason and Cabell Counties, West Virginia. Private collection. Rodney Roberts photograph. Smaller teeth, each **$15.00 – 25.00;** large undrilled bear tooth, **$35.00;** tally-marked teeth, each **$50.00.**

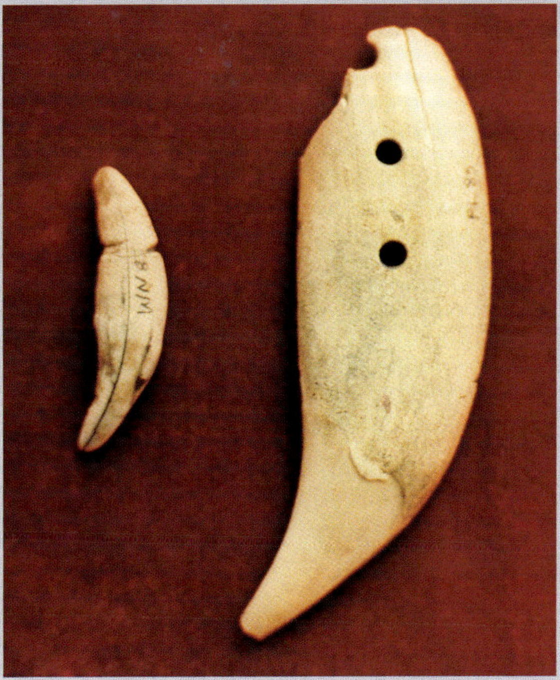

Animal teeth, worked, grooved tooth on left is 1⅜" long, Brown County, Illinois. Right, bear tooth, 3" long, with drill holes, Pike County, Illinois. Tim Liehr collection, Illinois. Small tooth, **$75.00;** large tooth, unlisted.

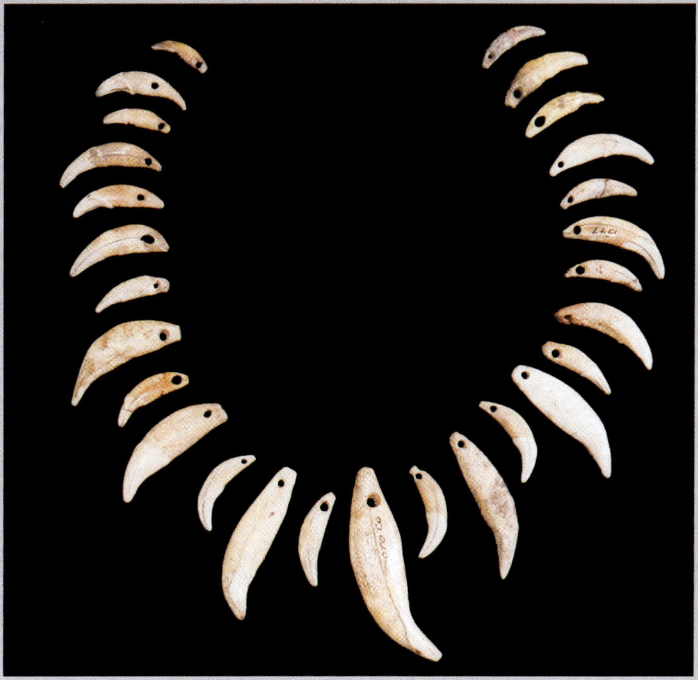

Necklace, 21 wolf teeth and bear canines (six largest). All teeth are drilled for suspension from both sides. The largest tooth is 8 cm long and is from Scioto County, Ohio. Other teeth are from Ohio, Tennessee, and Kentucky. Private collection. Each, **$15.00 – 20.00** (smaller wolf teeth) to **$200.00 to $225.00** (large drilled bear teeth).

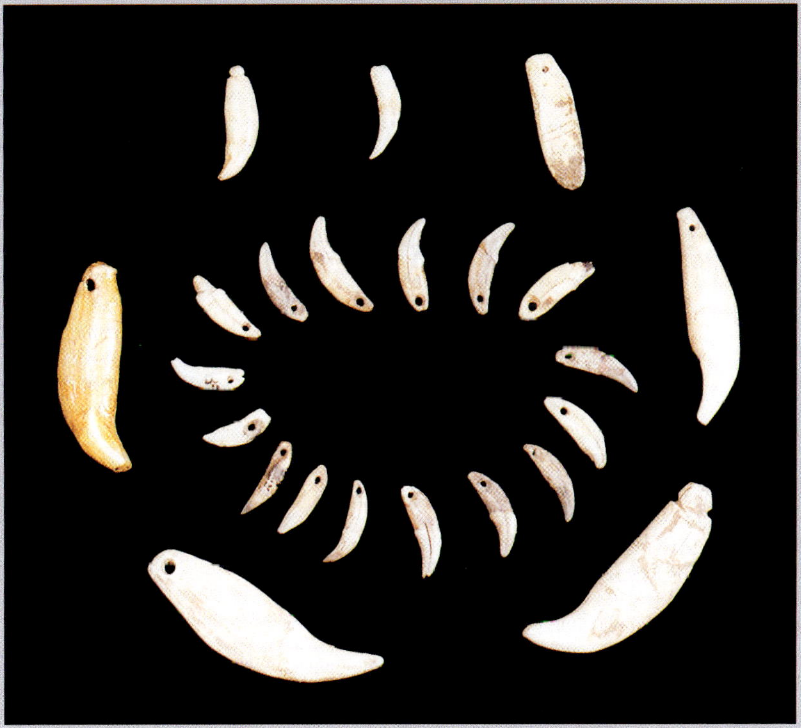

Teeth and bone effigy, notched bear tooth at bottom right is 7 cm long. Top row, left to right: notched seal tooth, Washington state; bobcat canine, a personal find of the owner in eastern Tennessee; tooth effigy made from deer bone, drilled, two etched lines. Center, 16 drilled dog or wolf canine teeth, all holes showing wear. Lower outside, two large and two very large bear canines. Private collection. Each, **$15.00 – 20.00** (dog teeth) to **$200.00** (grooved bear tooth).

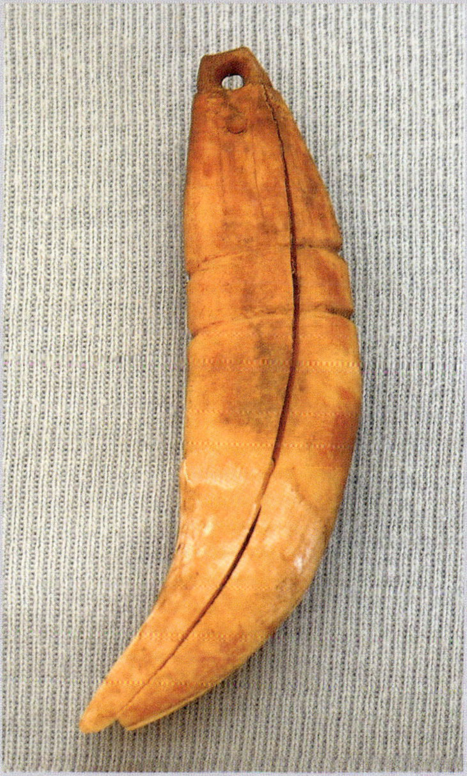

Pendant, bear tooth, 3" long. Judging by size and find region, this probably came from a grizzly bear. The tooth is drilled and has two incised decorative lines. Madison area, South Dakota. Rod Fuller collection, Nebraska. **$175.00 – 200.00.**

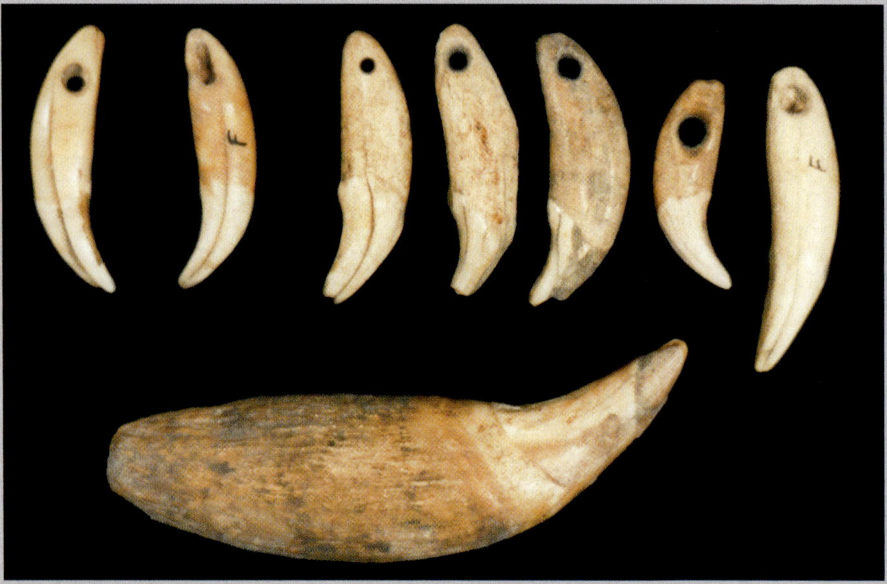

Pendants, wolf canines at top and a large black bear tooth at bottom. All came from a site in Greene County, Indiana. First Mesa, Indiana. Wolf teeth, each **$50.00 – 85.00;** bear tooth, **$85.00.**

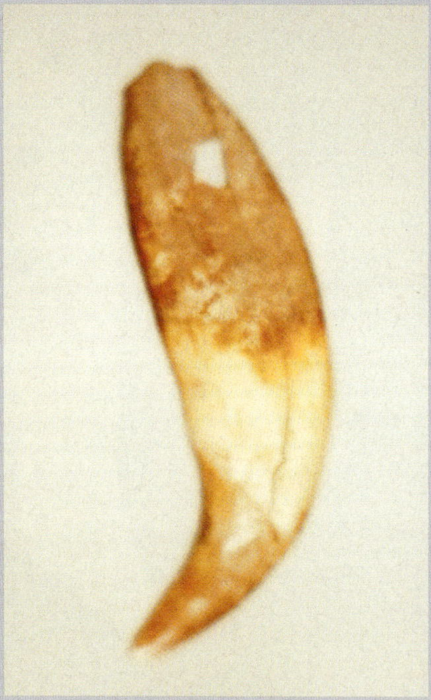

Bear tooth, suspension hole near top, 2¾". This tooth came from Nicholas County, Kentucky. Back to Earth. **$85.00.**

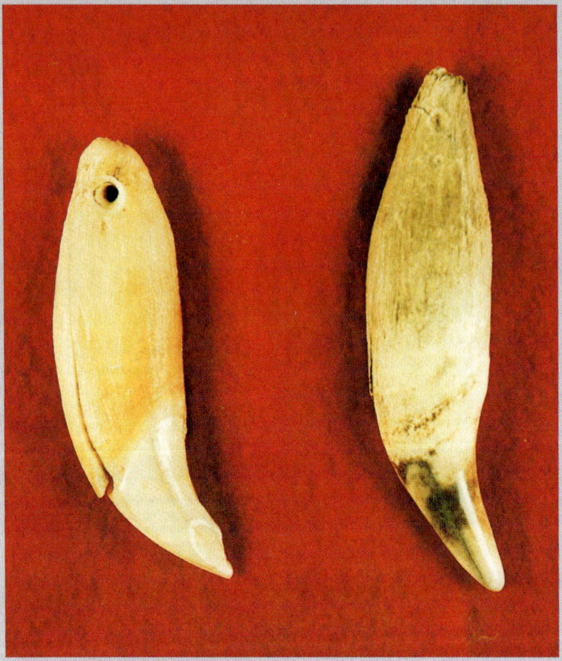

Bear teeth, both found in West Virginia. Left, drilled, 2¾". Right, drilling started. Private collection. Drilled tooth, **$85.00.** Other, **$45.00.**

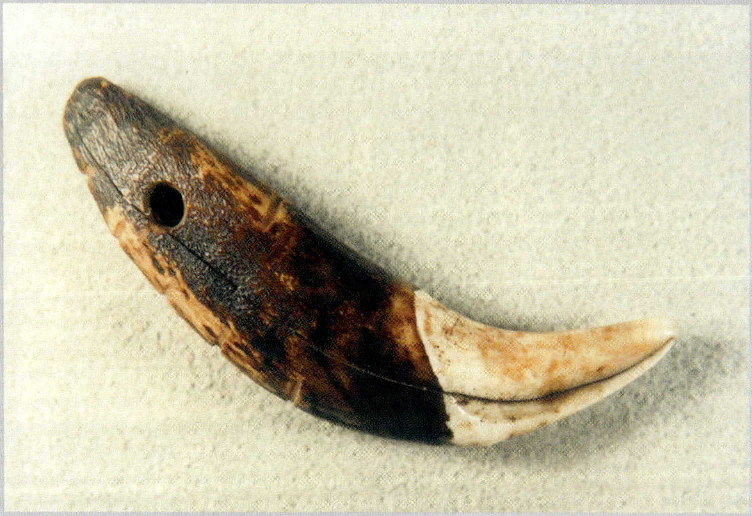

Black bear canine tooth, drilled for suspension, fracture crack from weather exposure. Tally marked on the edges, it was found along the Illinois River. La Salle County, Illinois. First Mesa, Indiana. **$85.00.**

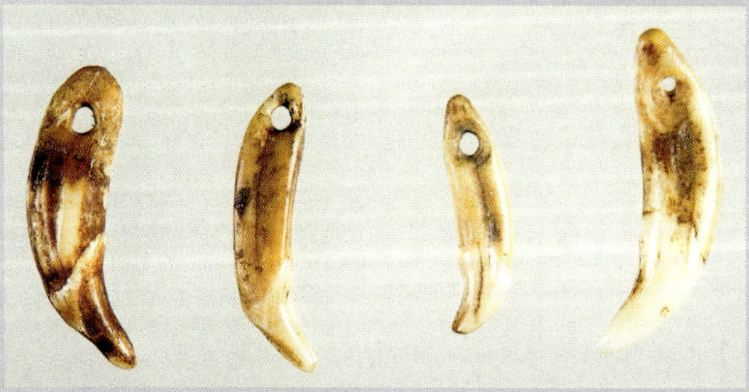

Pendants or necklace elements, dog or wolf judging by sizes, longest is 1⁷⁄₁₆". The example on left has been rounded at the top, and all are from the Vietzen collection. Ohio or Kentucky. Fred Winegardner collection. Each, **$15.00 – 20.00.**

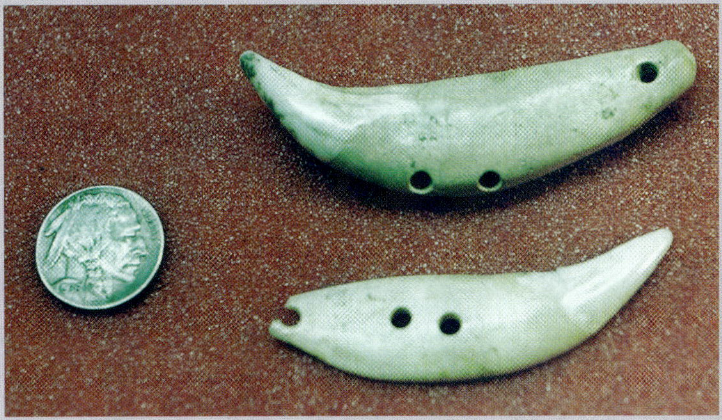

Drilled canine teeth, lower example a split mountain lion (cougar) tooth. The teeth have small drill-holes and may have been fastened to clothing. Origin unlisted. Fred Smith collection, Illinois. Each, **$125.00 – 175.00.**

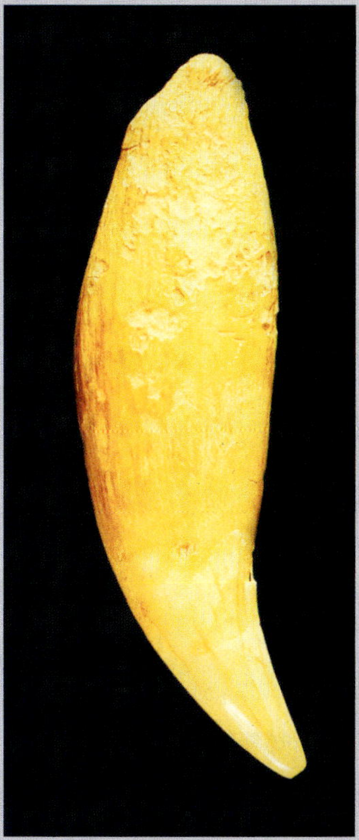

Bear tooth, quite large at 3⁵⁄₁₆". It was found on a prehistoric site in southeastern Illinois. Private collection. **$30.00.**

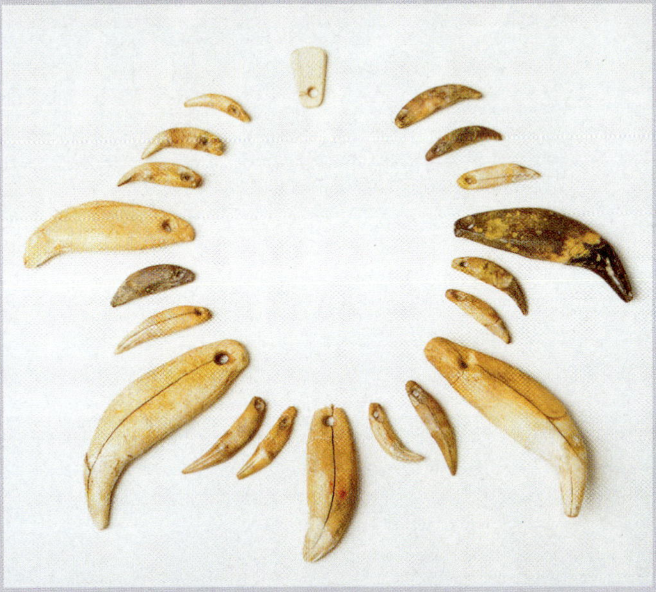

Necklace elements, bear and bobcat teeth. The largest bear tooth is 3" long and all teeth are drilled for suspension. These are from Tennessee. Robert Palmer collection, Georgia. Bear teeth, **$40.00 – 85.00;** bobcat teeth, **$20.00 – 30.00.**

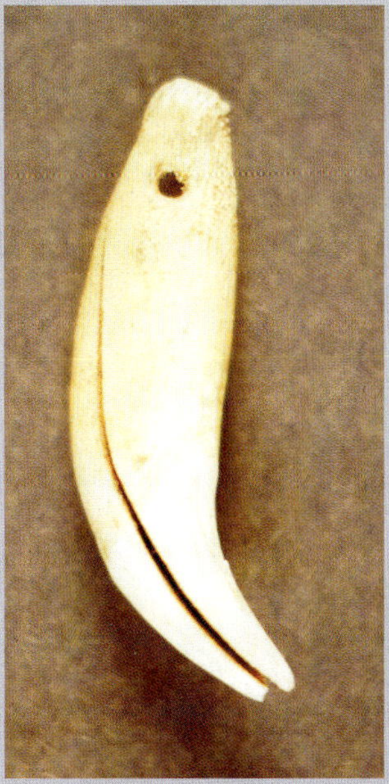

Bear tooth, drilled near root end, 2¼" long. It was found in Nicholas County, Kentucky. Larry Garvin collection. **$85.00.**

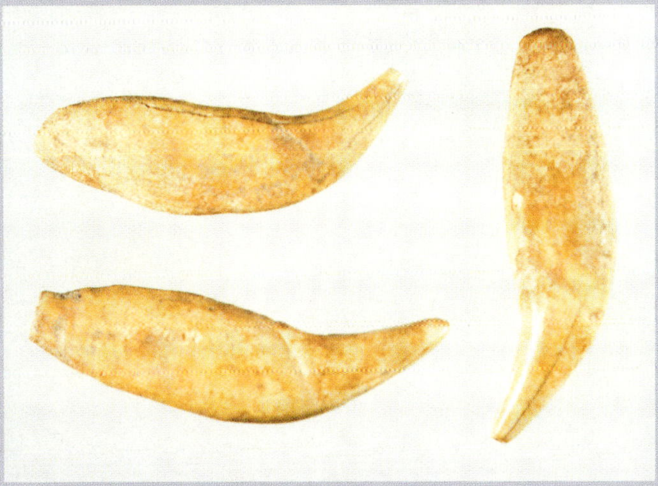

Bear teeth, longest is 2½", found on a late prehistoric site. The examples may have been for decorative objects, though there is a suggestion such teeth were used for delicate flint-knapping purposes. Ohio. Private collection. Each, **$15.00 – 20.00.**

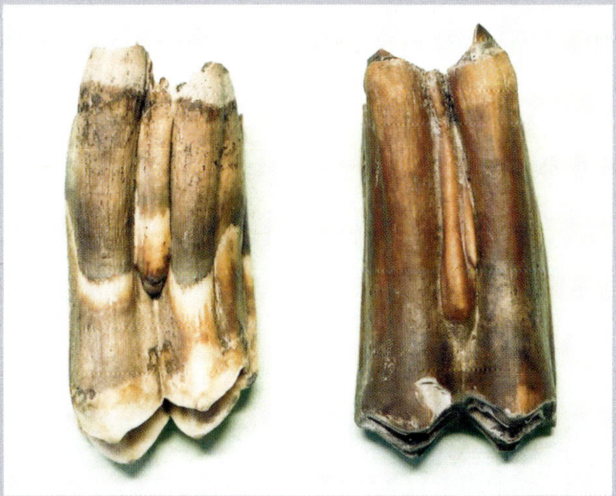

Bison teeth, from a medium-sized to large butchered bison, each tooth is 1¼ x 2½" long, ⅞" thick. The teeth were found in Box Elder County, northern Utah. Dann Russell collection, Utah. Each, **$25.00.**

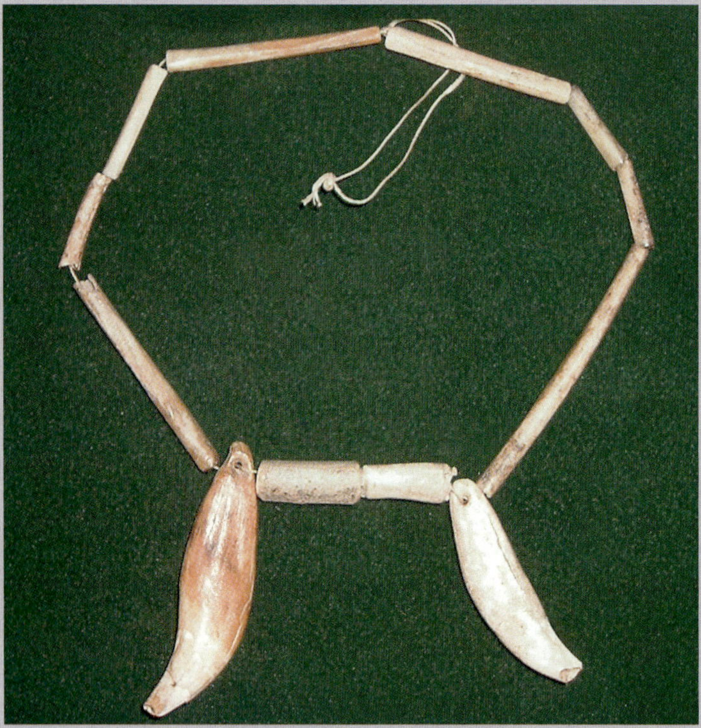

Necklace, hollow bird bones and bear teeth, 14" long. These have a Davis COA and came from Kentucky. Keith and Rhonda Dodge collection, Michigan. **$450.00.**

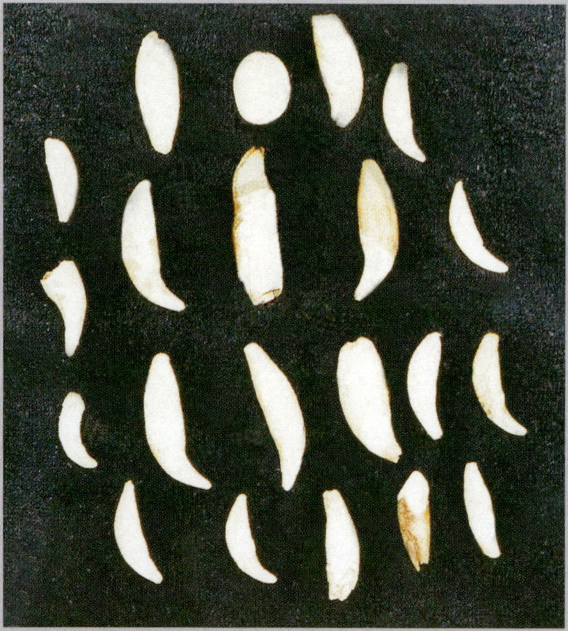

Teeth from Arkansas sites, bear teeth 2 to 2½" long and one alligator tooth (straighter tooth at upper center). All were found in northwestern Arkansas. Kenneth Hamilton collection, Arkansas. Unlisted.

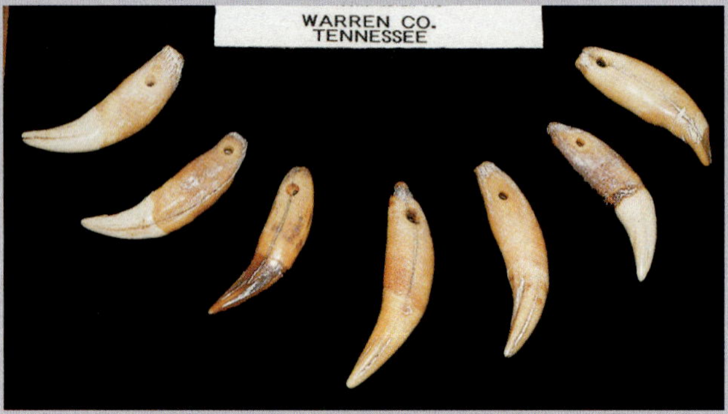

Bear teeth, all drilled for suspension and in fine condition. They were found in a rock shelter in Warren County, Tennessee. Back to Earth. Unlisted.

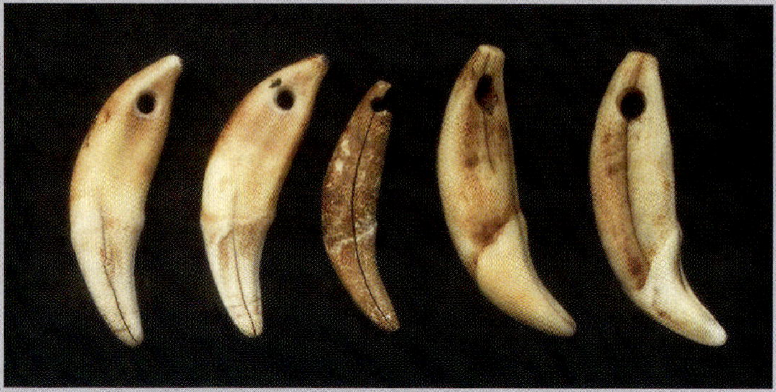

Pendants, Archaic to later, black bear canine teeth. The largest is ½ x 1¾". Ex-collection Levy, origin unknown. Collection of, and photograph by, Gary Henry, North Carolina. Each, **$25.00.**

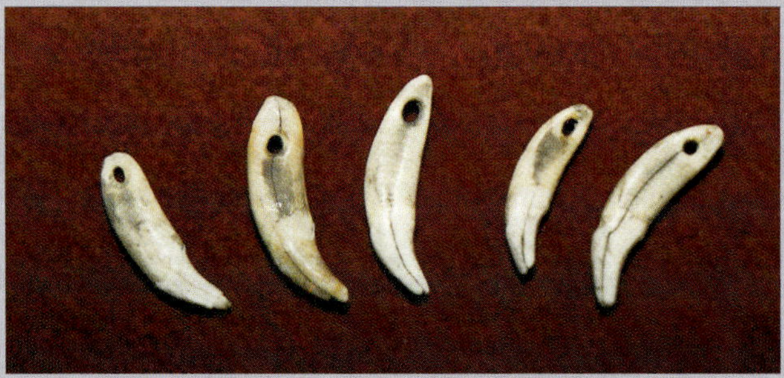

Canine teeth, drilled, frame size is 5 x 6". The teeth are ex-collection Vietzen, from Christian County, Kentucky. Back to Earth. **$145.00.**

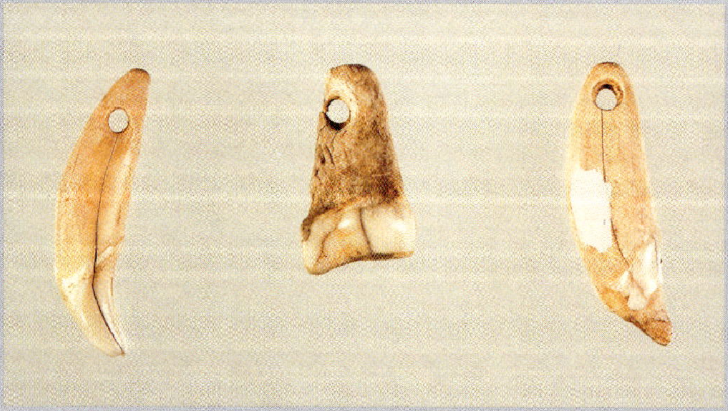

Drilled teeth, wolf or dog to left and right, deer or elk at center. The longest tooth is 1¼". All are from West Virginia. Doug Hooks collection. Each, **$15.00 – 25.00.**

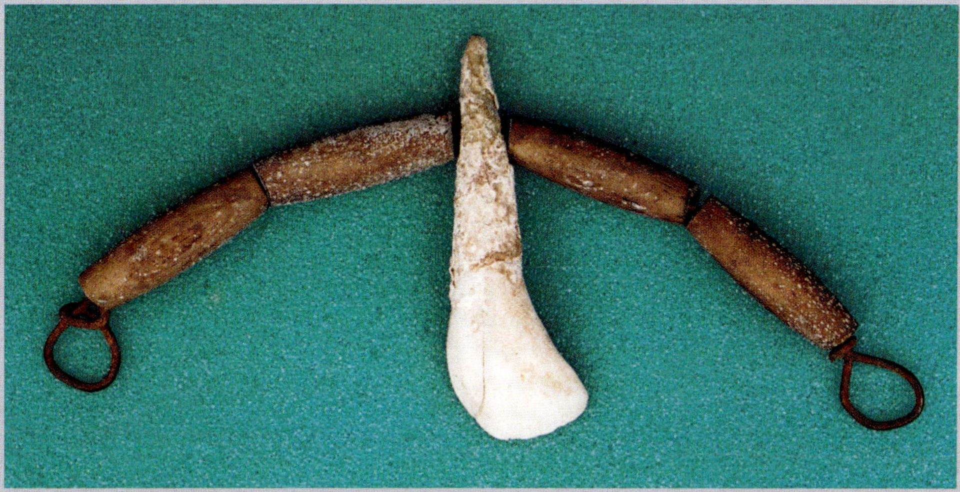

Decorative piece, four hair-pipe bone beads strung on wire and shell pendant, pendant size is 7/16 x 2". This is from historic times. Ex-collection Levy, origin unknown. Collection of, and photograph by, Gary Henry, North Carolina. **$75.00.**

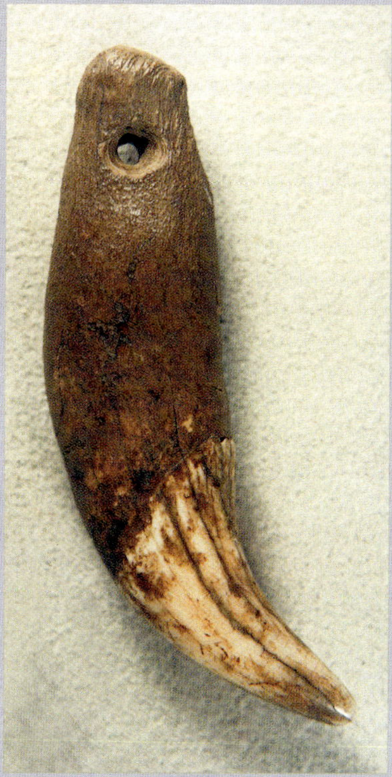

Black bear canine tooth, good age patina, drilled for suspension. It was found in the early 1900s. Posey County, Indiana. First Mesa, Indiana. **$185.00.**

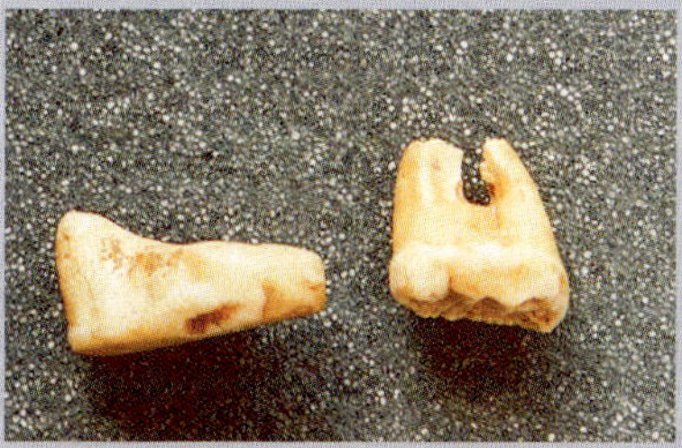

Bear molars, both worked, one ground flat to resemble a human foot and the other drilled at the roots. Once in the 1930s Whipple collection, these artifacts are Iroquois, ca. AD 1540-1560. The foot effigy is 1" long, and both were found near Richmond Mills. Ontario County, New York. Dave Summers collection, Victor, New York. Drilled tooth, **$60.00;** foot effigy, **$100.00.**

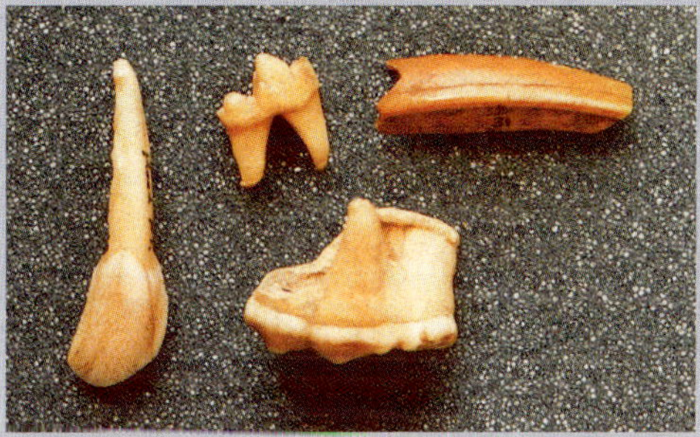

Animal teeth, ex-collection Wray, 5/8" to 1¼" long. They are, from the 9 o'clock position, deer, fox, beaver, and elk(?). All are from Iroquois sites (ca. AD 1540-1560), and were found near Richmond Mills, Ontario County, New York. Dave Summers collection, Victor, New York. Each, **$5.00.**

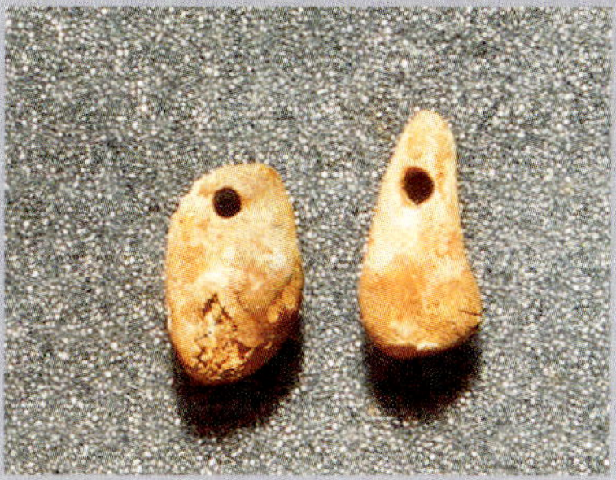

Elk canine teeth, drilled for suspension, historic Iroquois (Seneca), ca. AD 1675 – 1687, 7/8" and 1" long. These were found at a site near Victor, and were preserved by copper salts. Ontario County, New York. Dave Summers collection, Victor, New York. Each, **$40.00.**

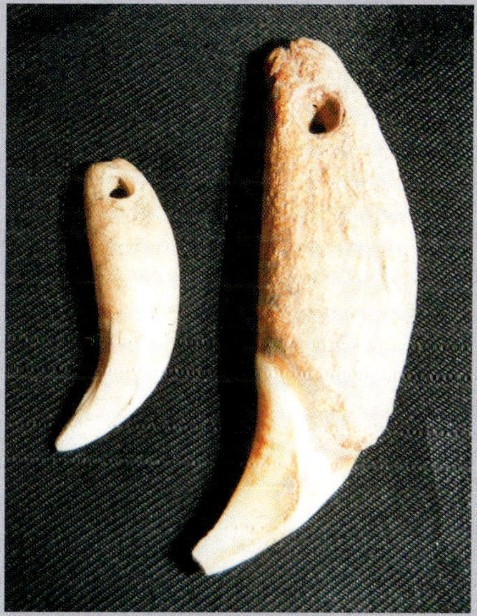

Canine teeth, the larger one is a bear tooth, drilled, Fort Ancient aspect. These were found in Mason County, Kentucky. Back to Earth. Each, **$125.00.**

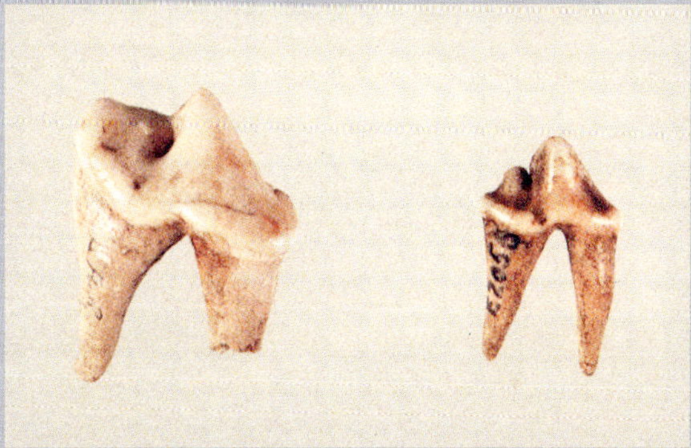

Teeth, village midden finds. The larger tooth is marked as a bear tooth and is 1 5/16" high. Both are Fort Ancient, from southern Ohio. Private collection. Each, **$2.00 – 5.00.**

Teeth and Ivory

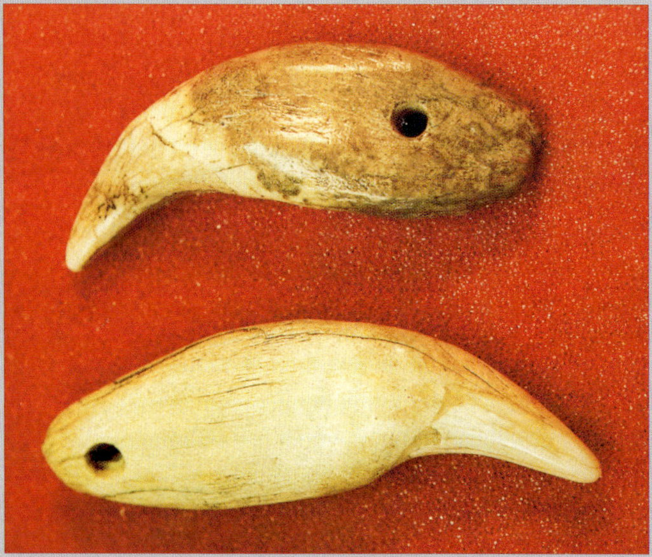

Pendants or necklace elements, drilled bear teeth. These are carefully drilled and the teeth are polished and in good condition. Fulton County, Illinois. Fred Smith collection, Illinois. Each, **$100.00 – 150.00.**

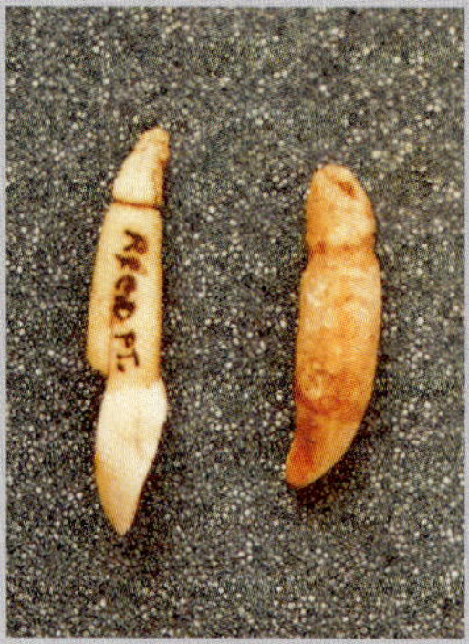

Pendants, grooved teeth, deer on left and dog(?) on right, they are 1½ and 1¼" long, respectively. Used by the Iroquois (ca. AD 1540-1560), the deer tooth is from near Richmond Mills, Ontario County, New York, while the dog canine is from near Canandaigua, also Ontario County. Dave Summers collection, Victor, New York. Each, **$30.00.**

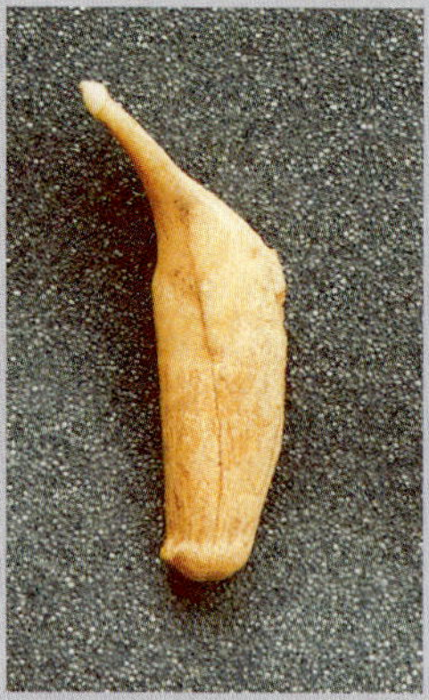

Bear incisor tool, much of tooth ground away, 2³⁄₁₆" long. Middle Archaic and Lamoka phase, it was found in Schuyler County, New York. Dave Summers collection, Victor, New York. **$50.00.**

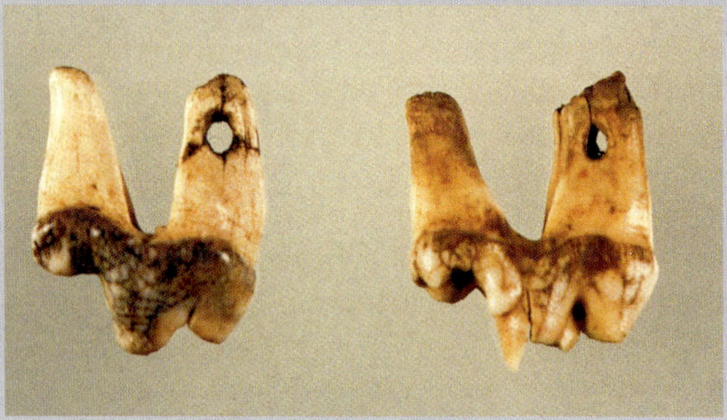

Black bear teeth, drilled for suspension, widest tooth is 1⅛". Ex-collection Tolliver, they are from Hocking County, Ohio. Private collection. Each, **$40.00 – 50.00.**

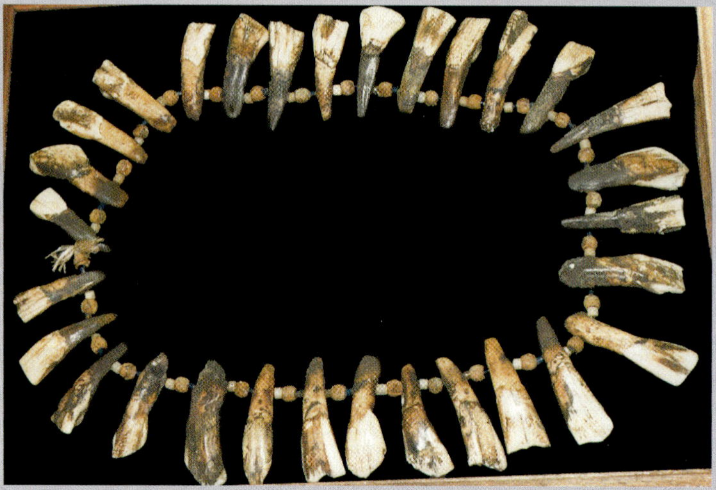

Plains Indian necklace, with bison front teeth and spacers of brass and glass beads. Frame size for this example is 9 x 12". Back to Earth. **$450.00.**

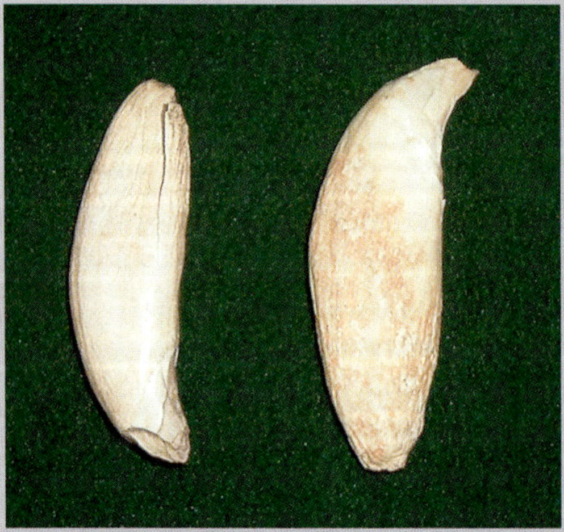

Bear teeth, 2 and 2½" long, respectively. Ex-collection Noel, the teeth were picked up in Kentucky. Keith and Rhonda Dodge collection, Michigan. Each, **$40.00 – 65.00.**

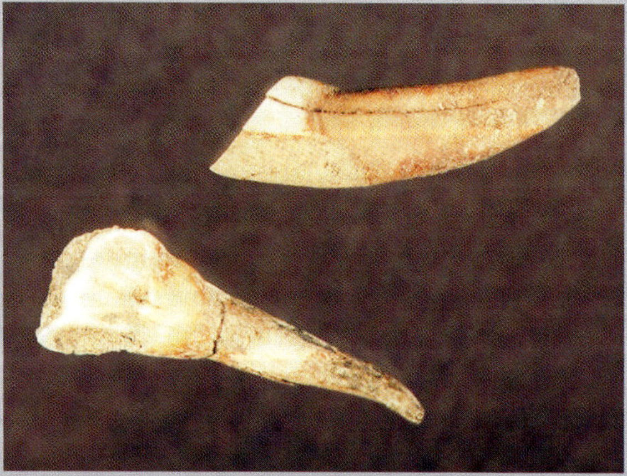

Deer teeth, unmodified, longer one is 1½". These were found at a Fort Ancient (late prehistoric) site in southern Ohio. Private collection. Each, **$1.00.**

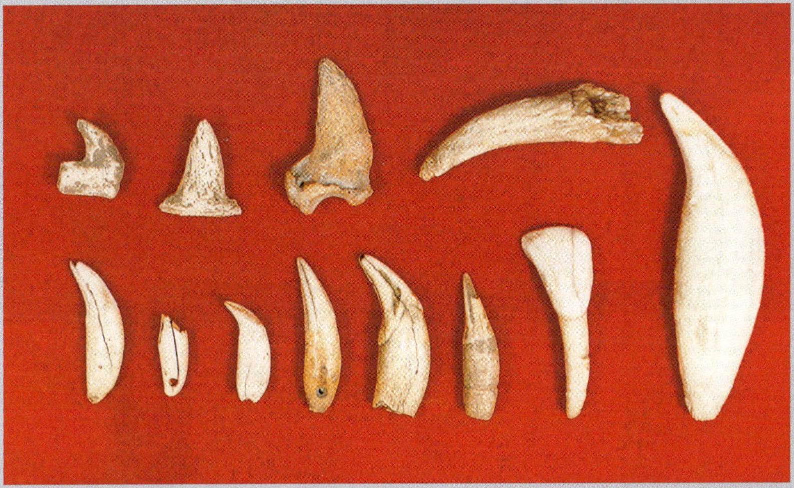

Pendant and necklace elements, Mississippian, from various sites in southern Ohio and Kentucky, all ex-collection Col. Raymond Vietzen. Top row, left to right: Cougar claw case; cut wild turkey spur; bear claw core; imitation bear tooth in antler; and, bear tooth, 3" long. Bottom row, left to right: Dog tooth with drilling started; unknown; unknown; drilled cougar tooth; cut and ground wolf tooth; cougar tooth which is cut, ground and grooved; grooved bison tooth. Pete Timoch collection. Each, **$25.00 – 50.00.**

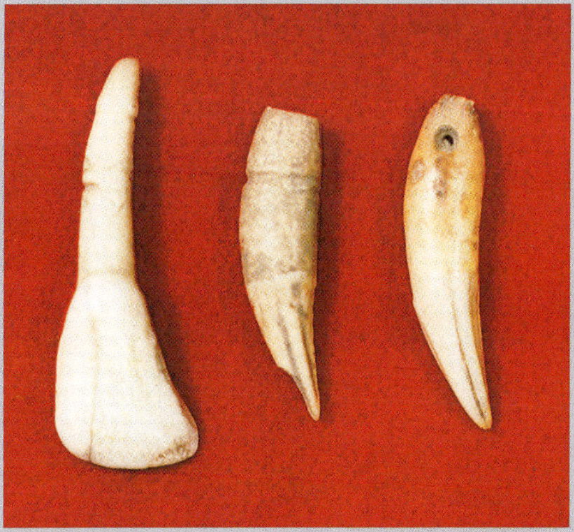

Closeup of grooved teeth, shown in previous photograph. All are ex-collection Vietzen, from southern Ohio and Kentucky. Left to right: Bison, $1\frac{3}{4}$"; cougar; and cougar, $1\frac{1}{2}$" long. Pete Timoch collection. Each, **$40.00 – 50.00.**

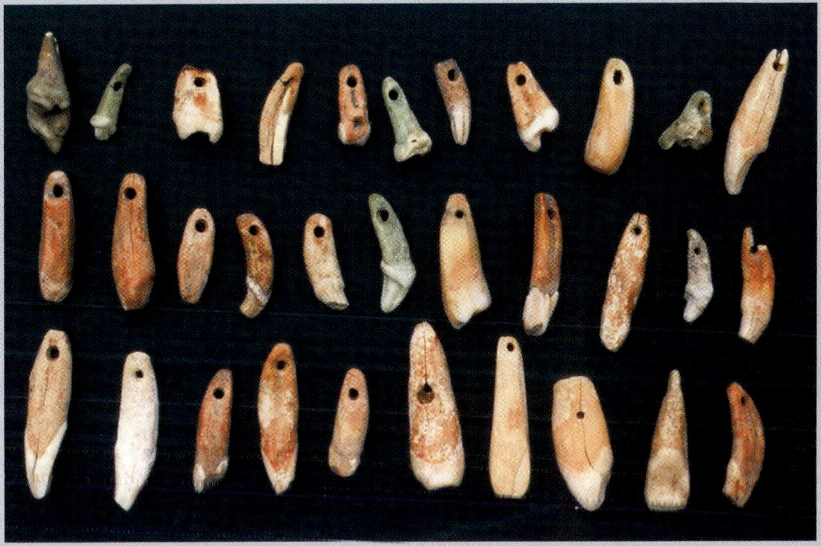

Pendants, mammal teeth, primarily incisors and canines, all drilled. Possibly Woodland period, the largest is $\frac{5}{16}$ x $1\frac{1}{16}$". These are ex-collection Levy, find-site unknown. Collection of, and photograph by, Gary Henry, North Carolina. Each, **$10.00 – 15.00.**

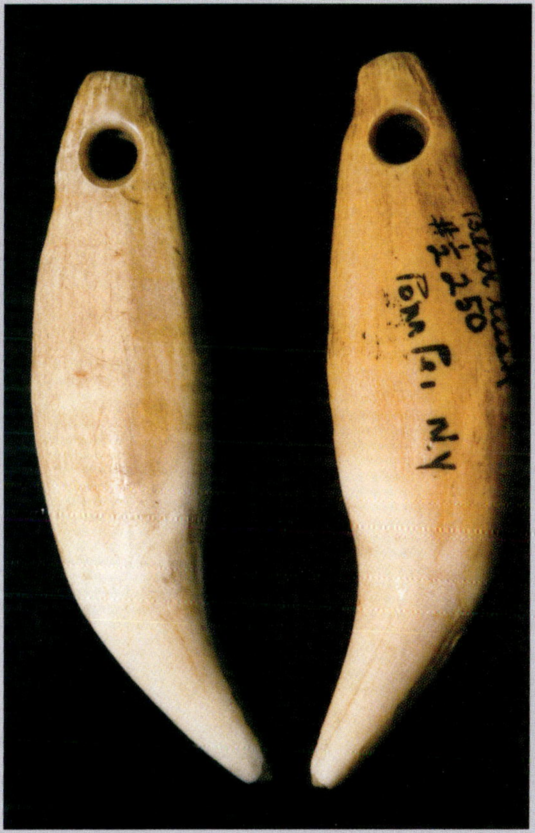

Bear tooth, drilled, front and back view, $2\frac{7}{8}$" long. This pendant was found at Pompey, Onondaga County, New York. Back to Earth. **$180.00 – 200.00.**

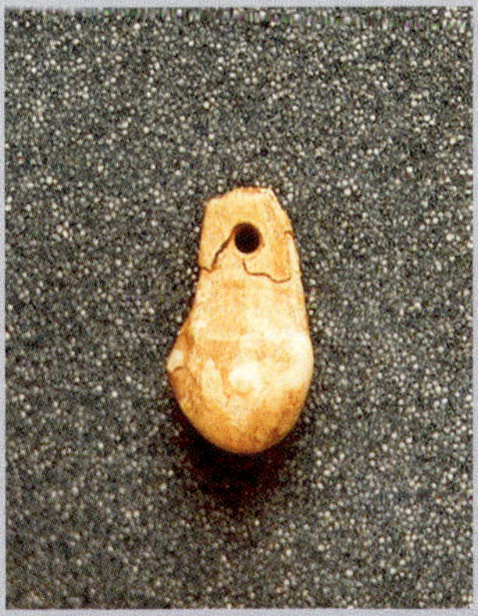

Imitation elk canine, bone, drilled near top, $1\frac{1}{8}$" long. It is Iroquois, ca. AD 1540-1560, and was found near Richmond Mills. Elk canines, two per animal, were sometimes scarce and copies were made in bone. This specimen is from near Richmond Mills, Ontario County, New York. Dave Summers collection, Victor, New York. **$65.00.**

Teeth and Ivory

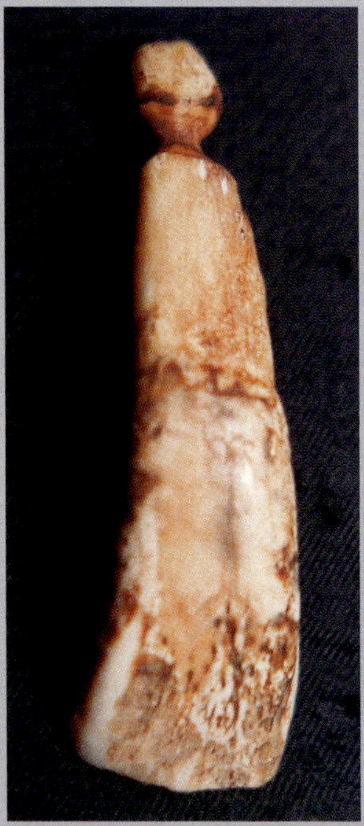

Pendant, bear incisor, grooved at top for cord attachment. Some example are drilled instead of being grooved. Back to Earth. Unlisted.

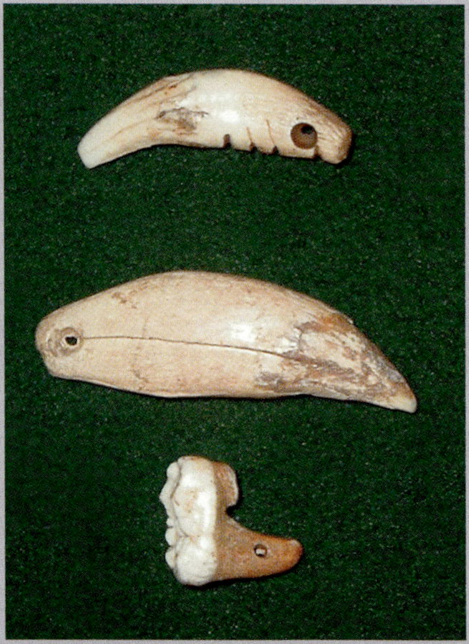

Drilled animal teeth, example at top (which may be a cougar tooth) shown below, this page. The others are bear teeth, drilled for suspension, and lengths are ¾" and 3½". Casey County, Kentucky. Keith and Rhonda Dodge collection, Michigan. Small tooth, **$50.00;** large canine, **$150.00;** cougar(?), **$150.00.**

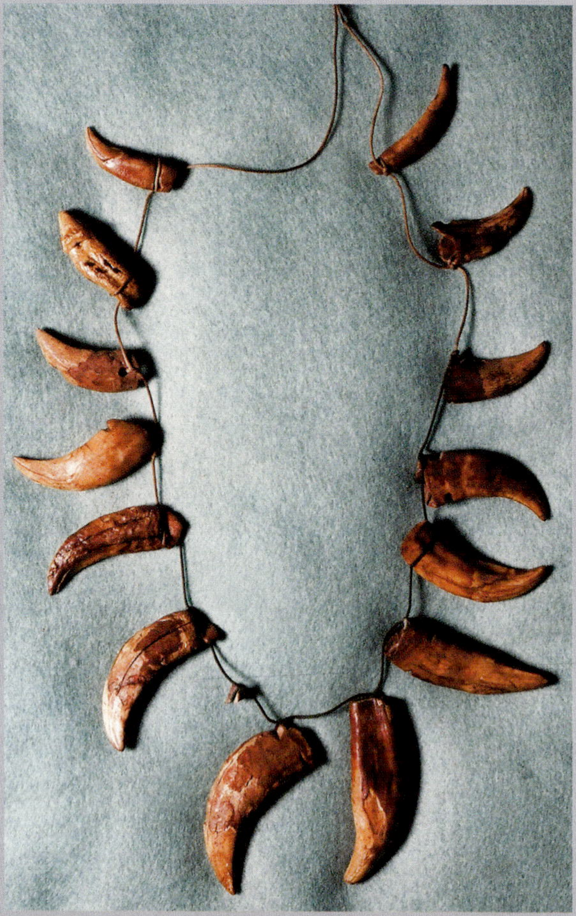

Teeth used as pendants or necklace elements, 13 bear canines and one (smallest) a dog or wolf tooth. One tooth is drilled and ten are notched. All were found in New York state. Private collection. Each, **$20.00 – 100.00.**

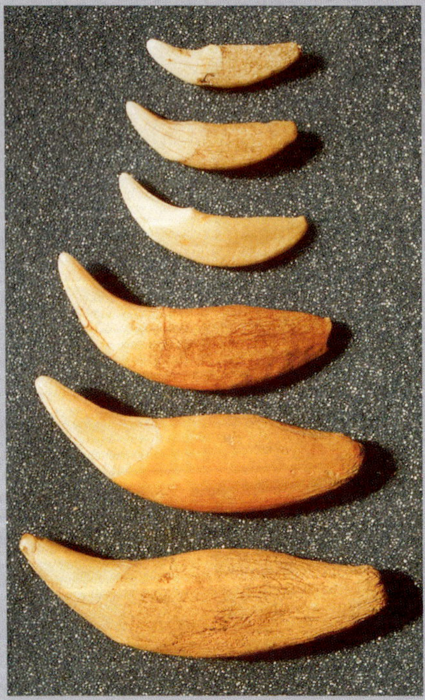

Bear canines, undrilled, from an historic Iroquois (Seneca) site dated AD 1650 – 1675. Bear teeth (these are from 1⅜ to 3" long) are often found on sites from Archaic to Contact times. They came from near Honeoye Falls, Monroe County, New York. Dave Summers collection, Victor, New York. Each, **$5.00 – 50.00.**

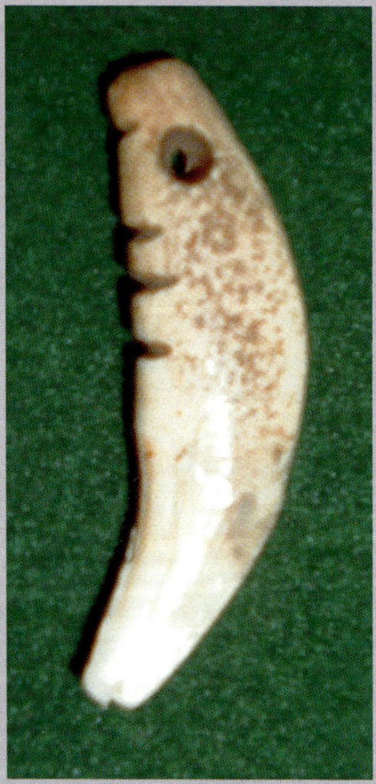

Drilled and tally marked animal tooth, 1¾" long. This pendant was found in Casey County, Kentucky. Keith and Rhonda Dodge collection, Michigan. **$150.00.**

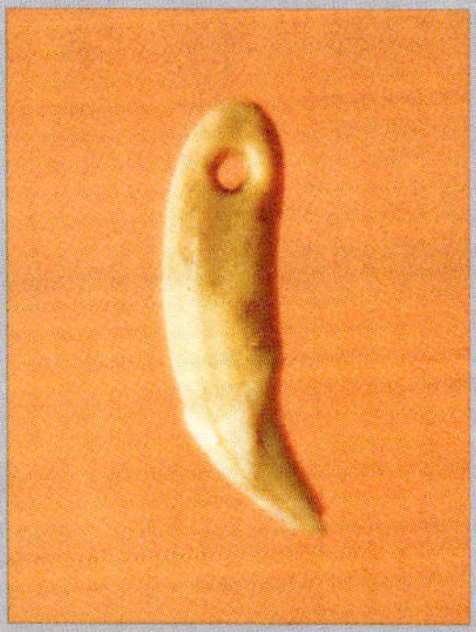

Lynx canine pendant, drilled for suspension, Late Archaic period, ex-collection Burch. The pendant is 1³⁄₁₆" long and was found near Cayuga Lake. Cayuga County, New York. Dave Summers collection, Victor, New York. **$55.00.**

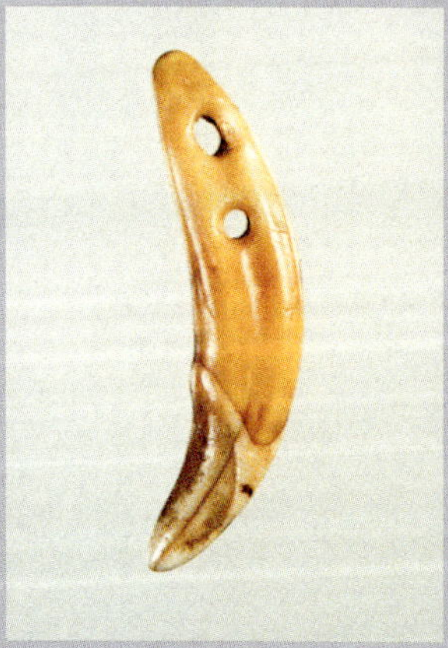

Pendant or necklace element, dog or wolf tooth, 1⁵⁄₁₆". This is an unusual example, with two drilled holes instead of one. It was once in the Vietzen collection and was found in Ohio or Kentucky. Fred Winegardner collection. Museum grade.

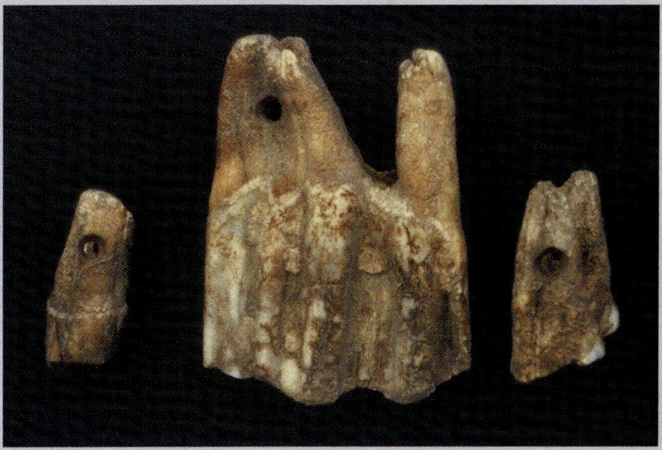

Pendants, possibly Woodland period, mammal molar teeth. The largest example is 1¾ x 2¼" and ⅝" thick. Drilled for attachment, they are ex-collection Levy. Origin is unknown. Collection of, and photograph by, Gary Henry, North Carolina. Each, **$25.00 – 50.00.**

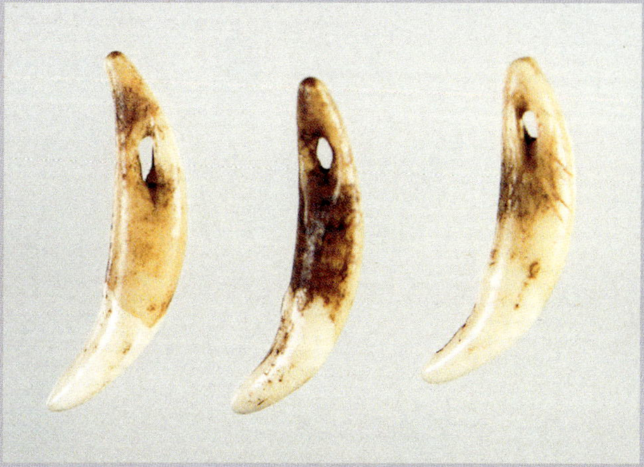

Pendant or necklace elements, average length just over 1⅜", elongated suspension holes instead of the typical round drill-mark. The holes have also been cut to create a wider surface opening. They are from the Vietzen collection, and were obtained in Ohio or Kentucky. Fred Winegardner collection. Each, **$15.00.**

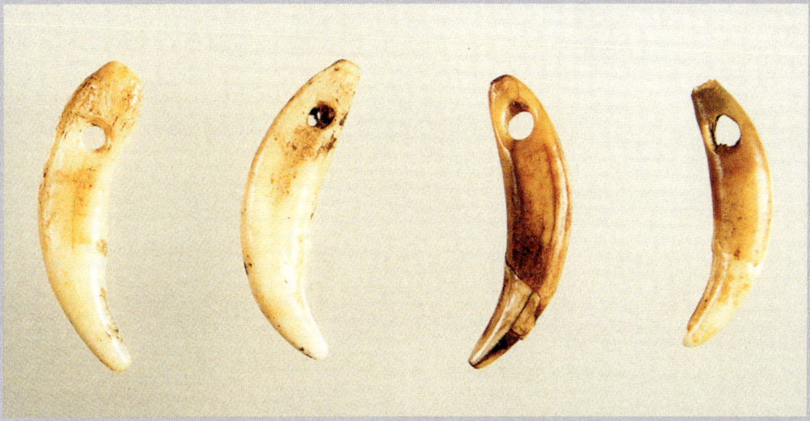

Pendant or necklace elements, longest is 1½". The different patination on the examples is of interest, also the varied drill-hole sizes. All are from the Vietzen collection. Ohio or Kentucky. Fred Winegardner collection. Each, **$15.00.**

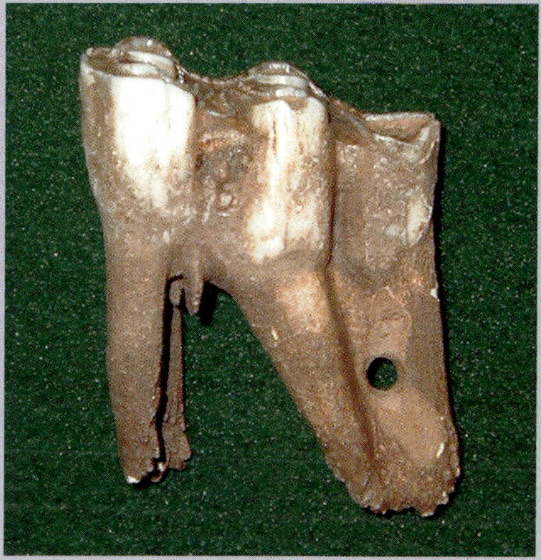

Mammal tooth, drilled for suspension, ex-collection Noel. It is 1½ x 2", from Kentucky. Keith and Rhonda Dodge collection, Michigan. **$75.00.**

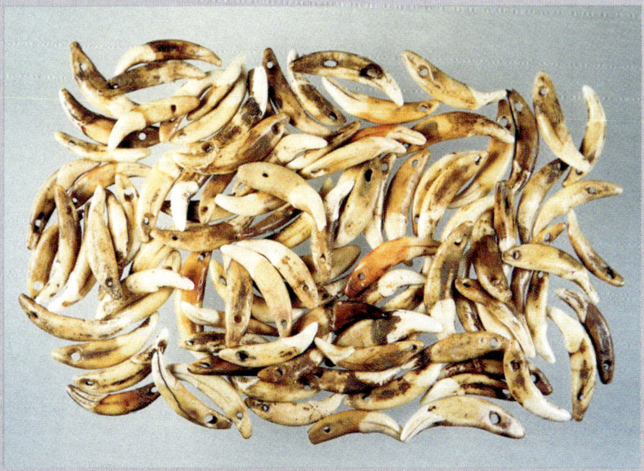

Pendants or necklace elements, probably dog or fox, longest is 1⅜". Despite the number shown, drilled animal teeth are not common. These were formerly in the Vietzen collection and are from Ohio or Kentucky. Fred Winegardner collection. Each, **$15.00 – 25.00.**

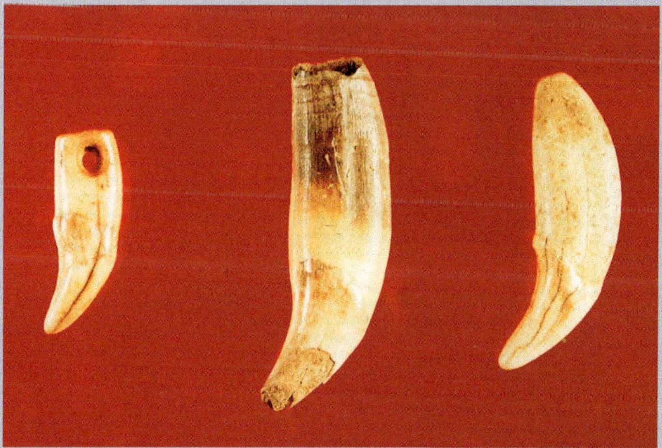

Prehistoric site material, all in a private collection and from Illinois. Left, drilled dog or wolf tooth, 1⅛" long, **$15.00.** Center, bear tooth, **$10.00.** Right, probably a wolf tooth. **$5.00.**

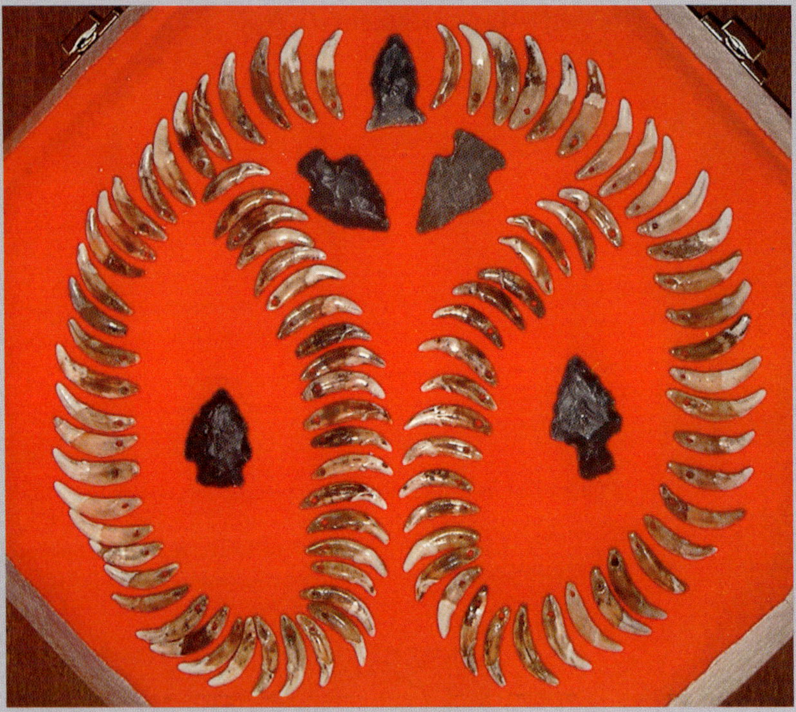

Canine tooth pendants or necklace elements, each 1½ to 1¾" long. They are ex-collection Vietzen and Parker, and came from Glover's Cave. Christian County, Kentucky. Keith and Rhonda Dodge collection, Michigan. Each tooth, **$15.00 – 20.00.**

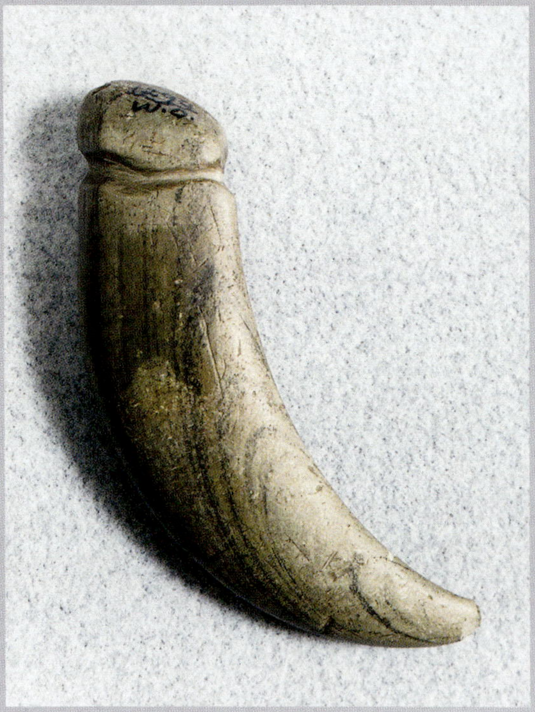

Effigy of a claw or talon, banded slate, 7 cm long. It was probably salvaged from a broken bannerstone. Manchester area, Ohio. Private collection. **$175.00.**

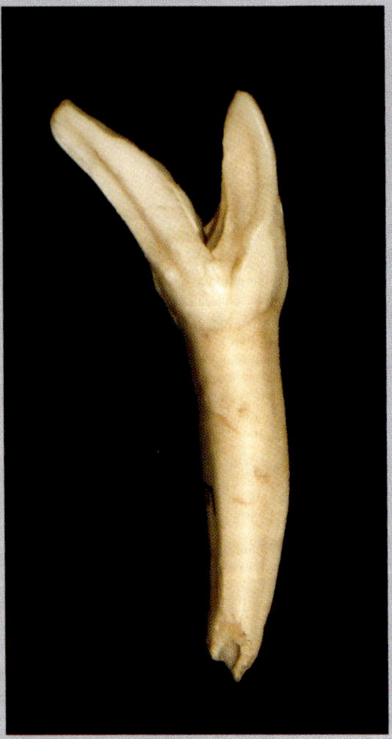

Tooth, 1½", ex-collection Beck. This highly different tooth has a root about an inch long and the tip was worked on an angle. Possibly a woods buffalo incisor, it is from the Bedford area, Pennsylvania. Tom Sekula collection, Pennsylvania. Unlisted.

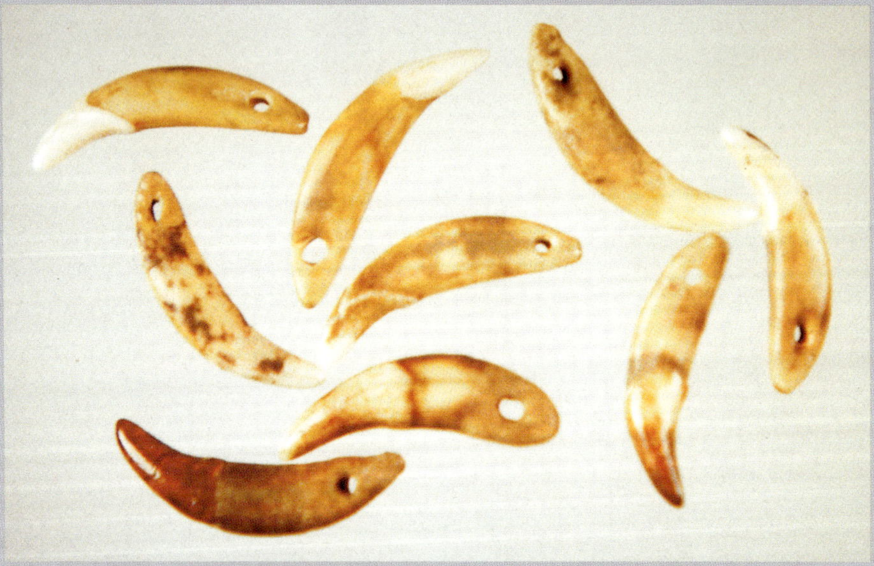

Drilled canine teeth, wolf or large dog, ex-collection Vietzen. The teeth average 1½" long and came from Christian County, Kentucky. Back to Earth. Each, **$15.00 – 20.00.**

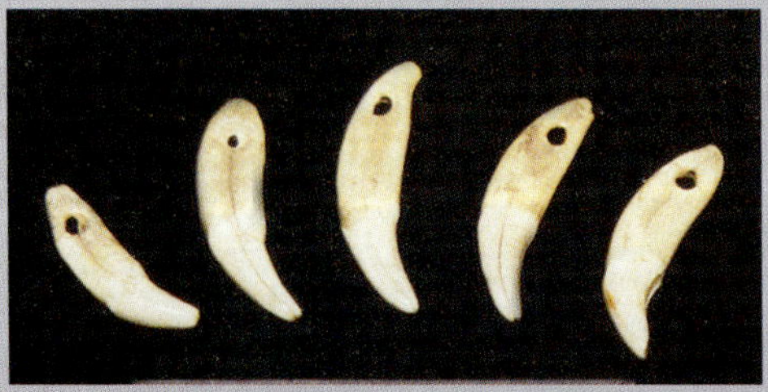

Drilled canine teeth, ex-collection Vietzen, frame size is 5 x 6". The artifacts were found in Christian County, Kentucky. Back to Earth. **$145.00.**

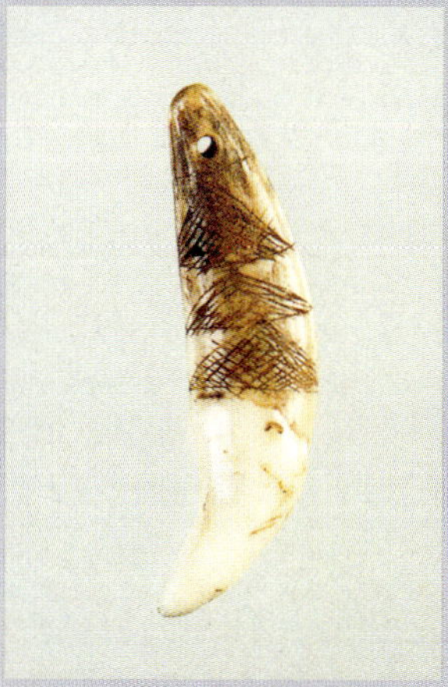

Pendant or necklace element, dog or wolf tooth, 1⁵⁄₁₆" long. This is a rare example, with incised and cross-hatched wide triangles on each face. It is from the Vietzen collection and came from Ohio or Kentucky. Fred Winegardner collection. Museum grade.

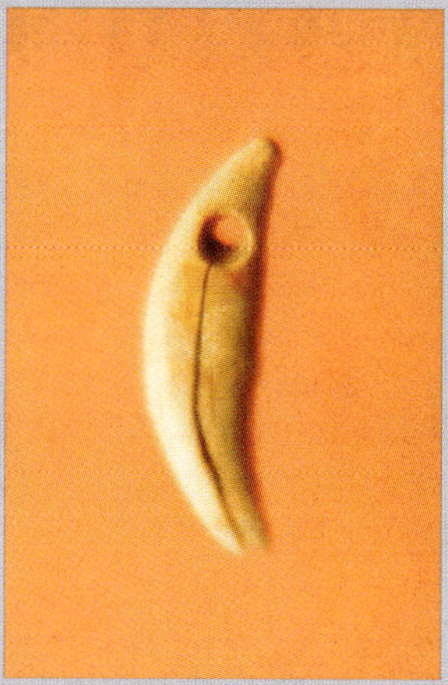

Wolf canine pendant, perforated, Frontenac phase of the Late Archaic, ca. 2000 BC. It is 1⁵⁄₁₆" long, ex-collection Burch, from near Cayuga Lake, Cayuga County, New York. Dave Summers collection, Victor, New York. **$60.00.**

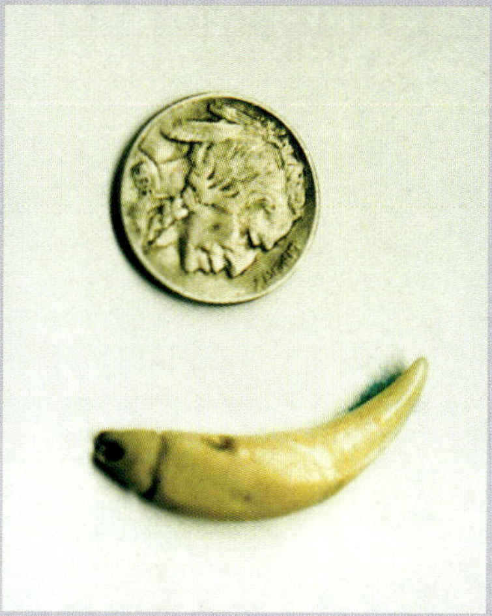

Dog or coyote canine tooth, unusual because it is both drilled and grooved for suspension. It is 1⅝" long. Fulton County, Illinois. Fred Smith collection, Illinois. **$50.00.**

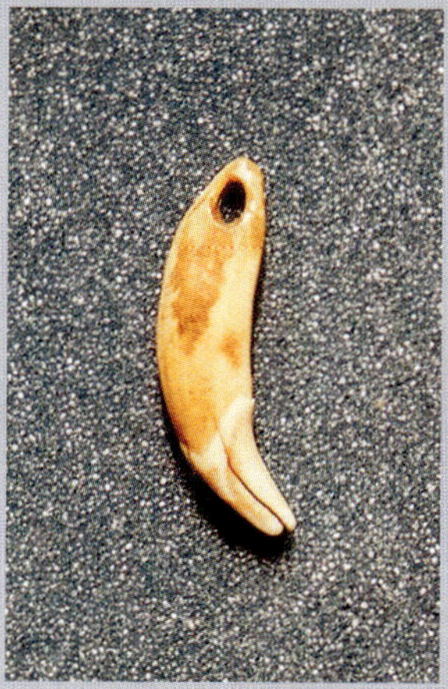

Black bear canine tooth, perforated, 1⅜" long, ex-collection Burch. Point Peninsula and Hopewell phases of the Middle Woodland, it is from near Van Buren, Onondaga County, New York. Dave Summers collection, Victor, New York. Unlisted.

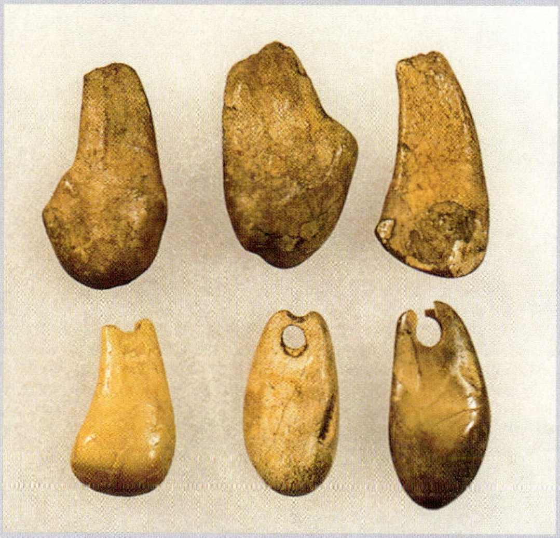

Elk teeth, lower examples drilled and polished, longest is 1¹⁄₁₆". These were in the Vietzen collection and are Mississippian in time. Northern Ohio. Pete Timoch collection. Drilled teeth, each **$25.00 – 50.00.**

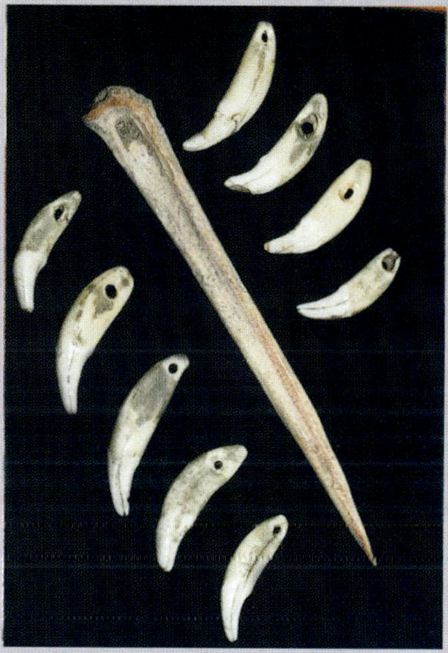

Drilled canine teeth and fine bone awl, 5" long. These were found by Col. Vietzen and came from Christian County, Kentucky. Back to Earth. **$350.00.**

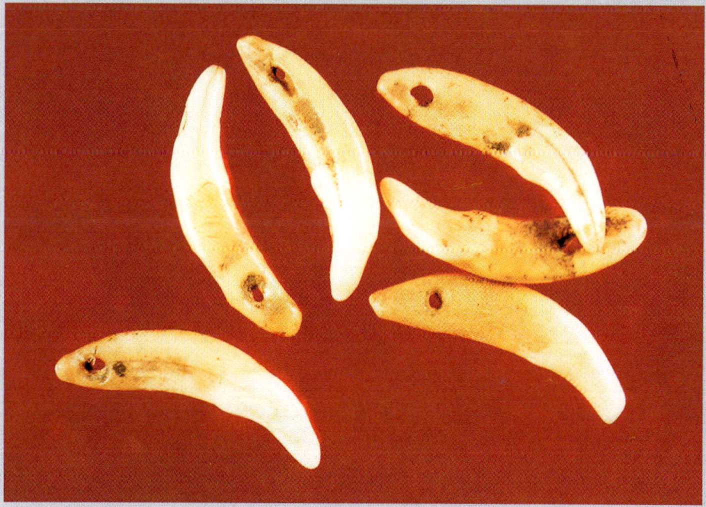

Animal teeth, drilled for suspension as pendants or necklace elements, longest is 1¼". Most specimens have a high polish. Kentucky. Private collection. Each, **$15.00.**

Eskimo (Inuit) Artifacts

The people of the North probably used bone, antler, and ivory more than any other American cultural group. The materials were a major part of the Inuit way of life, and had been for thousands of years. This continues to the present, and native artists and cooperatives turn out fine work. Older artifacts, both from prehistoric and historic times, are in great demand by astute collectors. This is because the material is somewhat different, the work is high quality, and the style is both individual and culturally distinct.

Bones, teeth, and tusks of land and sea animals were used, including deer, caribou, seal, whale, and walrus, among others. The artifacts, some of them unique to the Inuit, include many fittings for watercraft, food preparation, hunting and fishing gear, and tools for coping with a sometimes-harsh environment. These might be bone drill bows and shafts, harpoons of an almost endless variety, spear and arrow points, clothing buttons and fasteners, reindeer and caribou tooth decorations, ivory and bone labrets (lip ornaments), Atl-atl hooks or stops, combs made of bone and ivory, bundle and box handles, box lids, walrus tusk pipes, spoons and ladles, plain and decorated awls, ulu (household knife) handles, gambling pieces, small effigies of birds and animals, fish lures and hooks, and even bone strips for armor and sled runner edges.

Other Inuit artifacts, in bone and occasionally ivory, are earrings and pendants, bag and bladder plugs, snow knives, hunting and butchering knife handles, net mesh gauges, boat hooks, and snow goggles. Walrus tusk cribbage boards were made in more recent times, and many are etched with hunting scenes. Inuit art and artifacts are both easily recognized and readily appreciated.

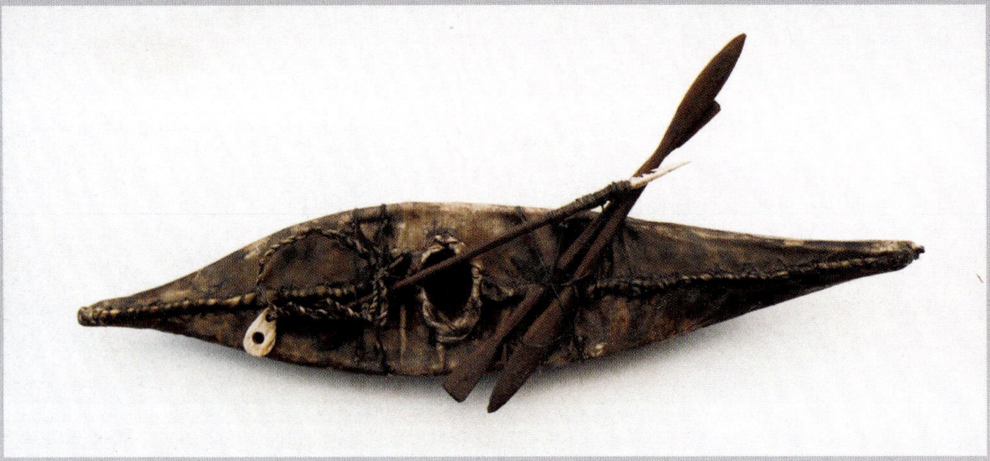

Toy kayak, historic, sealskin and sinew. The harpoon point and float are made of ivory, and the kayak is 2⅞ x 14". It is from Alaska. Collection of, and photograph by, Gary Henry, North Carolina. **$150.00.**

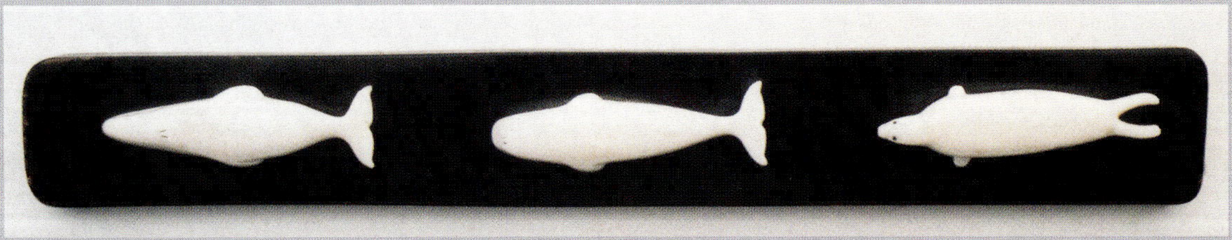

Ivory animals on wood, recent or contemporary. The animals are, left to right, bowhead whale, Pacific bottlenose dolphin, and a bearded seal. The plaque is 1⅛ x 9⅛" long and the animals are 2⅛" long. Eskimo, from Alaska. Collection of, and photograph by, Gary Henry, North Carolina. **$100.00.**

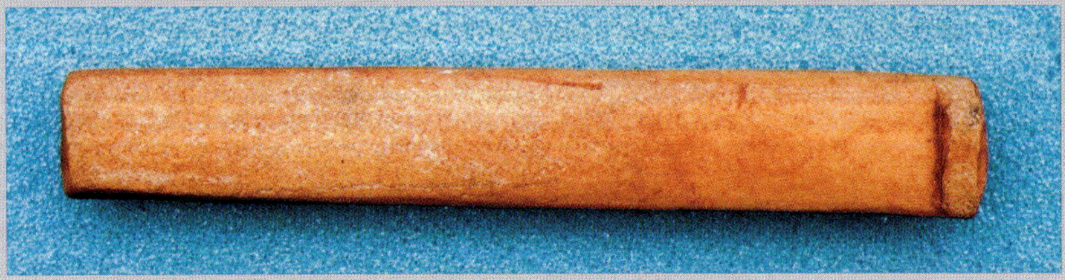

Bone artifact, prehistoric(?), incised on one side, ½ x 3 7/16". Of unknown use, it is ex-collection Cantrell and came from Alaska. Collection of, and photograph by, Gary Henry, North Carolina. **$20.00.**

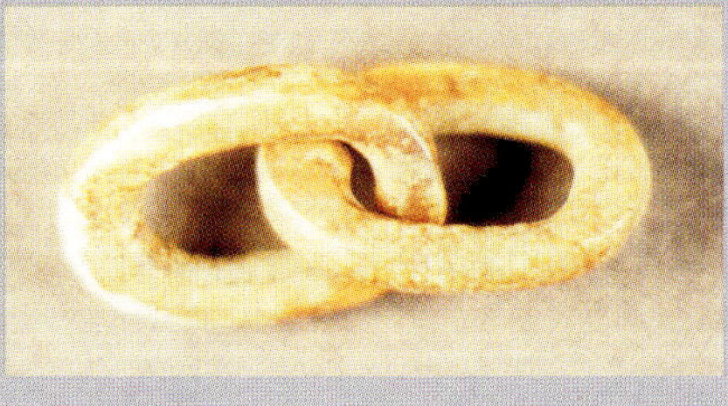

Ivory links, perhaps for sled dog harness or for pulling game, total length is 1¾". This artifact came from Alaska. Larry Garvin collection. **$45.00.**

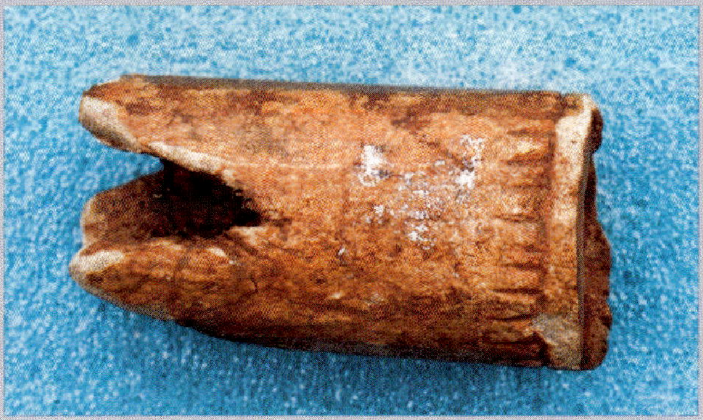

Notched bone bead, prehistoric(?), engraved around opposite end, ⅝ x 1¼". Ex-collection Cantrell, it is from Alaska. Collection of, and photograph by, Gary Henry, North Carolina. **$20.00.**

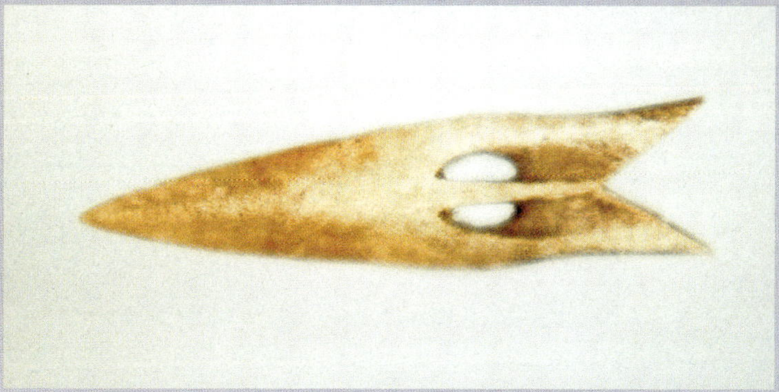

Harpoon tip, stained bone, 2½" long. With opposing barbs and cord holes, this piece came from Alaska. Larry Garvin collection. **$85.00.**

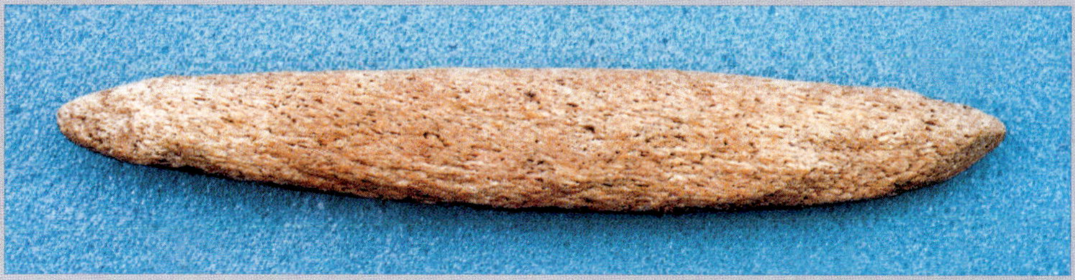

Bone pin or flaking tool, prehistoric(?), 9⁄16 x 3 15⁄16", 5⁄16" thick. This piece is ex-collection Cordeiro and came from Alaska. Collection of, and photograph by, Gary Henry, North Carolina. **$15.00.**

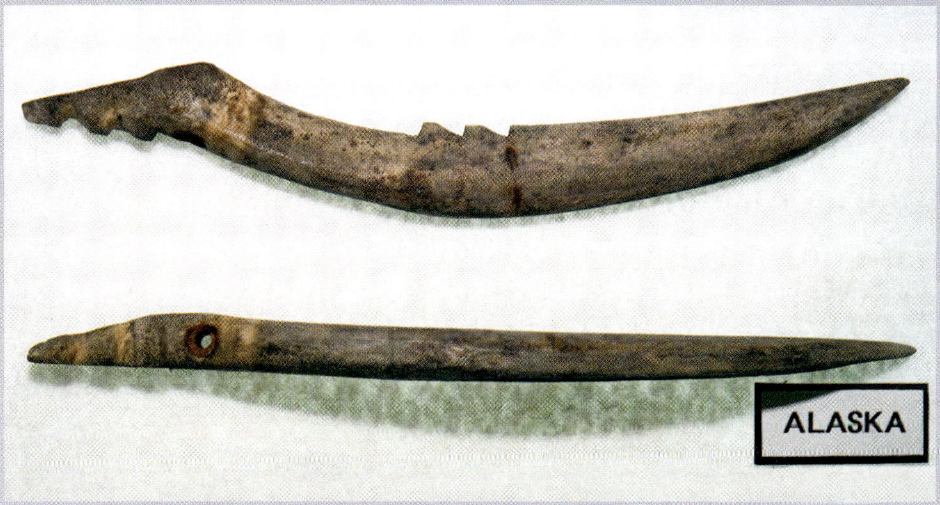

Artifact of unknown use, side and bottom views, with notches on the incurvate edges plus fastening notches and a single drilled hole at the non-pointed end. A possible ice pick head, it is 7½" long. (Note the similarities of this piece to the four much-smaller artifacts (single photograph) from Pennsylvania shown on page 215.) St. Lawrence Island, Alaska. Back to Earth. **$135.00 – 150.00.**

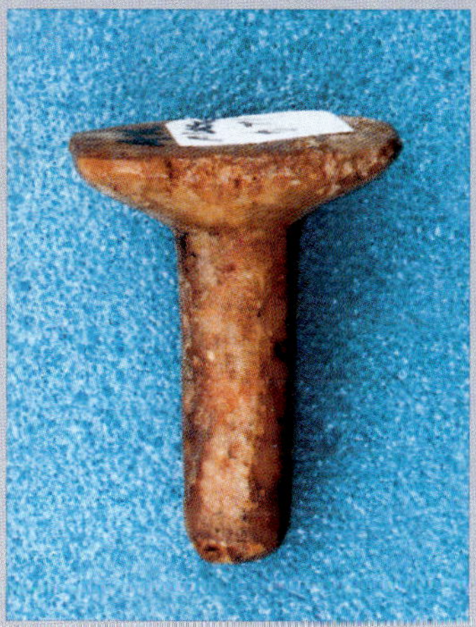

Lip plug (labret), prehistoric(?), walrus ivory, ¾ x 1" long. This piece is ex-collection Cordeiro, from Alaska. Collection of, and photograph by, Gary Henry, North Carolina. **$50.00.**

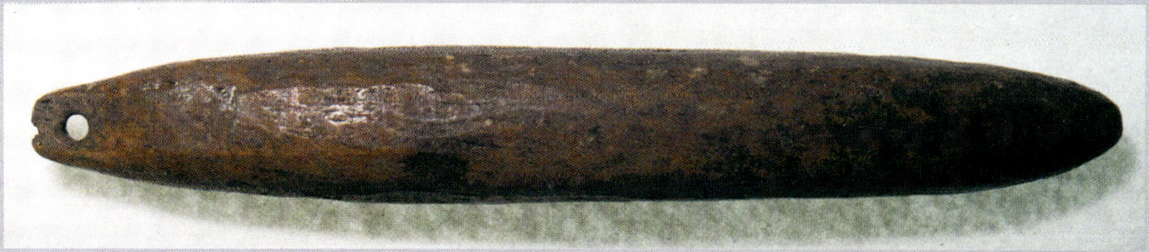

Bone artifact, 6¾" long, mineralized and patinated. This may have been a bolas weight, sinker, or part of a lure. St. Lawrence Island, Alaska. Back to Earth. **$145.00 – 160.00.**

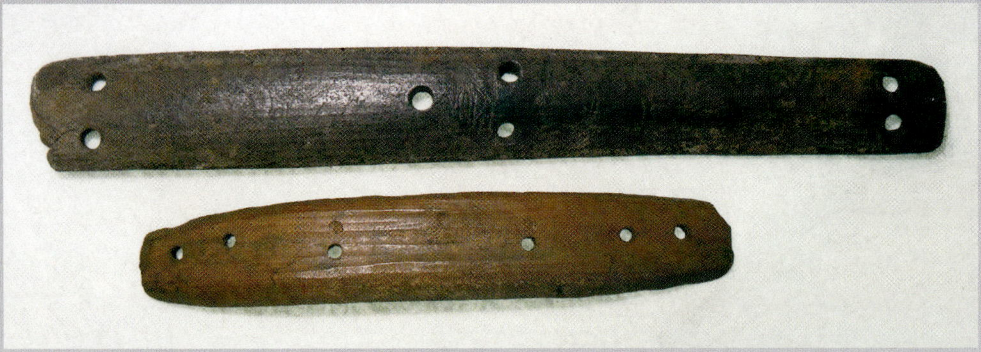

Body armor, with multiple drilled attachment holes, both mineralized to different degrees. The example with seven holes is 9⅝" long while the section with six holes is 6¼" long. Both are from St. Lawrence Island, Alaska. Back to Earth. Larger, **$135.00 – 150.00;** smaller, **$80.00 – 100.00.**

Bone body armor, section is 5" long, with large drilled attachment holes. Prehistoric, it is from St. Lawrence Island, Alaska. Back to Earth. **$125.00 – 150.00.**

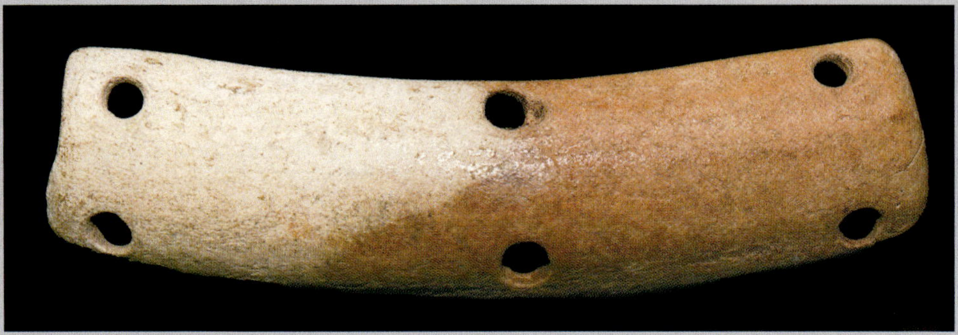

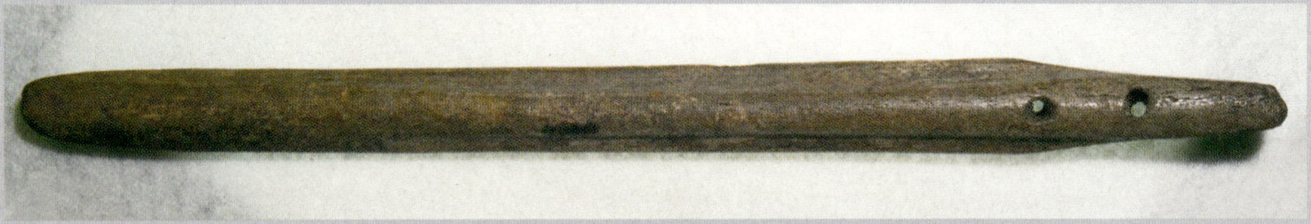

Ice probe, mineralized bone, two drilled attachment holes. It has good use wear and polish. St. Lawrence Island, Alaska. Back to Earth. **$145.00 – 160.00.**

Barbed harpoon heads, top bone example is 6⅛" long and bottom ivory harpoon is 4⅛". St. Lawrence Island, Alaska. Back to Earth. Bone harpoon, **$125.00 – 140.00;** ivory harpoon, **$110.00 – 125.00.**

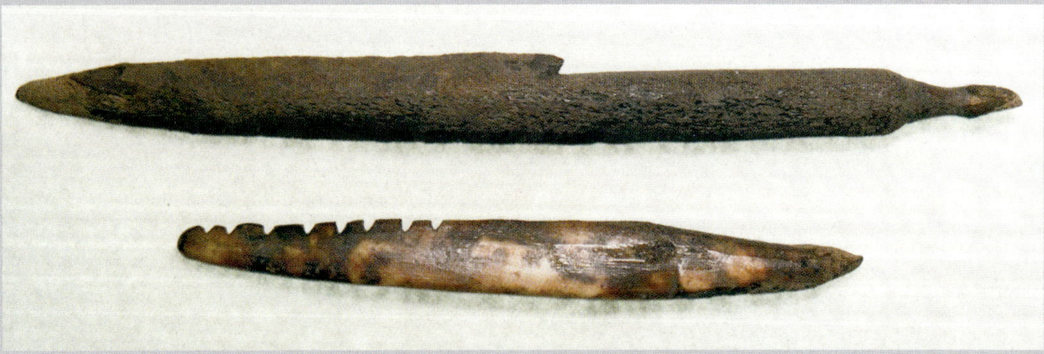

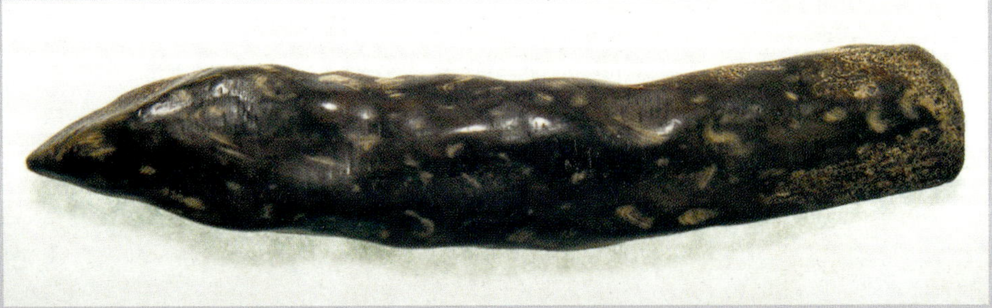

Fleshing tool, blunt working edge, length is 5¼". Heavily patinated, the artifact is from St. Lawrence Island, Alaska. Back to Earth. **$195.00.**

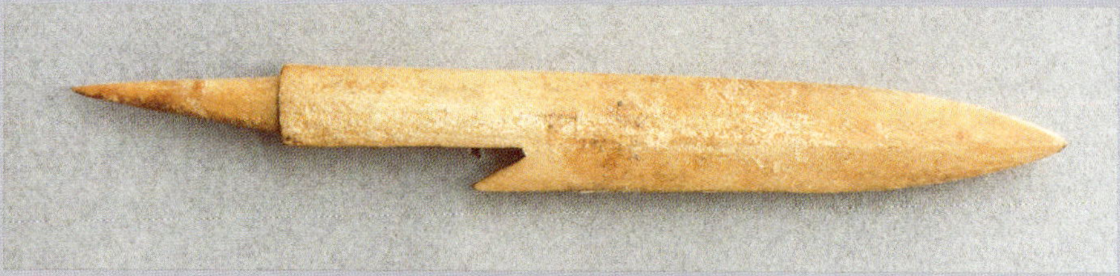

Projectile point or single-barb harpoon, 4½" long, Thule culture. This piece is ex-collection A. E. Hill, from Alaska. H. B. Greene II collection, Naples, Florida. **$125.00.**

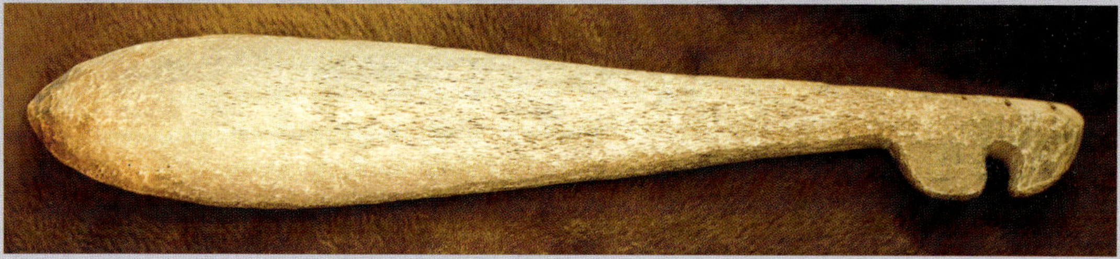

Club, whalebone, 3 x 17¾". ex-collection Ahlstrom. Well-carved and in good condition, it is from the Northwest Coast. Dale and Betty Roberts collection, Iowa. Unlisted.

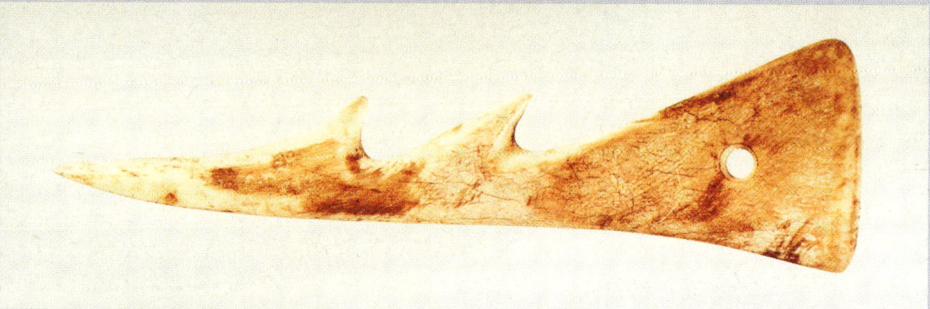

Harpoon tip, two barbs on one side and cord hole, 4⅜" long. Made of sturdy bone, this piece is from Alaska. Robin Fiser collection. **$175.00.**

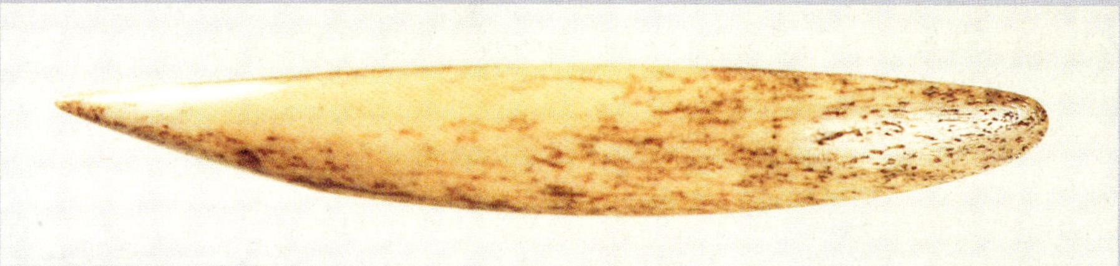

Awl, thick bone or ivory, 3¾" long. It is nicely shaped and highly polished. Alaska. Robin Fiser collection. **$55.00.**

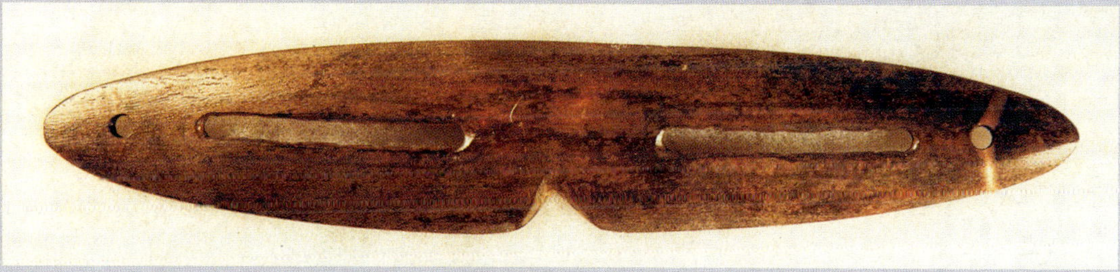

Snow goggles, carved bone, 8⅞" wide. Made of heavy bone, the goggles have a rich brown patina. Eskimo, the artifact is from Alaska. Robin Fiser collection. **$375.00.**

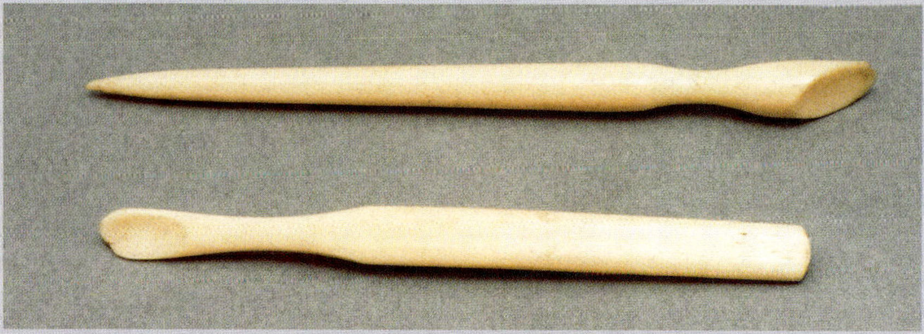

Pipe-cleaning tools, walrus ivory, 3⅜ and 4" long. Pre-1895, they are from the A. E. Hill collection. These tools were obtained in the St. Michael area, Alaska. H. B. Greene II collection, Naples, Florida. The pair, **$100.00.**

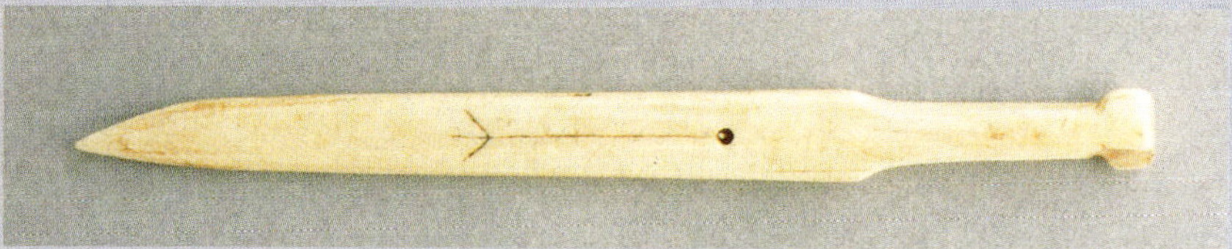

Awl, 5⅞" long, made in the form of a snow knife. It was found at a site on the Kobuk River, and is from the A. E. Hill collection. Alaska. H. B. Greene II collection, Naples, Florida. **$200.00.**

Eskimo Artifacts

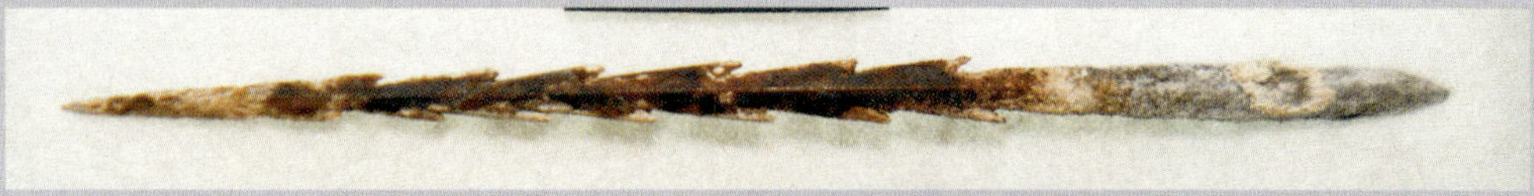

Bone fish spear, multiple barbs, long and delicate, 6¾". It is from St. Lawrence Island in the Bering Sea. Alaska. Back to Earth. **$185.00.**

Ivory tool, Eskimo, 5¼" long. This is a well-made piece with a single serrated edge, use unknown. Victor T. Trujillo collection, Nevada. **$90.00.**

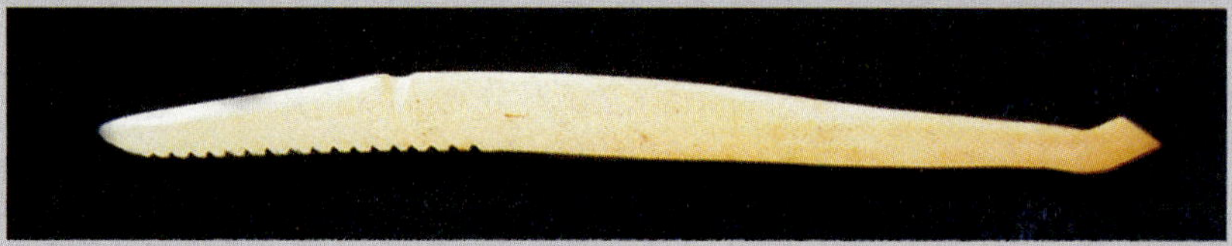

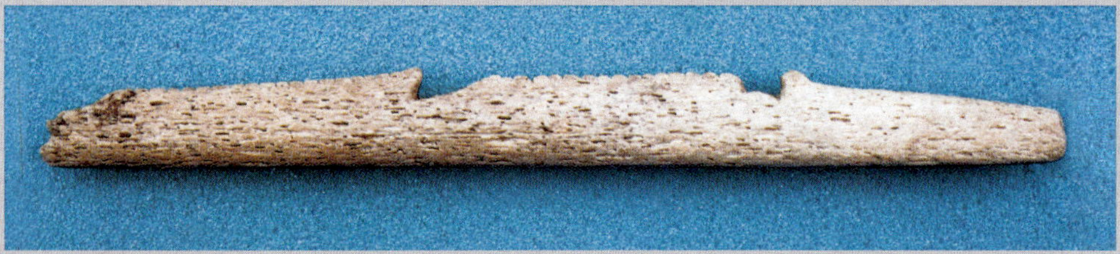

Bone harpoon, prehistoric(?), with barb and 35 tally marks. It has the tip damaged and now measures 7/16 x 5 1/16" long. The harpoon point is ex-collection Cordeiro, from Cook Inlet, Alaska. Collection of, and photograph by, Gary Henry, North Carolina. **$30.00.**

Slat armor, prehistoric(?), walrus bone, 1 5/16 x 8⅛", ⅛" thick. Armor strips like this were fastened to clothing. Ex-collection Cordeiro, it is Eskimo and from Alaska. Collection of, and photograph by, Gary Henry, North Carolina. **$75.00.**

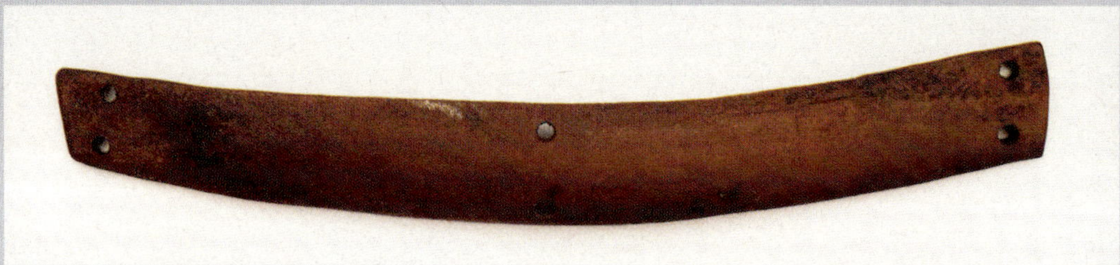

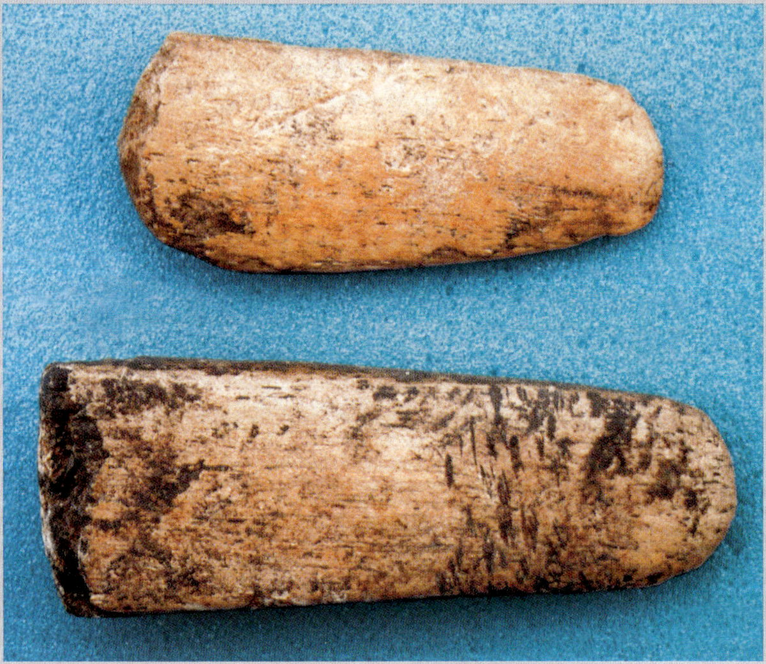

Bone chisels, both from Alaska, prehistoric(?), largest is 1⅛ x 3 7/16", ¾" thick. Ex-collection Cordeiro, the larger piece is from an island and the smaller one is from Cook Inlet. Collection of, and photograph by, Gary Henry, North Carolina. Each, **$50.00.**

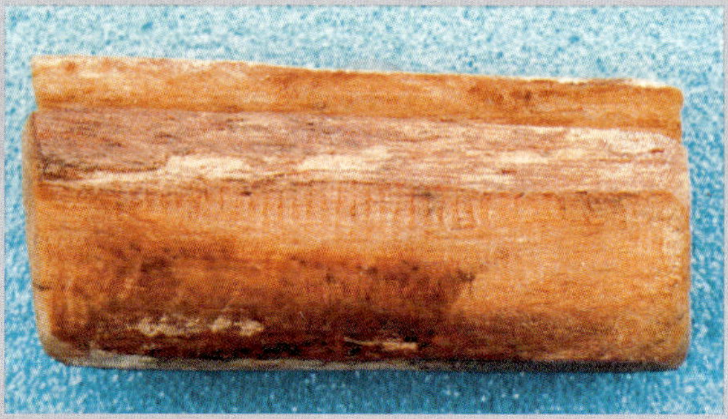

Slotted bone artifact, of unknown use, prehistoric(?), ¾ x 1⅝". Ex-collection Cantrell, it was found in Alaska. Collection of, and photograph by, Gary Henry, North Carolina. **$15.00.**

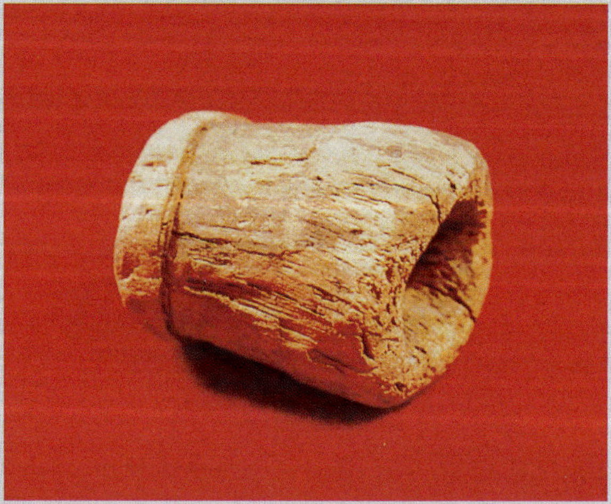

Wooden artifact, a form sometimes found in bone or ivory. A possible game call, it is 1⅞" in diameter at the wider end. Alaska. Pete Timoch collection. **$50.00.**

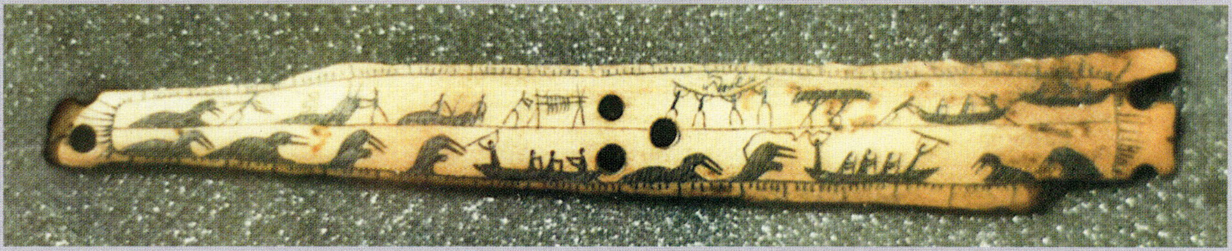

Walrus tusk, with panel of hunting expedition in two rows. Ca. 1800s, it has attachment holes at the ends and was probably an ornamental piece. This example, 8" long, is ex-collection Davis and from the Aleutian Islands. Jon Boyes collection, Illinois. **$750.00.**

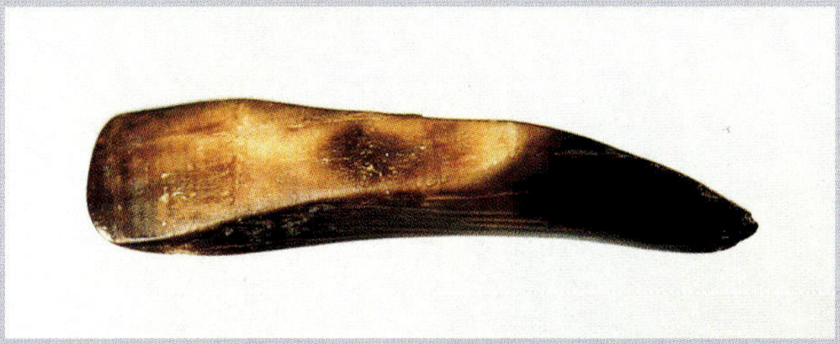

Gouge, ivory chip that is mineralized and patinated, 2³⁄₁₆" long. The curved and shallow-scooped blade edge is to the left. Alaska. Private collection. **$15.00.**

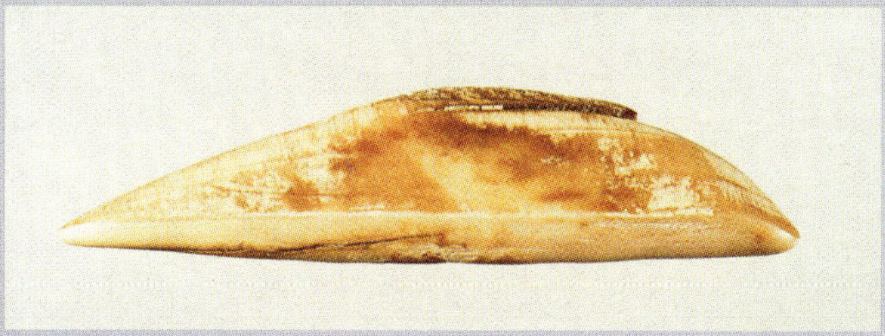

Awl or perforator, ivory chip that is mineralized, 2¾" long. With a tip polished from use, this was probably once set in a wood or bone handle. Alaska. Private collection. **$12.00.**

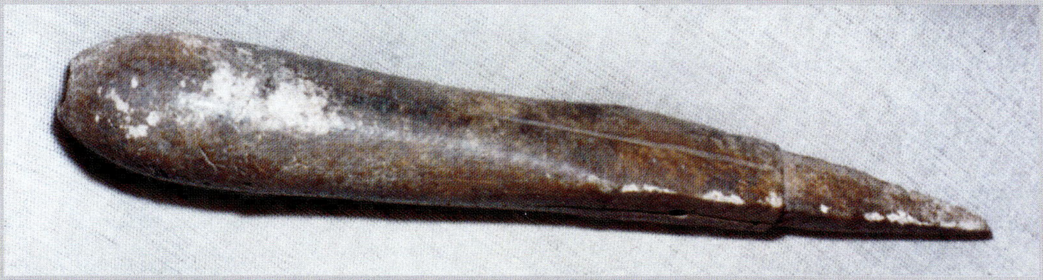

Harpoon foreshaft, Inuit from Bering Sea; Old Bering Sea culture, ca. AD 1000. It is whalebone with incised designs near the small end. The foreshaft is 8" long and was obtained from a San Pedro, California, collection in 2000. J. Steve and Anita Shearer collection, California. **$150.00.**

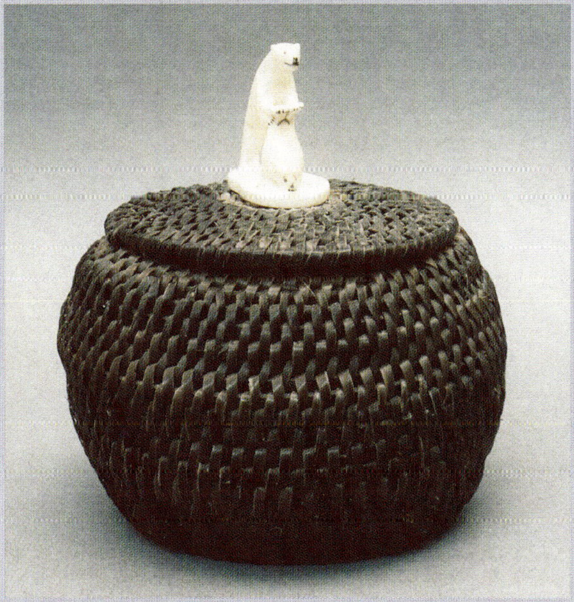

Basket, baleen with handle depicting a walrus ivory polar bear holding a seal. The basket is 3" high and 3⅞" in diameter, and the finial is 1½". Made in the 1950s by Eunice Hanks, the basket was collected by Richard Goulden. Northern Alaska. H. B. Greene II collection, Naples, Florida. Museum grade.

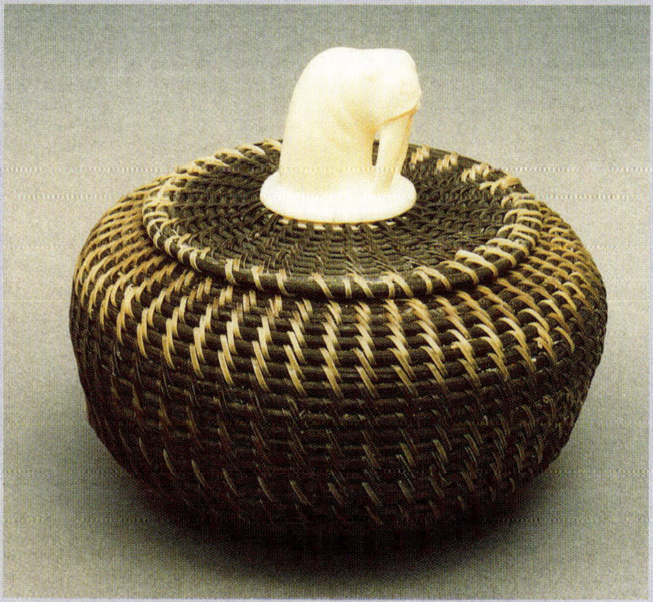

Basket, baleen with walrus ivory handle, basket 3½" high and 4¼" in diameter. The baleen is both light and dark, and the basket was made in 1998 at Point Barrow. The owner obtained this attractive work at the Native Hospital, Anchorage, Alaska. H. B. Greene II collection, Naples, Florida. **$1,250.00.**

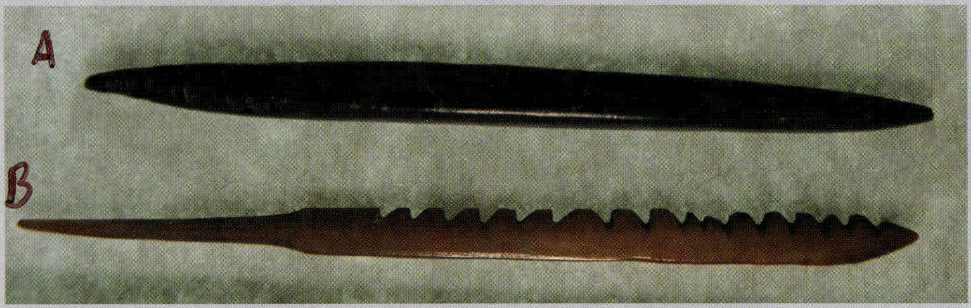

Alaskan artifacts, bone or ivory, both from St. Lawrence Island. Upper (A), pin or point, 3⅜". Fish spear (B), serrated edge, very fine. Back to Earth. Pin, **$90.00;** spearpoint, **$165.00.**

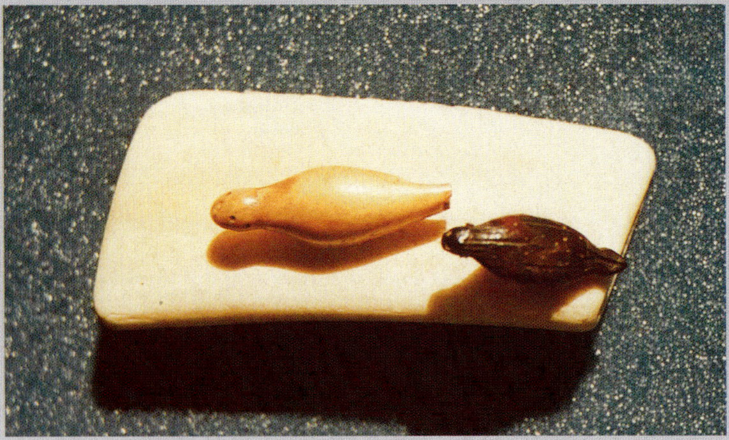

Prehistoric ivory bird effigy beads on rib bone, base is 3½" long. Found in Alaska. Dave Summers collection, Victor, New York. **$300.00.**

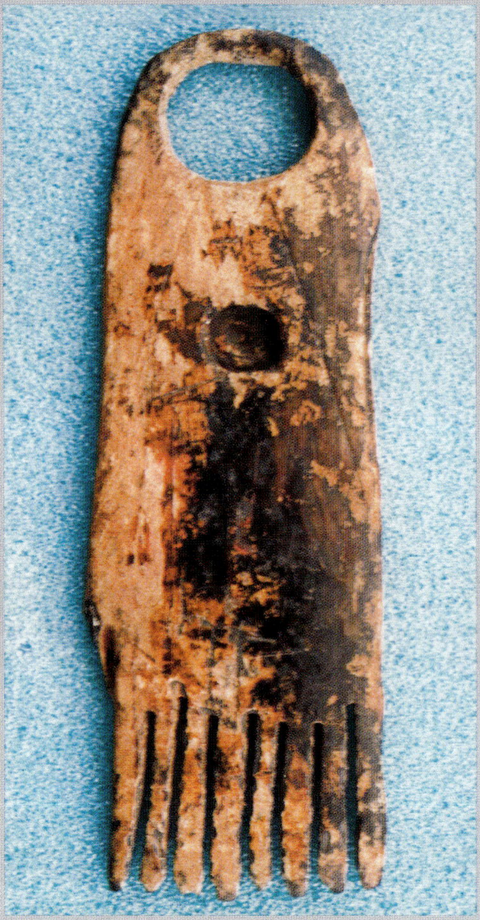

Comb, prehistoric(?), walrus bone or ivory, 1⅛ x 3¼", ⅛ " thick. Ex-collection Cordeiro, it is from St. Lawrence Island, Alaska. Collection of, and photograph by, Gary Henry, North Carolina. **$250.00.**

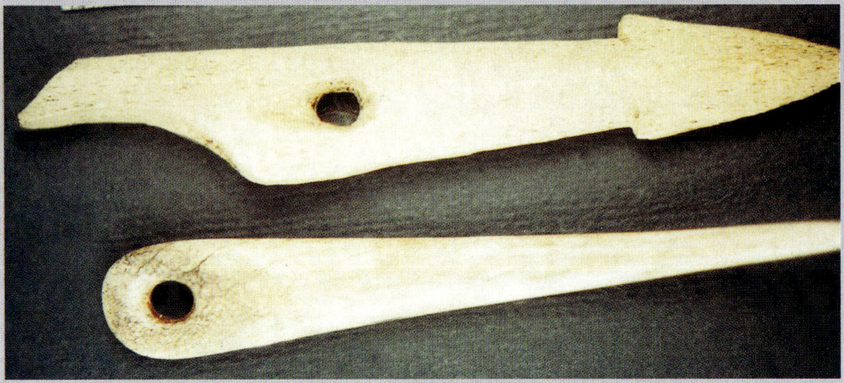

Bone artifacts, both from Alaska. Top, harpoon with cord hole. Bottom, eyed bodkin or dagger. Lee Hallman collection, Pennsylvania. Harpoon, **$150.00.** Bodkin, **$100.00.**

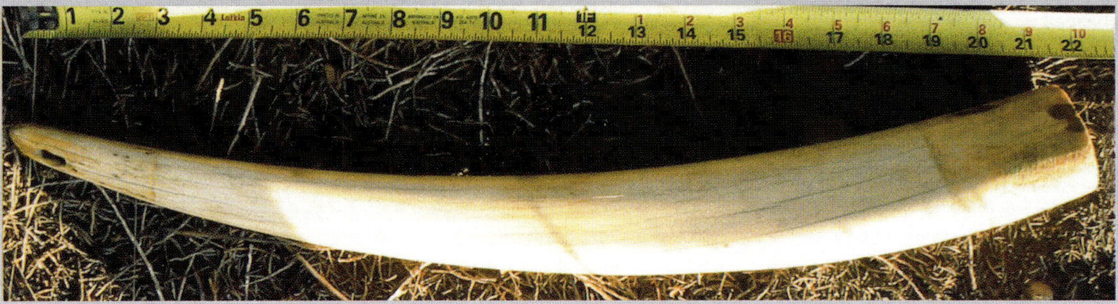

Halibut club, walrus tusk ivory, size as indicated. This large artifact has a hole near the small end, probably for a wrist loop. Alaska. John and Susan Mellyn collection, Texas. **$500.00.**

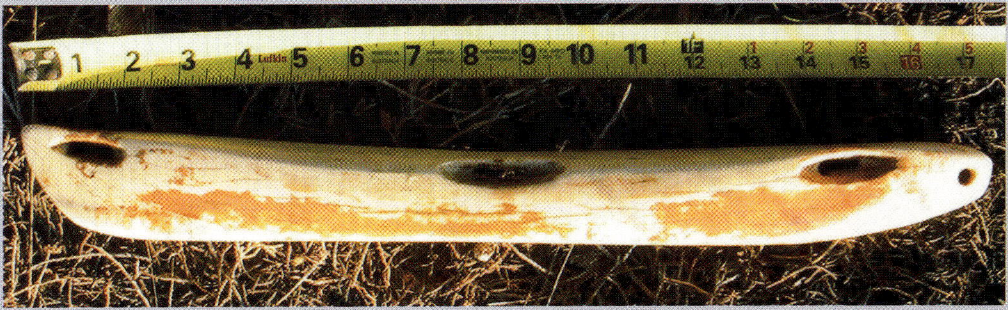

Ivory sled runner, size as indicated. The runner is Eskimo and came from St. Lawrence Island. John and Susan Mellyn collection, Texas. **$425.00.**

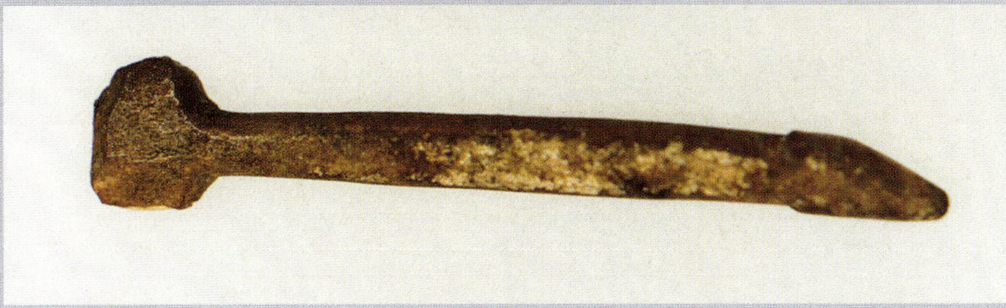

Hairpin, polished whalebone, 4¾" long. Well-shaped, it has a fantail base. Alaska. Brenda Rivers collection. **$75.00 – 100.00.**

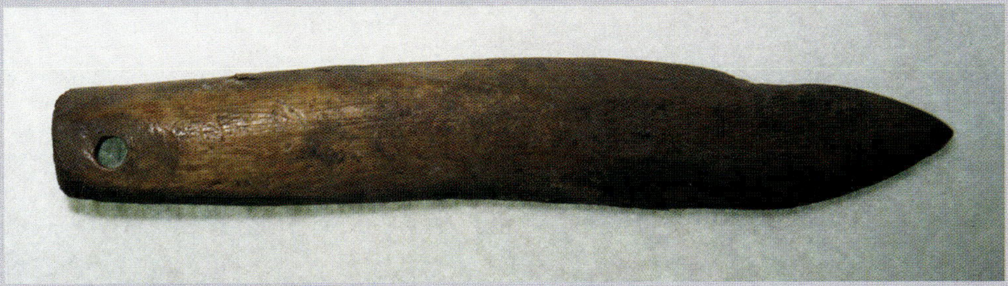

Bone knife, 6⅝" long, mineralized, drilled handle hole. This piece is about 2000 years old and was found on St. Lawrence Island, Alaska. Back to Earth. **$200.00 – 225.00.**

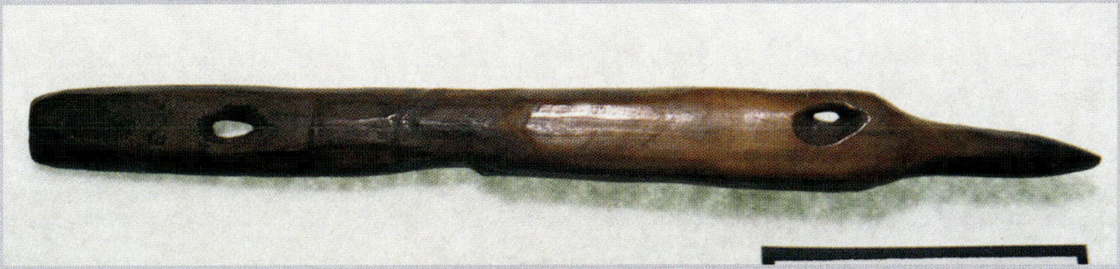

Harpoon foreshaft, mineralized ivory and highly polished, 5⅛" long. There are two attachment holes on this piece, found on St. Lawrence Island, Alaska. Back to Earth. **$160.00 – 175.00.**

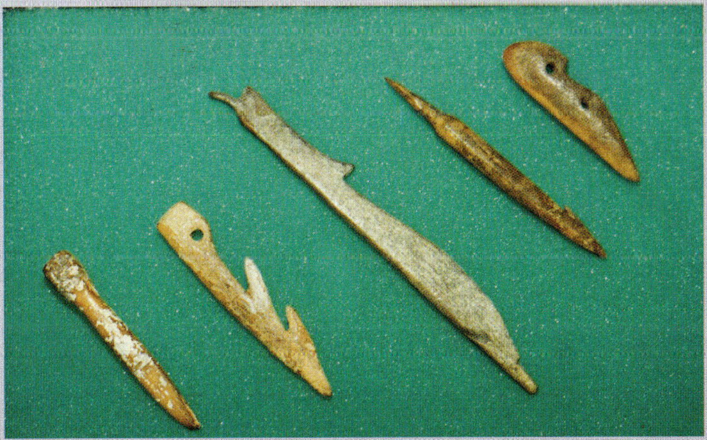

Bone harpoon and projectile points, evidencing a range of styles. All are from Alaska. Back to Earth. Unlisted.

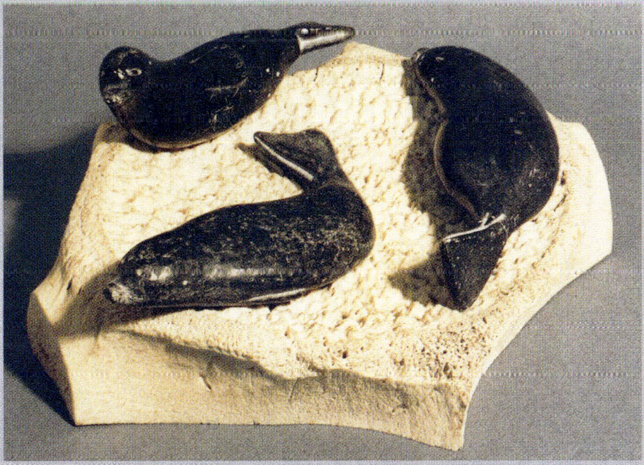

Carvings, steatite seals on whalebone ice floe, longest seal is 5¼" and bone base is 8" long. Ex-collection Paul A. Clifford, this group was carved by Matiusie, ca. 1947 – 1949. Most Eskimo stone carvings were done after WW-II and are Canadian North. H. B. Greene II collection, Naples, Florida. **$800.00.**

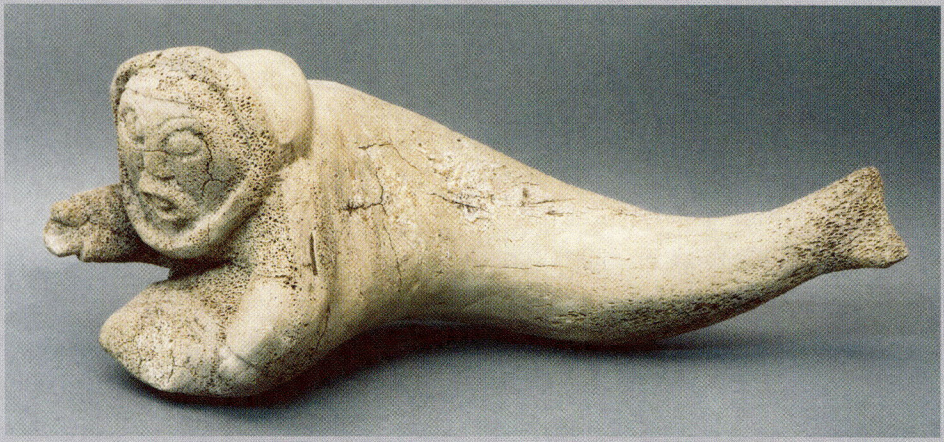

Whalebone fish person figure, 5½ x 17" long, ex-collection Quevlon. Recent, this piece was acquired about 1977 and represents an entity from the mythology of coastal people in northern Alaska. Elizabeth A. Greene collection, Naples, Florida. Museum grade.

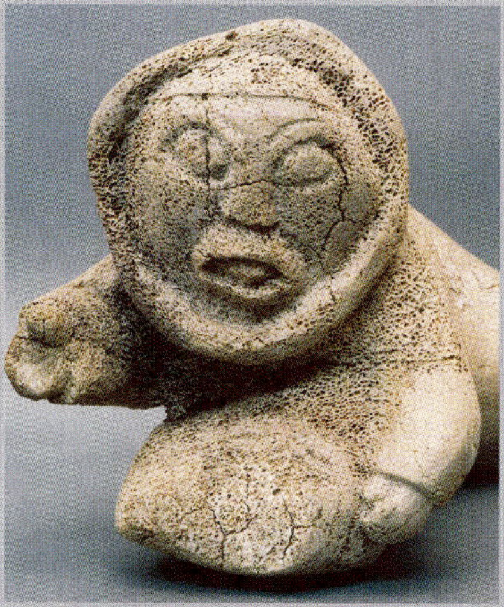

Fish person figure, closeup view of face. Overall length of piece is about 17". Northern Alaska. Elizabeth A. Greene collection, Naples, Florida. Museum grade.

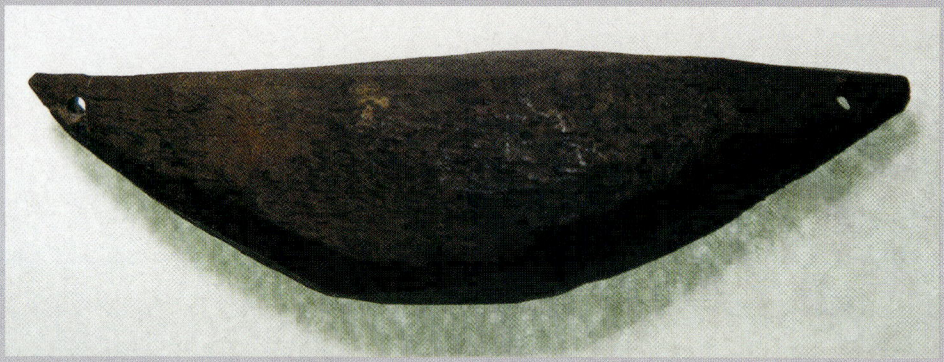

Net-sinker with two drilled attachment holes, 5⅞" long. About 2000 years old, this mineralized artifact came from St. Lawrence Island, Alaska. Back to Earth. **$140.00 – 150.00.**

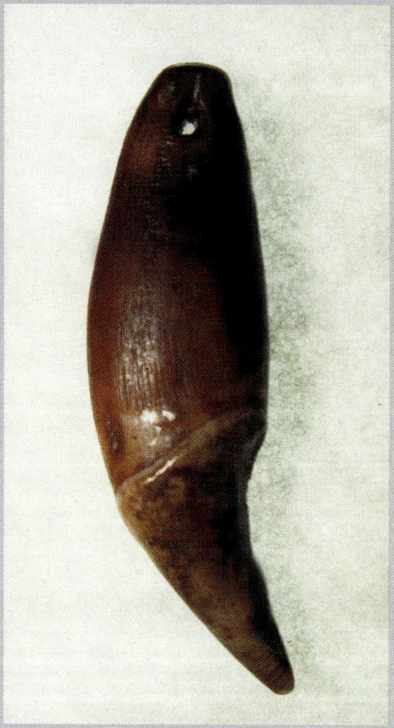

Pendant, grizzly bear tooth, fine, drilled. It is from the Kotzebue area, Alaska. Back to Earth. **$250.00.**

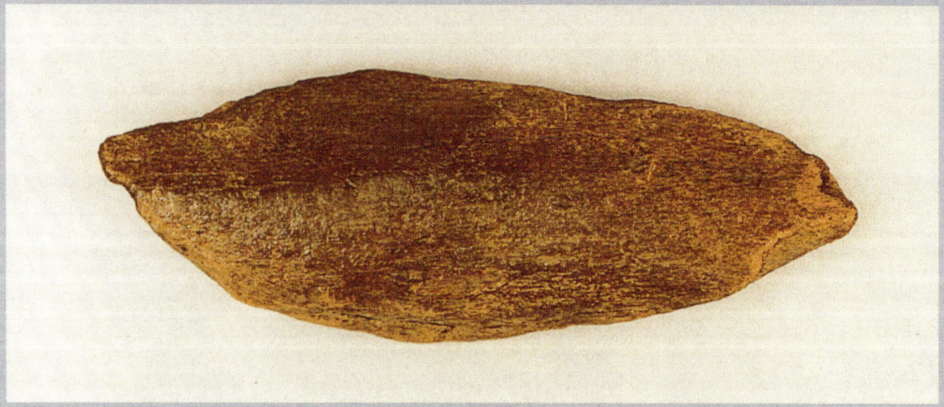

Whalebone chopper, 7¼" long. One face has hand polish and there is heavy wear overall. Alaska. Pete Timoch collection. **$100.00.**

Needle, thin bone, possibly for net weaving, 10⅛" long. In cross-section it is flat and only about 1⁄16" thick at midlength. The needle has wear around the two holes. Alaska. Pete Timoch collection. **$200.00.**

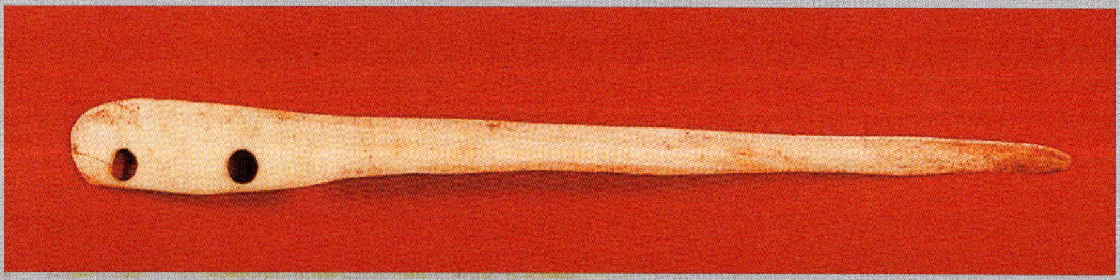

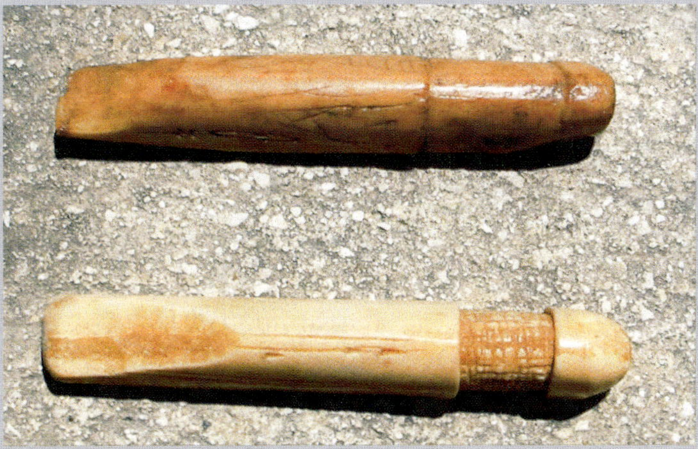

Ivory adz heads, each is 3" long. Such pieces had either wood or bone handles. They are Eskimo, from St. Lawrence Island. John and Susan Mellyn collection, Texas. Each, **$150.00.**

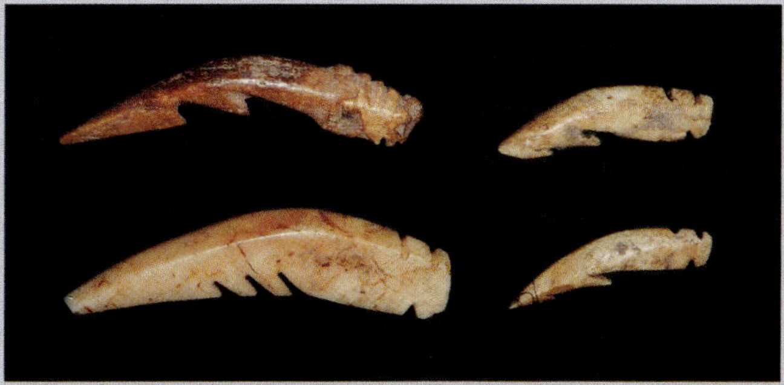

Harpoon-like hooks, antler or bone, lengths range from 1 to 1⅞". Beautifully made and highly polished, all have fastening notches and barbs on the incurvate edge. The purpose of these artifacts is unknown. Provenance unlisted. Private collection. Each, **$75.00 – 175.00.**

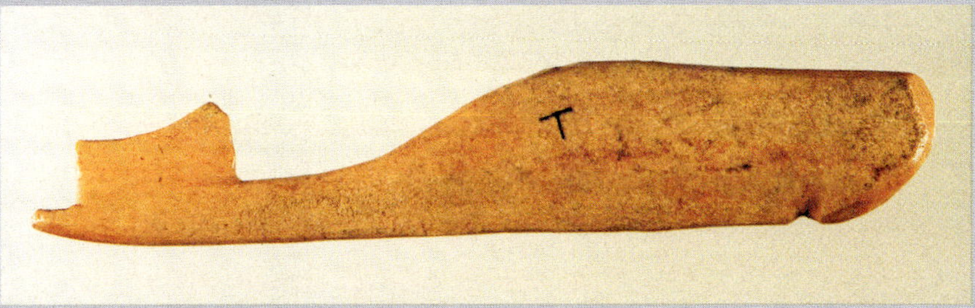

Net sizer or gauge, Eskimo, 4⅜" long. It has overall polish from use and came from Alaska. Don Casto collection. **$45.00.**

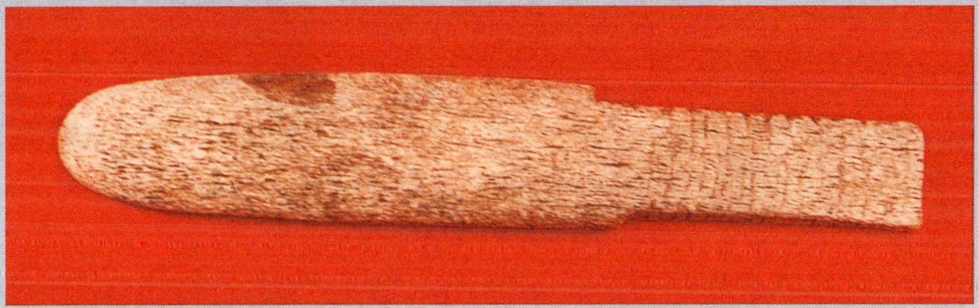

Whalebone dagger(?), 5¾" long. In cross-section the piece tapers toward the tip and also toward the hilt end, making it thickest near the center. The handle also has incised lines that encircle the handle for lashing purposes. Alaska. Pete Timoch collection. **$200.00.**

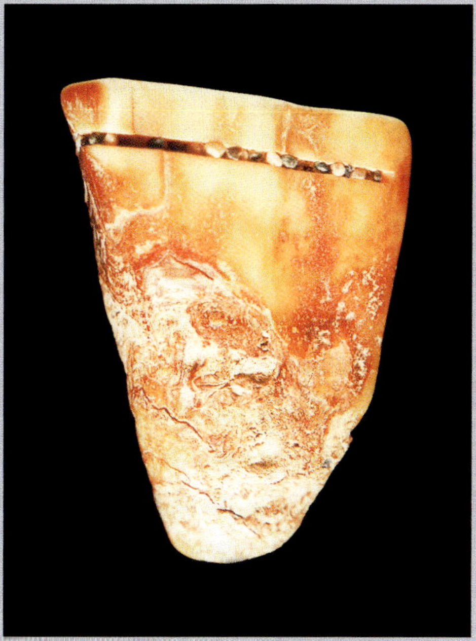

Ivory section, with edges polished by sand and wave action, 1½" long. The partial cut has beach sand wedged in the opening. Alaska. Private collection. **$10.00.**

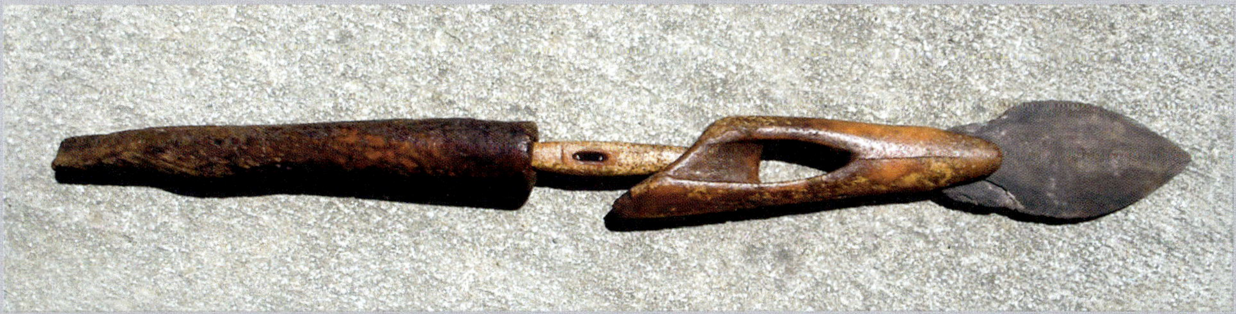

Bone harpoon outfit, three-piece with slate blade, overall length is 18". This sturdy piece is Eskimo, from St. Lawrence Island. John and Susan Mellyn collection, Texas. Museum grade.

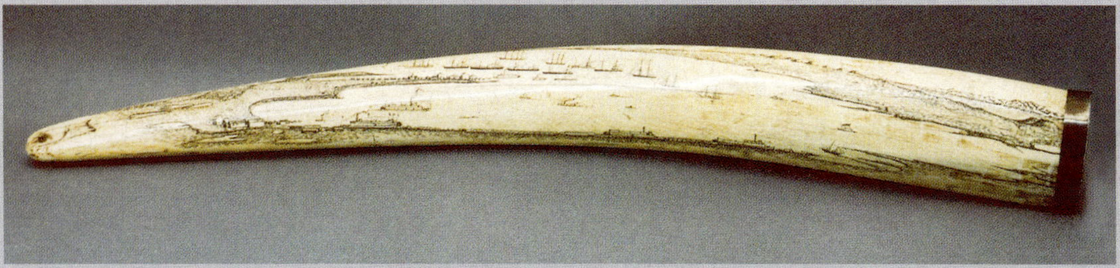

Walrus tusk, full view, very large at 30½", with well-executed scene of St. Michael Bay. It is dated 1897 and is attributed to Guy Kakarook. This superb example was traded to the owner from a museum. Alaska. H. B. Greene II collection, Naples, Florida. Museum grade.

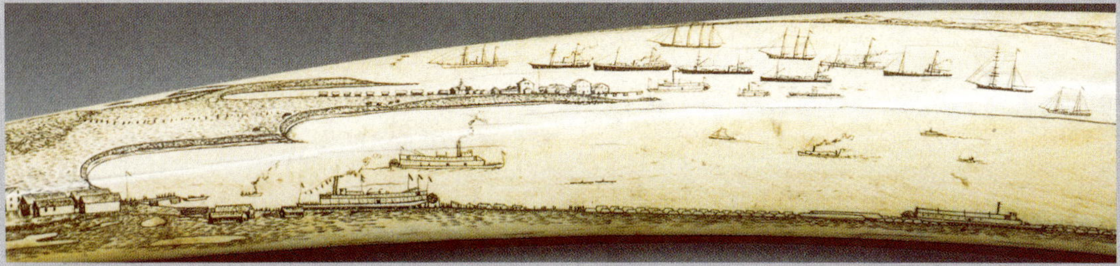

Closeup of walrus tusk, detail of St. Michael Bay, town and ships, overall length of ivory is 30½". This is a superb early (AD 1897) artwork in all respects. Alaska. H. B. Greene II collection, Naples, Florida. Museum grade.

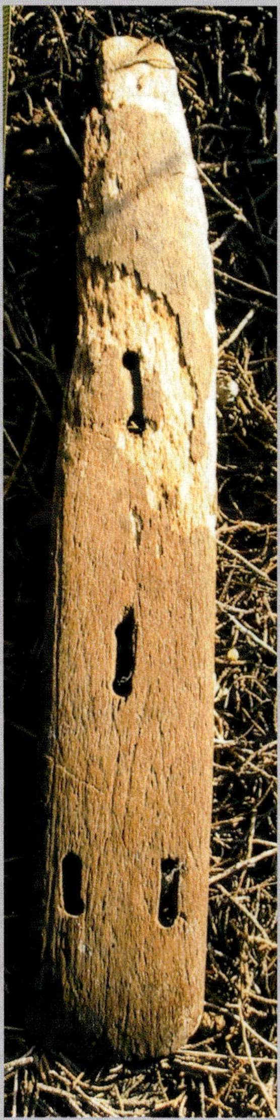

Bone tool or equipment part, Eskimo. The artifact was found on St. Lawrence Island. John and Susan Mellyn collection, Texas. Unlisted.

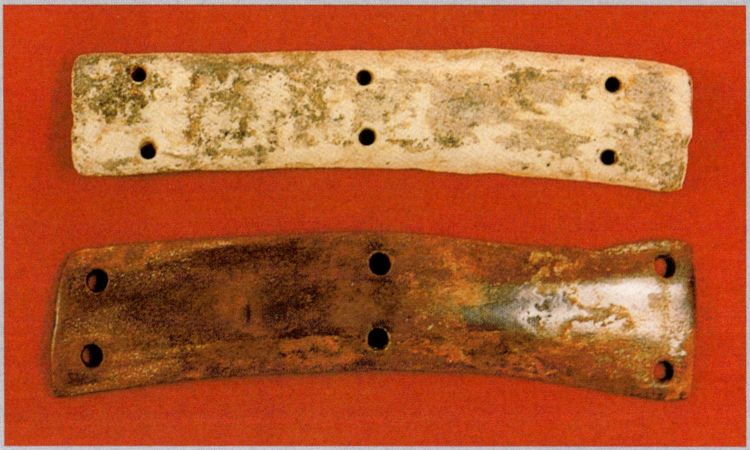

Armor slats, polished bone, northwest Alaska. Pete Timoch collection. Top, light-colored. **$75.00 – 100.00.** Bottom, 6¼". **$125.00.**

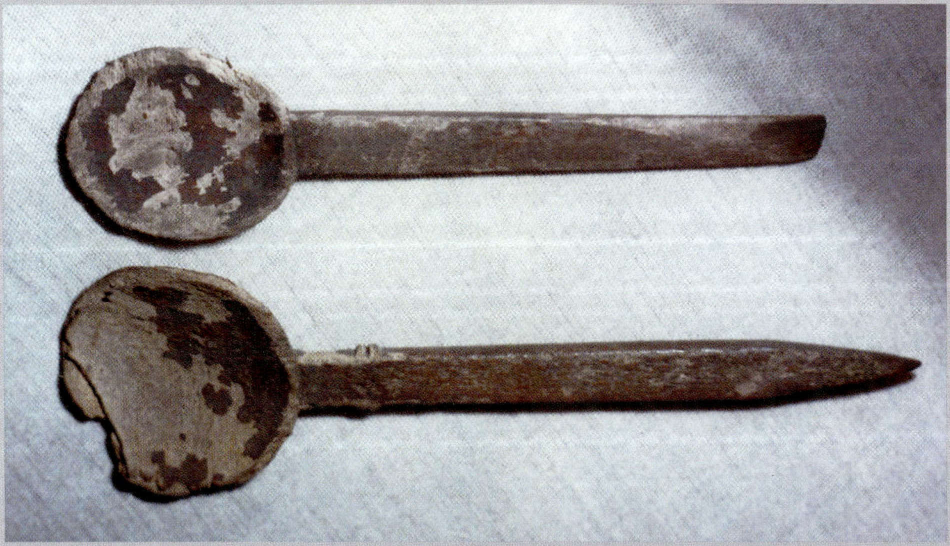

Bone spoons, Old Bering Sea culture, ca. AD 1000. The top example is 6" long while the bottom is 7". They were collected from a shop in Skagway, Alaska, in 1990. J. Steve and Anita Shearer collection, California. Top, **$100.00;** bottom, **$150.00.**

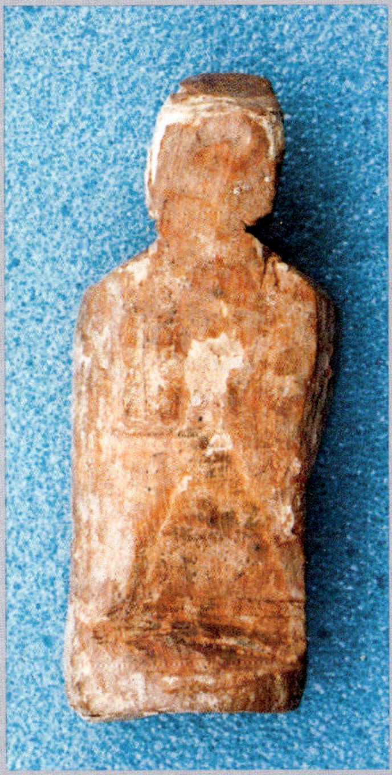

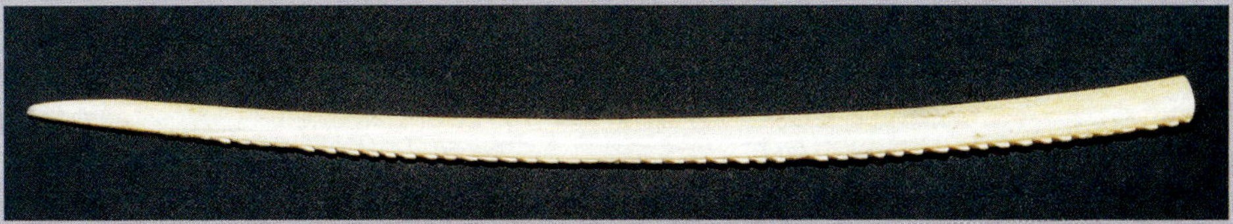

Needle or awl, probably for boat or kayak covers, 10¼". Made of bone or ivory, it is from the Nome area, Alaska. Back to Earth. **$145.00.**

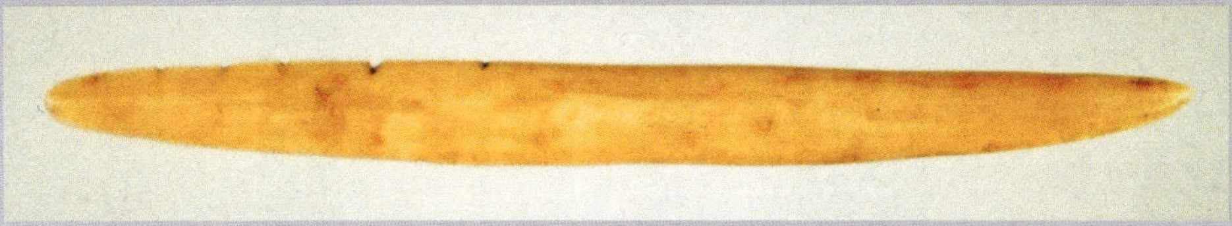

Ivory or bone artifact, possible fishing gig part, 3⅜" long. It has five notches or tally marks near one end. Alaska. Larry Garvin collection. **$30.00.**

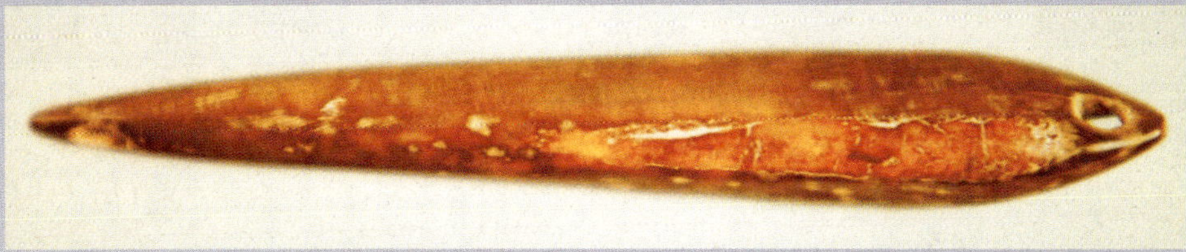

Polished ivory artifact, possible fishing lure body, 4" long. There is a drilled hole at each end of this piece. Found in Alaska. Larry Garvin collection. **$125.00.**

Bone carved human effigy figure, prehistoric(?), 1 1/16 x 1 9/16", 3/8" thick. It is ex-collection Cantrell and was found in Alaska. Collection of, and photograph by, Gary Henry, North Carolina. **$25.00.**

Awl or perforator, mineralized ivory with beach polish, 3⅝" long. It has high overall smoothing and came from Alaska. Lar Hothem collection. **$15.00.**

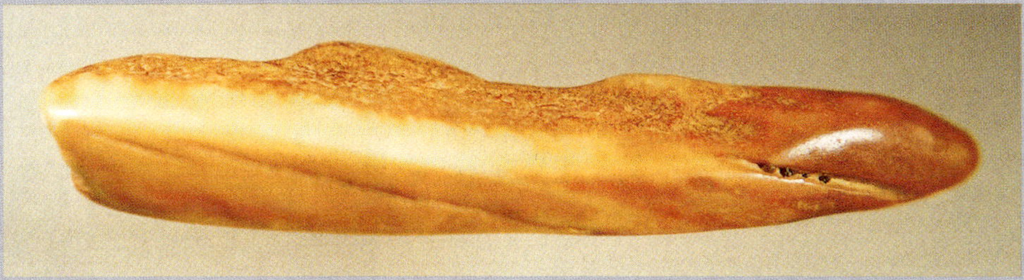

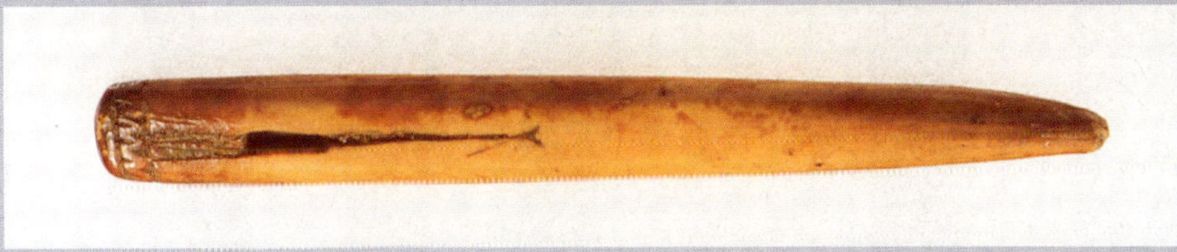

Ivory hairpin, highly polished with decorated thick end, 4⅜" long. Somewhat triangular in cross-section, the three thick end sides have a crosshatch design. Alaska. Pete Timoch collection. **$200.00.**

Walrus oosik (penis bone), made into a club, 16" long. It is from Alaska. John and Susan Mellyn collection, Texas. **$300.00.**

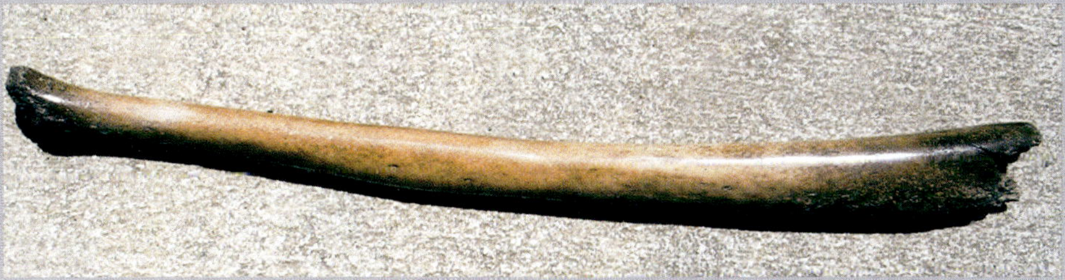

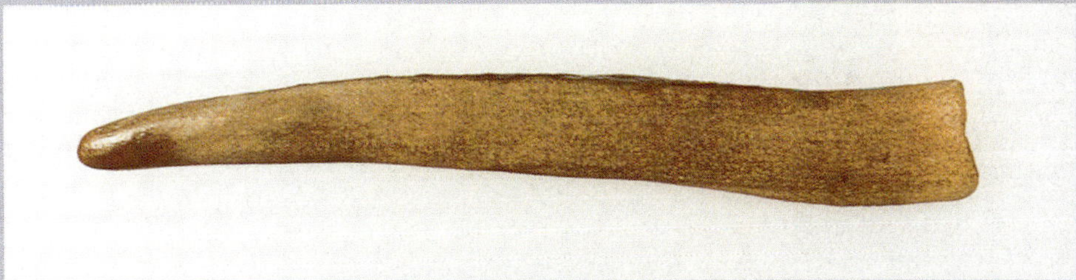

Awl or perforator, antler with polish at the tip, 9" long. The tip has a chiseled, not rounded, configuration. Alaska. Pete Timoch collection. **$100.00.**

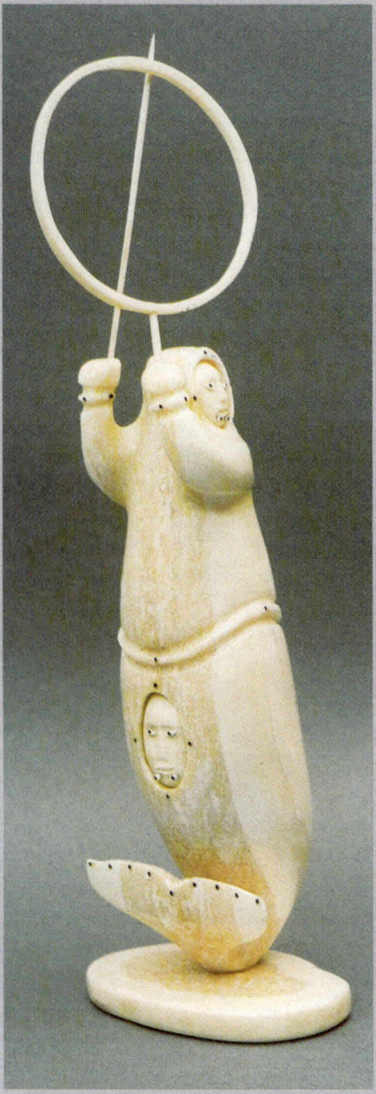

Figure, standing Whale-Man drummer, 10⅛" high. It is made of walrus ivory and whale baleen. Carved in 1998 by Levi Titpon, Shagtulik. The owner purchased this fine piece in 1999 at the Native Hospital, Anchorage, Alaska. Elizabeth A. Greene collection, Naples, Florida. **$1,350.00.**

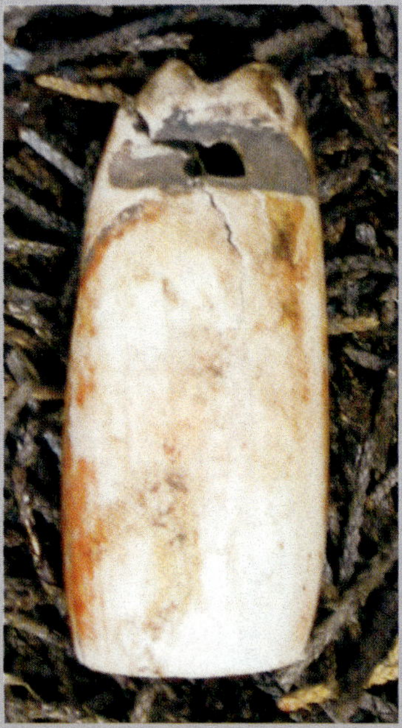

Shell bead, Eskimo, 1⅜" long. With a suspension hole, the artifact is from St. Lawrence Island. John and Susan Mellyn collection, Texas. **$35.00.**

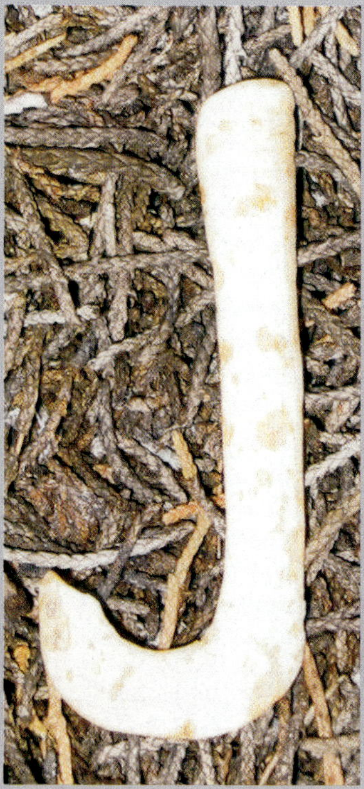

Bone fishhook, 1⅝" long. This is an Eskimo piece, from St. Lawrence Island. John and Susan Mellyn collection, Texas. Unlisted.

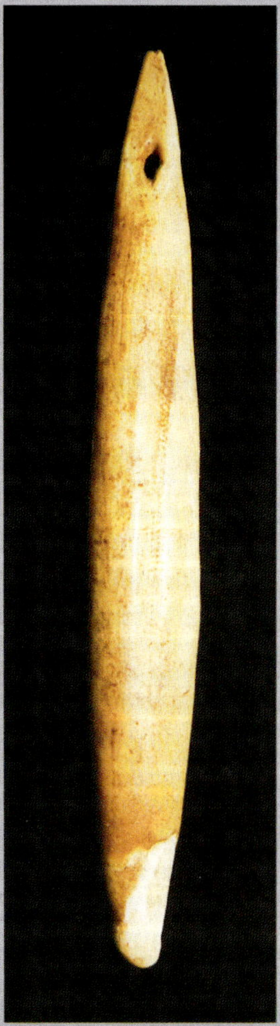

Walrus tusk, mineralized ivory, 5⅜" long. One end was drilled so the tusk could serve as a pendant. St. Lawrence Island, Alaska. Back to Earth. **$175.00 – 200.00.**

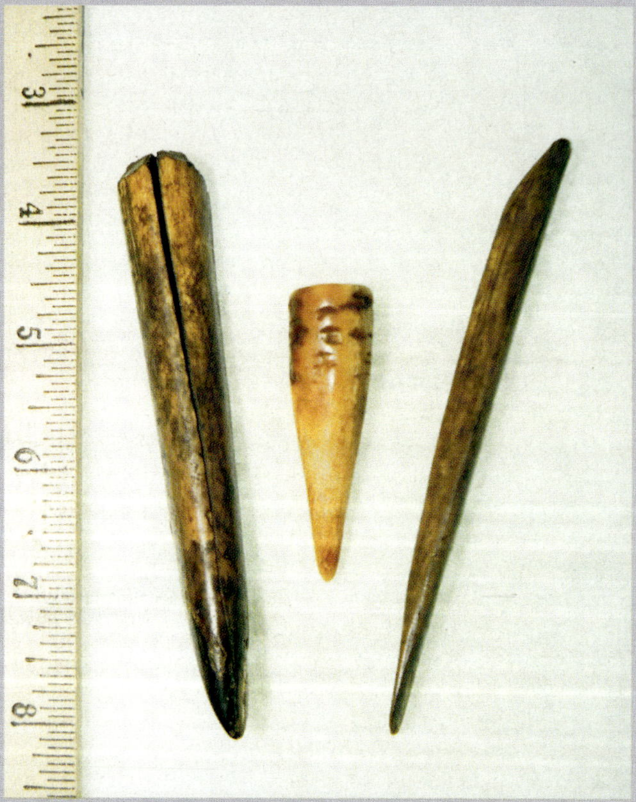

Bone and ivory pointed tools, all from St. Lawrence Island, Alaska. Back to Earth. The three, **$125.00.**

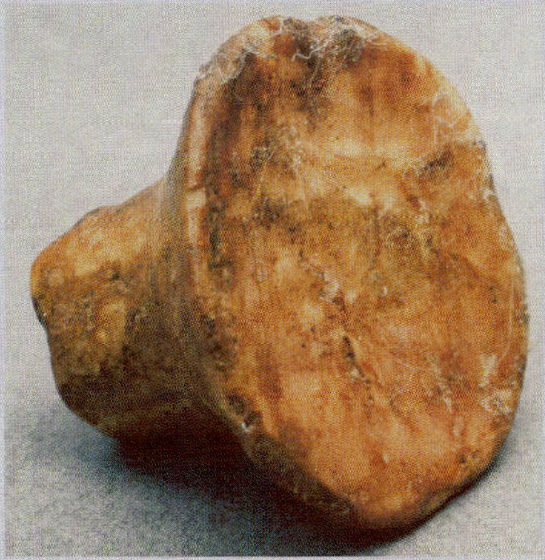

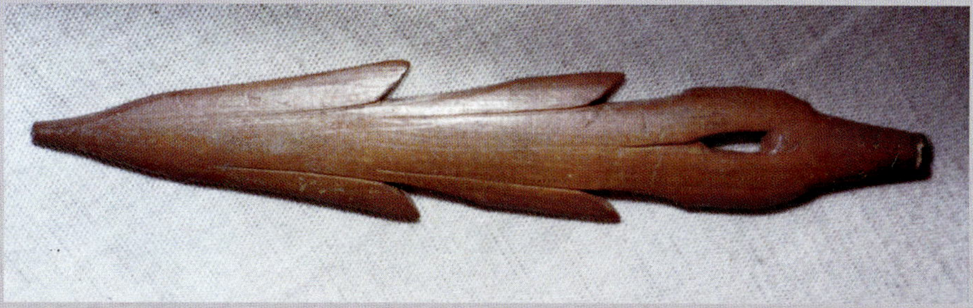

Bone harpoon head, Eskimo, from St. Lawrence Island. Thule culture, ca. AD 800, 6" long. Well-balanced with a brown patina, the harpoon head was obtained from a dealer in Pasadena, California. J. Steve and Anita Shearer collection, California. **$250.00.**

Labret or lip plug, fossil ivory, ½ x 1". Prehistoric, it came from a midden on the Kobuk River and was formerly in the A. E. Hill collection. Alaska. H. B. Greene II collection, Naples, Florida. **$95.00.**

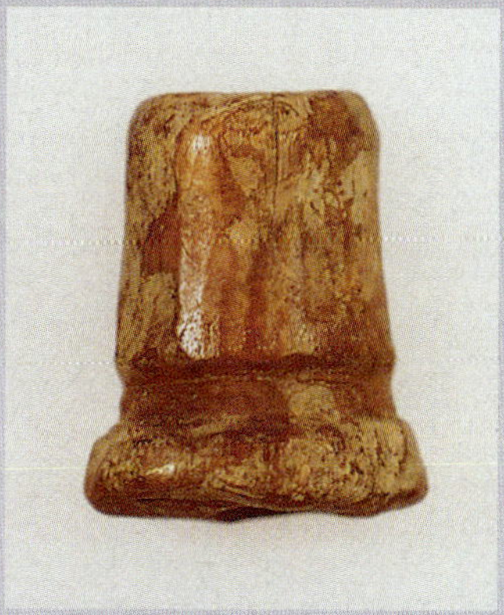

Ivory plug or short pipe, spool-shaped, 1⅜" long. It is drilled from both ends with tapering holes, 5/16" across at the smaller end and ½" across at the wide end. Since the holes meet near the center, it may be either a smoking pipe or a bladder plug. Alaska. Private collection. **$125.00 – 200.00.**

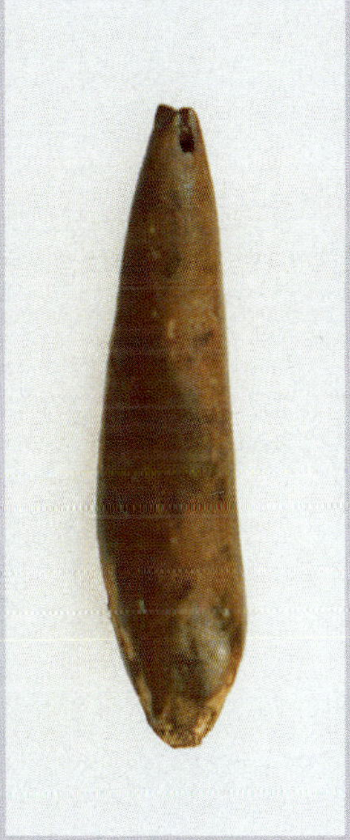

Net sinker, polished bone, 2⅞" long. This plummet-like object is from Alaska. Tony Napier collection. **$50.00.**

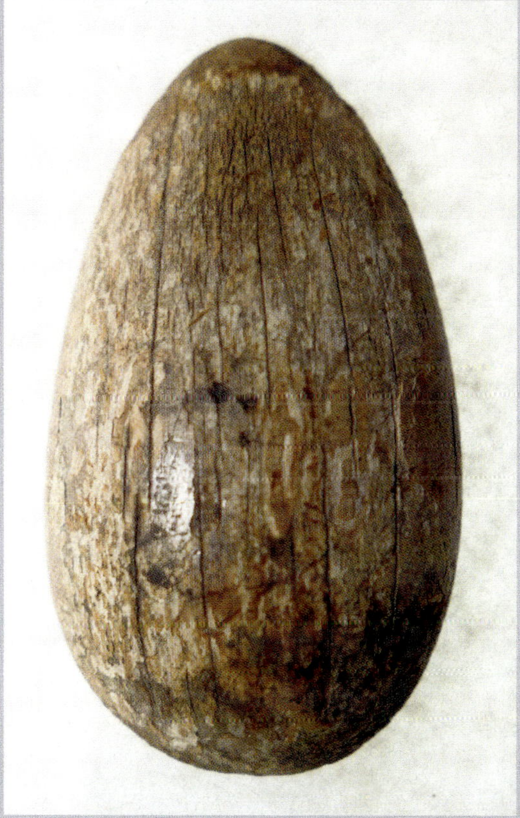

Ivory gorget or pendant (front view), 2⅞" long. The artifact is egg-shaped and the front is rounded and smoothed. St. Lawrence Island, Alaska. Garvin collection, Ohio. **$160.00 – 175.00.**

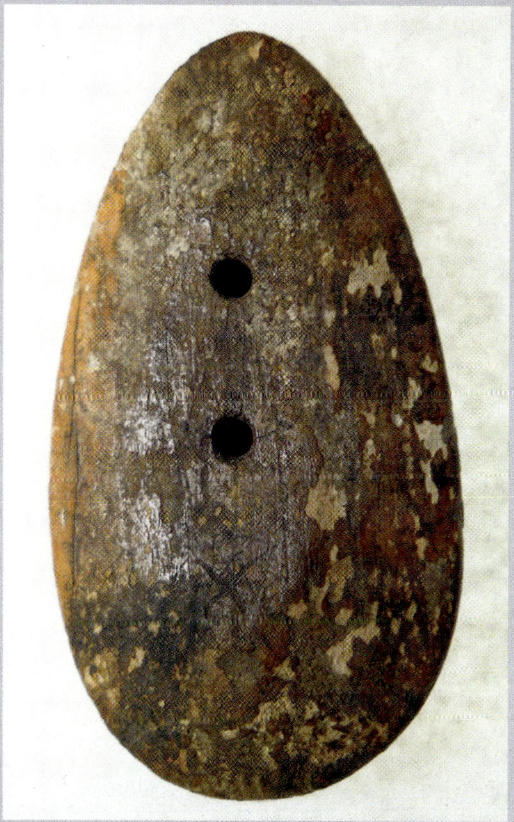

Ivory gorget or pendant (back view), 2⅞" long. This face is drilled with two deep holes which do not connect at the bottoms. St. Lawrence Island, Alaska. Garvin collection, Ohio. **$160.00 – 175.00.**

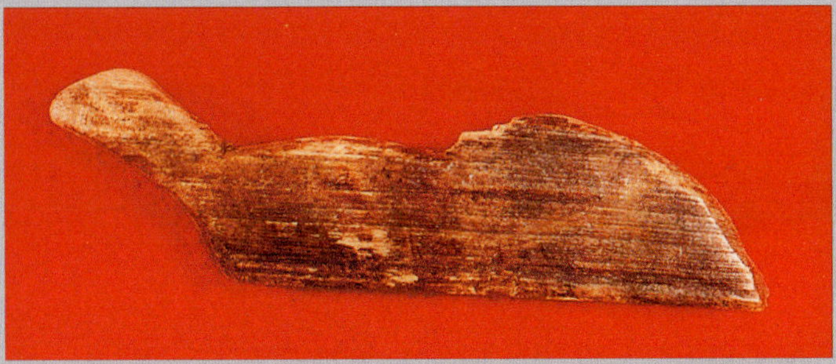

Seal effigy, polished wood, 4⅛" long. Though usually made of bone, ivory, or antler, many effigies were also crafted in wood. Alaska. Brenda Rivers collection. **$75.00.**

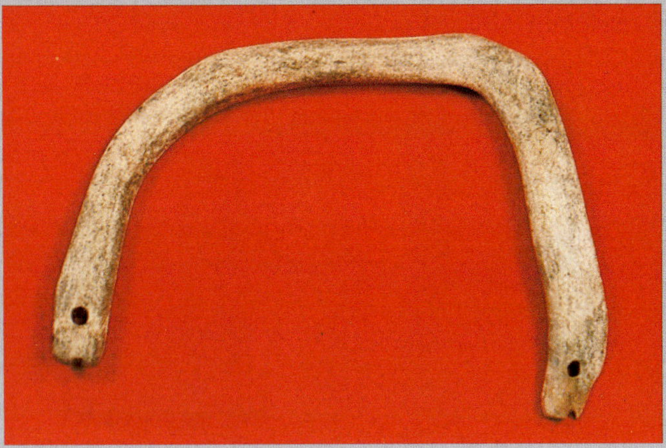

Caribou antler handle, 5⅝ x 7¾". It has an oversized grip so that heavy gloves could be used for dragging or carrying meat or other items. Alaska. John Timoch collection. **$50.00.**

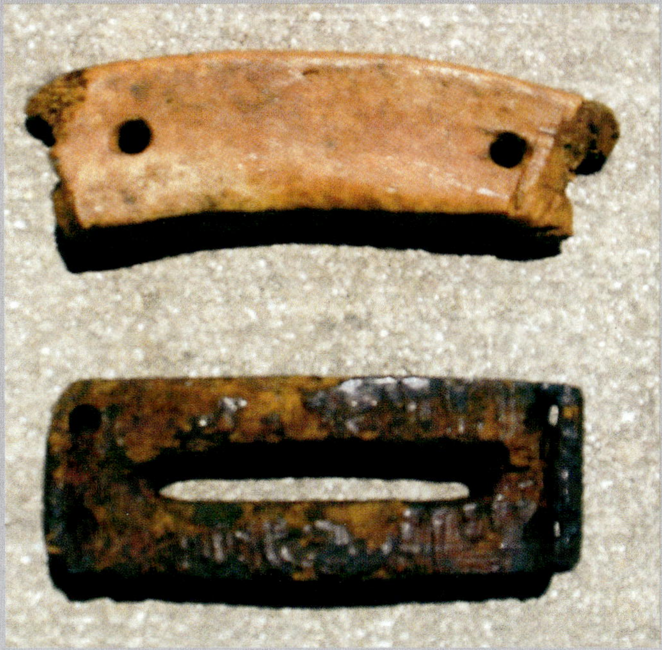

Bone tool or equipment parts, Eskimo. The top piece is 4¼" long and the bottom is 3½". They were found on St. Lawrence Island. John and Susan Mellyn collection, Texas. Unlisted.

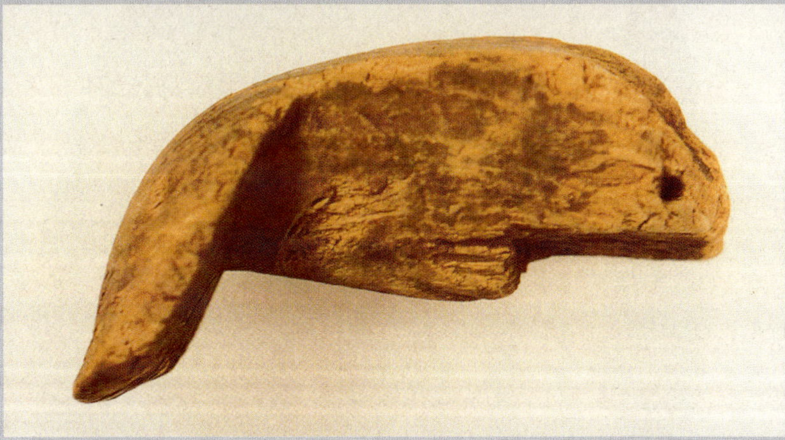

Whale effigy, probably driftwood, 4½" along the outside curve. Alaska. Brenda Rivers collection. **$100.00.**

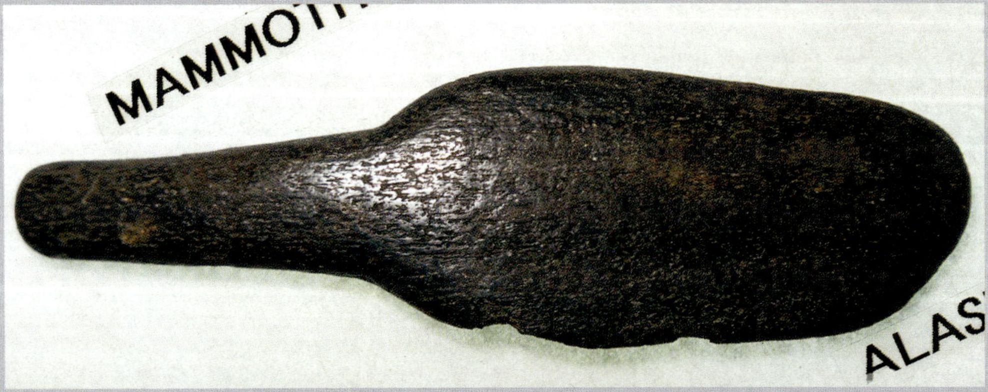

Spatula-shaped tool, 6½" long, polished mammoth bone. It was found at Delta Junction, Alaska. Back to Earth. **$165.00.**

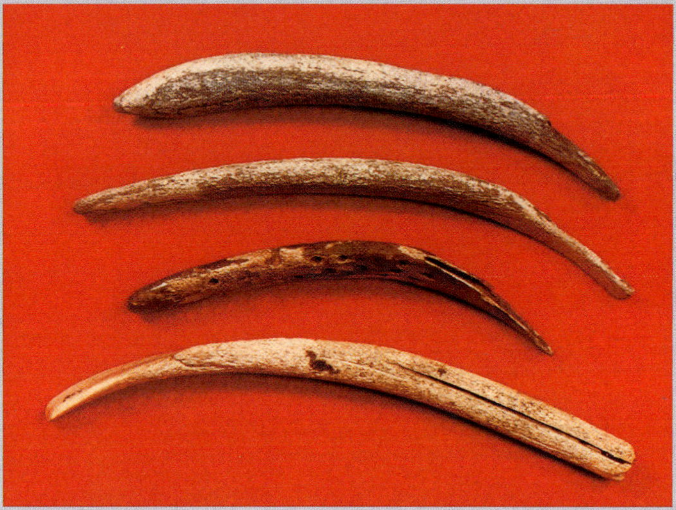

Whalebone harpoon barbs, longest is 7⅛" around the outside curve. These were the barb components of very large harpoons such as were used for whale hunting. The barb attached to the harpoon head and both remained in the flesh. This in turn secured the target prey to a strong cord that went to the hunter or a bladder float. Alaska. Pete Timoch collection. Each, **$50.00 – 75.00.**

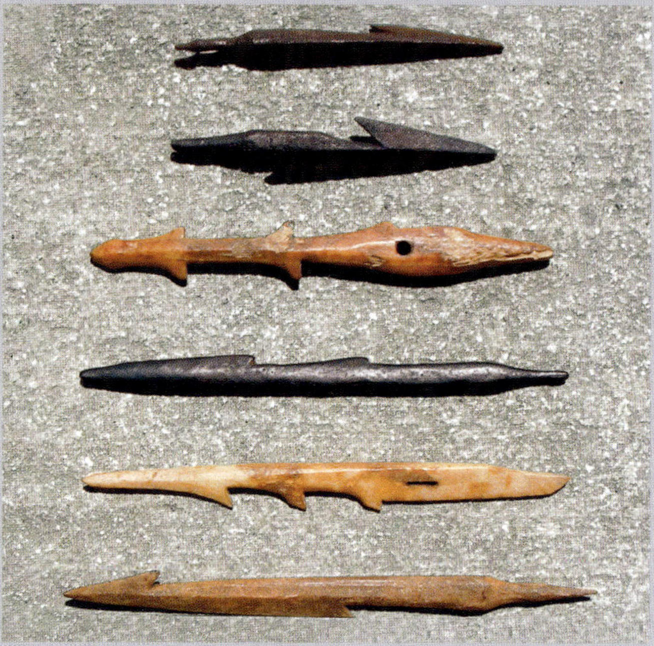

Bone harpoon tips, 3 to 5" long. These are Eskimo, from St. Lawrence Island. John and Susan Mellyn collection, Texas. Each, **$125.00 – 250.00.**

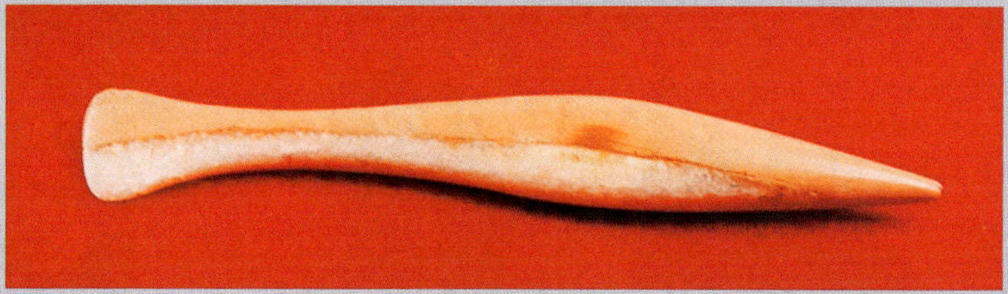

Fish effigy, polished ivory, 4⅛" long. This is likely a later piece since it does not have much weathering. It may be from contact or early historic times. Alaska. Brenda Rivers collection. **$150.00.**

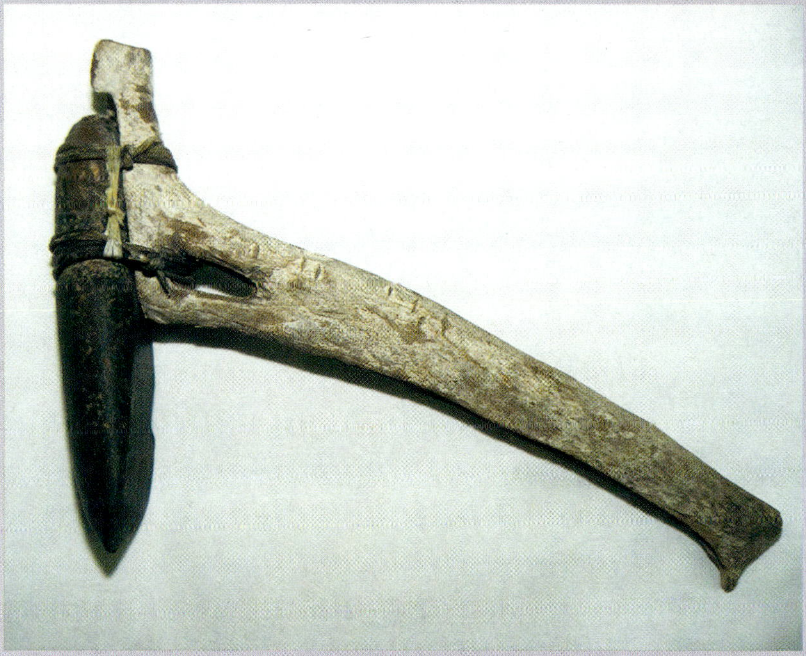

Stone adz, 5⅜" long, attached to a bone handle, 11" long. The adz came from Queen Charlotte Island, British Columbia, Canada. Back to Earth. **$400.00.**

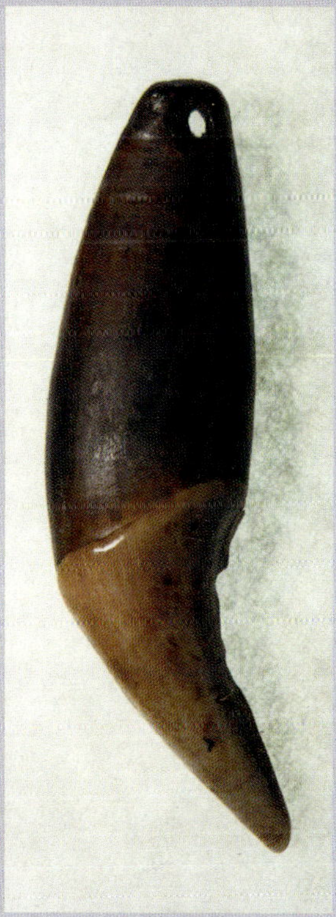

Brown bear tooth pendant, dark and mineralized. The artifact was found in the Kotzebue area, Alaska. Back to Earth. **$250.00.**

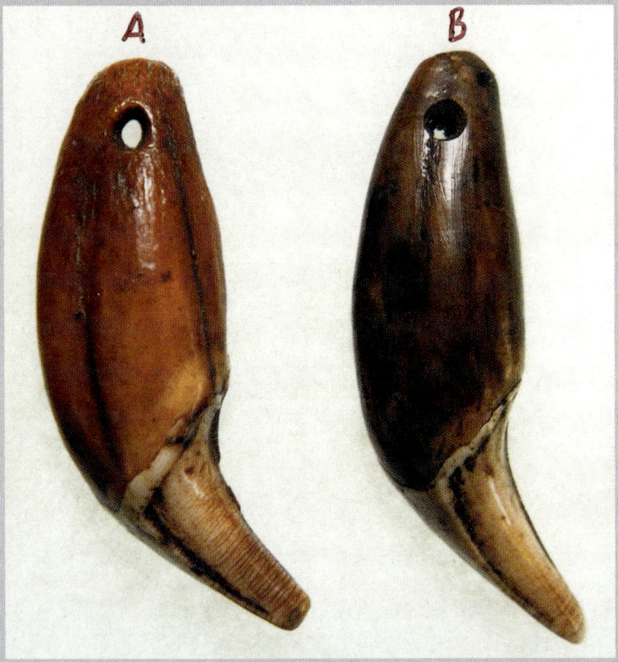

Brown bear canine pendants, ca. AD 500 or earlier. The teeth were found in the Kotzebue area, Alaska. Back to Earth. Each, **$250.00.**

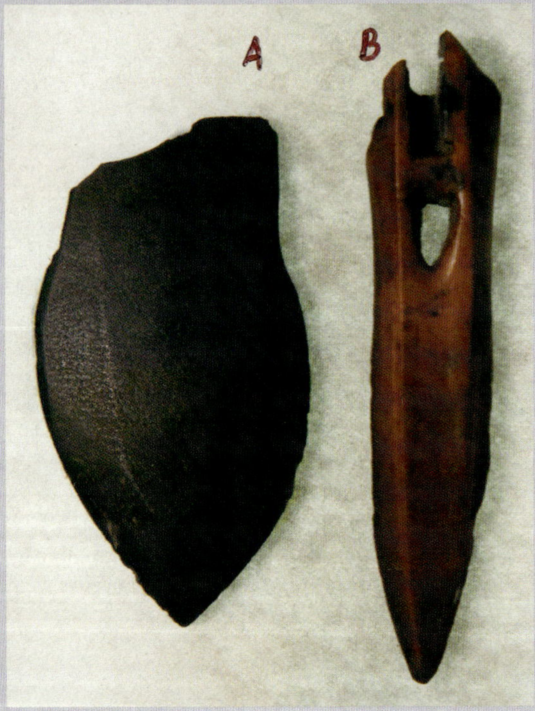

Alaskan artifacts, Bering Sea region. There is a polished slate blade (A) and an ivory toggle harpoon head (B) 3¼" long. Back to Earth. Blade, **$95.00;** harpoon, **$100.00.**

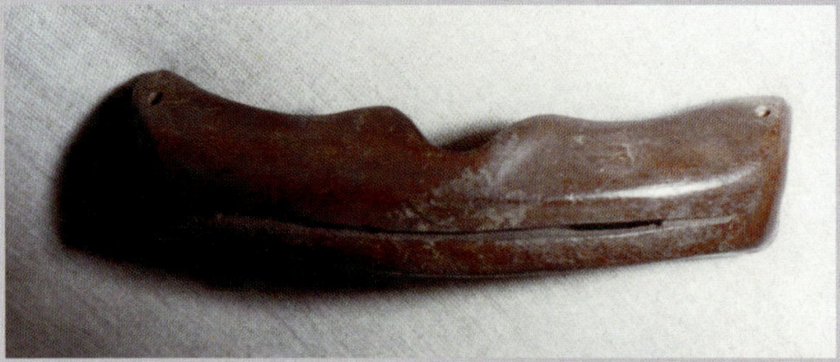

Bone snow goggles, 5" long. Known as I-gank', the narrow slit opening blocks glare from ice and snow to prevent blindness, ca. AD 800. Bering Sea Eskimo, Thule culture phase, the goggles were collected at a Portland, Oregon, antiques show in 1997. J. Steve and Anita Shearer collection, California. **$,1200.00.**

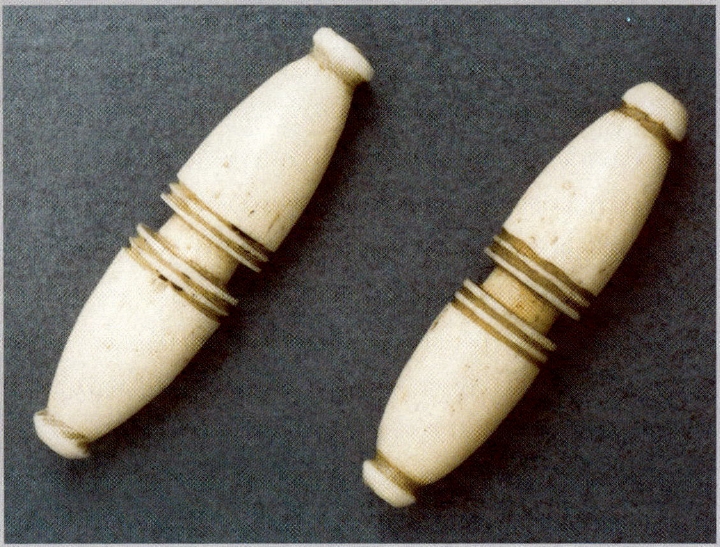

Buttons or toggle fasteners, each 1¼" long, walrus ivory. They are from the A. E. Hill collection, ca. 1880s – 1900. Northern Alaska. H. B. Greene II collection, Alaska. Each, **$60.00.**

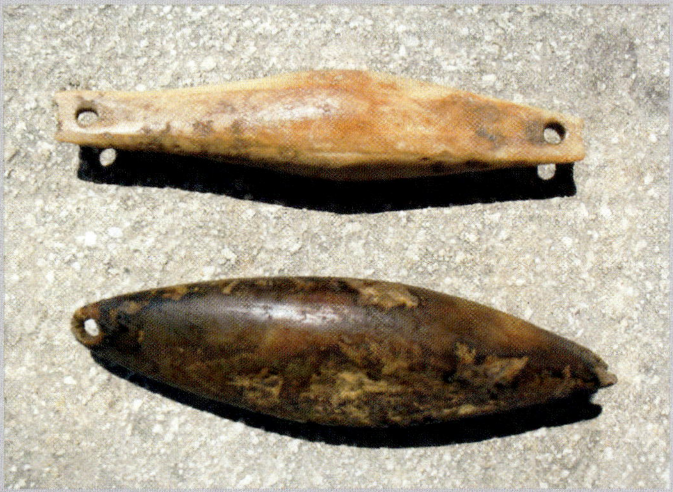

Fishing sinkers, top example is 3½" long, bottom is 3⅜". They are nicely carved from bone or ivory. Eskimo, St. Lawrence Island. John and Susan Mellyn collection, Texas. Each, **$75.00 – 125.00.**

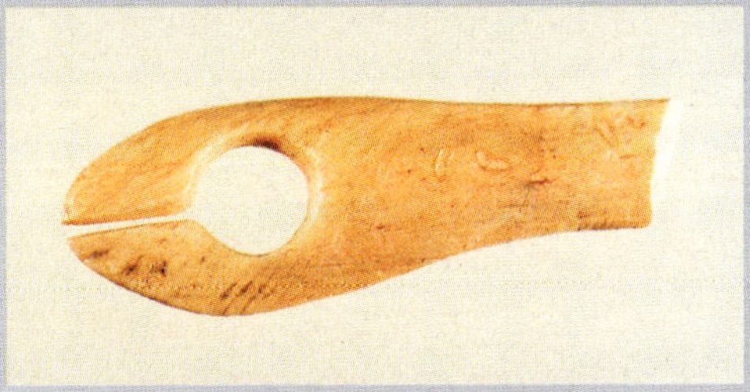

Tool part, broken, 2" long. Probably made of ivory, this is Eskimo (Inuit) from Alaska. Don Casto collection. **$20.00.**

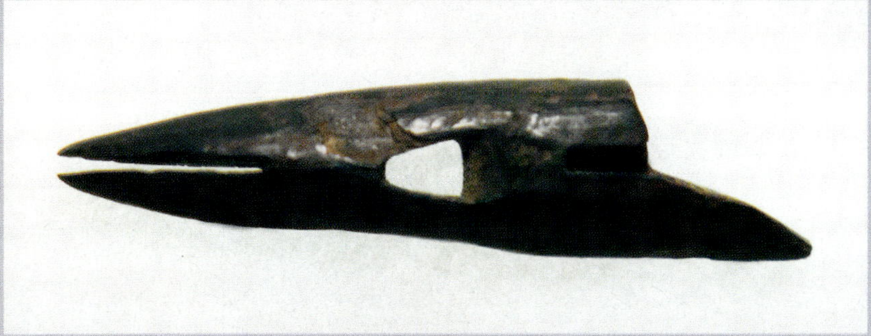

Bone harpoon head, 3⅛" long, dark patination. It has a Perino COA and came from Penuk Island, Alaska. Back to Earth. **$95.00.**

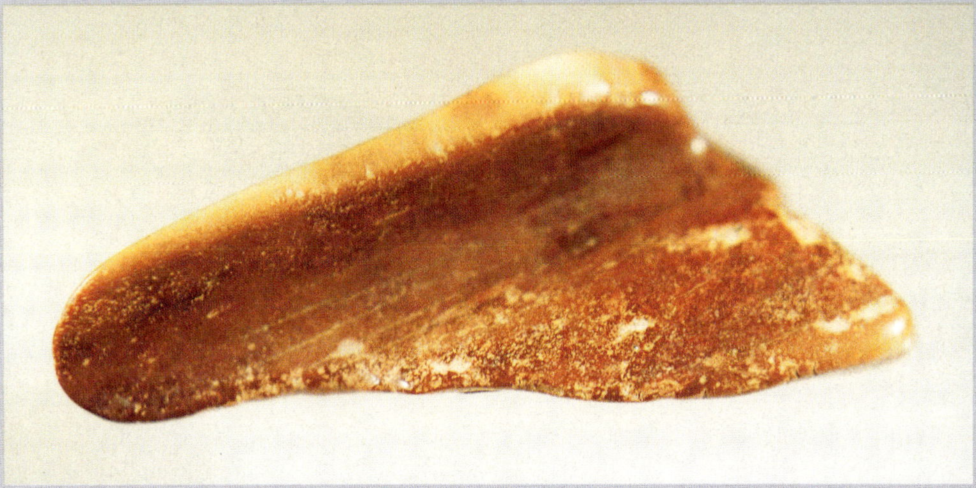

Chisel-like tool head, mineralized ivory with beach polish, 2¾" long. This piece was found in Alaska. Private collection. **$8.00.**

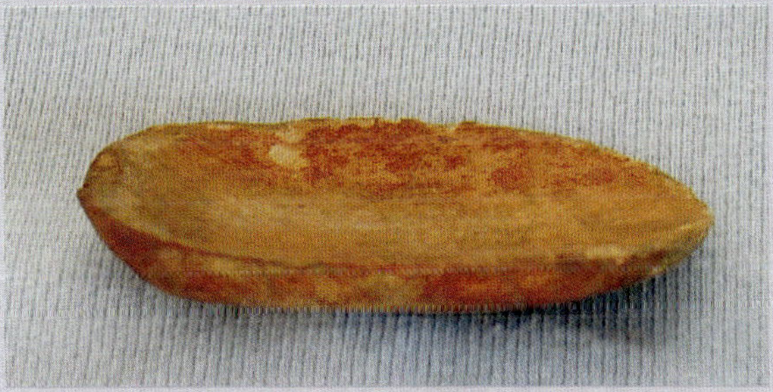

Bone spoon or shallow container, 2⅜" long. It is Eskimo, from Elim, Alaska. Rod Fuller collection, Nebraska. **$75.00 – 100.00.**

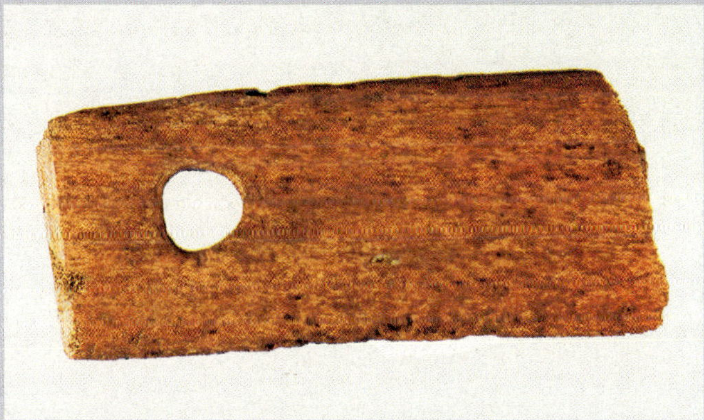

Tool or weapon part, thick drilled bone, 2¾" long. Inuit (Eskimo), it is from Alaska. Don Casto collection. **$12.00.**

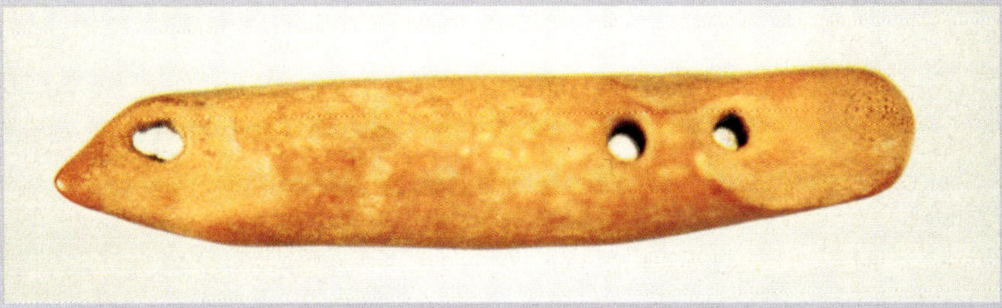

Bone artifact, with three holes, purpose not known, 3" long. It was found in Alaska. Back to Earth. **$40.00.**

Eskimo Artifacts

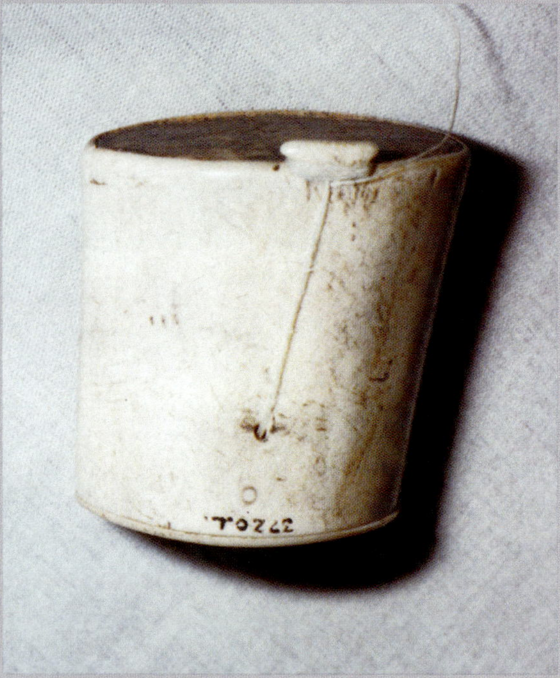

Snuff container, made from caribou antler, Inuit, 3" high and 2½" in diameter. It has a wooden base. The lid is removable and is held in place with a sinew line that goes through the side and attaches to the inside of the lid. This rare example is Bering Sea Eskimo, and was collected in Skagway, Alaska, in 1990. J. Steve and Anita Shearer collection, California. **$1,500.00.**

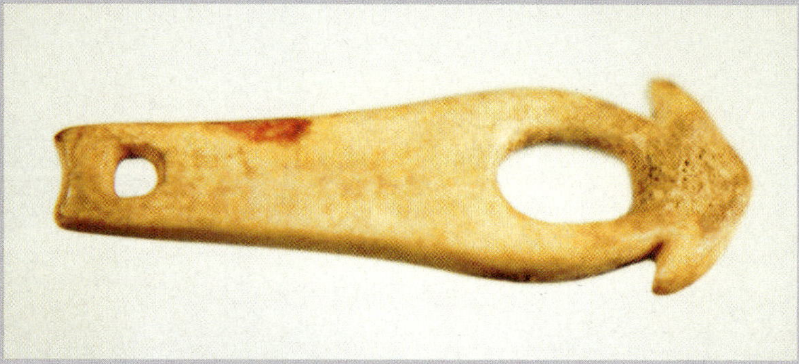

Artifact, weathered bone, 2⅝" long. Of unknown purpose, it came from the Aleutian Islands, Alaska. Larry Garvin collection. **$100.00.**

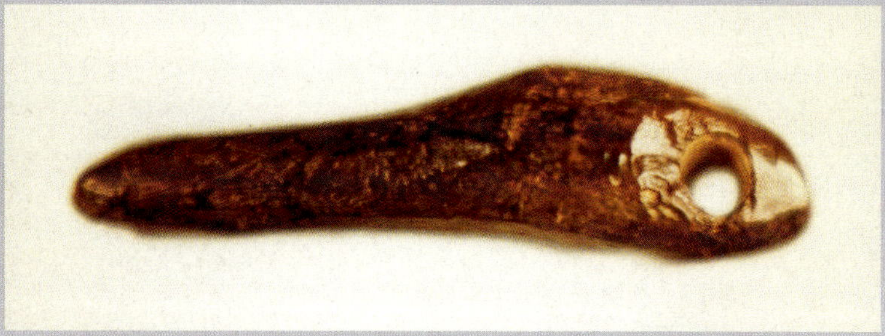

Bone artifact or part, carved bone with drilled hole, mineralized, 2⅝". The use of the object is not known. Alaska. Back to Earth. **$25.00.**

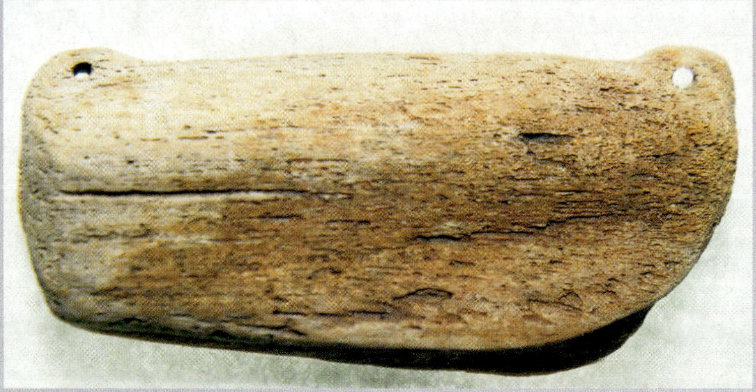

Sinker for a drift net, 4½" long, drilled at top corners. The sinker was found in Alaska. Back to Earth. **$85.00.**

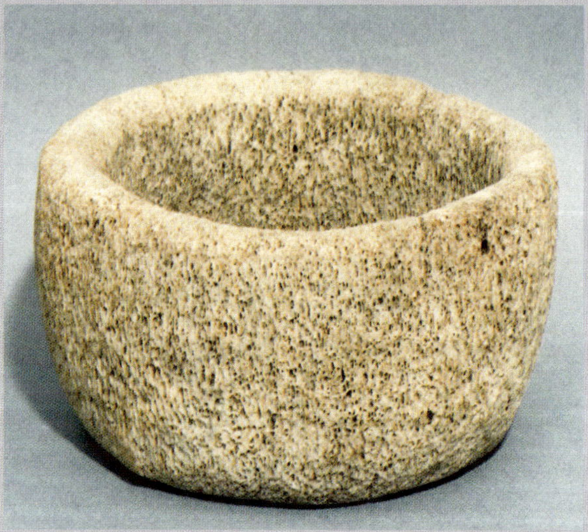

Whalebone bowl, 2¾ x 4⅞". The porous material is still impregnated with grease. This prehistoric bowl was obtained near the Ugasek River, Alaska. H. B. Greene II collection, Naples, Florida. **$225.00.**

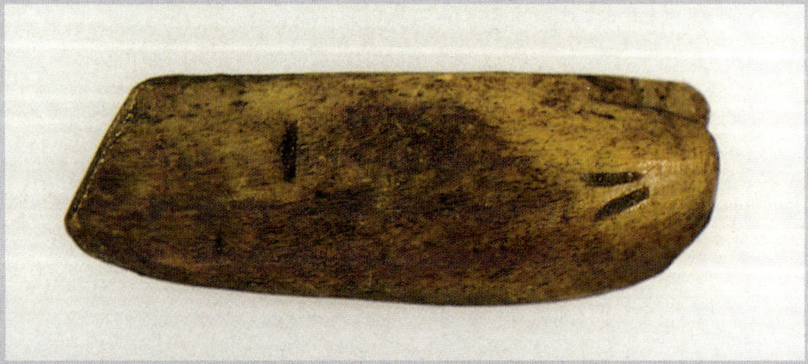

Seal effigy knife handle, top view shows nostrils to right, 3½" long. Made of polished antler, it is a salvaged piece. The blade slot was originally to the left, but it broke out; a new blade slot was then made in the other end. Alaska. Pete Timoch collection. **$200.00.**

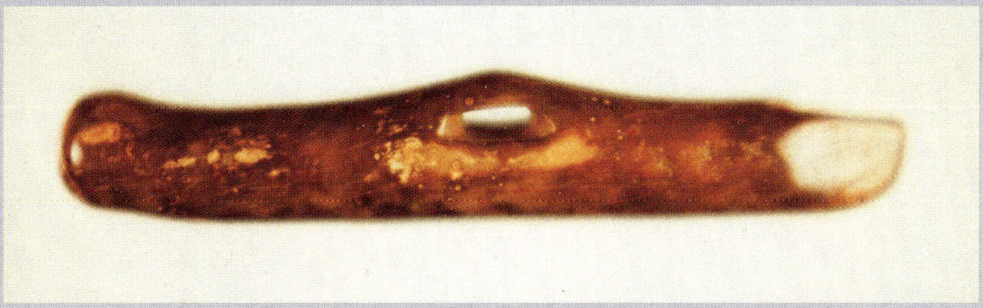

Bone artifact, mineralized and darkened, 3" long. A possible fishing lure part, it came from Alaska. Larry Garvin collection. **$60.00.**

Leister or fishspear tip, dense bone or ivory, 5⅜" long. The small and regular barbs give it a serrated appearance. Alaska. Larry Garvin collection. **$75.00.**

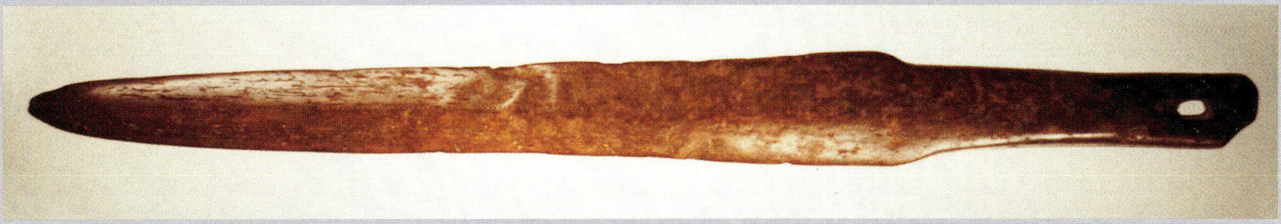

Dagger(?), heavy bone or ivory, handle with hole for suspension or for anchoring the handle wrap. This fine example is 10½" long and came from Alaska. Larry Garvin collection. Museum grade.

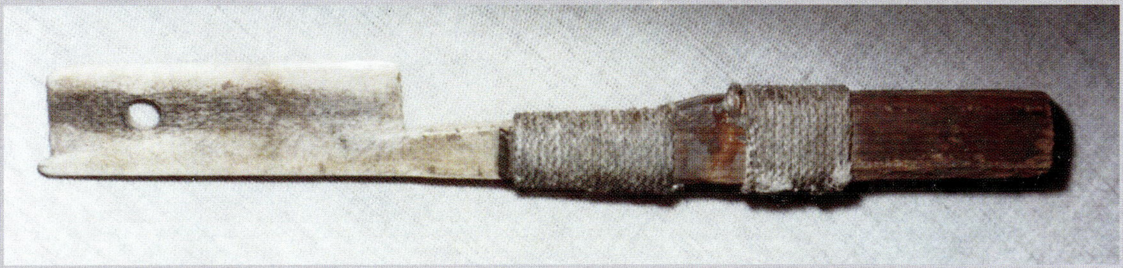

Net or mesh gauge, bone section, 5" long, and wooden handle, 4½" long. The carved bone gauge has trade cord wrapping. Overall length is 8½". Ca. 1850 – 1900, it was obtained from a dealer at a Portland, Oregon, antique show. J. Steve and Anita Shearer collection, California. **$300.00.**

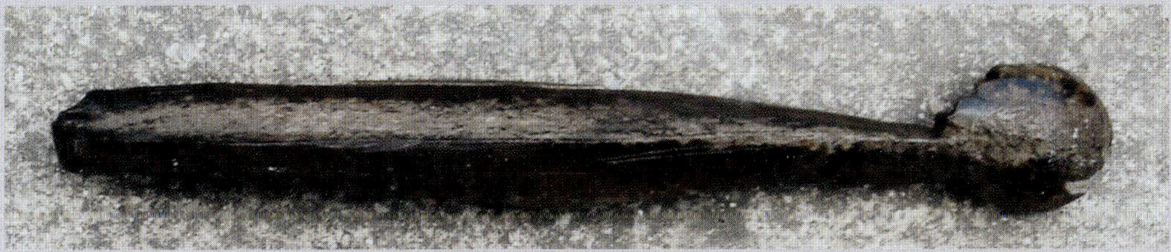

Bone artifact, Atl-atl part(?), 3⅞" long. This piece is Eskimo, from Alaska. John and Susan Mellyn collection, Texas. **$90.00.**

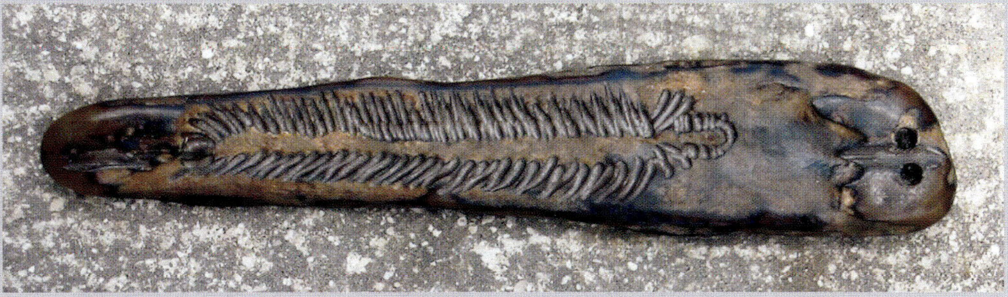

Bone unknown object, 3¼" long, Eskimo. This artifact is from Alaska. John and Susan Mellyn collection, Texas. Unlisted.

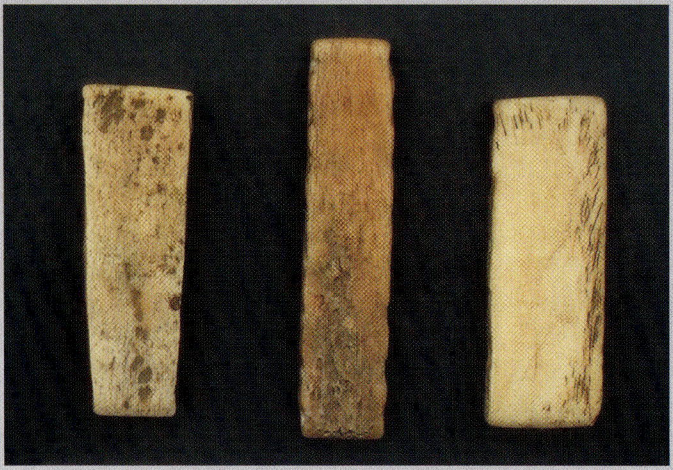

Bone gaming pieces, prehistoric(?), side view (top view photo of same pieces at right). They are from 1$\frac{15}{16}$ to 2$\frac{5}{16}$" long and all are $\frac{5}{16}$" thick. Ex-collection Levy, they are probably Eskimo from Alaska. Collection of, and photograph by, Gary Henry, North Carolina. Each, **$50.00.**

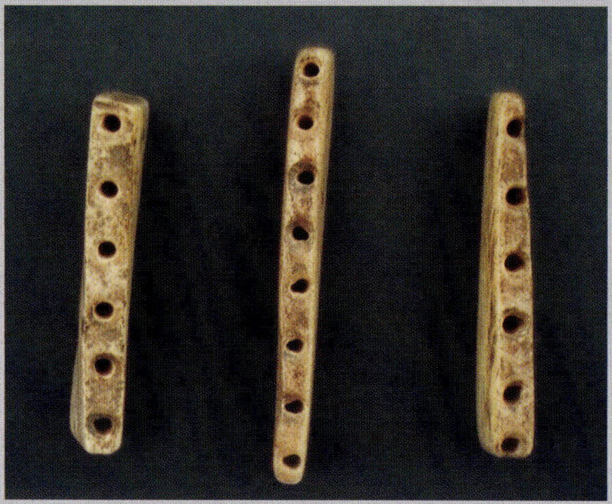

Bone gaming pieces, prehistoric(?), top view showing drilled holes. The center example is 2$\frac{5}{16}$" long, and all are ex-collection Levy. Alaska. Collection of, and photograph by, Gary Henry, North Carolina. Each, **$50.00.**

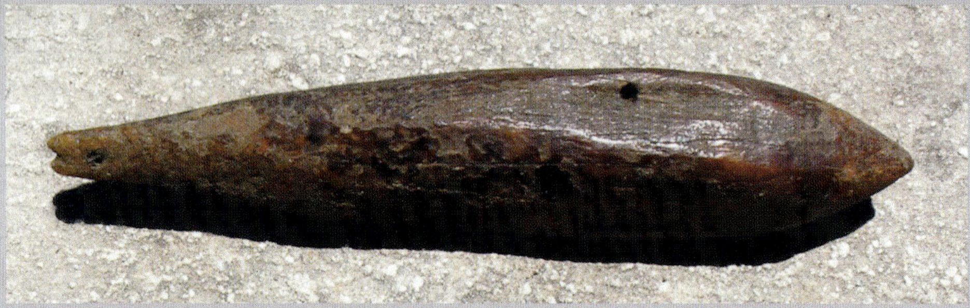

Fishing sinker(?), carved bone, 5⅛" long. Eskimo, it is from St. Lawrence Island. John and Susan Mellyn collection, Texas. **$85.00.**

Bone harpoon head, double opposing barbs, 5½" long. This example is from the Aleutian Islands, Alaska. Larry Garvin collection. **$175.00.**

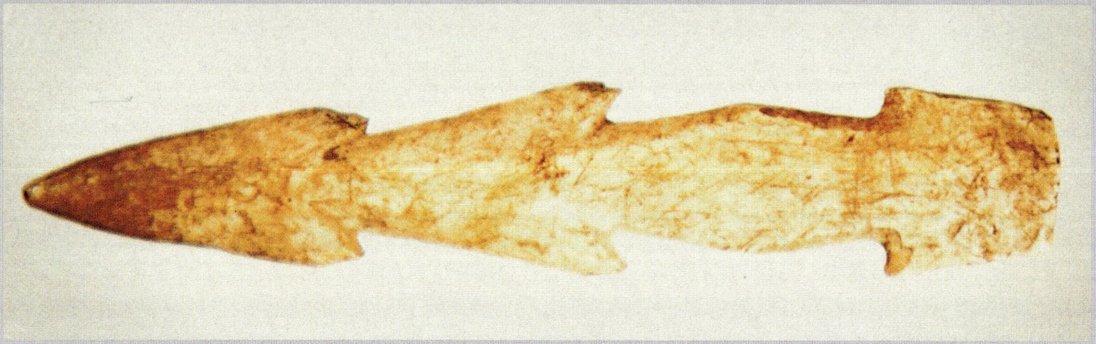

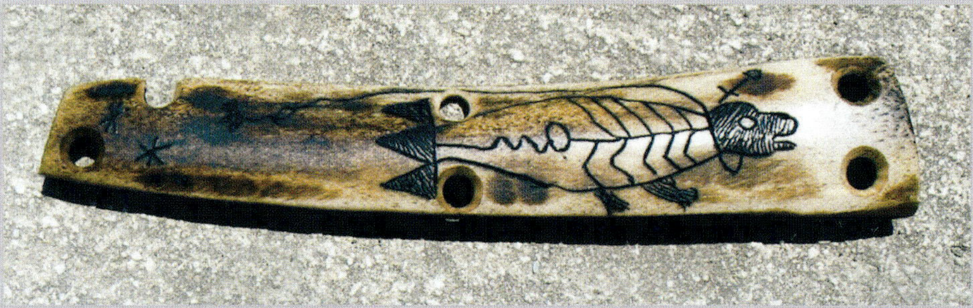

Armor slat or rectangular plate, Eskimo, incised effigy figure, slat is 4¾" long. This is a fine piece, from Alaska. John and Susan Mellyn collection, Texas. Museum grade.

Bone pin or fishing prong, mineralized and dark with age, 4⅜". This example was found in Alaska. Back to Earth. **$25.00.**

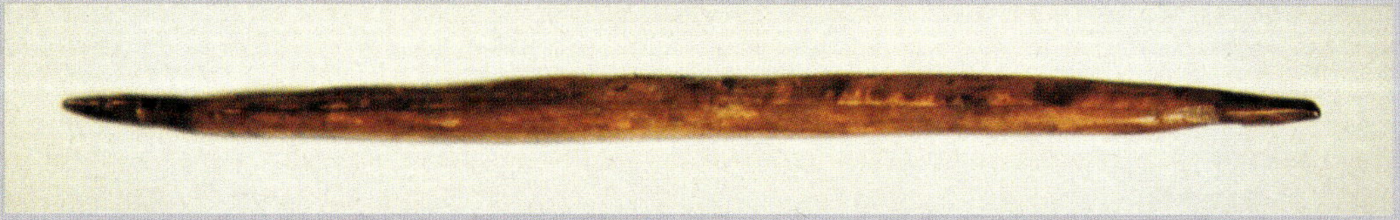

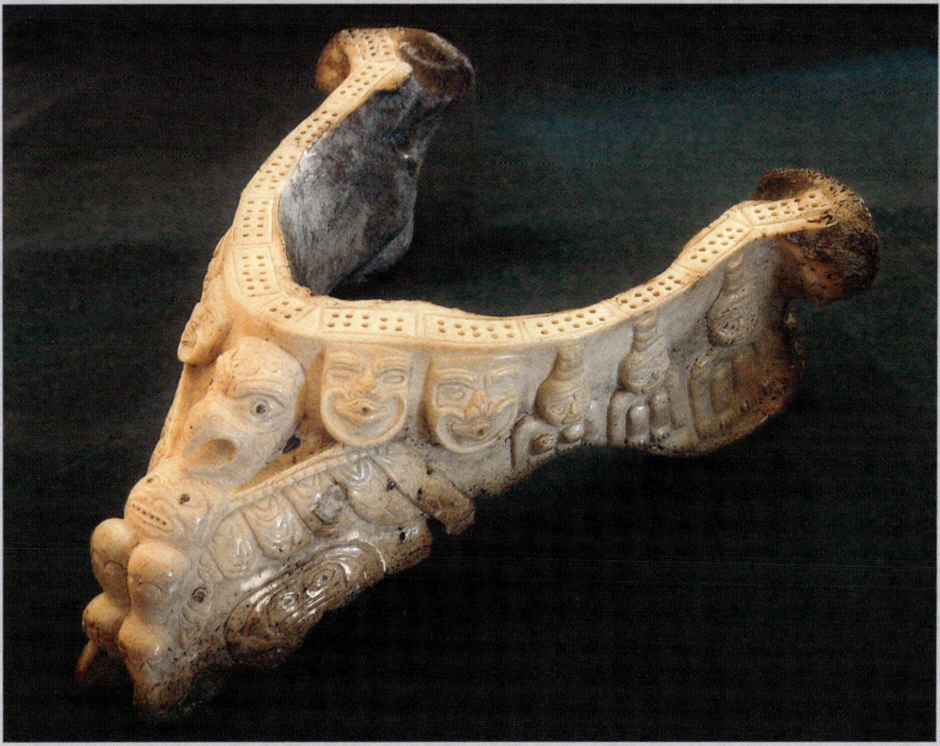

Cribbage board, Eskimo, fossilized lower walrus jaw bone carved with various figures, length is 8". This fine piece is carved with artistry and care. Keyuk, Alaska. Rod Fuller collection, Nebraska. Museum grade.

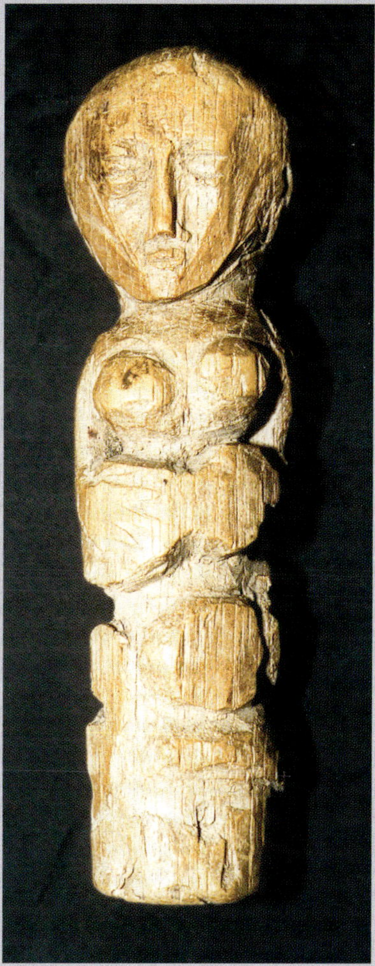

Human female effigy figure, fibrous bone, 6⅞" high. This rare object is from the collection of William Stowell, Arctic explorer and author. Alaska. Larry Garvin collection. Museum grade.

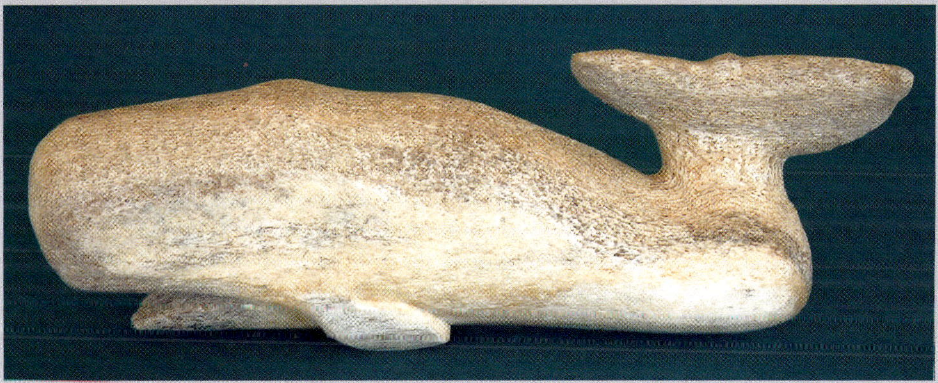

Whale carved in whalebone, Eskimo, 10" long. This is a well-done piece, from Unalakleet, Alaska. Rod Fuller collection, Nebraska. Museum grade.

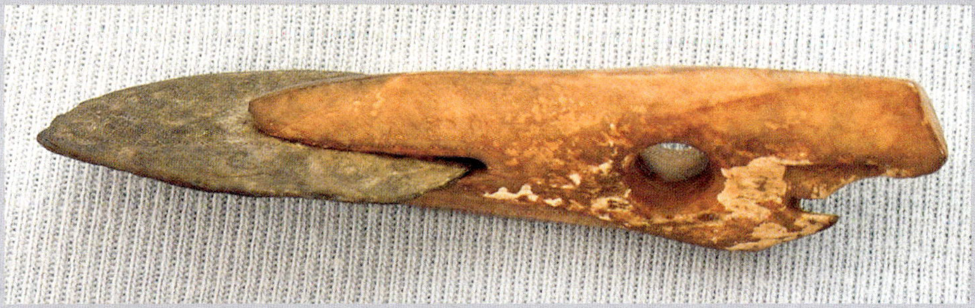

Harpoon head, Eskimo, with stone (probably slate) point, length is 3½". It is made of fossilized ivory and came from Keyuk, Alaska. Rod Fuller collection, Nebraska. **$175.00.**

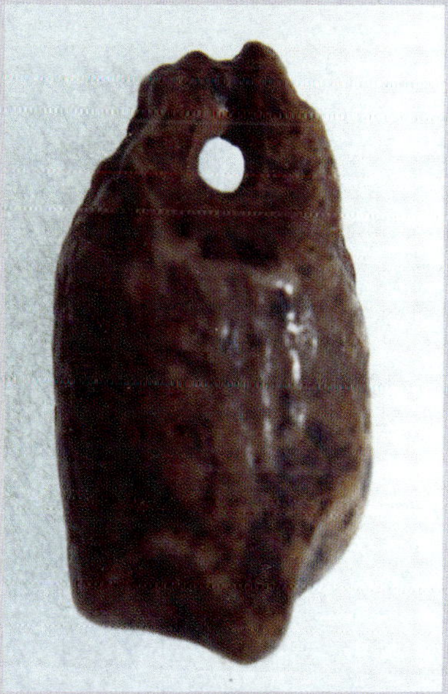

Seal tooth, drilled for cord, found in Alaska. Back to Earth. Unlisted.

Eskimo Artifacts

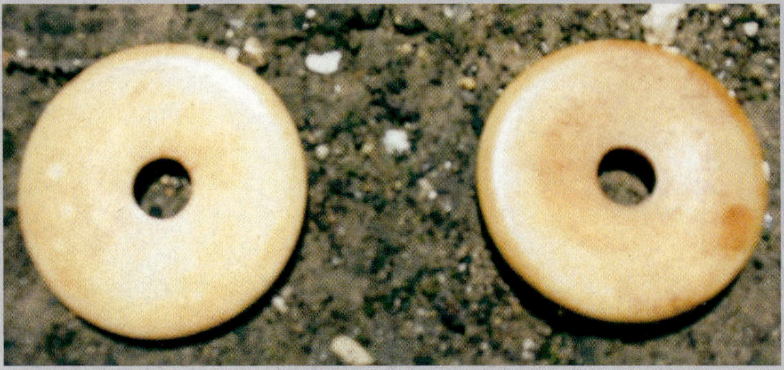

Bone spools, Eskimo, each is 1¹⁄₁₆" in diameter. Carefully made, they are from Alaska. John and Susan Mellyn collection, Texas. Each, **$45.00.**

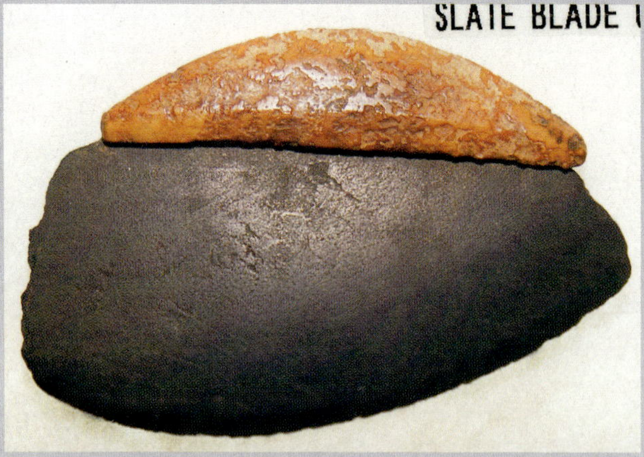

Ulu, or women's knife, large slate blade, overall size is 2¾ x 4½". The handle is walrus ivory and the knife came from St. Lawrence Island, Alaska. Back to Earth. **$250.00.**

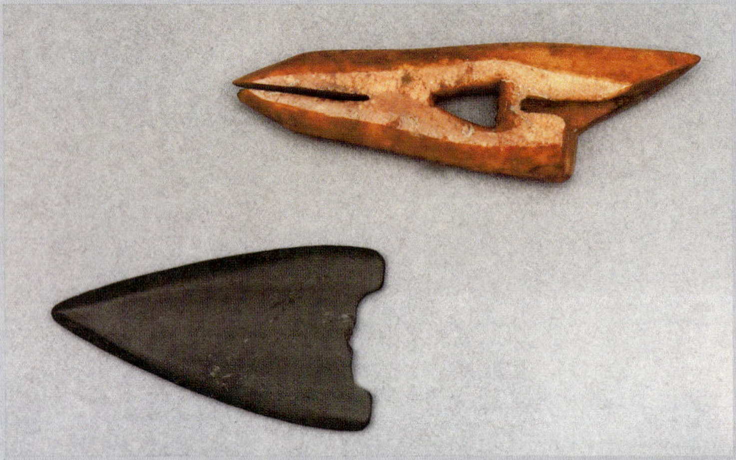

Harpoon set, fossil walrus ivory and slate blade, ivory is 2⅝" long and blade is 2" long. The blade is grooved near the center for insertion in the narrow slot of the ivory portion. Alaska. H. B. Greene II collection, Naples, Florida. **$300.00.**

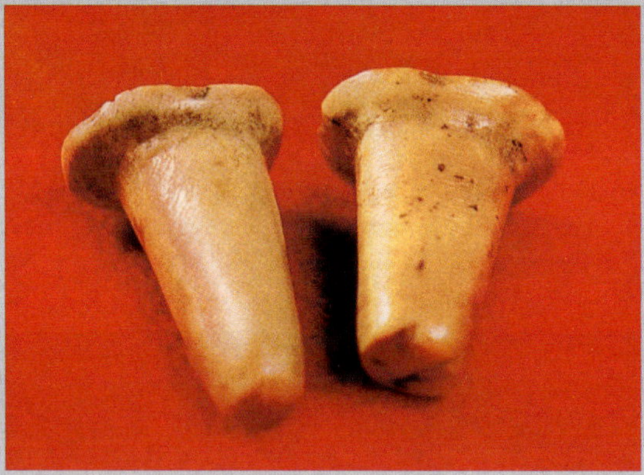

Labrets (lip decorations), well-carved in ivory with good polish, longest is 1". They were found in Alaska. Brenda Rivers collection. Each, **$100.00.**

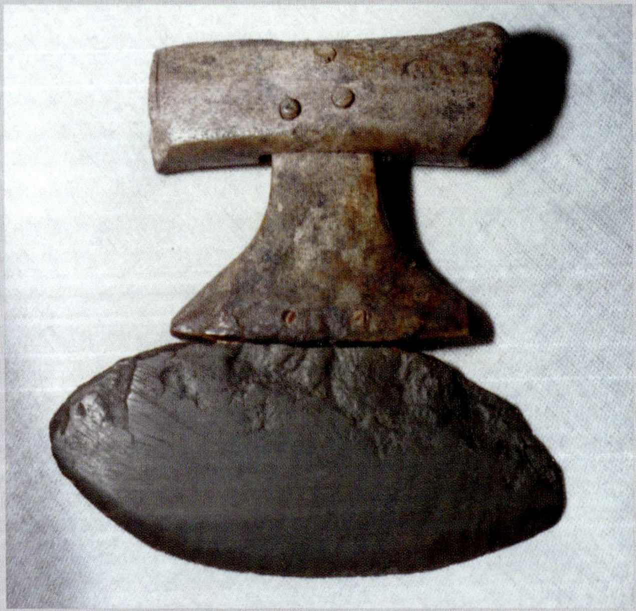

Ulu or household knife, with a slate blade and pegged bone handle made of seal or walrus bone. Eskimo (Inuit), ca. 1700 – 1800. Obtained from a dealer in Long Beach, California. J. Steve and Anita Shearer collection, California. **$450.00.**

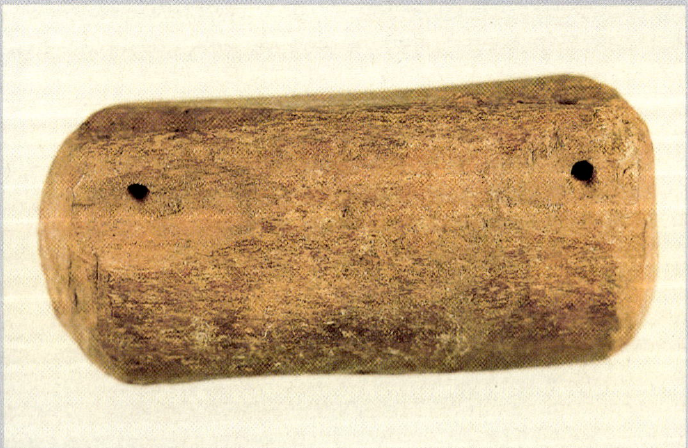

Fishing weight, mineralized material, 3½" wide. It has two sets of small line holes that go through the ridged top, and the weight is smoothly finished. Eskimo, from Alaska. Back to Earth. **$125.00.**

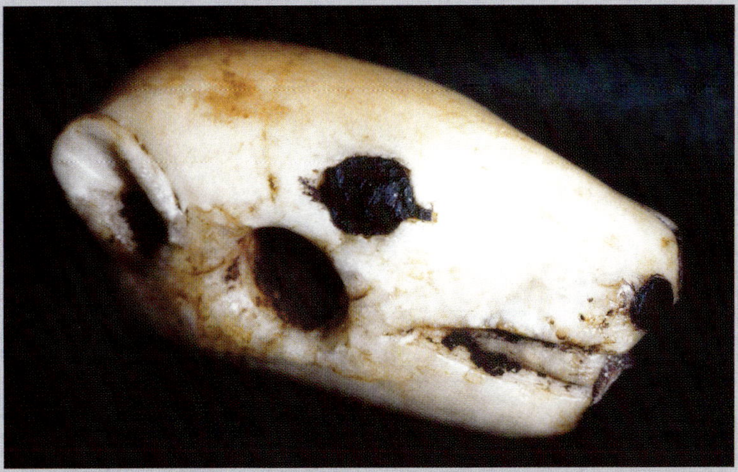

Polar bear head toggle, ivory, 1½" long. This beautiful example was collected in 1886 by a sailor on a whaling ship. Formerly in the Greene collection, present owner is unknown. Alaska. H. B. Greene II photograph, Naples, Florida. Unlisted.

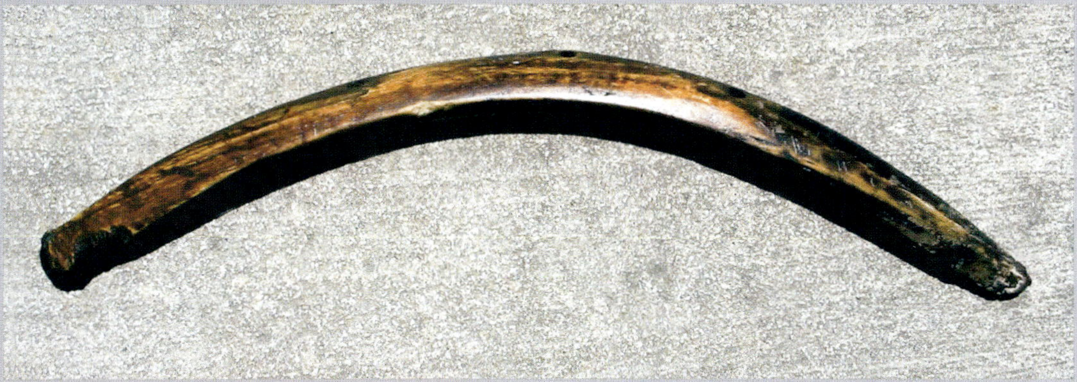

Tool or equipment part – probably made from the rib bone of a large sea mammal, 16¾" long. Found in Alaska. John and Susan Mellyn collection, Texas. **$175.00.**

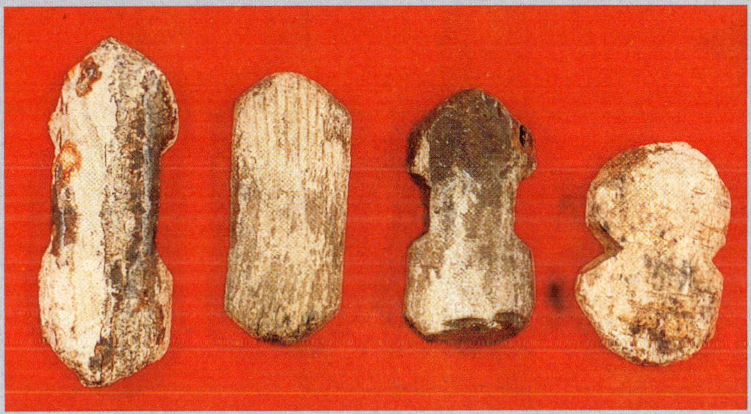

Hammer heads, whalebone and antler, longest is 3⅛". Once with handles, these hammers may have been used for flint-knapping and other light pounding tasks. Alaska. Pete Timoch collection. Each, **$25.00 – 40.00.**

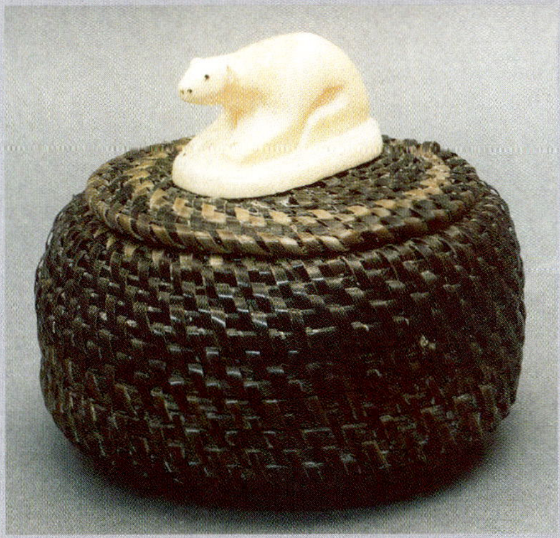

Baleen basket, with walrus ivory polar bear on top, basket is 3" high and 3⅞" in diameter. The basket was made by Herbert Koonuk of Point Hope, Alaska, in 1961, and was obtained by the owner at a Fairbanks antiques shop in 1999. Alaska. H. B. Greene II collection, Naples, Florida. Museum grade.

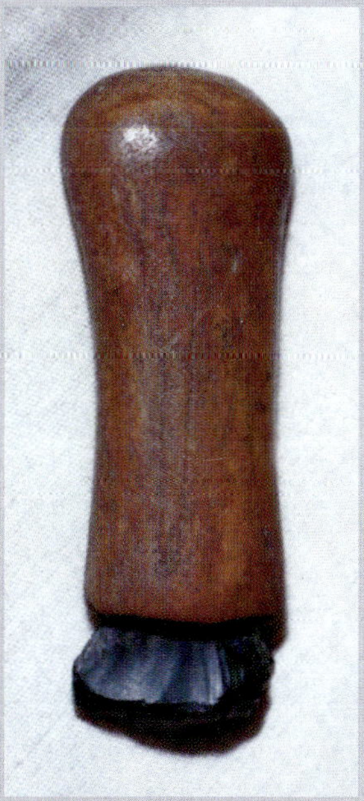

Scraper, bone handle with black flint blade, historic period, ca. AD 1850. This is a tool of the Bering Sea Eskimos of Alaska and is 4" long. It came from the Goulden collection in 2003. J. Steve and Anita Shearer collection, California. **$250.00.**

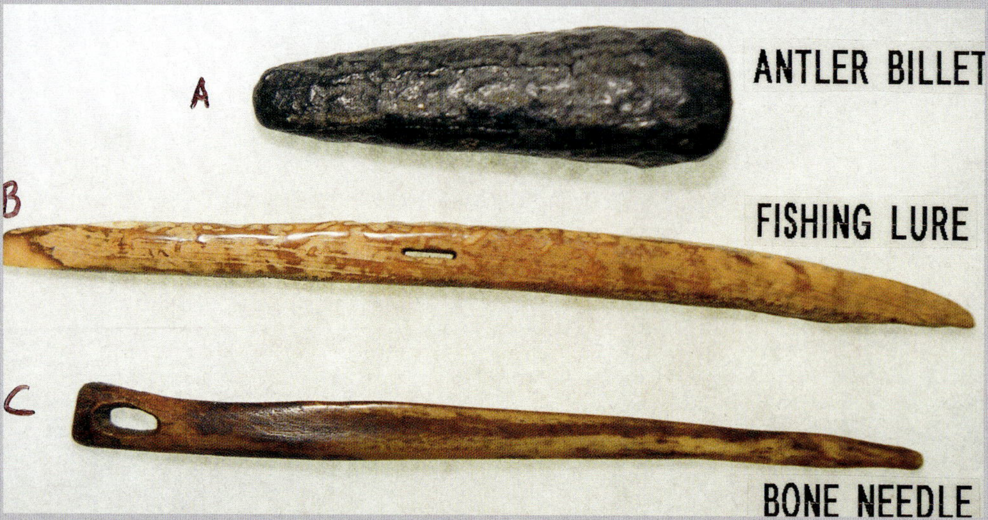

Alaskan artifacts, top to bottom: Antler billet, 3½", mineralized bone or ivory; lure or pin, 7¾", polished bone or ivory; bone needle, golden-brown patination, polished. Back to Earth. Billet, **$45.00;** lure, **$160.00;** needle, **$160.00.**

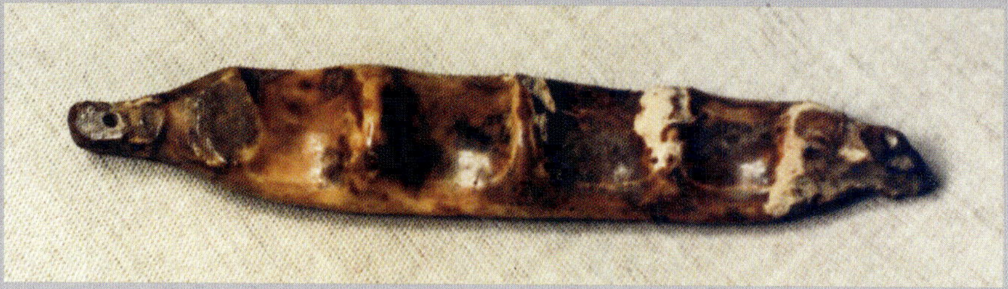

Handle, ivory or bone, Eskimo, probably for a wooden tool box. It is Old Bering Sea culture, ca. AD 1000. This piece is 5" long and was collected at a shop in Skagway, Alaska, in 1997. J. Steve and Anita Shearer collection, California. **$250.00.**

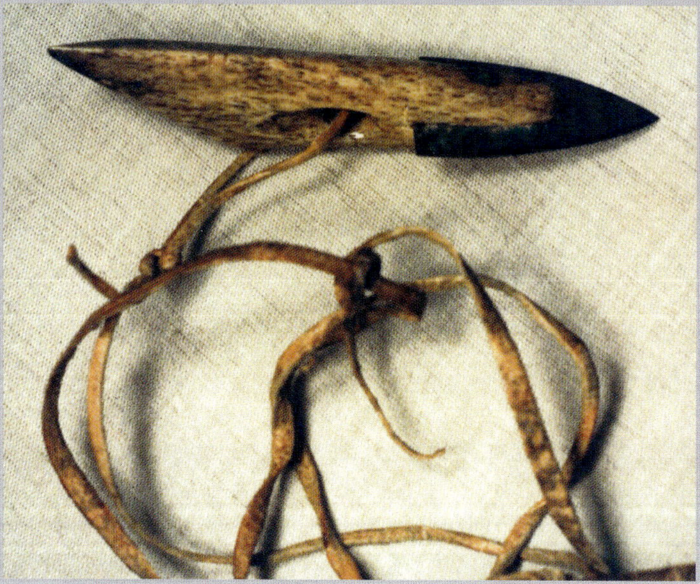

Harpoon head with seal hide rigging, Eskimo, ca. 1870 – 1880s. The head is 5" long, Bering Sea Inuit, Alaska. The head is bone and the blade is copper. It was obtained from a collector in Fallbrook, California, in 1984. J. Steve and Anita Shearer collection, California. **$400.00.**

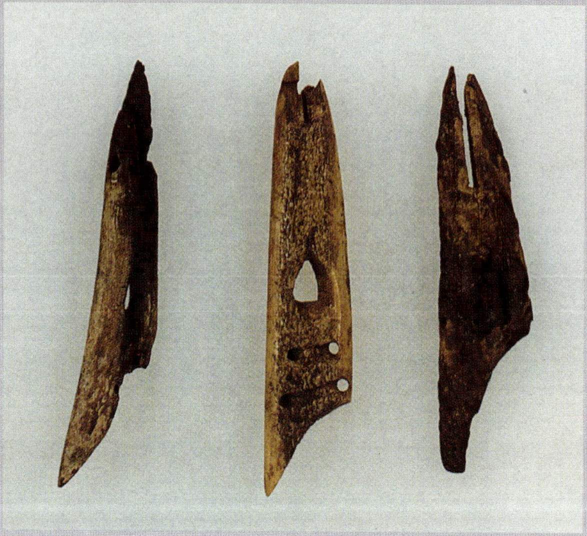

Bone harpoon heads, longest is 3⅝". One has a rusty iron or steel tip, indicating it came from contact or trade. A blade was fitted into the end slot and the head was fastened to a fore-shaft. Alaska. John Timoch collection. Each, **$75.00 – 125.00.**

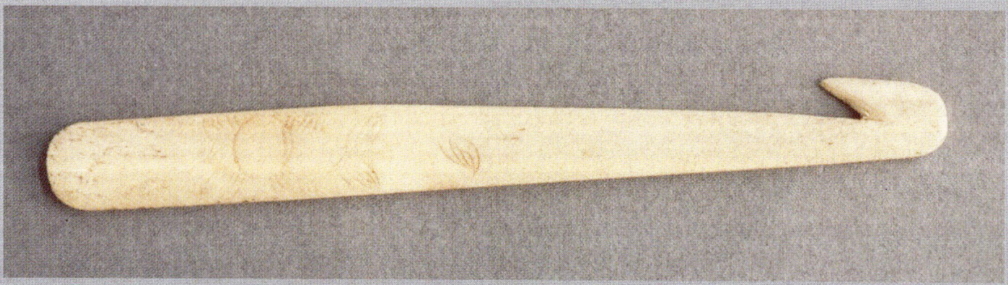

Hook, historic, light scrimshaw on handle, 4¾" long. It is from the A. E. Hill collection and came from St. Michael, Alaska. H. B. Greene II collection, Naples, Florida. **$225.00.**

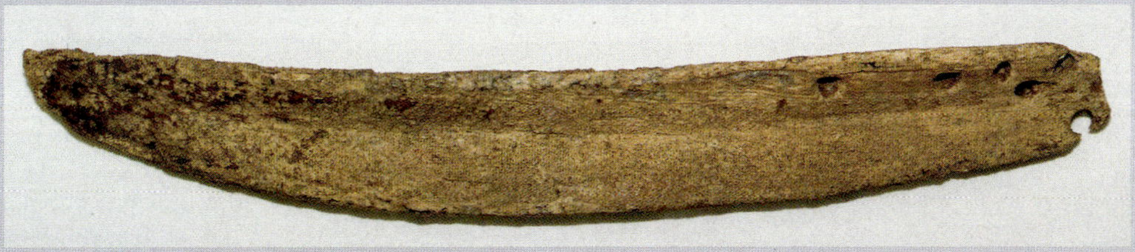

Ivory sled runner, 13½" long, and approximately 2000 years old. It has drilled lashing holes at one end and some are worn through by long use. Sleds were used to pull possessions and game across snow and ice. East Coast of Alaska. Back to Earth. **$225.00 – 250.00.**

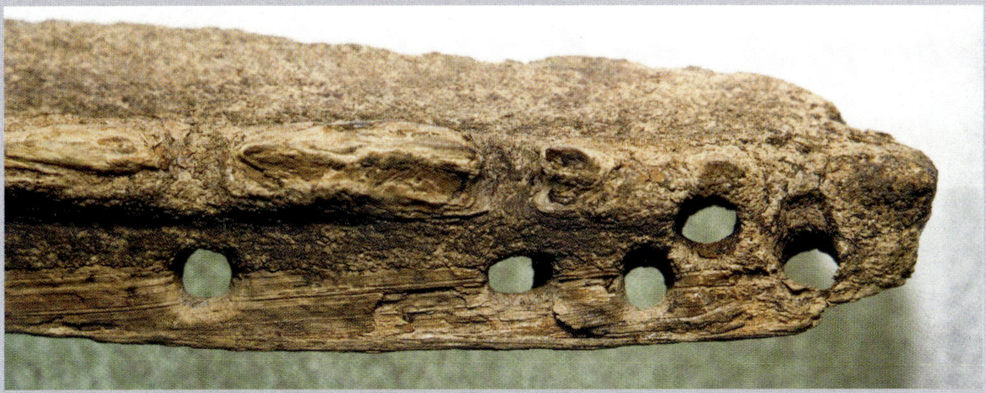

Closeup view, of drilled holes at one end of the ivory sled runner. The material is mineralized from much time in the earth. East Coast of Alaska. Back to Earth. **$225.00 – 250.00.**

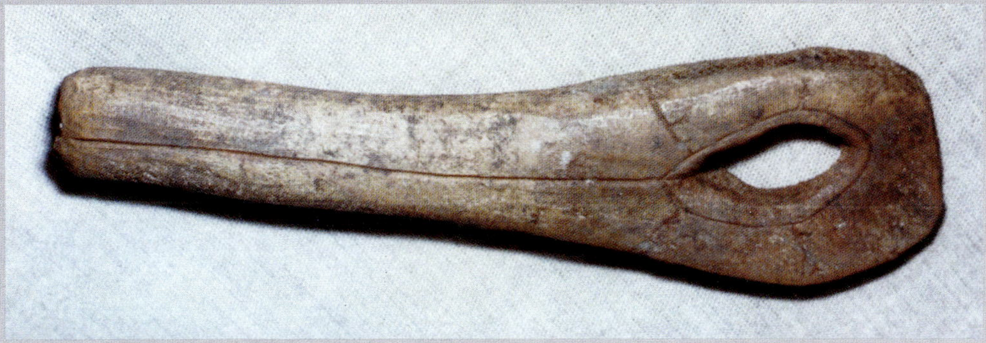

Arrow straightener (shaft wrench), Eskimo, caribou antler. The simple line incising is typical of the Old Bering Sea culture, ca. AD 1000. It is 6½" long and was collected at the village of Brevig Mission, Alaska. The tool was purchased at a shop in Skagway, Alaska, about 1997. J. Steve and Anita Shearer collection, California. **$150.00.**

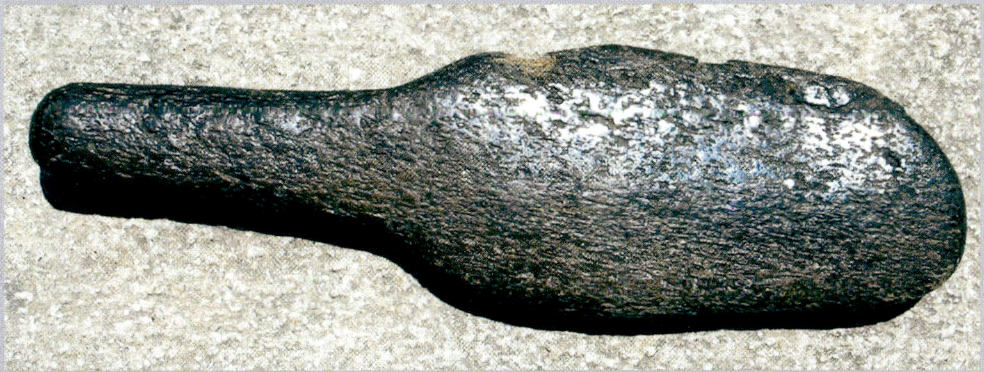

Spatula-like artifact, Eskimo, heavy animal bone, 6½" long. It is from Alaska. John and Susan Mellyn collection, Texas. **$150.00.**

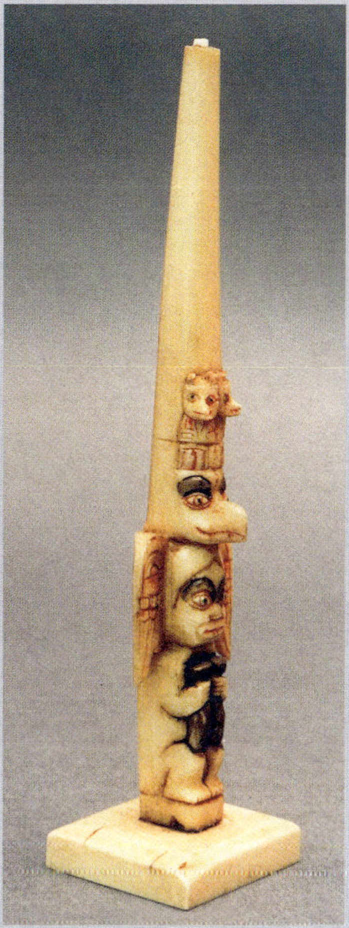

Whale totem pole, walrus ivory, miniature, top missing, 4¼" high. Marked "Johnson" on the bottom, it was exhibited at both the St. Louis World's Fair and the Smithsonian Institution. Southern Alaska. H. B. Greene II collection, Naples, Florida. Museum grade.

Eskimo Artifacts

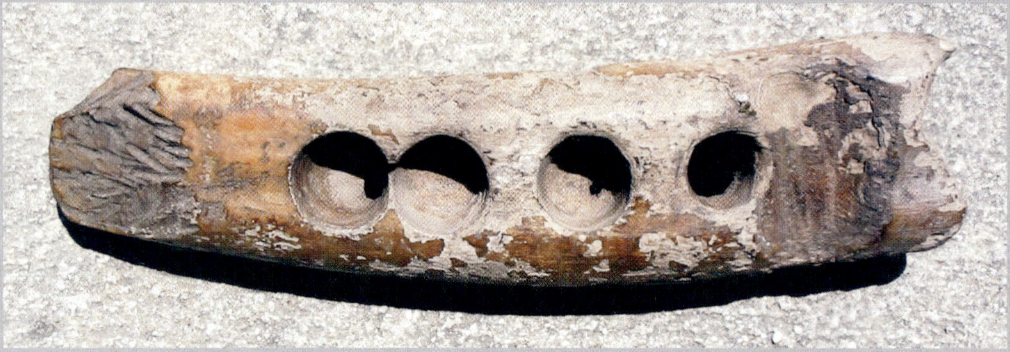

Bone hearth for bow-drill and fire-making, 7⅝" long. This interesting Eskimo piece is from Alaska. John and Susan Mellyn collection, Texas. **$175.00.**

Harpoon head, bone that has turned brown with age and weathering, six barbs. The head is 5" long and it was found in Alaska. Larry Garvin collection. **$125.00.**

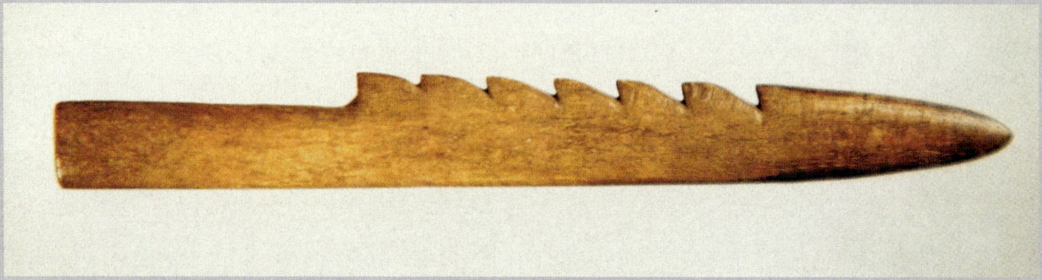

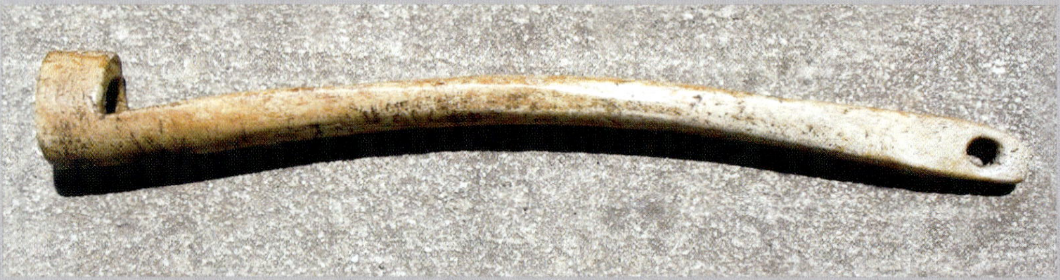

Tool or equipment part, bone, 12½" long. Nicely finished, it is Eskimo and from St. Lawrence Island. John and Susan Mellyn collection, Texas. **$200.00.**

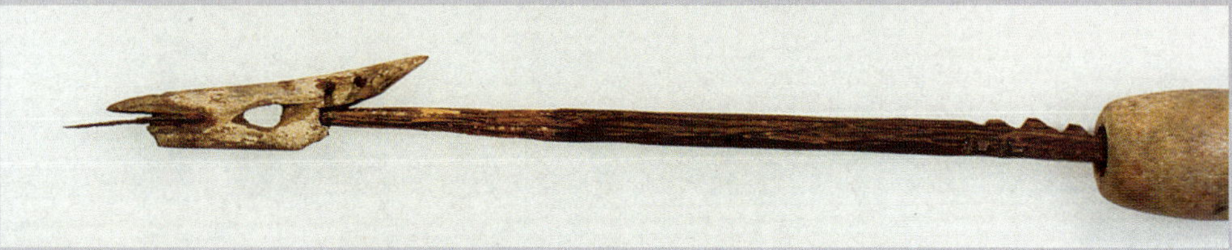

Harpoon, all parts old and authentic. An iron tip is fastened to the bone harpoon head, which in turn is secured to a narrow foreshaft fastened to a bone connector at the end of a wooden shaft. In use, the foreshaft easily released the harpoon head, which itself was fastened to a long cord. Some of the cords were made of walrus-hide leather. Alaska. John Timoch collection. Unlisted.

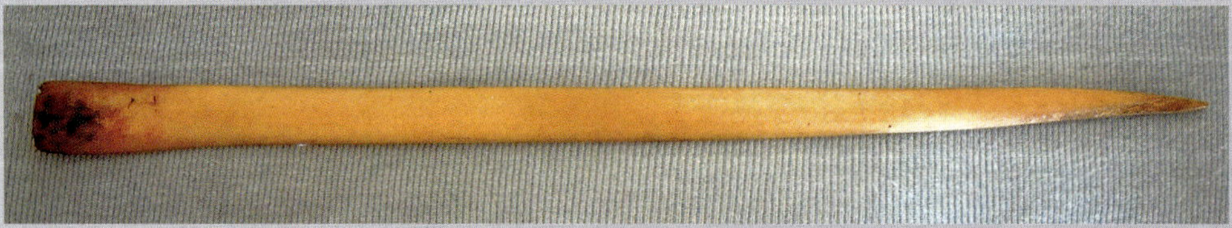

Bone pin, polished surface, 10⅝" long. It is Eskimo, from Elim, Alaska. Rod Fuller collection, Nebraska. **$150.00.**

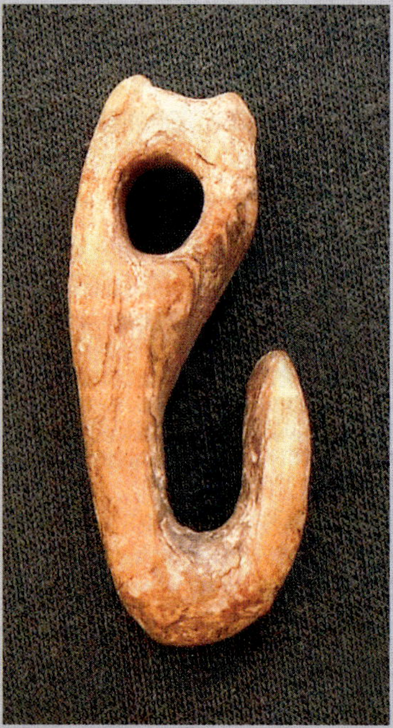

Bone hook, pleasingly carved, 1⅝" long, purpose unknown. This example is Eskimo. Eek, Alaska. Rod Fuller collection, Nebraska. **$45.00.**

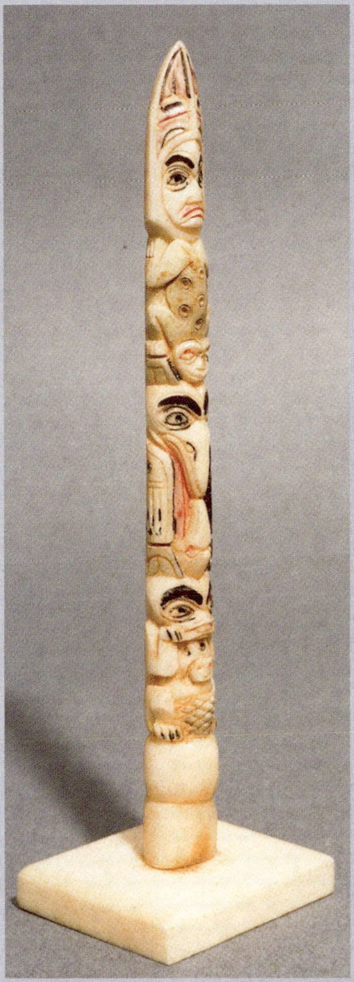

Frog totem pole, miniature, walrus ivory, 4" high. Exhibited at the St. Louis World's Fair, it is marked "Kahlteen" on the platform bottom. Southern Alaska. H. B. Greene II collection, Naples, Florida. Museum grade.

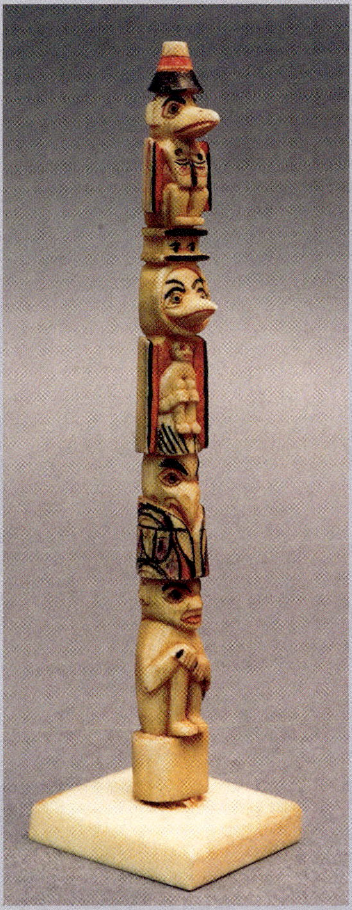

Raven totem pole, miniature, walrus ivory, 4⅛" high, displayed at the St. Louis World's Fair. Colorful and intricate, it was made in southern Alaska. H. B. Greene II collection, Naples, Florida. Museum grade.

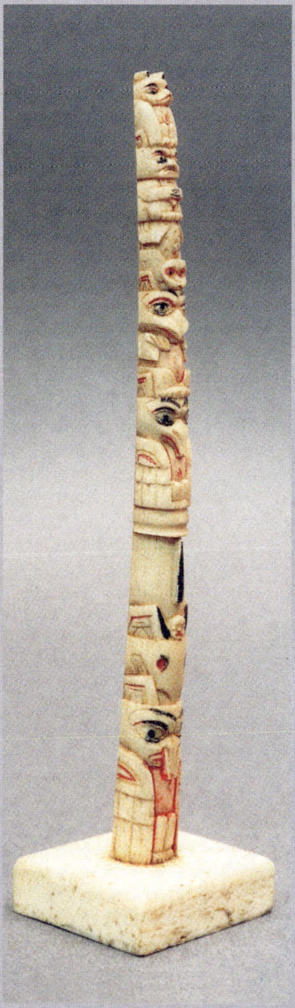

Owl totem pole, miniature, walrus ivory, 4⅞" high. Displayed at the St. Louis World's Fair, it is marked "Sitka" on the bottom. Southern Alaska. H. B. Greene II collection, Naples, Florida. Museum grade.

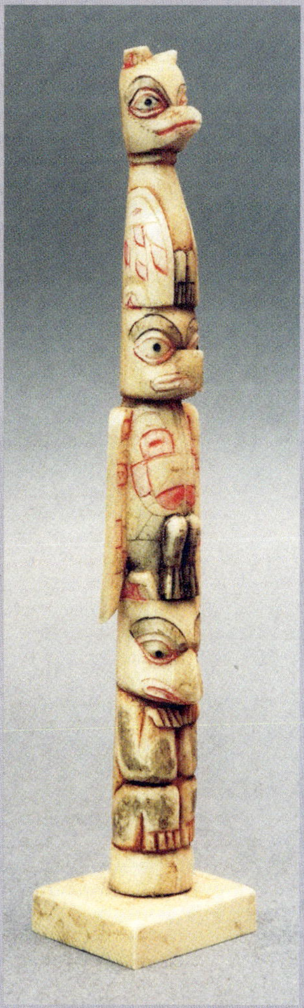

Eagle totem pole, walrus ivory, 5¼" high. Exhibited at the St. Louis World's Fair and the Smithsonian Institution, it was carved in southern Alaska. H. B. Greene II collection, Naples, Florida. Museum grade.

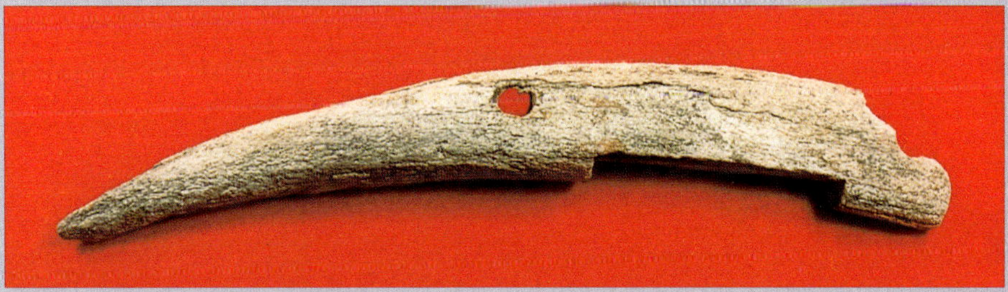

Whalebone pick, 14½" along the outside curve. The handle would have been mounted at about right angles to the cutout, and was secured through the hole and indented end. This piece is quite scarce. Alaska. Pete Timoch collection. **$350.00.**

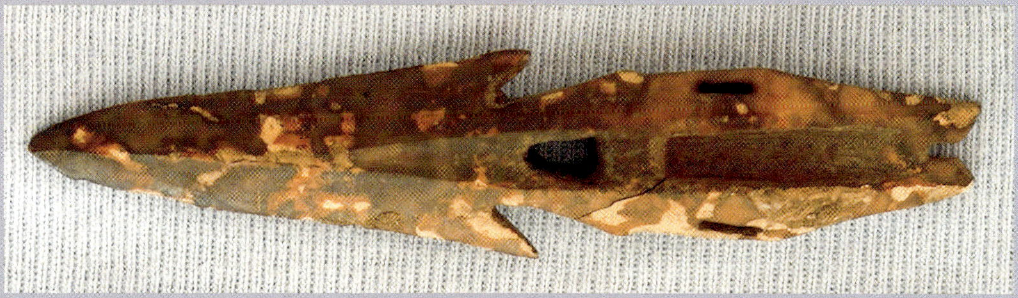

Harpoon point, fossilized ivory, 3¾" long. This Eskimo piece is streamlined and would have been an effective hunting tool. Elim, Alaska. Rod Fuller collection, Nebraska. **$200.00.**

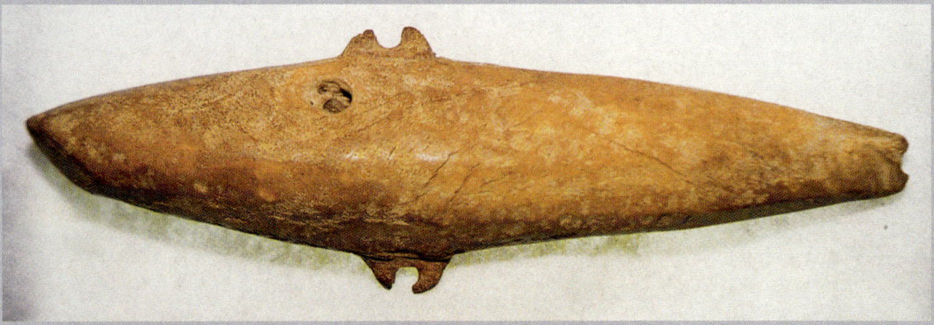

Fishing lure, mineralized bone or ivory, drilled hole through body. It was found on St. Lawrence Island, Alaska. Back to Earth. **$225.00.**

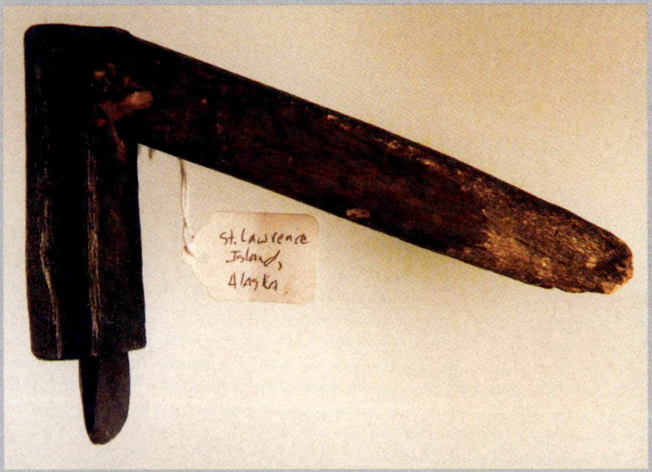

Eskimo adz, bone sockets, bone handle, and slate blade. The socket and blade arrangement is 4¾" high. The adz was found on St. Lawrence Island, Alaska. Back to Earth. **$425.00.**

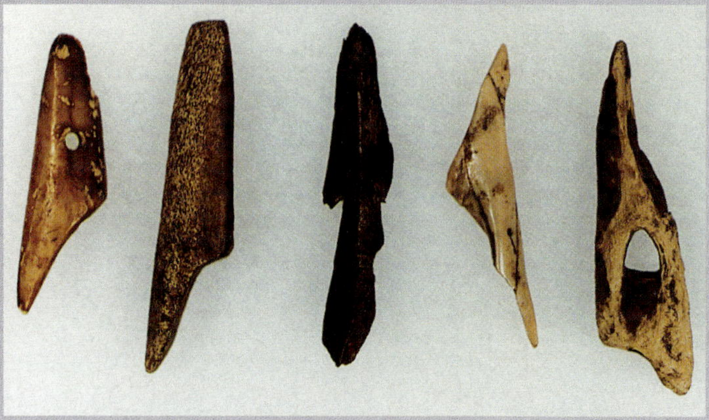

Harpoon heads, bone and ivory, longest is 2¾". These tipped a multi-part weapon, and were fastened to a foreshaft. A line was usually attached at or near the heads. Alaska. James Timoch collection. Each, **$25.00 – 40.00.**

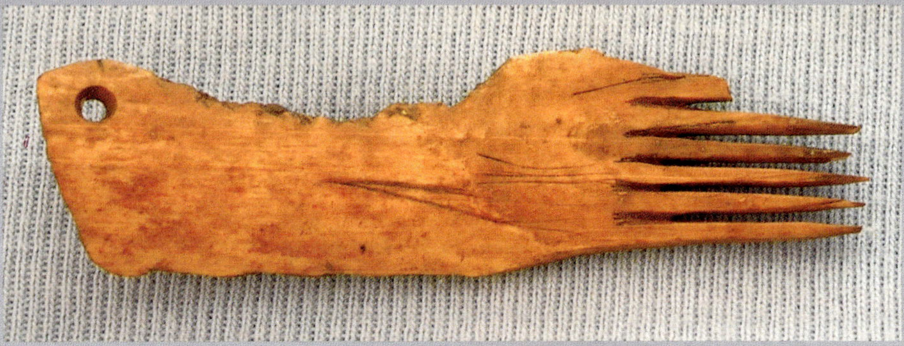

Bone comb, Eskimo, 3" long. This artifact was found at Keyuk, Alaska. Rod Fuller collection, Nebraska. **$125.00.**

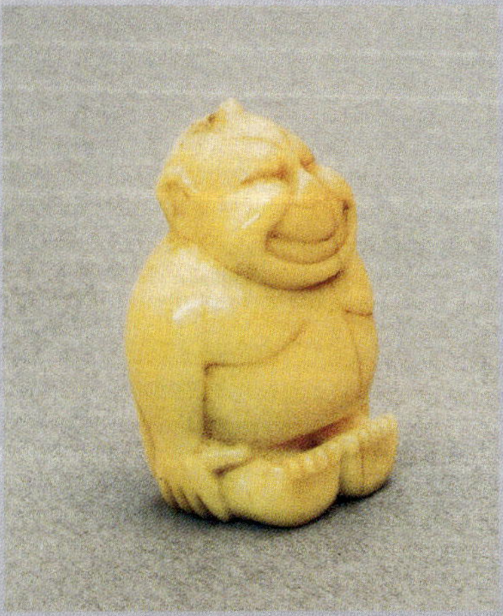

Walrus ivory billiken, ¾ x 1". Said to have been made by the native artist Happy Jack in 1909 or 1910, it is from Nome, Alaska. This Billiken was purchased by the owner from a California dealer. Elizabeth A. Greene collection, Naples, Florida. **$125.00.**

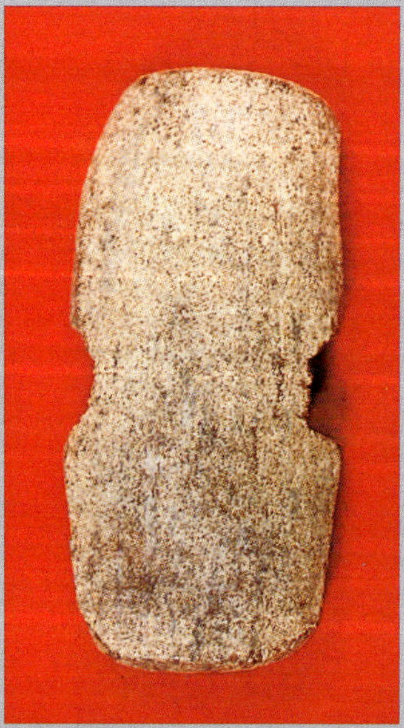

Whalebone hammer head, with side notches, 3" long. This head was hafted and possibly used for tasks like flint-knapping. Alaska. Pete Timoch collection. **$100.00.**

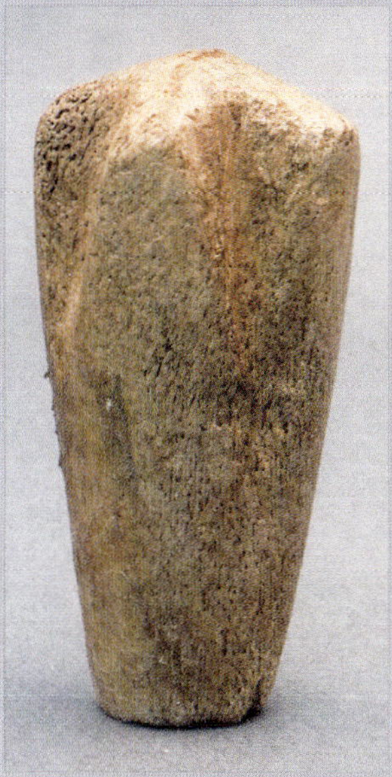

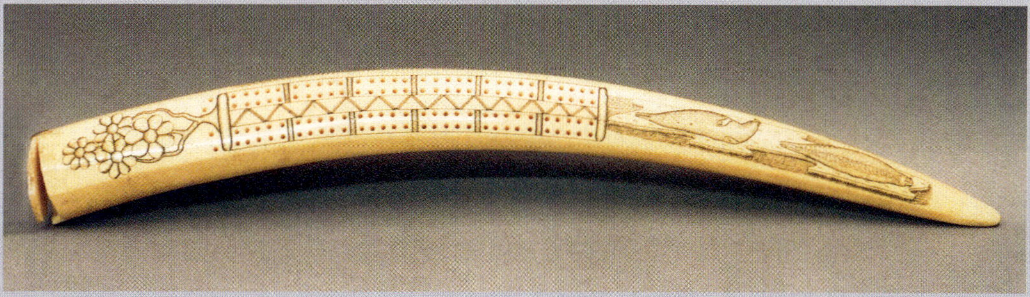

Cribbage board, walrus ivory, 18¾" long. Made in the 1890s, note the hinged lid at left that opens a storage compartment for game pins. Nome, Alaska. Elizabeth A. Greene collection, Naples, Florida. **$700.00.**

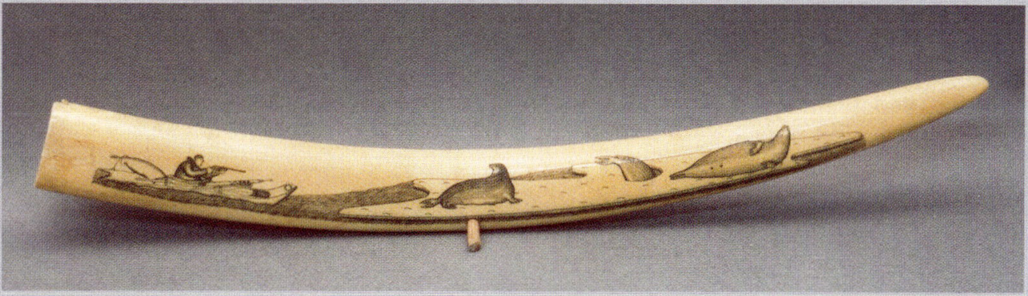

Blunt projectile point, 1 x 1⅞", prehistoric. It was found in a midden along the Kobuk River and is from the A. E. Hill collection. Alaska. H. B. Greene II collection, Naples, Florida. **$65.00.**

Cribbage board, scrimshawed back showing hunter shooting seals on an ice floe. Walrus ivory, from Nome, Alaska. Elizabeth A. Greene collection, Naples, Florida. **$700.00.**

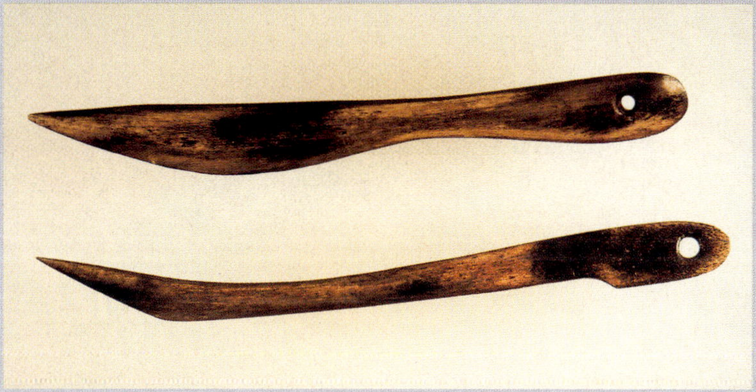

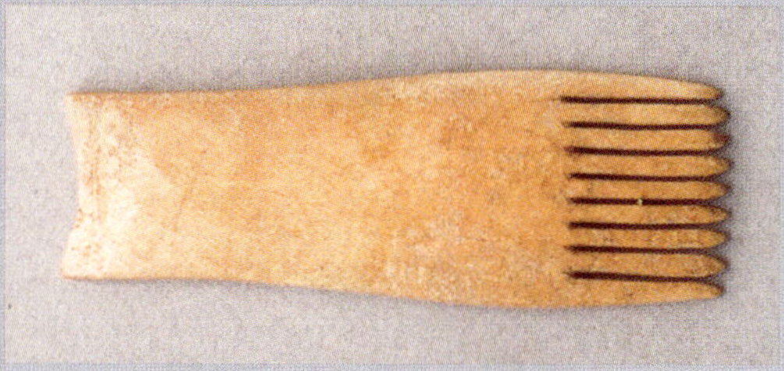

Bone comb, 3½" long, prehistoric. From the A. E. Hill collection, it was found in a midden along the Kobuk River, Alaska. H. B. Greene II collection, Naples, Florida. **$200.00.**

Bone tools, ornate examples with perforated handles, top example is 7 1/16" long. On both artifacts, the lower section (to left) has a sharp edge. These are Eskimo, from Alaska. Robin Fiser collection. Each, **$65.00.**

Loon figurine, 1⅝ x 3¾", walrus ivory, red glass bead eyes. Theresa Mayac carved this recent piece in the 1980s. Alaska. Elizabeth A. Greene collection, Naples, Florida. **$450.00.**

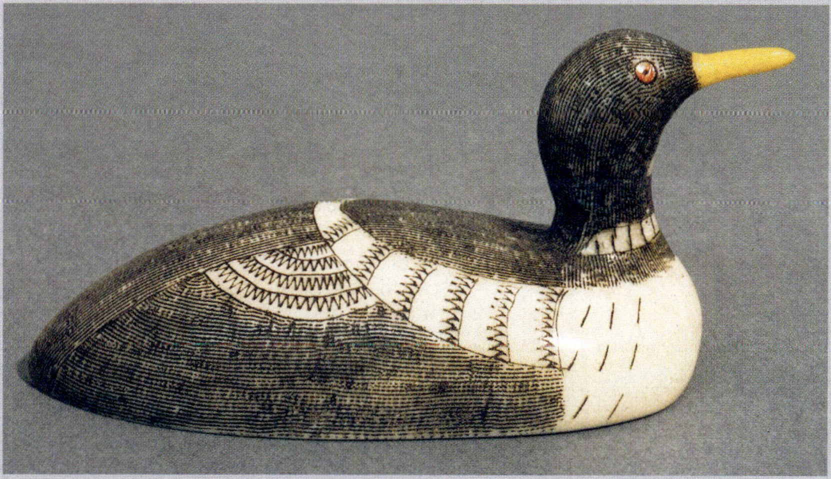

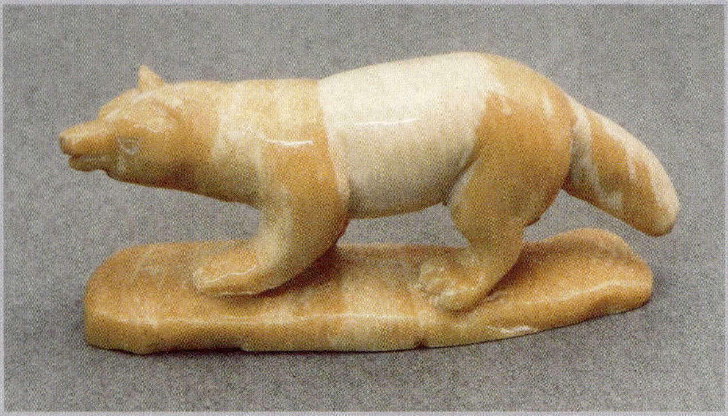

Arctic fox figurine, ⅝ x 1⅝", fossilized mastodon ivory. Made ca. 1967, it is from Alaska. Elizabeth A. Greene collection, Naples, Florida. **$100.00.**

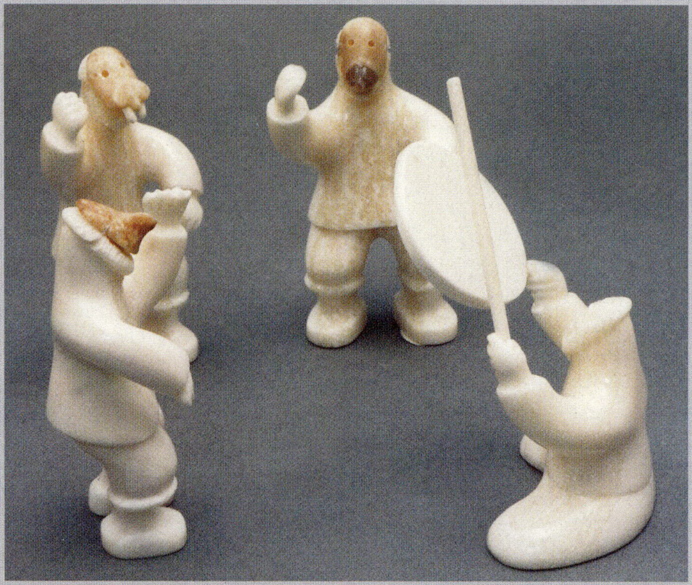

Drummer and dancers, walrus ivory, dancers are 2¾" high. Carved by Isaac Koyuk of King Island, the masks are Raven, Walrus, and Seal. The owner obtained this set in Alaska. Elizabeth A. Greene collection, Naples, Florida. Set, **$1,300.00.**

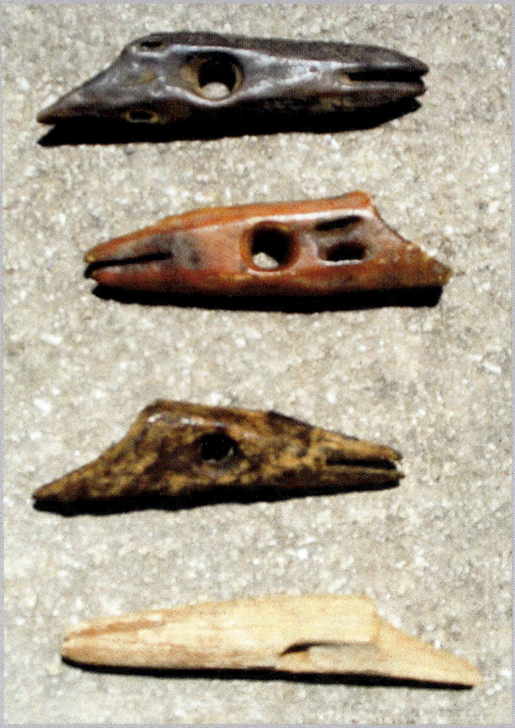

Toggle harpoon heads, 3 to 3⅝" long, carved from ivory. These are Eskimo, from Alaska. John and Susan Mellyn collection, Texas. Each, **$125.00 – 175.00.**

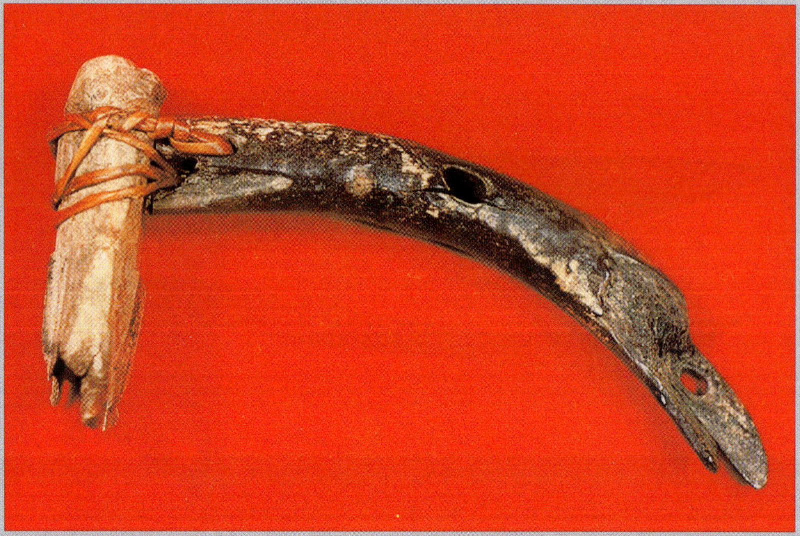

Adz, bone head, 5" long, and large rib bone handle, 12" long. Modern lashing is used to illustrate how the two parts were fastened together. The handle has drilled holes for holding a cord. Alaska. Pete Timoch collection. Unlisted.

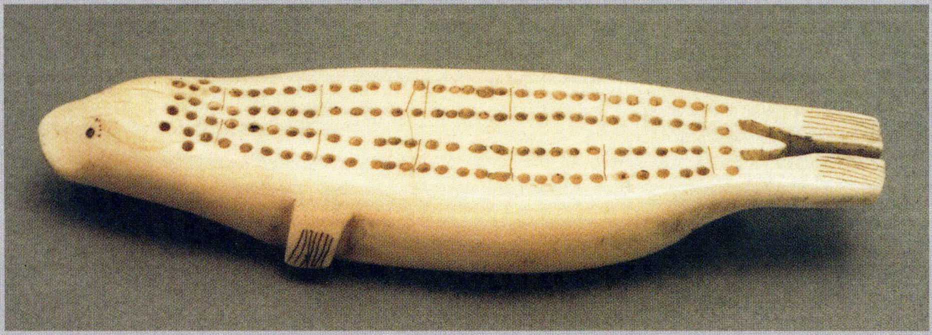

Seal-shaped cribbage board, 1½ x 5⅜". Made in the 1890s, such objects were often carried by gold miners during the Nome gold rush of the same period. Alaska. H. B. Greene II collection, Naples, Florida. **$500.00.**

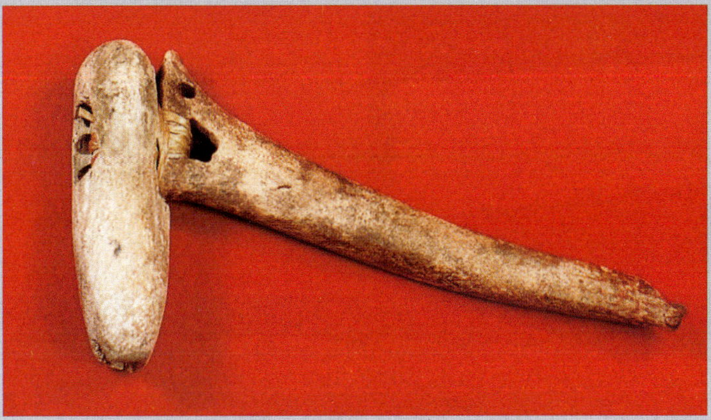

Adz or celt holder, antler handle and bone tool head receptacle, handle 7½" long. Modern sinew was used to fasten the two pieces together for photographic purposes. Artifacts like these can survive many centuries in permafrost. Alaska. Pete Timoch collection. Unlisted.

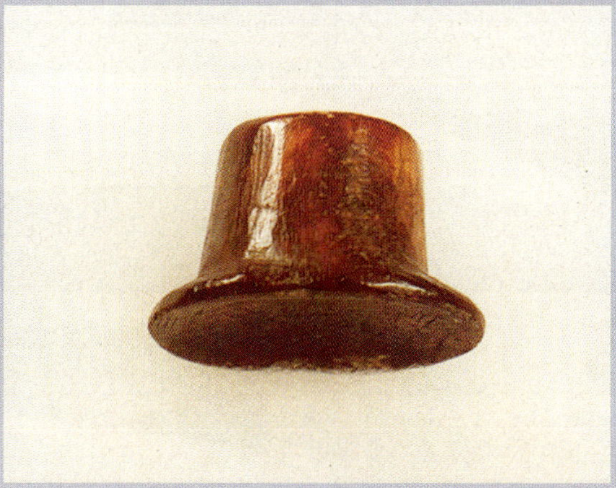

Labret, basal diameter 1¼", height ¾". It has age patina and high overall polish. Alaska. Private collection. **$100.00.**

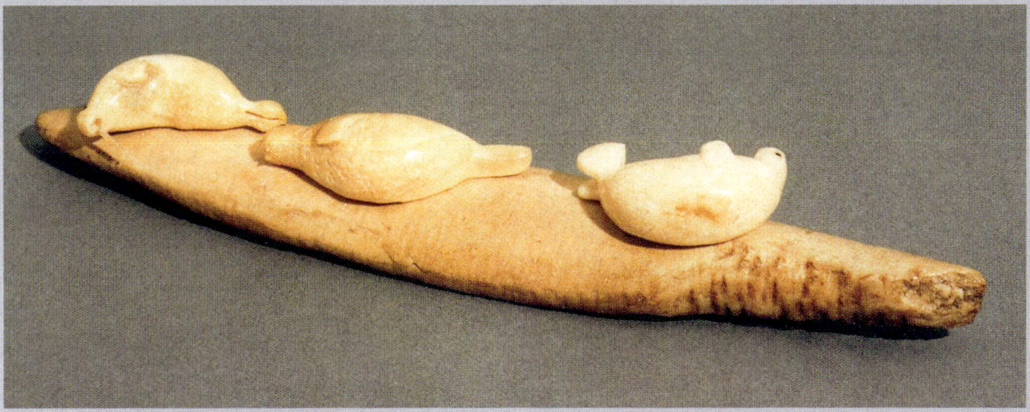

Walrus ivory seals on whalebone ice floe, 9⅛" long. Probably from the 1940s, the carvings are from Alaska. Elizabeth A. Greene collection, Naples, Florida. **$550.00.**

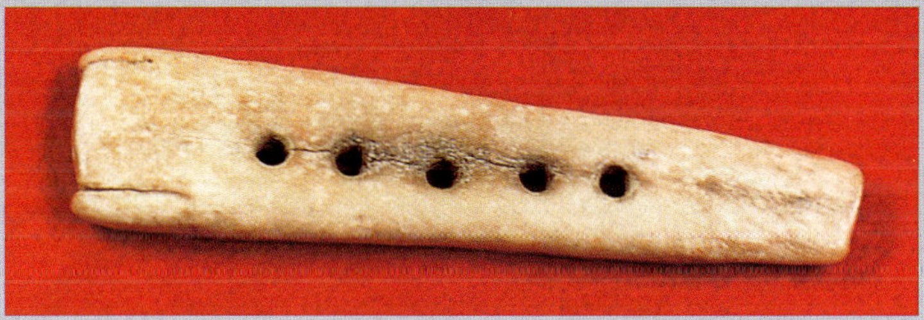

Bone knife handle, 4½" long. The handle has five drilled holes and the wider end has a slotted blade receptacle, plus a blade access hole drilled in the side. With use and hand polish, the bone is solid and heavy. Alaska. Pete Timoch collection. **$200.00.**

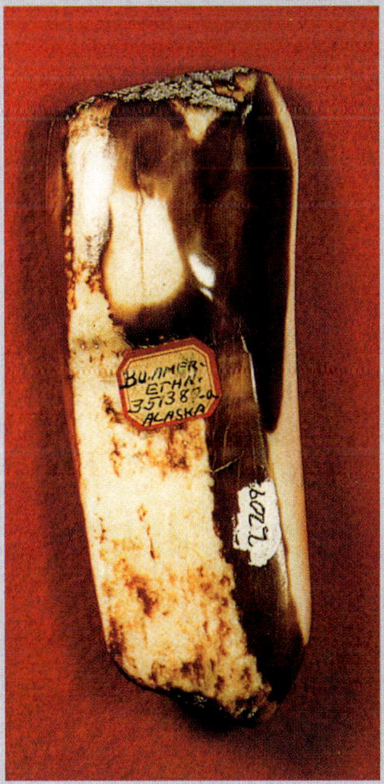

Adz head, highly polished ivory, 5½" long, quite colorful. The poll end (top) has slight battering, and the blade is nearly flat on one face. Alaska. Pete Timoch collection. **$250.00.**

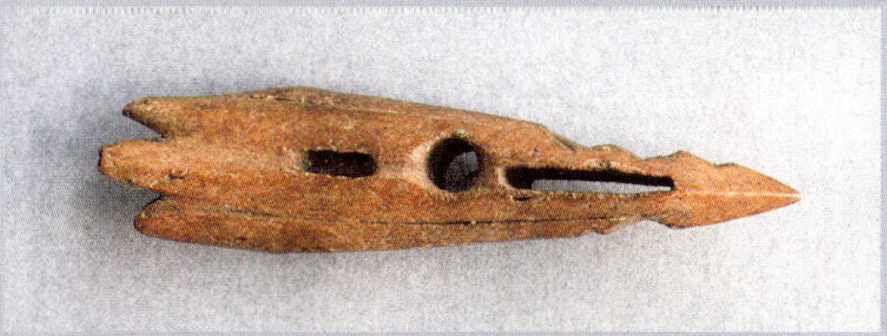

Bone harpoon head, 3" long. Ca. 500 BC, it is from the A. E. Hill collection and came from the Aleutian Islands. Alaska. H. B. Greene II collection, Naples, Florida. **$90.00.**

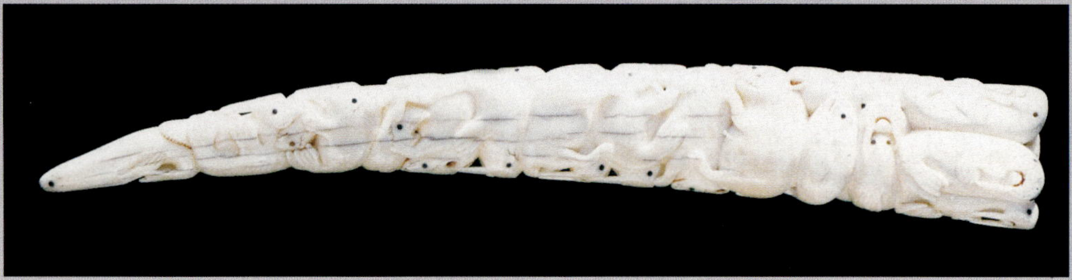

Carved walrus tusk, about 26" long, carved in the 1920s on Nunivak Island. This ivory was formerly in the Greene collection. Alaska. H. B. Greene II photograph, Naples, Florida. Museum grade.

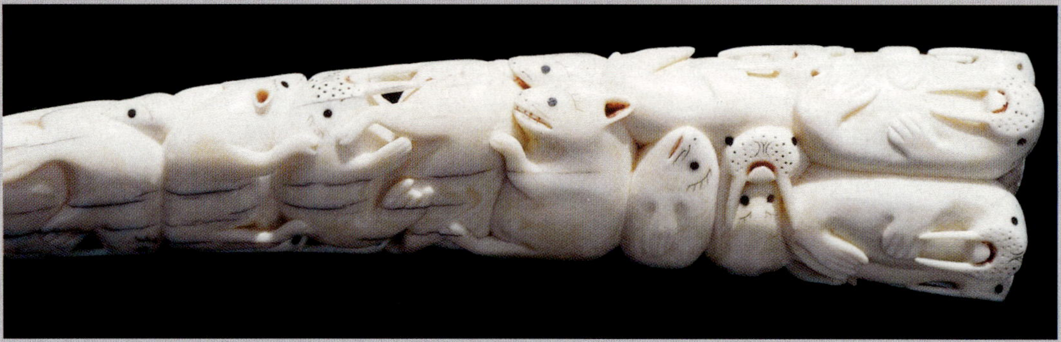

Carved walrus tusk, (close-up of base), overall length, about 26". Among the creatures depicted are fish, lemmings, seals, and walrus. Nunivak Island, Alaska. H. B. Greene II photograph, Naples, Florida. Museum grade.

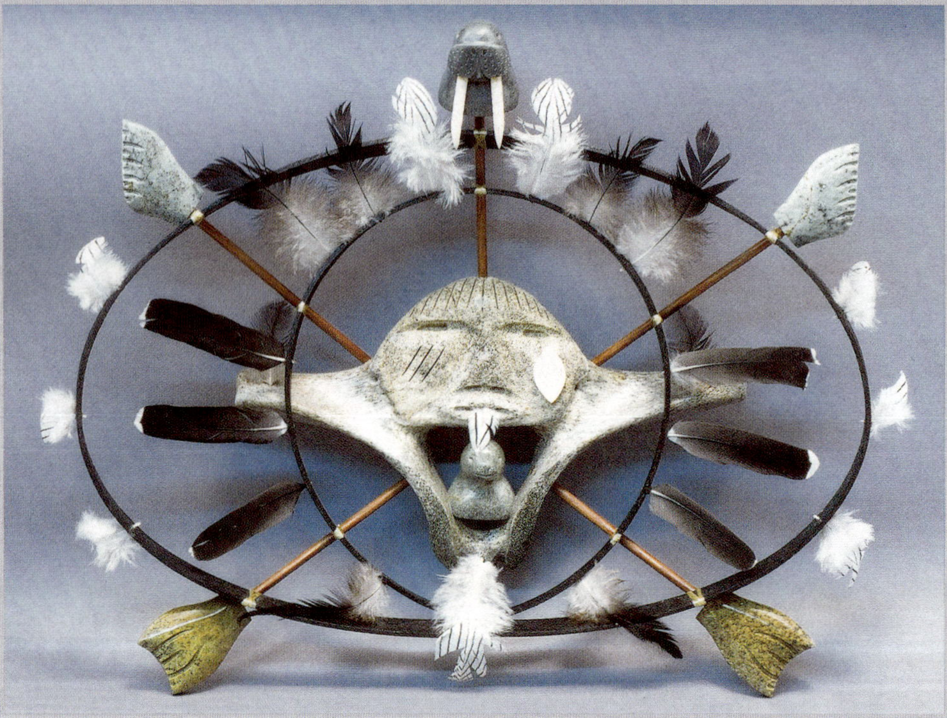

Contemporary Eskimo mask, 16½ x 22", bone and baleen. Made in 1999, it was purchased from K. Komakkoy. This represents the traditional mask worn to celebrate a walrus hunt. Nome, Alaska. Elizabeth A. Greene collection, Naples, Florida. Museum grade.

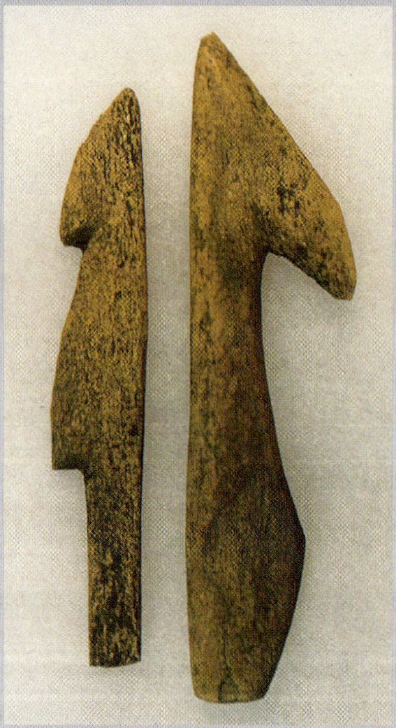

Bone harpoon heads, longest is 3⅞", socketed bases for attachment to long shafts. Northwest Coast. Pete Timoch collection. Smaller, **$200.00.** Larger, **$300.00.**

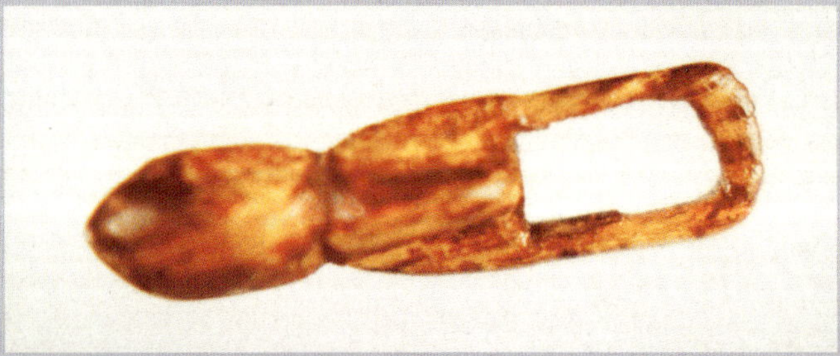

Swivel or toggle, for use with cord or thin rope, carved ivory, 1¾" long. It came from Alaska. Back to Earth. **$50.00.**

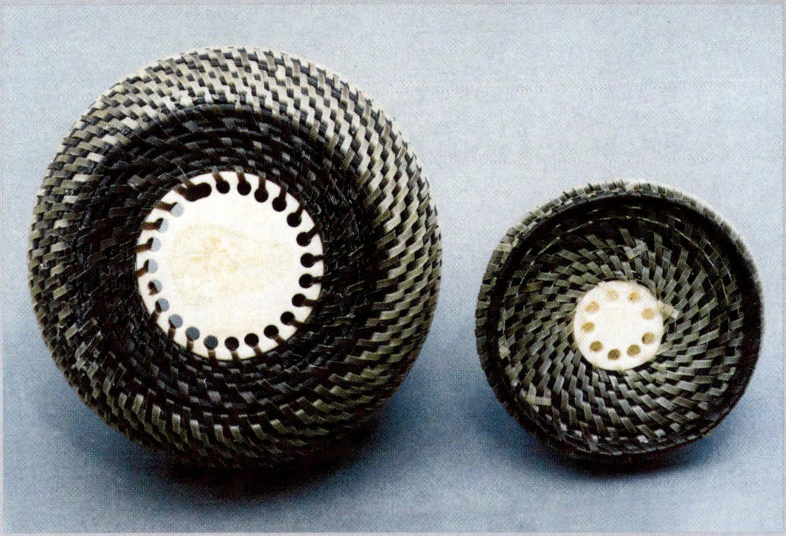

Basket, showing the bottom and top interior, basket is 3½" in diameter. Baleen, also known as whalebone, is the tough, fiberous material in the mouths of certain whales; it helps filter seawater to remove edible plankton. This basket view shows the round ivory weaving centerpieces. Alaska. H. B. Greene II collection, Naples, Florida. **$800.00.**

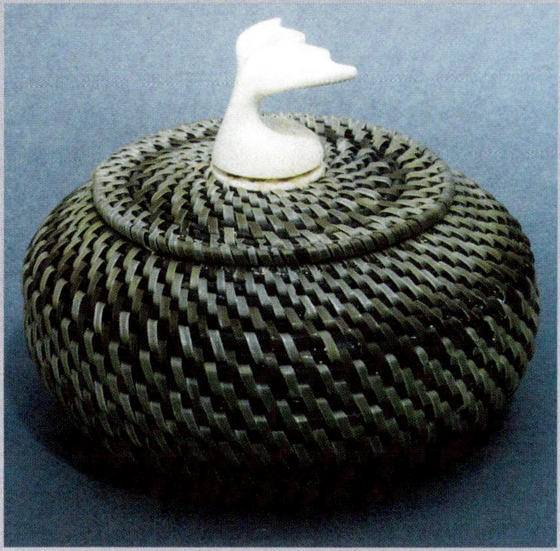

Basket, baleen and walrus ivory, 1¾" high plus ¾" whale fluke finial. The basket is made of light and dark baleen. This small work of art was made by Ekayuke, Point Hope, and was obtained by the owner at the Native Hospital, Anchorage, Alaska. H. B. Greene II collection, Naples, Florida. **$800.00.**

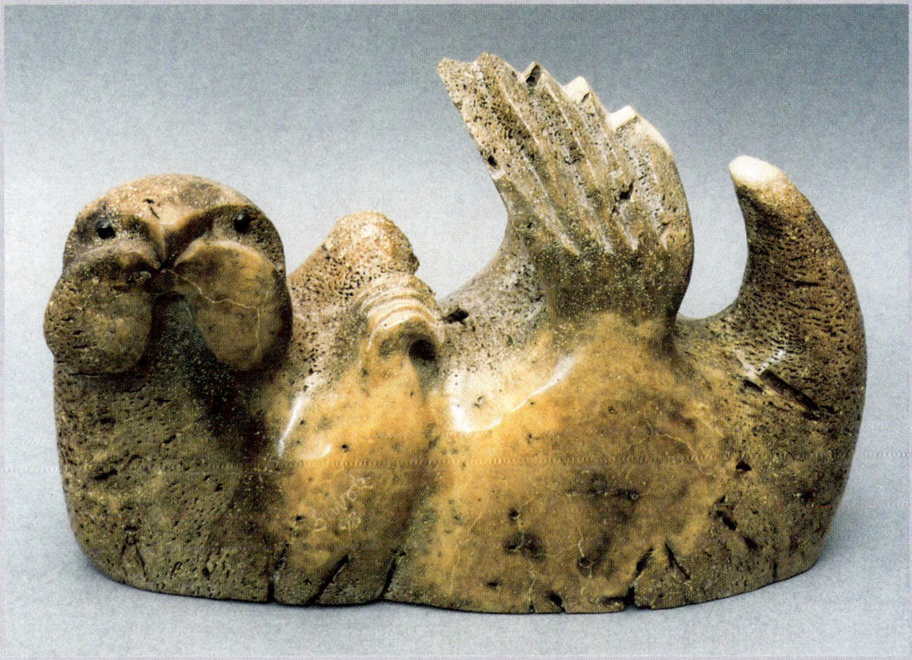

Sea otter figurine, fossil bone, 4½ x 7⅛". This contemporary artwork was carved by Savok who used glass beads for the eyes. It was obtained by the owner at the Native Hospital, Anchorage, Alaska. Elizabeth A. Greene collection, Naples, Florida. **$500.00.**

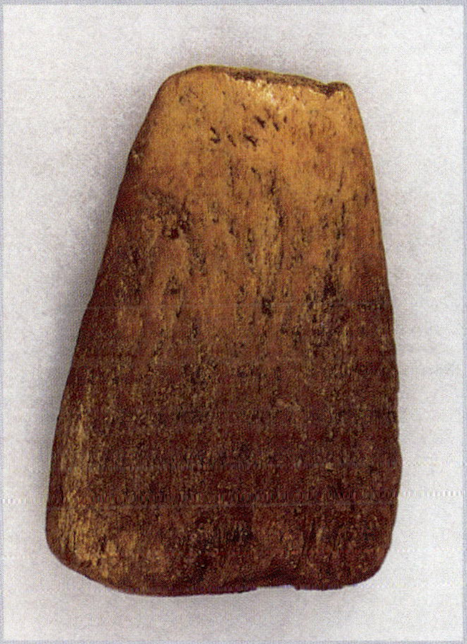

Adz blade, polished antler with brown patina, 3" long. Sometimes small blades like this were mounted as butchering tools for food preparation, like separating a joint. Alaska. Pete Timoch collection. **$125.00.**

Dogsled runner, prehistoric(?), curved whalebone, 25" long. It has drilled attachment holes and the excurvate surface has high polish from ice and snow. This unusual piece came from St. Lawrence Island. Back to Earth. **$200.00.**

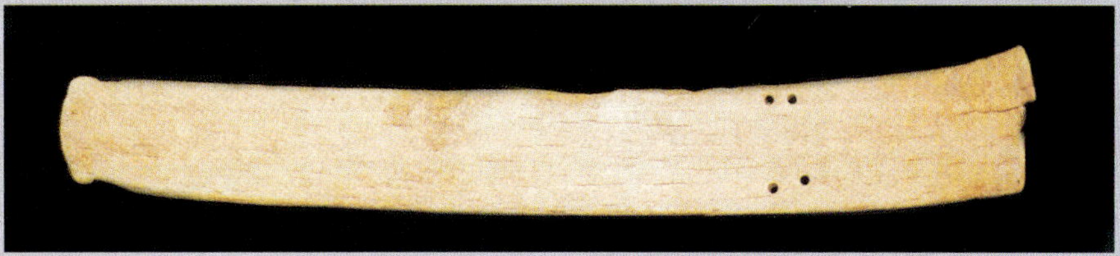

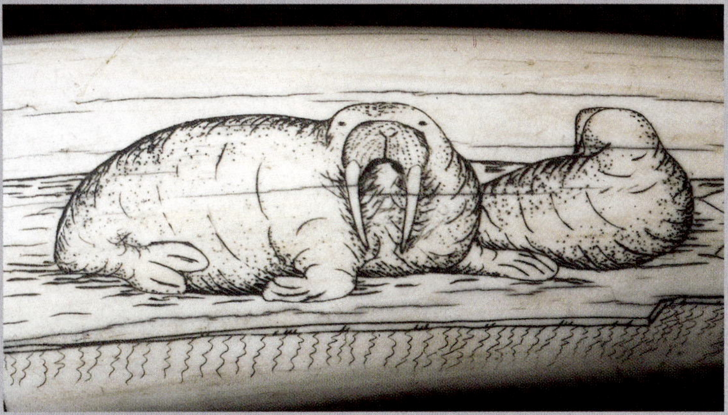

Walrus ivory scrimshawed tusk, scene of two walrus on ice floe, pre-1900. Once in the Greene collection, the present owner of the tusk is unknown. Alaska. H. B. Greene II photograph, Naples, Florida. Unlisted.

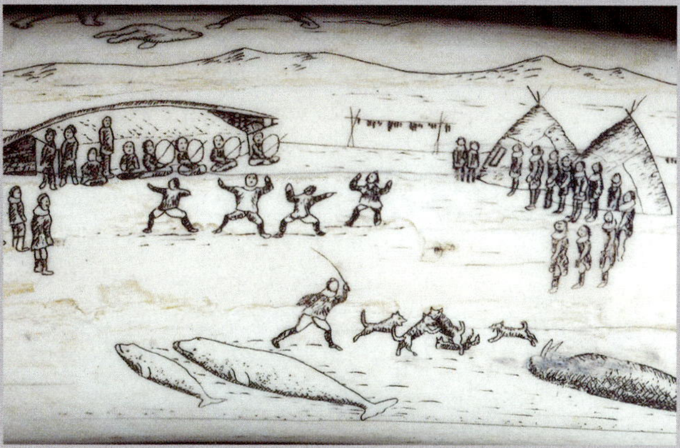

Walrus ivory scrimshawed tusk, native village, pre-1900. This tusk was formerly in the Greene collection. Alaska. H. B. Greene II photograph, Naples, Florida. Unlisted.

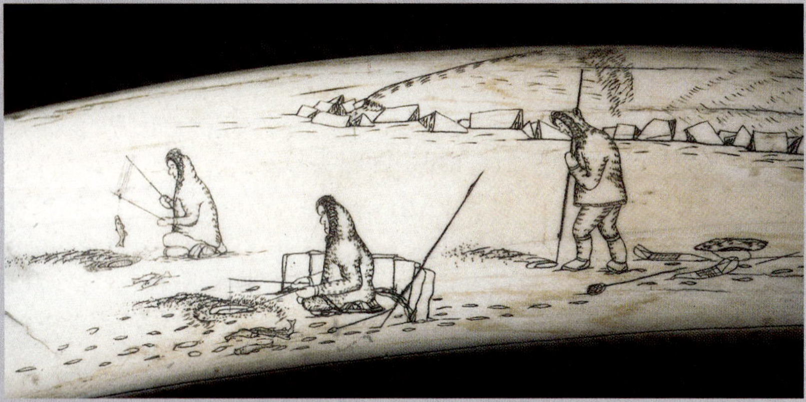

Walrus ivory scrimshawed tusk, three men ice-fishing, pre-1900. This tusk was once in the Greene collection, and present owner is unknown. Alaska. H. B. Greene II photograph, Naples, Florida. Unlisted.

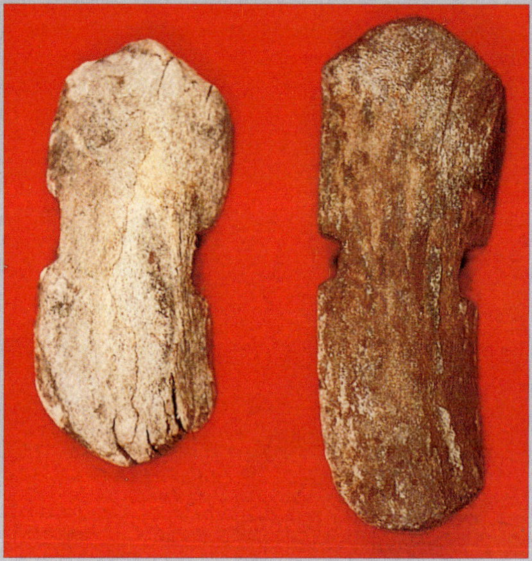

Notched hammer heads, longest is 4⅛", both made of whalebone. General purpose tools, these show some weathering. Alaska. Pete Timoch collection. Each, **$60.00 – 75.00.**

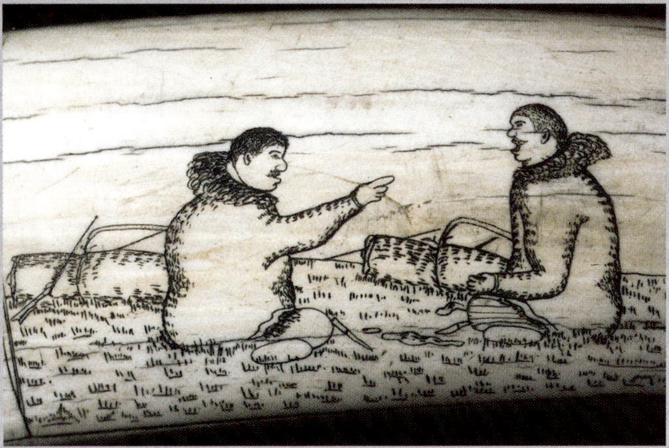

Walrus ivory scrimshawed tusk, two hunters conversing, pre-1900. The tusk was formerly in the Greene collection. Alaska. H. B. Greene II photograph, Naples, Florida. Unlisted.

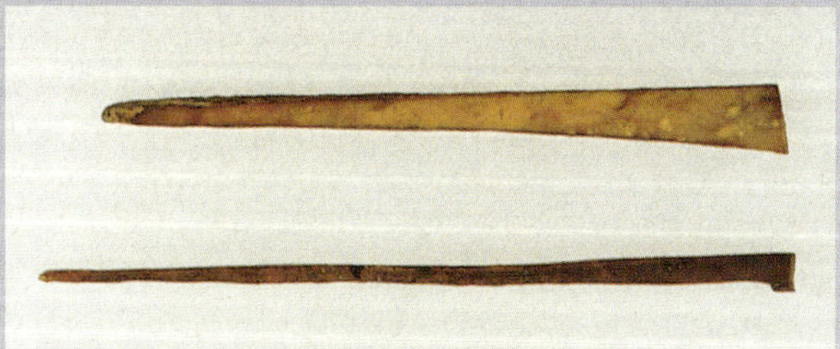

Bone sliver wedges, longest is 3⅛". One side is fairly straight on each while the opposite side tapers. Such tool parts had many uses, mainly tightening heads in sockets and knives in handles. Alaska. Pete Timoch collection. Each, **$30.00.**

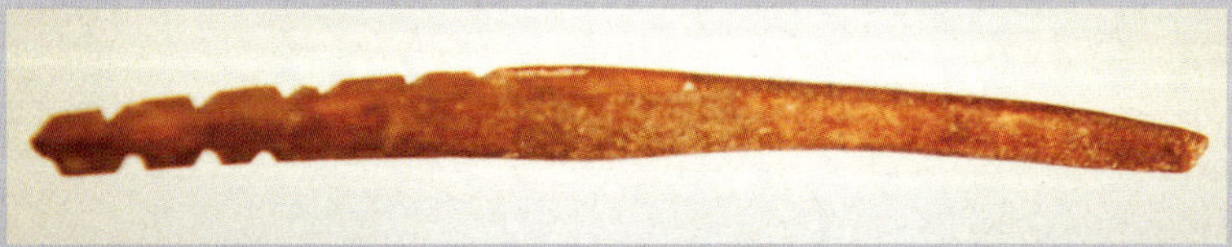

Artifact, mineralized animal bone, unknown use, 3¾" long. This piece is from Alaska. Back to Earth. **$40.00.**

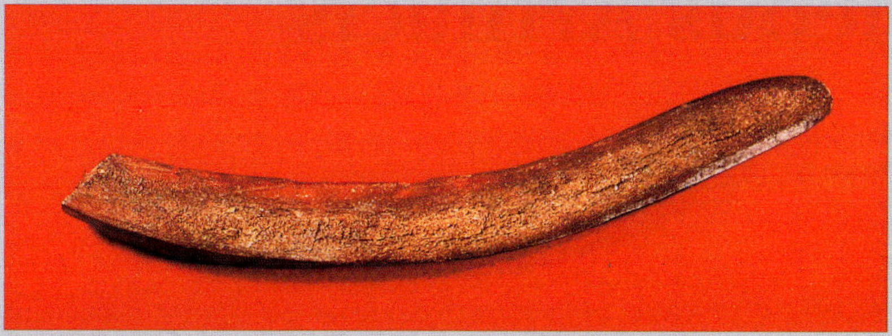

Snow knife, split bone, 11½" around the outside curve. Often used for cutting snow blocks to build wind-breaks and temporary shelters, it is well-shaped and has a beautiful brown patina. Alaska. Pete Timoch collection. **$200.00.**

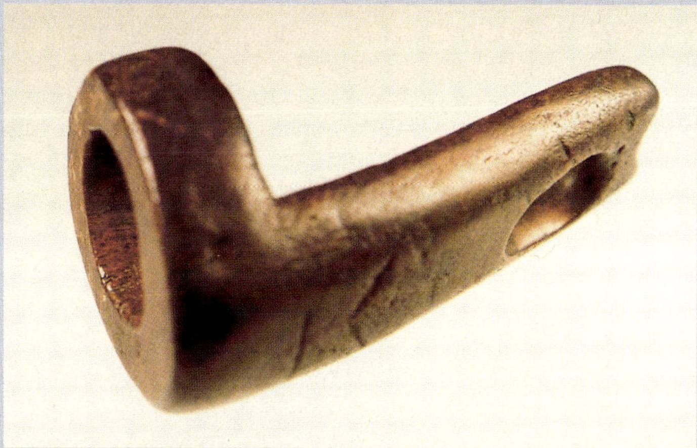

Artifact, uncertain use, dark mineralized bone, 3⅛" long. Ex-collection Stowall, it is from Alaska. Larry Garvin collection. **$100.00.**

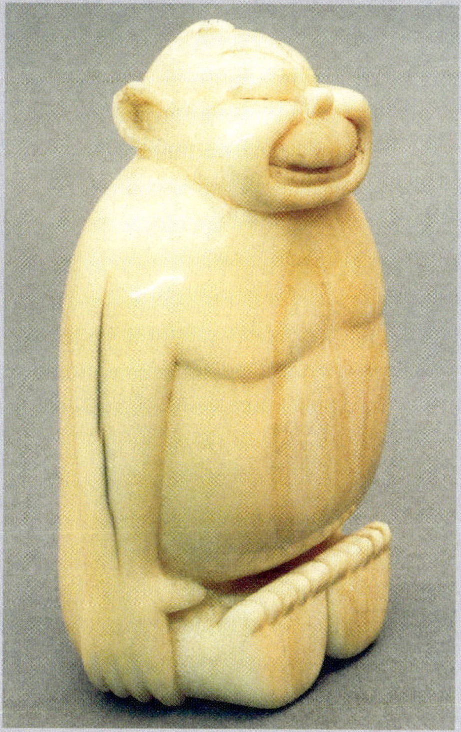

Billiken, walrus ivory, 2⅜ x 3½". Billikens are mirthful and mischievous entities in native folklore. This example is reputed to have been carved by the artist Happy Jack in 1909 or 1910 in Nome, Alaska. The owner obtained this piece from a dealer in California. Elizabeth A. Greene collection, Naples, Florida. **$300.00.**

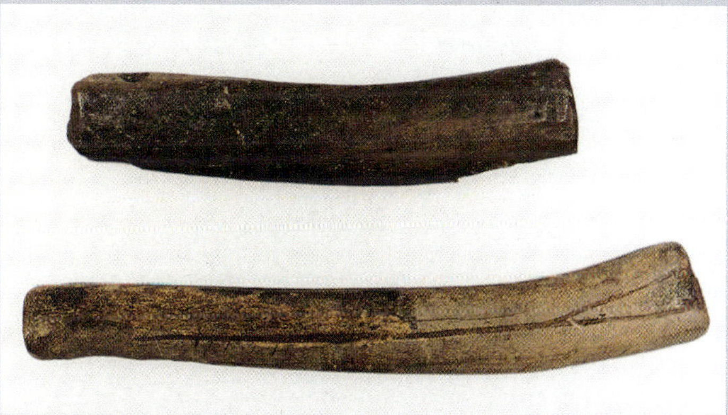

Antler tool handles, longer example is 4 15/16". Both are drilled through at the smaller ends, perhaps for carrying thongs. The longer handle is decorated on all four sides with incised lines, and it has an elongated side slot for wedging or for removing the blade. Alaska. Pete Timoch collection. Smaller, **$100.00 – 125.00.** Larger, **$200.00.**

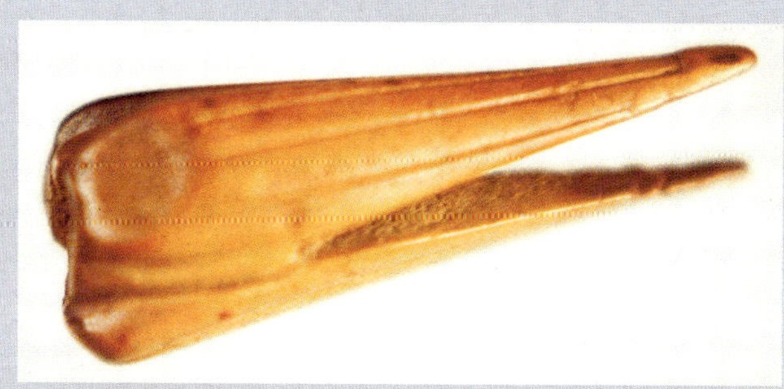

Artifact, carved bone with decorative lines, 2⅜" long. This is probably part of another tool or weapon. Alaska. Larry Garvin collection. **$75.00.**

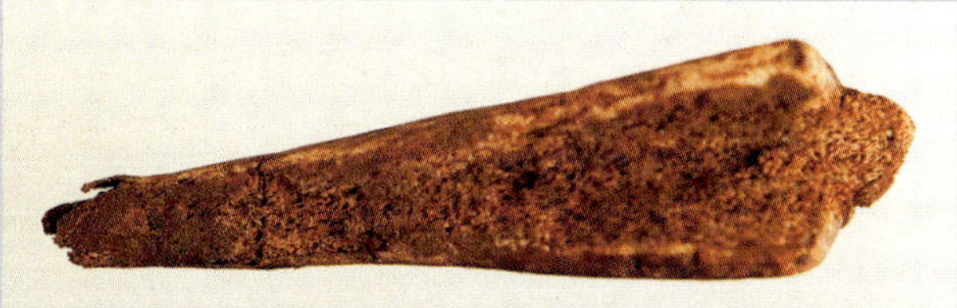

Projectile point, bone, small tapered stem, point is 2 15/16" long. It is four-sided, Inuit, from Alaska. Don Casto collection. **$20.00.**

Miscellaneous Artifacts

Beyond the major artifact classes covered in this book, there are also minor classes and many few-of-a-kind objects made of antler, bone, and shell. The range is very wide, covering (as it does) various cultural regions of North America and great expanses of time. A non-comprehensive listing follows:

Elk and deer antler and bone wedges; polished sandhill crane beak awls; wooden fishing spears with bone barbs; beaver teeth set in long antler handles; bone gaming pieces and counters; elk antler purses; antler combs; dice made of animal teeth; bone chisels and gouges; incised bone cylinders of unknown use; shell pendants of many kinds; bone projectile and harpoon points; rectangular marine shell gorgets that copied those made of glacial slate; large Late Archaic shell gorgets or pendants; drilled fossil shark teeth; mat-weaving needles of flat bone; short and double-pointed fish gorges; antler Atl-atl handles and hooks; sectional shell Atl-atl weights; antler and bone chisels with beveled edges; shell earrings and ear danglers; thin bone or antler anklets and bracelets; antler digging stick handles; antler picks; shoulder bone scoops and shovels; clamshell hoes; elk antler spoons and dippers; elk antler hide-scrapers; and, hollow bone paint containers.

Other artifacts include: Bison rib shaft-straighteners; antler arrowshaft wrenches; conch whorl pendants and pick heads made from the same material; shell two-piece fishhooks; shell pulley-type earplugs; deer toe dice; bone net-spacers(?); wild turkey spur perforators; historic ornate shell buttons or fasteners; awls made from woodpecker beaks; deer jawbone scrapers; animal mandible pendants; snowshoe needles; pendants of bear claw cores; oyster shell beads; wampum beads and message belts; historic copper and iron nail awls in antler and bone handles; worked porcupine teeth; antler base paint cups; and small bone pestles.

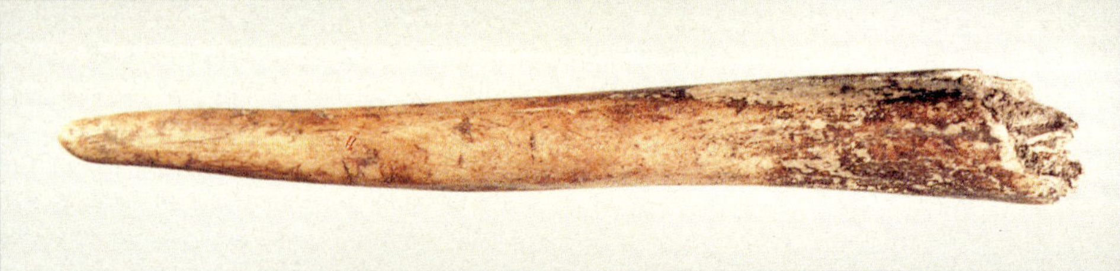

Antler perforator or punch, snapped base, 6¾". Largely unmodified, the tip has some probable use polish. Kentucky or Tennessee. Private collection. **$8.00.**

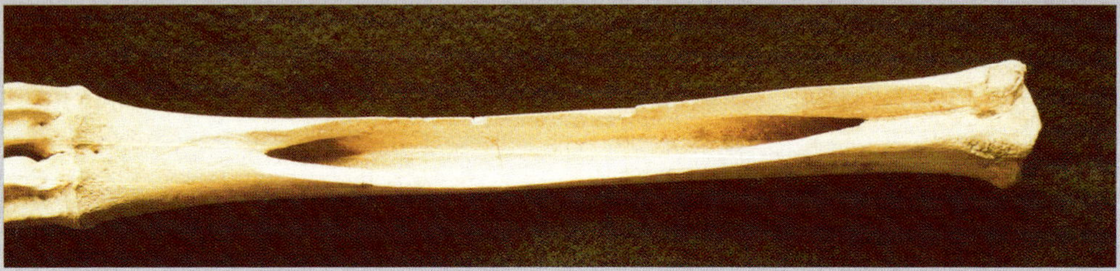

Beamer or drawshave, deer metapodial bone, 9¾" long, from the Whipple collection assembled in the 1930s. This example is Iroquois, ca. AD 1540-1560. Most examples are worn through or broken near the center, so this intact artifact is very collectible. It came from near Richmond Mills, Ontario County, New York. Dave Summers collection, Victor, New York. **$175.00.**

Double-pointed pin, polished walrus ivory, just over 3" long. A small amount of such ivory has been found in the Northeast, but examples are quite rare. This piece is Algonquian phase of the Late Woodland, ca. AD 1000 – 1600. St. Lawrence County, New York. Dave Summers collection, Victor, New York. Museum grade.

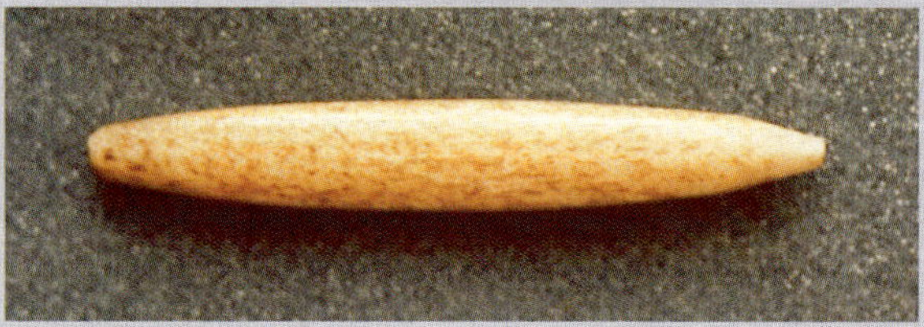

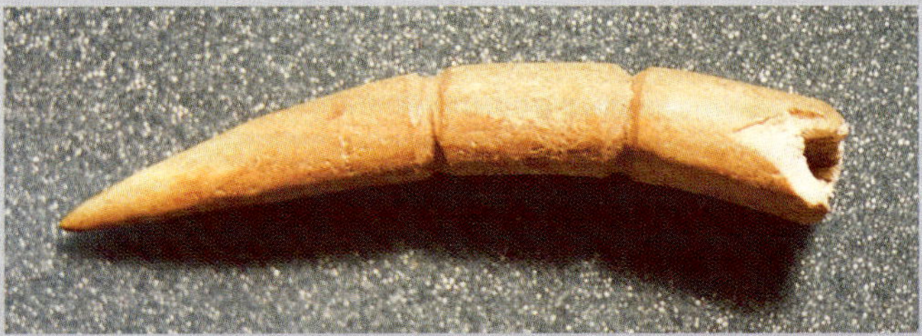

Deer antler tine with grooves, possibly part of headdress, 4" long. It is Early Woodland, Adena phase, ca.1000 – 1 BC. Western New York. Dave Summers collection, Victor, New York. **$150.00.**

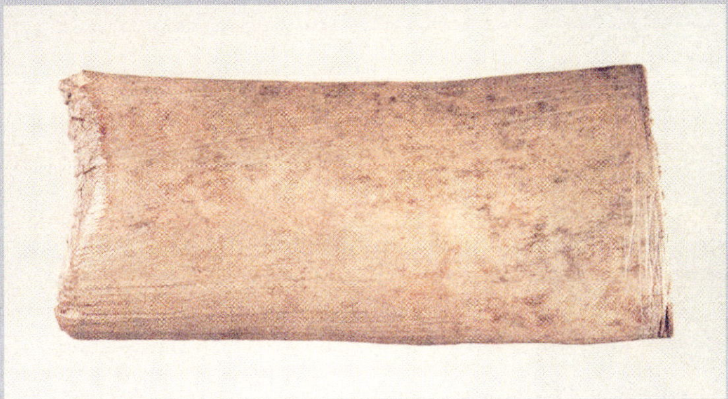

Preform, thinned bone section from a large animal, 1⅜ x 3¼". Ex-collection Copeland, it is from a Fort Ancient site in southern Ohio. Private collection. **$15.00.**

Bone artifact preforms, large bird bones, both Fort Ancient from southern Ohio. Private collection. Longer one is 4⅜" and chemically stabilized, left end cut and the right snapped. **$7.00.** Smaller, one end sawed while the other is cut off. **$5.00.**

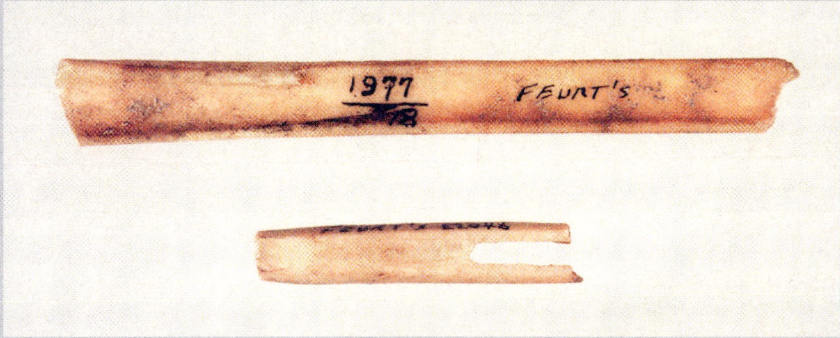

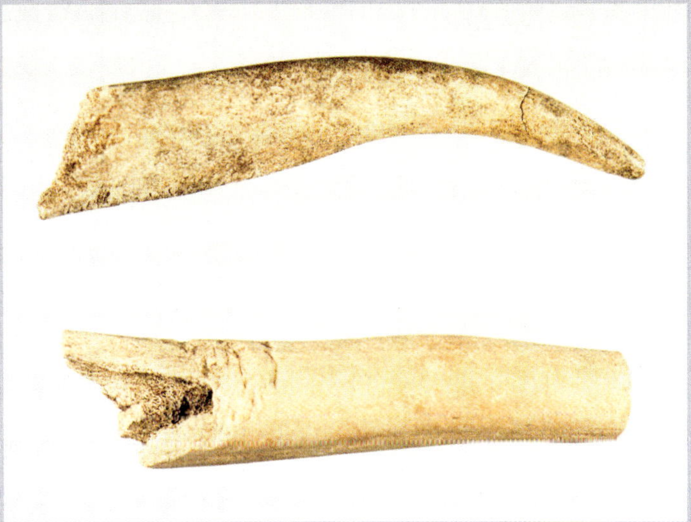

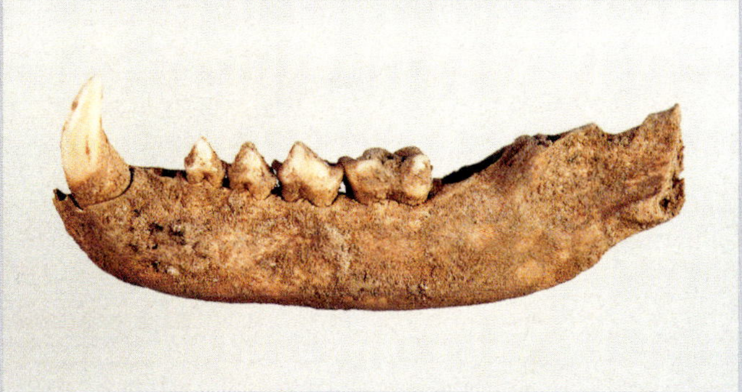

Animal jawbone, raccoon mandible, 2¾" long. It has several teeth missing and came from a village midden. Kentucky. Fred Winegardner collection. **$10.00.**

Antler tools, longer one is 3⅝". The pointed perforator has a polished tip, while the other has the tip cut off. Both Kentucky. Private collection. Each, **$7.00.**

Antler handle, Late Archaic to Woodland, 4¼" long, with wear polish. The smaller end has been worked down and flattened, perhaps to receive a scraper and binding. Ex-collection Vietzen, Christian County, Kentucky. Pete Timoch collection. **$175.00 – 200.00.**

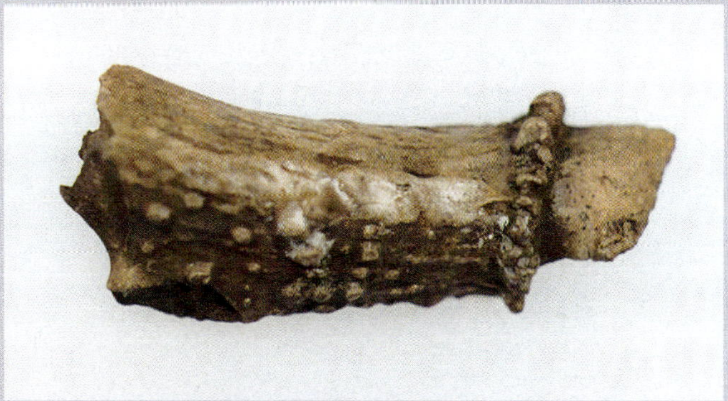

Miscellaneous Artifacts

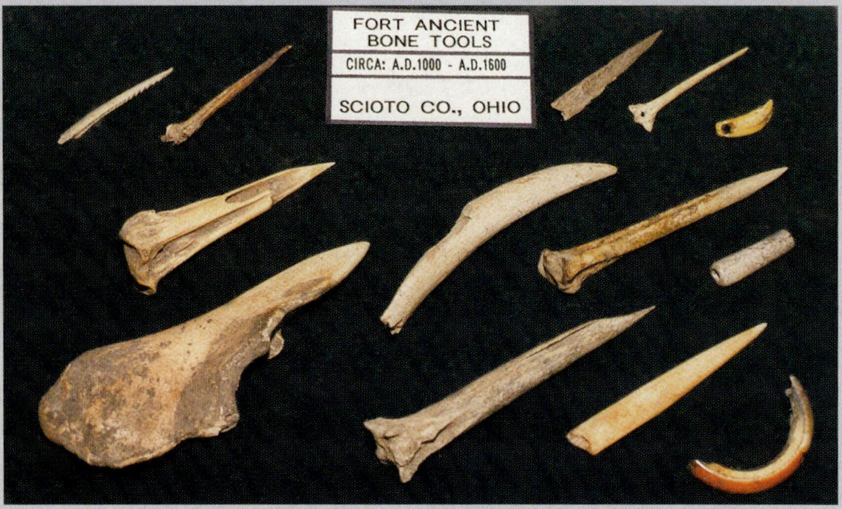
FORT ANCIENT
BONE TOOLS
CIRCA: A.D.1000 - A.D.1600
SCIOTO CO., OHIO

Bone tools and animal teeth, all found on a Fort Ancient site in southern Ohio. Back to Earth. **$200.00.**

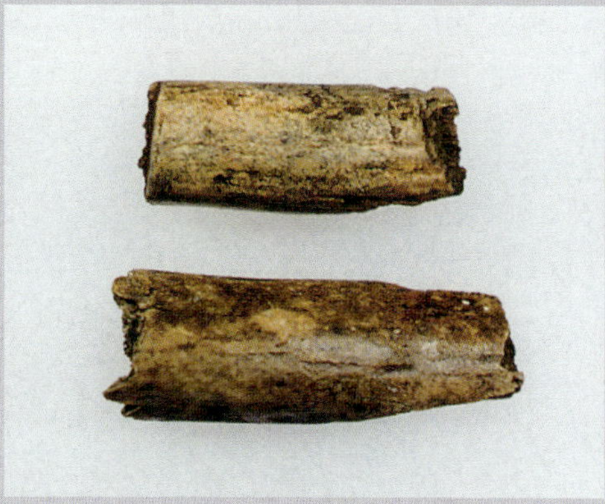

Antler tool handles, Late Archaic to Woodland, shorter piece is 2⅛", longer one is 2¹³⁄₁₆". The top specimen has shallow grooves at the smaller end, perhaps as a hafting aid. Both were worked down to have reduced diameters at one end, and both have high polish. Ex-collection Vietzen, Christian County, Kentucky. Pete Timoch collection. Each, **$75.00.**

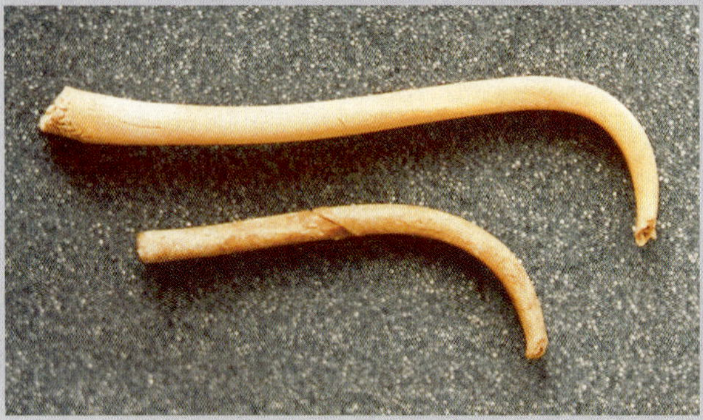

Perforators, raccoon penis bones, 2½ and 3⅝" long, respectively. They are Iroquois, ca. AD 1540 – 1560, and were found near Richmond Mills. Ontario County, New York. Dave Summers collection, Victor, New York. Smaller, **$20.00;** larger, **$30.00.**

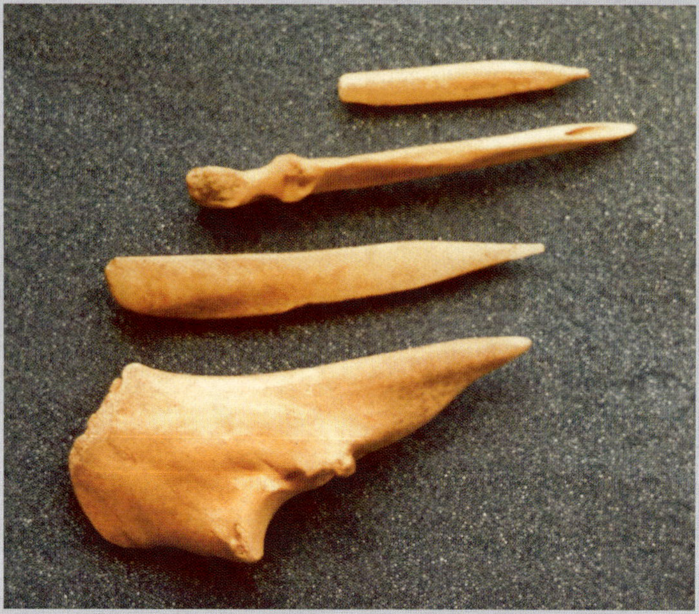

Bone tools, all Transitional period, ca. 1300 – 1000 BC. Top, split bone awl, 1⅞". Next, joint bone awl, 3⅜" long. Next, Split bone awl, 3½". Bottom, trigger awl, deer ulna, 3½" long. All are from near Cayuga Lake, Cayuga County, New York. Dave Summers collection, Victor, New York. Top to bottom: **$15.00; $30.00; $25.00; $30.00.**

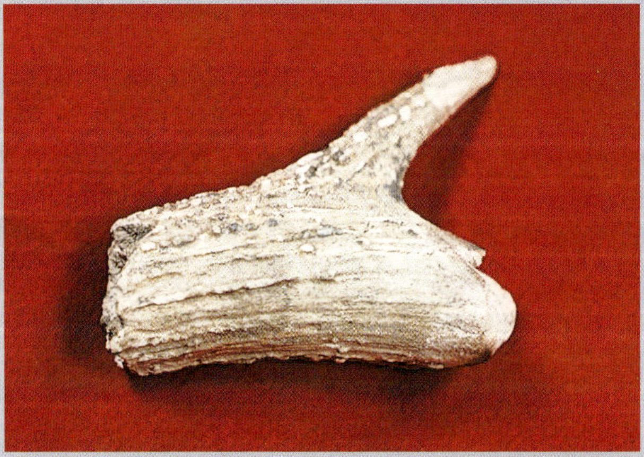

Antler celt or tool holder, Late Archaic to Woodland, handle is 6" long. A hole at the larger end (on right) is 2½" deep, and the tool head could have been glued in position using asphalt as an adhesive. Kentucky was a major center for the use of asphalt in prehistoric times. Ex-collection Vietzen, Christian County, Kentucky. Pete Timoch collection. **$300.00 – 500.00.**

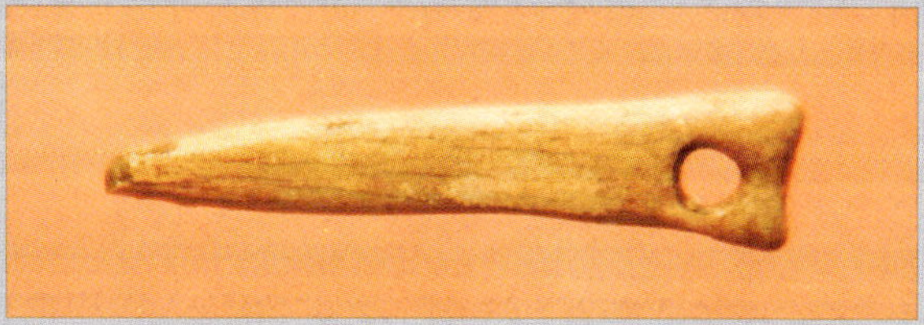

Deer bone, perforated for plume holder(?), 2⁵⁄₁₆" long. It is Middle Archaic, Lamoka phase (ca. 3000 – 2500 BC), and was picked up in Schuyler County, New York. Dave Summers collection, Victor, New York. **$100.00.**

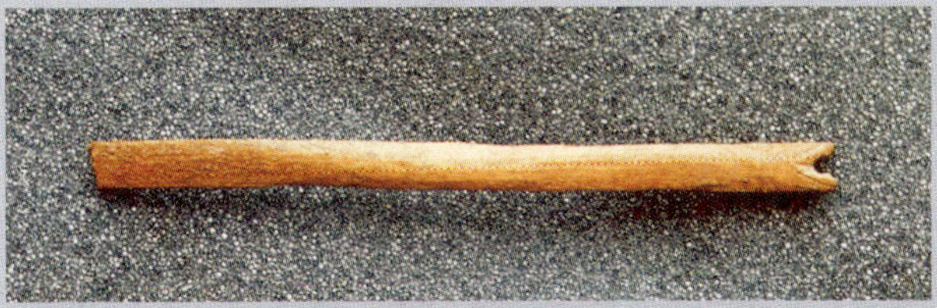

Bone needle, one-half of original artifact with hole in center, 4" long. Possibly a matting needle, it is Brewerton phase, Late Archaic period. The needle was found in Cayuga County, New York. Dave Summers collection, Victor, New York. **$50.00.**

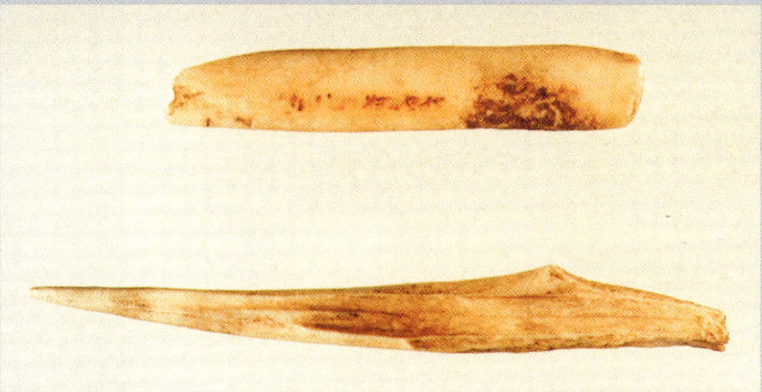

Bone artifacts, possibly a fishhook blank and an awl, both Midwestern. Don Casto collection. Top, polished bone, **$20.00.** Bottom, awl, 3⅜". **$15.00.**

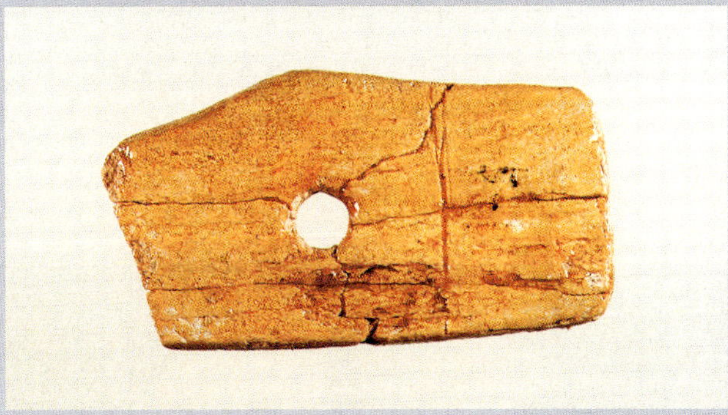

Tool or ornament, flat bone, 2" long. This artifact of unknown use is Midwestern. Don Casto collection. **$20.00.**

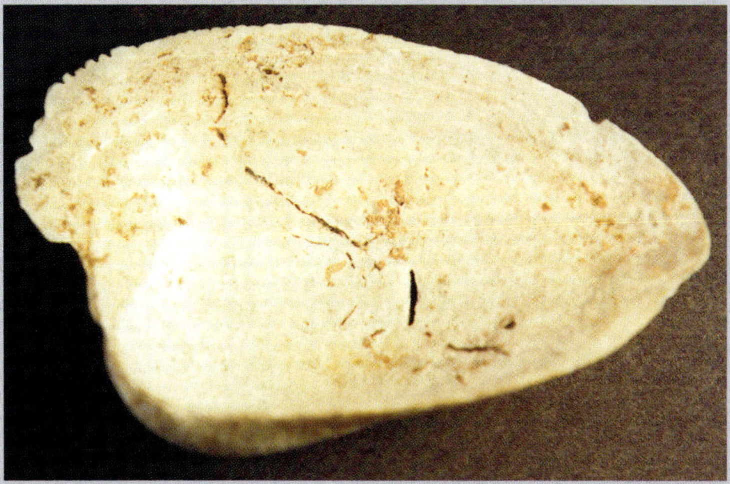

Spoon or dipper, mussel shell, 4⅝" long. The edge is ground and fringed on this artifact, which also has a slot and small hole cut in the bottom. Ex-collection Bingman, it is from southeastern Illinois. Private collection. Unlisted.

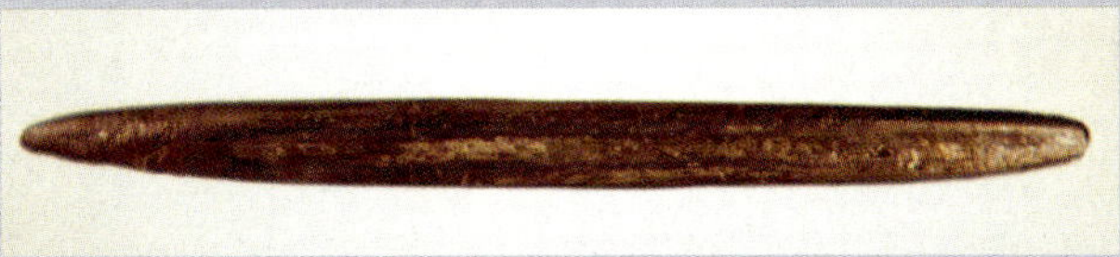

Bone point or pin, mineralized black, 4¼" long. Bone pins of this kind are frequently found near prehistoric Indian sites in the Southeast. Jefferson County, Florida. Back to Earth. **$75.00.**

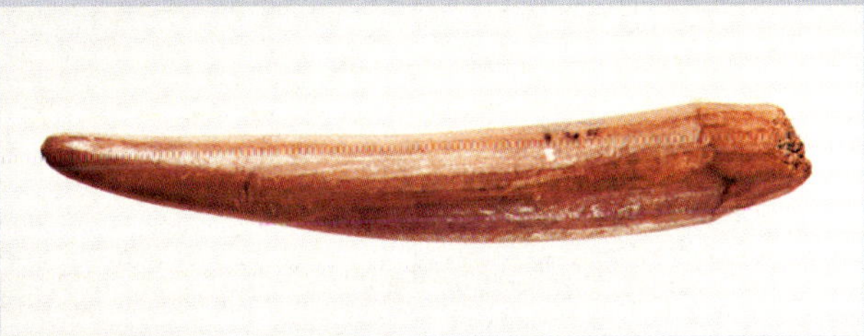

Awl, antler tine, base whittled to a smaller diameter for insertion into a bone, antler or wood handle. The tine is 2⅜" long and has a light brown patina. Polished at the tip and base, it is obvious that the knife used was razor-sharp and likely a flake knife or bladelet made in Middle Woodland times. Lar Hothem collection. **$20.00.**

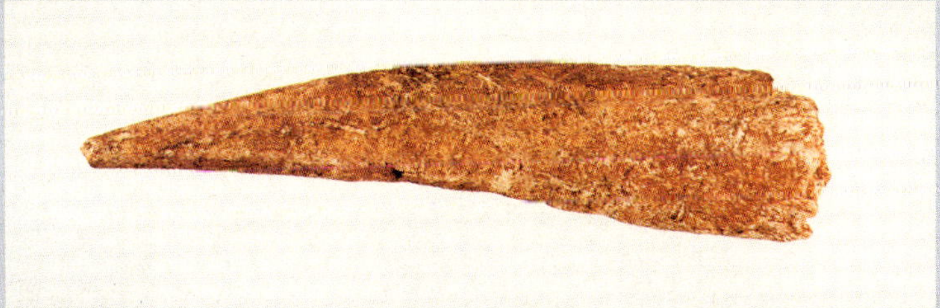

Awl, flattened bone splinter, 3" long. The tip is broken on this example, which has a weathered surface. Eastern Midwest. Private collection. **$3.00 – 6.00.**

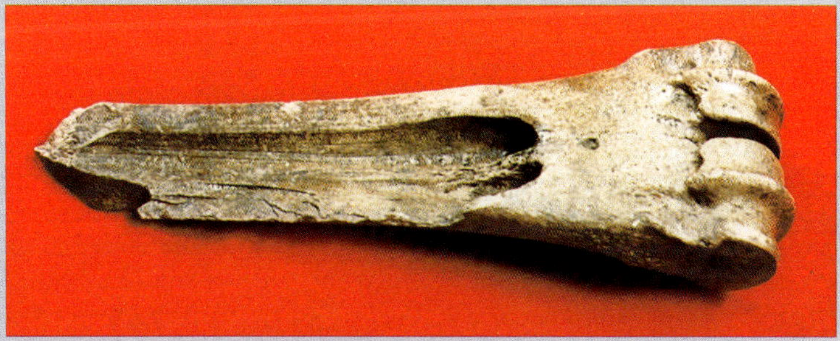

Gouge, elk bone (judging by size), Mississippian period, 6¼" long. Ex-collection Vietzen, it is pictured in his *The Immortal Eries*, page 317. Northern Ohio. Pete Timoch collection. **$125.00.**

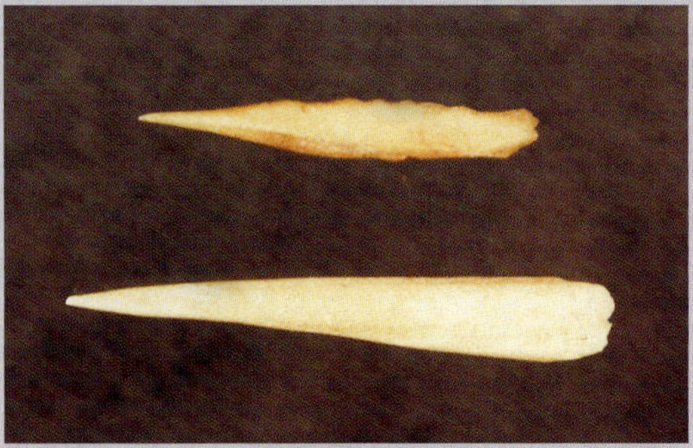

Bone artifacts, longer one is 1¾". These are thin and highly polished bone splinters, and the smaller piece is quite fragile. Probably tattooing needles, they are Fort Ancient of the Mississippian (AD 800 – 1500) period. Southern Ohio. Private collection. Each, **$8.00 – 15.00.**

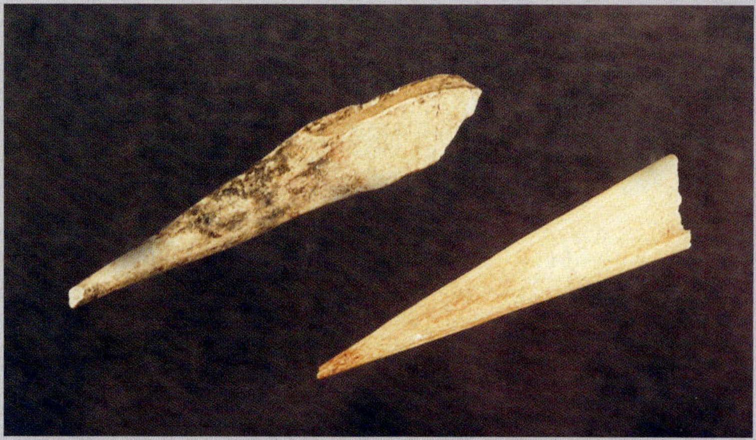

Awls, bone splinters, longer one is 2⅙". The awls are Mississippian period, Fort Ancient people. Southern Ohio. Private collection. Each, **$4.00 – 6.00.**

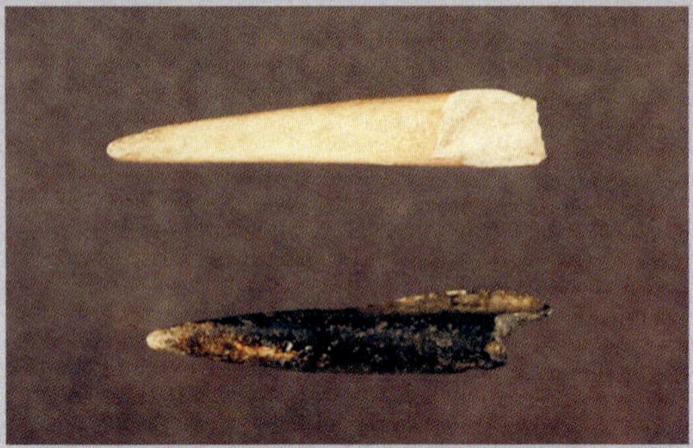

Awls, broken, bone splinters, longest is 1½". They have polish and the darker example is fire-scorched. Fort Ancient culture, southern Ohio. Private collection. Each, **$2.00 – 4.00.**

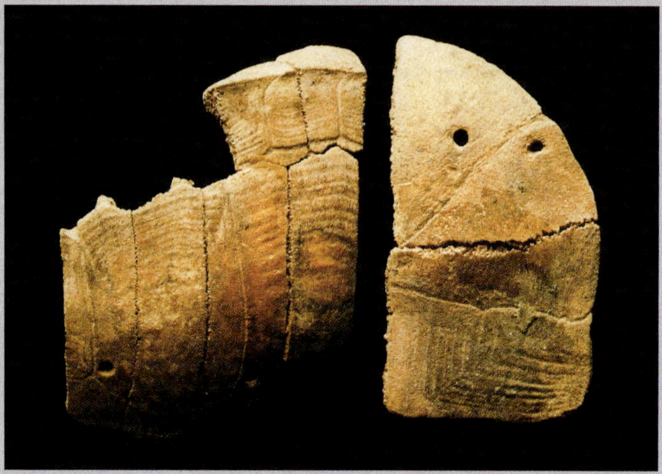

Box turtle or woods turtle (tortoise) rattle fragments, Frontenac phase of the Late Archaic (ca. 2000 BC). These were found in Cayuga County, New York. Dave Summers collection, Victor, New York. **$200.00.**

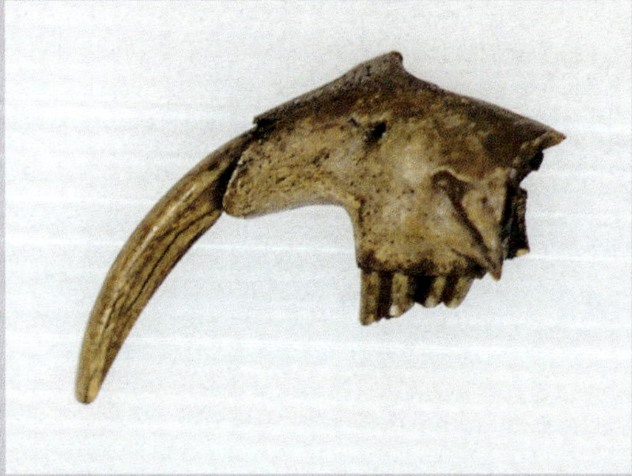

Beaver tooth crooked knife or gouge, Mississippian, 4" around the outside curve. The tooth was split longitudinally and reinserted in the lower jaw to serve as a graving or gouging tool. A rare piece, this original set is ex-collection Vietzen, from northern Ohio. Pete Timoch collection. **$300.00 – 500.00.**

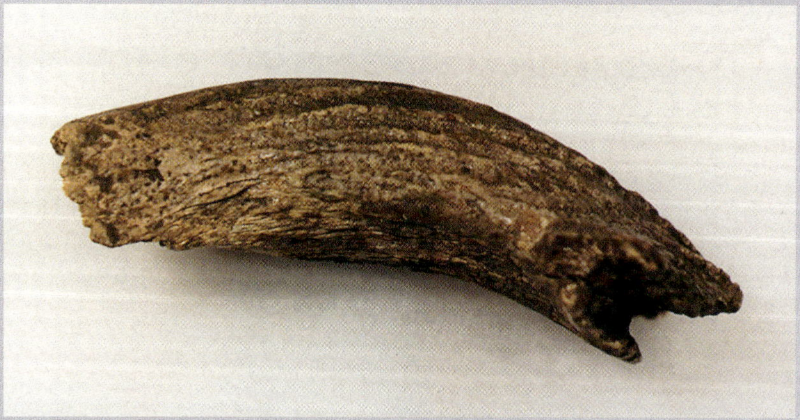

Antler celt or adz holder, 7" along the outside curve. It has a hole at each end: the celt hole measures 1 x 1¼", while the smaller and opposite hole is ¾ x 1⅛". Perhaps the connected holes were designed so that a punch could knock out a damaged or worn hardstone blade. Ex-collection Vietzen, Christian County, Kentucky. Pete Timoch collection. **$250.00.**

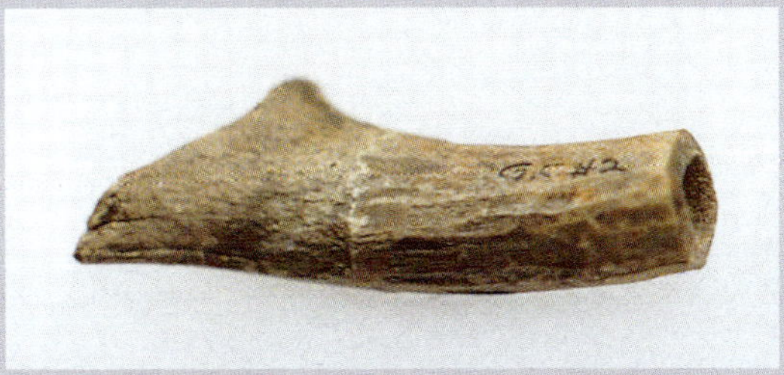

Antler tool handle, Late Archaic to Woodland times, 3" long. It has good use-polish and the end hole is ½" deep and 5⁄16" across. This size would fit a rounded-end bone awl or flint drill. It was once in the Vietzen collection and similar handles are pictured in his book, *The Saga of Glover's Cave*, page 213. Christian County, Kentucky. Pete Timoch collection. **$250.00.**

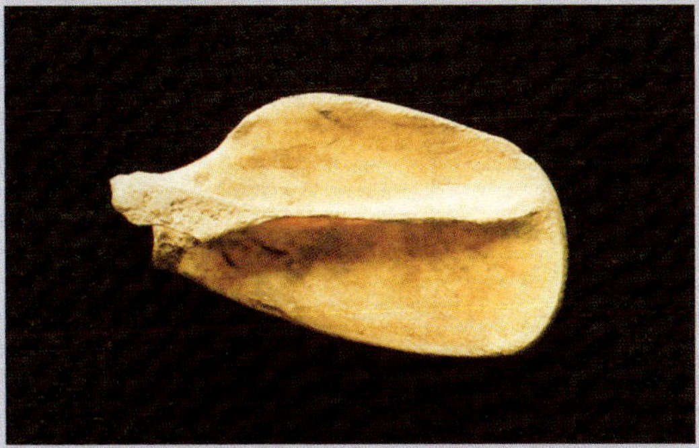

Bone scraper, scapula, 2½" long. It is Frontenac phase, Late Archaic, ca. 2000 BC. Cayuga County, New York. Dave Summers collection, Victor, New York. **$60.00.**

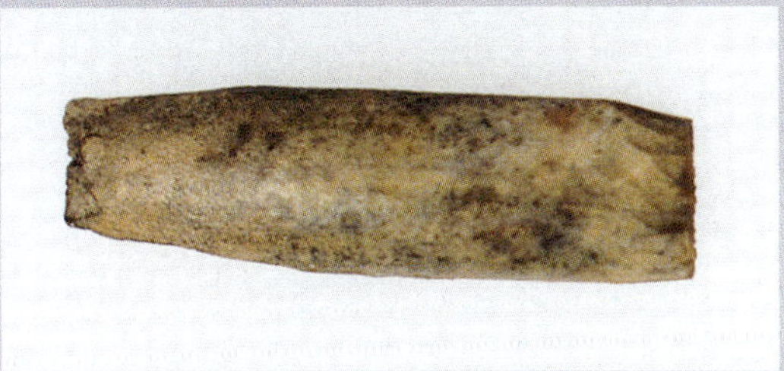

Antler tool handle, Late Archaic to Woodland, 3 9⁄16". The right end is worked down and the left end is tapered, perhaps for a scraper or knife blade. The smaller end does not have a blade slot, so this piece may not be in the final stage of completion. Once in the Vietzen collection, it is from Christian County, Kentucky. Pete Timoch collection. Unlisted.

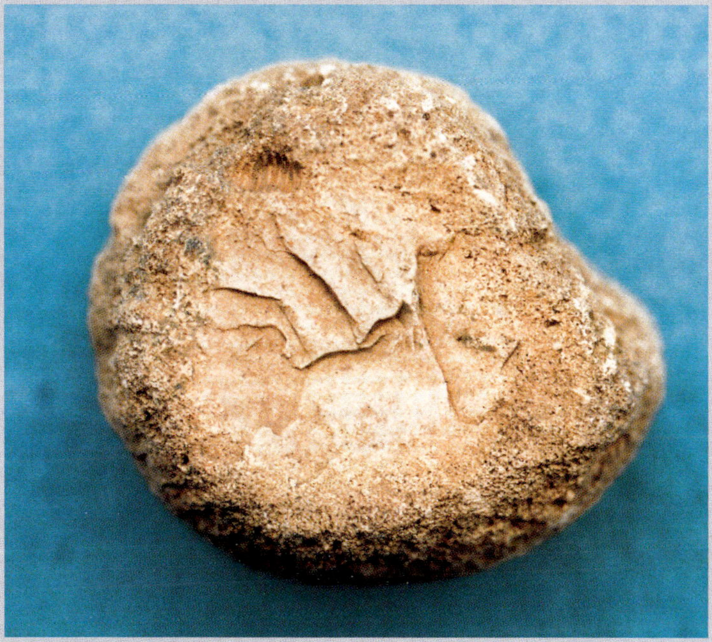

Gamestone(?), mineralized antler, Woodland period or later. It measures 1½ x 1 11⁄16" and is 1 3⁄16" thick. Found by Harwood in 1954 or 1961, it is from Limestone County, Alabama. Collection of, and photograph by, Gary Henry, North Carolina. **$50.00.**

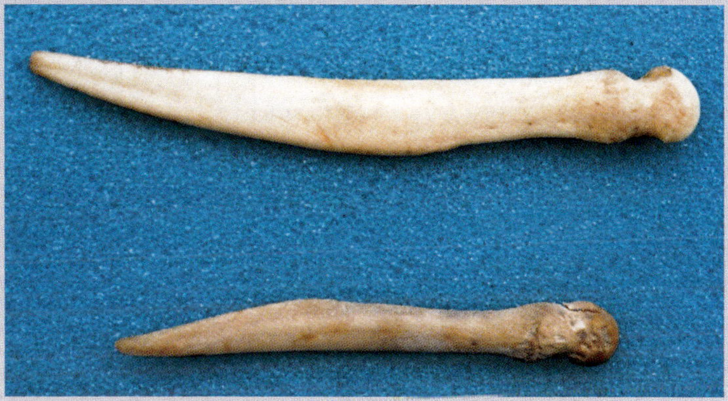

Awls or toothpicks, Archaic or later, deer dew claw bones. The largest specimen here is ¼ x 2 5⁄16". Such bones are not often seen. These are ex-collection Snyder, Meigs County, Tennessee. Collection of, and photograph by, Gary Henry, North Carolina. Each, **$20.00.**

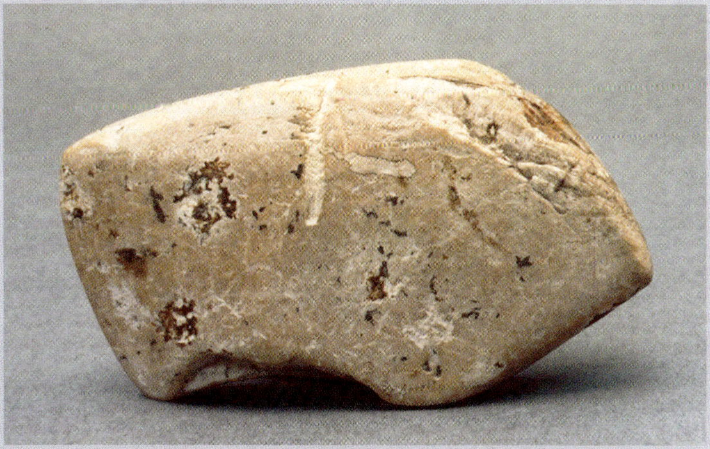

Shell scraper or cutting tool, heavy marine shell, 1⅜ x 2⅜". It came from a village midden or debris dump along the St. Johns River. Orange County, Florida. H. B. Greene II collection, Naples, Florida. **$25.00.**

Miscellaneous Artifacts

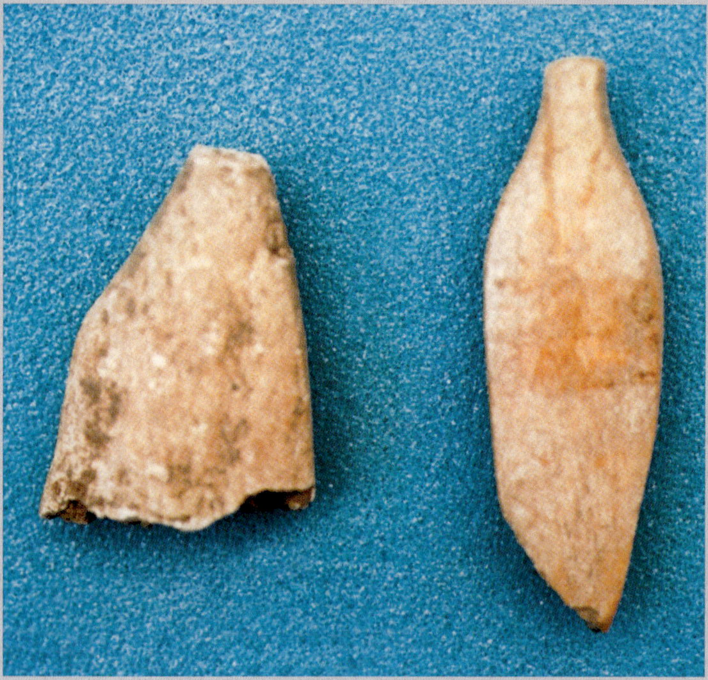

Bone flaking tools, Archaic or later, longest example (right) is ½ x 1$^{11}/_{16}$". These are ex-collection Snyder, from Meigs County, Tennessee. Collection of, and photograph by, Gary Henry, North Carolina. Each, **$5.00 – 10.00.**

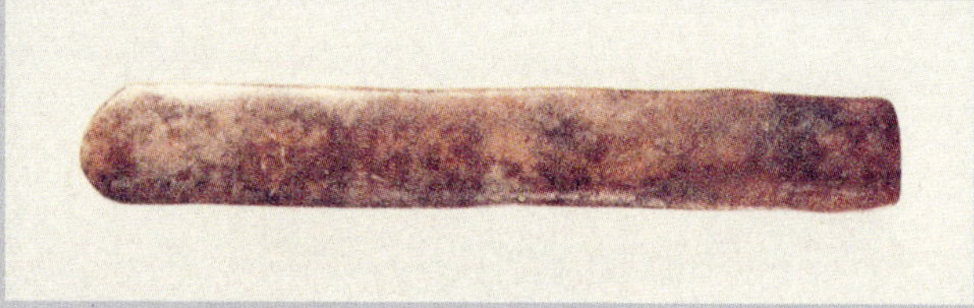

Tool, thin bird bone, high total polish, 2¼". The rounded end is beveled on the reverse to make a miniature gouge edge. Found in 1977, it is ex-collection Copeland. Fort Ancient, Mississippian period, it is from southern Ohio. Private collection. **$20.00.**

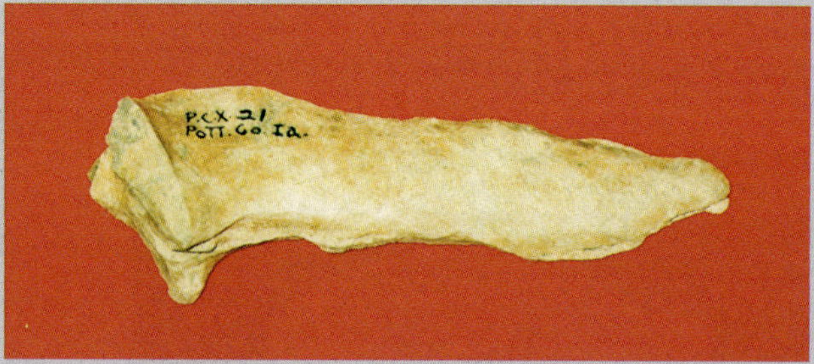

Bone digging tool, ca. AD 1 – 1200, 7½" long. This sturdy artifact was found in southwestern Iowa. Richard Krueger collection, Iowa; Sandra Krueger photograph. **$45.00.**

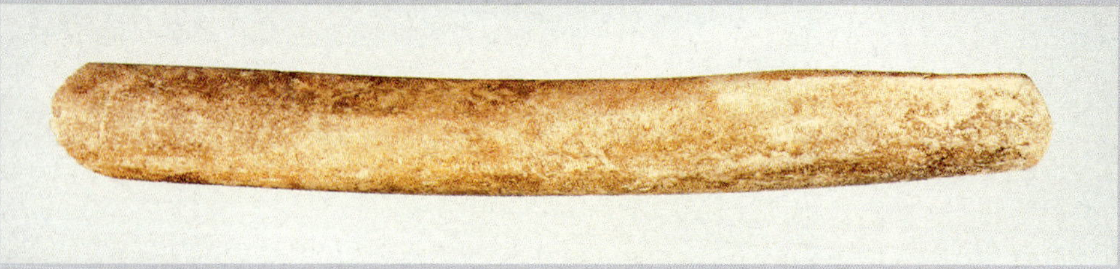

Tool, bison or elk bone, 5½" long. This may have been a hide-working tool. Four Corners area, Arizona. Don Casto collection. **$20.00.**

Tool, spatula end, 6⅛" long. Elk or bison bone, the green stain at midlength suggests contact with a copper artifact. Four Corners area, Arizona. Don Casto collection. **$25.00.**

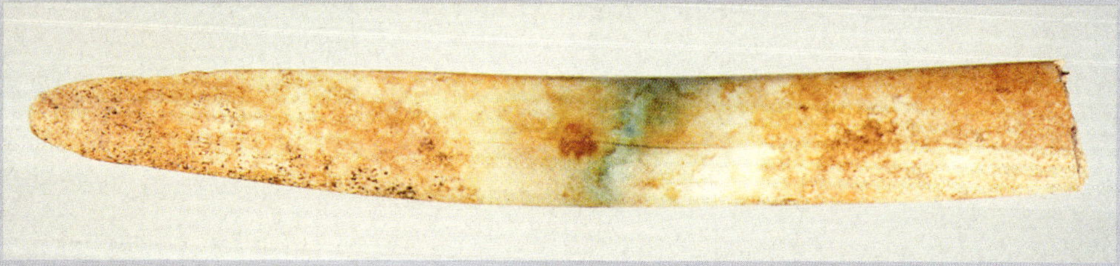

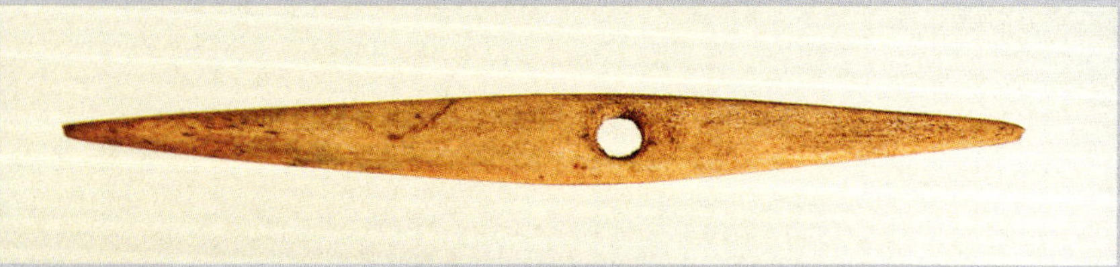

Needle or awl, double-tipped, 3½" long, Such examples have been called mat needles and snowshoe needles; this example is well-made and precisely drilled. Midwestern. Don Casto collection. **$45.00.**

Spatulate artifact, possibly a pottery working tool, 4$^{3}/_{16}$". It has very high handle polish as if from long-term use. The tool is ex-collections Copeland and Hooks. Southern Ohio. Fred Winegardner collection. **$100.00.**

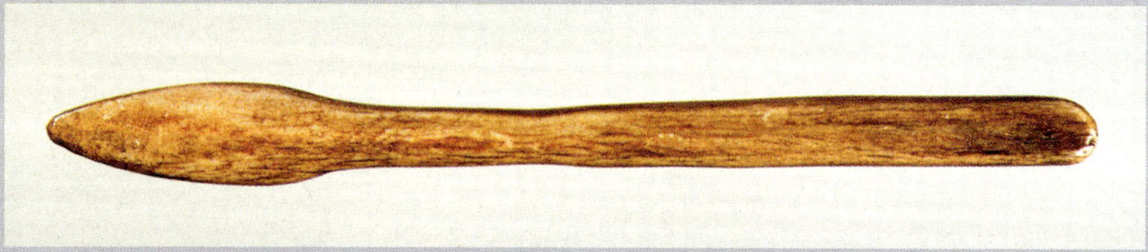

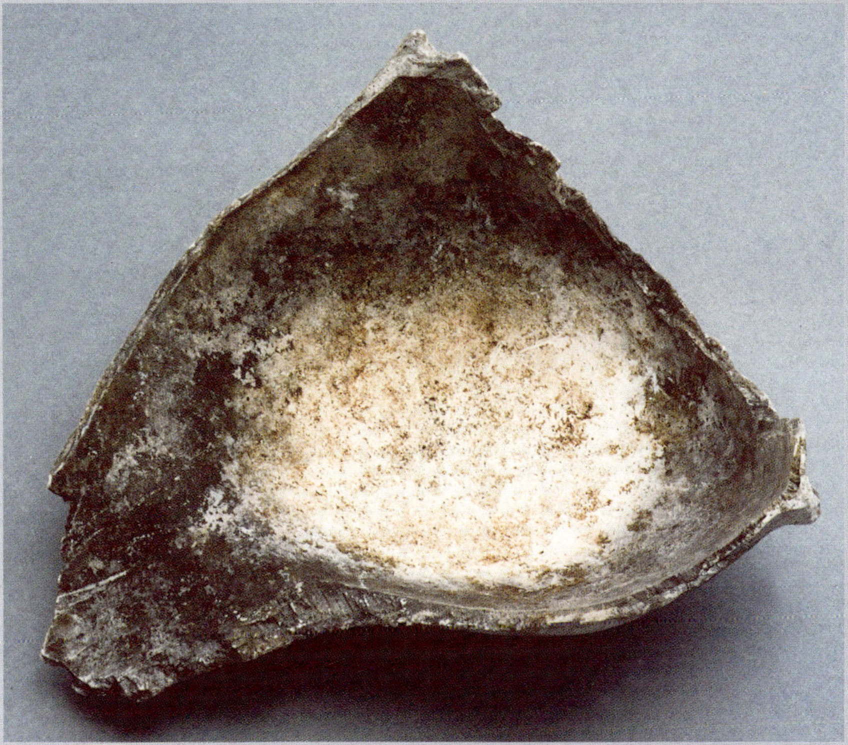

Shell spoon or small bowl, 6" long, AD 1450 or earlier. It is Calusa culture and came from Key Marco, Collier County, Florida. H. B. Greene II collection, Naples, Florida. **$75.00.**

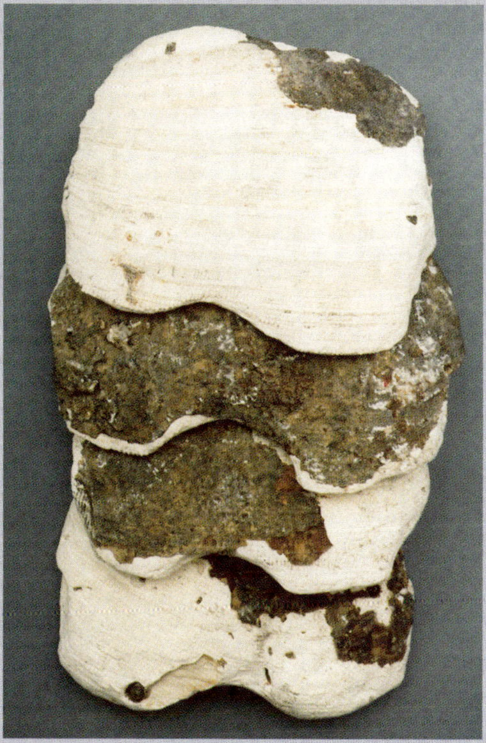

Net sinkers, clam shell, 3 to 3½" wide. They are AD 1450 or earlier, Calusa culture. All came from the south end of Key Marco, Collier County, Florida. H. B. Greene II collection, Naples, Florida. Each, **$10.00.**

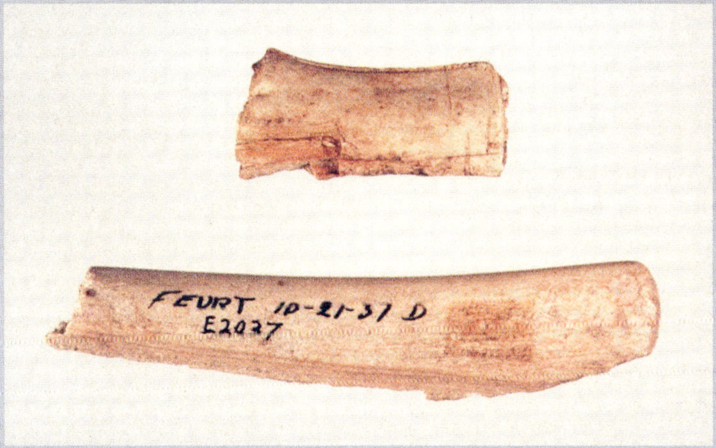

Animal bone, cut and worked, from a Fort Ancient site in southern Ohio. Private collection. Top, bead, deer rib bone, 1½", hollowed for length. **$10.00.** Bottom, 3⅝", found in 1937, handle(?) for tool. **$5.00.**

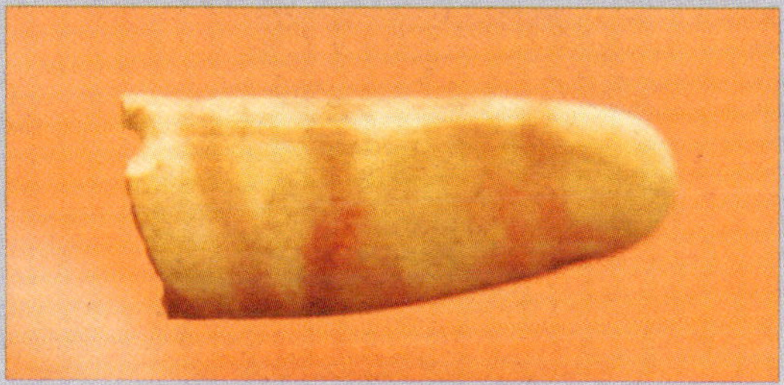

Bone tool with horizontal bands of red paint, scarce example, Lamoka phase of the Middle Archaic period. It is ground, drilled, and polished and was possibly used to weave nets. It is 2¹⁄₁₆" long, from Schuyler County, New York. Dave Summers collection, Victor, New York. **$150.00.**

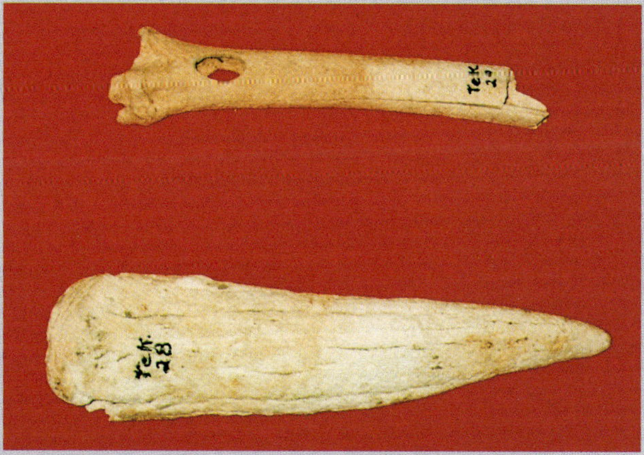

Plains artifacts, digging tool and shaft wrench. The digger is made of buffalo (bison) horn core and is 8¼" long. The shaft wrench is buffalo bone and is 6½" long. Eastcentral Nebraska. Richard Krueger collection, Iowa. Sandra Krueger photograph. Digger, **$50.00;** wrench, **$90.00.**

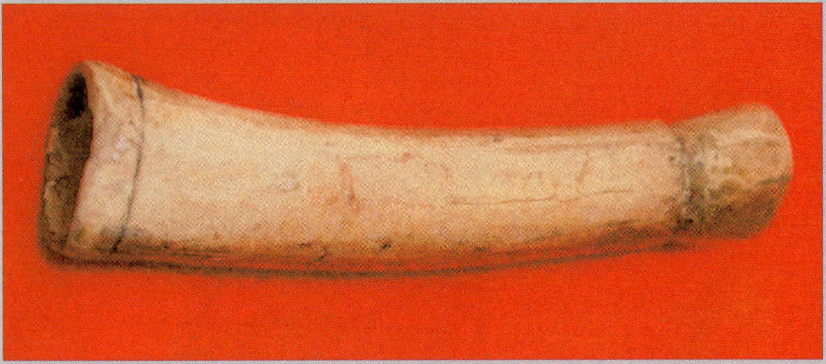

Bone sucking tube, 7⁄16 x 5⁄8", 2⅞" long. Such objects were sometimes used in ceremonies. This example is historic period and Chippewa. Michigan. Michael F. Slasinski collection, Michigan. **$150.00.**

Bone needle case, strap with trade beads, 5⁄16 x 2" long. This historic period artifact is Potawatomi, from Michigan. Michael F. Slasinski collection, Michigan. **$225.00.**

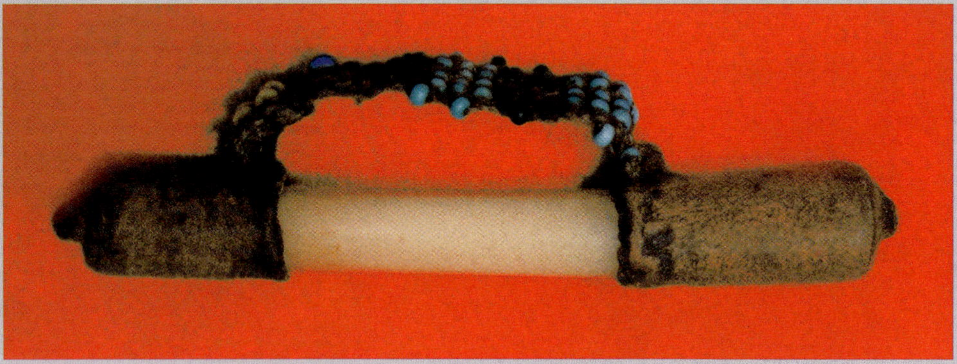

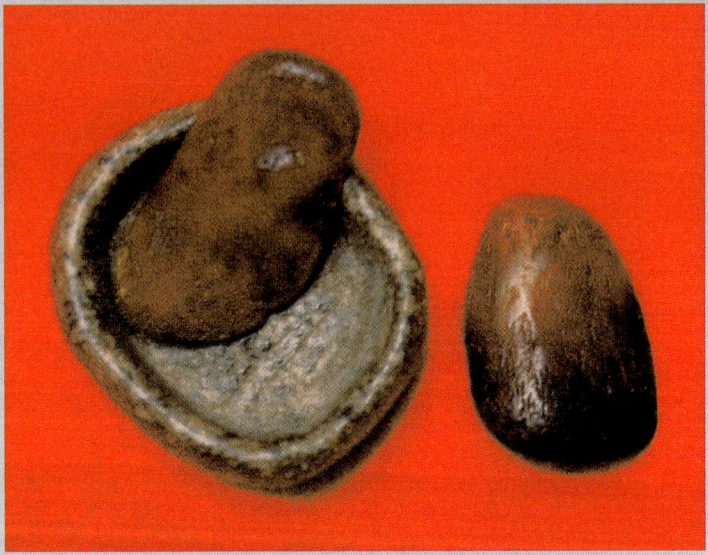

Paint bones, ¾ x 1⅛", 3⁄16" thick. Used to apply paint, the spongy bone interiors held pigment well. They are from historic times and are shown with a stone paint container. Wisconsin. Michael F. Slasinski collection, Michigan. All, **$150.00.**

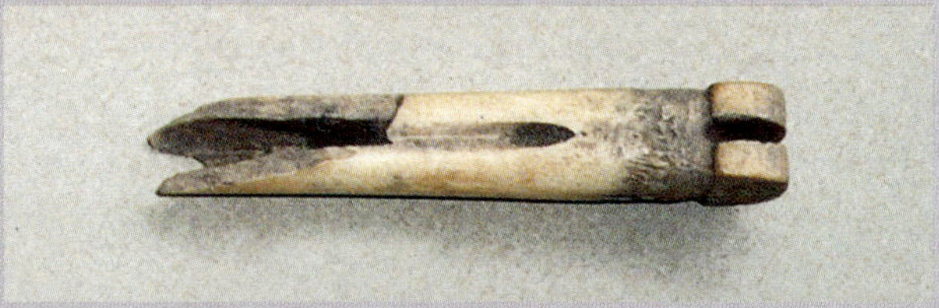

Bone tool, with double tip and much carving and shaping, 3¾" long. This interesting piece was found in Arkansas. Wilfred Dick collection, Mississippi. **$65.00.**

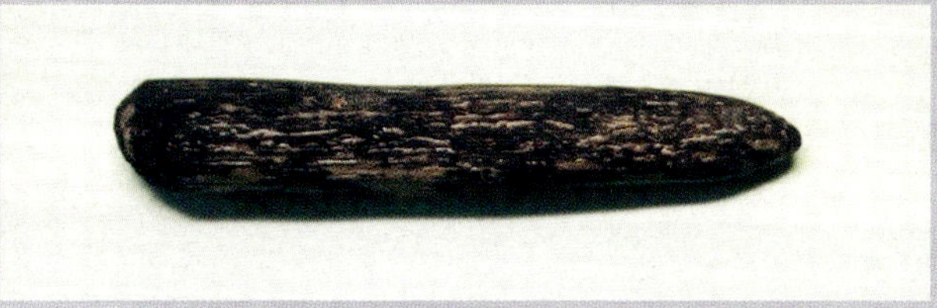

Antler tip flaking tool, probably mule deer, ⅜ x 2½" long. This example was found in Box Elder County, northern Utah. Dann Russell collection, Utah. **$30.00.**

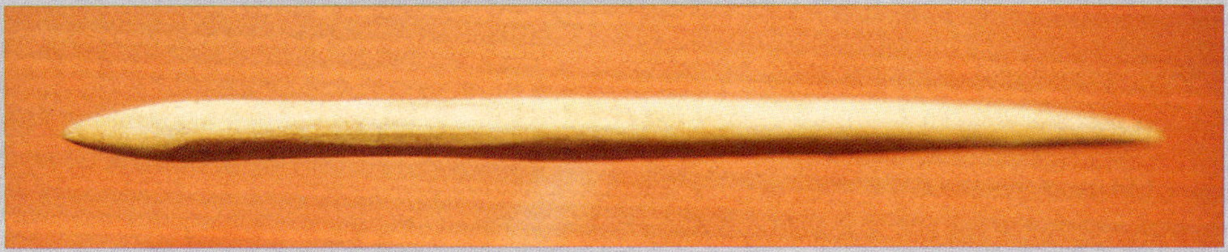

Double-pointed rod or weaving tool, Lamoka phase (3000 – 2500 BC), 6½" long. This Archaic tool is from Schuyler County, New York. Dave Summers collection, Victor, New York. **$50.00.**

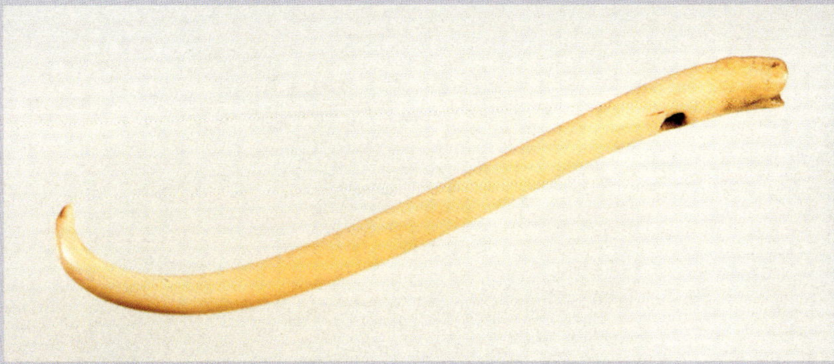

Raccoon penis bone pendant, 3½" long. The thick end is drilled and the smaller end has been worked as well. Ex-collections Copeland and Hooks, the artifact is from southern Ohio. Fred Winegardner collection. **$95.00.**

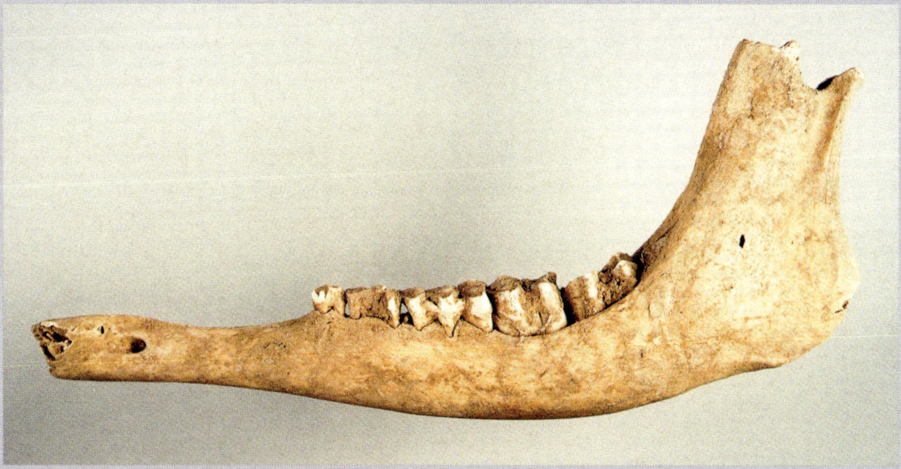

Deer jawbone, from village debris, 6½" long. Such objects were sometimes used as corn scrapers or thatch sickles. Kentucky. Fred Winegardner collection. Unlisted.

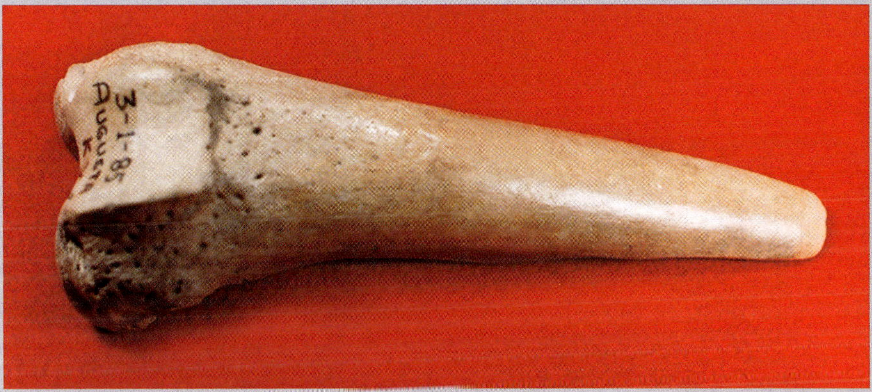

Dagger or gouge, elk or moose leg bone, a very impressive artifact, 7⅝" long. Late Woodland to Mississippian in time, it has high polish on 80% of the surface, good symmetry, and a sharp edge. It was found near Augusta, Kentucky. Pete Timoch collection. **$200.00 – 300.00.**

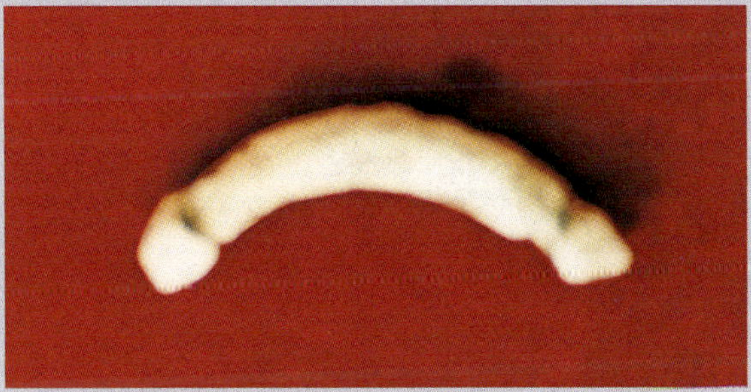

Bone ornament, nose ring(?), 1⅜" long. It was found in the 1980s, location unknown. Darin Liehr collection, Illinois. Unlisted.

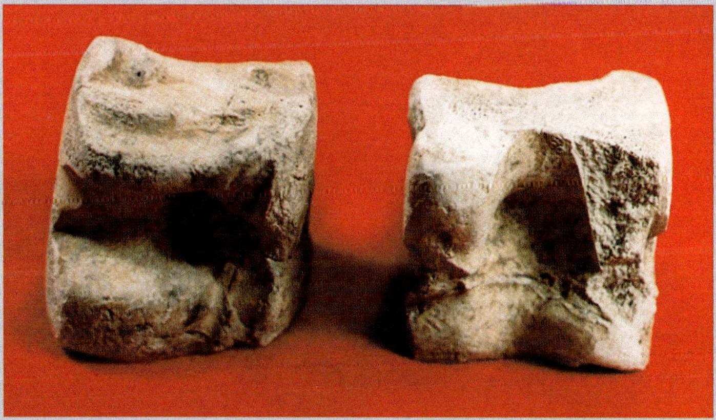

Gaming pieces or dice, ankle bones from very large animals, possibly buffalo. They were ground into cubes and the sides are 2" long. Unusual artifacts, they are ex-collection Hovan and were found in Arkansas. Pete Timoch collection. Each, **$100.00.**

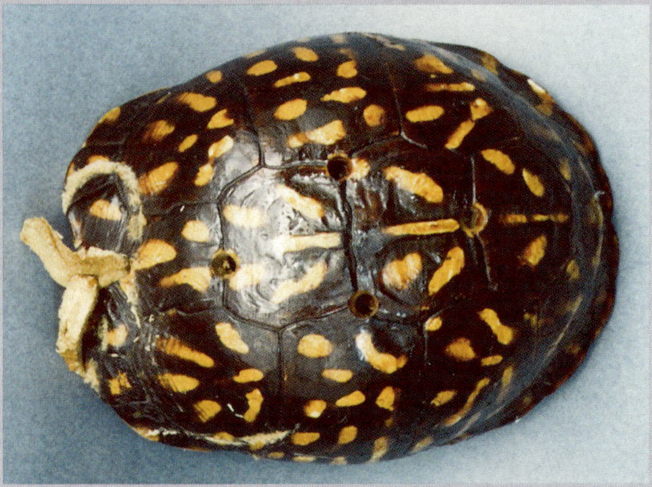

Ceremonial rattle, tortoise shell, 3½ x 4⅝", From the mid-1900s, the shell has drilled holes so that the sound can escape. This was a gift to the owner from O. B. Osceola, Seminole, from southern Florida. H. B. Greene II collection, Naples, Florida. Unlisted.

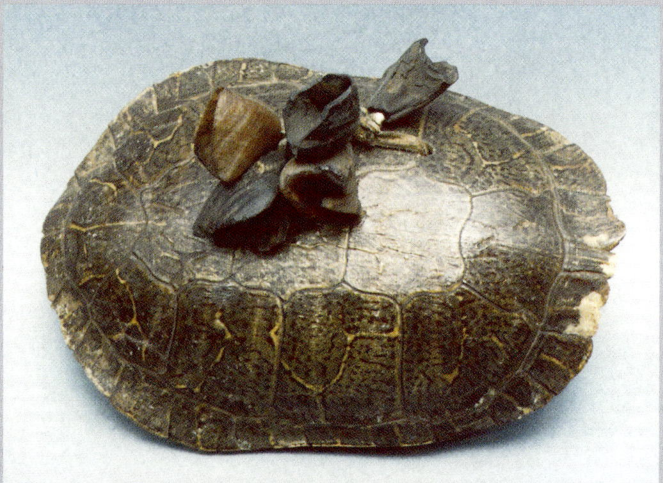

Ceremonial rattle, tortoise shell, 4¼ x 6¼". Deer dewclaws are attached with leather to the shell. This rattle was collected in 1879 by the owner's great-grandfather. Northeastern Woodland. H. B. Greene II collection, Naples, Florida. Unlisted.

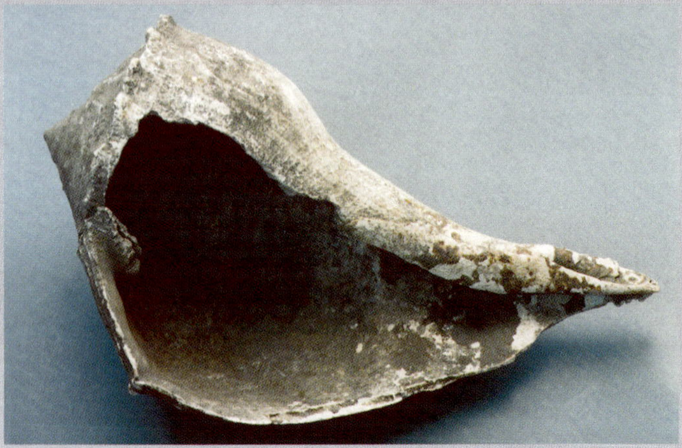

Bowl or dipper, busycon shell, 11½" long, AD 1450 or earlier. This large artifact is Calusa culture and was found on Key Marco, Collier County, Florida. H. B. Greene II collection, Naples, Florida. **$185.00.**

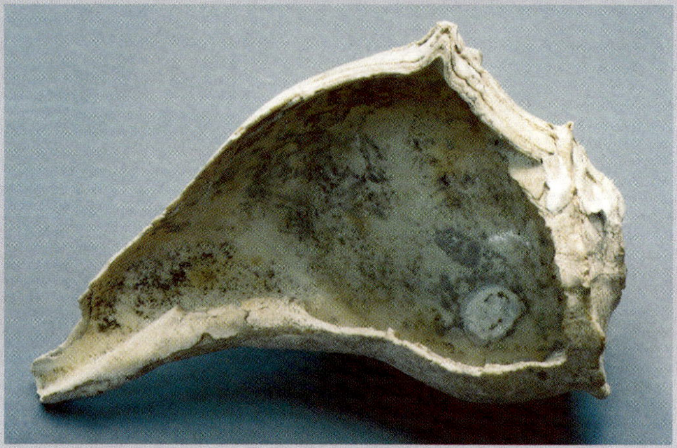

Bowl or dipper, busycon shell, 10¼" long, AD 1450 or earlier. It was made by the Calusa people and was found at Key Marco, Florida. H. B. Greene II collection, Naples, Florida. **$165.00.**

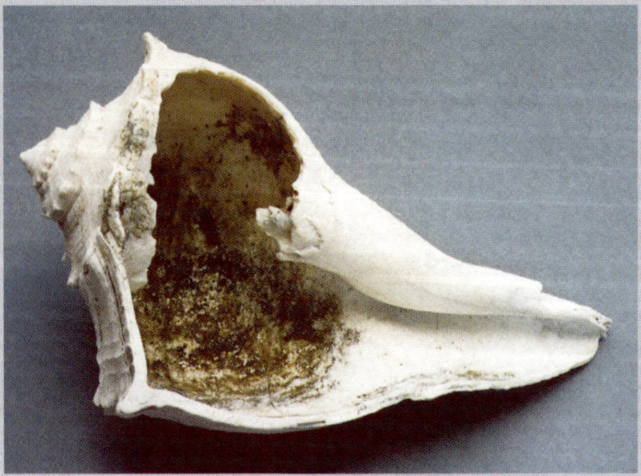

Spoon or dipper, busycon shell, 7⅜" long, AD 1450 or earlier. It is Calusa culture and came from Key Marco, Collier County, Florida. H. B. Greene II collection, Naples, Florida. **$60.00.**

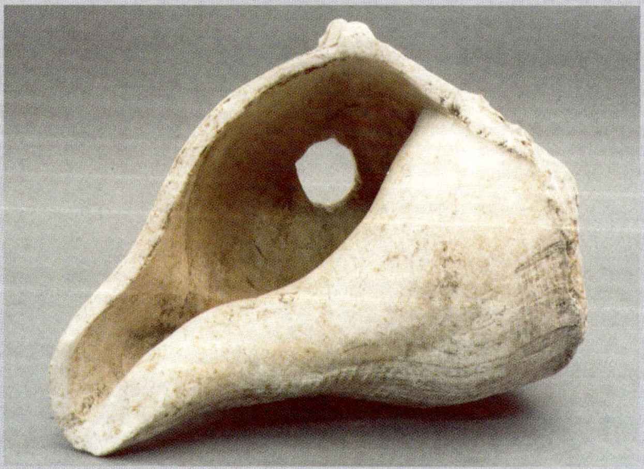

Pick, busycon shell, 7¼" long, AD 1450 or earlier. Calusa culture, it was found on Key Marco, Collier County, Florida. H. B. Greene II collection, Naples, Florida. **$85.00.**

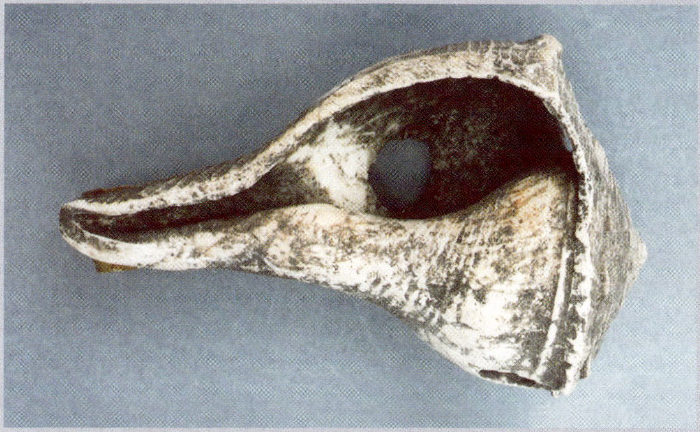

Shell pick, 7" long, AD 1450 or before. It has two handle holes and the tool head came from Marco Island, Collier County, Florida. H. B. Greene II collection, Naples, Florida. **$75.00.**

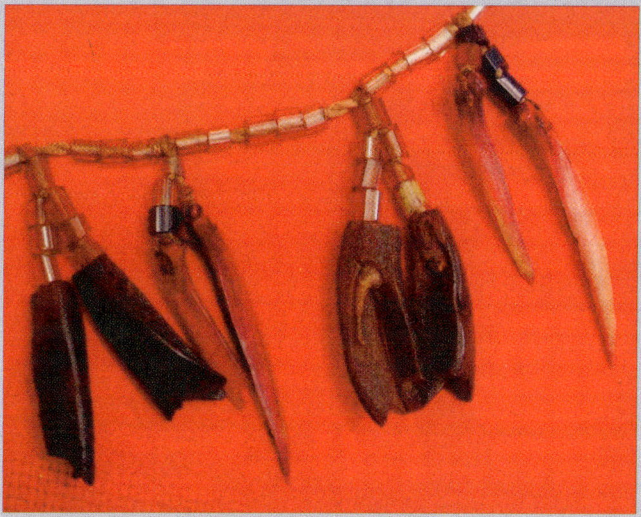

Closeup of Cherokee necklace elements, (whole necklace is shown on page 278), deer dew claws, bone imitation claws, and cut glass trade beads. The dew claws are about 1¼" long. North Carolina. Michael F. Slasinski collection, Michigan. Necklace, **$400.00.**

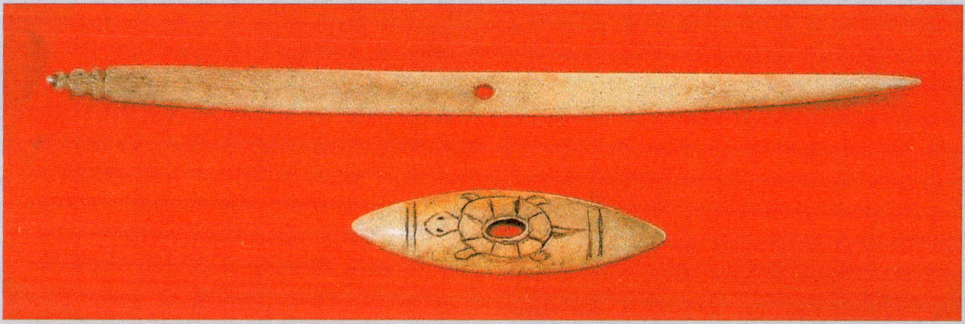

Mat needle and snowshoe needle, (also shown on page 260), mat needle is 7⁄16 x 9", 3⁄32" thick. Mats made of reeds served as floor coverings, bedding, windbreaks and more, and this is a fine historic example. Michigan. Michael F. Slasinski collection, Michigan. Mat needle, **$175.00;** snowshoe needle, **$250.00.**

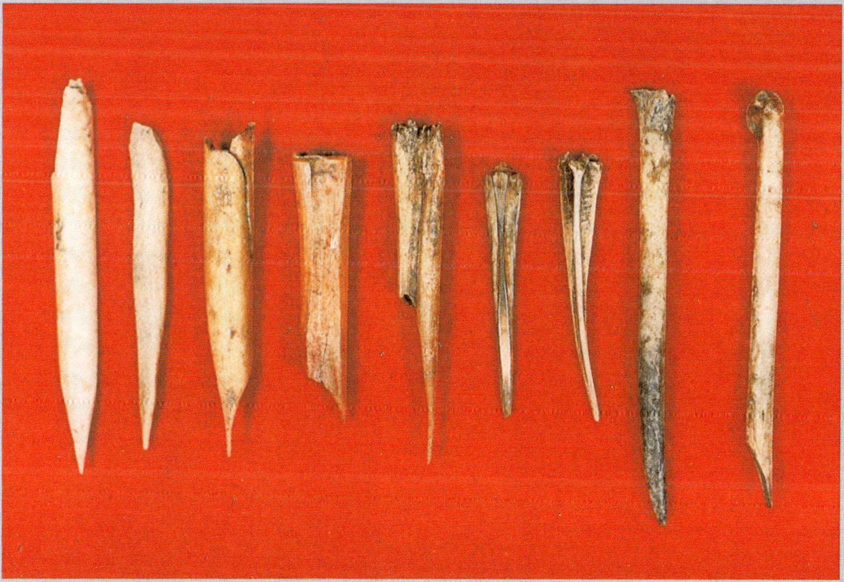

Awls, bird bones, Late Archaic to Woodland, longest is 4 1⁄16". Some have been cut at the bases and a few have specialized needle tips. The left two examples were split from larger bones. All were formerly in the Vietzen collection and came from Christian County, Kentucky. Pete Timoch collection. Each, **$20.00 – 50.00.**

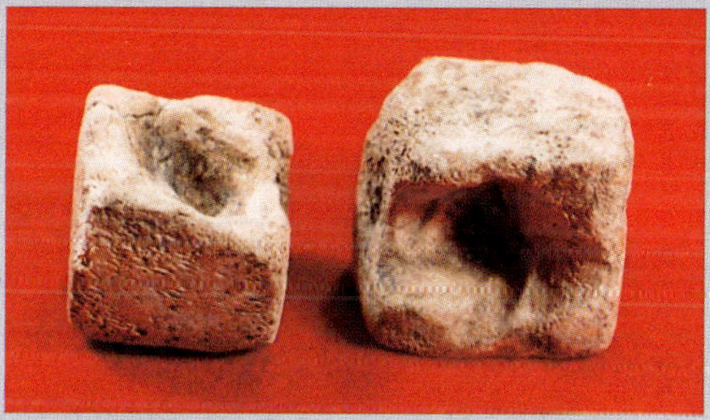

Gaming pieces or dice, ankle bones ground into cube shape, largest is 1½" across. From Mississippian times, they are ex-collection Hovan and came from Arkansas. Pete Timoch collection. Each, **$75.00.**

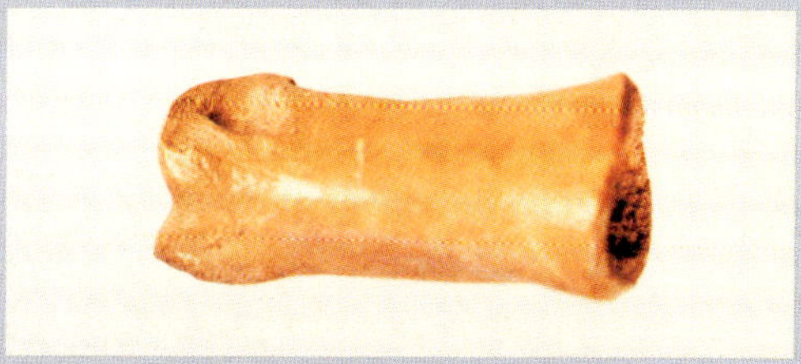

Handle or receptacle, interior hollowed, 1⅜". Of unknown use, this Fort Ancient piece came from southern Ohio. Fred Winegardner collection. **$20.00.**

Miscellaneous Artifacts

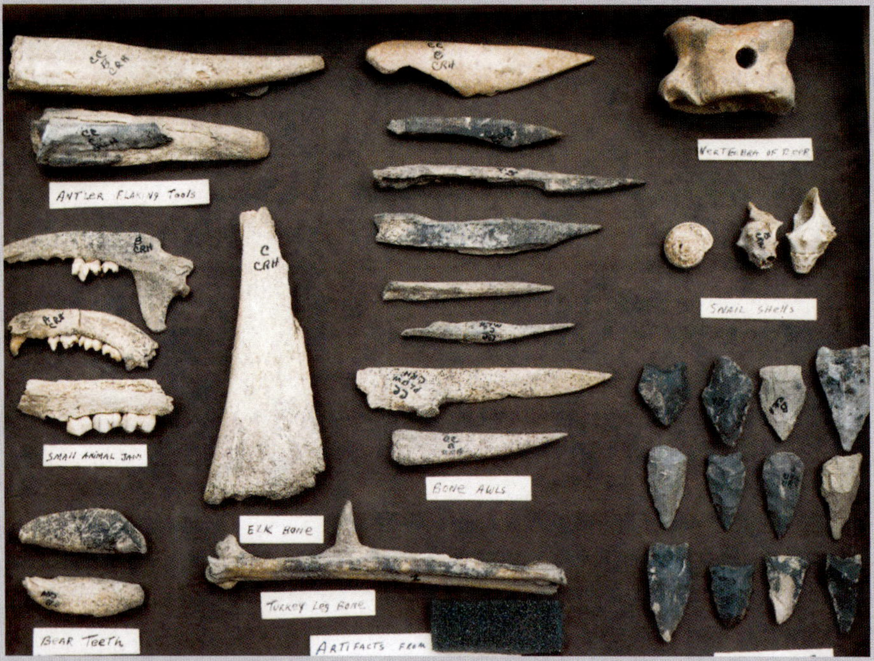

Village midden artifacts, bone, teeth, shell and chert. These objects include mammal jawbones with teeth, awls, flaking tools, turkey leg bone with spur, bear canines, snail shells, a perforated deer vertebrae pendant, an elk bone, and twelve chipped points or blades. Harwood found all in 1957. Greene County, Tennessee. Collection of, and photograph by, Gary Henry, North Carolina. Group, **$1,000.00.**

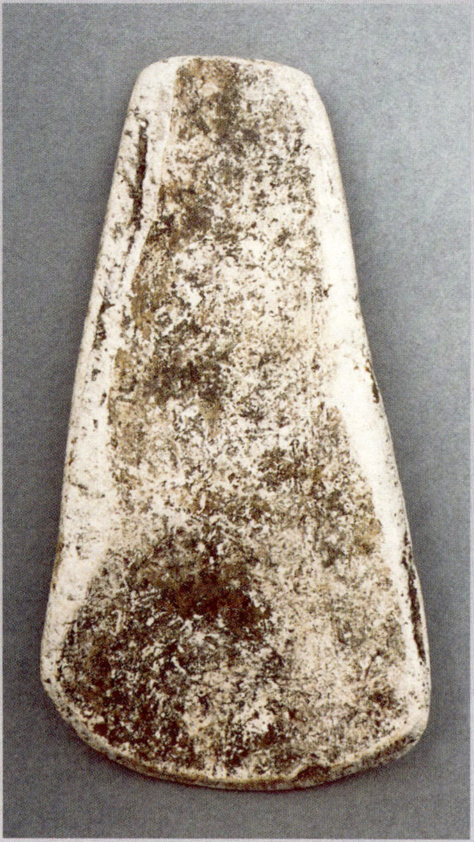

Shell adz blade, 1⅝ x 2⅜", AD 1450 or earlier. This tool was found on Marco Island, Florida. H. B. Greene II collection, Naples, Florida. **$60.00.**

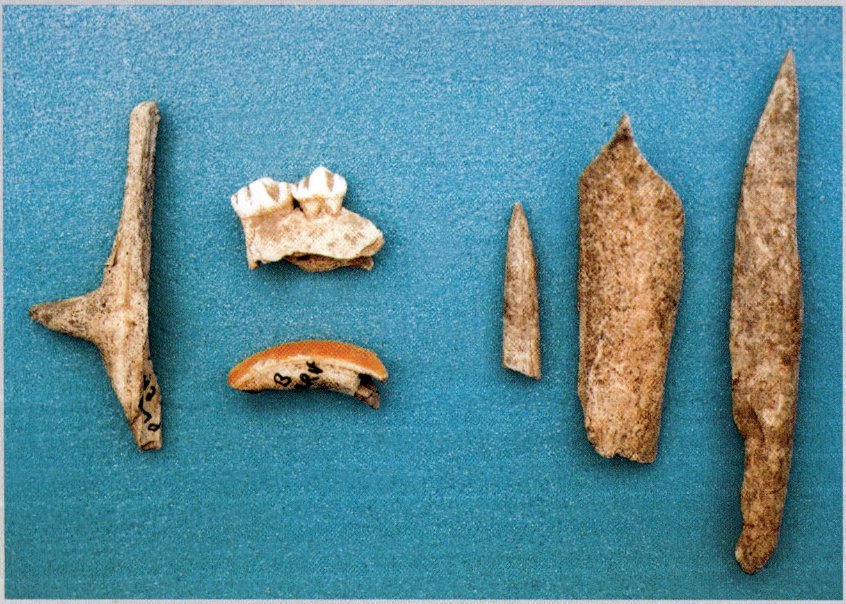

Village midden artifacts, bone and teeth, Archaic or later. The objects include three awls, a turkey leg bone with spur, and a worked beaver incisor. The largest awl (far right) is ½ x 3⅞". Harwood found all in 1957. Greene County, Tennessee. Collection of, and photograph by, Gary Henry, North Carolina. Group, **$100.00.**

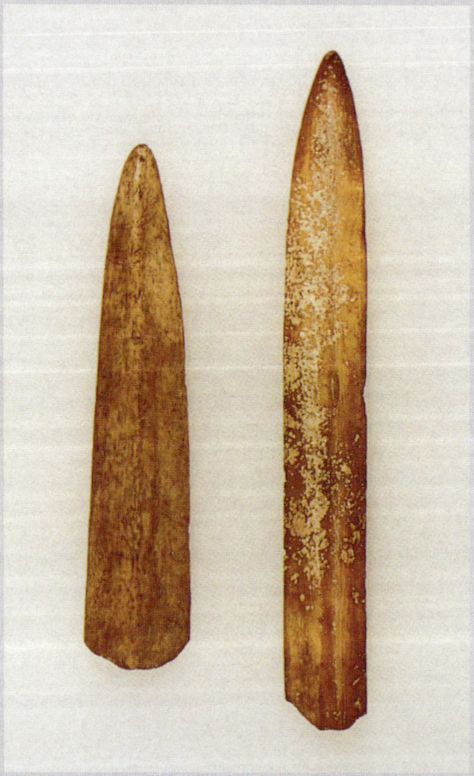

Spearpoints, which could be put in a shaft socket, both from Alaska. James Timoch collection. Left, whalebone, 5" long. **$60.00.** Right, ivory, 6 7/16". **$100.00.**

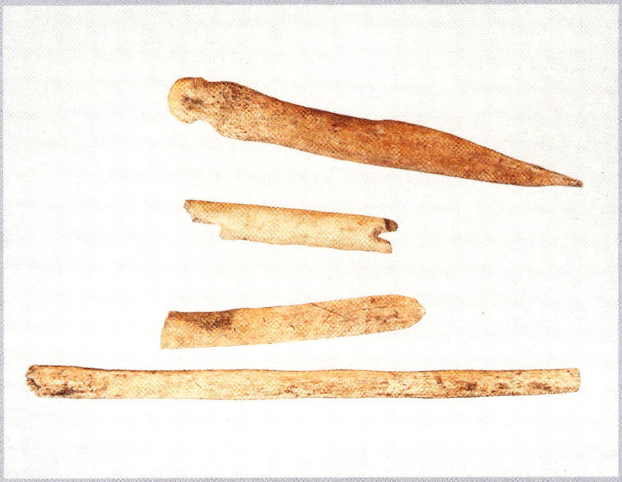

Bone artifacts, bottom three bones extremely thin, longest is 3⅛". These came from a village midden near East Bloomfield, New York. Fred Winegardner collection. All, **$30.00.**

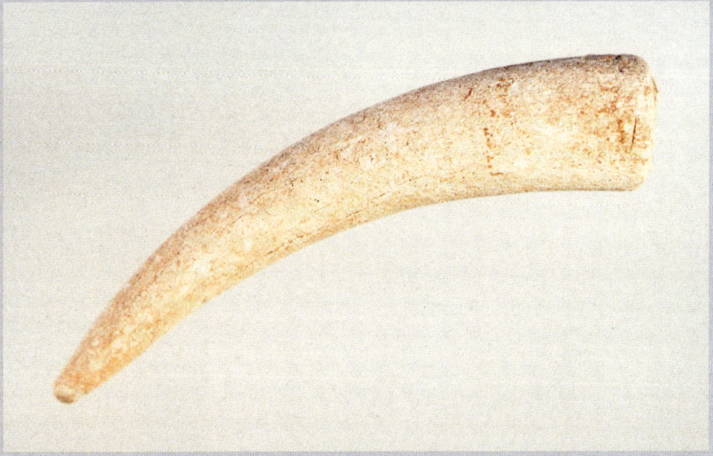

Awl or perforator, antler, thicker end sawed and snapped. It is 3½" long and is marked "1878." The artifact was found in the eastern Midwest. Fred Winegardner collection. **$15.00.**

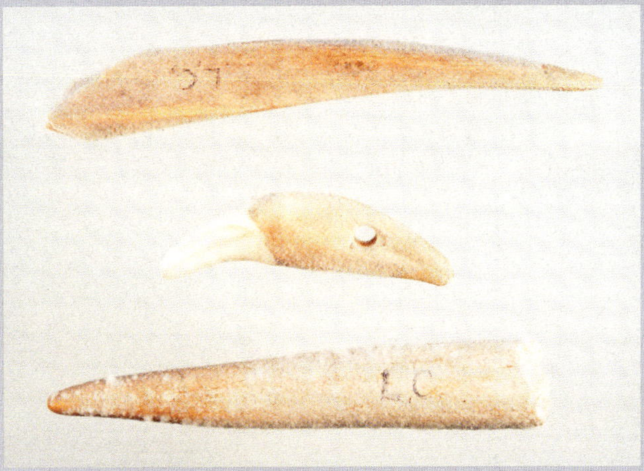

Storage - an important aspect of collecting bone and other artifacts of organic material. The objects shown in the photo may have been cleaned with water by a previous collector and placed in the frame while still damp. A cotton-like mold has developed; this growth should be wiped off, the artifacts completely dried, and the frame matting replaced with new. Spencer County, Kentucky. Private collection. Top, splinter bone awl, 3¼". Center, drilled tooth. Bottom, deer antler pin. All, **$50.00.**

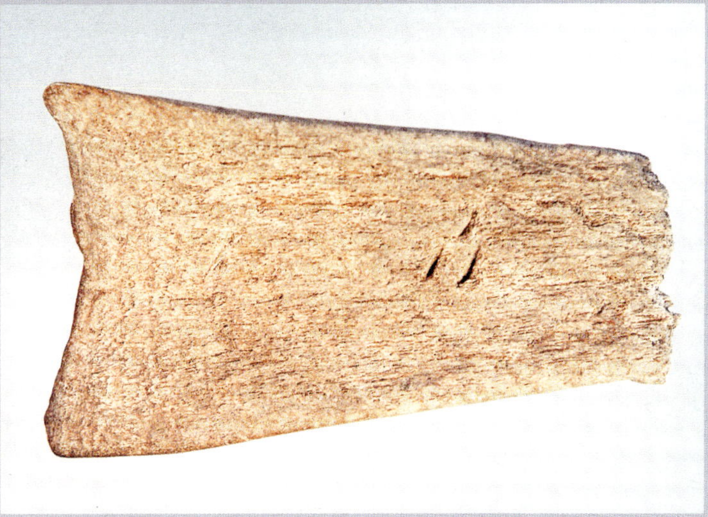

Hoe, elk antler, 3⅛ x 5⅝". A very scarce artifact type, it is Fort Ancient, from southern Ohio. Fred Winegardner collection. Museum grade.

Bone projectile heads, with blunt tips, holes drilled about ½" deep. The 2-inch specimen (right) has a diameter of ¾" while the other has a ½" diameter. Provenance unlisted. Private collection. Each, **$50.00 – 75.00.**

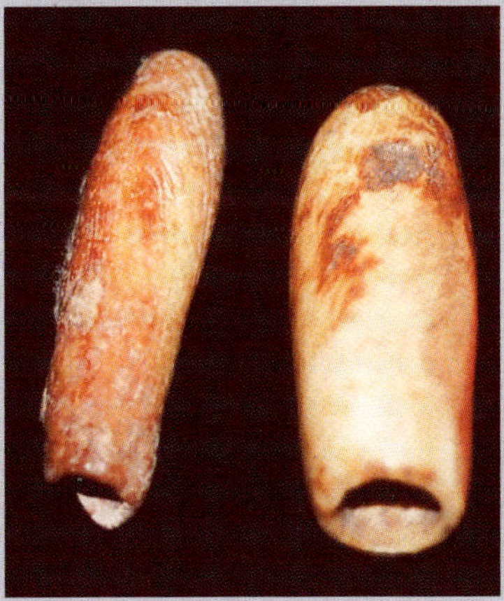

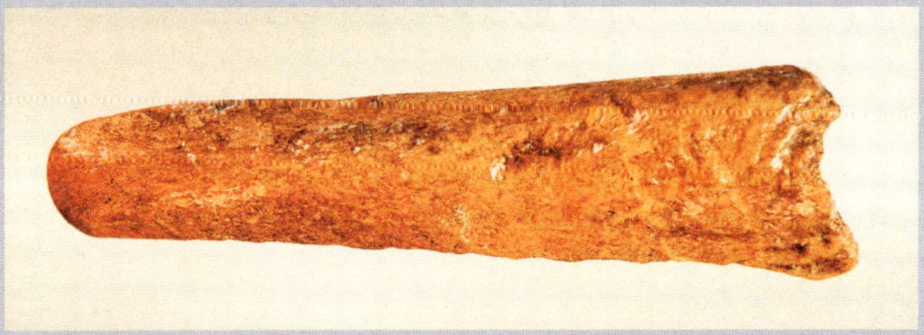

Chisel, heavy animal (elk?) bone, 4½". It has a thin shellac layer and the edge is finely shaped. Mississippian period, the chisel came from southern Ohio. Fred Winegardner collection. **$100.00.**

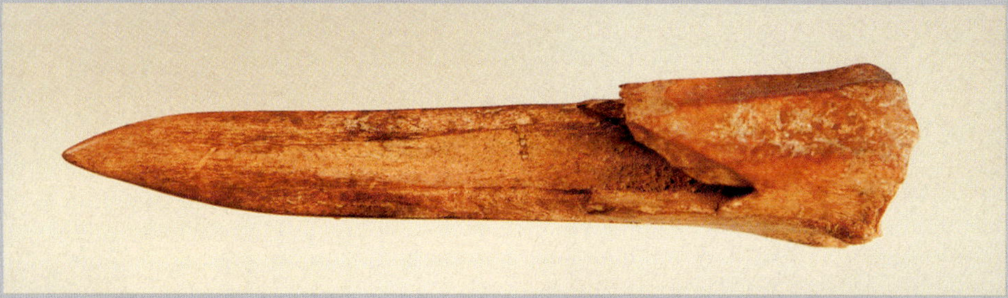

Dagger or knife, deer bone, ground and polished lower blade, 4⅝". It is Fort Ancient, from southern Ohio. Fred Winegardner collection. **$85.00.**

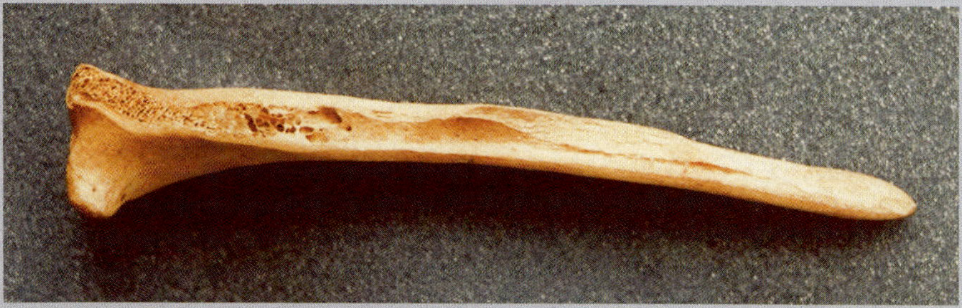

Dagger, triangular cross-section, Middle Archaic period, 6" long. This Lamoka phase artifact was found in Schuyler County, New York. Dave Summers collection, Victor, New York. **$50.00.**

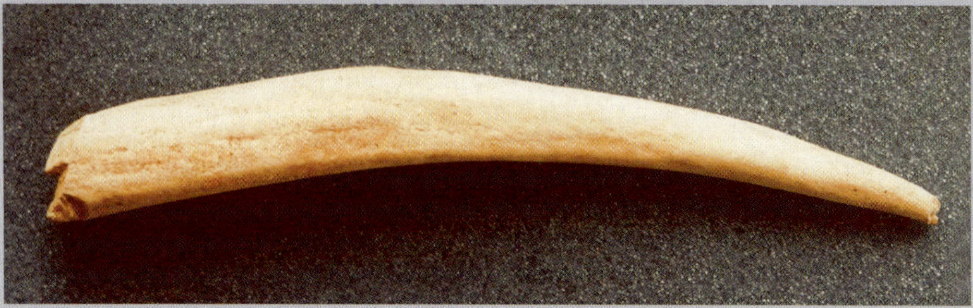

Bone chisel, Lamoka phase of the Middle Archaic, 6¾" long. It is from Schuyler County, New York. Dave Summers collection, Victor, New York. **$50.00.**

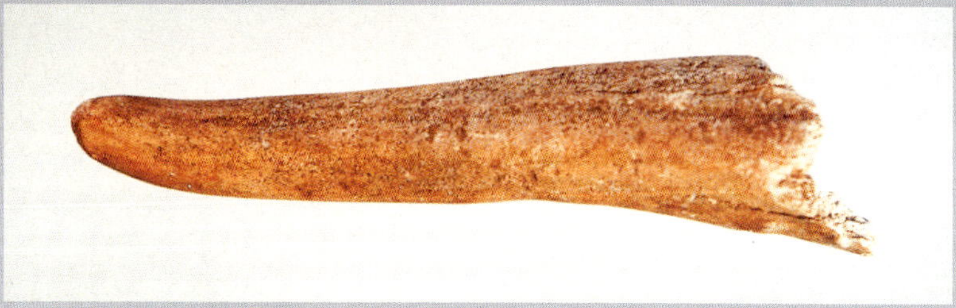

Antler tool, 3⅞" long. It was found on a Mississippian site in southern Ohio. Fred Winegardner collection. **$12.00.**

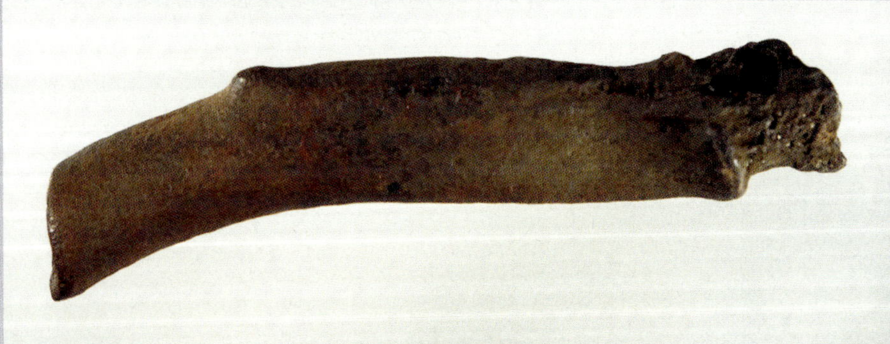

Antler tool or knife handle, heavily mineralized, 6¼". Waterworn, it came from a river in Florida. Dwight Wolfe collection. **$55.00.**

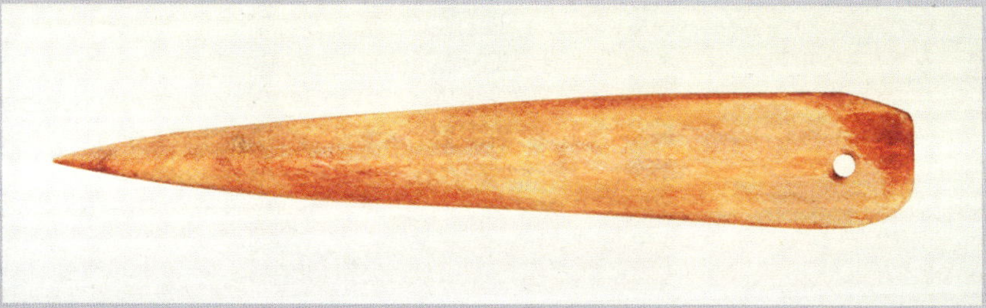

Awl or wide needle, amber patination in several shades, 3½" long. This piece was found near Elizabethtown, Kentucky. Robin Fiser collection. **$40.00.**

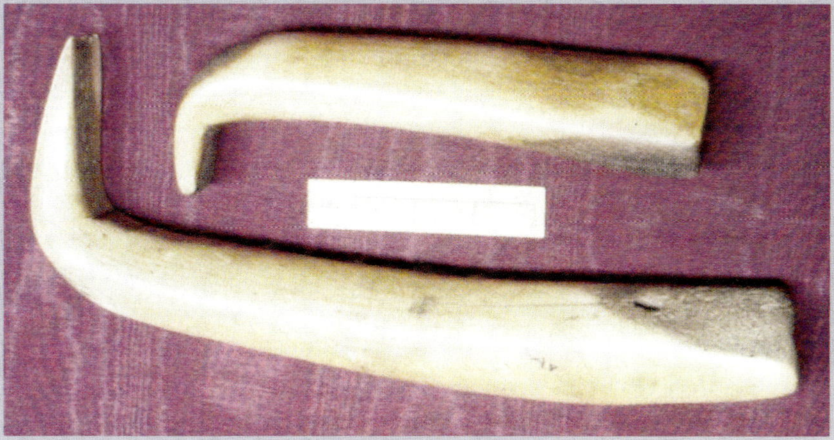

Plains Indian hide-scrapers, historic period, made from elk antler. A flint or steel working edge was fastened to the inside of the angled end, and the heavy tool could be used for many years. Montana. Ben Thompson collection, Missouri. Small handle, **$125.00;** large handle, **$175.00.**

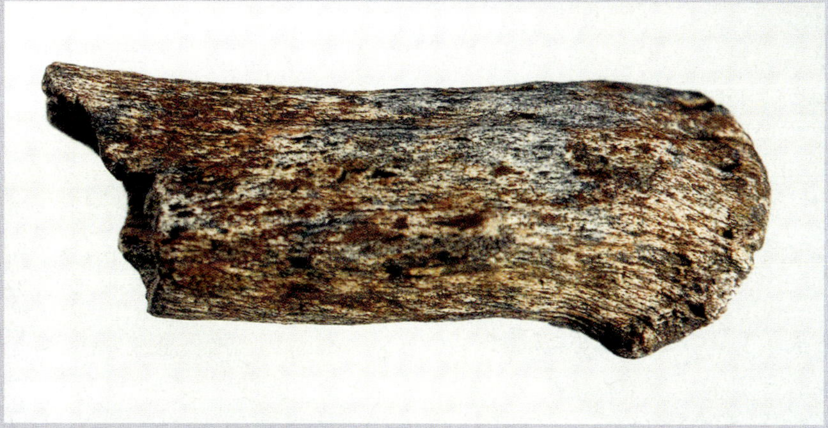

Antler handle, large deer or small elk, 4¼". Waterworn in shades of brown, the handle came from the Tennessee River in Kentucky. Dwight Wolfe collection. **$20.00.**

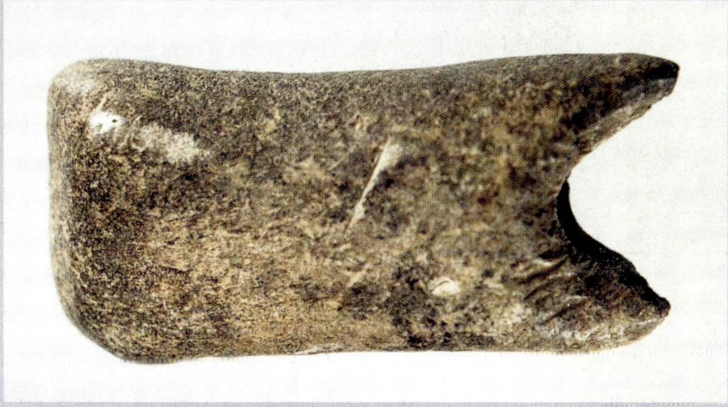

Handle, rectangular, probably an Atl-atl grip from the Early Woodland people, 3¼" long. The surface is polished and both short sides have zigzag incised lines, while the U-shaped end has an oval hole. This rare artifact came from eastern Tennessee. Dwight Wolfe collection. Museum grade.

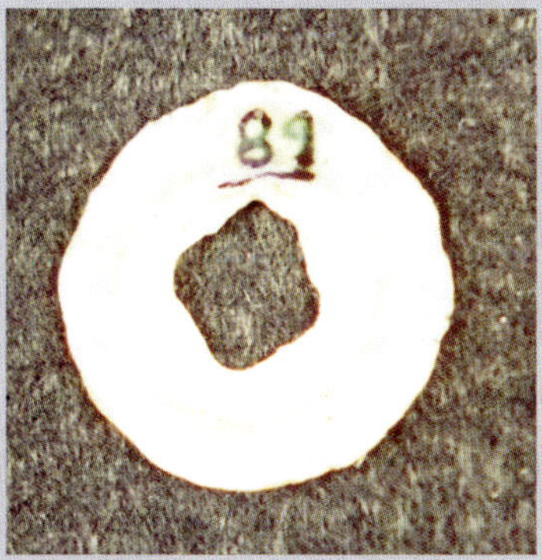

Shell button, large squared opening. The owner found it on a site in Pennsylvania. Lee Hallman collection, Pennsylvania. **$15.00.**

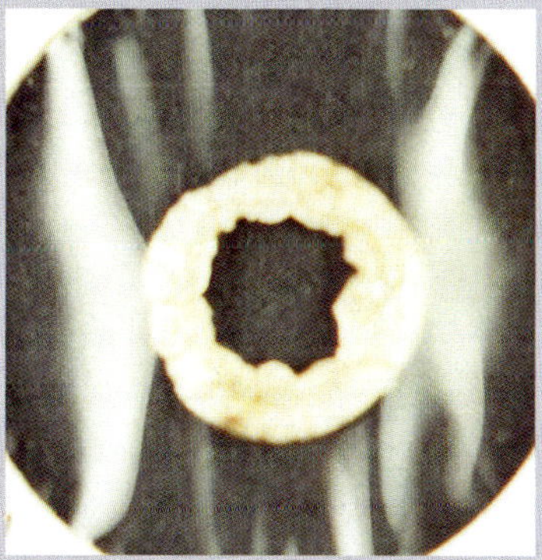

Shell button, large opening. Found at Site 48 in Pennsylvania. Lee Hallman collection, Pennsylvania. **$15.00.**

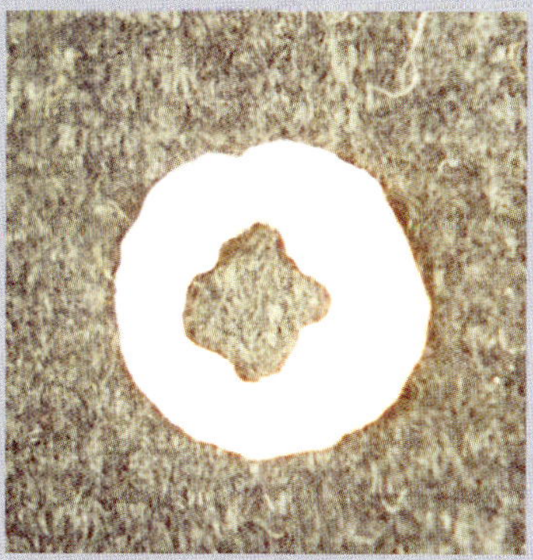

Shell button, large and irregular center hole. The owner picked it up on a Pennsylvania site. Lee Hallman collection, Pennsylvania. **$10.00.**

Miscellaneous Artifacts

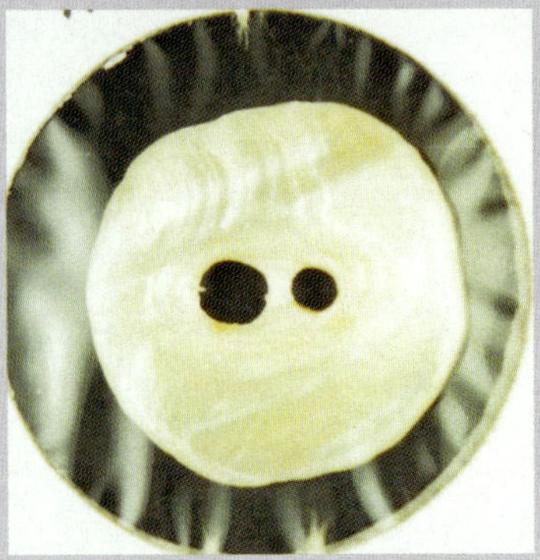

Shell button, two drilled holes, fine condition. Found by the owner, it is from Site 48, Pennsylvania. Lee Hallman collection, Pennsylvania. **$20.00.**

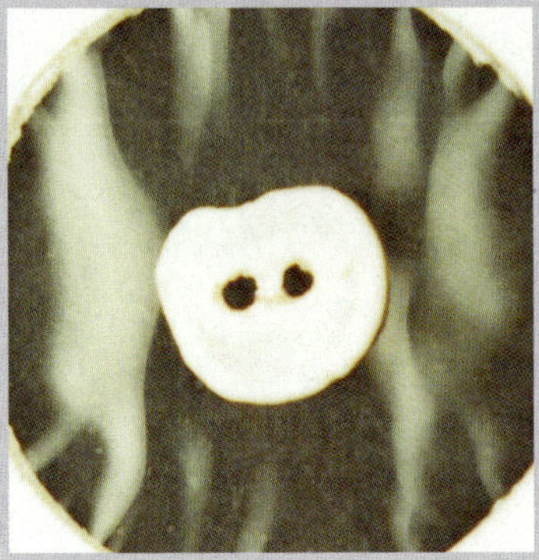

Shell button, two attachment holes, found by the owner at Site 48 in Pennsylvania. Lee Hallman collection, Pennsylvania. **$10.00.**

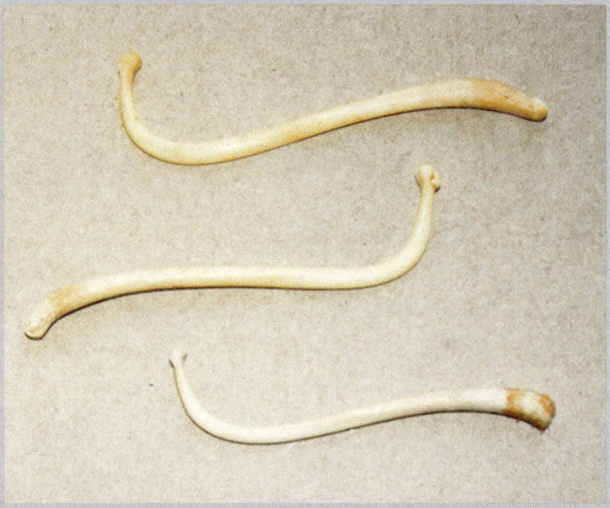

Raccoon penis bones, polished but undrilled. Find-locations unknown. Wilfred Dick collection, Mississippi. Unlisted.

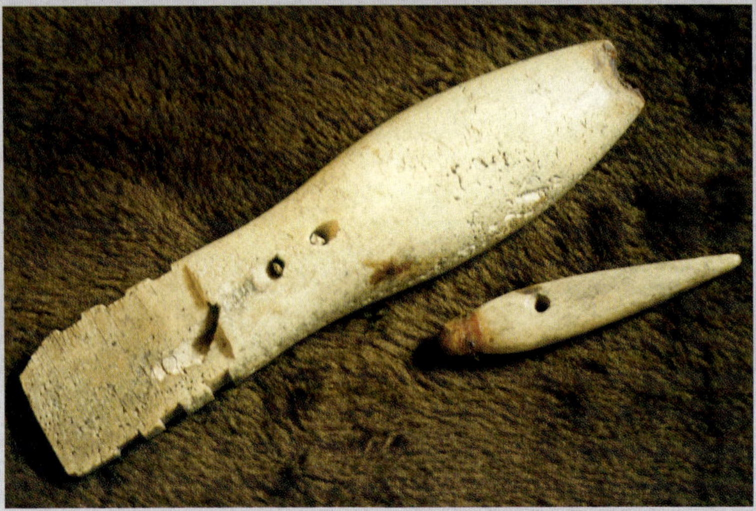

Two-piece harpoon, walrus tusk, 12" long. The large section has hafting notches on the base (bottom left) and the tip is detachable. Northwest Coast. Dale and Betty Roberts collection, Iowa. **$500.00.**

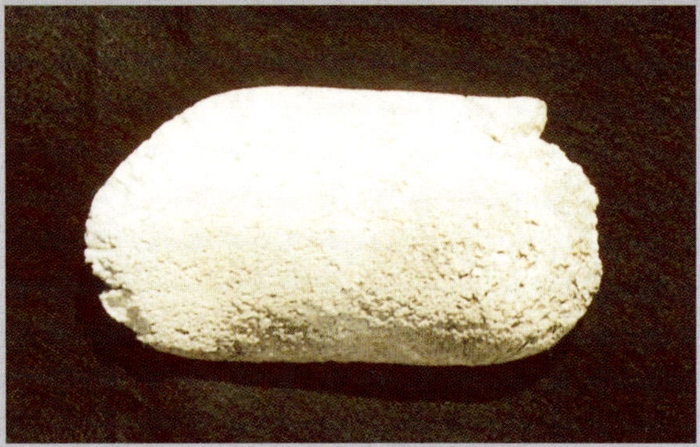

Mastodon or mammoth bone, with scrape marks, Pleistocene (Ice Age) times, 3½ x 6½". It was found in Orange County, New York. Dave Summers collection, Victor, New York. **$25.00.**

Shell dipper, large marine conch, found in 1935 at a major Mississippian site in Oklahoma. It is ex-collections Braecklein and Cheeseboro and is signed by the former. Oklahoma. Dale and Betty Roberts collection, Iowa. Unlisted.

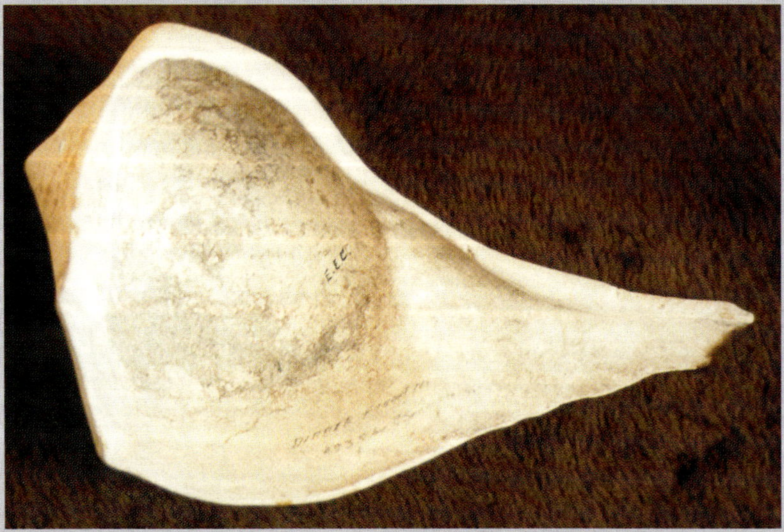

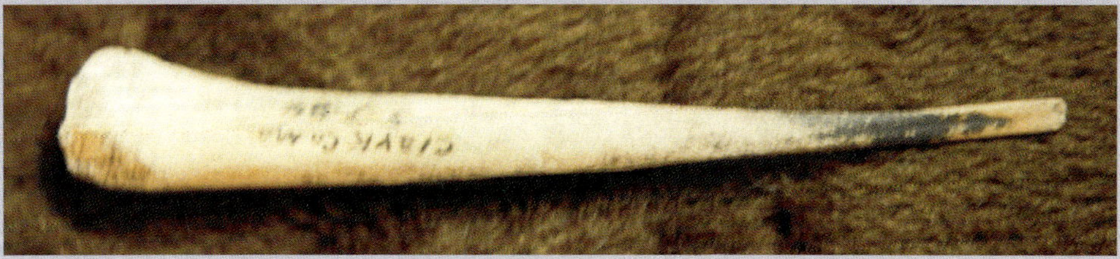

Bone weaving(?) tool, with a large rounded end and a thin flat tip, length is 6⅝". The artifact was found by the owners and came from Clark County, Missouri. Dale and Betty Roberts collection, Iowa. **$175.00.**

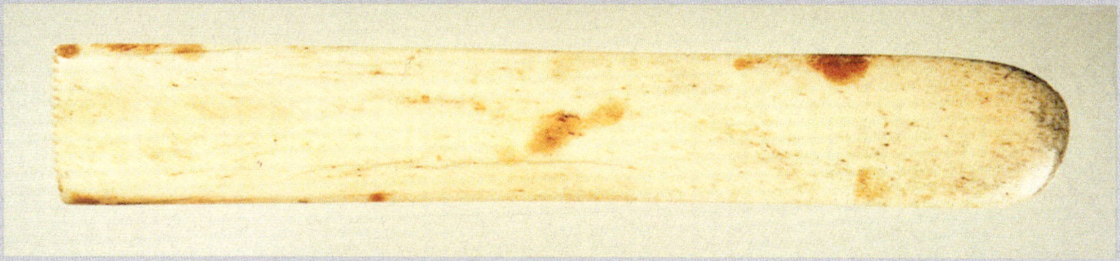

Skinning or hide-working tool, heavy bone or ivory, 6⅞" long. This example has a toothed end and a spatula end. Alaska. Robin Fiser collection. **$75.00.**

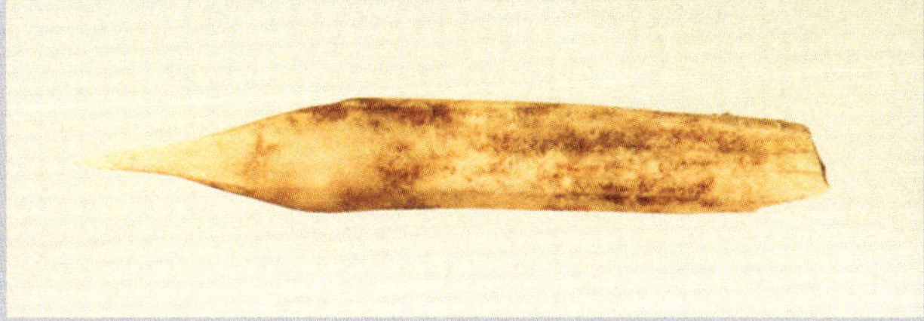

Awl, bird bone splinter, 2⅜" long. This example is from the eastern Midwest. Robin Fiser collection. **$15.00 – 20.00.**

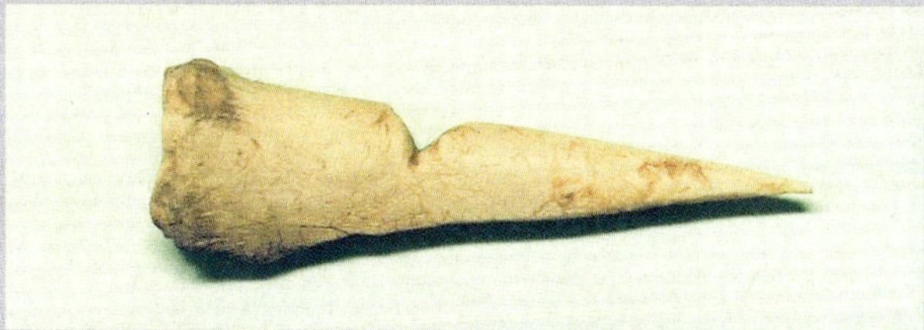

Awl, mammal bone, 1 5/16 x 3¼". It has been notched, possibly for suspension around the neck. This awl came from Weber County, northern Utah. Dann Russell collection, Utah. **$40.00.**

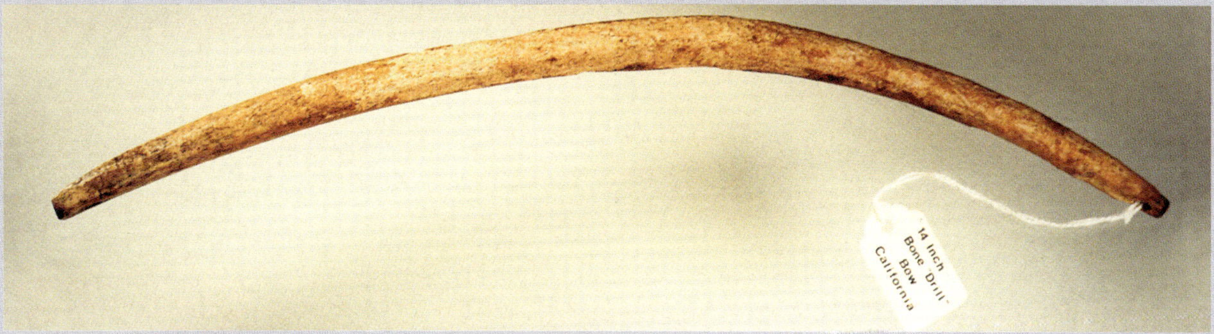

Bone bow drill handle, 14" long. There is a cord hole at each end of this scarce artifact which was found in California. Robin Fiser collection. Museum grade.

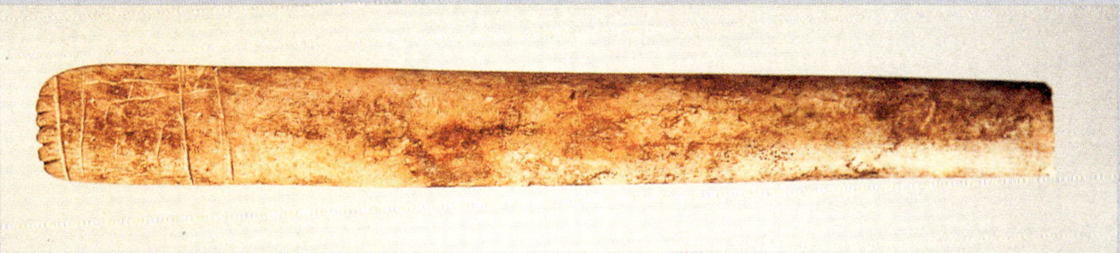

Bone hide-working tool, bison or elk 7" long. One end has a toothed edge and is decorated with incised lines. Four Corners area, Arizona. Don Casto collection. **$50.00.**

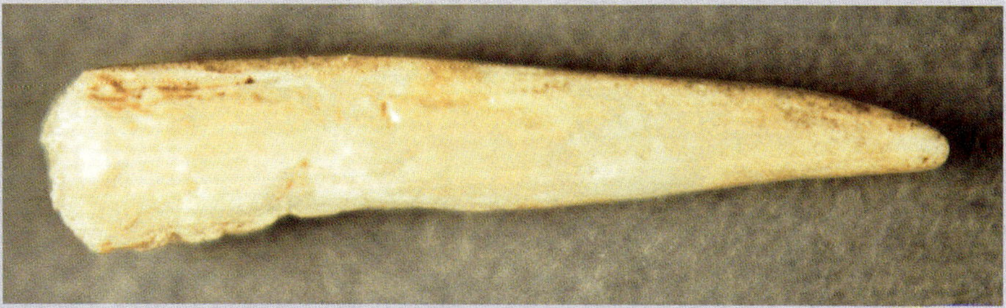

Antler tine cut from a larger section, possibly for an awl or projectile point. This example is 2¾" long, from Mississippi County, Arkansas. Back to Earth. **$15.00.**

Miscellaneous Artifacts

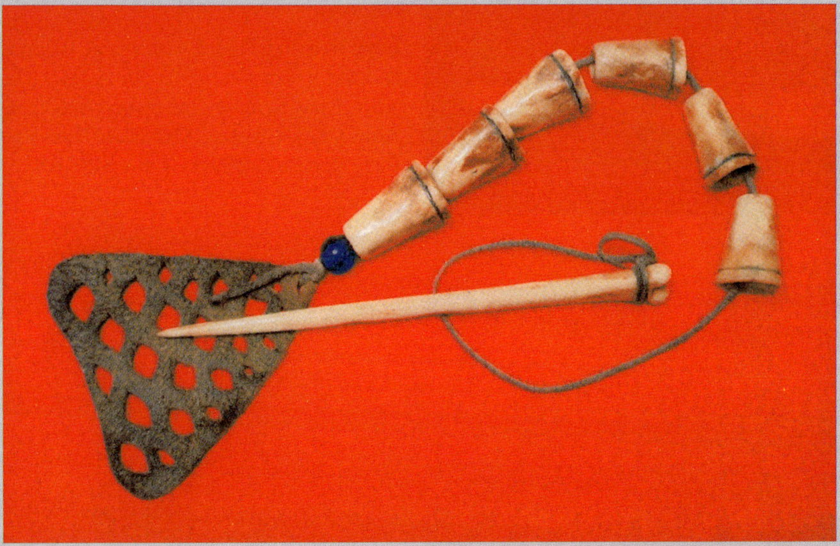

Cup and pin game set, historic, bone cups ⅝ x ⅞" and bone pin 5" long. It has a decorative leather flap and a glass trade bead. Well-made, this unusual set is Chippewa, from Michigan. Michael F. Slasinski collection, Michigan. **$400.00.**

Snowshoe needle, bone, 1³⁄₁₆ x 3⅛", ⅛" thick. Historic, it is decorated with incised lines and a turtle figure. Michigan. Michael F. Slasinski collection, Michigan. **$250.00.**

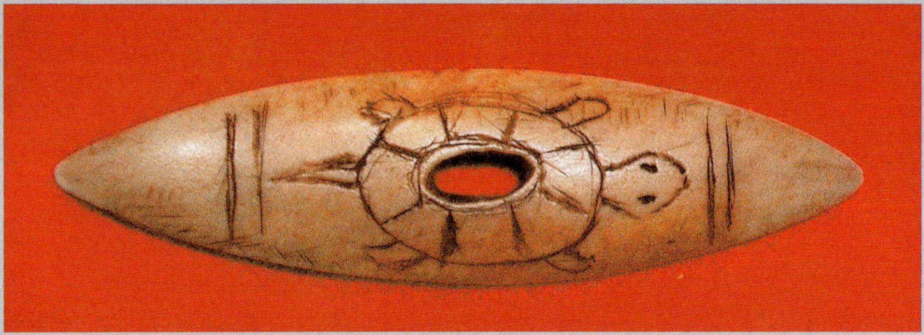

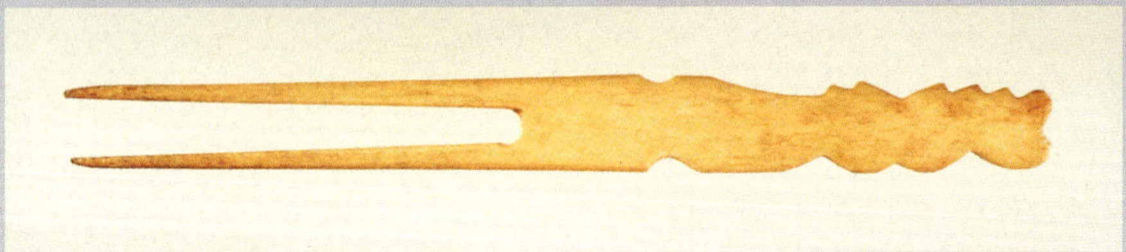

Hairpin(?), double shafts, 4⅝" long. This piece is nicely carved and in fine condition. Limestone County, Alabama. Robin Fiser collection. **$125.00.**

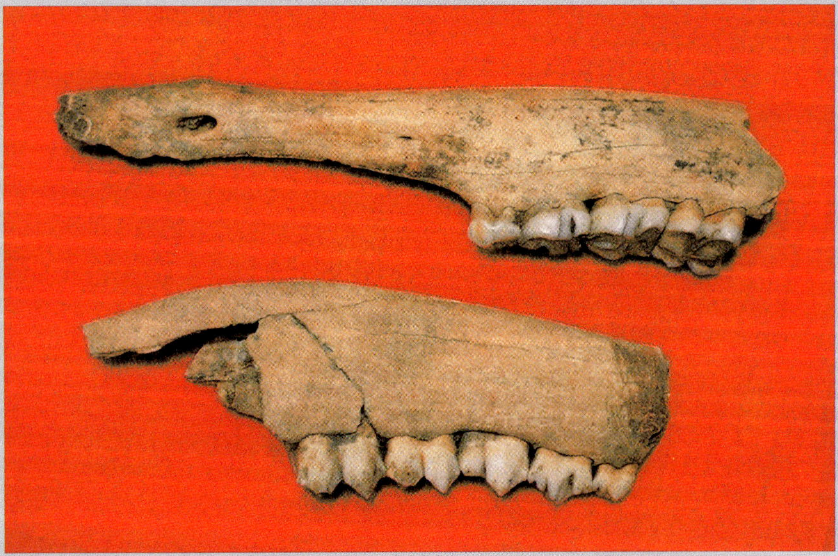

Corn scrapers, deer jawbones, 1⅛ x 5" long, ⁷⁄₁₆" thick. The Iroquois used these in New York state. Michael F. Slasinski collection, Michigan. Each, **$25.00 – 75.00.**

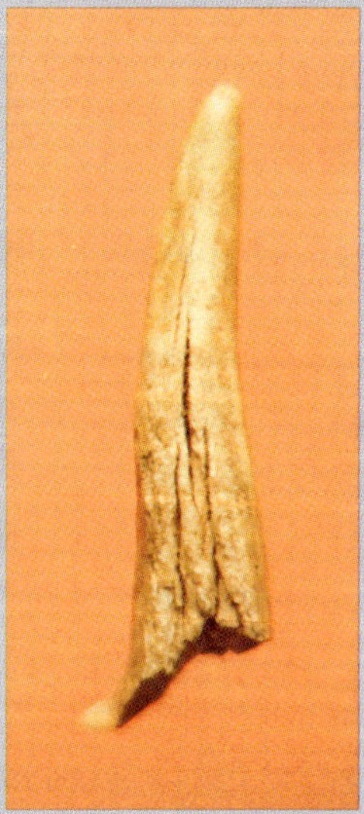

Flaker, antler tine, 2¼" long. Lamoka from the Middle Archaic. It was found in Schuyler County, New York. Dave Summers collection, Victor, New York. **$20.00.**

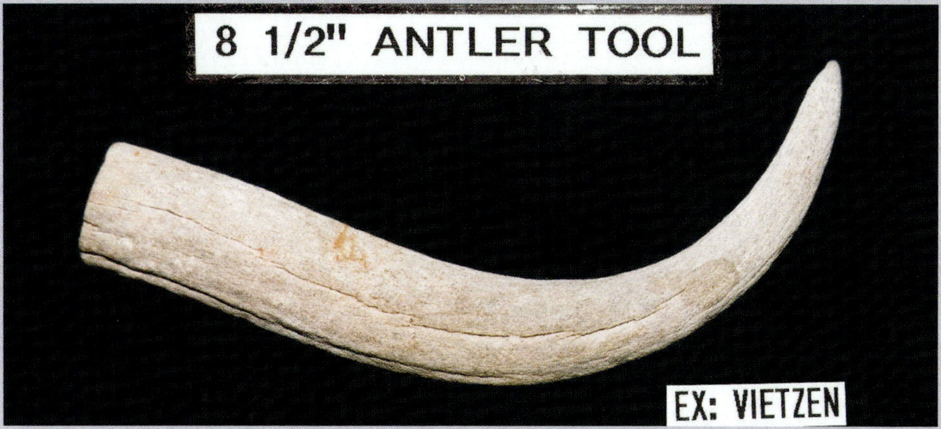

Antler flaking tool or short club, found by Col. Vietzen in 1942 and formerly in his museum collection, 8½" long. It is from Erie County, Ohio. Back to Earth. **$165.00.**

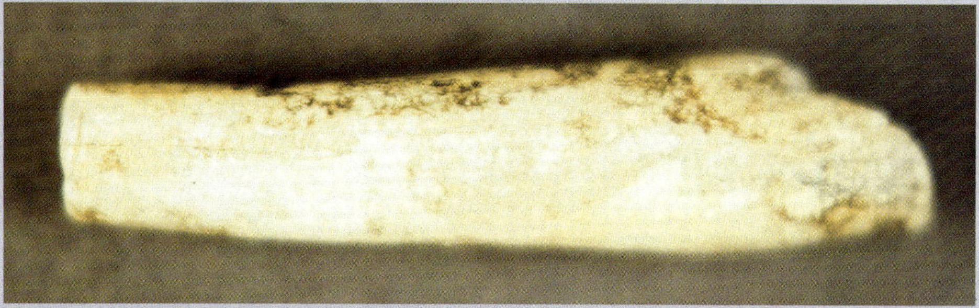

Antler tine, with smaller end cut off, 2¾" long. This piece came from Mississippi County, Arkansas. Back to Earth. **$10.00.**

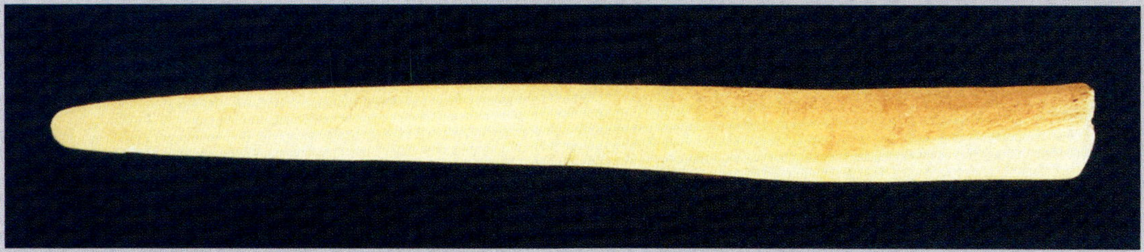

Tool, elk or bison bone, spatulate small end and cut wide end, 8$^{15}/_{16}$" long. This large tool was found in the Four Corners region of the Southwest. Don Casto collection. **$40.00.**

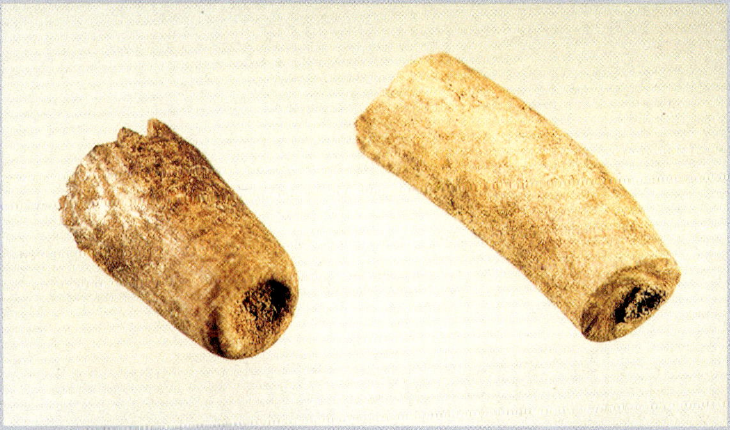

Antler sections cut off at the tips, the larger example, 2" long, is cut in the usual way. The smaller has an indented thimble-like end. Both are from Kentucky. Private collection. Unlisted.

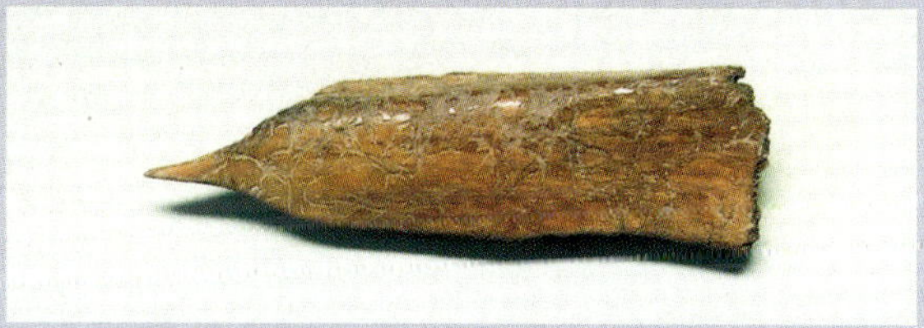

Awl, mammal bone, $^{9}/_{16}$ x 2⅛" long. It has a short but sharp tip and the awl is broken at the base. Weber County, northern Utah. Dann Russell collection, Utah. **$30.00.**

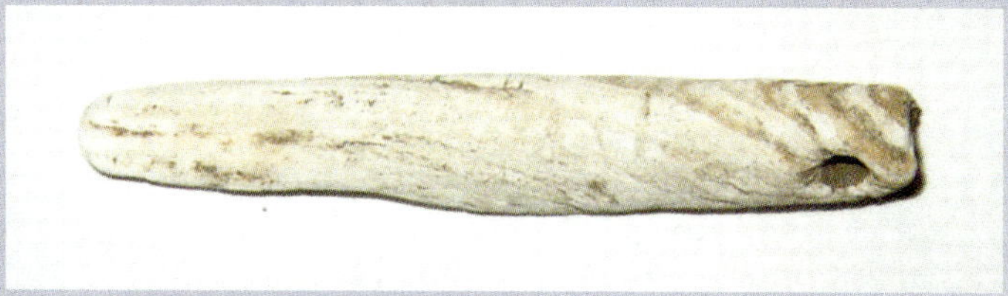

Pendant or elongated bead, drilled at top, 1$^{15}/_{16}$" long. The owner found it in April of 2003 along the Ohio River in Mason County, West Virginia. Private collection. Rodney Roberts photograph. **$40.00.**

Miscellaneous Artifacts

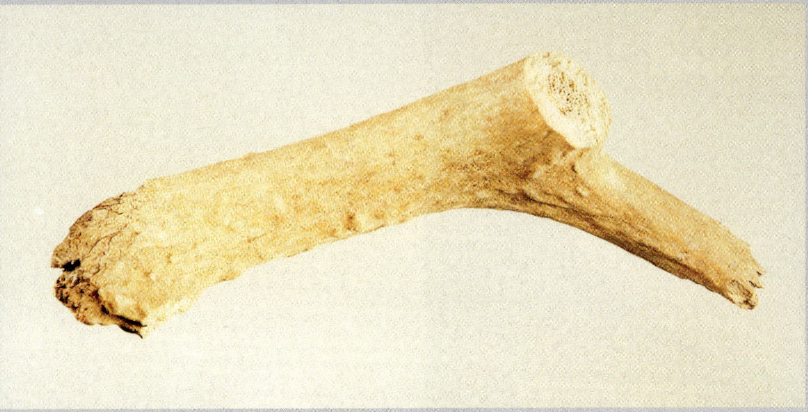

Antler branch from village midden – raw material for tools, $6\frac{1}{16}$" long. Several tines were broken off. Kentucky. Private collection. Unlisted.

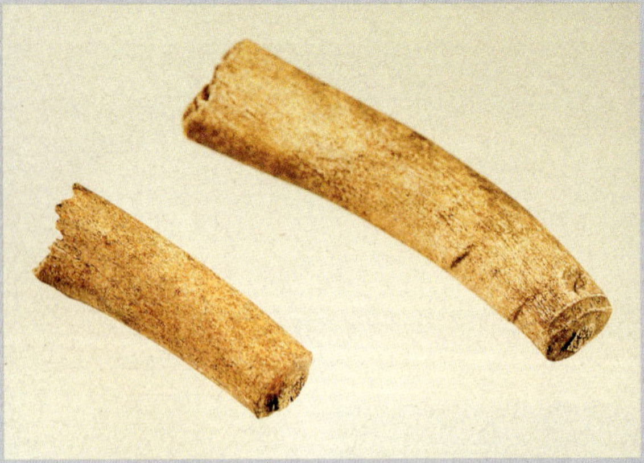

Antler sections, tips cut off for tools or points, longer one is 3". Existing marks indicate that the antler was cut all around before the small remaining central section was snapped off. Kentucky. Private collection. Unlisted.

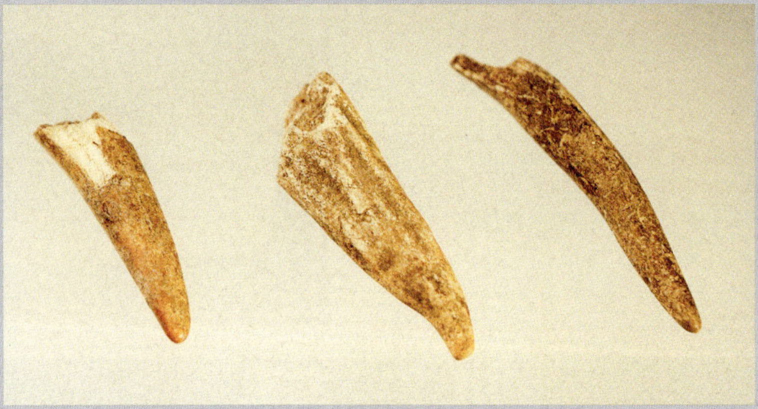

Antler tips, from village midden, longest is $2\frac{9}{32}$". The two on left and right are deer tines, while the larger center piece is elk antler. These were probably intended for projectile points, and all are from Kentucky. Private collection. Unlisted.

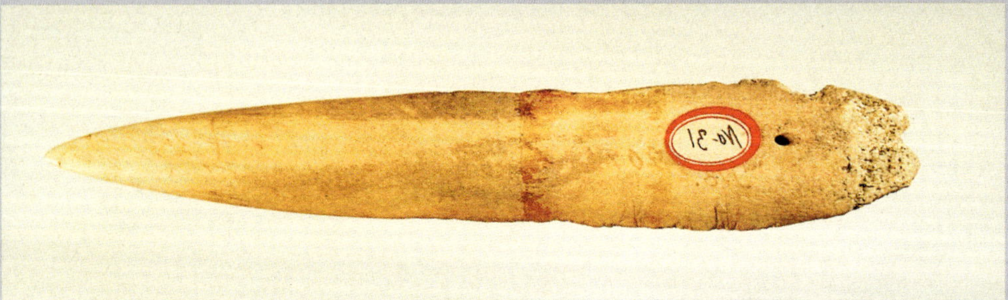

Dagger or knife, V-notch at hilt center, split deer bone. It is $4\frac{5}{8}$" long and the lower blade is well-shaped and polished. This tool or weapon was found in southern Ohio. Lar Hothem collection. **$60.00.**

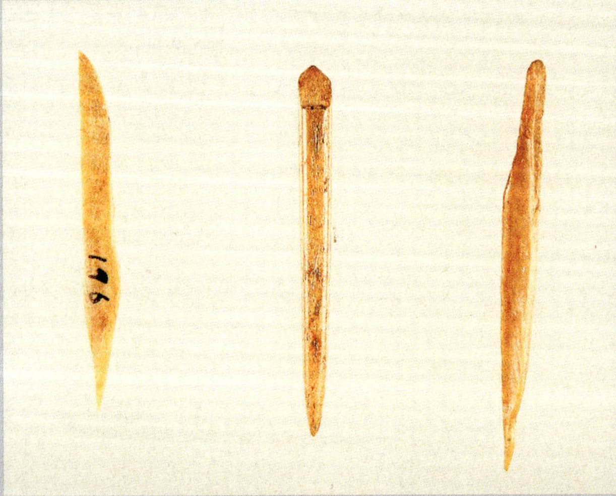

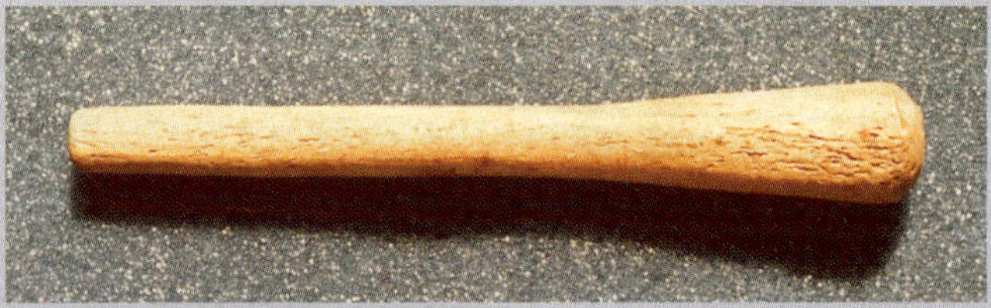

Bone billet, with narrow handle and expanded end, ex-collection Burch. It is historic Iroquois and came from a site dated AD 1625 – 1645. Of uncertain use, this well-made artifact is $4\frac{1}{2}$" long. Livingston County, New York. Dave Summers collection, Victor, New York. **$175.00.**

Perforators, now coated with shellac, deer bone splinters, center example is $2\frac{1}{8}$". Probably hafted when in use, they are Fort Ancient, from southern Ohio. Private collection. All, **$25.00.**

Bone tool, highly polished spatulate blade, perhaps used for pottery shaping. The tool is historic Iroquois and came from a site dating ca. 1650 – 1765. It is 6⅞" long and was found near Honeoye Falls, Monroe County, New York. Dave Summers collection, Victor, New York. **$150.00.**

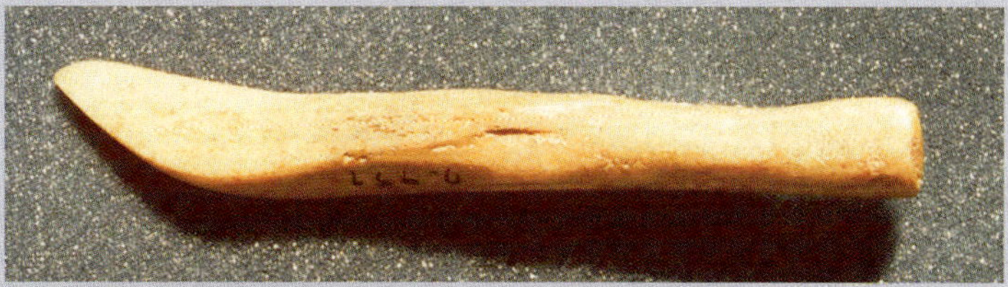

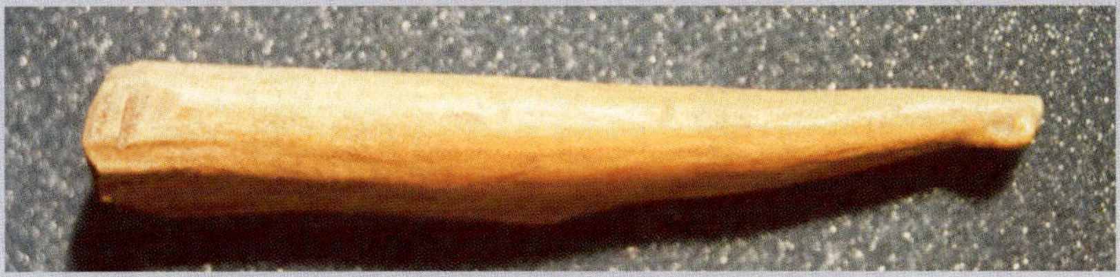

Flaker, deer antler, historic Seneca site dated ca. 1650 – 1675, 6¾" long. It was found near East Bloomfield, Ontario County, New York. Dave Summers collection, Victor, New York. **$35.00.**

Unknown artifact, bird bone, 5" long. It has part of the shaft cut out in a manner similar to beamers, and one end of the bone has been cut off. Bracken County, Kentucky. Robin Fiser collection. **$75.00.**

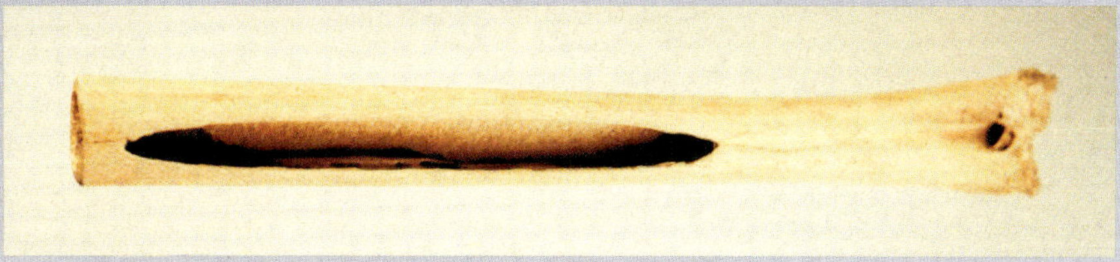

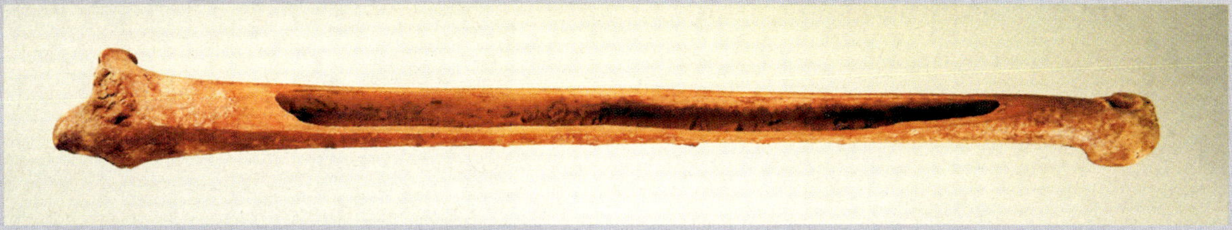

Beamer, wild turkey bone with red ochre staining, 9" long. It is highly unusual to find beamers made from bird bones rather than the typical deer or elk bones. Quite fragile, this piece came from Union County, Kentucky. Robin Fiser collection. **$225.00 – 250.00.**

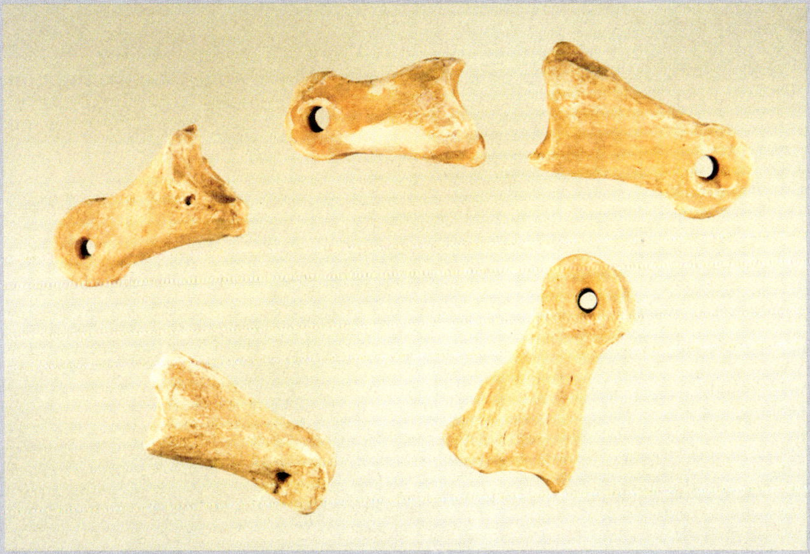

Danglers, deer toe bones, longest is 1⅝". Besides such decorations, these deer bones were also used for beads and fishhooks. Mason County, Kentucky. Robin Fiser collection. Each, **$20.00.**

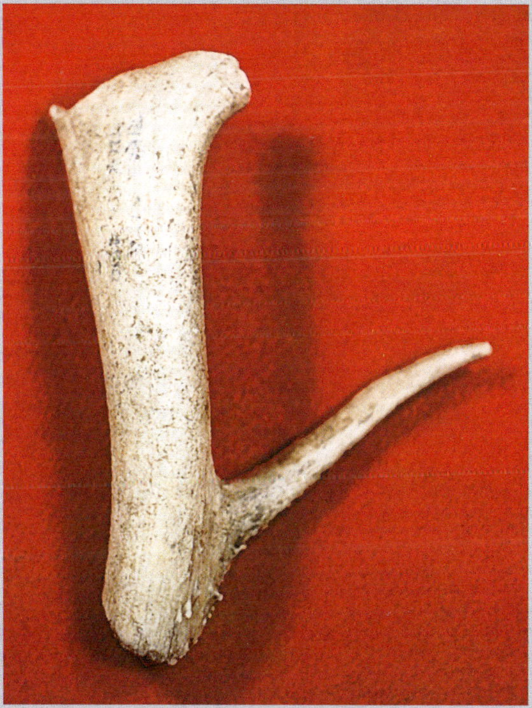

Antler celt or blade holder, Mississippian, 8" long. The smaller, bottom end has a hole for insertion of the blade. Ex-collection Vietzen, the tool handle was found in Ohio. Pete Timoch collection. Museum grade.

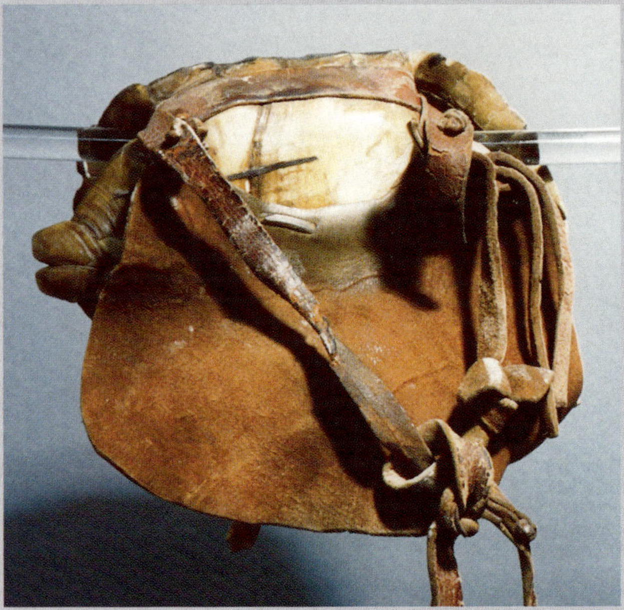

Ceremonial rattle, tortoise shell, leather, and deer hoofs, etc. Ca. 1930s, it measures 5½ x 7⅞". Hopi culture. H. B. Greene II collection, Naples, Florida. Museum grade.

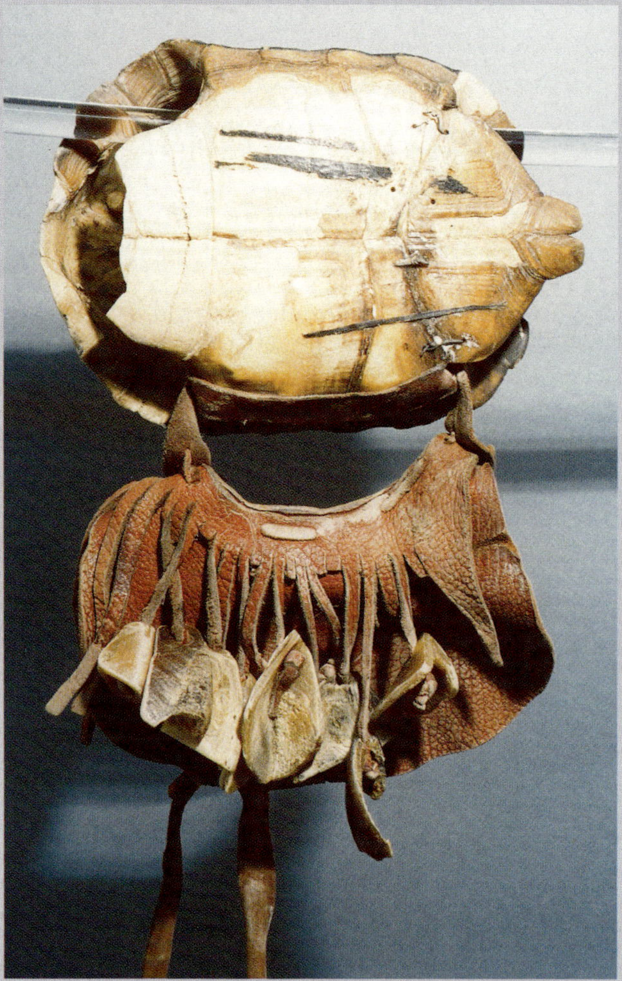

Ceremonial rattle, opened to show parts. Closed, it was tied behind the right leg and movement caused the hoofs to strike the shell. This was a gift to the owner from a Hopi friend. H. B. Greene II collection, Naples, Florida. Museum grade.

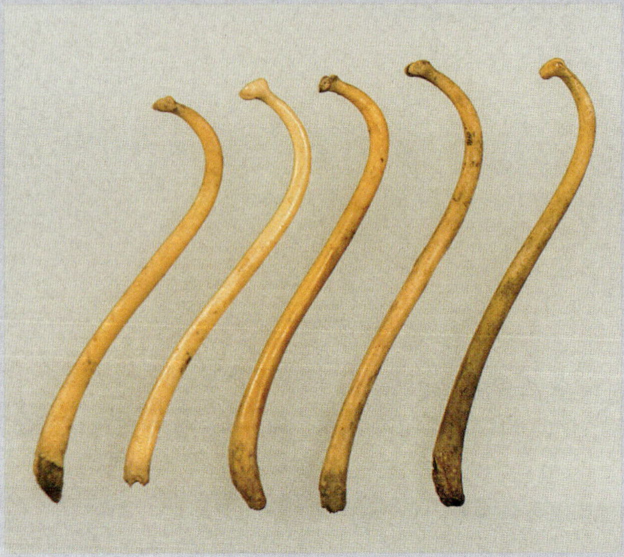

Pendants, raccoon penis bones, Woodland period, longest is 4¼". All are ex-collection Vietzen and came from Christian County, Kentucky. Pete Timoch collection. Unlisted.

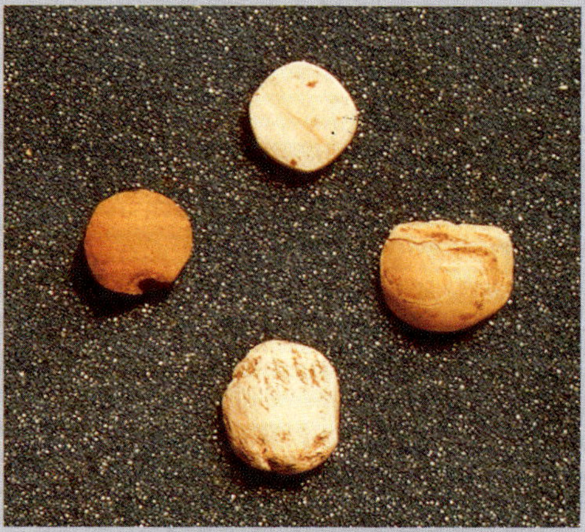

Gaming discs of various materials, from 12 o'clock: Shell, turtle plate, shell, and bone. They are from ⅝ to ¾" in diameter and historic Iroquois (Seneca), ca. AD 1650 – 1675. These were found near East Bloomfield, Ontario County, New York. Dave Summers collection, Victor, New York. Each, **$30.00.**

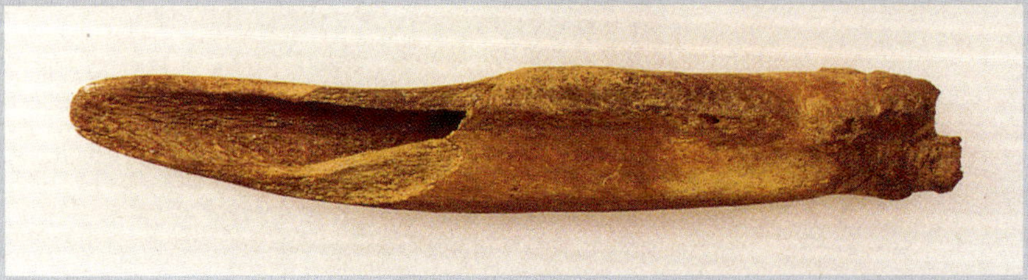

Bone knife, Mississippian, surface polish from handling and use-wear, 6½" long. Ex-collection Vietzen, it is pictured in his 1945 book, *The Immortal Eries*, page 317. Probably Ohio. Pete Timoch collection. **$250.00.**

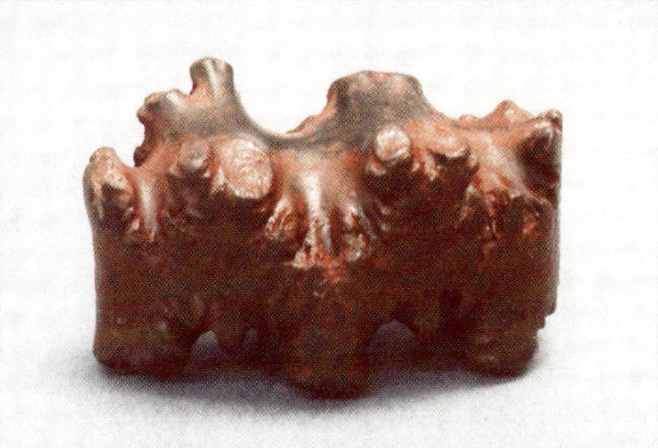

Shell section, baculite fossil, about 60 million years old and 2" long. This is from a Blackfoot medicine bundle and is called an *Iniskim* or Buffalo Calling stone, to be used in hunting ritual. (See Scriver's *The Blackfeet Artists of the Northern Plains*, page 178.) Plains region. H. B. Greene II collection, Naples, Florida. Unlisted.

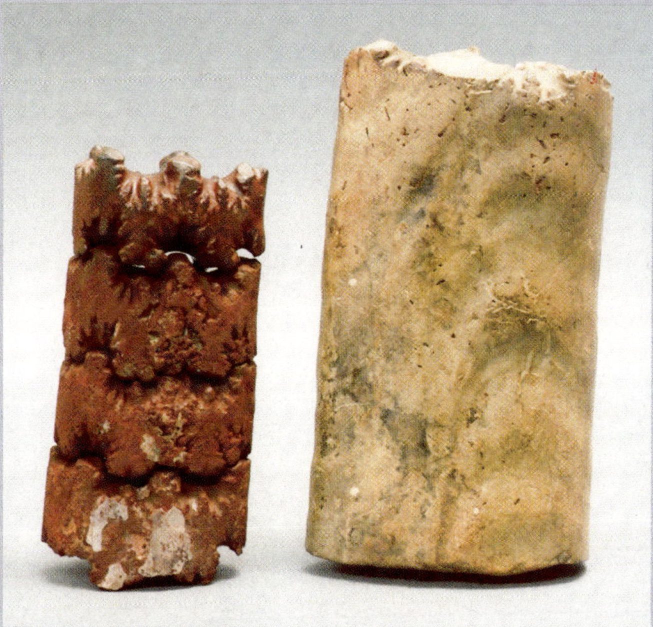

Fossil baculite shells, left example with four interlocking sections. At right is a shell that does not have the sections and sutures exposed. Left example, about 2" in diameter. These are *Iniskim*, rare pieces, often used in Blackfoot medicine bundles because they look somewhat like buffalo. Plains region. H. B. Greene II collection, Naples, Florida. Unlisted.

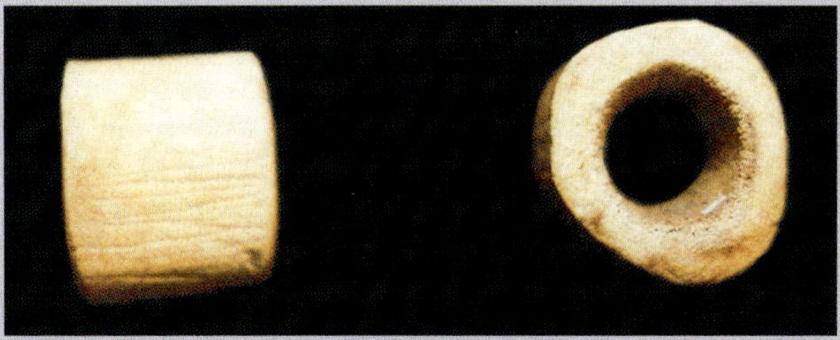

Bone bead, two views, ⅝" in diameter. This cut and drilled bead was a personal find of the owner. Mississippi County, Arkansas. Garvin collection. **$35.00.**

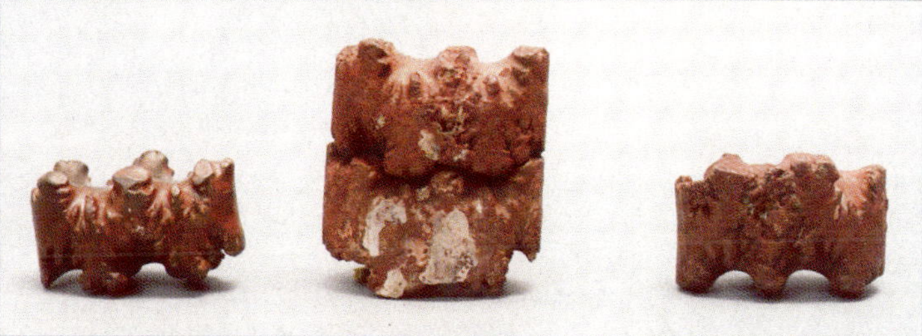

Buffalo calling stones, fossil baculite shells, examples about 2" across. Often used in Blackfoot medicine bundles, they are from the Plains region. H. B. Greene II collection, Naples, Florida. Unlisted.

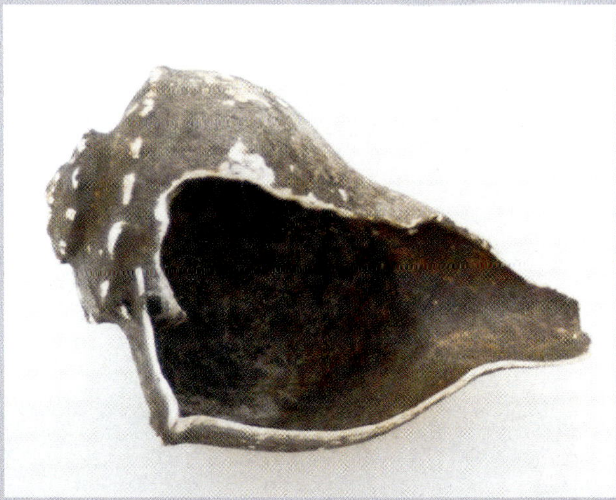

Conch shell cup, possibly used in Black Drink rituals, 6¾" long. It came from Bartow County, Georgia. Jim Maus collection, North Carolina. Unlisted.

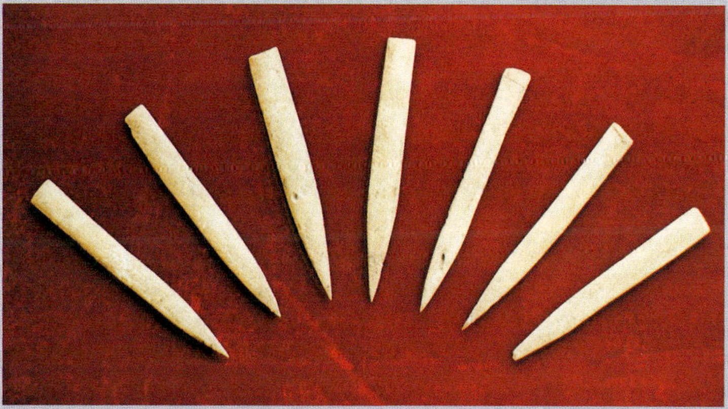

Bone needles or pins, ¼" wide and 2¼ to 2⅜" long. Judging by their shapes, these may have had a special purpose. The artifacts were found in Brown County, Illinois. Tim Liehr collection, Illinois. Each, **$25.00 – 40.00.**

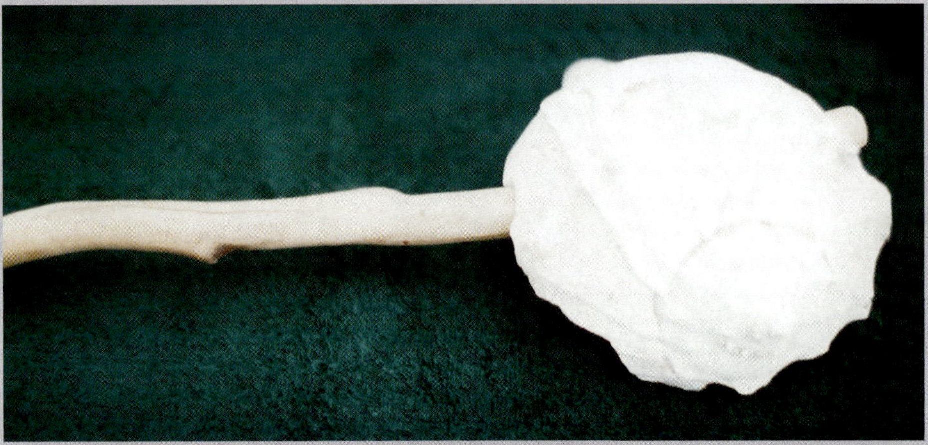

Conch shell hammer, head (with hole for handle) is 5¼ x 7". This artifact is ex-collection Dr. Gish and was found in Florida. Bob Hess collection, Indiana. **$100.00.**

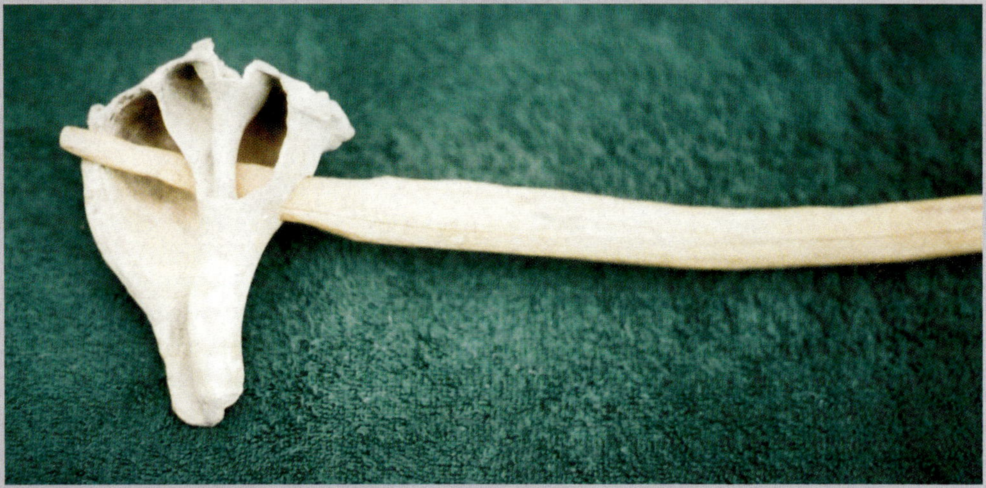

Conch shell hammer or pick, head size is 3½ x 4¼", shell is holed for handle. Ex-collection Dr. Gish, it came from a shell midden in Florida. Bob Hess collection, Indiana. **$75.00.**

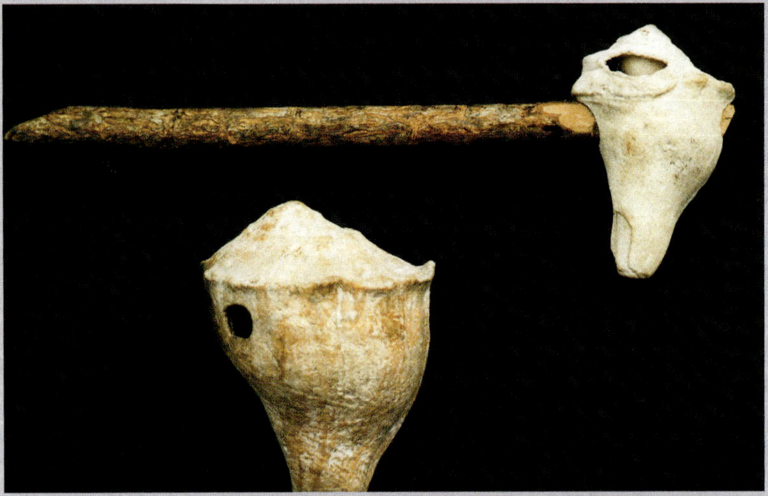

Conch shell hoes or picks, Mississippian period, ca. AD 1200 – 1600, drilled in two places for hafting. The bottom shell is 4¼ x 5¼" and the top shell (with modern wood handle) is 2½ x 4¼". These came from the Gulf Coast of Florida. Dave Summers collection, Victor, New York. Top, **$30.00;** bottom, **$50.00.**

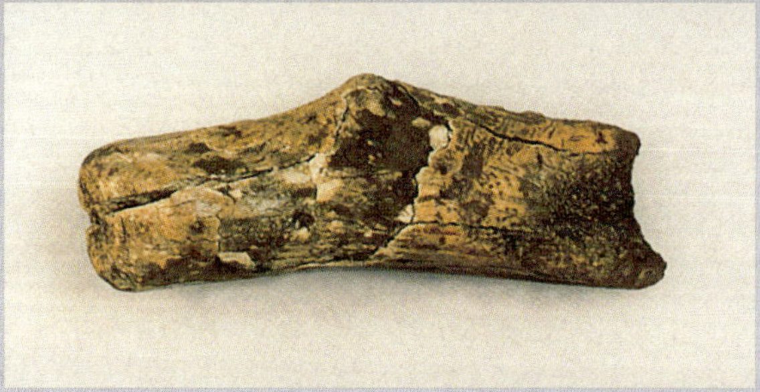

Antler celt socket, Late Archaic to Woodland, 5⅛" long. A scarce tool part, the stone celt was inset at one end (right) and the rounded opposite end may have been fitted into a wooden handle. Christian County, Kentucky. Pete Timoch collection. **$125.00 – 200.00.**

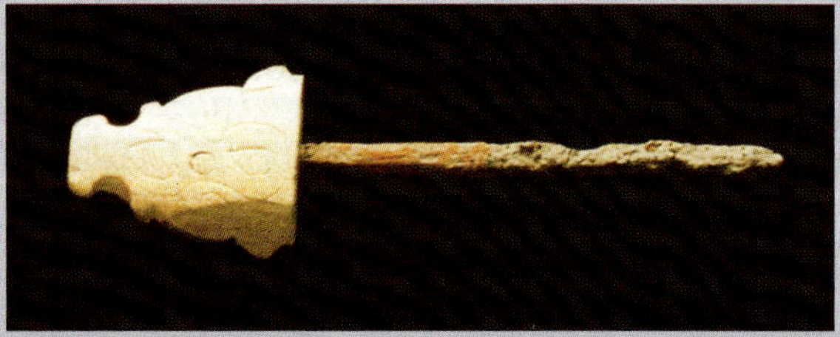

Awl, steel blade inserted into the hilt of an European bone handle, 3" overall length. This is historic Iroquois (Seneca) and was used sometime before AD 1779. It was found near the town of Canandaigua, Ontario County, New York. Dave Summers collection, Victor, New York. **$60.00.**

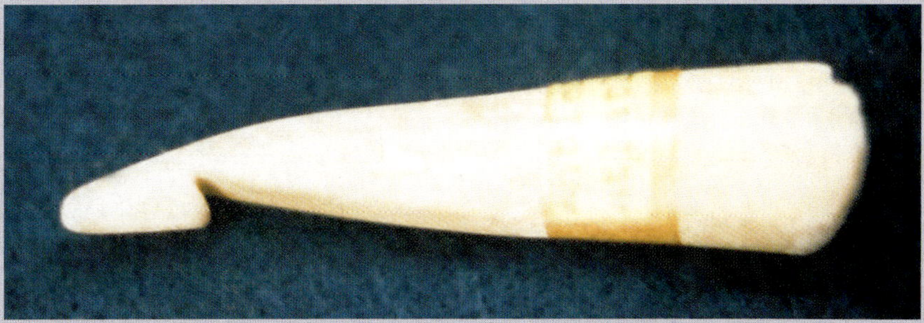

Bone Atl-atl hook, 3" long. This well-carved and rare artifact is ex-collection Morast. Central Tennessee. Bob Hess collection, Indiana. Museum grade.

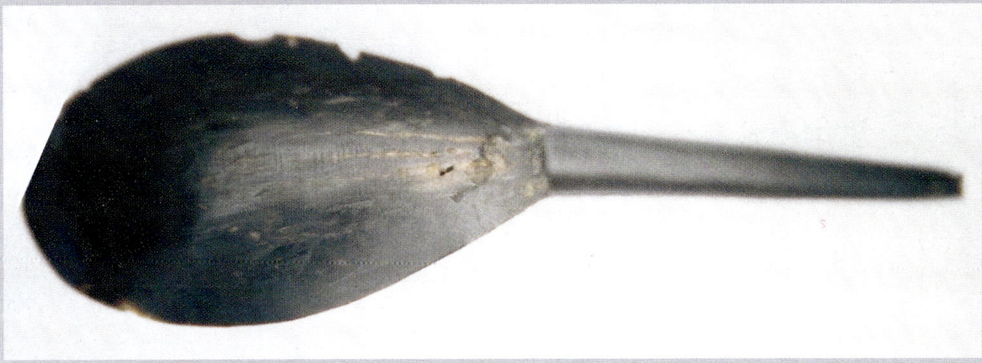

Buffalo horn spoon, 2¼ x 7" long. This historic item is ex-collection Miller, from Wyoming. Bob Hess collection, Indiana. **$275.00.**

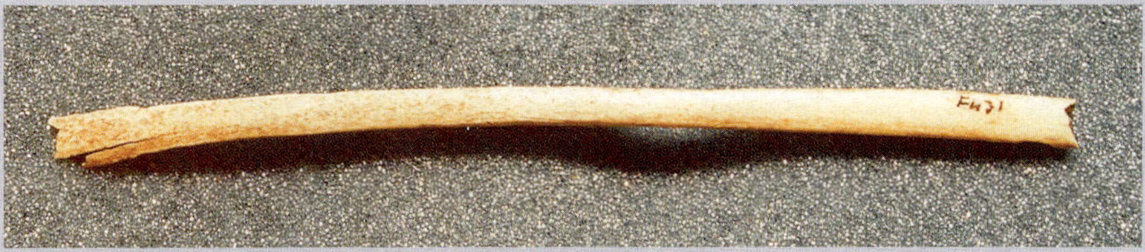

Mat-weaving needle section, poor condition, 6½" long. The needle is historic Iroquois (Seneca), ca. AD 1590 – 1610. It is from a site near East Bloomfield, Ontario County, New York. Dave Summers collection, Victor, New York. **$10.00.**

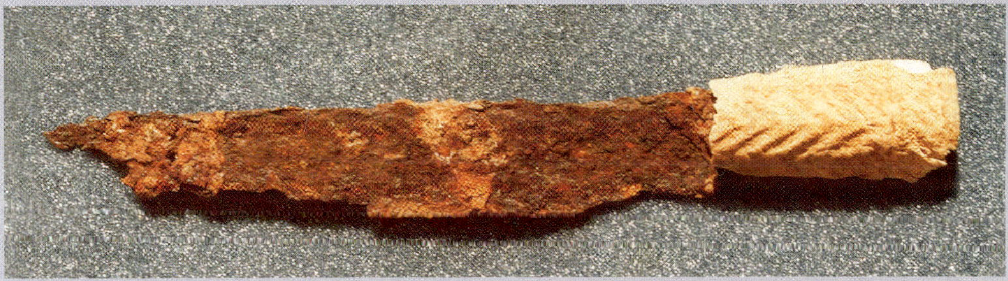

European knife, with engraved bone handle, 8½" long, ex-collections Schroff (ca. 1930) and Wray. It is historic Iroquois (Seneca) and dates ca. AD 1675 – 1687. The knife came from near Victor, Ontario County, New York. Dave Summers collection, Victor, New York. **$200.00.**

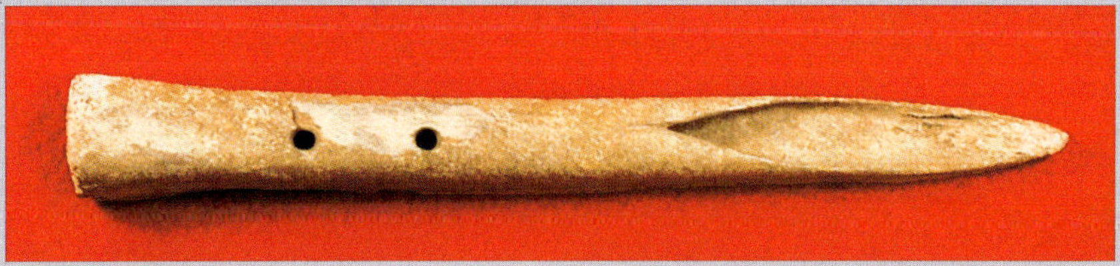

Bone dagger, Mississippian, elk leg bone, 9⅝". This piece has two flute or flageolet holes and might be termed a "flute-dagger." This rare piece is ca. AD 1300 – 1400, and the purpose or use is unknown. Ohio. Pete Timoch collection. Museum grade.

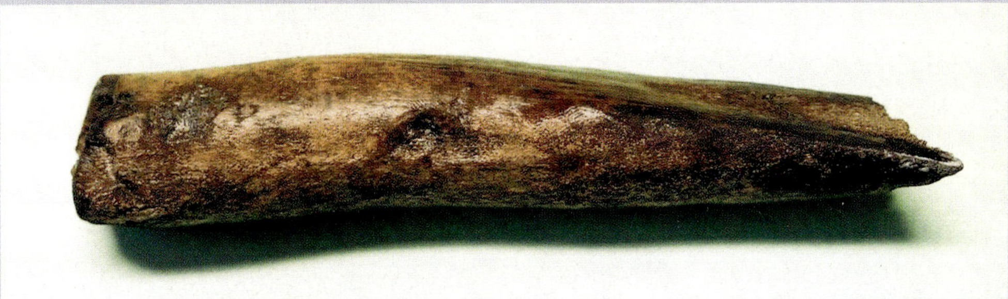

Antler scraper, tine cut from main beam, 1¼ x 7¼". The tip was ground to a wedge shape and the artifact has heavy polish. It came from Box Elder County, northern Utah. Dann Russell collection, Utah. **$75.00.**

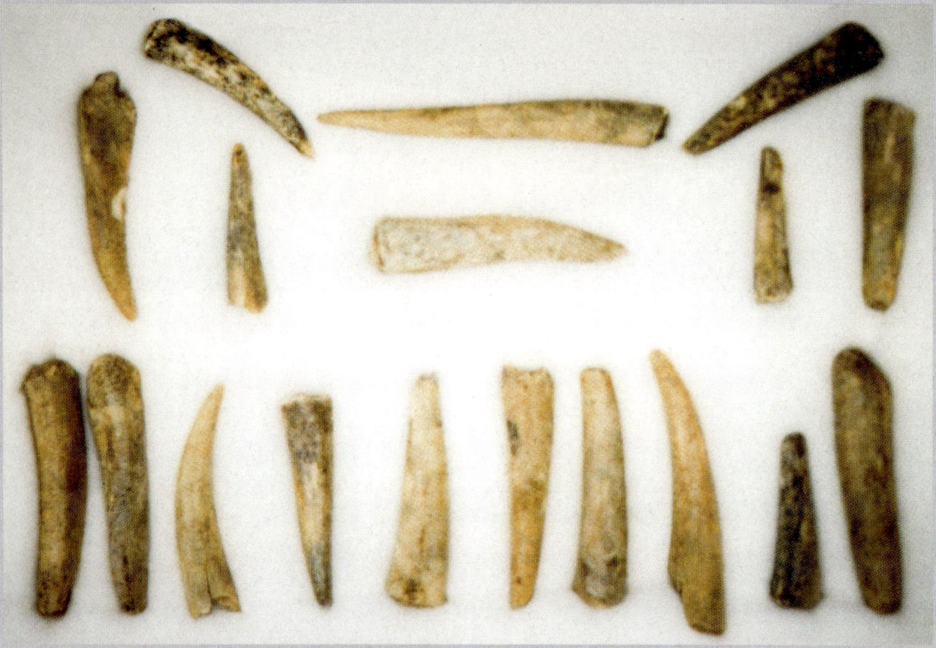

Antler flaking tools,18 shown from a cache of 34, lengths are 1¾ to 4". The cache was found in Mississippi County, Arkansas. Bob Hess collection, Indiana. Each, **$5.00 – 15.00.**

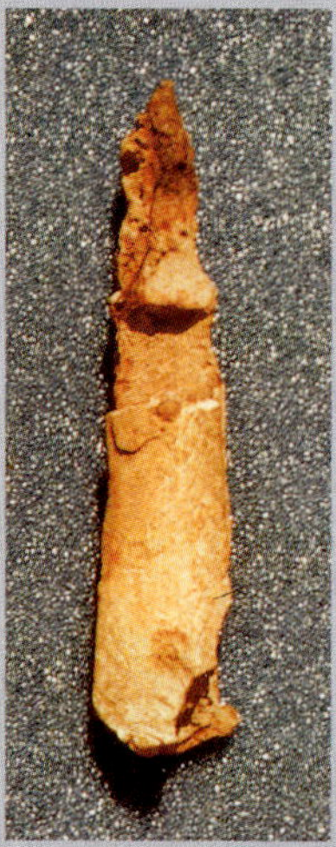

European knife, with carved bone handle, 3" long. The blade is nearly rusted away on this general purpose knife, found on an historic Iroquois (Seneca) site which dated to AD 1650 – 1675. It is from near East Bloomfield, Ontario County, New York. Dave Summers collection, Victor, New York. **$100.00.**

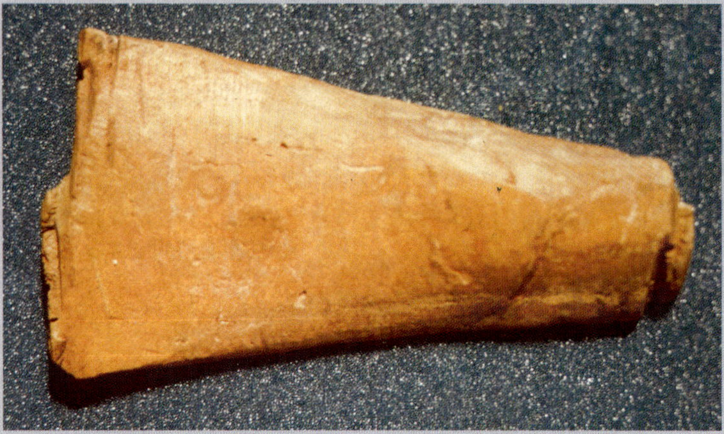

Moose antler section, roughed out to make a comb, historic Iroquois (ca. AD 1550 – 1700), 5⅝" long. It came from a site in Saratoga County, New York. Dave Summers collection, Victor, New York. **$225.00.**

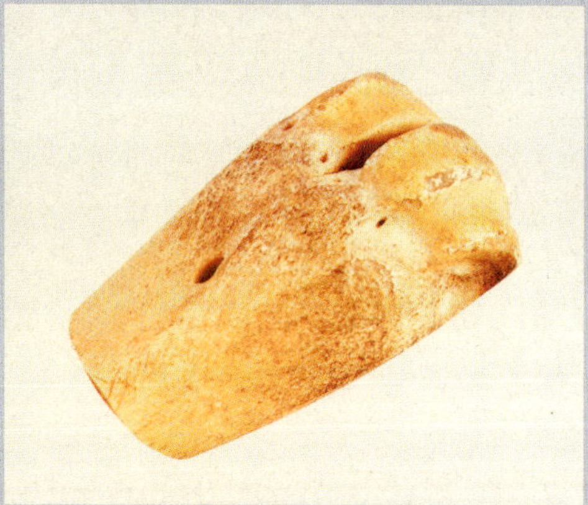

Tool, deer bone joint, 1¾". The shorter edge is beveled and the reverse face is ground flat. Southern Ohio. Fred Winegardner collection. **$25.00.**

Box turtle rattle, ex-collection Wray, 3¾" long. Both bottom and top have drilled holes for fastening together. The rattle is historic Iroquois (Seneca), ca. AD 1630 – 1650. It came from near East Bloomfield, Ontario County, New York. Dave Summers collection, Victor, New York. **$250.00.**

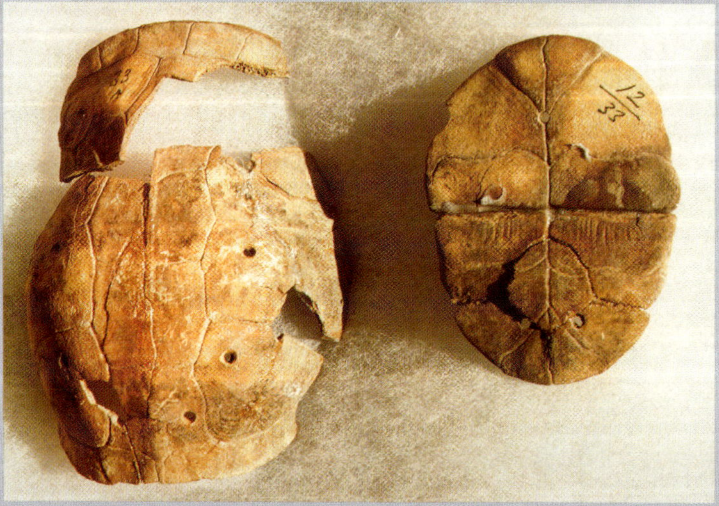

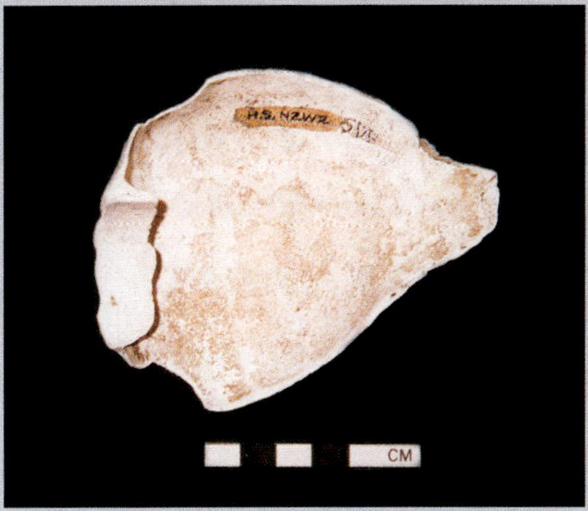

Drinking cup, whelk shell, 3¼ x 4½". This was a 1970 find by Alan Lowry in Haley Shelter on the periphery of the Wamsutta Archaeological Site. The cup, protected by the rock shelter and well-drained sandy soil, was in direct association with about 50 stone artifacts diagnostic of the terminal Paleo through initial Archaic. The owner reports that Wamsutta produced over 4500 artifacts including 50-plus fluted points. Canton area, Massachusetts. Joe Finneran collection, Massachusetts. Unlisted.

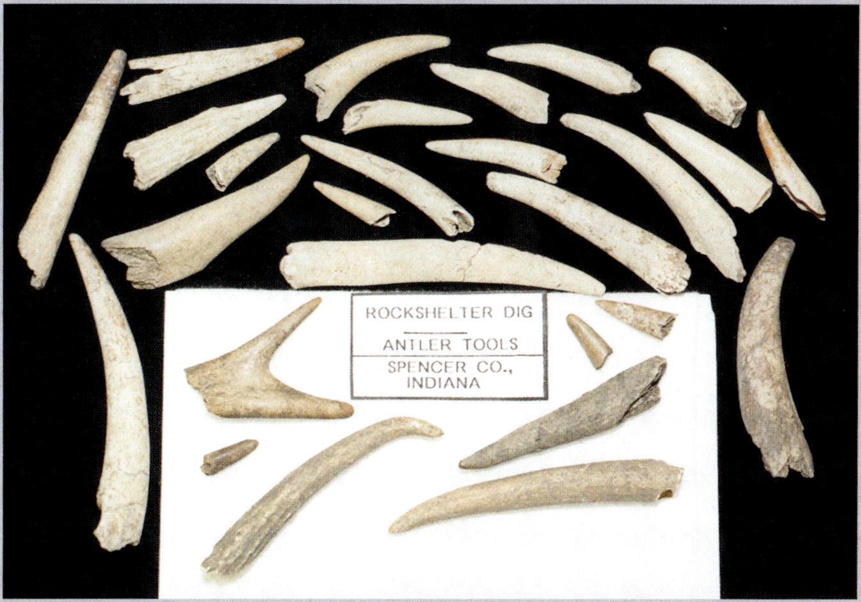

Antler tools, group of 27, ex-collection Darland. The longest piece is 5". All came from a rock shelter in Spencer County, Indiana. Back to Earth. Group, **$155.00.**

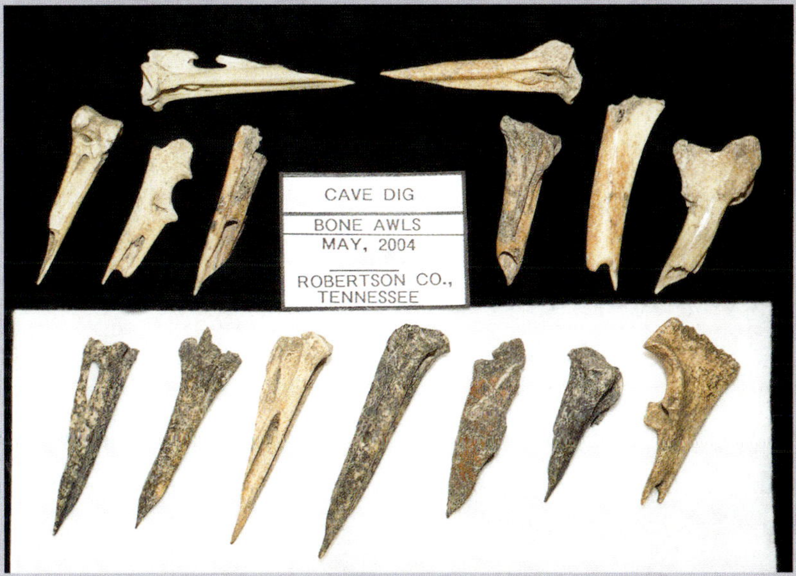

Bone awl group, longest piece is 3⅝". Exceptional examples found in a rock shelter in Robertson County, Tennessee. Back to Earth. Group, **$250.00.**

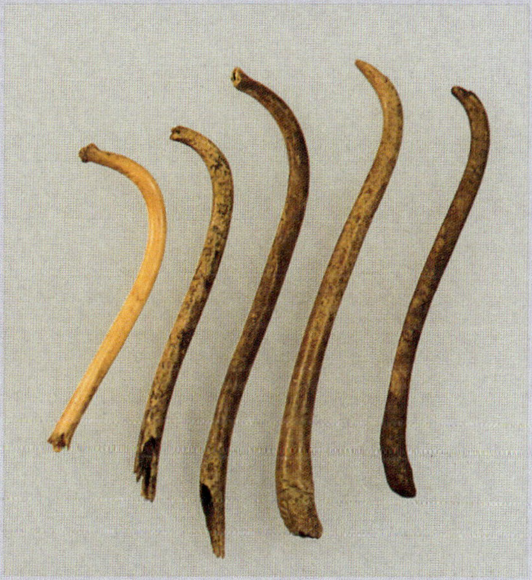

Pendants, raccoon penis bones, Mississippian, longest is 3⅞". They are ex-collection Vietzen, and the two longest examples are shown in his 1945 book, *The Immortal Eries*, page 315. They are from Ohio and Kentucky sites. Pete Timoch collection. Each, **$20.00 – 40.00.**

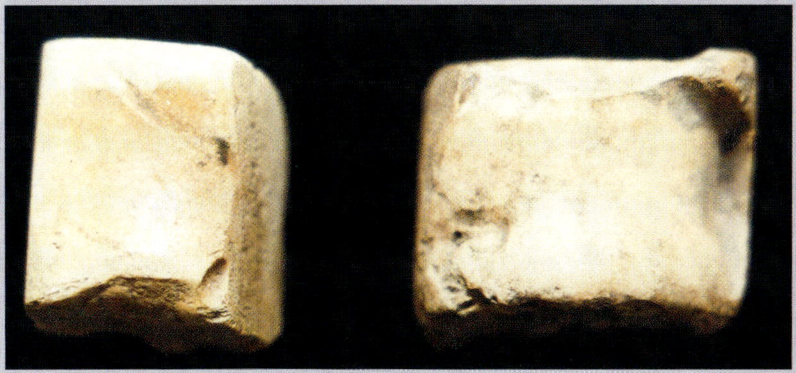

Bone dice, 1" and 1¼" across, made by grinding flat surfaces on deer foot bones. These were personal finds by the owner in Mississippi County, Arkansas. Garvin collection. Each, **$25.00 – 35.00.**

Miscellaneous Artifacts

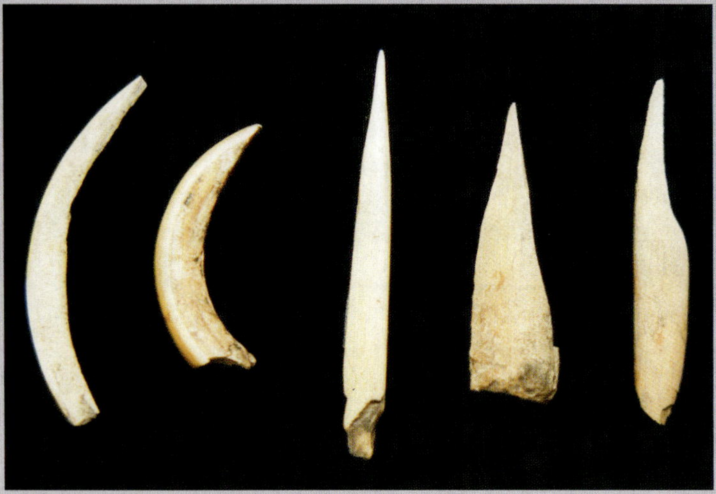

Group of five bone tools, Left to right: two beaver teeth, a highly polished bone needle, and two splinter awls. Found in Mississippi County, Arkansas. Garvin collection. Group, **$95.00.**

Sheath knife – with antler handle, historic period, 11" long overall. The knife has a nickel-silver handguard and sheath is held together with lead rivets. Back to Earth. Set, **$300.00 – 350.00.**

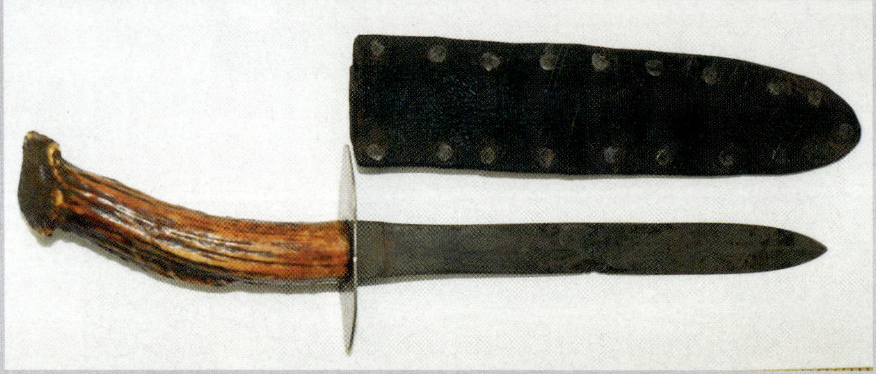

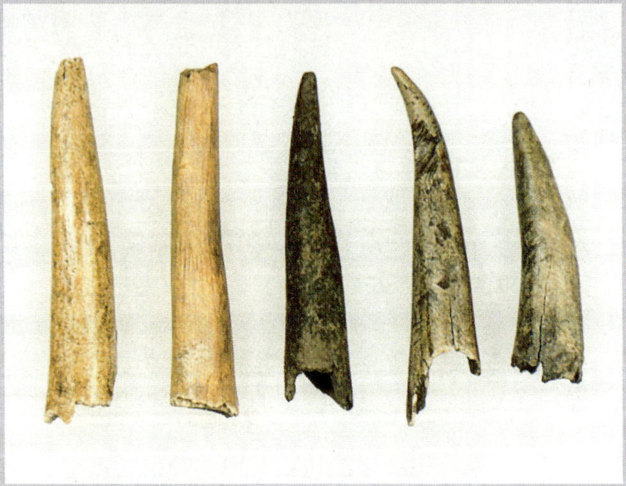

Antler socketed projectile tips, Woodland to Mississippian. These may be Atl-atl or spear points judging by size, and the longest is 3⅞". Ex-collection Vietzen, they are from Ohio and Kentucky. Pete Timoch collection. Each, **$50.00 – 75.00.**

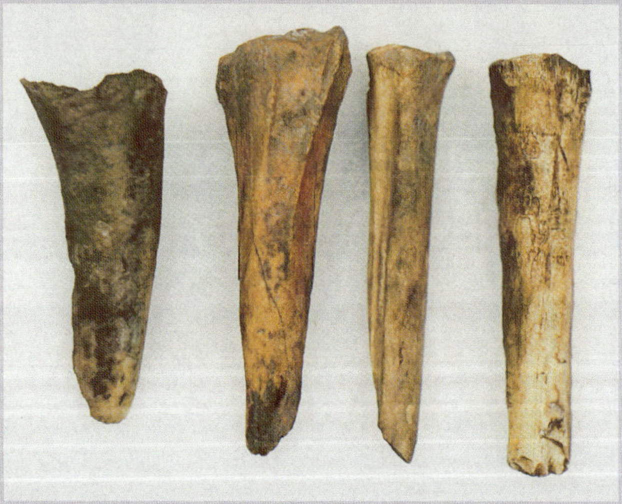

Chisels or gouges, heavy bone, Late Archaic to Woodland, The longest is 4¼" and all are ex-collection Vietzen. Rock shelter finds, the artifacts are from Christian County, Kentucky. Pete Timoch collection. Each, **$25.00 – 30.00.**

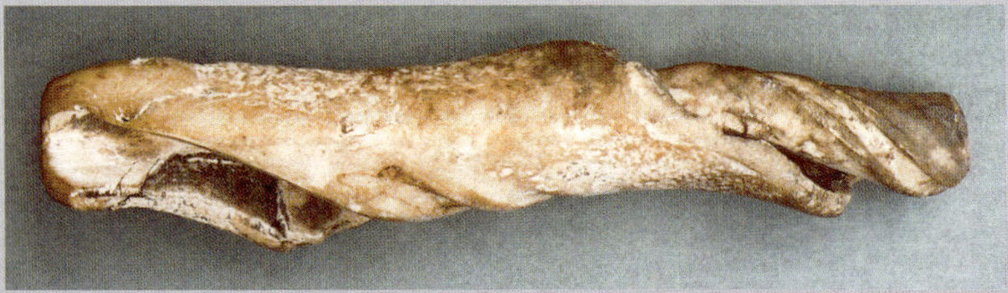

Shell tool, 6½" long, Calusa culture, pre-1450. It was found on Key Marco (now Marco Island), Collier County, Florida. H. B. Greene II collection, Naples, Florida. **$65.00.**

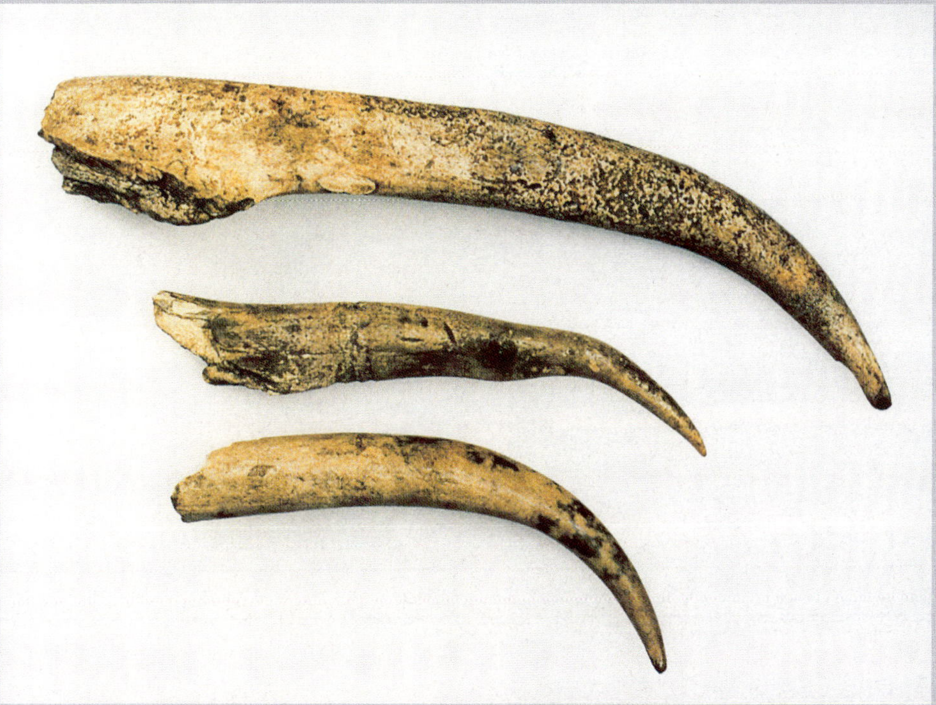

Antler tools, perhaps used as diggers, longest is 12". From the Late Archaic to Woodland, they are ex-collection Vietzen. Christian County, Kentucky. Pete Timoch collection. Each, **$50.00 – 75.00.**

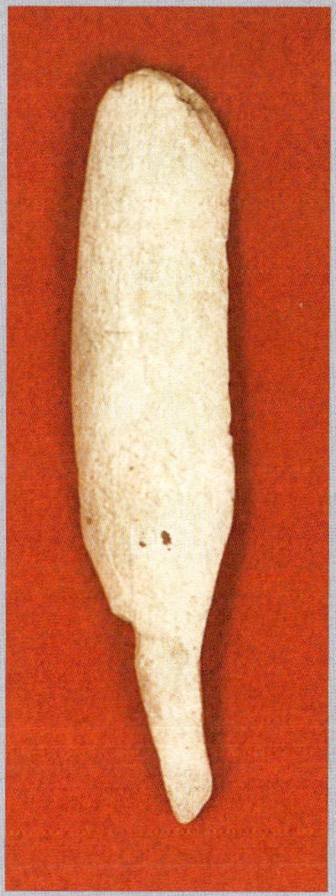

Chisel tip awl – split bone, Mississippian, 3 9/16" long. The handle is worn smooth from long use. The awl is from Ohio. Ex-collection Vietzen. Pete Timoch collection. **$50.00.**

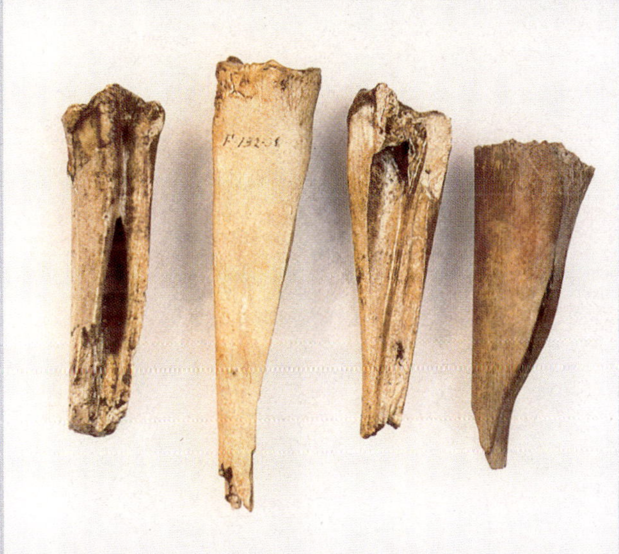

Beamer or hide-scraping tools, made into gouges, deer or elk leg bones, longest is 5½". All were once in the Vietzen collection and came from Fort Ancient sites in Ohio and Kentucky. Pete Timoch collection. Each, **$10.00 – 20.00.**

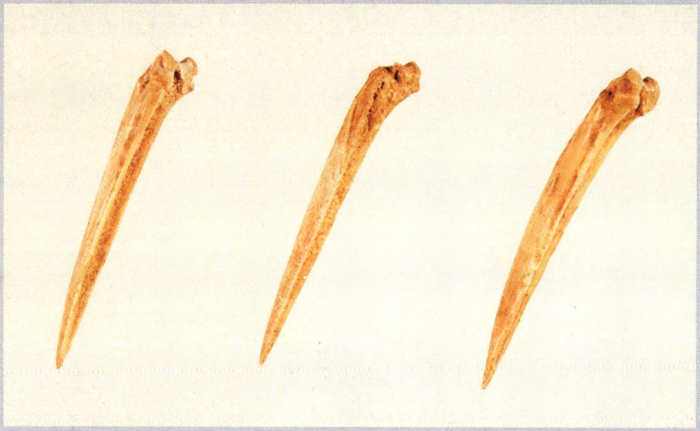

Necklace elements, fish spines, longest is 2⅛". They are ex-collection Vietzen and were found in Ohio or Kentucky. Fred Winegardner collection. Each, **$5.00.**

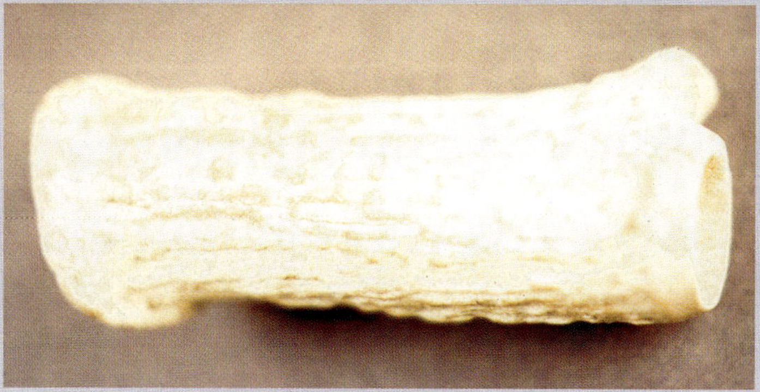

Antler artifact, hollowed, 2½" long. The purpose or use is unknown, but it may be a tool handle. Warren County, Tennessee. Larry Garvin collection. **$150.00.**

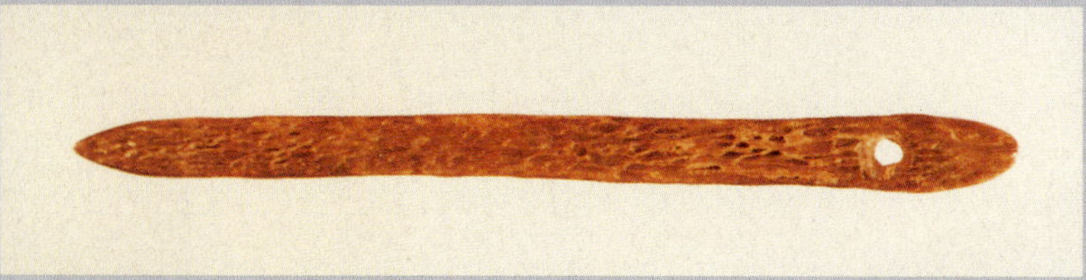

Antler strip, highly polished, drilled near one end, 3¼". Fort Ancient in origin, it is from southern Ohio. Fred Winegardner collection. **$50.00.**

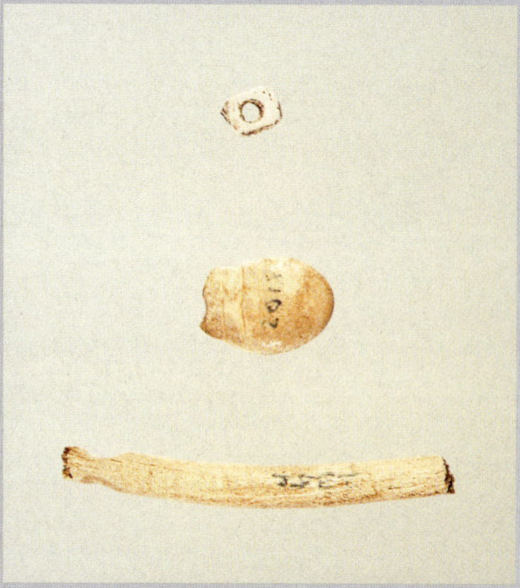

Midden artifacts, all Mississippian period from northern Ohio. Fred Winegardner collection. They are: Notched bone, 2⅛" long, an elk tooth with incised lines, and a small shell bead. All, **$45.00.**

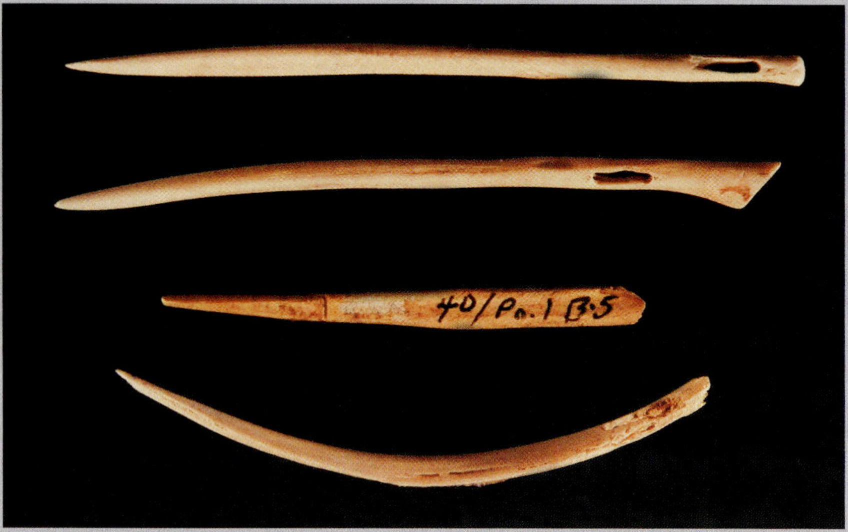

Bone artifacts, two awls or perforators and two needles with eyes. They were found in 1958 and are Dallas culture, from eastern Tennessee. Collection of, and photograph by, Ron Harris, North Carolina. Eyed needles, each **$150.00 – 175.00;** awls, each **$10.00 – 15.00.**

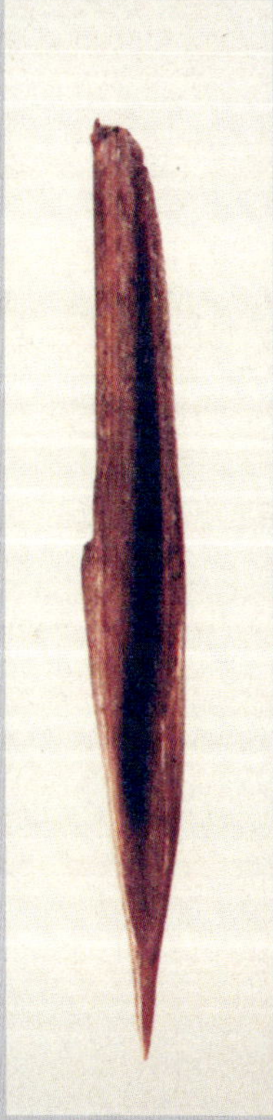

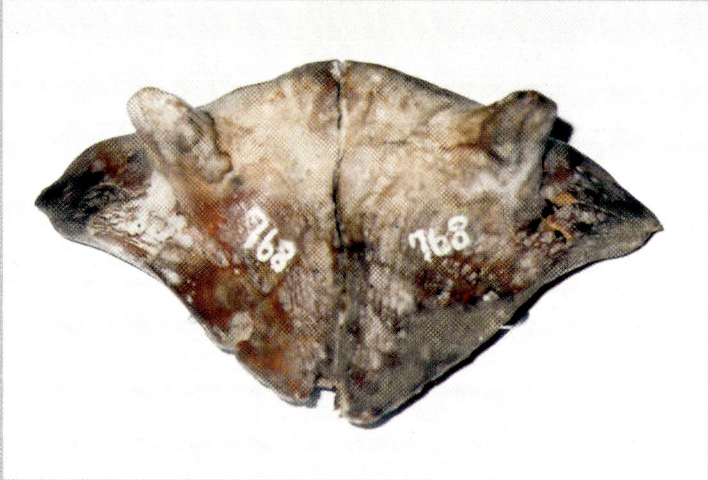

Rattle(?), upper jawbone of a drumfish, about 3" across. Some grinding was done to shape this piece, perhaps into an effigy form. Ex-collections Dickson and Fraser, it was found in Fulton County, Illinois. Joseph Sulka collection, Illinois. Unlisted.

Tattooing(?) needle, bird bone, very pointed tip, 3" long. It has patinated to a medium chocolate color and is a delicate tool. Kentucky or Tennessee. Private collection. **$15.00.**

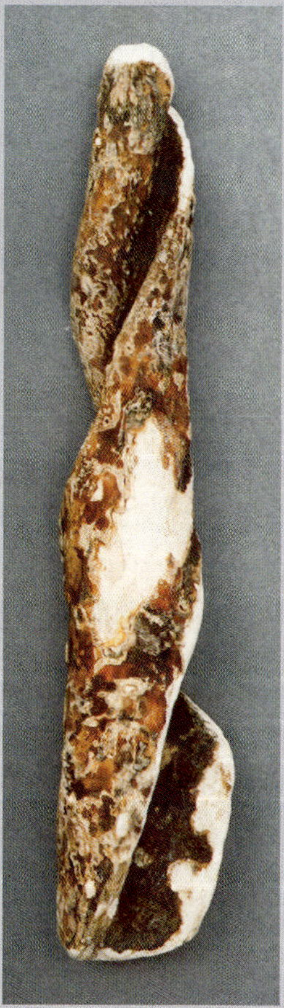

Shell tool, conch columella, 5½" long. It is AD 1450 or earlier, Calusa culture, and was found on Key Marco. Now known as Marco Island, it is in Collier County, Florida. H. B. Greene II collection, Naples, Florida. **$65.00.**

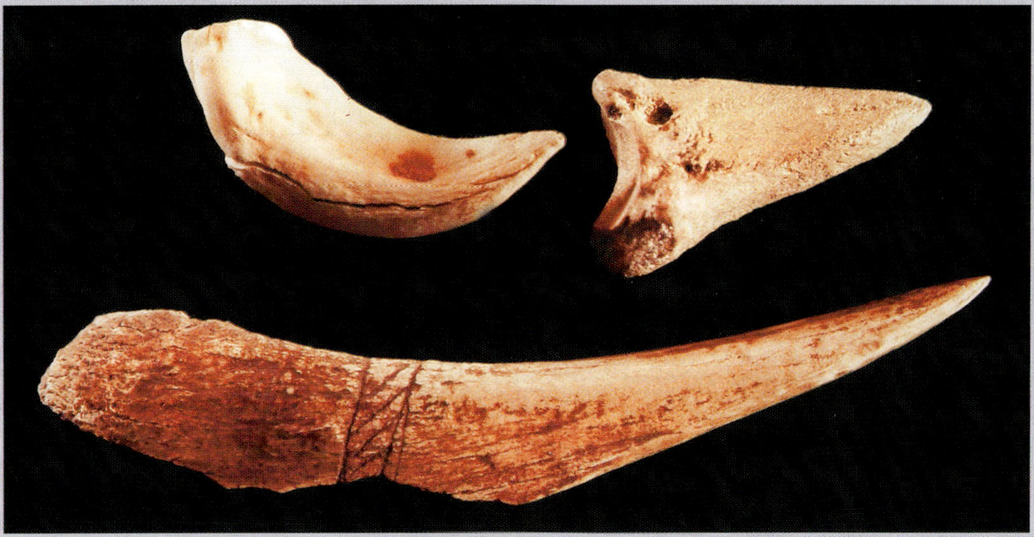

Bone artifacts, an animal claw; a triangular bone point(?); and a curved bone perforator, 3" long. The last is decorated with incised lines. These are ca. AD 1450 – 1600, from a site on the east side of the Yadkin River, Davidson County, North Carolina. Collection of, and photograph by, Ron Harris, North Carolina. Claw, **$10.00;** point, **$30.00;** perforator, **$100.00.**

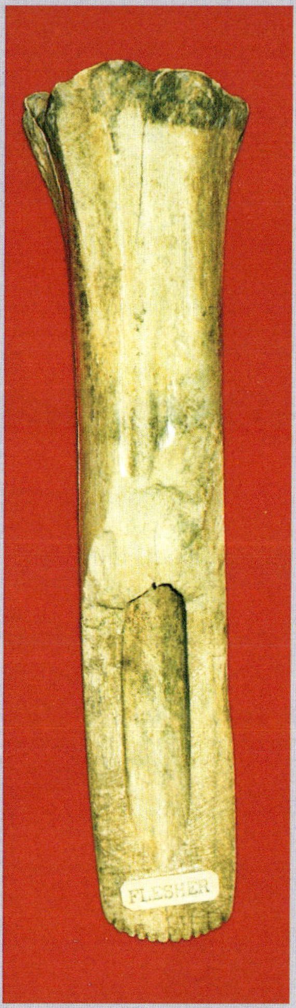

Bison bone flesher, serrated edge, 7" long, historic Pawnee. Eastcentral Nebraska. Richard Krueger collection, Iowa. Sandra Krueger photograph. **$250.00.**

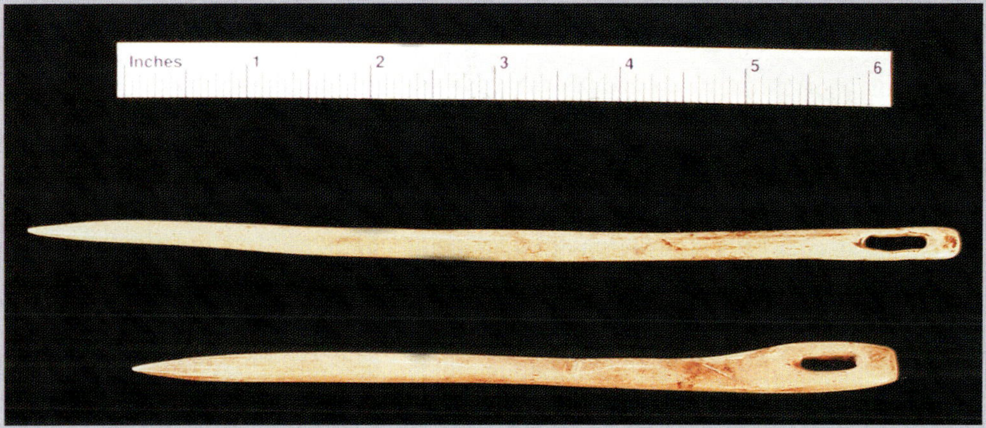

Bone needles with elongated eyes, top example is 7¾" long, bottom example is 6¼" long. They were found in a rock shelter and are exceptional specimens in length and finish. The needles are from near the headwaters of North Fork Holston River, Smyth County, Virginia. Collection of, and photograph by, Ron Harris, North Carolina. Each, **$225.00 – 250.00.**

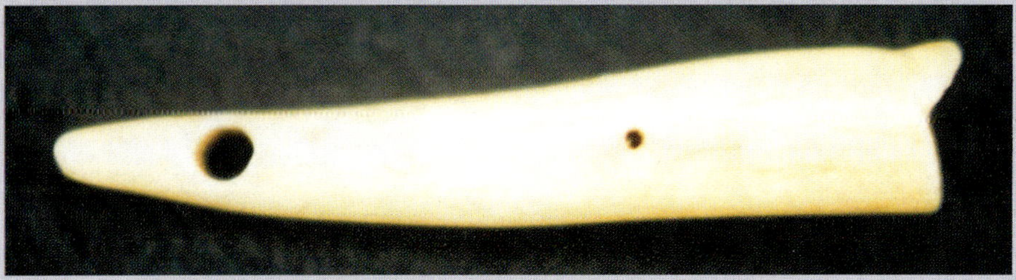

Antler artifact, drilled, 2¾" long. It was found in Kentucky. Bob Hess collection, Indiana. Unlisted.

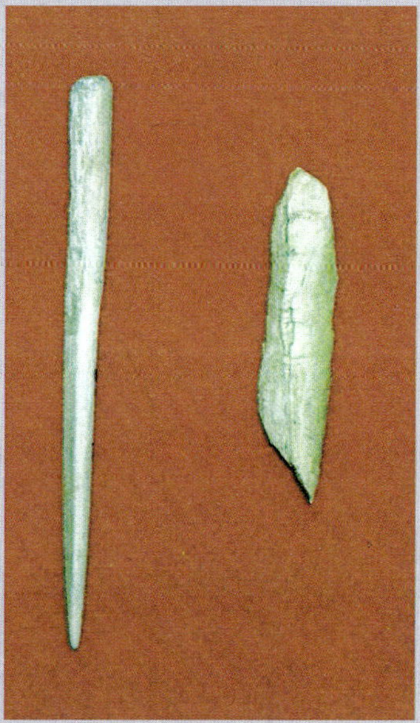

Bone awl and graver, historic Pawnee. The awl is 3½" long and the graver is 2" long. Eastcentral Nebraska. Richard Krueger collection, Iowa; Sandra Krueger photograph. Awl, **$20.00;** graver, **$15.00.**

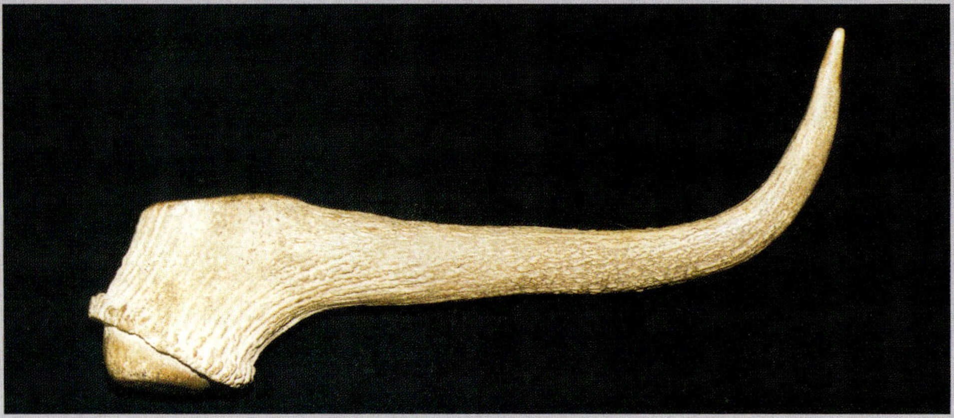

Elk antler warclub, mineralized material, 18½" long. An extremely rare artifact, it was found in 1926 in a gravel pit. The original collector retained the club until 1975, when the present owner acquired it. The weapon (Carbon-14 dated) was made about AD 1440, placing it in the Fort Ancient timespan. This is the same culture that built the Panther and the Serpent effigy mounds in the state. Hamilton County, Ohio. Larry Garvin collection. Museum grade.

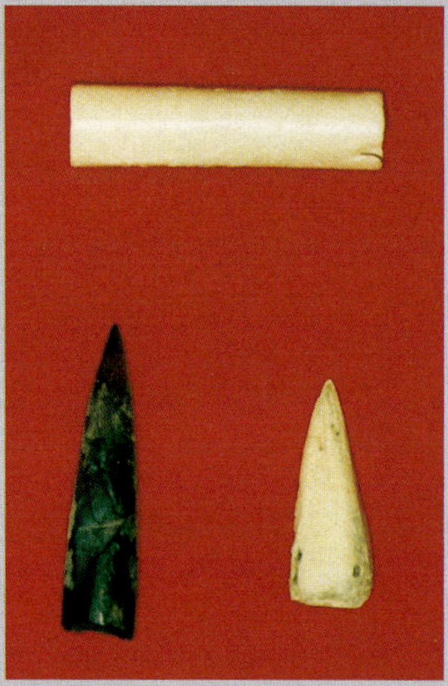

Bone bead, bone point and antler point, historic Pawnee. The bead is 1⅜" long, the antler point is the same length, and the bone point is ⅞" long. Eastern Nebraska. Richard Krueger collection, Iowa. Sandra Krueger photograph. Bone bead, **$40.00;** antler point, **$25.00;** bone point, **$25.00.**

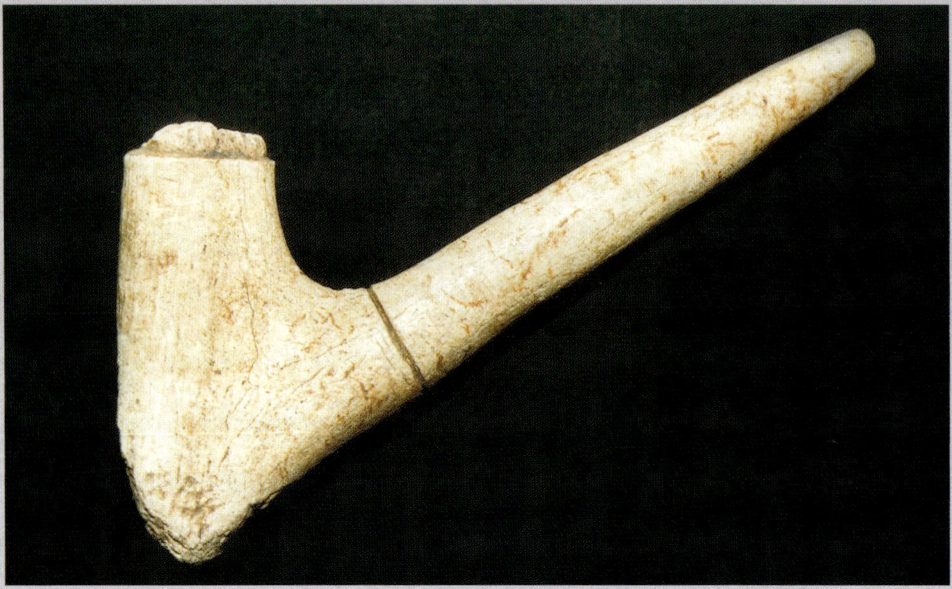

Antler tool, 6¾" long. One tine has been cut off and the other has been grooved at the base so it could be broken away. The tine itself may have been intended for a flint-knapping tool or projectile point. This piece might be considered a work in progress, interrupted by the centuries. Back to Earth. Unlisted.

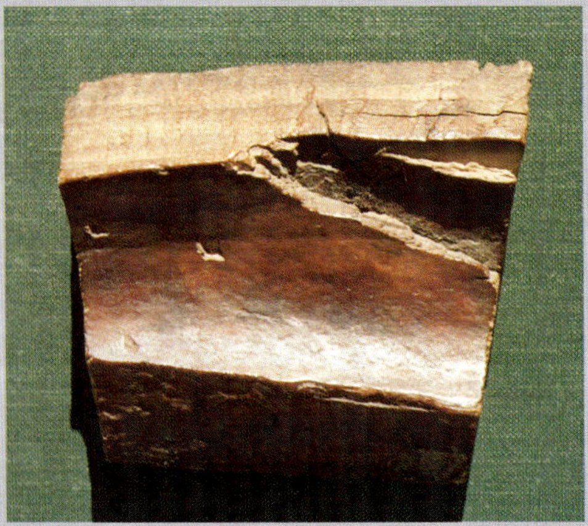

Woolly mammoth tusk section, Ice Age (Pleistocene), 3½" long. The tusk was found in Wayne County, New York. Dave Summers collection, Victor, New York. **$50.00.**

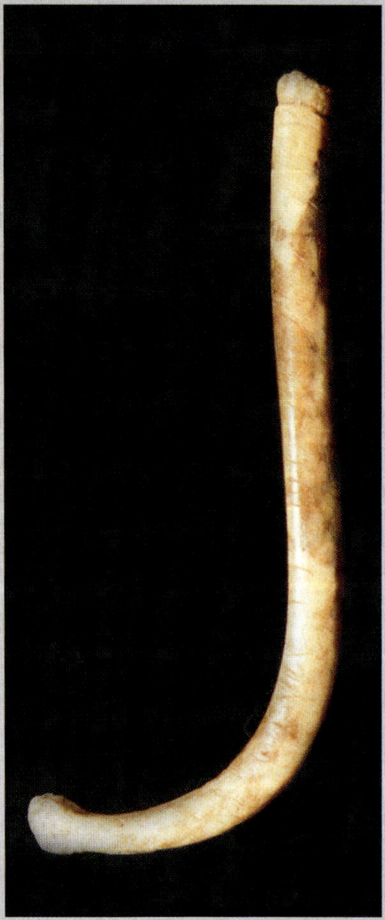

Racoon penis bone pendant, grooved at top, 2⅝" long. It was a personal find of the owner in Mississippi County, Arkansas. Garvin collection. **$95.00.**

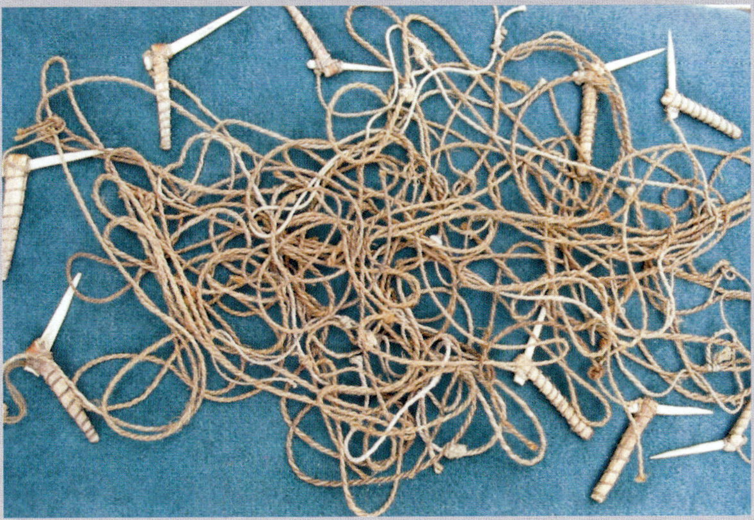

Trotline, fiber cord and bone pin hooks. This rare artifact was found in a dry cave or rock shelter. Four Corners area, Colorado. John and Susan Mellyn collection, Texas. Museum grade.

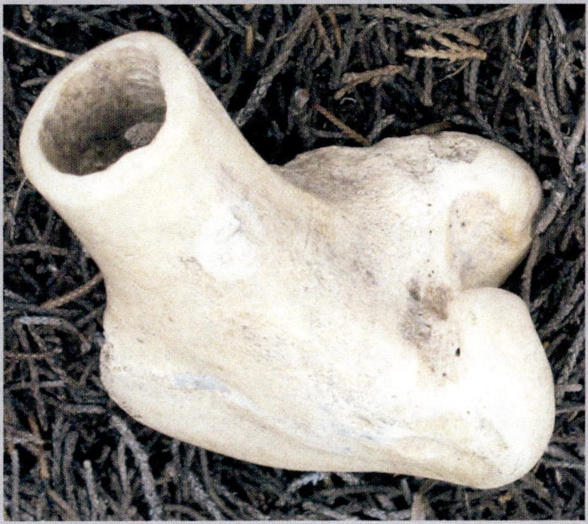

Ring bone, large bone which served as the source for cutting off bone rings, 3⅛" long. Origin unknown. John and Susan Mellyn collection, Texas. Unlisted.

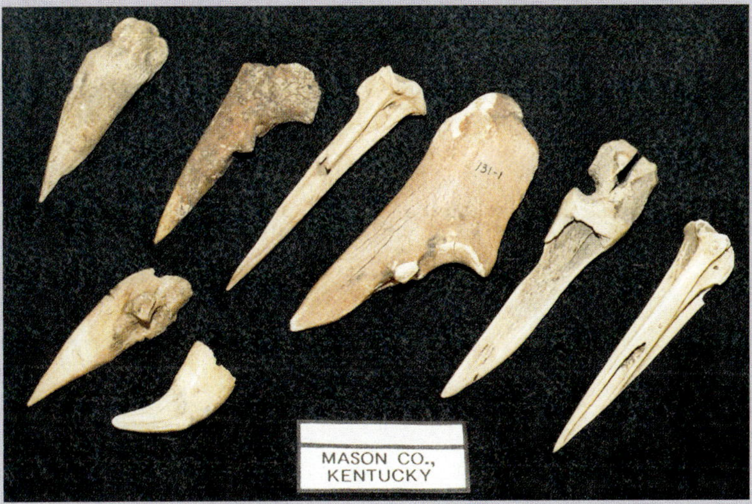

Awls, Mississippian period, from a major site near the Ohio River, sizes as indicated. All are made of bone except for the tip of a large bear's tooth (bottom left). Ex-collection Matthews, the awls are from Mason County, Kentucky. Garvin collection, Ohio. Group, **$185.00.**

Double-pointed awl, bone, high polish and wear at tips and holes, 5⅞". From Alaska. Private collection. **$100.00.**

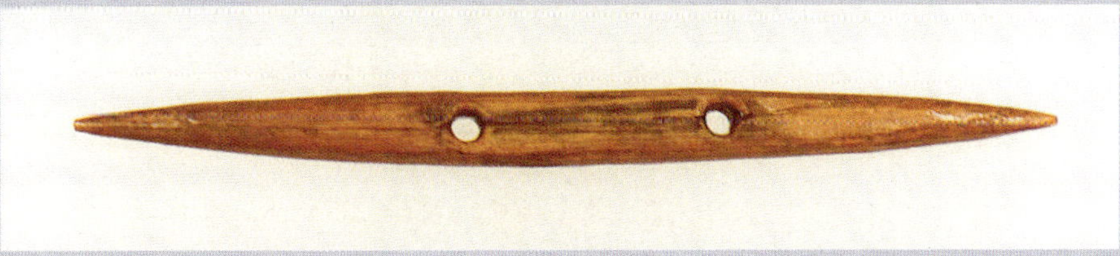

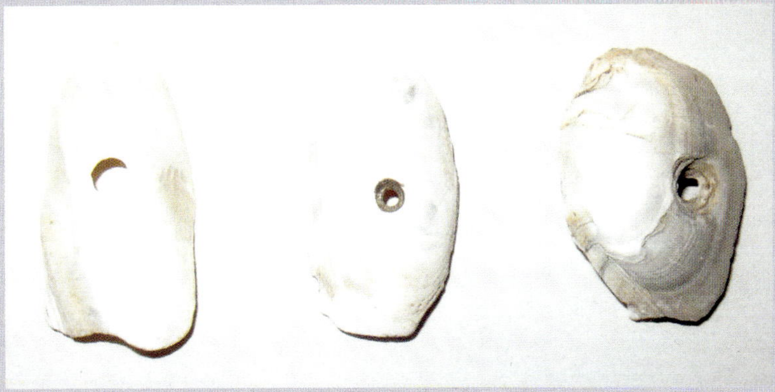

Shell pendants, Mississippian, longest example is 2¼". The iridescence of such shells made them attractive ornaments. Mason County, West Virginia. Private collection. Rodney Roberts photograph. Each, **$12.00 – 20.00.**

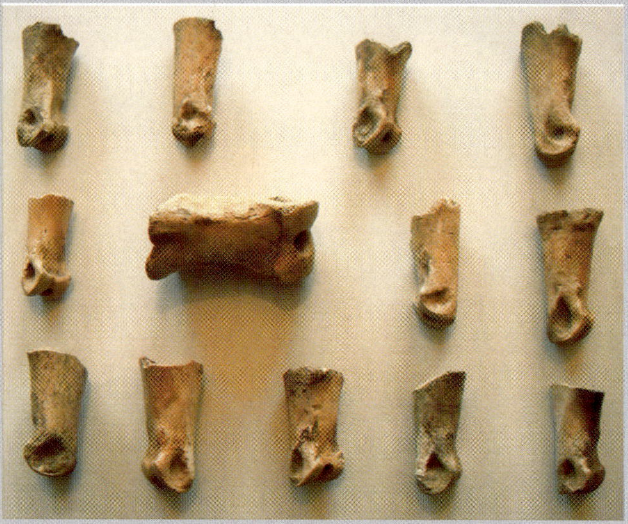

Deer toe bone tinklers, all cut and with drilled bases. Lengths range from 1$\frac{3}{16}$ to 1$\frac{7}{8}$", largest is an elk toe bone. These were found in Mason and Cabell Counties, West Virginia. Private collection. Rodney Roberts photograph. Each deer bone, **$15.00;** elk bone, **$30.00.**

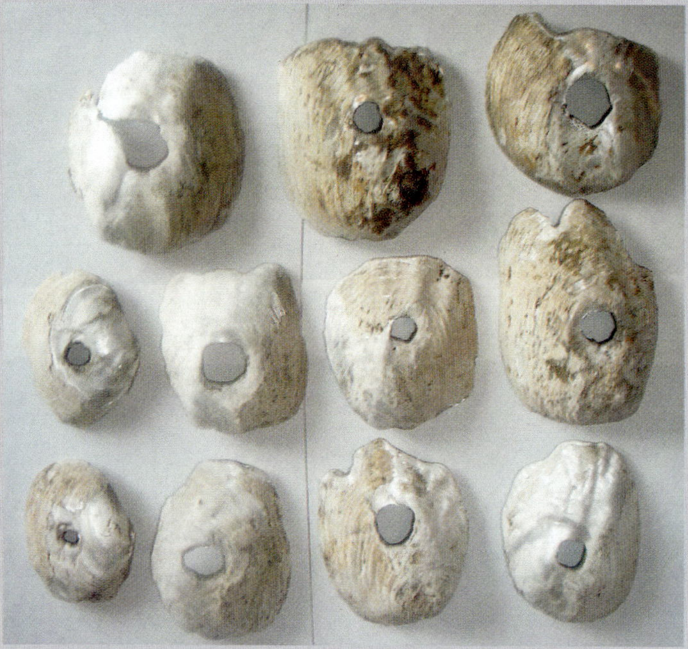

Clamshell hoe blades, Mississippian period with handle holes, size range from 2$\frac{1}{4}$ to 3$\frac{1}{2}$" long. The owner found these in March to May in 2003. Mason County, West Virginia. Private collection; Rodney Roberts photograph. Each, **$4.00 – 8.00.**

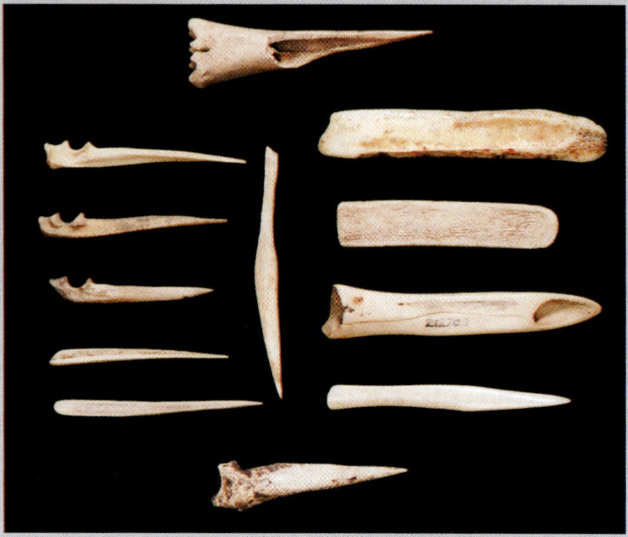

Bone artifacts, identification clockwise beginning at the 12 o'clock position: deer fibia awl; thick bone chisel; 12 cm long; thinner and more finished chisel; deer humerus gouge; bone splinter awl; 6 o'clock, deer radius awl; two bone splinter awls; and three trigger awls from small animals. These are all well-made tools. Private collection. Each, **$35.00 – 200.00.**

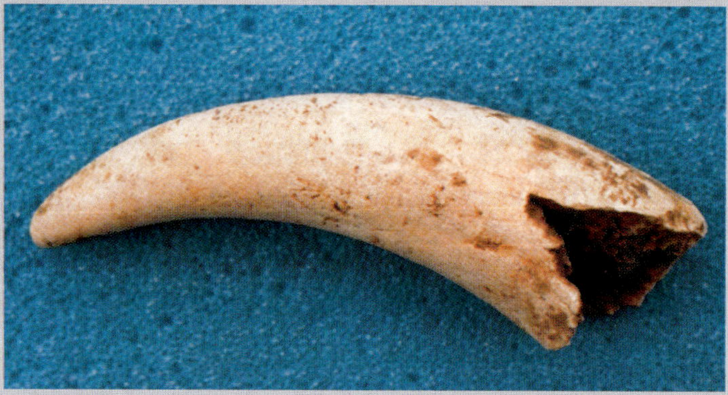

Antler flaker, $\frac{5}{8}$ x 2", Woodland or Mississippian. Ex-collection Snyder and found by him between 1947 and 1958. It is from Polk County, Tennessee. Collection of, and photograph by, Gary Henry, North Carolina. **$10.00.**

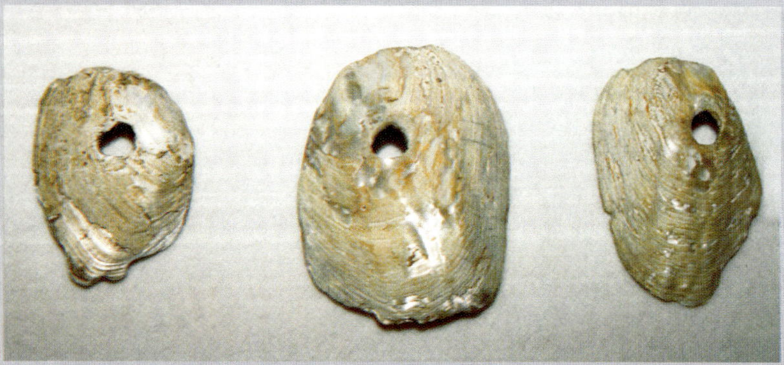

Clamshell hoe heads, Mississippian (Fort Ancient) period, with handle holes. The shells are from 3 to 3$\frac{3}{8}$" long and were found along the Ohio River. Mason County, West Virginia. Private collection. Rodney Roberts photograph. Each, **$5.00 – 10.00.**

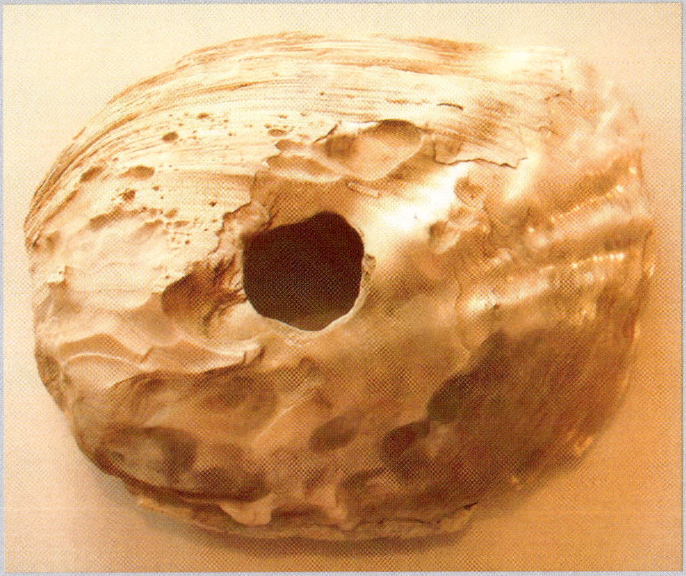

Clamshell hoe head, with handle hole, Mississippian, 4" long. Found in March of 2004 in the spill from a groundhog hole. Ohio River bank, Mason County, West Virginia. Private collection. Rodney Roberts photograph. **$12.00 – 15.00.**

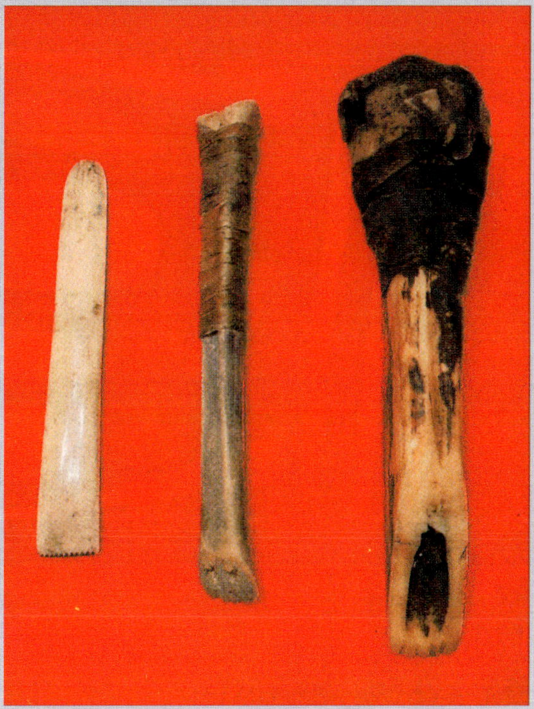

Bone hide scrapers, 6½ to 9" long. All have toothed hide-working edges (example on right is also shown on page 293). All are historic period, from Michigan. Michael F. Slasinski collection, Michigan. Left, **$175.00;** middle, **$250.00;** right, **$325.00.**

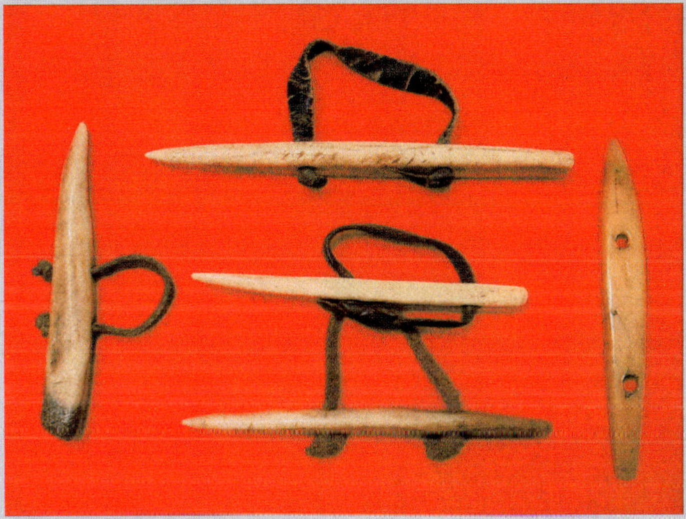

Corn-husking pegs, pioneer period, largest is ½ x 5¼", 5⁄16" thick. Made of bone, four have leather finger-thongs. Various U. S. states. Michael F. Slasinski collection, Michigan. Each, **$15.00 – 20.00.**

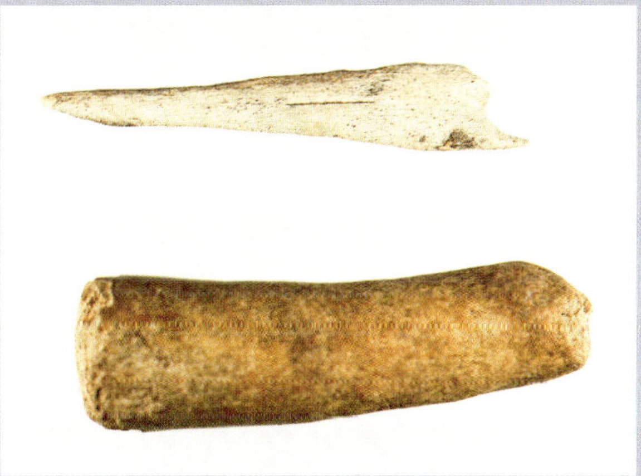

Artifacts, Fort Ancient of the Mississippian period, southern Ohio. Top, bone splinter awl. Private collection. **$5.00.** Bottom, antler drift or flaker 2¼", polished and with rounded ends. Private collection. **$10.00.**

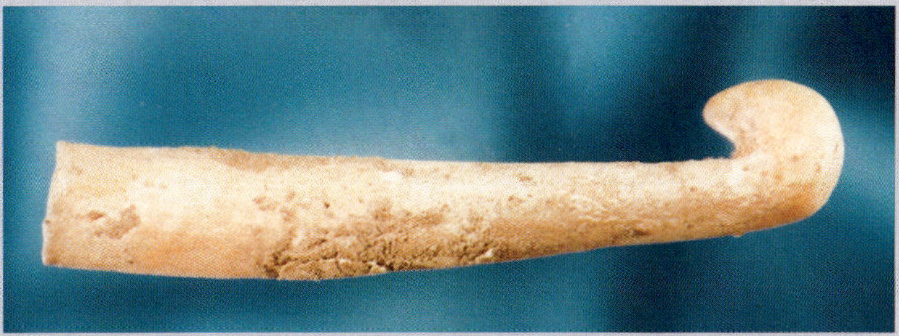

Atl-atl hook, carved antler, size as indicated in this Davis photograph. The inside of this hook is extensively reamed out, and the exterior is carefully carved and smoothed. This is a rare object, found by Col. Vietzen at Glover's Cave, Christian County, Kentucky. It is featured in his book *The Saga of Glover's Cave,* page 210. Private collection. Museum grade.

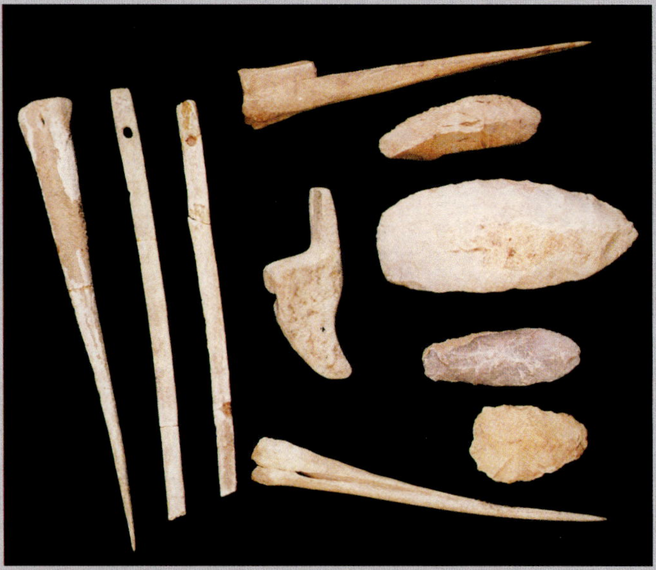

Cache of artifacts, possibly Hopewell (Middle Woodland), with bird of prey effigy pipe at near center made of limestone. It has an etched mouth and eye, and the stem hole is so small it may have been made with a copper drill. The bowl was drilled with the sand and stick method. Also shown are two mat-weaving needles (with eyes) and three fine awls up to 22 cm long. One (at top) uses part of the tibia as a finger-hold. There are four preform blades in this cache and the longest is 12 cm. Alexander County, Illinois. Private collection. Pipe, unlisted; mat needles, each, **$20.00 – 35.00;** awls, each, **$90.00 – 175.00.**

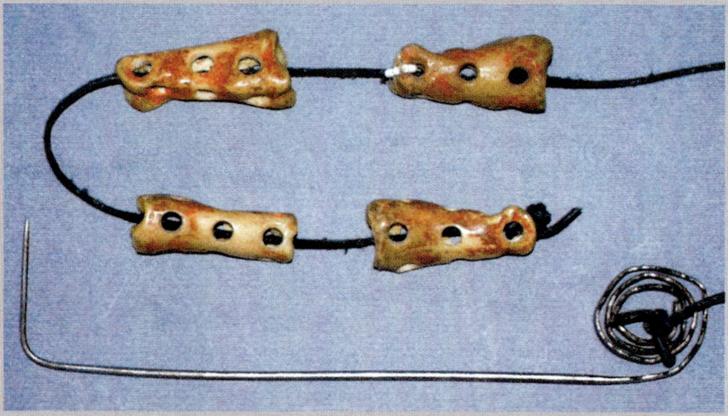

"Toss and catch" game, deer toe bones on cord and wire catcher. Each bone averages 1¾" long, has multiple holes, and one bone also has small white beads attached. Indians and Eskimos alike played this game. Provenance unlisted. H. B. Greene II collection, Florida. Museum grade.

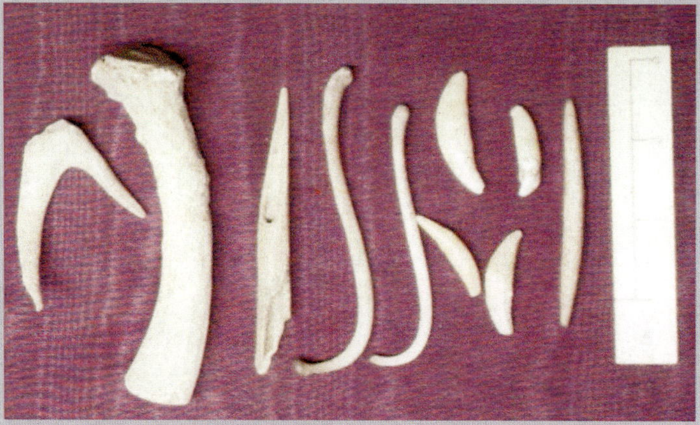

Bone and antler artifacts, found at the famous Bone Bank site in the 1940s. Posey County, Indiana. Ben Thompson collection, Missouri. Each, **$15.00 – 40.00.**

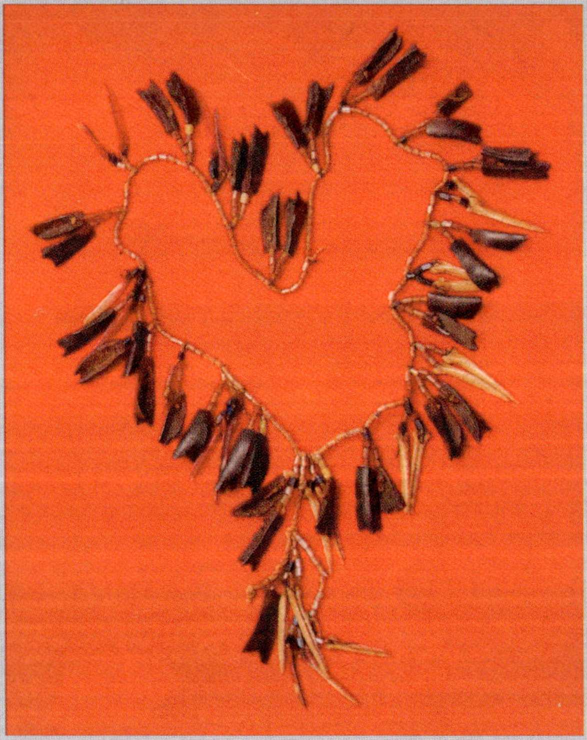

Necklace, historic, deer dew claws and bone imitation claws or talons, strand is 33" long (for closeup view, see page 253). Strung on natural fiber, it is Cherokee Indian. North Carolina. Michael F. Slasinski collection, Michigan. **$400.00.**

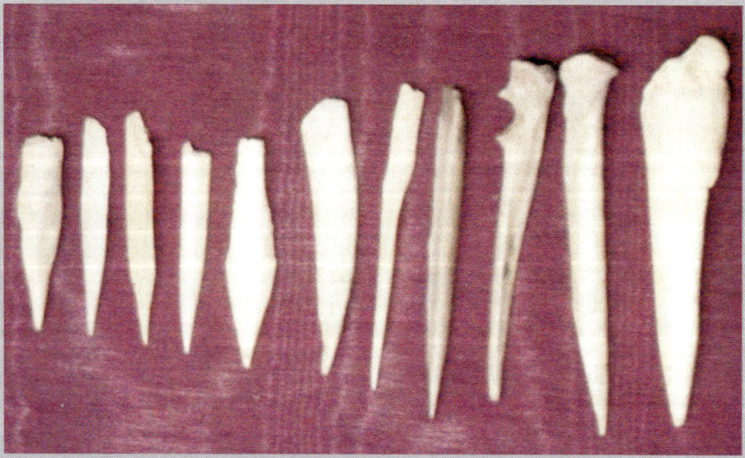

Awls, bone, a variety of piercing tools in different shapes and sizes. All were found in southern Indiana. Ben Thompson collection, Missouri. Each, **$10.00 – 50.00.**

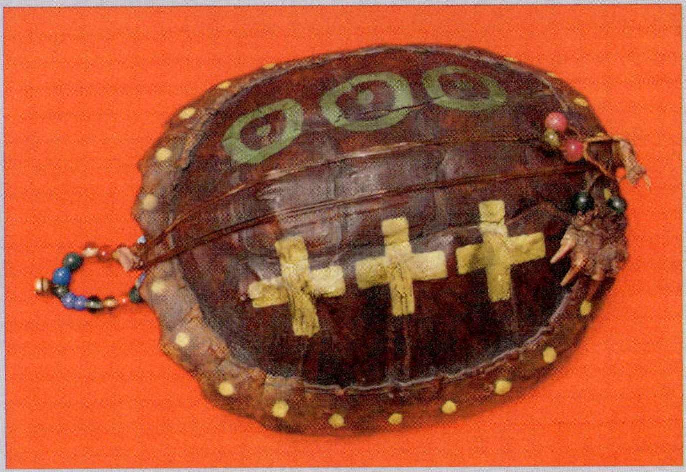

Turtle shell rattle, (top view) 8 x 9" long. It has painted designs and bead decorations. North Carolina. Michael F. Slasinski collection, Michigan. **$400.00.**

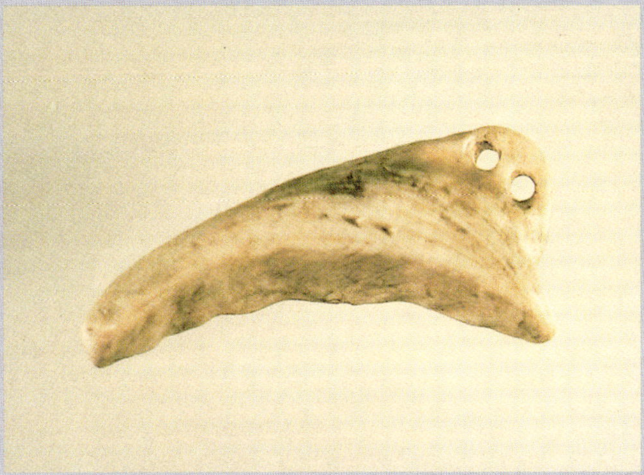

Two-hole pendant, 2⅛" long. Probably made of marine shell, it is cleanly drilled and highly polished. Decatur area, Alabama. Robin Fiser collection. **$75.00.**

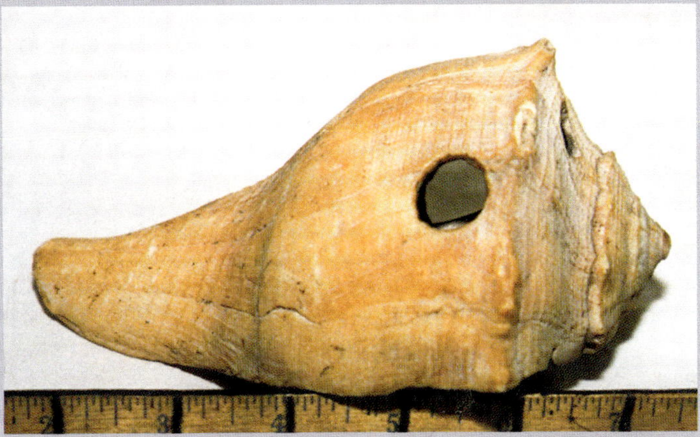

Conch shell pick(?) or tool, two large holes, probably late prehistoric. It would be from the southeast coastal region. Back to Earth. Unlisted.

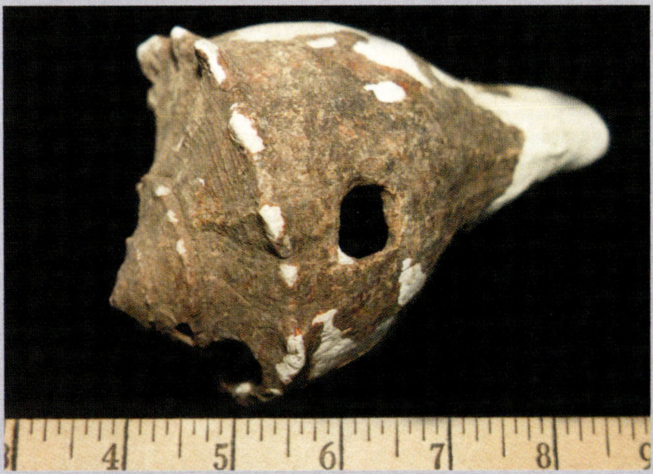

Conch shell tool, possibly a pick, size as indicated. It originated on the southeastern coastal area. Back to Earth. Unlisted.

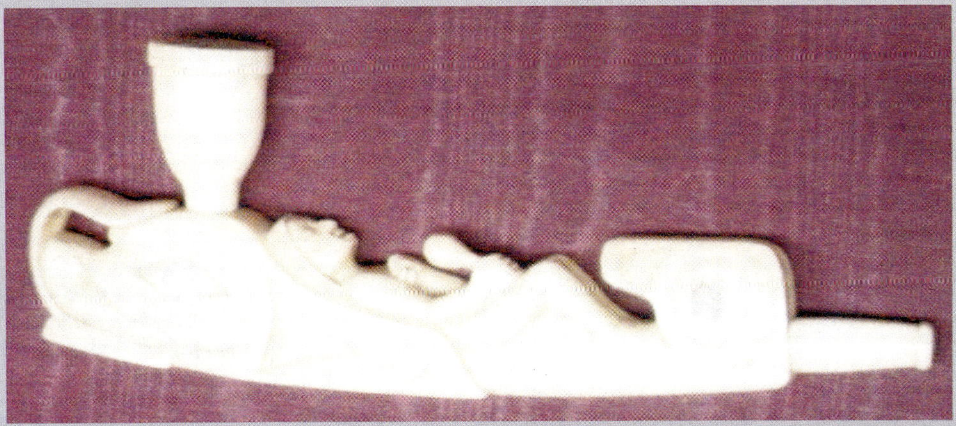

Pipe, carved walrus ivory, Tlingit Indian ca. 1920. This finely made example is done in the Northwest Coast style and is nicely detailed. Ben Thompson collection, Missouri. **$1,200.00.**

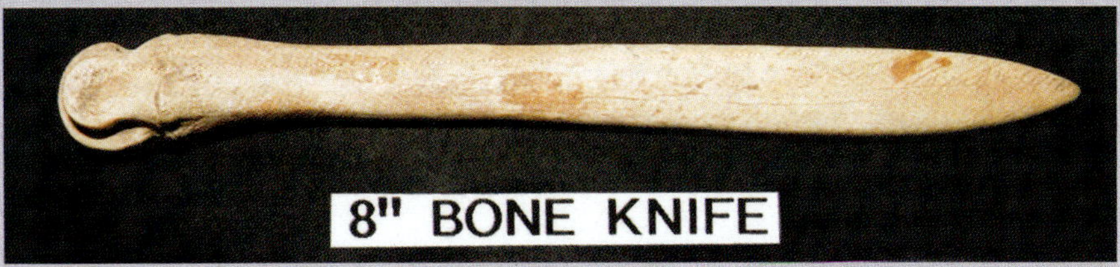

Bone knife, Fort Ancient, 8" long. This is a classic specimen, size, workmanship, and condition. Probably Ohio Valley region. Back to Earth. Unlisted.

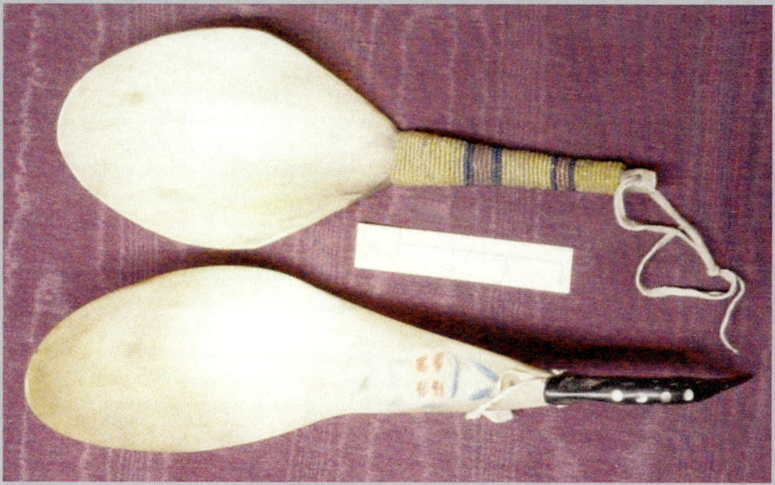

Horn spoons or dippers, bighorn sheep, ca. 1940. The upper example has a beaded handle, while the lower has a handle termination made of buffalo horn. Ben Thompson collection, Missouri. Each, **$750.00.**

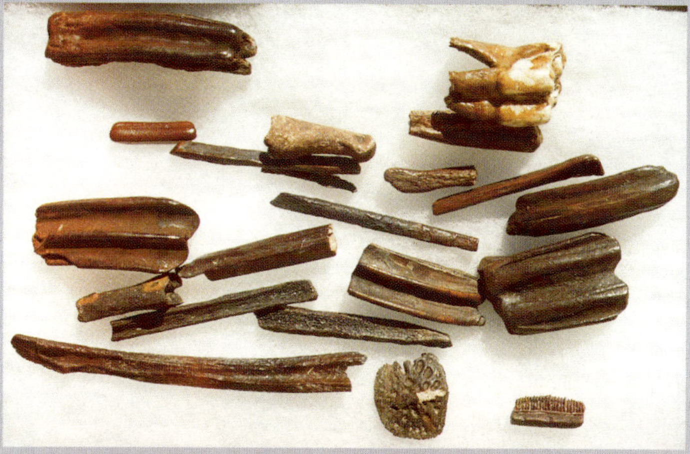

Pleistocene (Ice Age) animal parts and tools, made of ivory, frame size is 8 x 12". The bones are from alligators, turtles, deer and American camel, and these were recovered from the Caloosahatchee River in Lee County, Florida. Dave Summers collection, Victor, New York. Frame, **$300.00.**

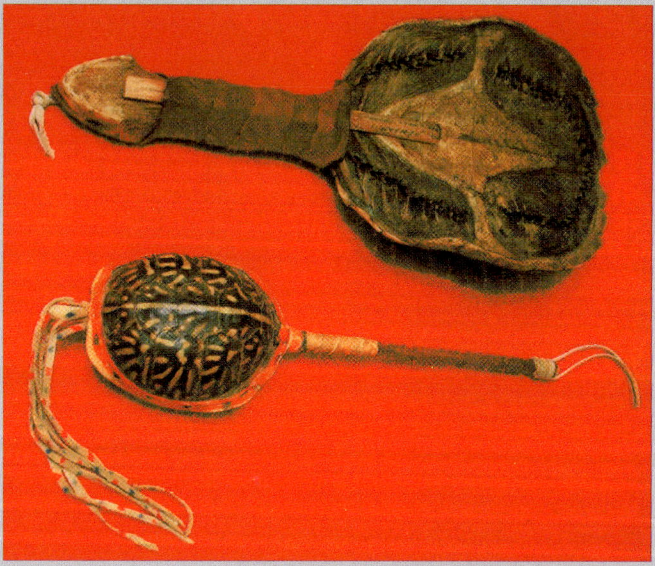

Rattles, longer one is approximately 15" long, smaller one is about 3½" wide. They are from Michigan and Canada. Michael F. Slasinski collection, Michigan. Upper, snapping turtle, **$250.00;** lower, land tortoise, **$200.00.**

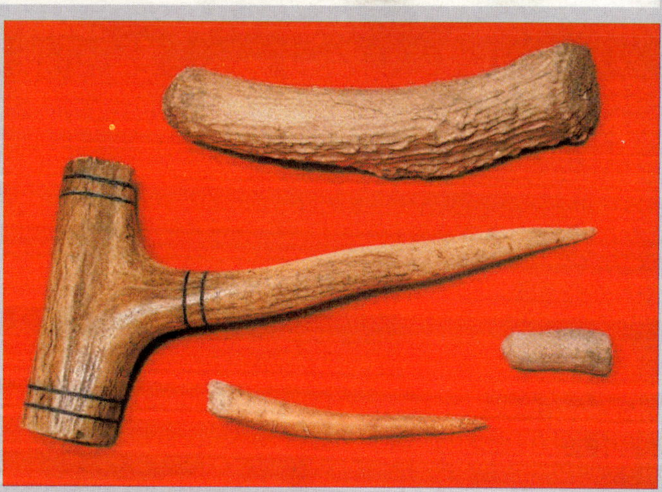

Antler flint-knapping tools, the baton (from Tennessee) is 6" long, the antler tine is 3¾", and the small antler chipping tool is 1½" long. Except for the baton, the others were found in Michigan. Michael F. Slasinski collection, Michigan. Each, **$10.00 – 125.00.**

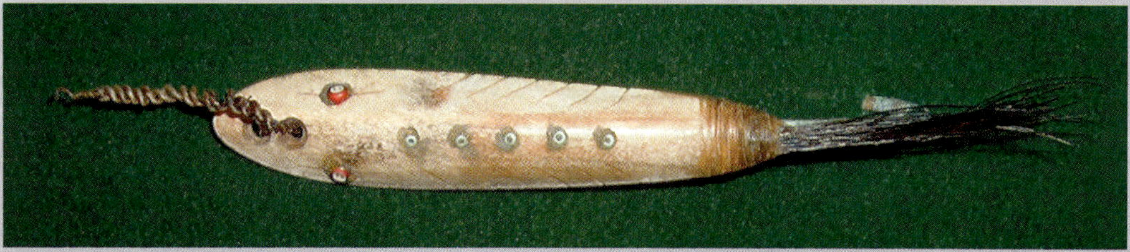

Bone fishing lure with hook, ¾ x 5½" long. The lure is from the Northwest Coast. Keith and Rhonda Dodge collection, Michigan. **$300.00.**

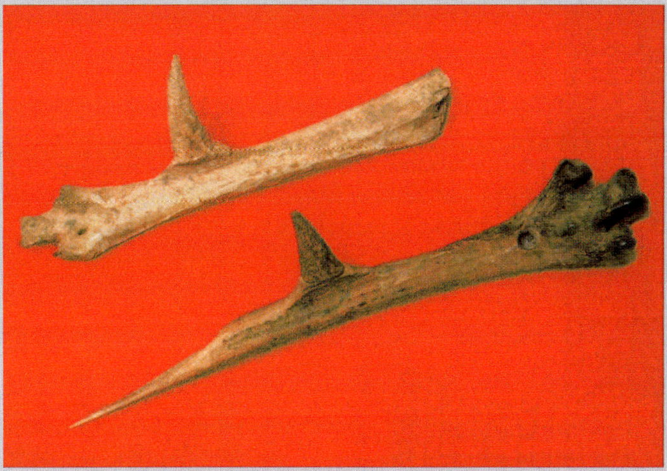

Awls, wild turkey legbones with spurs, average size is ⅜ x 5", width at spurs is 1¼". They are Woodland or Mississippian in time, and the bottom example combines a typical awl plus the spur tip. Tennessee. Michael F. Slasinski collection, Michigan. Top, **$50.00;** bottom, **$85.00.**

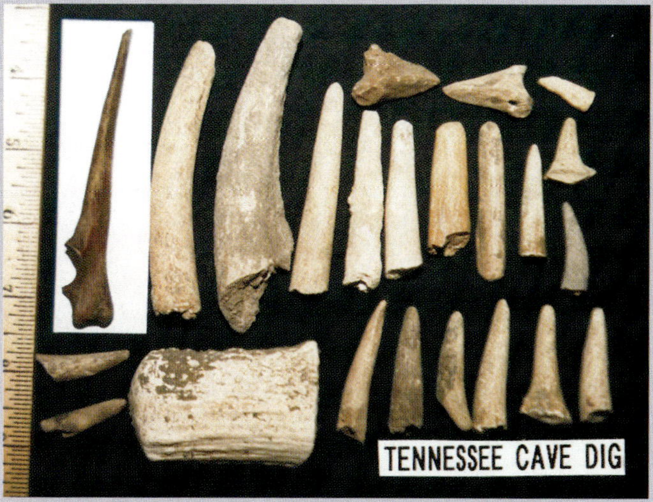
TENNESSEE CAVE DIG

Artifacts, antler and bone, longest is 4". They were found in a rock shelter. Gallatin County, Tennessee. Back to Earth. **$145.00.**

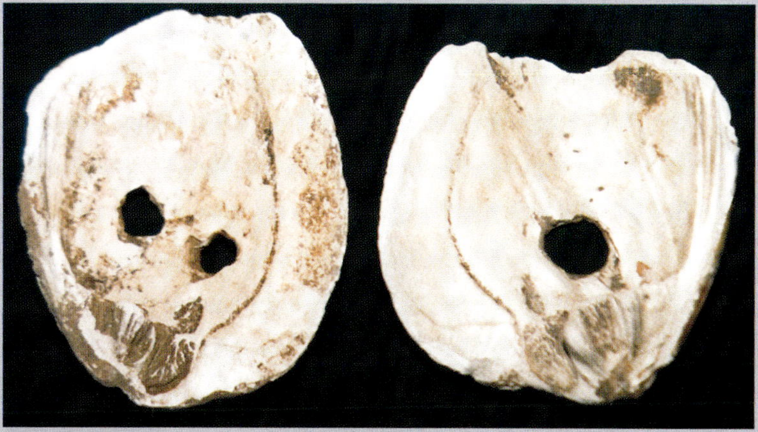

Shell hoes or scrapers, Fort Ancient (late prehistoric), single and double holes. the material is freshwater mussel. Back to Earth. Unlisted.

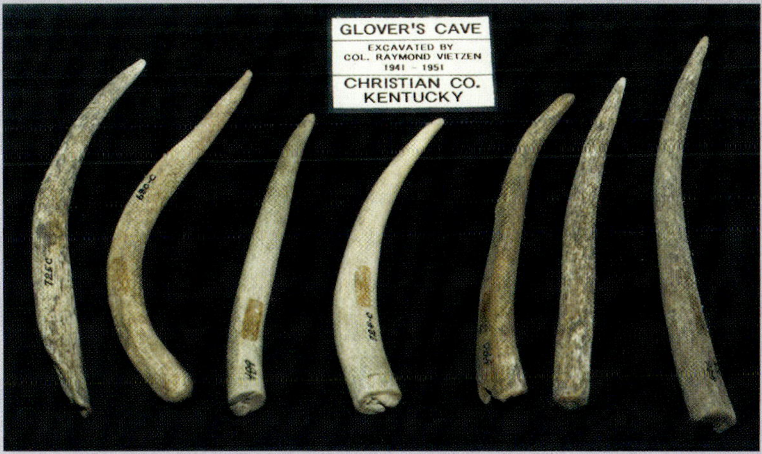
GLOVER'S CAVE
EXCAVATED BY
COL. RAYMOND VIETZEN
1941 - 1951
CHRISTIAN CO.
KENTUCKY

Antler tools, awls or flint-knappers, ex-collection Vietzen. These came from a rock shelter in Christian County, Kentucky. Back to Earth. Unlisted.

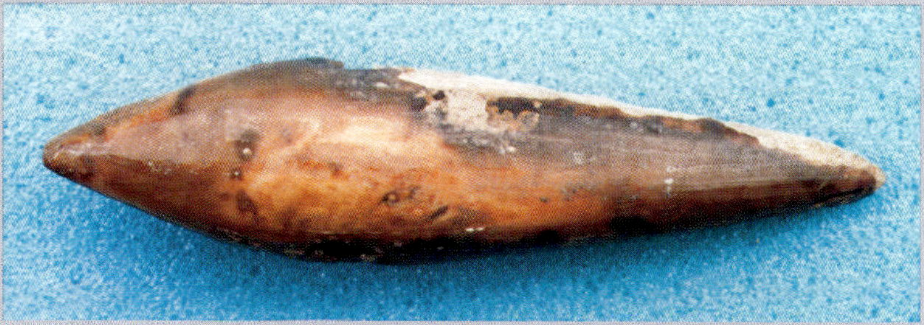

Charm or plummet-like artifact, prehistoric(?), ¾ x 3 7/16". Made of fossil bone. Ex-collection Levy, it is probably from California. Collection of, and photograph by, Gary Henry, North Carolina. **$34.00.**

Miscellaneous Artifacts

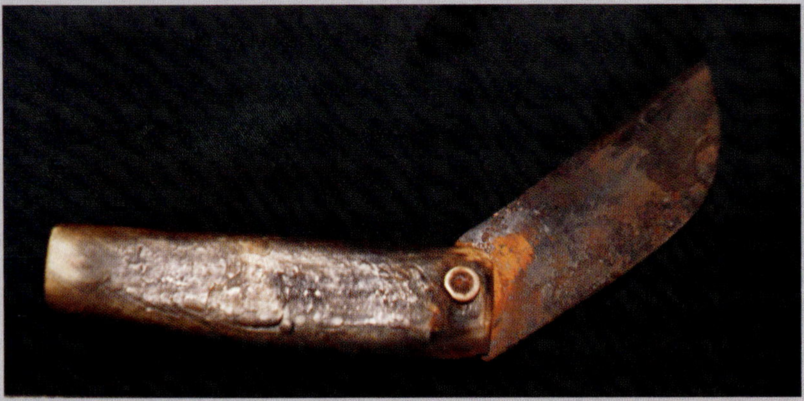

Antler-handled knife, metal blade and brass rivet. Antler was much-used by both Indians and Whites in early historic times. Back to Earth. Unlisted.

Tools, bone, two trigger awls, two split bone awls, one flint-knapping rod. They are Fort Ancient, from Kentucky. Back to Earth. Unlisted.

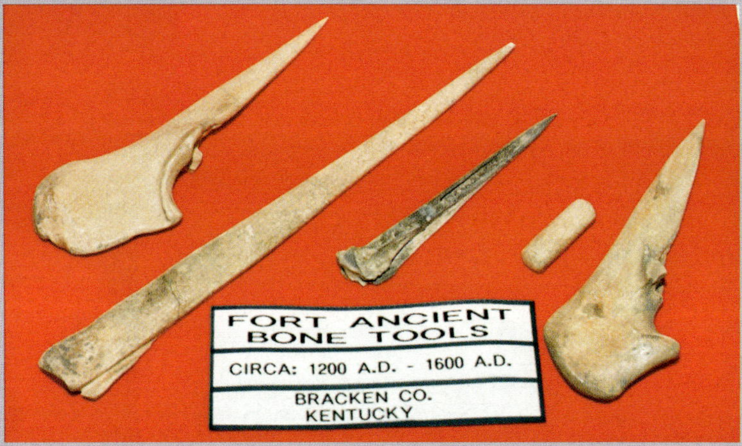

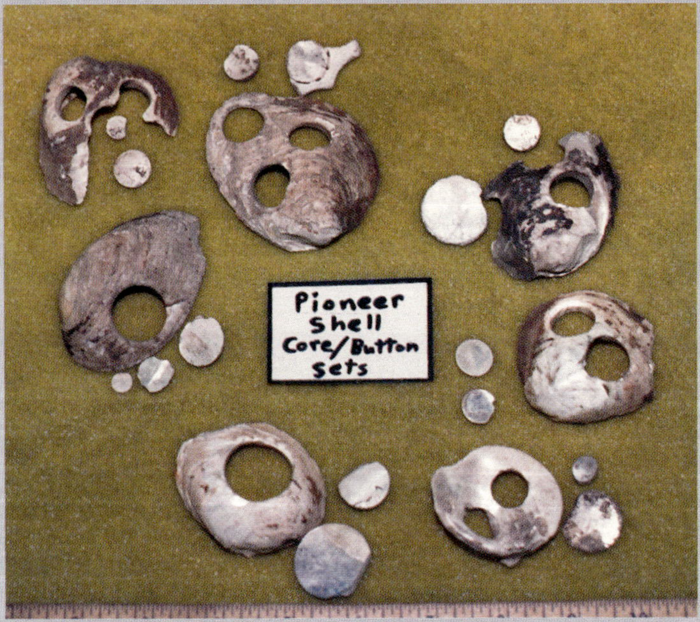

Shell artifacts, from the 1800s. These are freshwater mussel shell blanks with circular cutouts for buttons, and should not be mistaken for Indian artifacts. In the Upper Mississippi watershed many small factories near major streams produced shell buttons. Back to Earth. Unlisted.

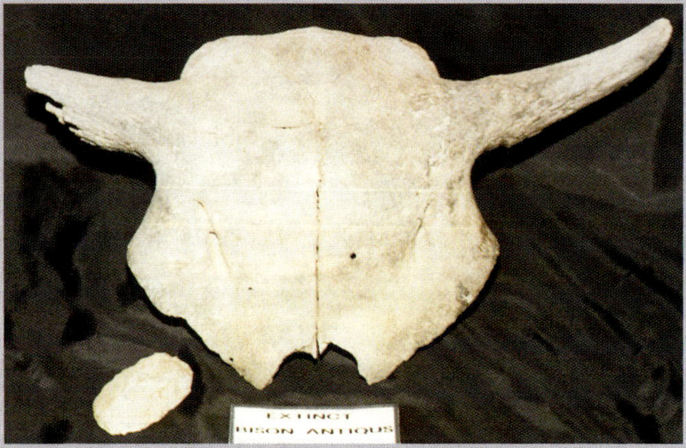

Bison skull, extinct animal form. Paleo people hunted such bison and occasionally their projectile points are found with the bones. Back to Earth. Unlisted.

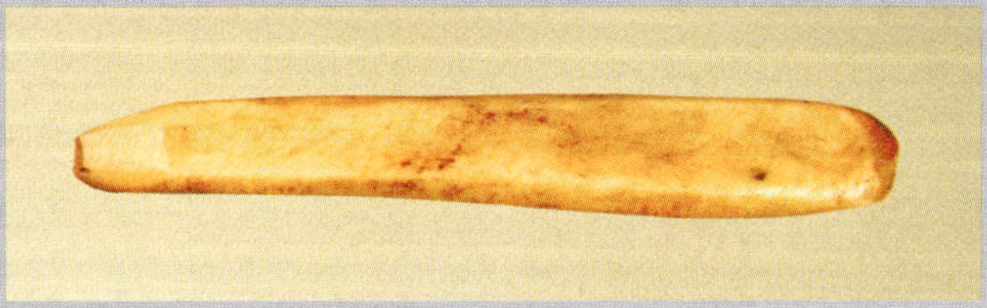

Spatulate bone tool, smaller end reground in recent times, ivory-like dense bone. The main reason a modern person would regrind the tip is to overwork a damaged section, so this hurts value. It is 2$^{11}/_{16}$", from Kentucky. Private collection. **$10.00.**

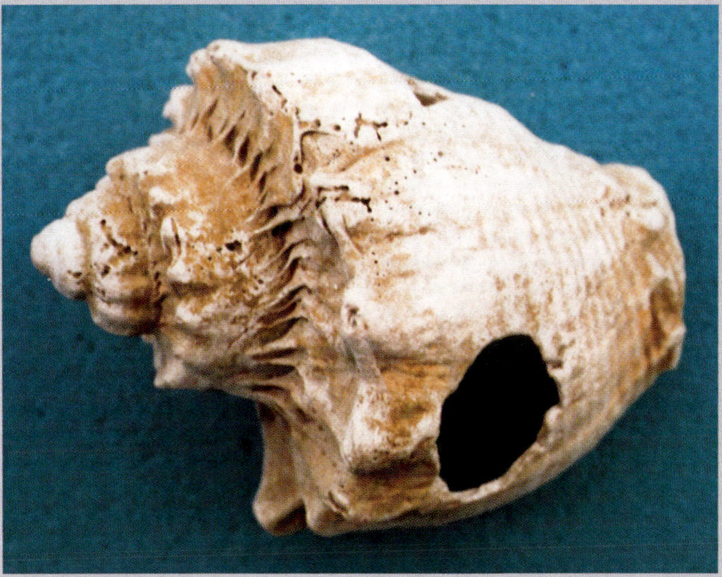

Conch shell pick, Archaic or later, shell size is 1¾ x 2⅛", 3" long. Ex-collection O'Neil, the pick is from Dixie County, Florida. Collection of, and photograph by, Gary Henry, North Carolina. **$20.00.**

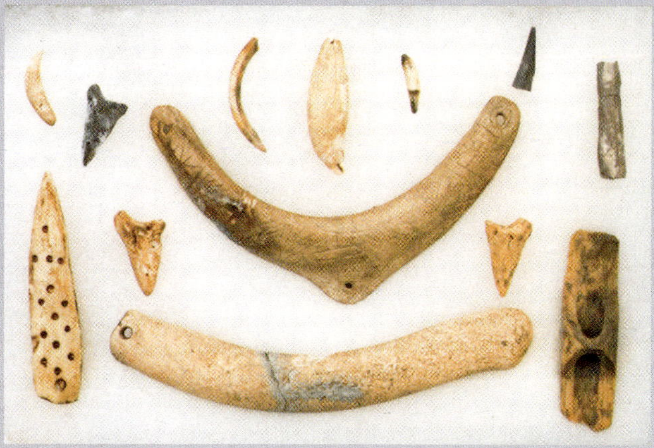

Frame containing pendants, a bead, an awl, and other objects. Woodland or later, there is an engraved three-hole bone gorget, a punctated antler pendant, a worked bone pendant, bobcat canine pendant, bear canine, bone bead, rodent incisor, bobcat canine, fossil bone awl, fossil bone piece and three deer toe bones. The long, drilled bone piece (bottom center) is 1 x 7". Ex-collection Snyder, Meigs County, Tennessee. Collection of, and photograph by, Gary Henry, North Carolina. Frame contents, **$500.00.**

Bone arrow foreshaft, prehistoric(?), one end slotted for point, 5/16 x 7" long. Ex-collection Cordeiro, it is from Alaska. Collection of, and photograph by, Gary Henry, North Carolina. **$50.00.**

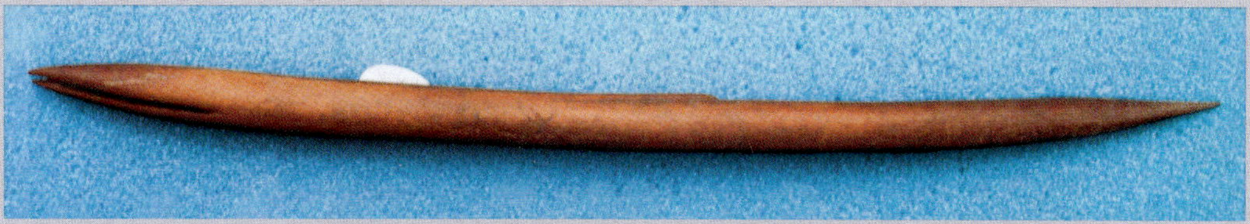

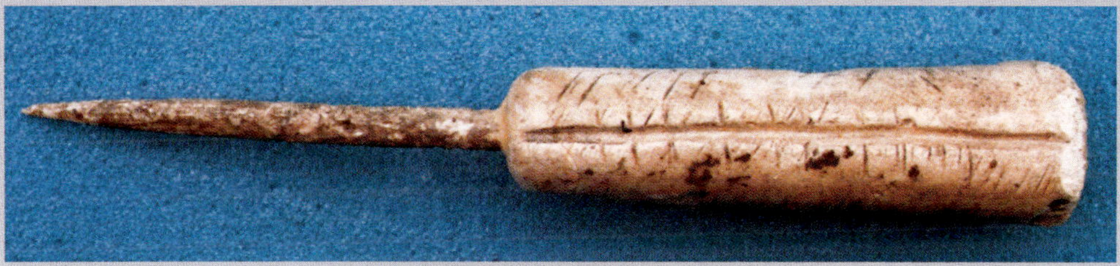

One-piece bone awl, handle with two grooves on opposite sides and randomly marked lines, Woodland or later, ¾ x 4⅝". Very unusual, the artifact is ex-collection Snyder. Morgan County, Tennessee. Collection of, and photograph by, Gary Henry, North Carolina. **$150.00.**

Bone punch or pin, drilled, Woodland or later, ½ x 2⅞". It is ex-collection Levy, origin unknown. Collection of, and photograph by, Gary Henry, North Carolina. **$50.00.**

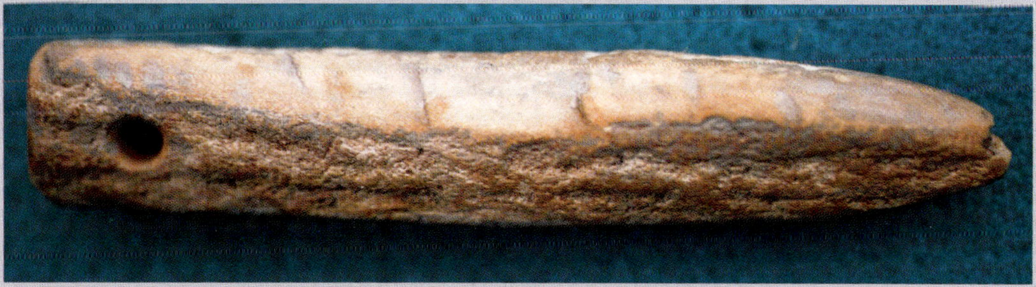

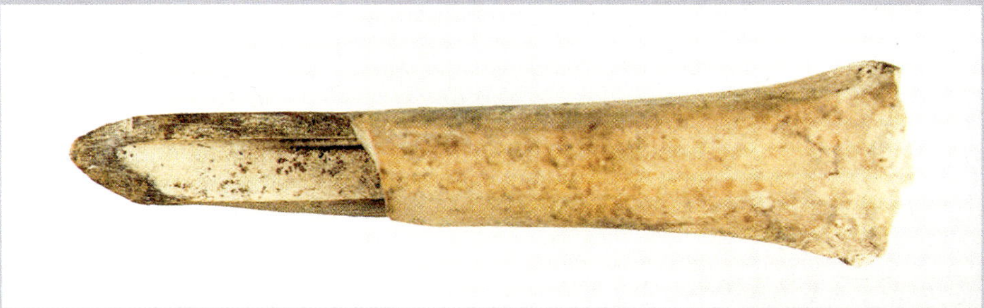

Dagger or knife, heavy long bone split and remaining section ground on both faces to form sharp edges and a rounded tip. The artifact is 4¾" long and from Fort Ancient times. Southern Ohio. Private collection. **$75.00.**

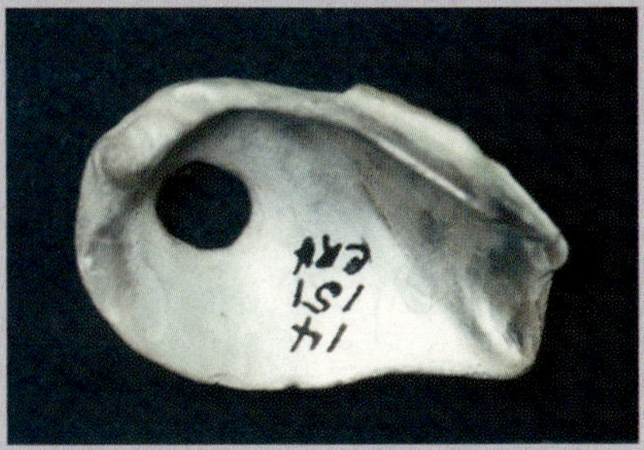

Pendant(?), mussel shell, Woodland or Mississippian, ⅞ x 1⅜". Harwood found it in 1958. Morgan County, Alabama. Collection of, and photograph by, Gary Henry, North Carolina. **$25.00.**

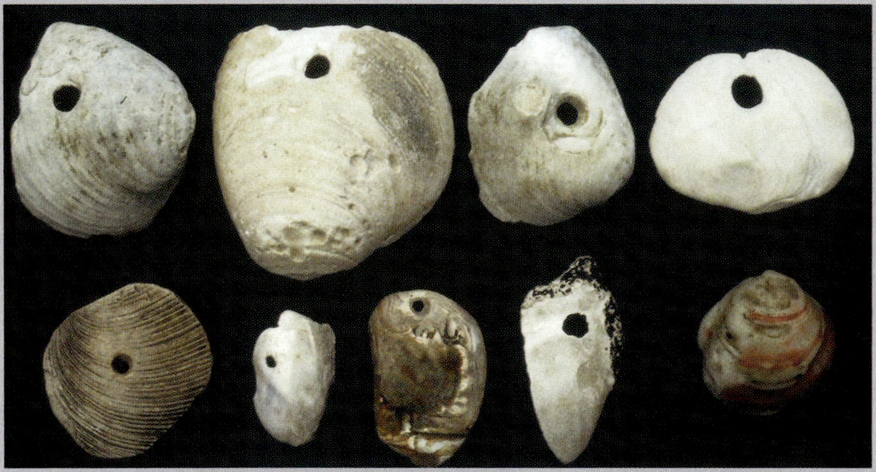

Pendants(?), mussel shells, Woodland and later, largest is 2 x 2". Ex-collection Levy, origin unknown. Collection of, and photograph by, Gary Henry, North Carolina. Each, **$25.00.**

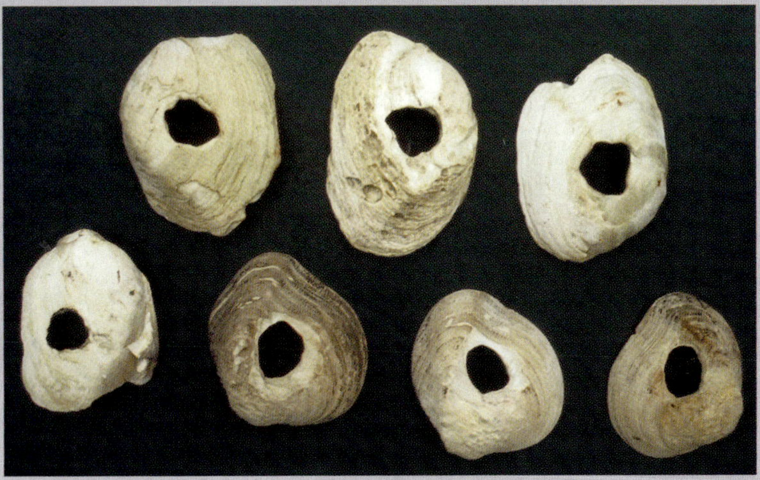

Scrapers or hoes, Woodland and later, mussel shell. The largest artifact is 2¼ x 3⅛". These are ex-collection Levy, origin unknown. Collection of, and photograph by, Gary Henry, North Carolina. Each, **$10.00.**

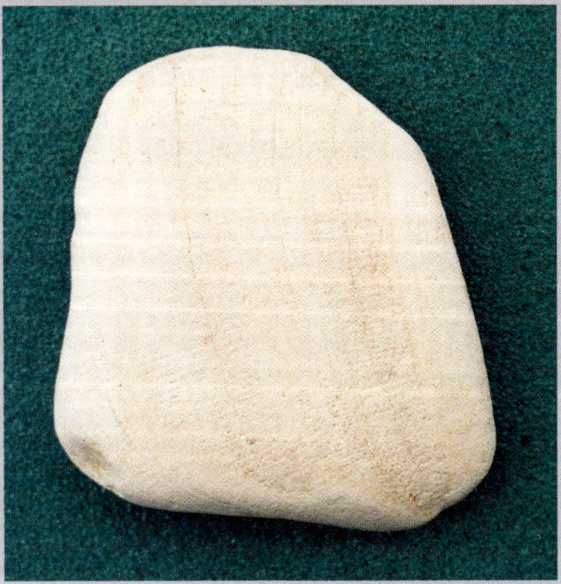

Pendant preform(?), ground but not drilled, mussel shell, 1⅜ x 1½". Woodland or later, the owner found it in 1986. Buncombe County, North Carolina. Collection of, and photograph by, Gary Henry, North Carolina. **$10.00.**

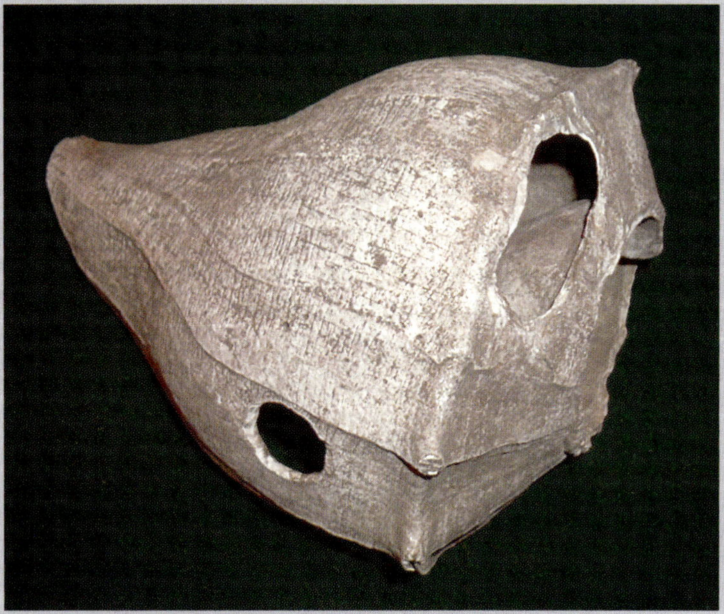

Shell pick or hoe, (holed for handle), 5½ x 7½". The artifact was found in Dade County, Florida. Keith and Rhonda Dodge collection, Michigan. **$90.00.**

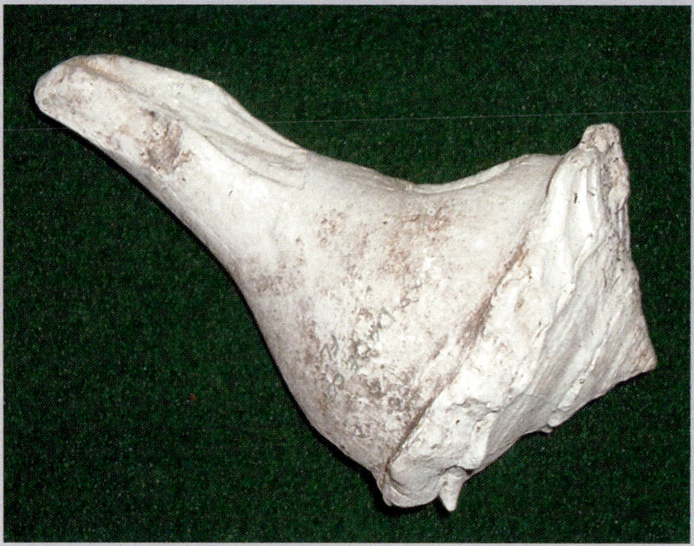

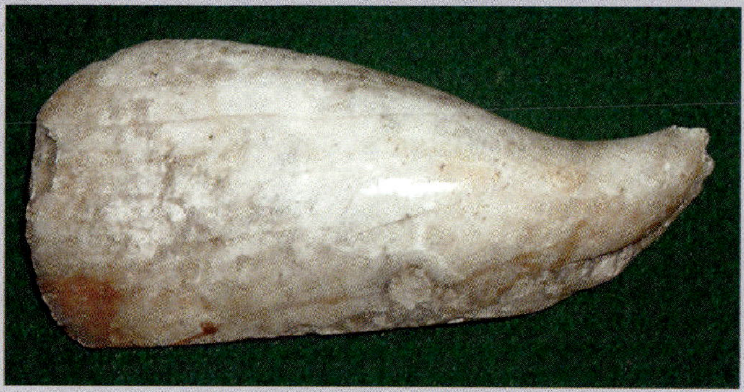

Tool, shell, 2 x 5", ex-collections Payne and Cooper. It was found in Lee County, Florida. Keith and Rhonda Dodge collection, Michigan.

Shell artifact, 2½ x 4½", Dade County, Florida. Keith and Rhonda Dodge collection, Michigan. **$65.00.**

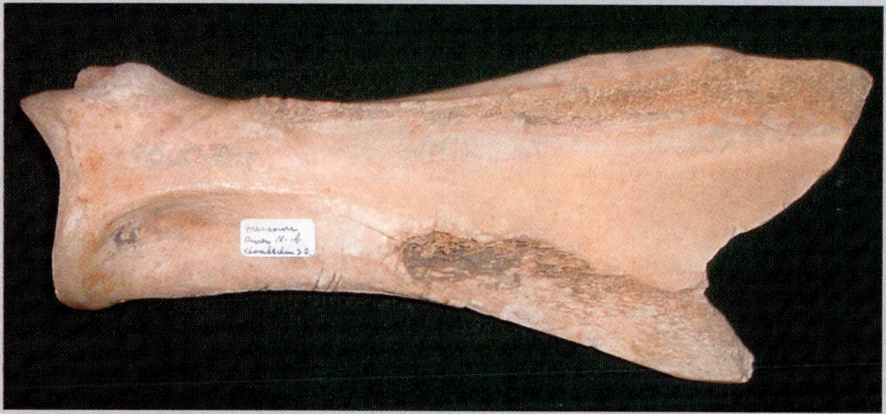

Bison shoulder bone spade, 4½ x 12½". This spade was found along the Missouri River north of Chamberlain, South Dakota. Keith and Rhonda Dodge collection, Michigan. **$125.00.**

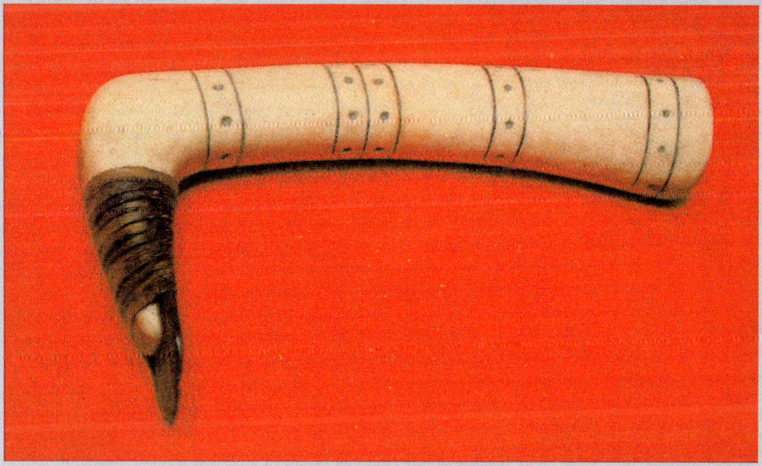

Elk antler hide-scraper, 9" long and 2" wide at the metal blade, with leather blade lashing. This beautiful piece has line-and-dot decoration. Provenance unknown. Michael F. Slasinski collection, Michigan. **$600.00.**

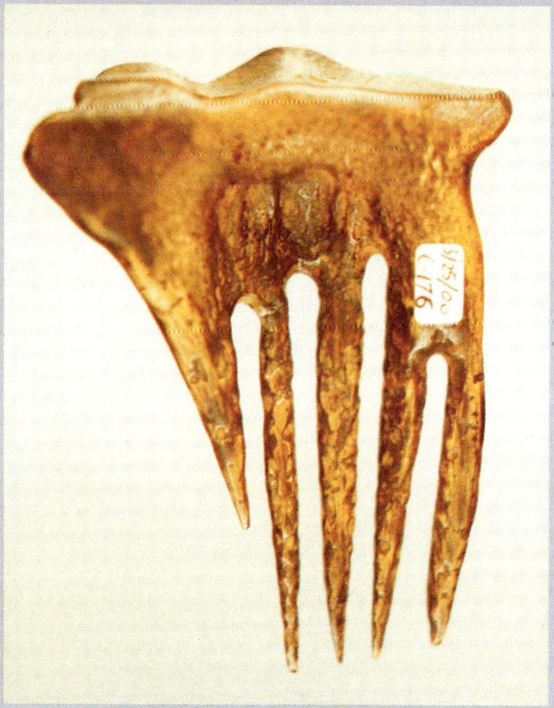

Antler comb, slight restoration, probably elk antler, 4" long. The comb was found in 1952 in Clay County, Arkansas. Larry Garvin collection. Museum grade.

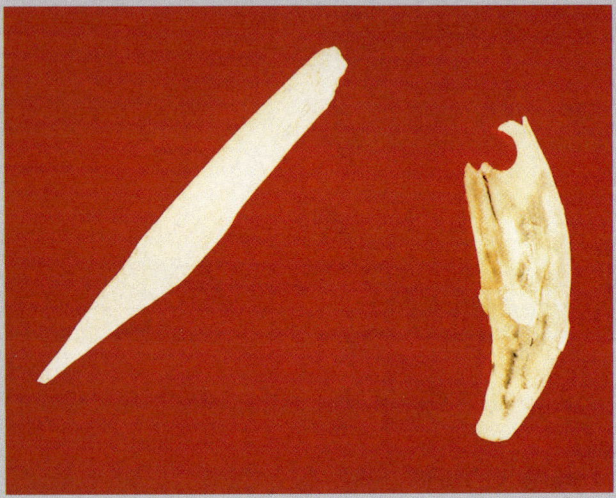

Prehistoric site material, private collection, Illinois. Left, splinter awl, thin, 2¼". Right, bear tooth, broken at the large suspension hole. **$8.00** and **$12.00,** respectively.

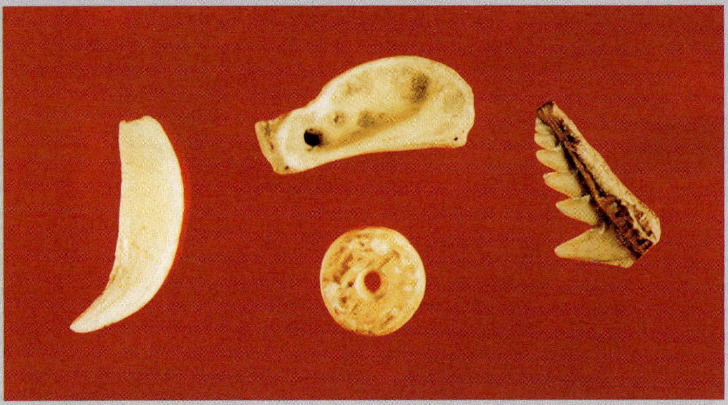

Prehistoric site material, private collection, all from Kentucky. Left, animal tooth, 1" long. Top center, drilled turtle bone. Bottom center, shell bead. Right, bone with teeth. **$2.00, $10.00, $3.00,** and **$2.00.**

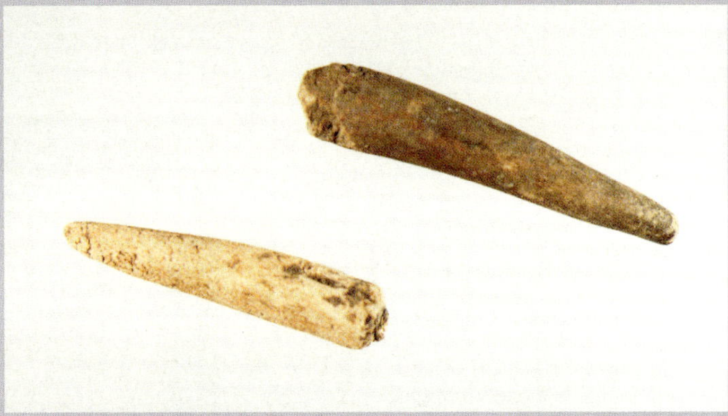

Antler tips, likely raw material for projectile points, longer piece is 1⅞". Both are from Kentucky. Private collection. Each, **$3.00.**

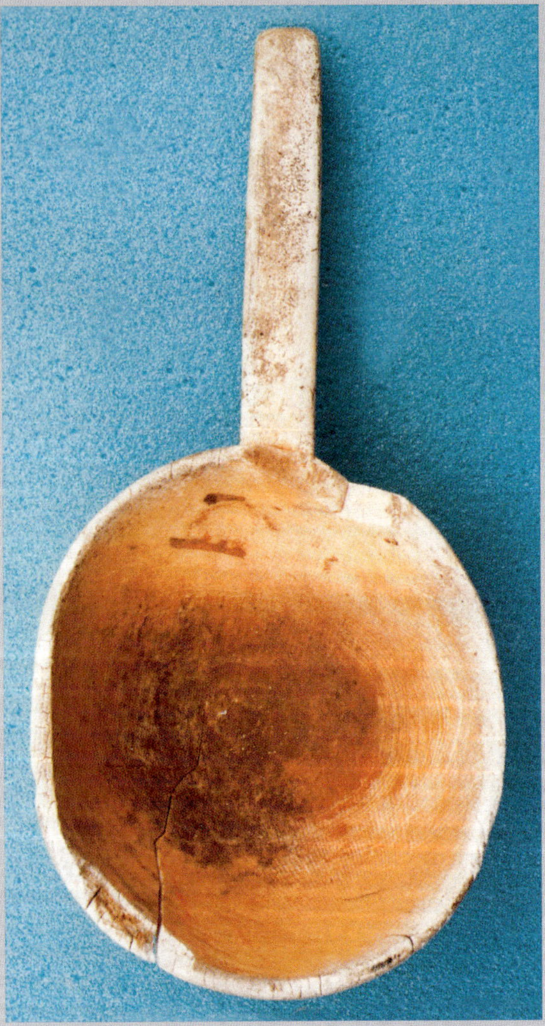

Ladle or horn, prehistoric(?), 3 x 6" and 1⅝" high. It was in the Levy collection and is probably from the Northwest. Collection of, and photograph by, Gary Henry, North Carolina. **$200.00.**

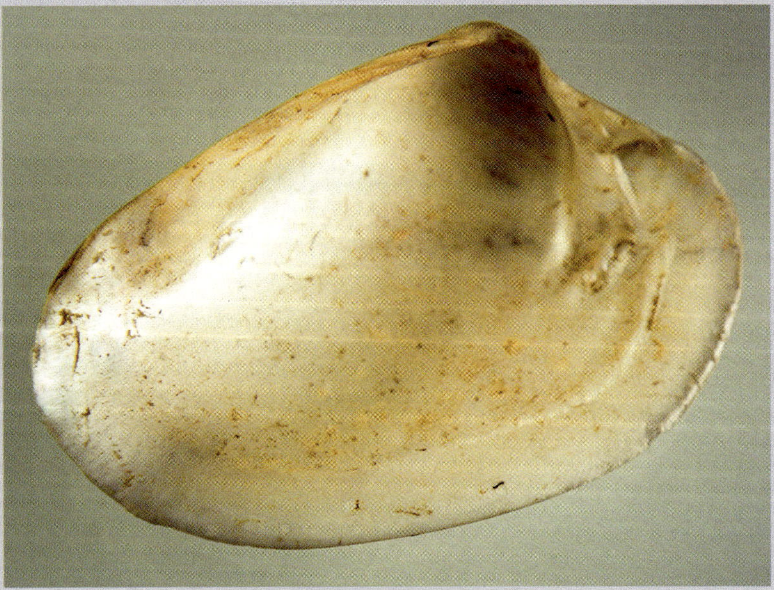

Spoon, ladle, or dipper, freshwater mussel shell, Mississippian period. The shell is 5" at longest dimension and the entire excurvate edge opposite the hinge has been ground smooth. Ex-collection Norbert Bingman, southeastern Illinois. Private collection. Unlisted.

Bison bone, broken section, $4\frac{1}{16}$" long, with $\frac{5}{16}$" average thickness. Probably fractured to obtain the marrow or raw material for artifacts. A campsite find on the Great Plains, private collection. Unlisted.

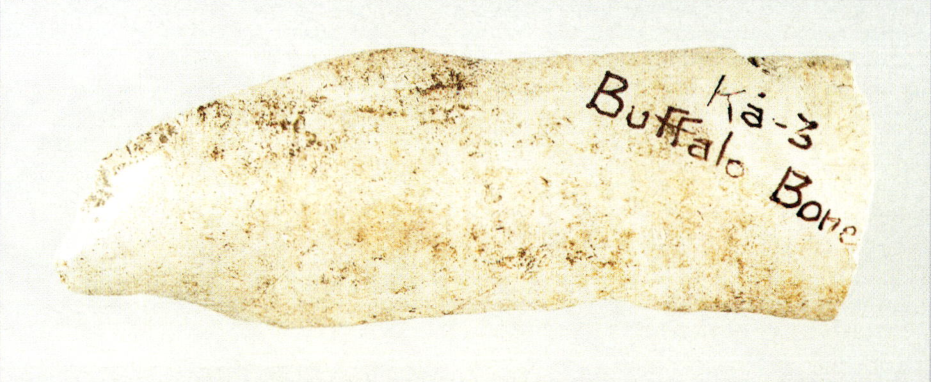

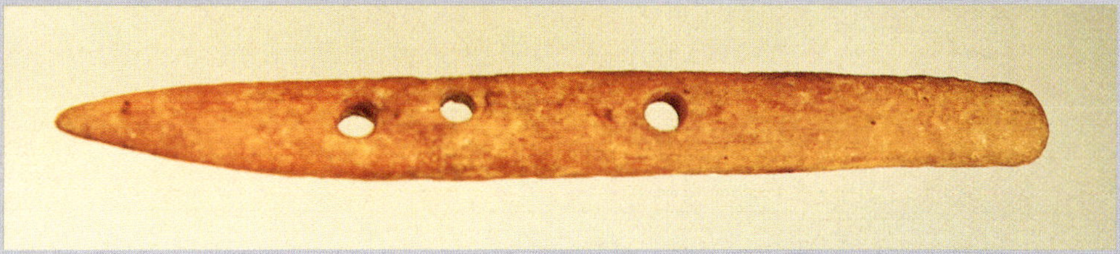

Bone artifact, three drilled holes, chemically stabilized, unknown use. It is $4\frac{3}{4}$" long and, while provenance was given as Florida, it is more like an Alaskan artifact. Private collection. **$25.00.**

Horn spoon with incised design, $5\frac{1}{2}$" long. Davis COA. The spoon is from the Northwest Coast. Keith and Rhonda Dodge collection, Michigan. **$550.00.**

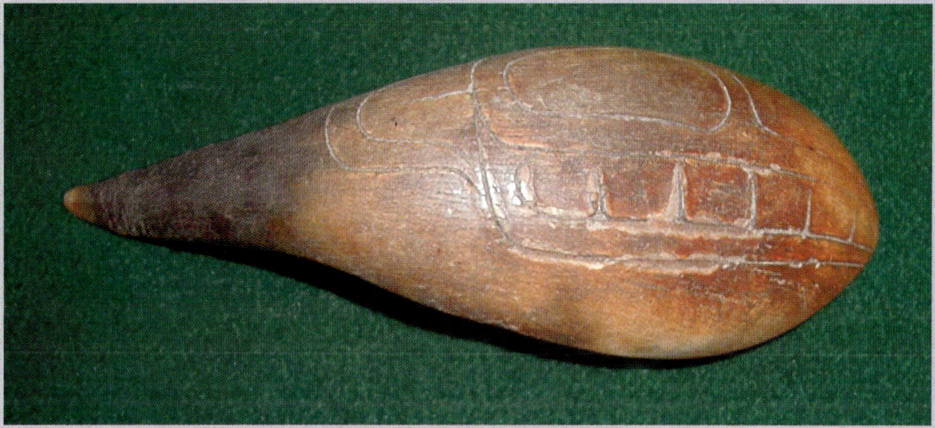

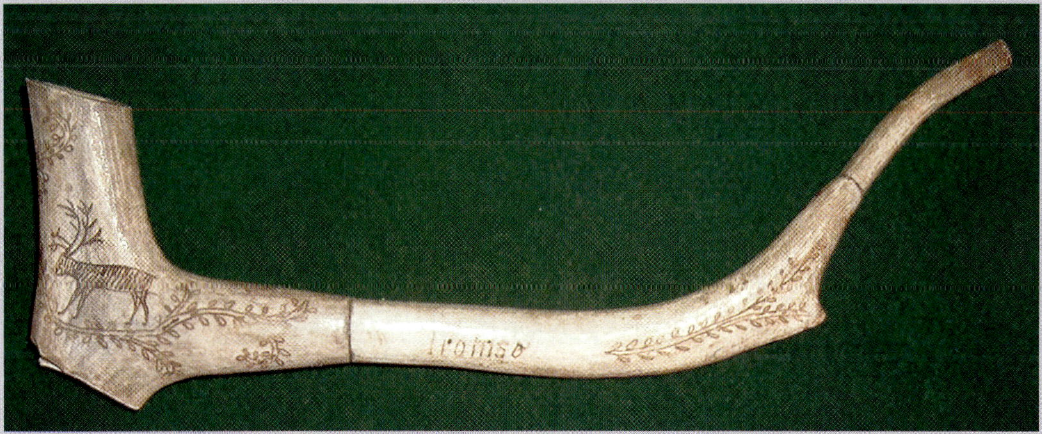

Antler sectional pipe, 3 x 12", incised designs. It has a Davis COA and came from Greenland. Keith and Rhonda Dodge collection, Michigan. Unlisted.

Perforator(?), double-tipped at one end, bird leg bone. A rare artifact type, it is $2\frac{11}{16}$" long and each tip has been sharpened from 360 degrees around. That portion of the bone is hollow while the opposite end is solid. Similar bone artifacts found in archaeological contexts have been suggested to be tattooing needles for making parallel rows of dots. Ex-collection Vietzen, Christian County, Kentucky. Pete Timoch collection. **$100.00.**

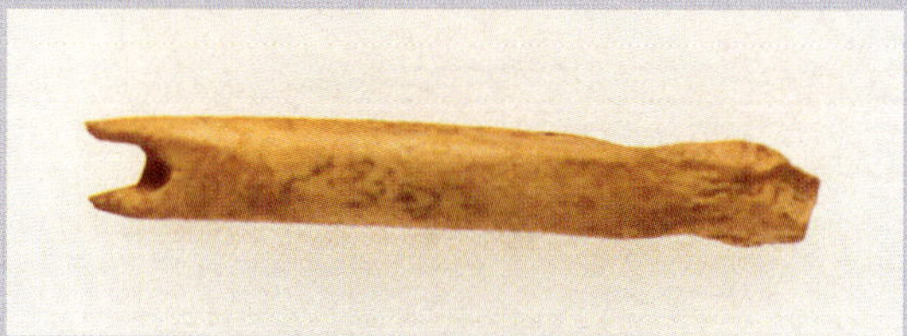

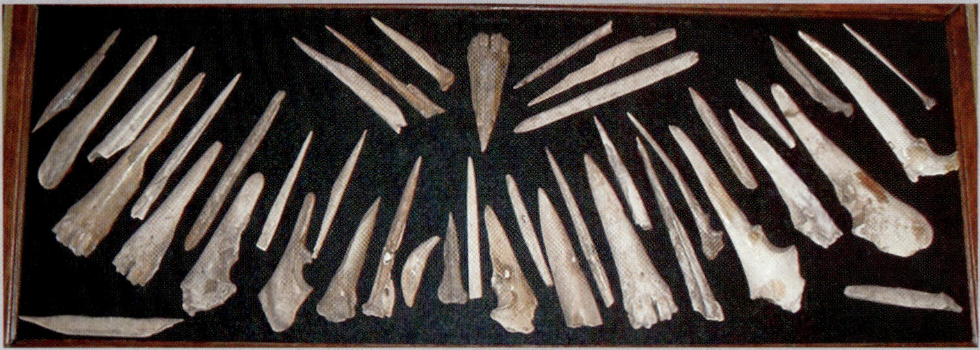

Bone artifacts, trigger awls, awls, hairpins, and a needle. They are 2 to 6" long and were found in Casey County, Kentucky. Keith and Rhonda Dodge collection, Michigan. Each artifact, **$10.00 – 60.00.**

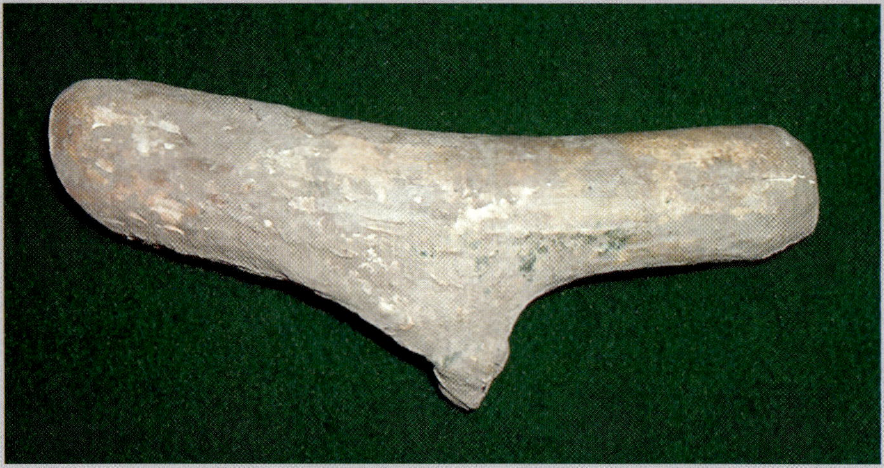

Bone tool, ex-collection Vietzen, 6" long. It has a Davis COA and was found in Glover's Cave, Christian County, Kentucky. Keith and Rhonda Dodge collection, Michigan. **$75.00.**

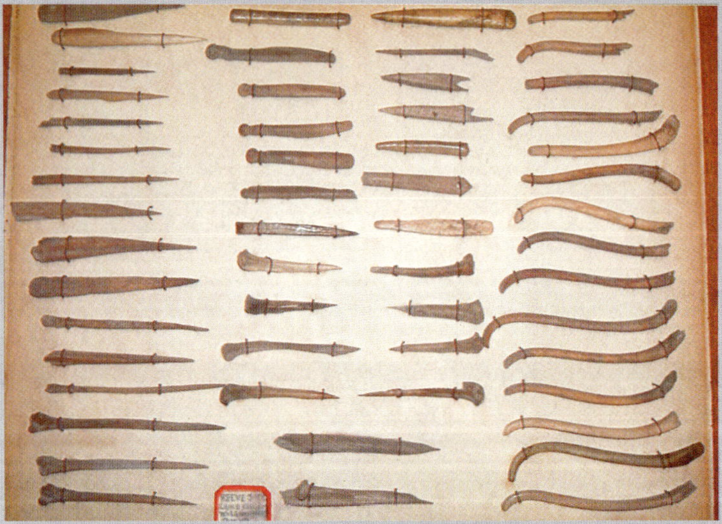

Bone artifacts, mainly awls and small tools, Reeve village. This was a Mississippian-era (late prehistoric) site in Lake County, Ohio. Keith and Rhonda Dodge collection, Michigan. Each piece, **$15.00 – 40.00.**

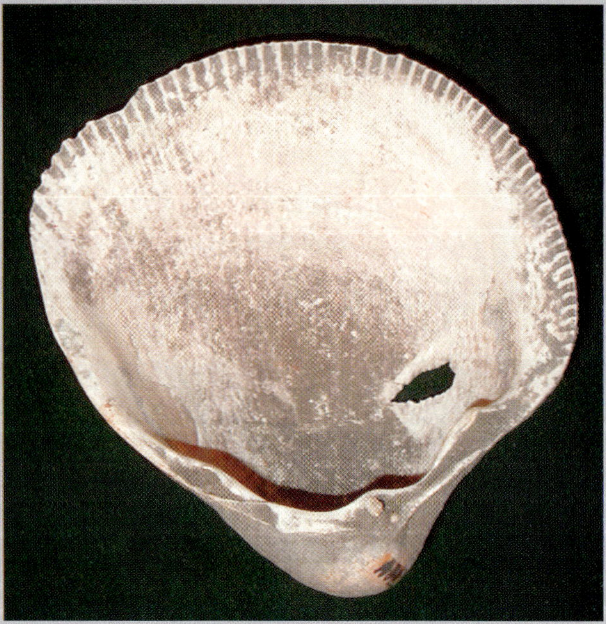

Marine shell dipper, ex-collection Cooper, $4\frac{3}{4}$ x $5\frac{1}{2}$". It is from Dade County, Florida. Keith and Rhonda Dodge collection, Michigan. **$175.00.**

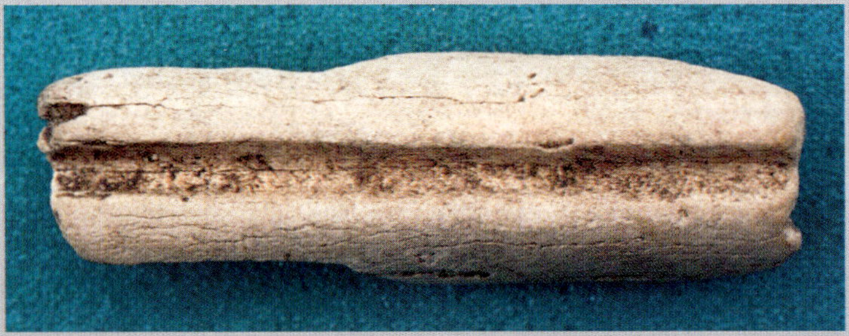

Antler tool, with $\frac{1}{8}$" wide groove. The artifact is $\frac{5}{8}$ x $2\frac{3}{16}$" long and the purpose is unknown. Woodland or later in time, Harwood found it between 1954 and 1956. Morgan County, Alabama. Collection of, and photograph by, Gary Henry, North Carolina. **$25.00.**

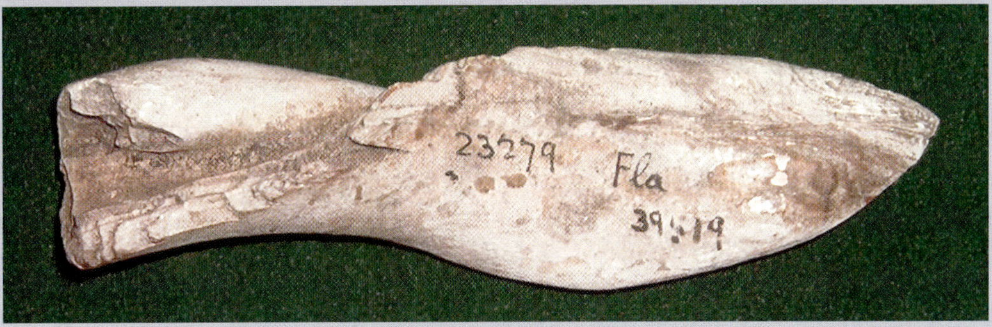

Tool, shell, 1½ x 5" long, blade-like end. This artifact is ex-collection Vietzen and from Florida. Keith and Rhonda Dodge collection, Michigan. **$85.00.**

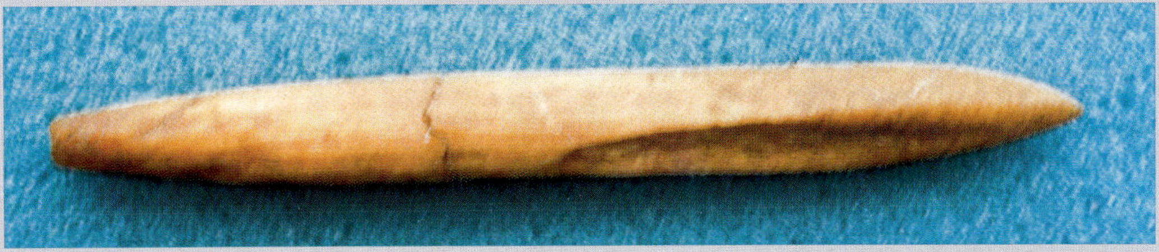

Pin, bone, Woodland or later, ¼ x 2³⁄₁₆". Such pins are often considered to be projectile points. Ex-collection Snyder, it came from Talladega County, Alabama. Collection of, and photograph by, Gary Henry, North Carolina. **$25.00.**

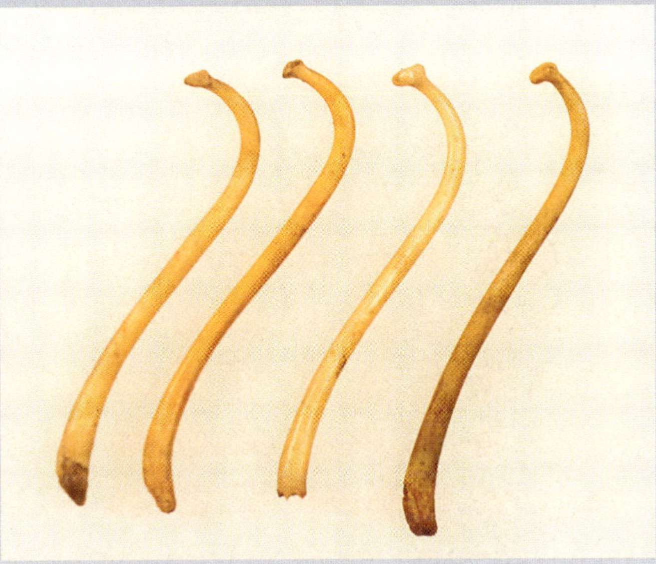

Raccoon penis bone pendants, Woodland period, longest is 4". Ex-collection Vietzen, the three examples on the left are pictured in his book *The Saga of Glover's Cave*. Christian County, Kentucky. Pete Timoch collection. Each, **$50.00.**

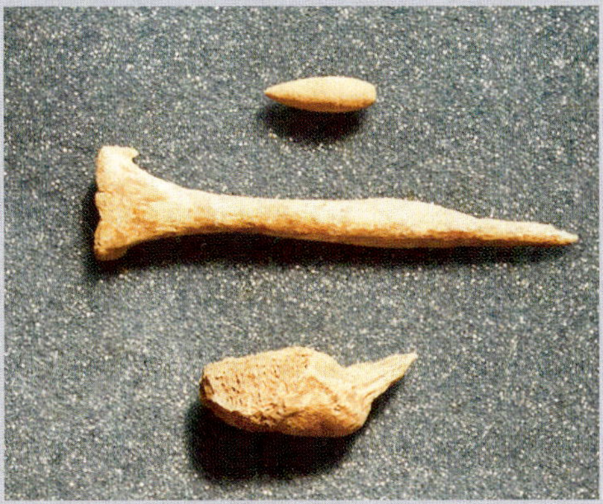

Pottery-making(?) tools, ¾ to 3" long. Probably used for finishing pottery vessels, they are (top to bottom), for puncturing, engraving and smoothing, and, engraving. The bone artifacts are historic Iroquois (Seneca), ca. 1650 – 1675. These were found near East Bloomfield, Ontario County, New York. Dave Summers collection, Victor, New York. The three, **$50.00.**

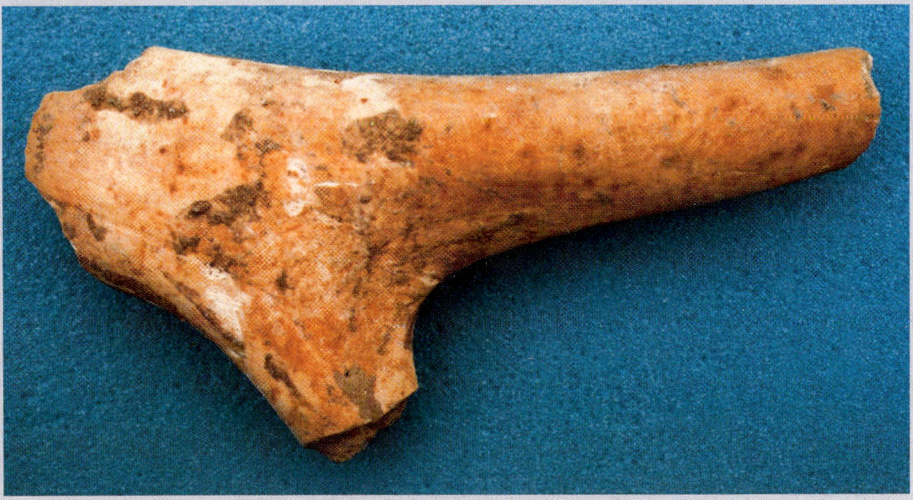

Antler preform(?) or material stock for artifacts, Woodland or Mississippian. Two of the tines have been removed and the remaining section is 2 x 4⅜". Ex-collection Snyder, it is from Meigs County, Tennessee. Collection of, and photograph by, Gary Henry, North Carolina. **$15.00.**

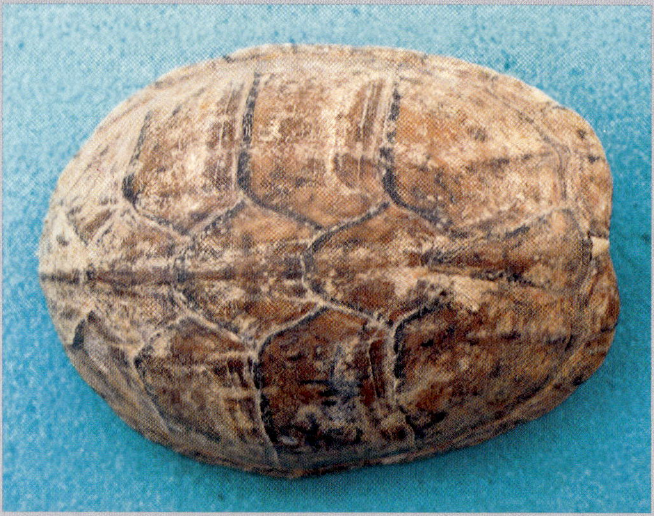

Rattle preform or rattle that has lost contents, (complete with plastron and carapace), 2¼ x 3⅛", 1⅜" high. Harwood found this land tortoise shell, Woodland or Mississippian, between 1954 and 1956. Collection of, and photograph by, Gary Henry, North Carolina. Unlisted.

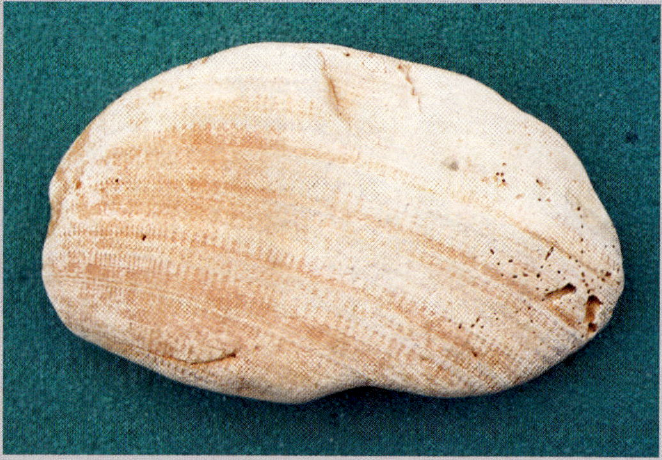

Pendant preform(?), mussel shell, Woodland or later, $1\frac{5}{16}$ x 2¼". The owner found this in 1987. Buncombe County, North Carolina. Collection of, and photograph by, Gary Henry, North Carolina. **$10.00.**

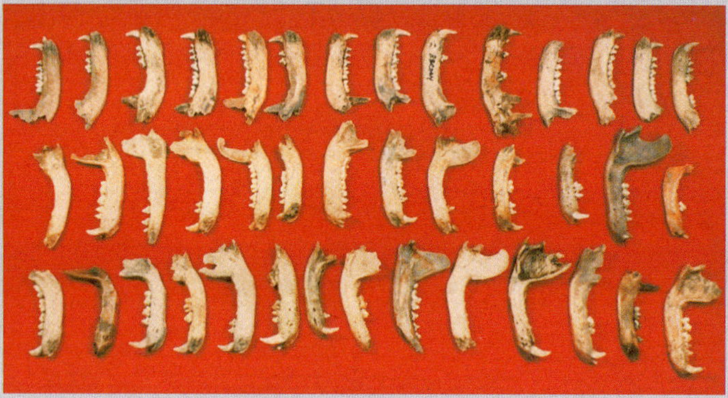

Mandible ornaments, mainly raccoon, longest is 3½". Many examples are notched as if for cord suspension, and comparable examples from Woodland to Mississippian times were drilled for the same purpose. Ex-collection Vietzen, Kentucky. Private collection. Unlisted.

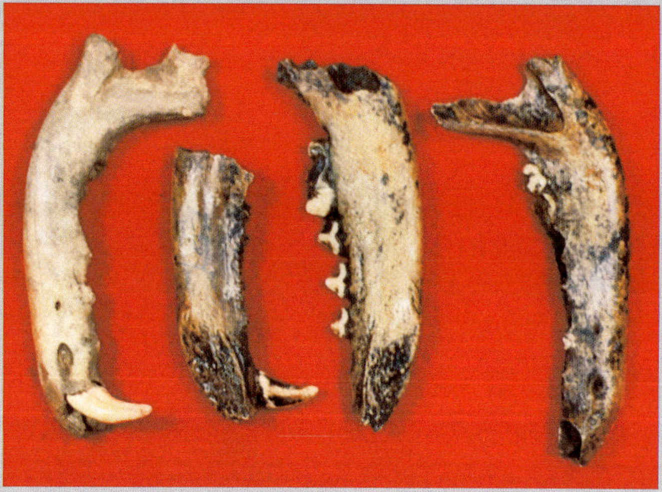

Ornaments or decorations, longest is 4¼", dog or wolf mandibles. Probably from the Woodland period, these have wear and polish. Ex-collection Vietzen, they are from Christian County, Kentucky. Private collection. Unlisted.

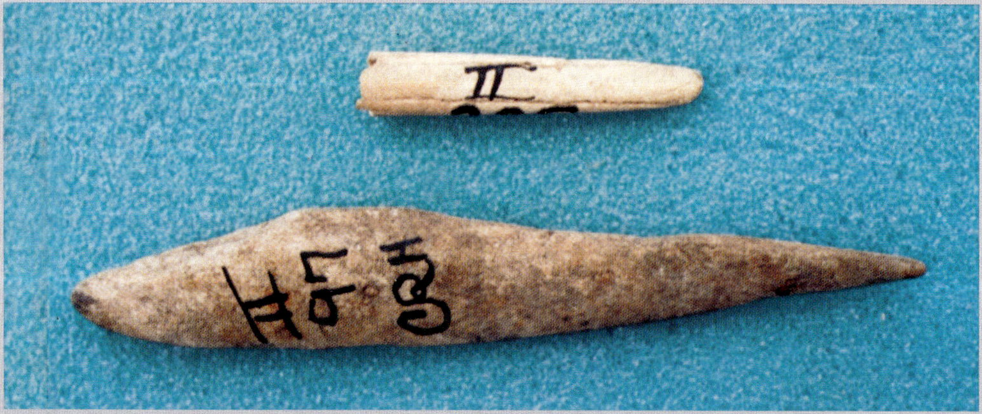

Bone tools, late prehistoric(?), both found by Harwood in 1954. At top is a flaker ⅜ x 1⅛"; bottom piece is an awl, ½ x $2\frac{7}{8}$". Morgan County, Alabama. Collection of, and photograph by, Gary Henry, North Carolina. Each, **$8.00 – 12.00.**

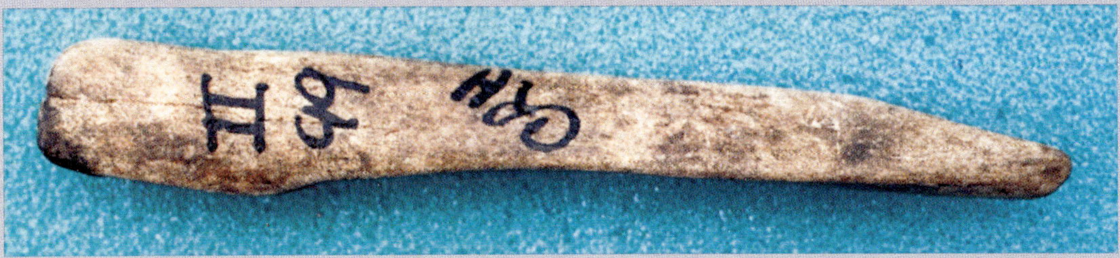

Bone flaker, Archaic or later, 3/8 x 27/8". Found by Harwood in 1954, it was picked up in Morgan County, Alabama. Collection of, and photograph by, Gary Henry, North Carolina. **$8.00.**

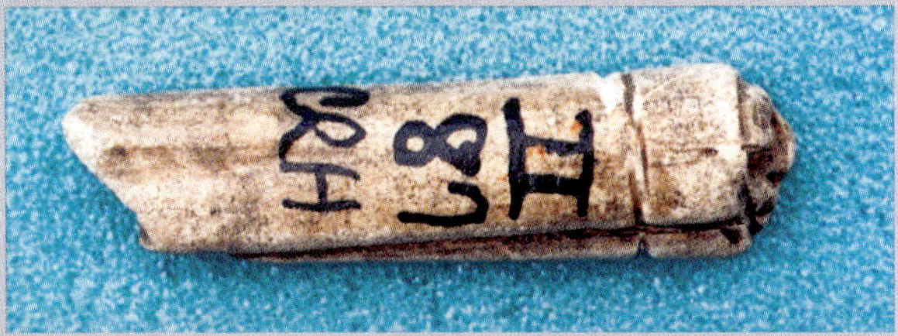

Bone fragment with cut marks, Woodland or later, 5/8 x 13/8". Found by Harwood in 1954, it is from Morgan County, Alabama. Collection of, and photograph by, Gary Henry, North Carolina. **$10.00.**

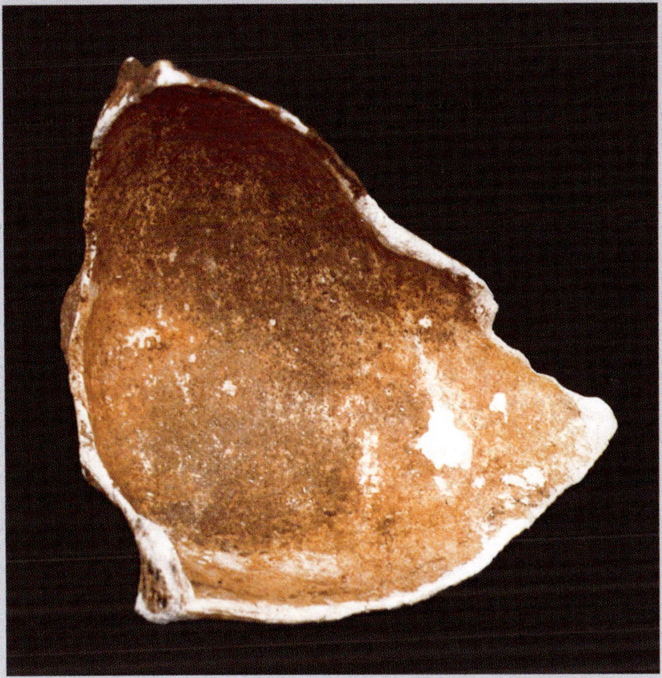

Conch shell dipper or bowl, Mississippian period, 57/8 x 65/8", 3½" deep. This example is ex-collection Snyder, who found it between 1947 and 1958 in Polk County, Tennessee. Collection of, and photograph by, Gary Henry, North Carolina. **$150.00.**

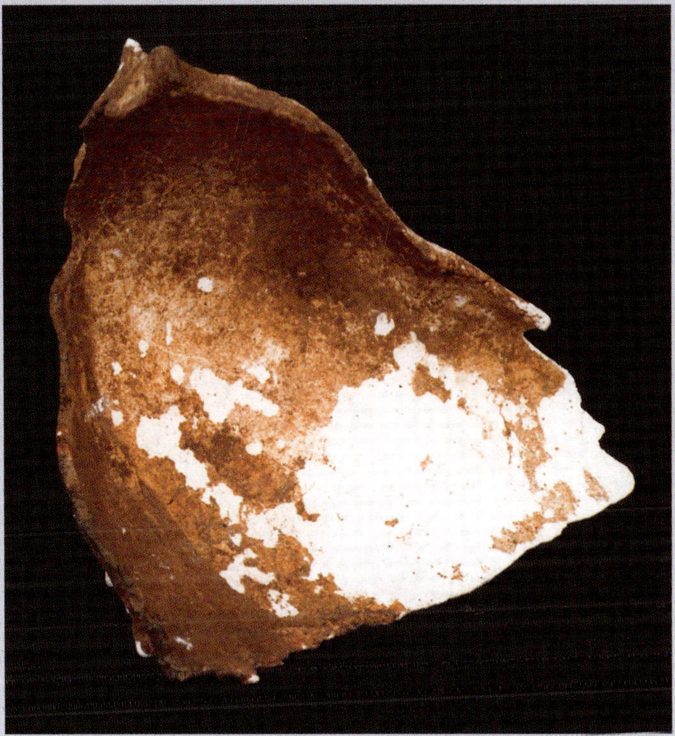

Conch shell dipper or bowl, Mississippian period. This large, cut example is 63/8 x 7½" and 3¾" deep. Once in the Snyder collection, it was found between 1947 and 1958 in Polk County, Tennessee. Collection of, and photograph by, Gary Henry, North Carolina. **$150.00.**

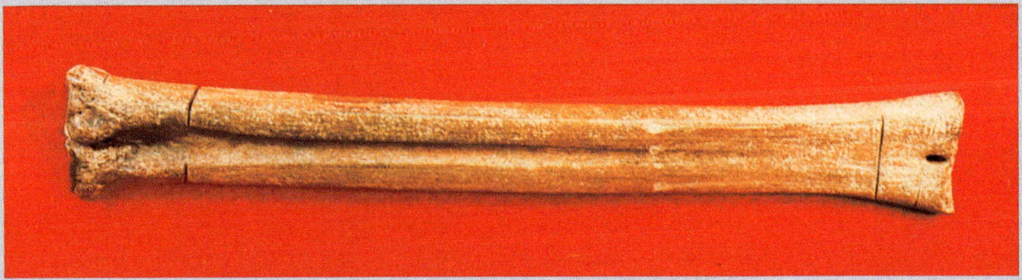

Beamer or hide-working tool, 71/8" long, deer leg bone. Mississippian in time, it is ex-collections Hovan and Sauer. This beamer has good form and wear, and there are cut-marks near each end. Most beamers were hard-used and are in broken condition. Ohio. Pete Timoch collection. **$200.00.**

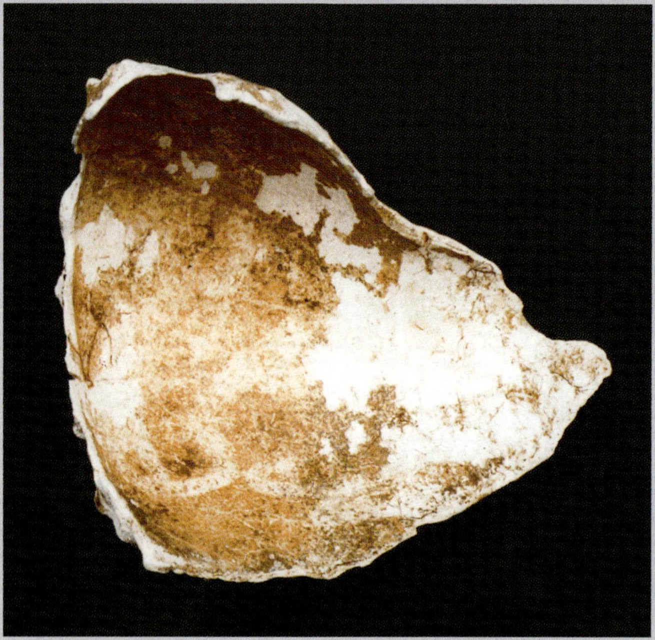

Conch shell dipper or bowl, Mississippian period. This utensil is 5¼ x 6¾" and 3" deep. Snyder found it between 1947 and 1958 in Polk County, Tennessee. Collection of, and photograph by, Gary Henry, North Carolina. **$150.00.**

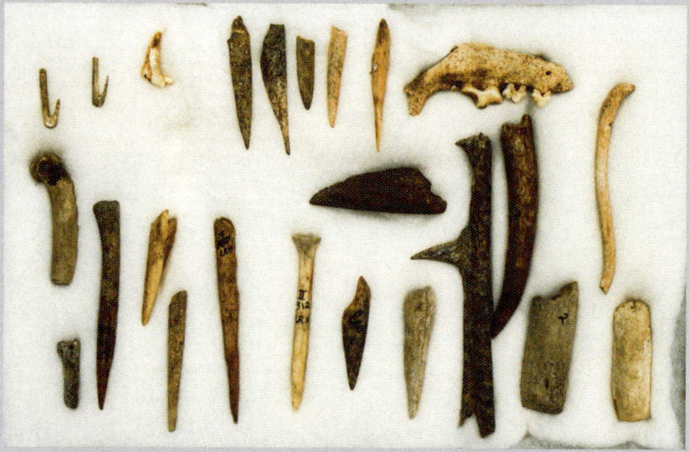

Bone and antler artifacts, Archaic or later, fishhooks, awls, a needle, a pendant, and other worked objects. This frame illustrates typical rock shelter and village midden contents. Harwood found all between 1954 and 1958. The artifacts came from Greene County, Tennessee, and Limestone and Morgan Counties, Alabama. Collection of, and photograph by, Gary Henry, North Carolina. Frame, **$600.00.**

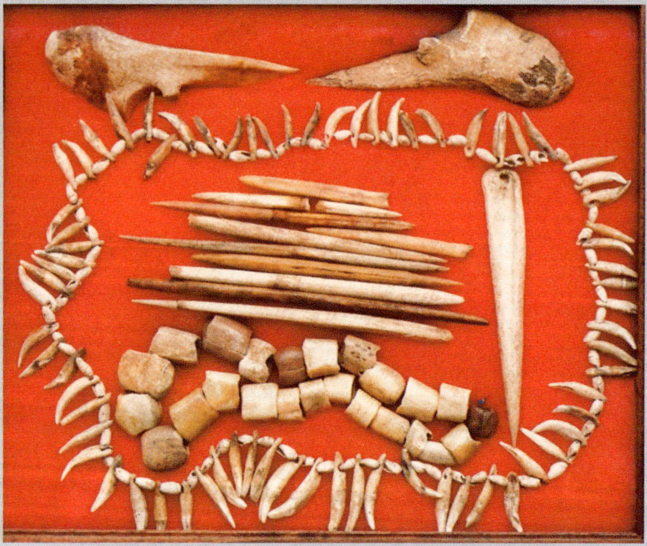

Artifacts, made of bone and teeth, Woodland or later. The beads consist of snail shells (72) and bobcat canines (72). The larger beads (24) are made of wild turkey leg bones and the largest bead is ⅜ x 1⁵⁄₁₆". The longest awl is 6", and the longest bobcat canine is 1¼ ". Ex-collection Snyder, this group is from Greene County, Tennessee. Collection of, and photograph by, Gary Henry, North Carolina. Group, **$1,500.00.**

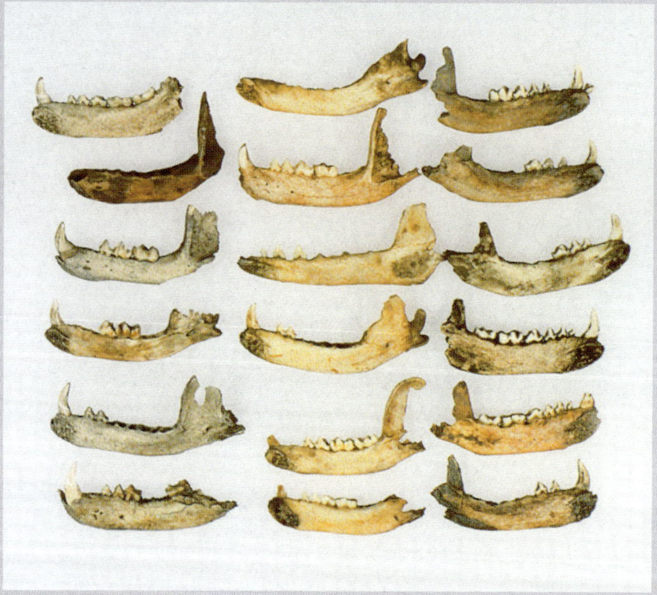

Ornaments or decorations, longest is 3½", mainly raccoon mandibles, Woodland or Mississippian period. Some are notched for cord suspension and all are from the Vietzen collection. Ohio and Kentucky. Private collection. Unlisted.

Marine shell disc beads, Frontenac phase of the Late Archaic, ca. 2000 BC. They are ¾" in diameter, nicely shaped, and polished. The beads were found near Cayuga Lake, Cayuga County, New York. Dave Summers collection, Victor, New York. Each, **$10.00.**

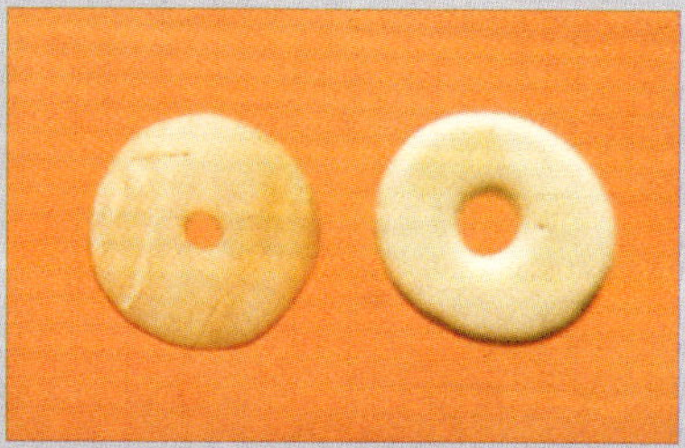

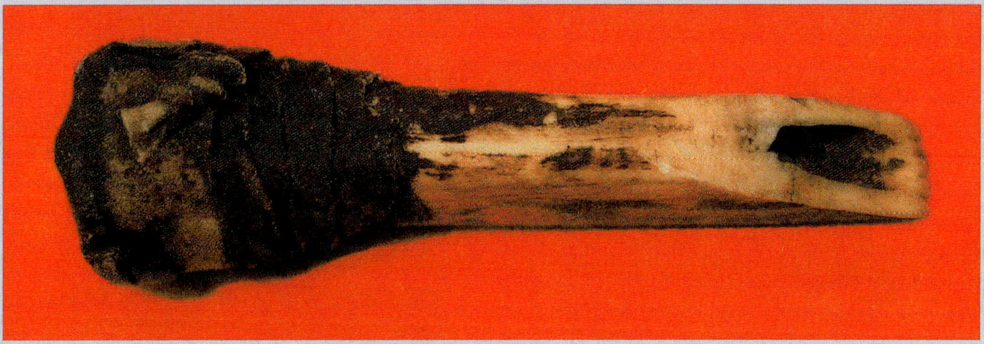

Bone hide-scraper, with rawhide handle wrap, size 2 x 9" long, 1¾" thick. This historic piece, with toothed working edge, is from Alpena, Michigan. Michael F. Slasinski collection, Michigan. **$325.00.**

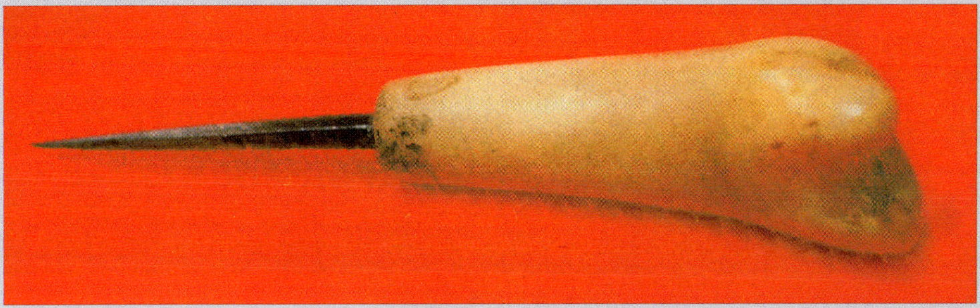

Awl, historic period, bone handle and metal tip, 3" long. It is from Ontario, Canada. Michael F. Slasinski collection, Michigan. **$125.00.**

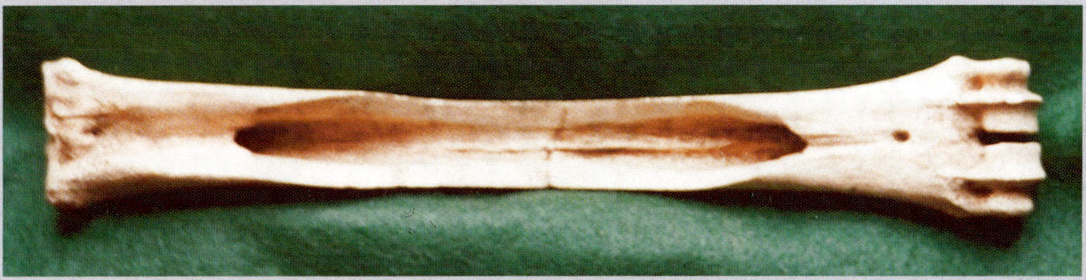

Beamer or drawshave, metapodial bone, 9" long. It is Mississippian in origin and was found in Page County, Virginia. Dave Summers collection, Victor, New York. **$150.00.**

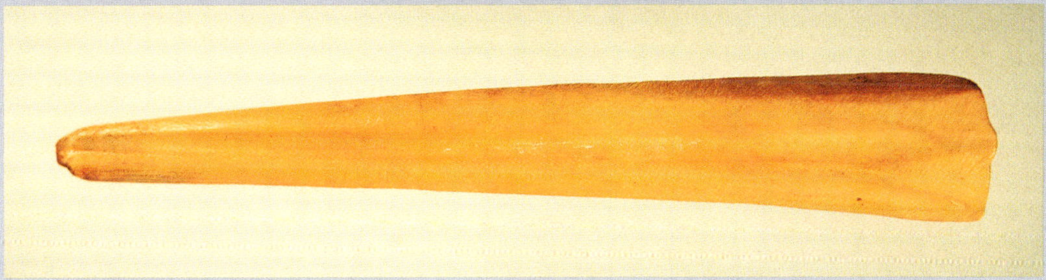

Awl or punch, blunted tip, ground section of large animal bone, chemically stabilized, 5⁵⁄₁₆" long. It is from Kentucky. Private collection. **$25.00.**

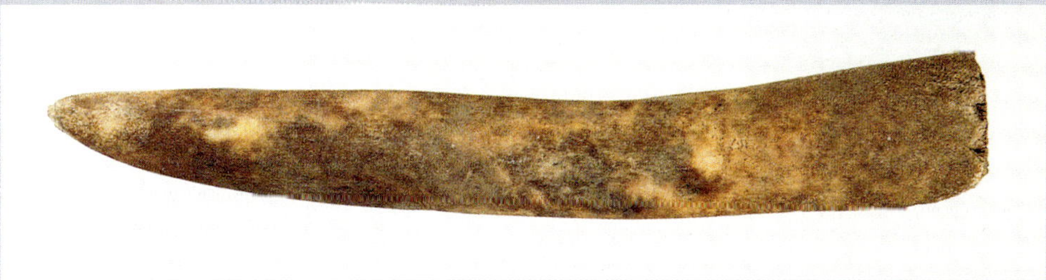

Dagger(?) or tool, animal bone, 4⅝". It has a mottled brown and cream patina and is ex-collection Hall. Wayne County, Kentucky. Private collection. **$15.00.**

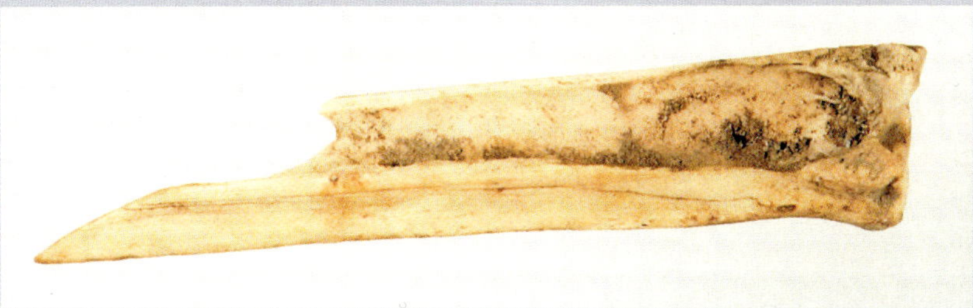

Awl, thick animal bone, tip formed along one side, 3⅝" long. It is ex-collection Hall. Wayne County, Kentucky. Private collection. **$12.00.**

Miscellaneous Artifacts

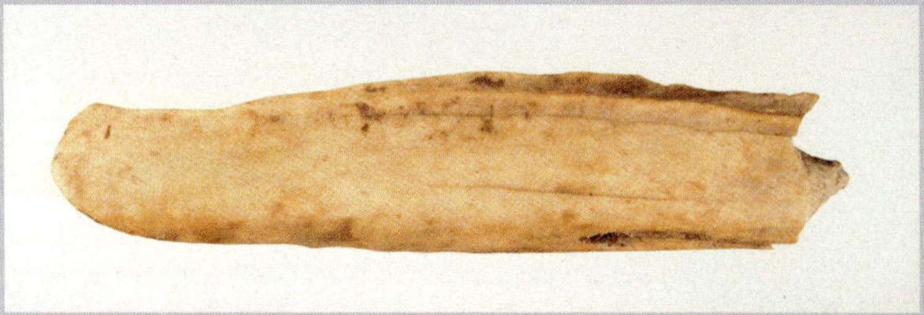

Tool, split animal bone, 3⅛" long. The working end is at bottom left and the blade edge is rounded. Ex-collection Hall, the artifact is from Wayne County, Kentucky. Private collection. **$15.00.**

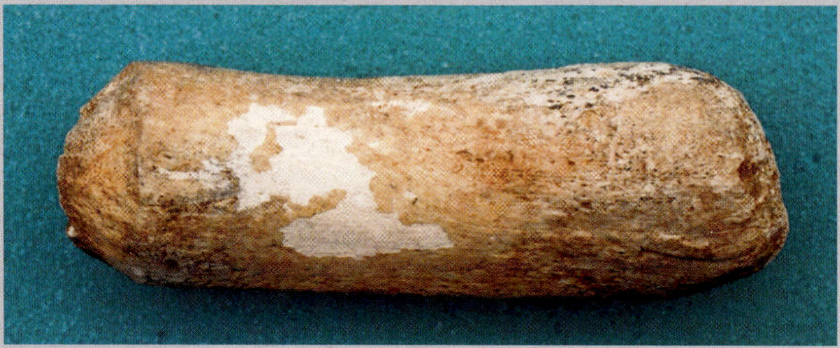

Bone handle with hole in one end, 1 x 3" long. Possibly an awl handle, it is Woodland or later in time. Ex-collection Snyder, it is from Talladega County, Alabama. Collection of, and photograph by, Gary Henry, North Carolina. **$40.00.**

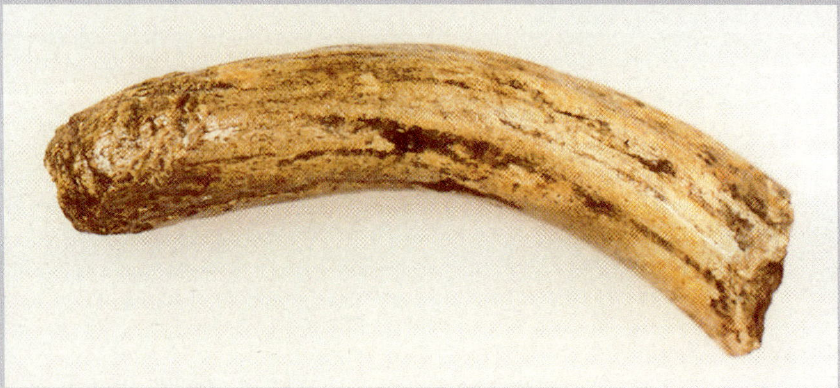

Antler effigy phallus, Late Archaic to Woodland, outside curve is 5½". Formerly in the Vietzen collection, it came from Christian County, Kentucky. Pete Timoch collection. Unlisted.

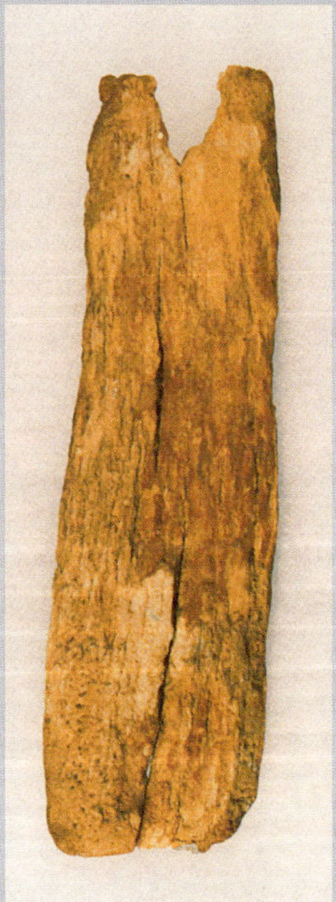

Bone hoe(?), Woodland or Mississippian period, 6⅛" long. A wooden handle would fit through the top hole, and the blade was perhaps lashed in position. Southwestern Kentucky. Pete Timoch collection. **$50.00 – 75.00.**

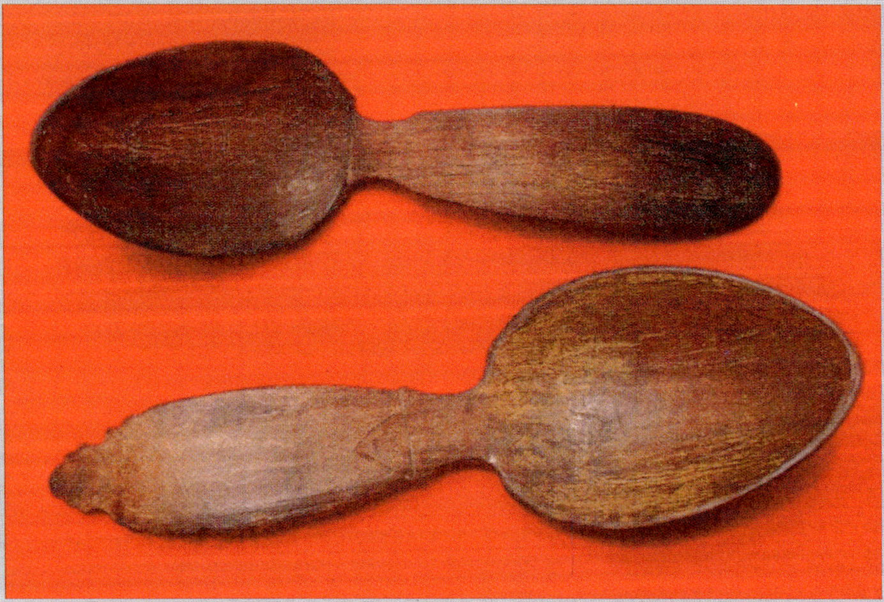

Horn spoons, larger specimen is 1¾ x 6½", ¾" deep. Probably historic Iroquois, these came from Pennsylvania. Michael F. Slasinski collection, Michigan. Each, **$225.00 – 300.00.**

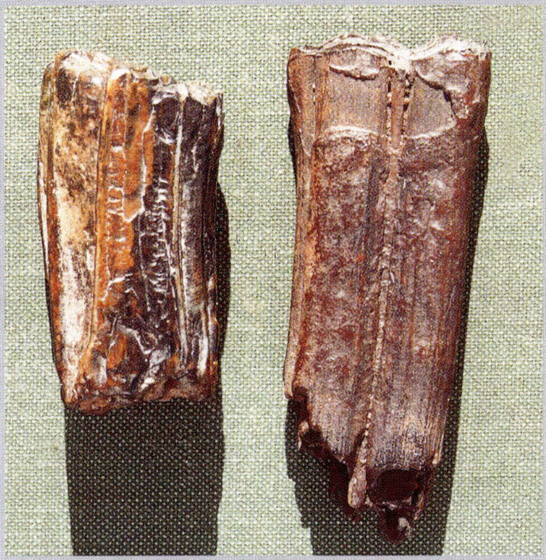

Large teeth, Pleistocene, water-stained. Paleo hunters probably lived at the same time as these Ice Age animals. Caloosahatchee River. Lee County, Florida. Dave Summers collection, Victor, New York. Each, **$50.00.**

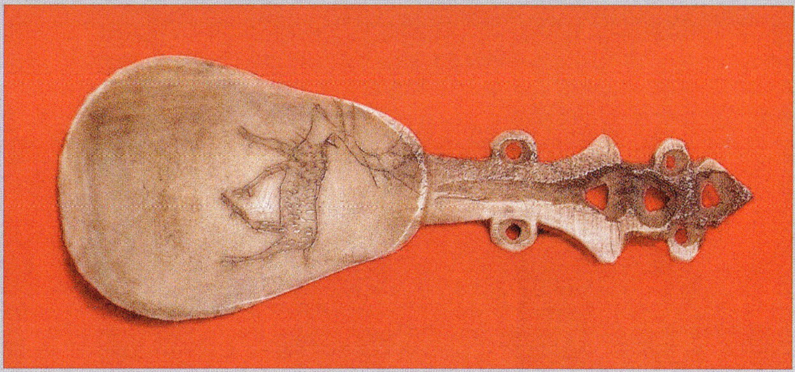

Horn spoon, 1 7/16 x 4" long, 5/32" thick. This artifact is well-made and decorated with an engraved animal, probably a caribou. The spoon is likely Cree Indian, from the North. Michael F. Slasinski collection, Michigan. **$500.00.**

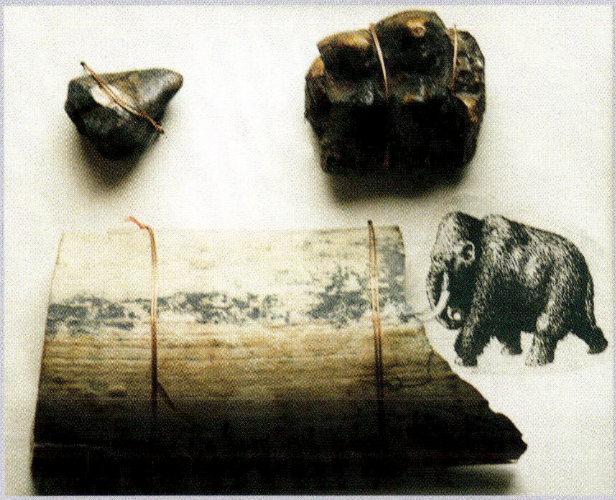

Pleistocene remains, mastodon tusk section and teeth, tusk is 10" long. Such Ice Age objects are rarely found, and these examples came from Orange County, New York. Dave Summers collection, Victor, New York. Three pieces in frame, **$400.00.**

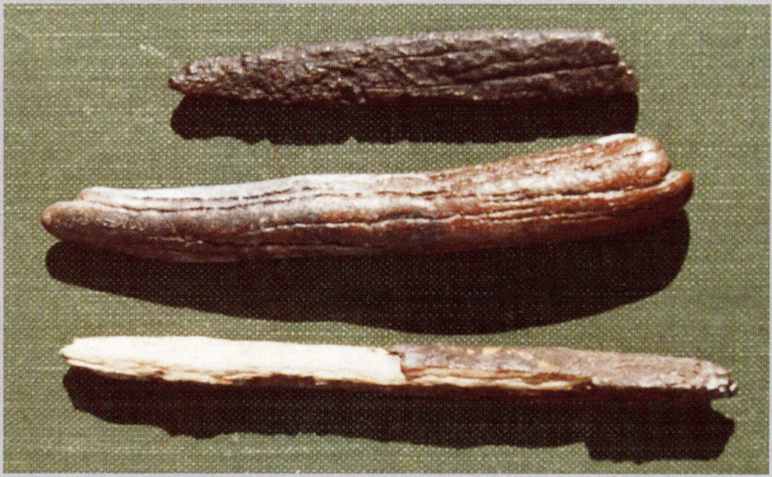

Pleistocene artifacts, rare, including a deer rib projectile point, bone awl, and bone chisel. From 3 1/8 to 4 1/2" long, these Ice Age objects are from the Caloosahatchee River, Lee County, Florida. Dave Summers collection, Victor, New York. All, **$500.00.**

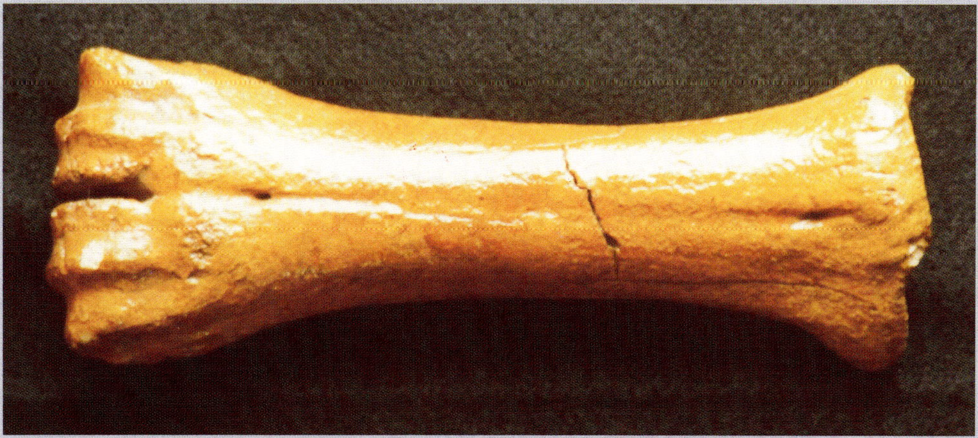

Pleistocene bison leg bone, 3 x 8". This Ice Age piece was found in Chautauqua County, New York. Dave Summers collection, Victor, New York. **$200.00.**

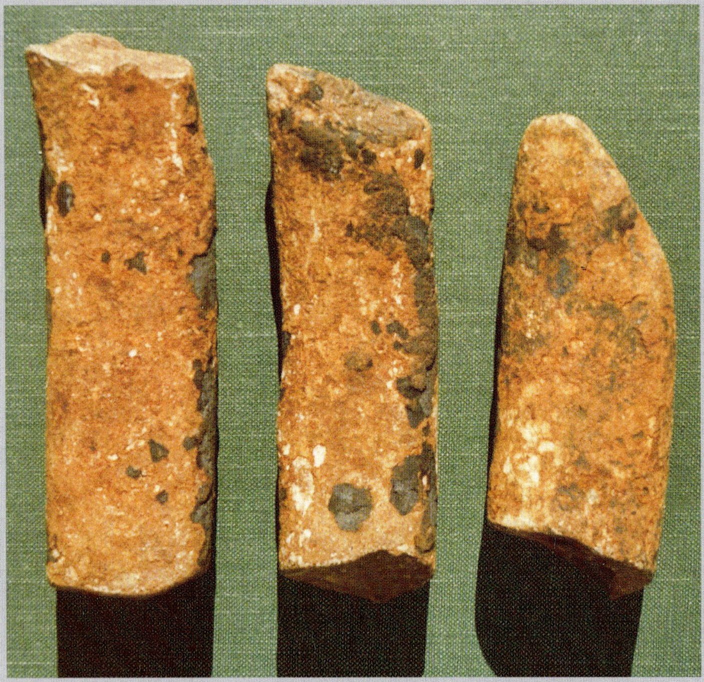

Pleistocene (Ice Age) mastodon rib sections, 4 to 4⅜" long. These were recovered in the Caloosahatchee River, Lee County, Florida. Dave Summers collection, Victor, New York. All, **$100.00.**

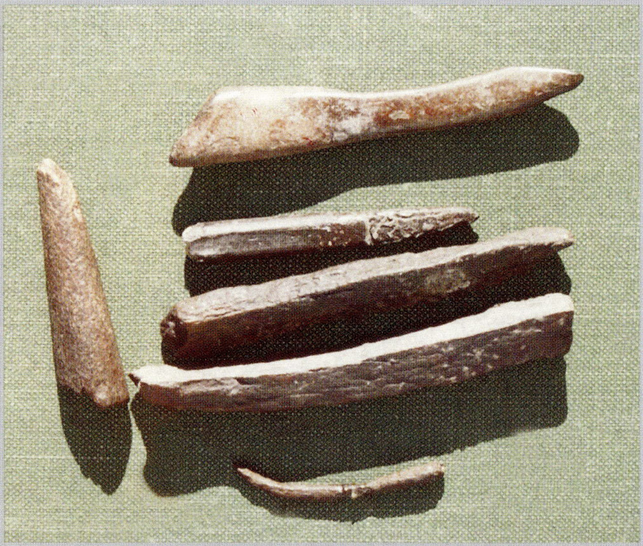

Pleistocene (Ice Age) bone, split bone awls and an antler tip, 1½ to 3" long. All were found in the Caloosahatchee River, Lee County, Florida. Dave Summers collection, Victor, New York. All, **$450.00.**

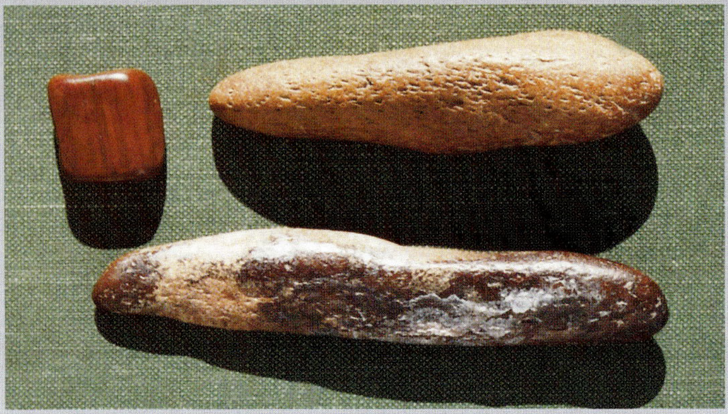

Pleistocene (Ice Age) ivory charmstone(?), plus two sections of mastodon bones, longest piece 4". These were recovered from the Caloosahatchee River, Lee County, Florida. Dave Summers collection, Victor, New York. Ivory charm, **$150.00;** bones, each **$25.00.**

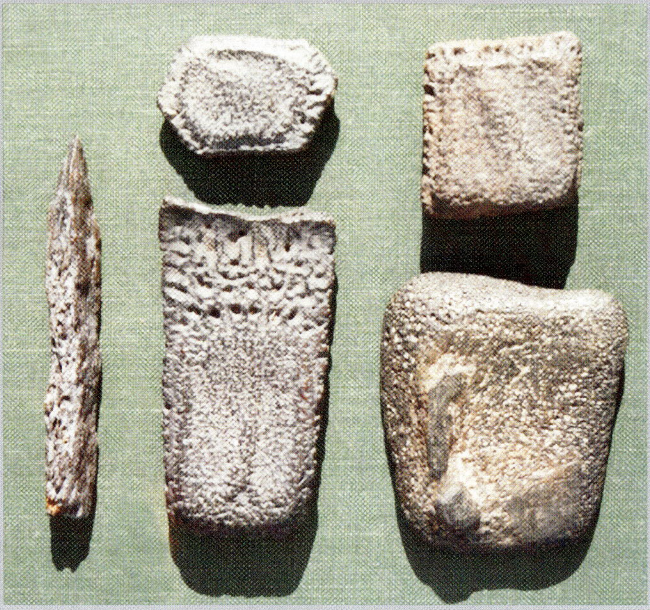

Pleistocene (Ice Age) animal remains, turtle bone and shell pieces plus a deer bone split to a point. The awl-like artifact is 3" long. All were found in the Caloosahatchee River, Lee County, Florida. Dave Summers collection, Victor, New York. All, **$70.00.**

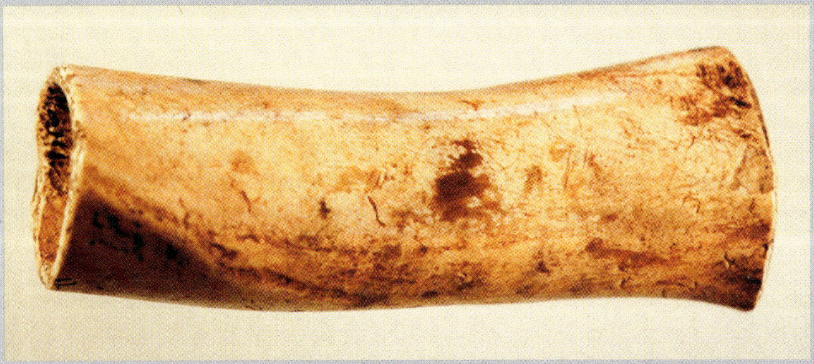

Handle, large animal bone, highly polished exterior, 3⅜" long. This tool part is ex-collection Tolliver and came from Hocking County, Ohio. Private collection. **$200.00.**

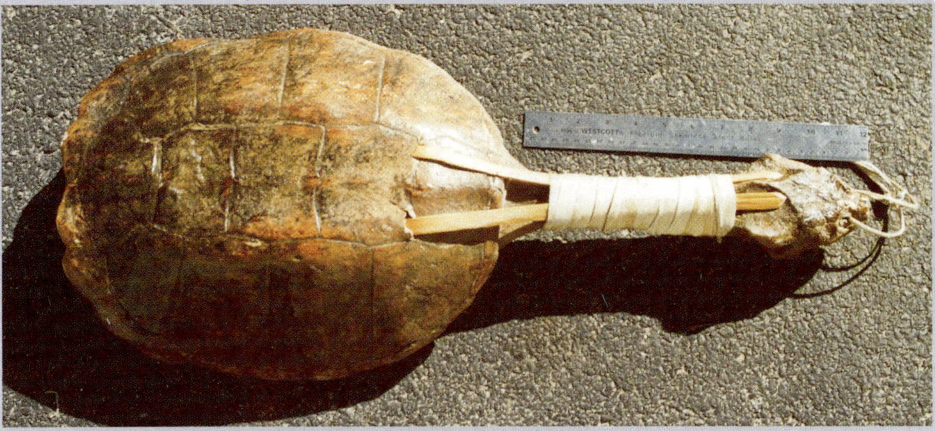

Snapping turtle rattle, large size at 27" long, late historic Iroquois. This well-made piece is from New York state. Dave Summers collection, Victor, New York. **$500.00.**

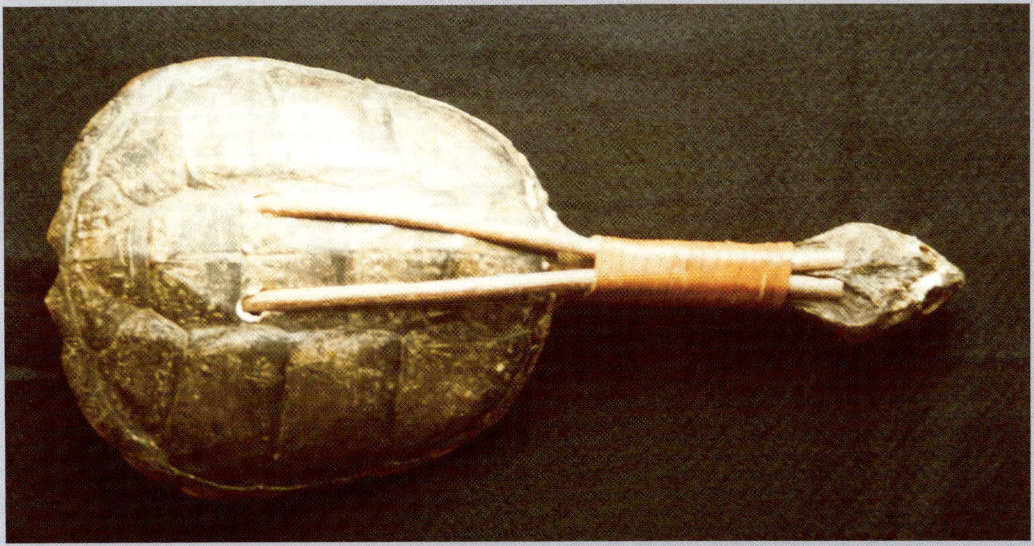

Snapping turtle rattle, 16" long. It is Mohawk, ca. 1950, from the St. Regis Reservation. Franklin County, New York. Dave Summers collection, Victor, New York. **$200.00.**

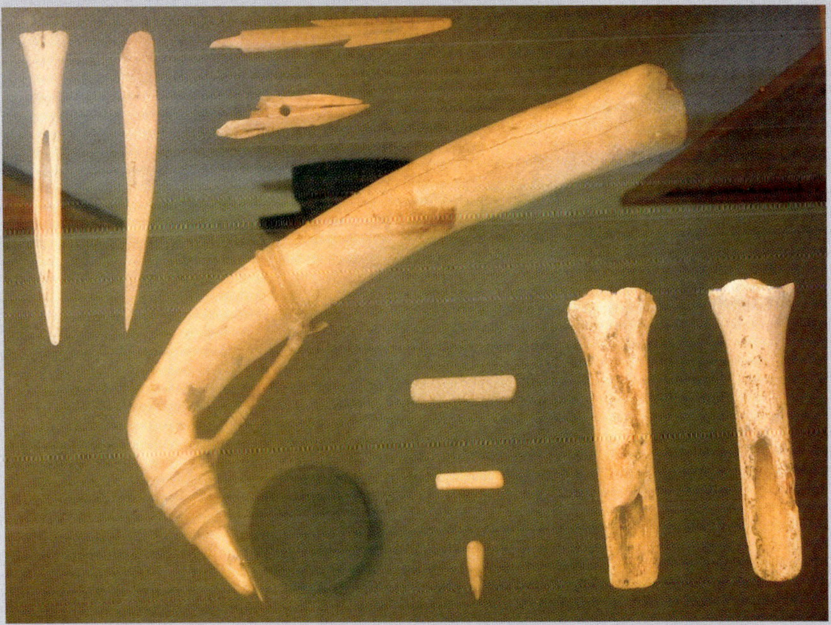

Frame of bone artifacts, pieces include awls, harpoon heads, flakers, gouges, and a large elk antler Plains-type scraper. Rod Fuller collection, Nebraska. Unlisted.

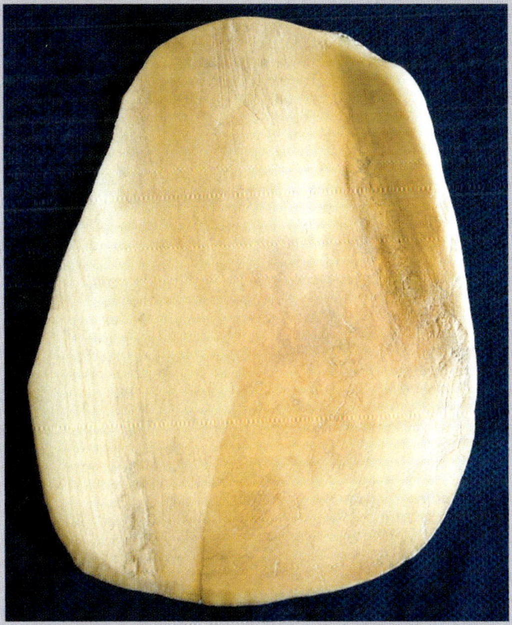

Squash knife, buffalo shoulder blade, widest end (at bottom) with thin blade edge. This specialized knife form is 4¾" high, from near Mobridge, South Dakota. Rod Fuller collection, Nebraska. **$100.00 – 125.00.**

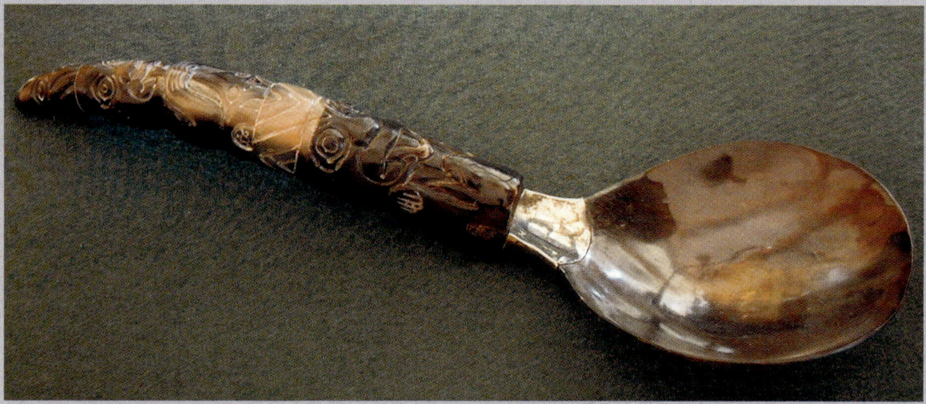

Spoon or ladle, bison or bighorn sheep, 11" long. This artistic example in Northwest Coast style has a silver fastening/ornamental band. Unalakleet, Alaska. Rod Fuller collection. Museum grade.

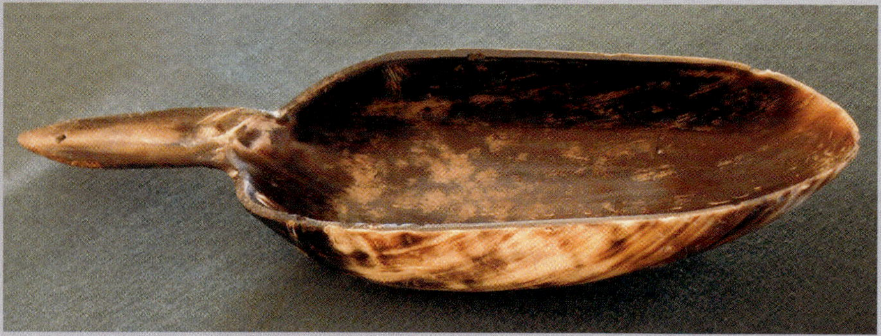

Buffalo (bison) horn scoop, well-made, fine condition, 11½" long. From the Conrad area, Montana. Rod Fuller collection, Nebraska. **$350.00 – 400.00.**

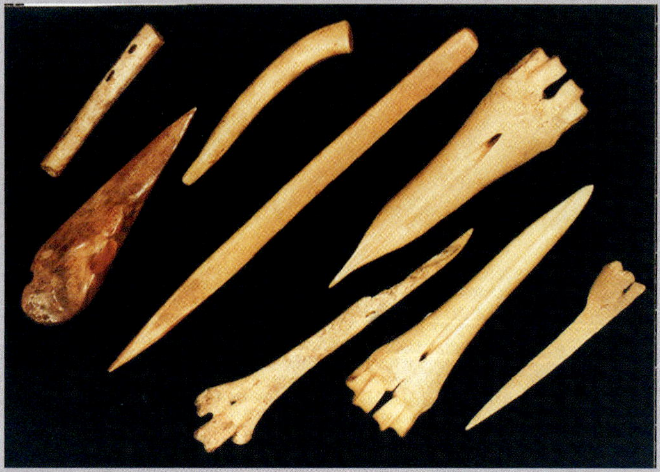

Bone artifacts, including awls, punches, reamers, and flint-knapping tools. There is also a three-hole flute at upper left. These came from a Fort Ancient site in Madison County, Kentucky. First Mesa, Indiana. Each, **$50.00 – 250.00.**

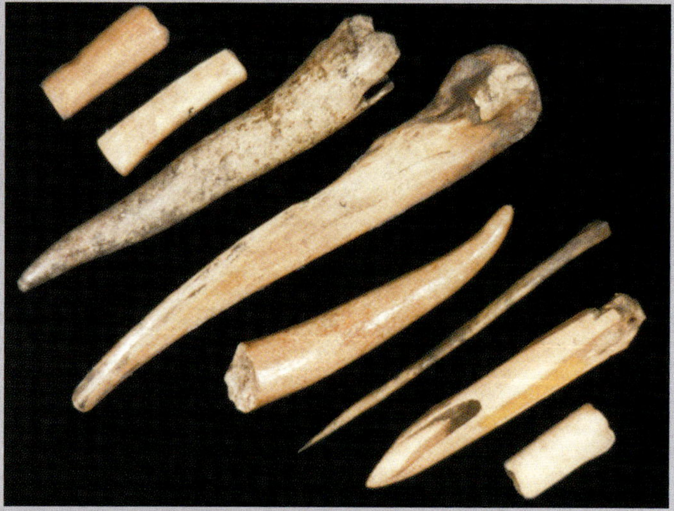

Bone artifacts, including beads, awls, needles, and flaking tools. Most have high use polish. These came from sites in Greene and Sullivan Counties, Indiana. First Mesa, Indiana. Each, **$20.00 – 95.00.**

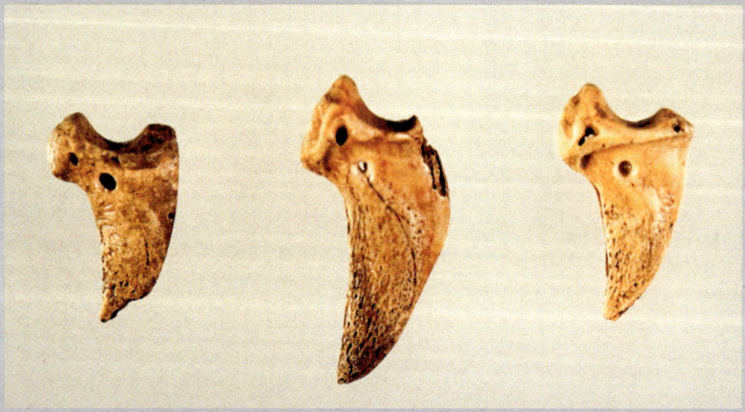

Bear claw cores, longest is 1⅜", each is drilled for suspension. These are rare pieces. Ex-collection Tolliver from Hocking County, Ohio. Private collection. Each, **$20.00 – 30.00.**

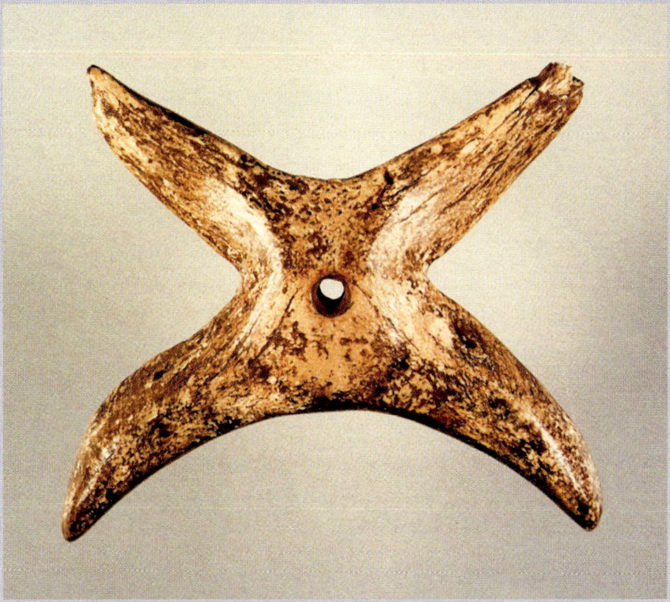

Ornament, probably a section of elk shoulder bone. The piece is 3⅝" wide, ⅜" thick. Of unknown purpose or use, it is ex-collection Tolliver. Hocking County, Ohio. Private collection. Museum grade.

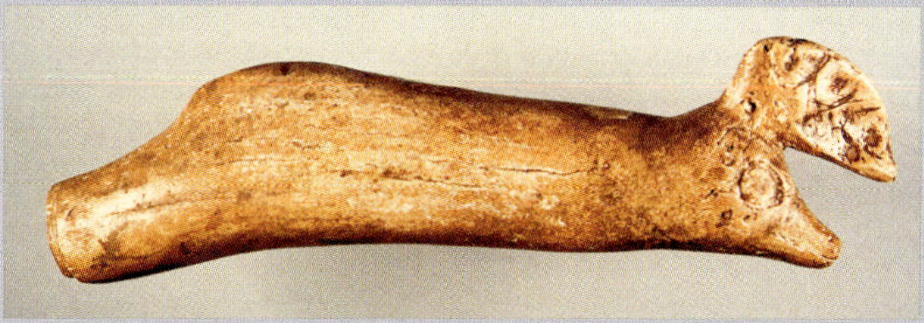

Elk antler effigy handle or staff finial, central hole in base, 7⅛" long. It probably represents an elk; antlers are depicted on both sides of the crest-like projection over the head. Ex-collection Tolliver, Hocking County, Ohio. Private collection. Museum grade.

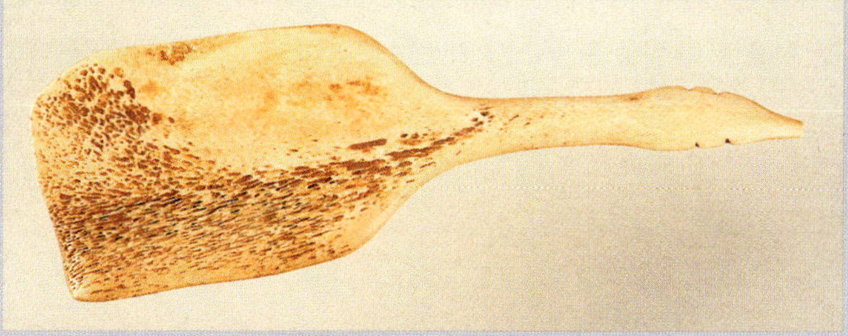

Awl or fork and spoon combination, 5³⁄₁₆" long, handle with notched decoration. Bone or antler, it is a rare artifact type. Ex-collection Tolliver, Hocking County, Ohio. Private collection. Museum grade.

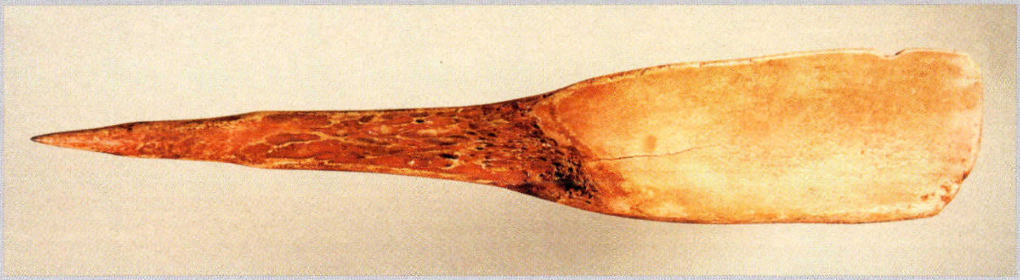

Awl or fork and spoon combination, large size at 8⅝". The spoon bowl (if that is what it is) has smoothness from wear. This piece is ex-collection Tolliver, who explored many sandstone rock shelters years ago. Hocking County, Ohio. Private collection. Museum grade.

Flaker, elk antler, 5⅝" long. It is ex-collection Selb, from West Virginia. Doug Hooks collection. **$25.00.**

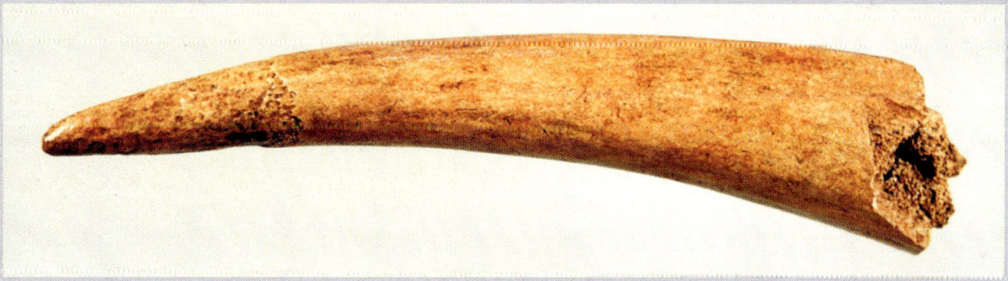

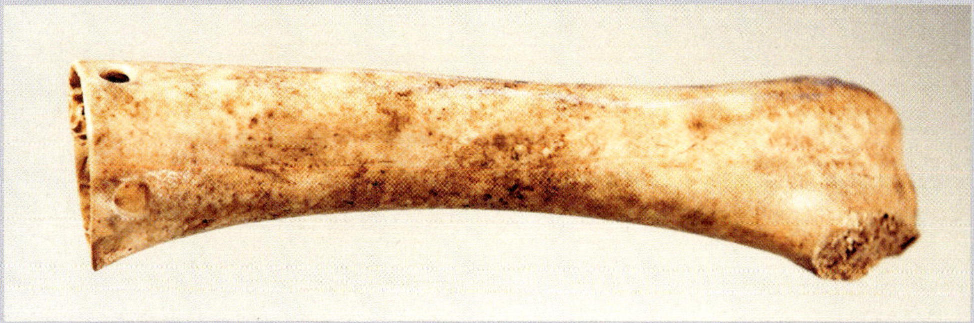

Handle(?), glossy animal bone, 4⅝" long. It has three drilled holes near the cut end, two close together. This polished example is ex-collection Tolliver, Hocking County, Ohio. Private collection. **$225.00.**

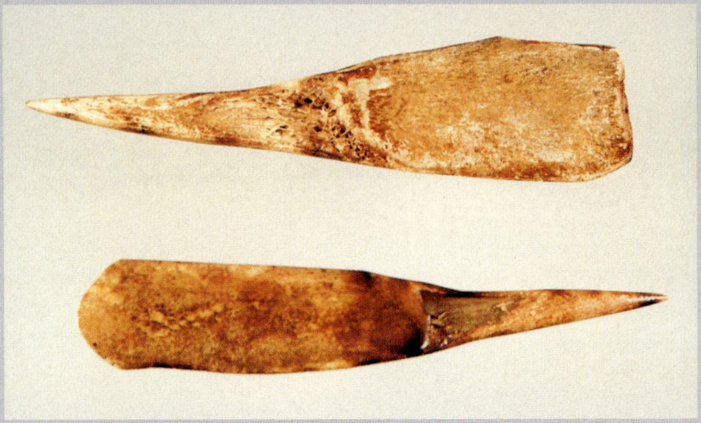

Awl or fork and spoon combinations, longest 4½". These are very unusual tools that may have been eating utensils. Possibly a spoon and one-tine fork, they are ex-collection Tolliver, Hocking County, Ohio. Private collection. Museum grade.

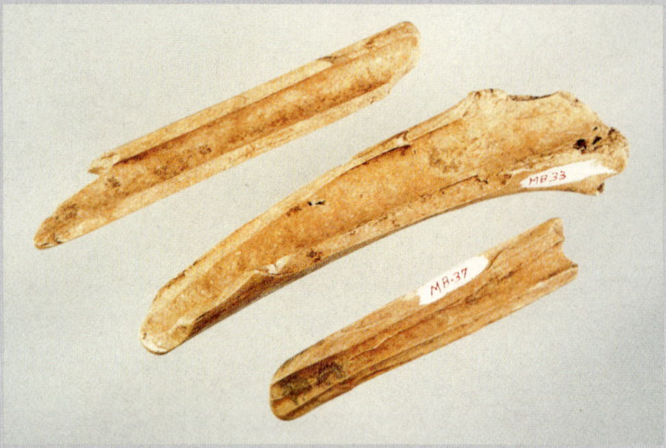

Splinter tools, elk bones, center example is 5¼" long. These have extensive use-wear at one end. West Virginia. Doug Hooks collection. Each, **$15.00 – 25.00.**

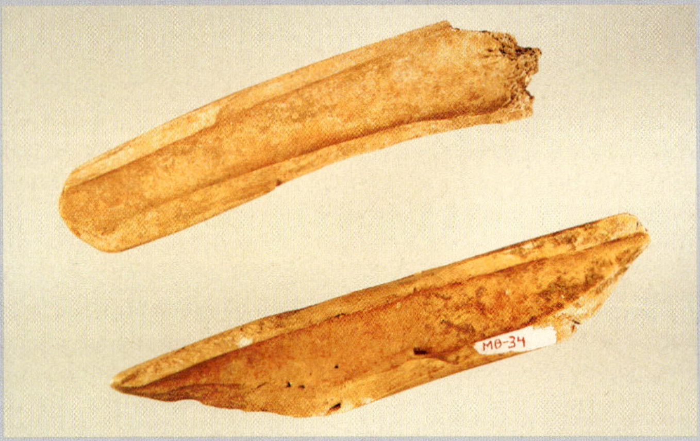

Elk bone splinter tools, (judging by size and wall thickness), longest is 5⅟₁₆". Heavily worn at one end, they are ex-collection, Selb, West Virginia. Doug Hooks collection. Top, **$20.00.** Bottom, **$12.00 – 15.00.**

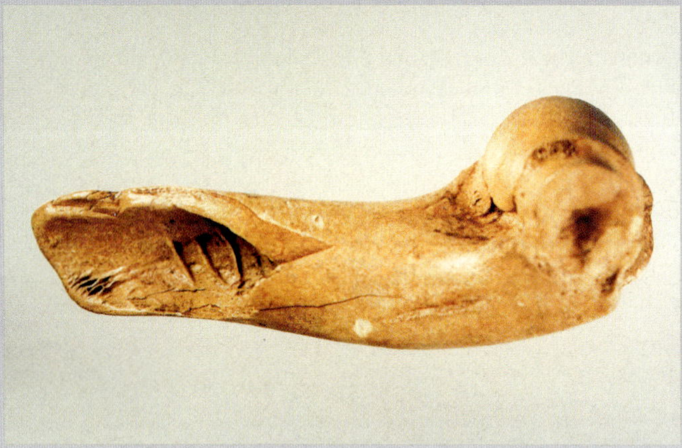

Gouge, joint and shaft of elk bone, smaller working end with much wear and polish. The tool is 5⅟₁₆" long. Ex-collection Selb, West Virginia. Doug Hooks collection. **$35.00 – 45.00.**

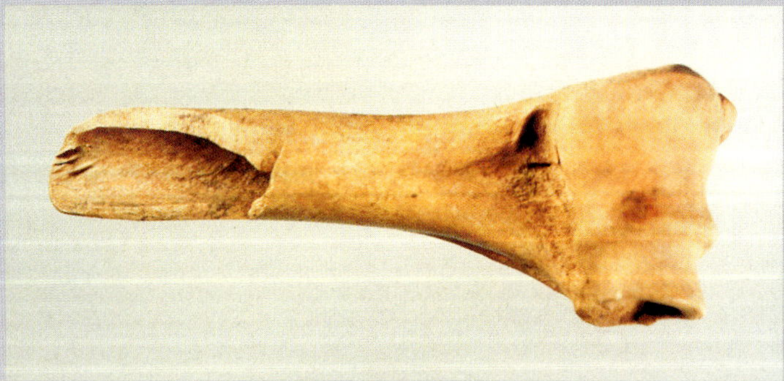

Gouge, joint and shaft of elk bone, rounded end with much wear, 4⅞" long. Ex-collection Selb, West Virginia. Doug Hooks collection. **$25.00 – 35.00.**

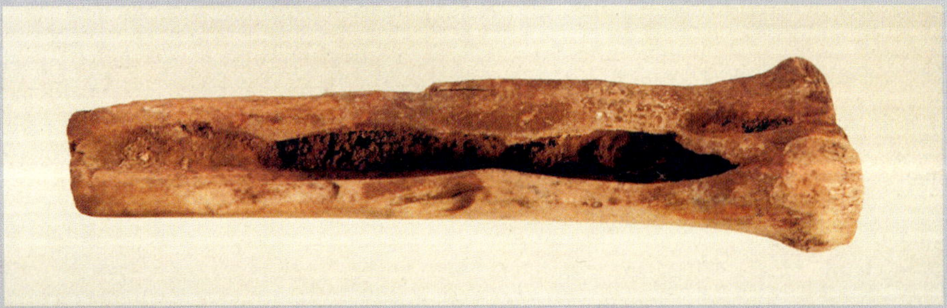

Deer bone gouge, squared and polished working edge, 4¼" long. It was found in Wayne County, Kentucky. Private collection. **$30.00.**

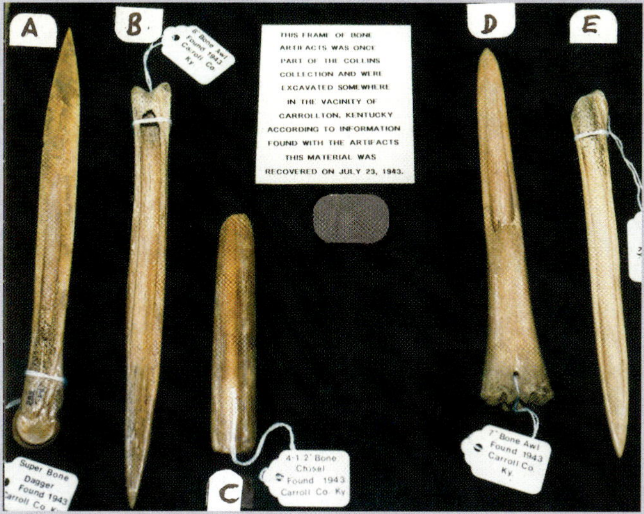
A
B
C
D
E
THIS FRAME OF BONE ARTIFACTS WAS ONCE PART OF THE COLLINS COLLECTION AND WERE EXCAVATED SOMEWHERE IN THE VACINITY OF CARROLLTON, KENTUCKY ACCORDING TO INFORMATION FOUND WITH THE ARTIFACTS THIS MATERIAL WAS RECOVERED ON JULY 23, 1943.
Super Bone Dagger Found 1943
8" Bone Awl Found 1943 Carroll Co Ky
4-1/2" Bone Chisel Found 1943 Carroll Co. Ky
7" Bone Awl Found 1943 Carroll Co. Ky

Fine bone artifacts, all ex-collection Garvin and found in July of 1943. A) is a fine bone dagger, and B) is another dagger 8" long. C) is a scarce bone chisel 4½" long. D) is a large bone dagger 7" long, while E) is a bone awl or dagger 7¼" long. All were found near Carrollton, Kentucky. Back to Earth photo, Robin Fiser collection. Each, **$100.00 – 225.00.**

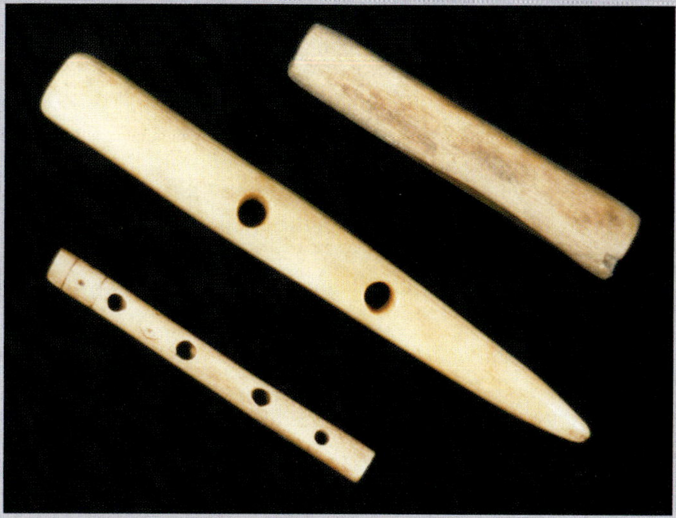

Bone artifacts, all with use polish and in top condition. There is a 2½" long bone bead, a 4½" long drilled, specialized tool of some sort, and a 2½" long engraved, four-hole flute or flageolet. All are from Greene County, Indiana. First Mesa, Indiana. Bead, **$50.00;** tool, **$225.00;** flageolet, **$300.00.**

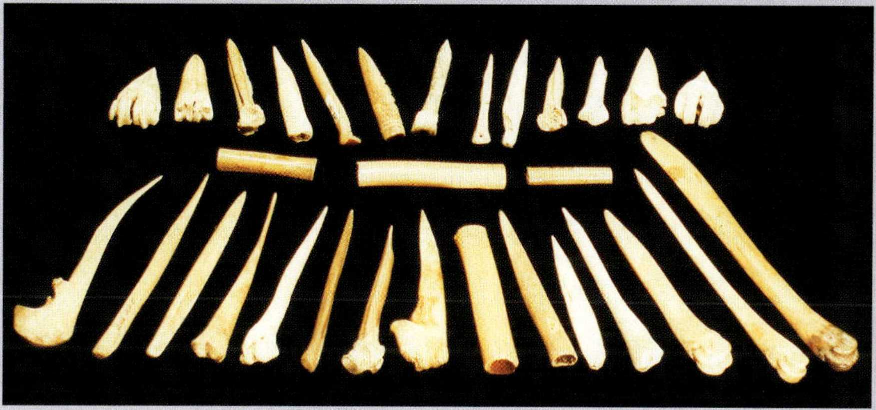

Bone artifacts, Fort Ancient culture, many pieces with use polish. Represented are deer leg bone awls, turkey leg bone awls, needles, beads, trigger awls, and split deer bone tools. Size range is from 2½ to 9", and all are from a site in Mason County, Kentucky. First Mesa, Indiana. Each, **$25.00 – 175.00.**

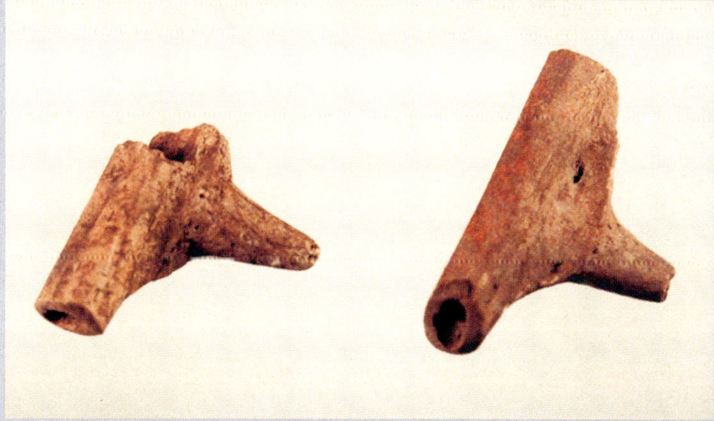

Wild turkey leg bone sections with spurs attached, (cut off at either side of spurs), longest example is 1½". These are tool parts or beads. Wayne County, Kentucky. Private collection. Each, **$10.00 – 15.00.**

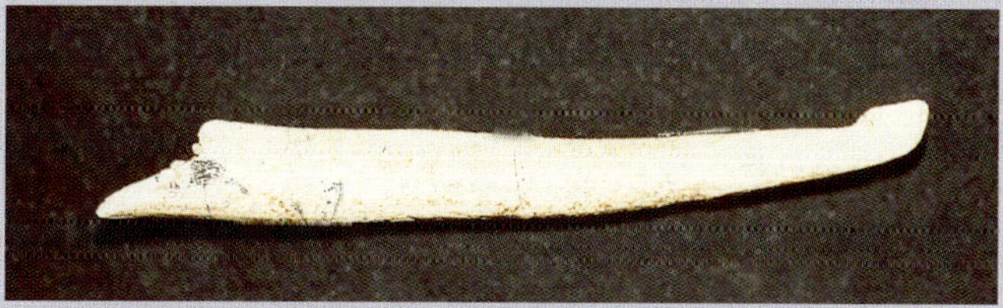

Deer antler Atl-atl hook, 8½" long. These artifacts are, perhaps, the rarest objects made from antler in prehistoric North America. Northwestern Arkansas. Kenneth Hamilton collection, Arkansas. Museum grade.

Miscellaneous Artifacts

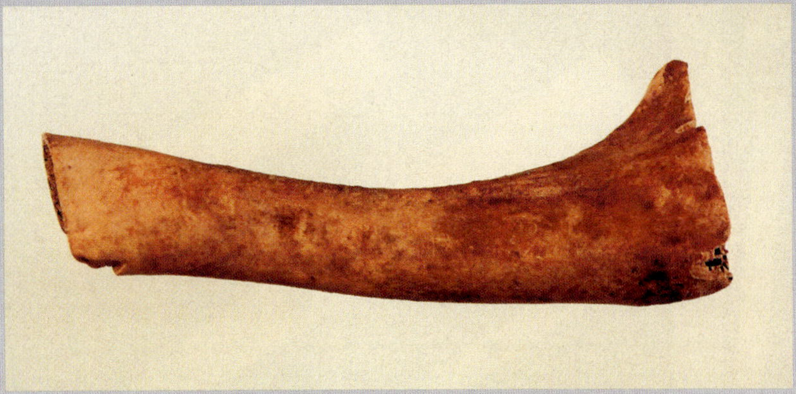

Handle(?), large bone with smaller end ground off, 4 1/16". The shaft is polished on this piece, found in Wayne County, Kentucky. Private collection. **$30.00.**

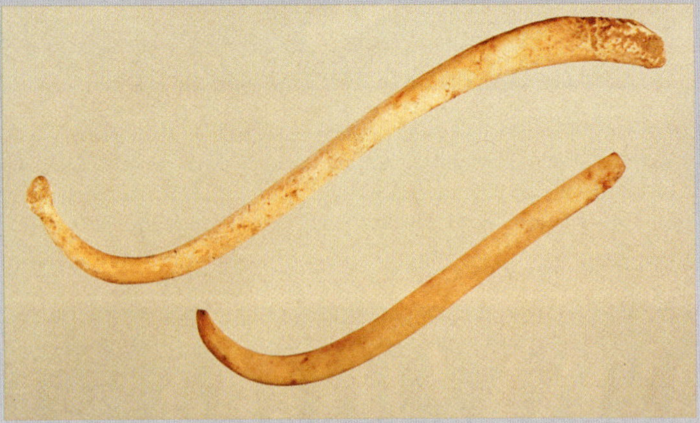

Raccoon penis bones, top specimen in natural form, 4" long. The bottom piece is worked, and the smaller end has been ground to a tip. Wayne County, Kentucky. Private collection. Top, unlisted; bottom, **$15.00.**

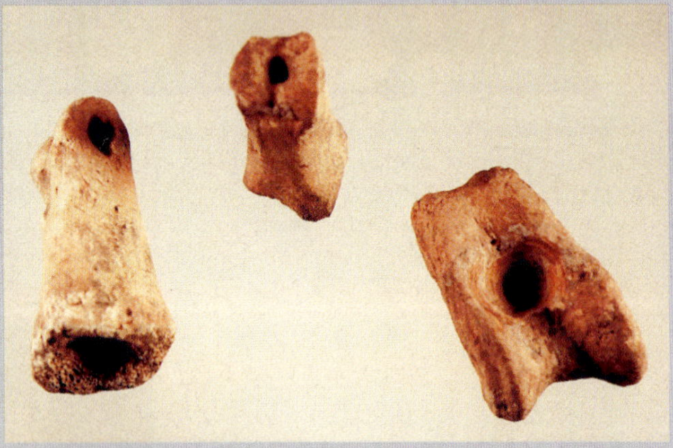

Deer foot bones, each drilled in a different manner, the longest is 1¾". They came from Wayne County, Kentucky. Private collection. Each, **$10.00 – 15.00.**

Antler tool, spike buck, 4¾" long. The tip on this antler has been ground at an angle. Wayne County, Kentucky. Private collection. **$20.00.**

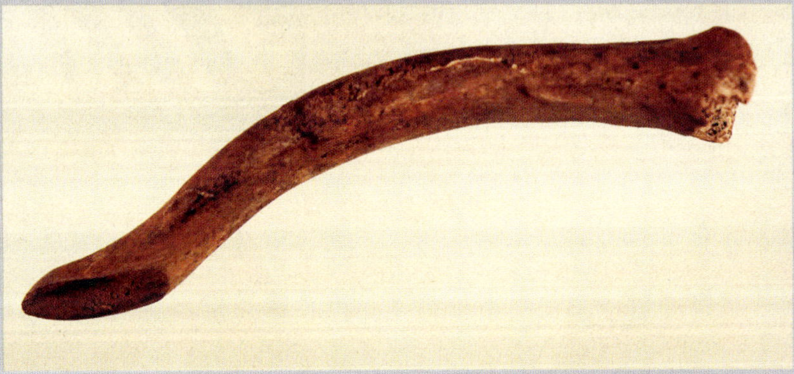

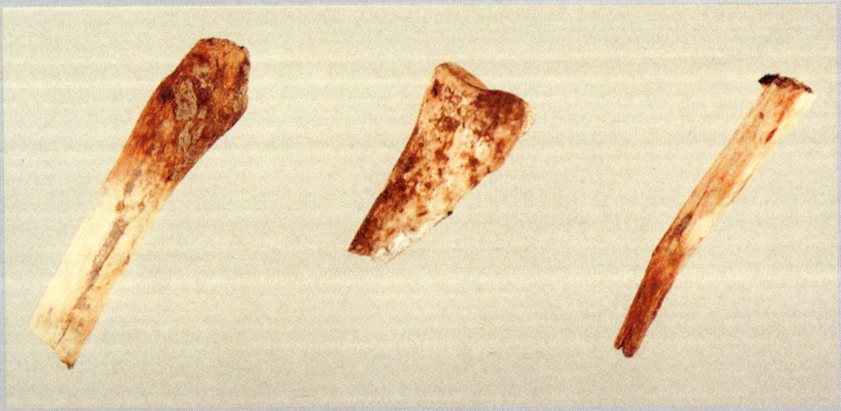

Broken bone artifacts, typical of many pieces found on prehistoric sites that are protected from the elements. The longest example is 1⅞". Wayne County, Kentucky. Private collection. Unlisted.

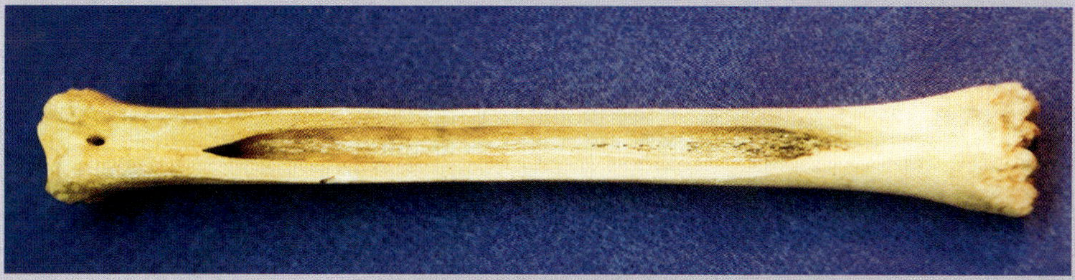

Deer legbone flesher or beamer, 9¼" long. These typically are found on Woodland and Mississippian sites, and complete examples are quite scarce. This fine example is drilled at one end, perhaps to be worn or transported. Fulton County, Illinois. Fred Smith collection, Illinois. **$250.00 – 300.00.**

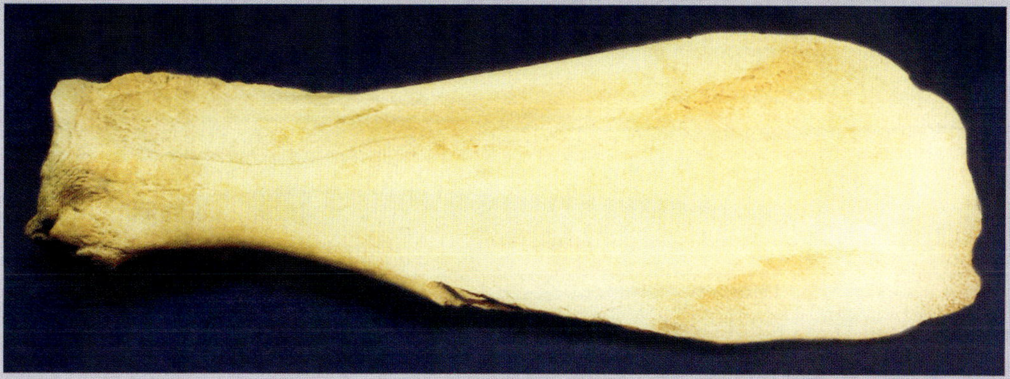

Bison scapula spade or shovel, (shoulder bone), used for digging trash or storage pits. This large piece is from a Mandan site, South Dakota. Fred Smith collection, Illinois. **$75.00 – 100.00.**

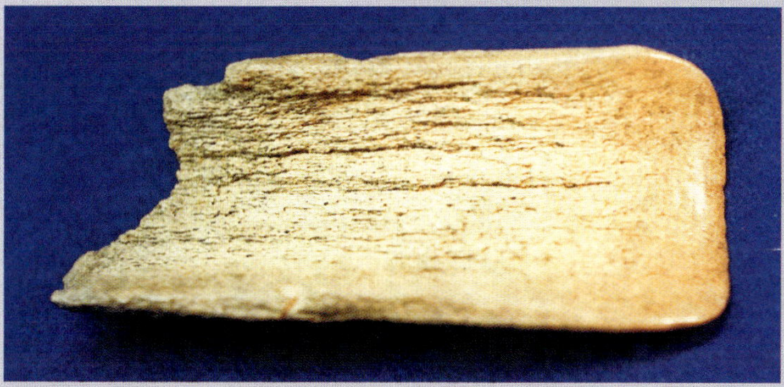

Gouge, moose or elk antler, well-used, 4½" long. It came from an Oneida site in Fulton County, Illinois. Fred Smith collection, Illinois. **$45.00 – 60.00.**

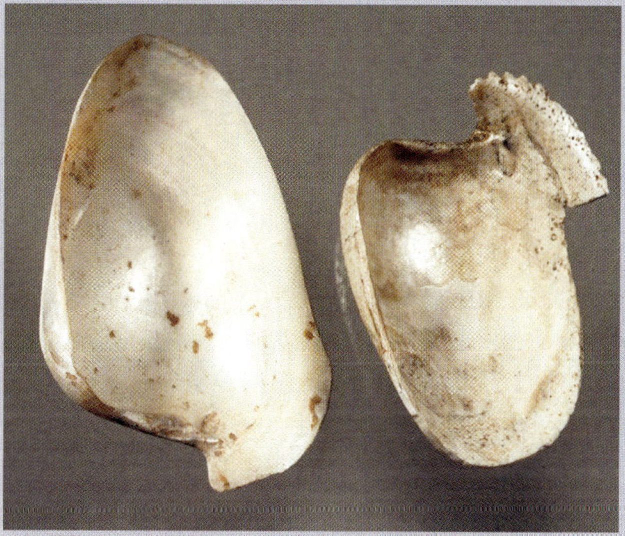

Shell spoons, freshwater mussel, Mississippian period, ca. AD 1330 – 1435. Values vary depending on condition and the presence of engraving. The pictured examples are ex-collection Dickson and were displayed in the early years of the Dickson Mounds Museum. Fulton County, Illinois. John Smith collection, Illinois. Each, **$75.00 – 125.00.**

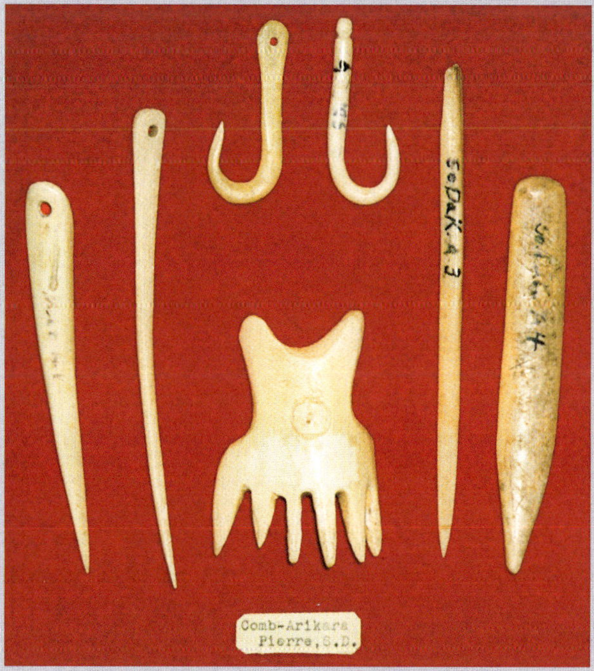

Bone artifacts, historic Arikara, longest eyed needle is 5". The items include two needles, two fishhooks, two awls, and a comb. These came from the Missouri River area, South Dakota. Richard Krueger collection, Iowa. Sandra Krueger photograph. Needles, each **$125.00 – 150.00;** fishhooks, each **$150.00 – 200.00;** awls, each **$35.00 – 45.00;** comb, **$250.00 – 300.00.**

Miscellaneous Artifacts

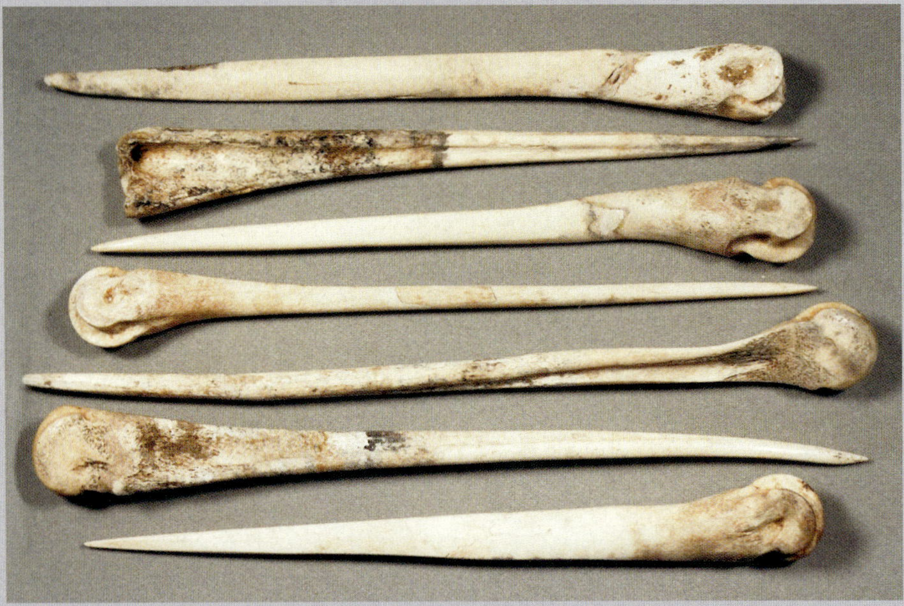

Bone pins, Hopewell of the Middle Woodland, longest example is 13". (A similar grouping of nine Hopewell pins was found in Scioto County, Ohio, many years ago. The longest of those was just less than 9".) These pins were found near Frederick, Schuyler County, Illinois. Private collection. Group, **$1,500.00.**

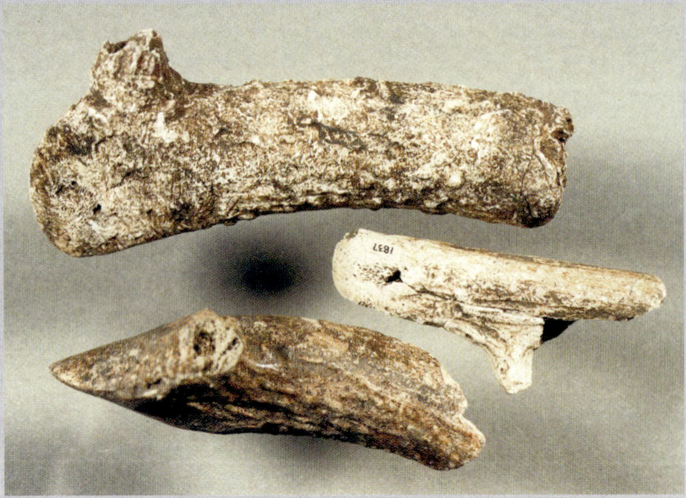

Antler gouges, Riverton people in Indiana and Illinois, Late Archaic period. Primarily living in the middle and lower Wabash River Valley, these Indians probably used the gouges to deflesh animal skins or even as wedges. All three were found in Crawford County, Illinois. Larger undamaged gouge, **$60.00;** others at about half.

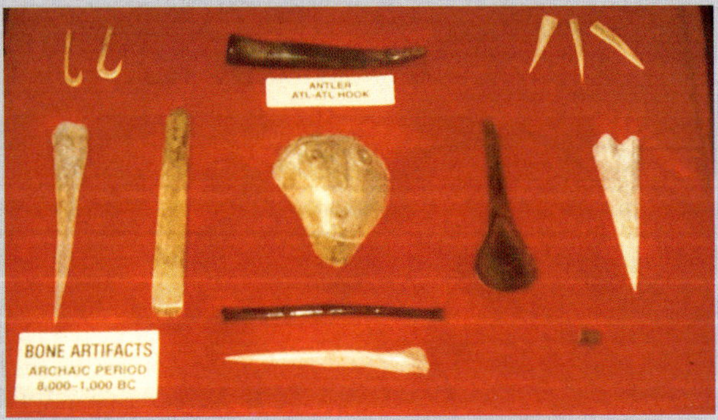

Bone artifacts, antler and shell (centerpiece). Top row: fishhooks (left), longest is 1⅝", probably Midwestern; polished antler Atl-atl hook, 4⅞" long, from Riley County, Kansas; points or short awls (right). Bottom row: fine bone awl, 5" long, from Kansas; flesher, ivory-like bone, 5½", incised V-shaped marks on reverse, widest end is toothed, from Missouri; shell mask gorget (center), 3¼" high, from Missouri. antler or bone spoon, dark patina, from Missouri; bone awl (right); flute or flageolet (bottom center), 4⅞", from Missouri; bone awl (bottom lower center). All are from the Tom Wyatt collection, Kansas. Unlisted.

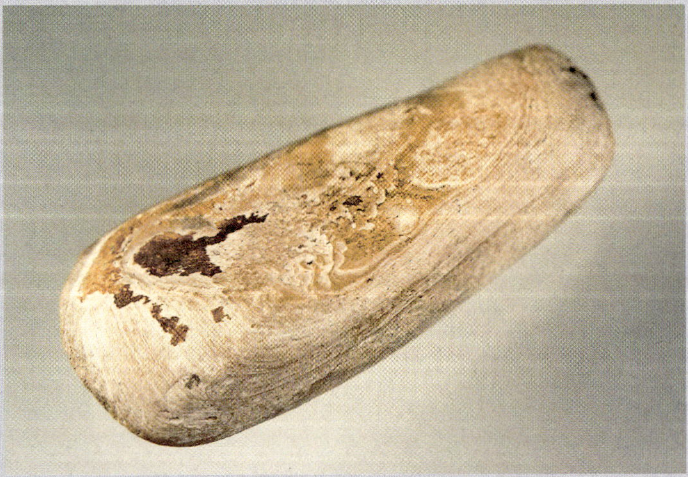

Shell adz, made from large marine shell, size 1⅝", ⅞" thick. It has a wide, beveled edge and was discovered years ago at Howe Key, Florida. Lar Hothem collection. **$85.00.**

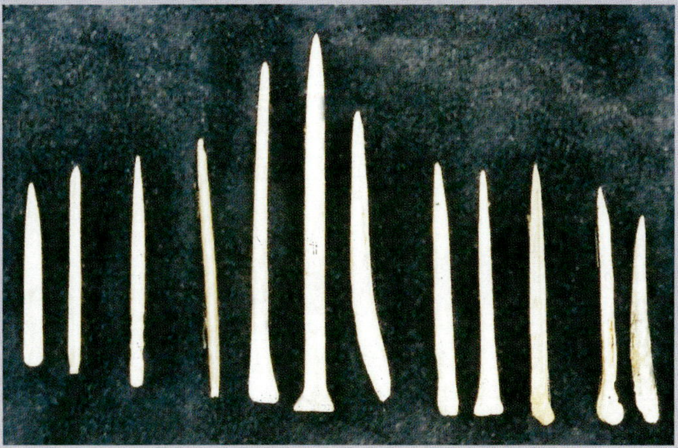

Bone hairpins, lengths to 8½". There are some fine examples in this grouping, found in northwestern Arkansas. Kenneth Hamilton collection, Arkansas. Each, **$35.00 – 300.00.**

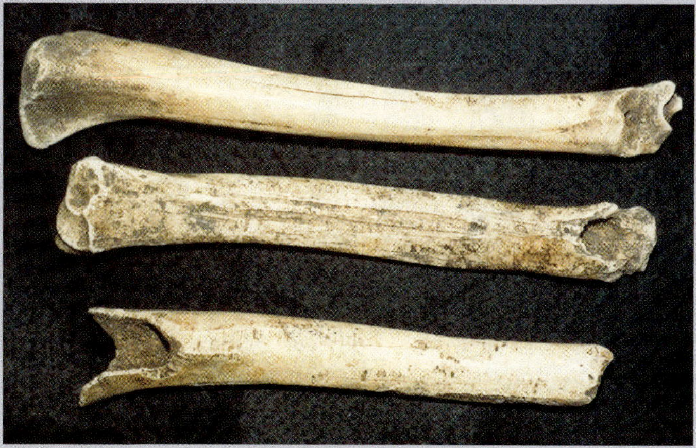

Worked bones from large animals, unknown uses. Length range is 8½ to 11", and all are from northwestern Arkansas. Kenneth Hamilton collection, Arkansas. Unlisted.

Tool, split deer bone, 9½" long. It is from northwestern Arkansas. Kenneth Hamilton collection, Arkansas. **$25.00.**

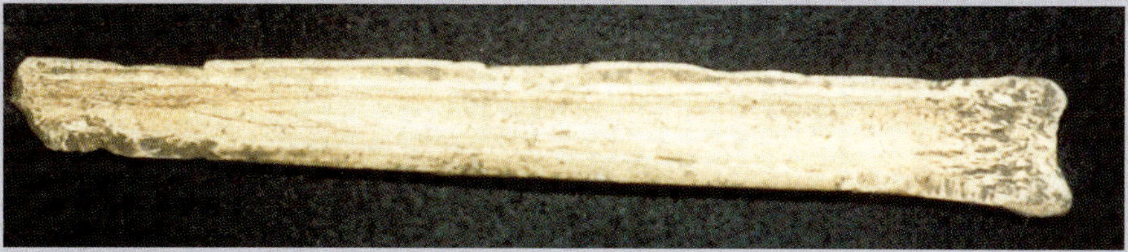

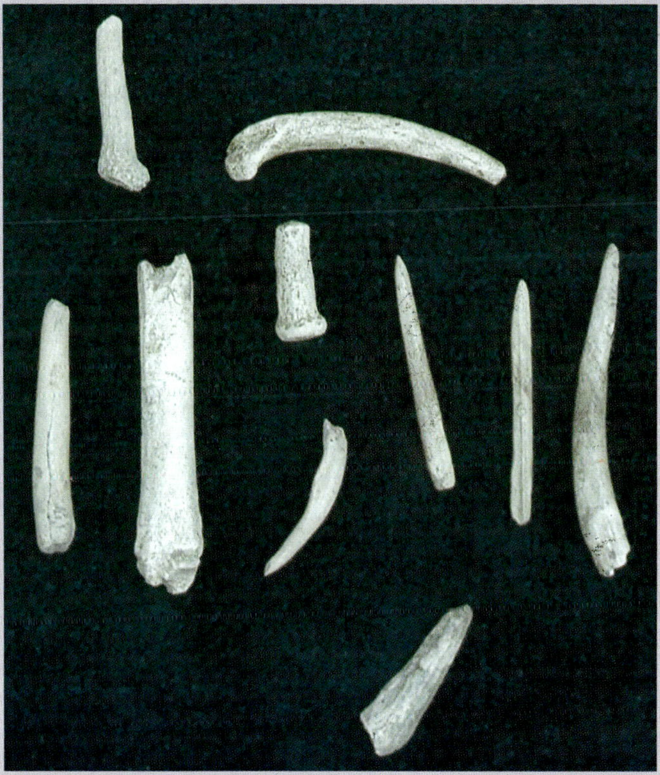

Antler chipping tools or flakers, 2½ to 5½" long. The largest artifact (second from left) is a bone handle. They are from northwestern Arkansas. Kenneth Hamilton collection, Arkansas. Flakers, **$10.00 – 20.00;** handle, **$25.00.**

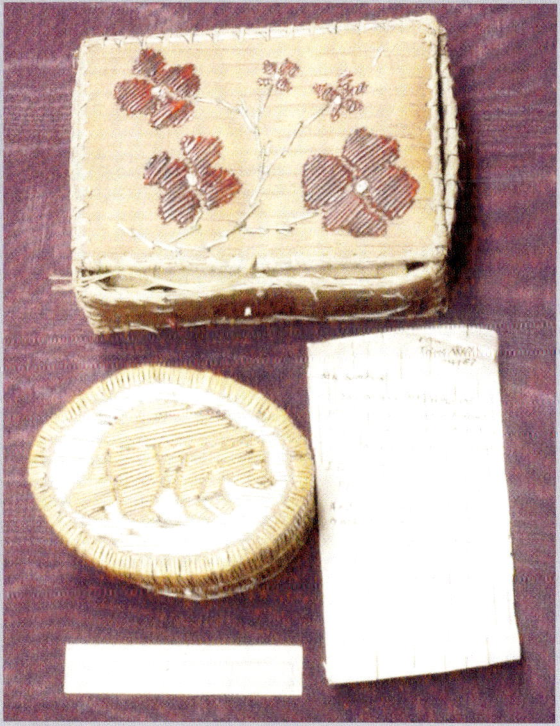

Organic material of a different sort, the birchbark basket and box are decorated with porcupine quills. An Indian in Maine made them in the 1970s, and the maker wrote a letter to the owner on a piece of birchbark. Ben Thompson collection, Missouri. Unlisted.

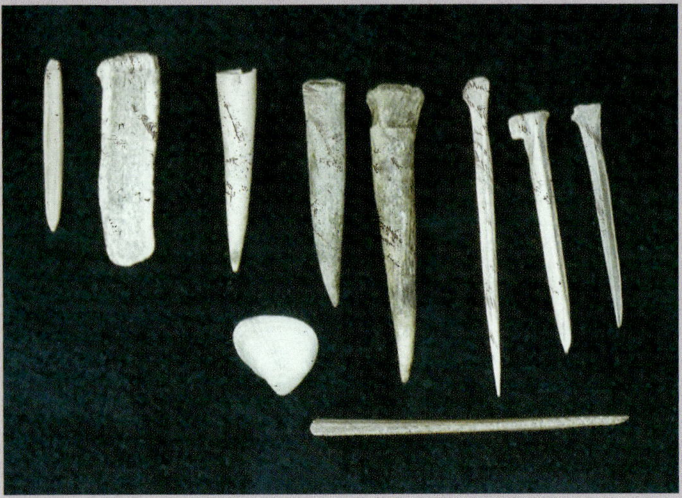

Deer antler artifacts, 5½ to 8½" long; bone awls up to 9" long. These are from northwestern Arkansas. Kenneth Hamilton collection, Arkansas. Antler artifacts, **$20.00 – 95.00;** awls, **$40.00 – 100.00.**

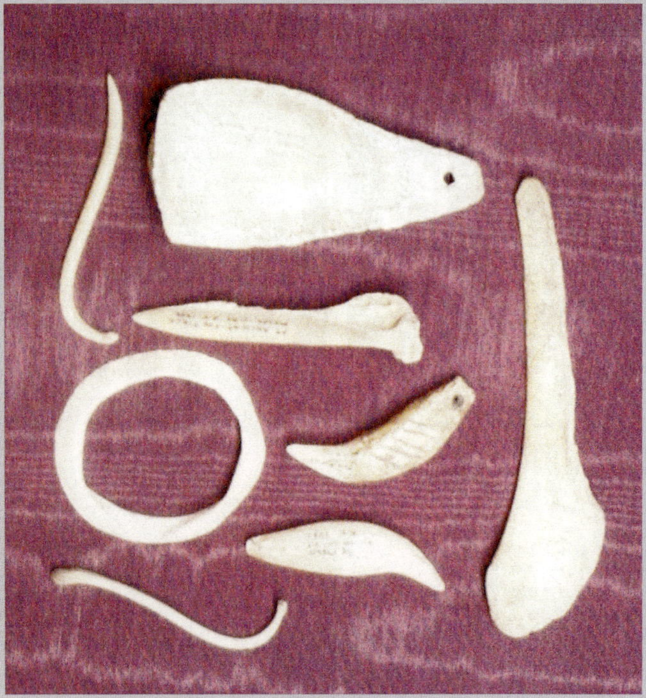

Bone artifacts, shell and teeth, all from a Fort Ancient site in Mason County, Kentucky. The owner's brother, Russell Thompson found them, in the 1970s. Ben Thompson collection, Missouri. Each, **$25.00 – 75.00.**

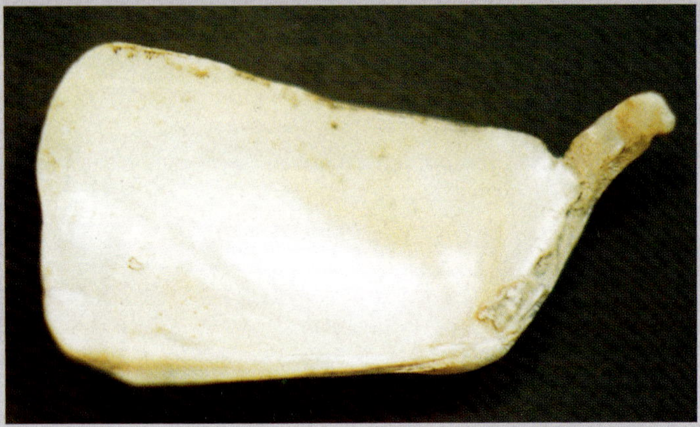

Shell spoon, 2½" long, probably historic period. It was found near Chamberlain, South Dakota. Mike Fox collection, Iowa. **$100.00.**

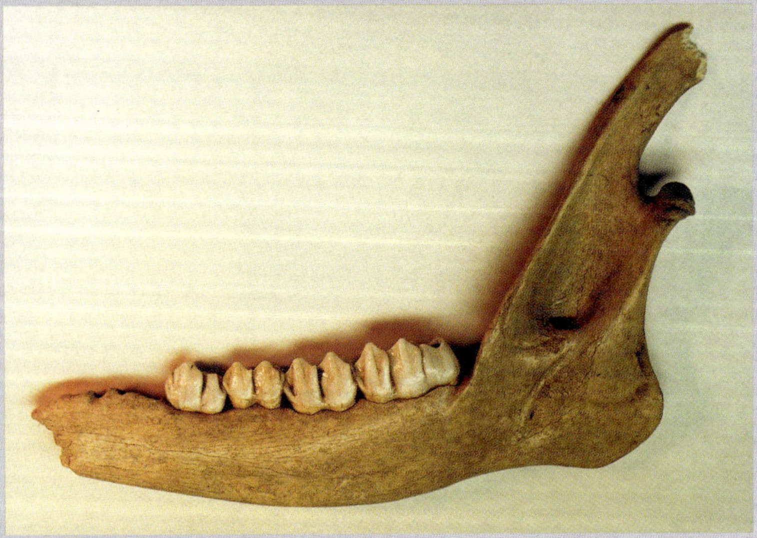

Deer jawbone corn sheller, 7⅜" long. Such examples were used into historic times. Fulton County, Illinois. Fred Smith collection, Illinois. **$40.00.**

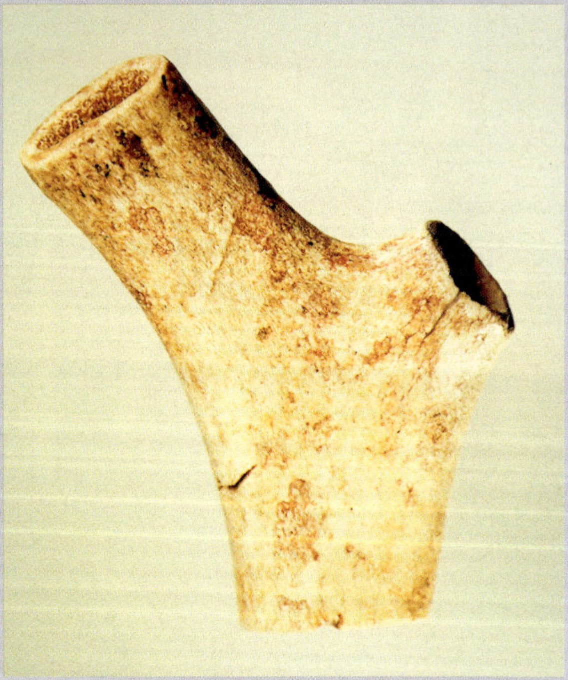

Antler pipe, one of the rarest antler artifacts made. This example is 3¼" high and is pictured in Hothem's *Collector's Guide to Indian Pipes*, page 63. Another example, from Arizona, is shown on page 250 of the same publication. When found by the owner, this pipe had touches of green, probably from contact with copper. Limestone County, Alabama. Robin Fiser collection. Museum grade.

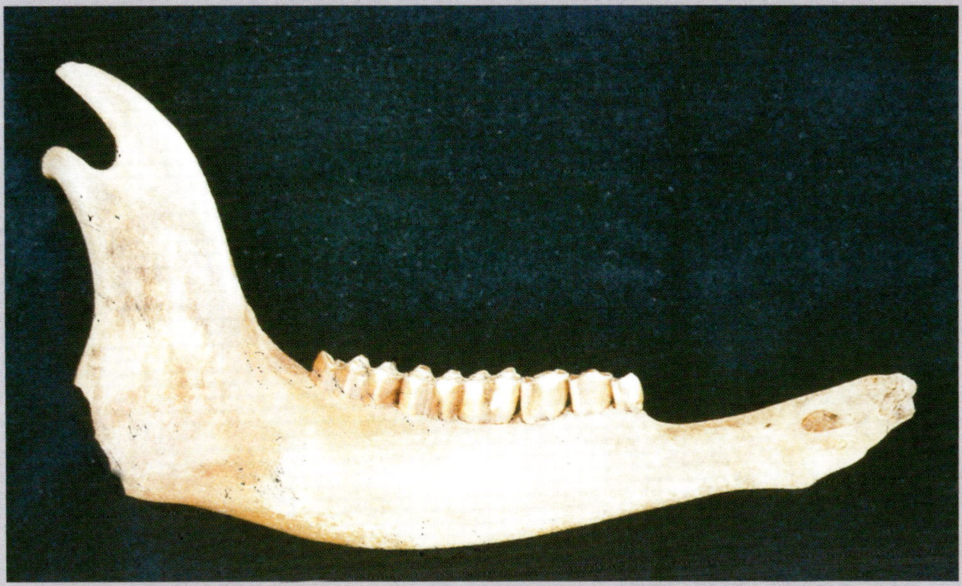

Buffalo (bison) jawbone tool, 4 x 14" long. This heavy bone may have had multiple uses. Oklahoma. Kenneth Hamilton collection, Arkansas. **$125.00.**

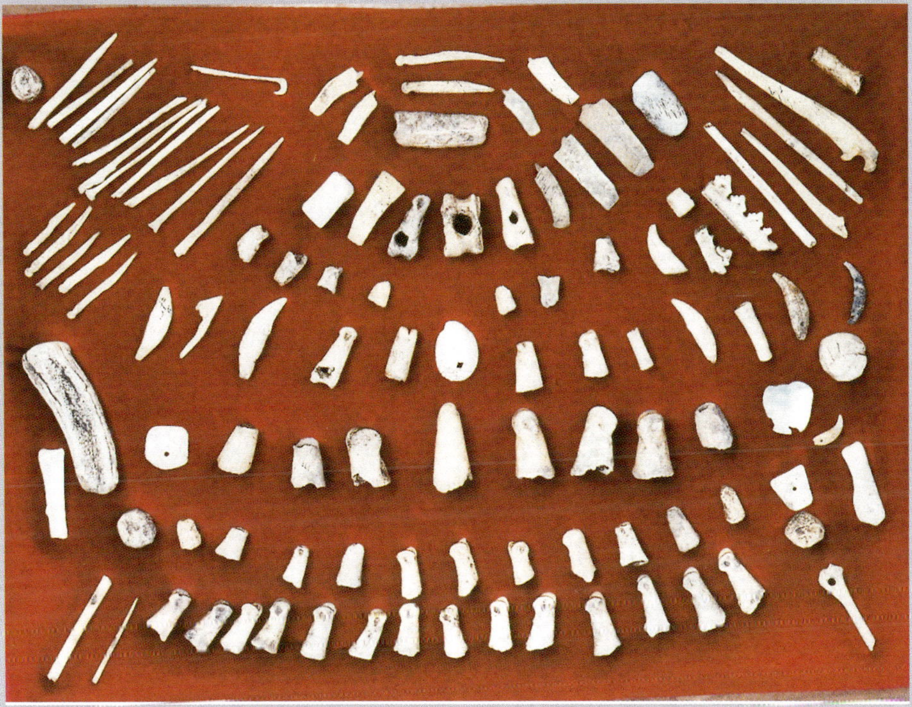

Bone artifacts, a fine range of objects including many drilled deer toe bones. The antler wedge at left is 5¼" long and the slender needles are 2½ to 3½" long. All the artifacts are from northwestern Arkansas. Kenneth Hamilton collection, Arkansas. Wedge, **$35.00;** needles, each **$5.00 – 20.00;** toe bones, each **$3.00 – 5.00.**

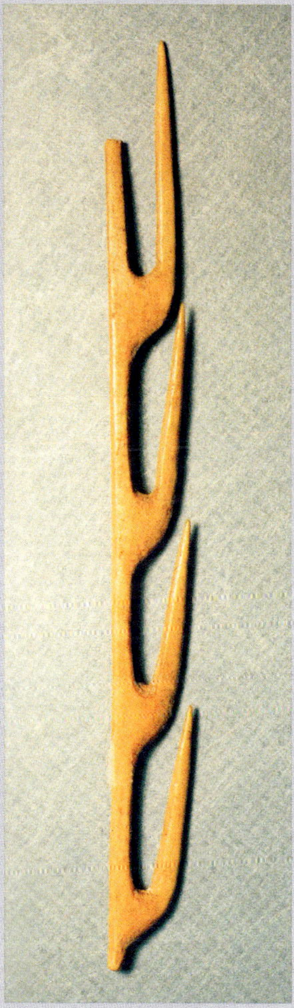

Fishhook, four barbs, historic period, ca. AD 1750. This rare artifact is 5" long and was picked up in Morton County, North Dakota. Private collection. Museum grade

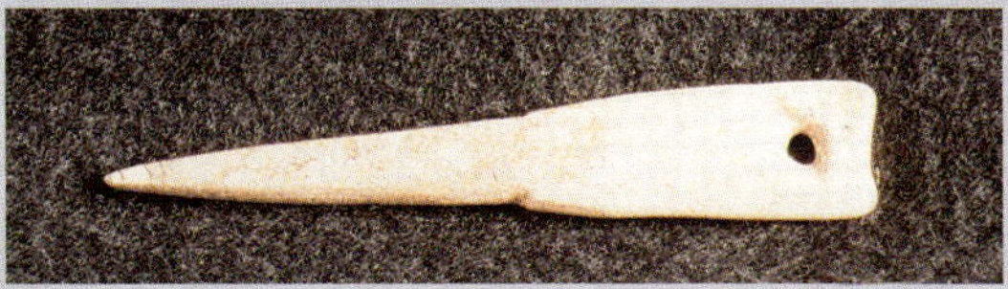

Hairpin, drilled at wide end, 2 15/16" long. The origin of this artifact is unknown. John F. Wubker collection, Illinois. **$75.00 – 100.00.**

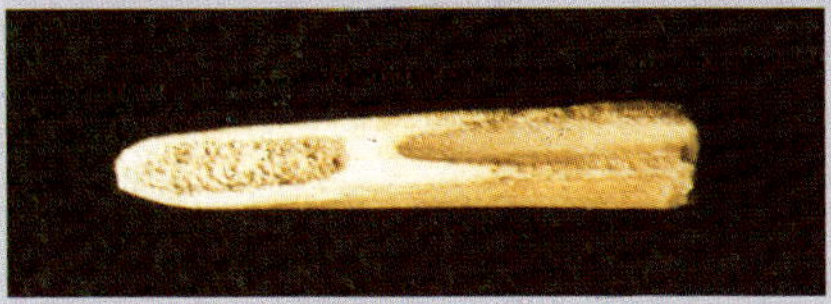

Snowshoe web spacer, caribou bone, used to regulate size of cord openings, 2½" long. It is from an historic Iroquois site, ca. AD 1700 – 1800. The spacer is from New York state. Dave Summers collection, Victor, New York. **$70.00.**

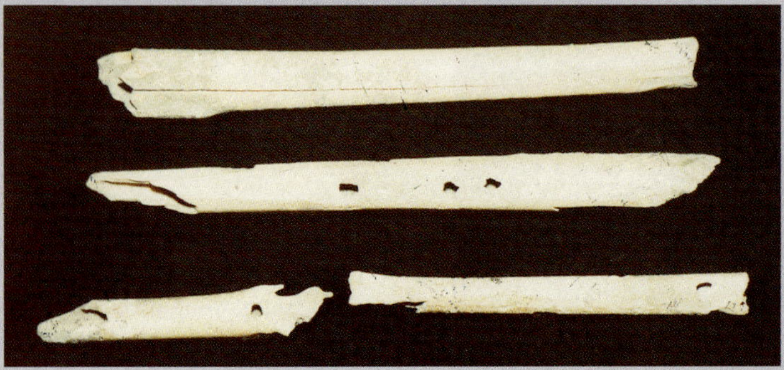

Flute-like objects, bone, longest 10½". All have drilled holes, and came from northwestern Arkansas. Kenneth Hamilton collection, Arkansas. Unlisted.

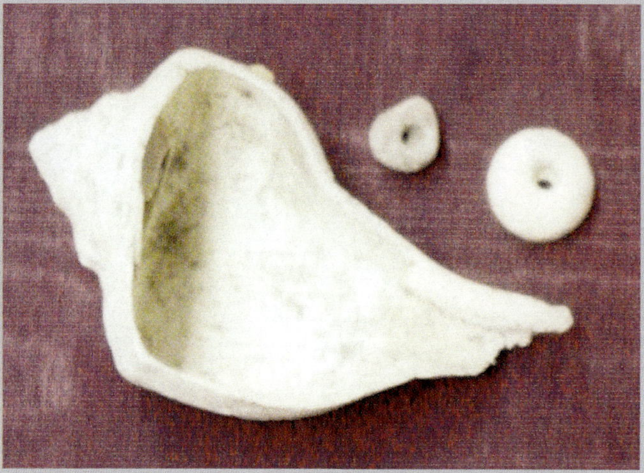

Cup or dipper and two shell beads, conch shell, all from Alabama. These are probably late prehistoric. Ben Thompson collection, Missouri. Unlisted.

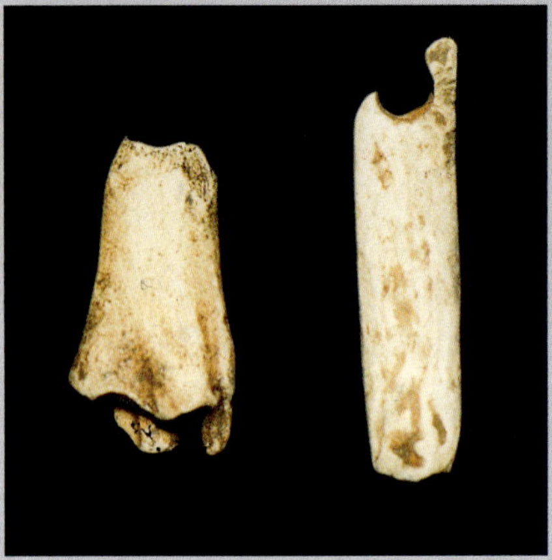

Artifacts, bone, handle at left 2½" long and object to right 3½" long. These were found in northwestern Arkansas. Kenneth Hamilton collection, Arkansas. Unlisted.

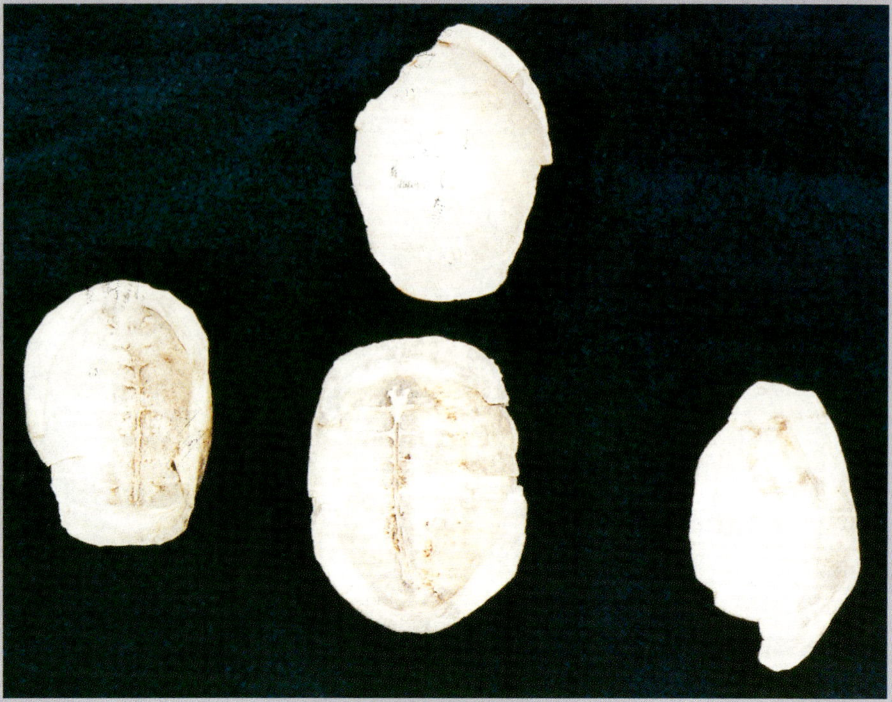

Tortoise shells bowls, lengths range from 6½ to 8½" long. All were found in northwestern Arkansas. Kenneth Hamilton collection, Arkansas. Unlisted.

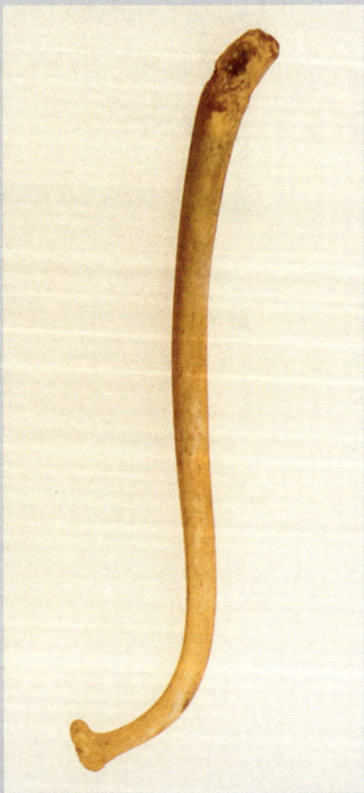

Raccoon penis bone pendant, Woodland, formerly in the Vietzen collection. This specimen is 4¼" long and is drilled at the base for suspension. Christian County, Kentucky. Pete Timoch collection. Unlisted.

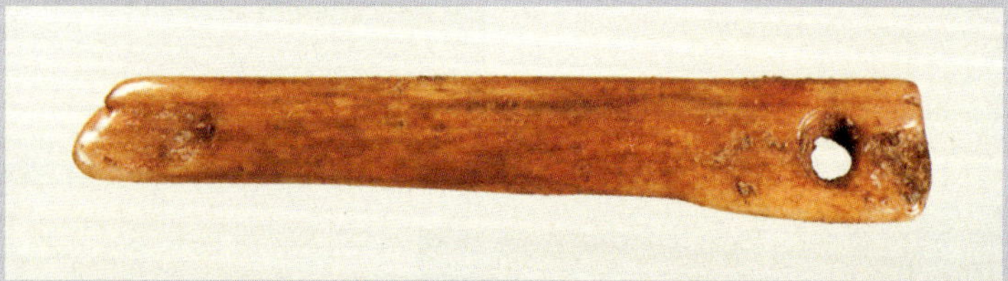

Awl or needle, broken tip area with much use-polish. This tool was heavily used as-is. Ex-collection Miller, it is from a rock shelter. Southern Tennessee. Lar Hothem collection. **$25.00.**

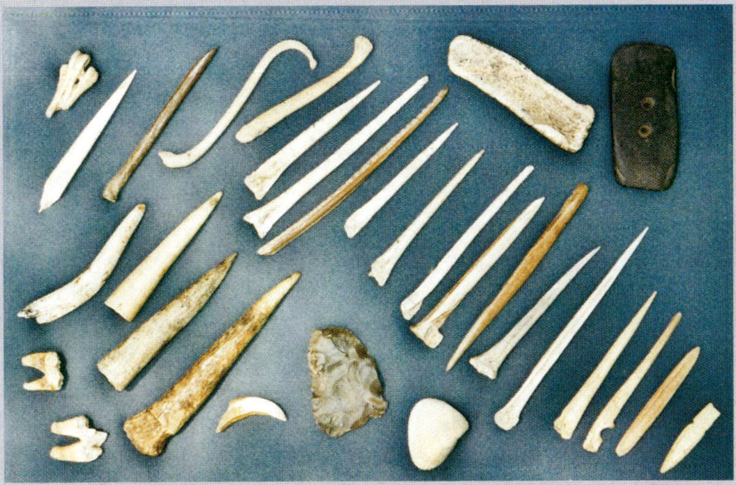

Bone awls and hairpins, and four deer antler points(?) (bottom left), 4½ to 6½" long. Everything is from northwestern Arkansas. Kenneth Hamilton collection, Arkansas. Awls and hairpins, each **$15.00 – 95.00;** antler objects, each **$20.00 – 75.00.**

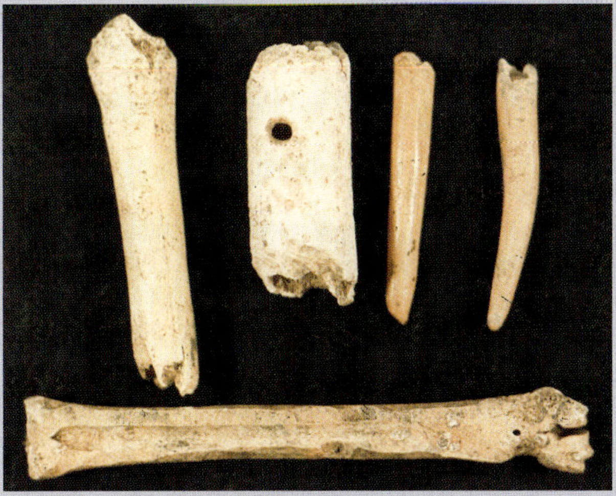

Bone artifacts, flakers are 2½" long. At bottom is a short beamer-like tool; unknown object (second from left) is drilled. All are from northwestern Arkansas. Kenneth Hamilton collection, Arkansas. Knappers, each **$25.00;** beamer, **$45.00;** others, unlisted.

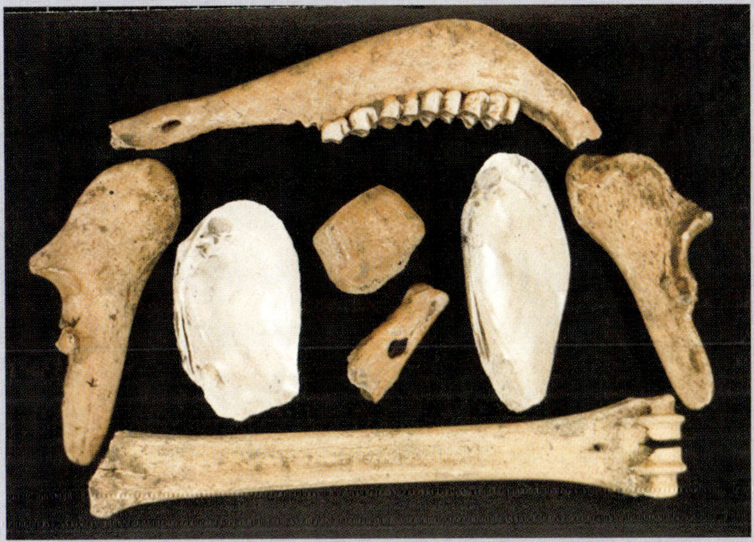

Bone and shell artifacts, cut deer jawbone (top) is 8" long. Also included are two well-worn trigger awls (perhaps, in this condition, used as flakers), and two shell spoons. Northwest Arkansas. Kenneth Hamilton collection, Arkansas. Jawbone, **$65.00;** trigger awls, each **$20.00;** long bone at bottom, **$25.00.**

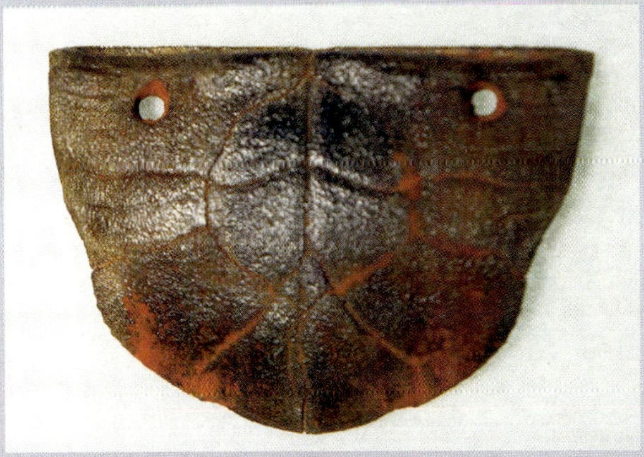

Plastron gorget, tortoise, drilled for suspension. It was found in a rock shelter in Union County, Illinois. Back to Earth. **$135.00.**

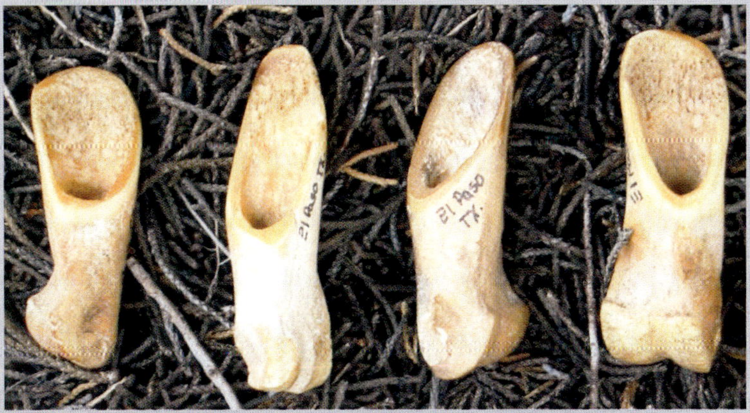

Bone scoops or adz blades, 1⅝ to 1⅞" long. All were found in the El Paso area, Texas. John and Susan Mellyn collection, Texas. Each, **$45.00.**

Miscellaneous Artifacts

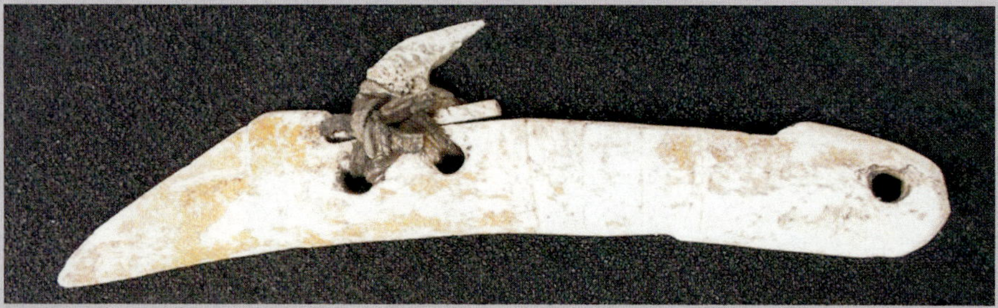

Bone hook, 5⅜" long. A dry cave find, the artifact came from the Northwest Coast. John and Susan Mellyn collection, Texas. **$175.00.**

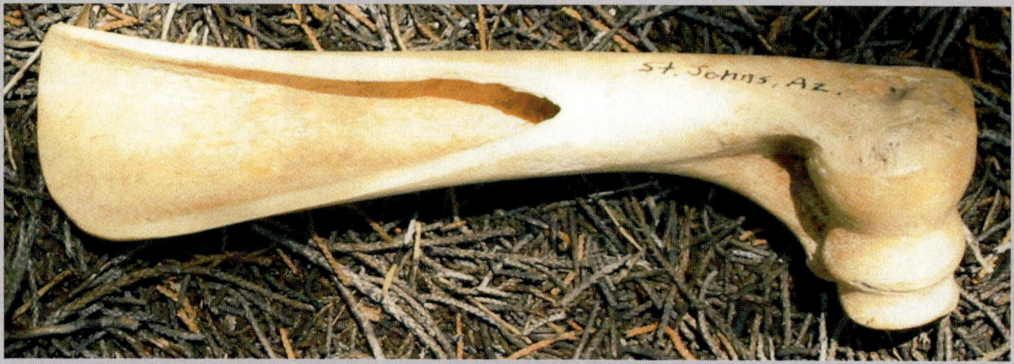

Adz or scoop, large animal bone, 5⅞" long. It is from the St. Johns area, Arizona. John and Susan Mellyn collection, Texas. **$150.00.**

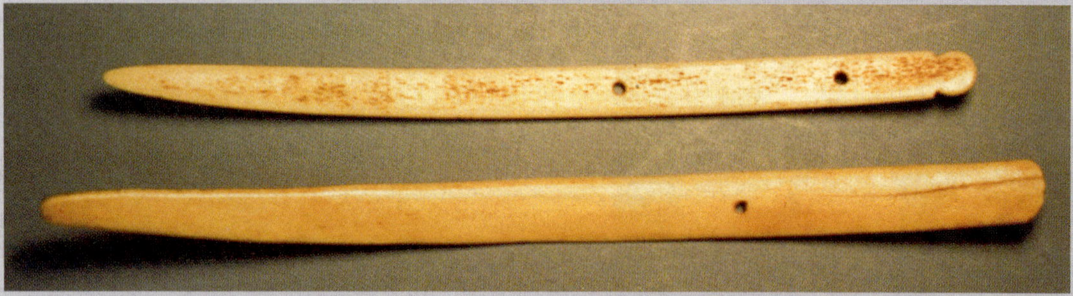

Bone mat needles, used for weaving rush mats together. The longest needle is 11½". Historic Mesquakie, ca. AD 1870. Iowa County, Iowa. Private collection. Each, **$250.00.**

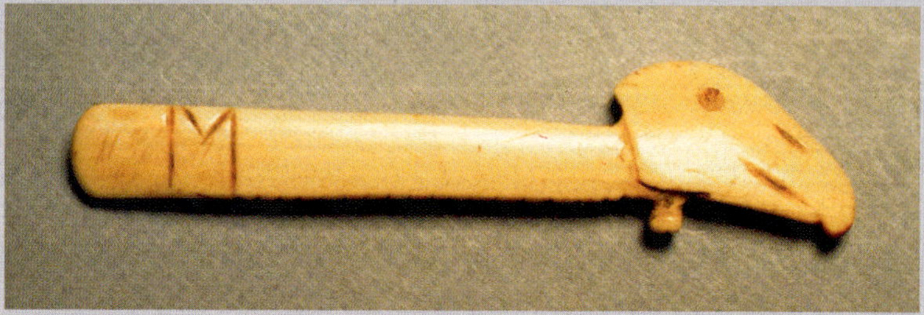

Bone bird effigy, a rare piece with incised "M" and tally marks, 3¼" long. This is one of about ten that were found in the 1970s on the Boley site, and the use or purpose is unknown. It is ca. AD 1750, from Morton County, North Dakota. Private collection. Museum grade.

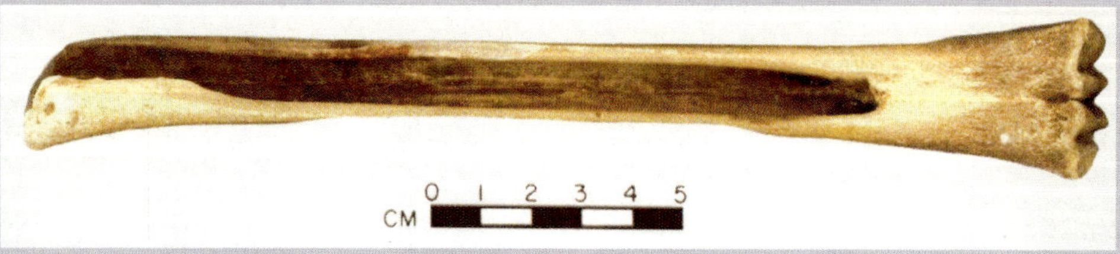

Beamer, deer leg bone, size as indicated by scale. Part of a late prehistoric cache, it was excavated at Stow Rockshelter in January of 1955. The artifact was reported in the *Ohio Archaeologist*, Vol. 50 No. 4, Fall 2000. Imaged by Thomas R. Pigott, Sofsky Archives. Unlisted.

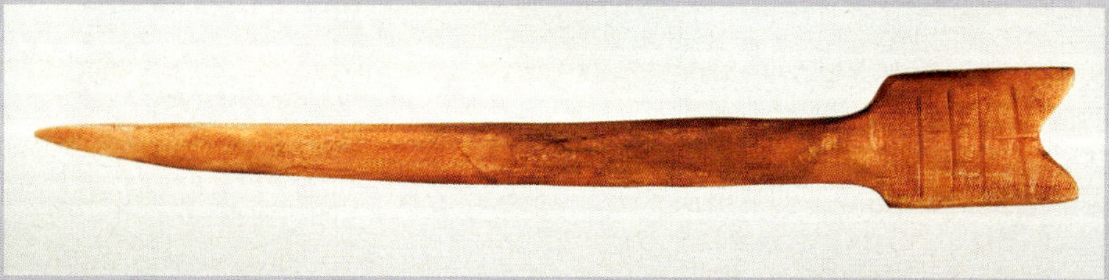

Reproduction (fake) hairpin, 4¾" long. This modern piece has brown dye, no patination or deposits, and machine marks are present. There are small, parallel abrasions and longitudinal facets in the bone from a power sander or grinder. Indiana. Private collection. Study value only.

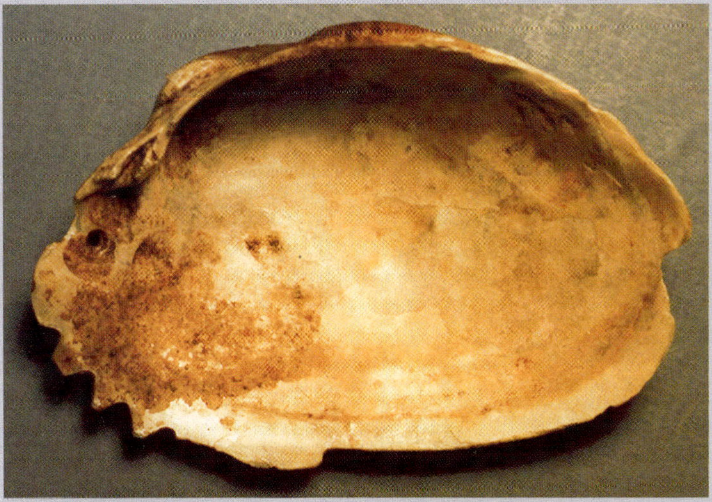

Shell spoon, freshwater mussel, 4" long. late prehistoric ca. AD 1000 – 1700. It is drilled and has a partial fringed edge. Middle Mississippi River Valley area. Private collection. **$125.00.**

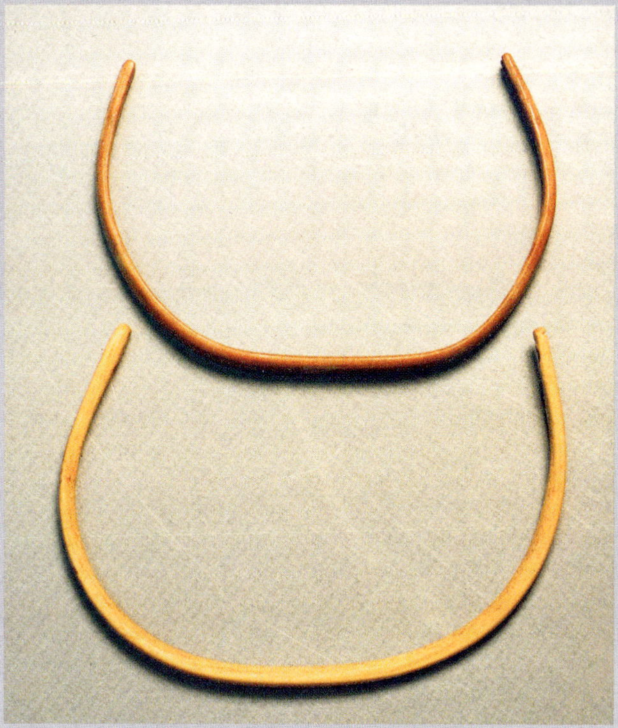

Arm bands, bone, drilled with holes at each end, 3½" in diameter. They are ca. AD 1750, from Morton County, North Dakota. Private collection. Each, **$150.00.**

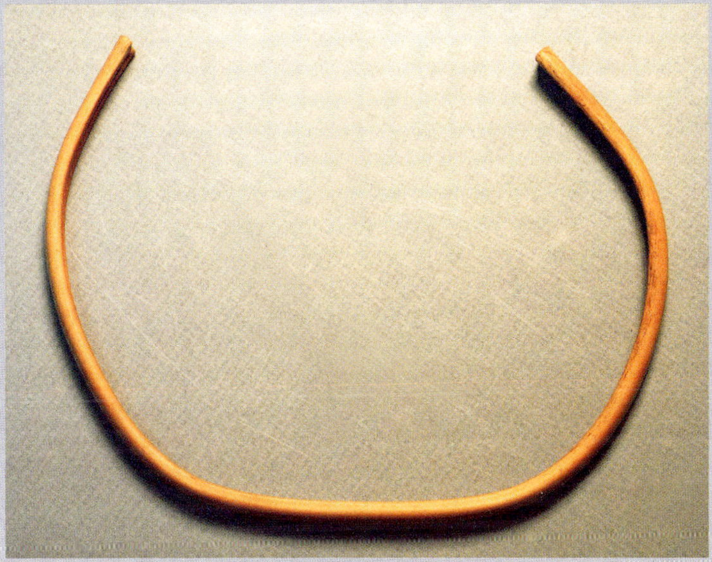

Bone arm band, drilled with holes at each end for cord ties, diameter is 5". It is historic, ca. AD 1750, and came from Morton County, North Dakota. Private collection. **$200.00.**

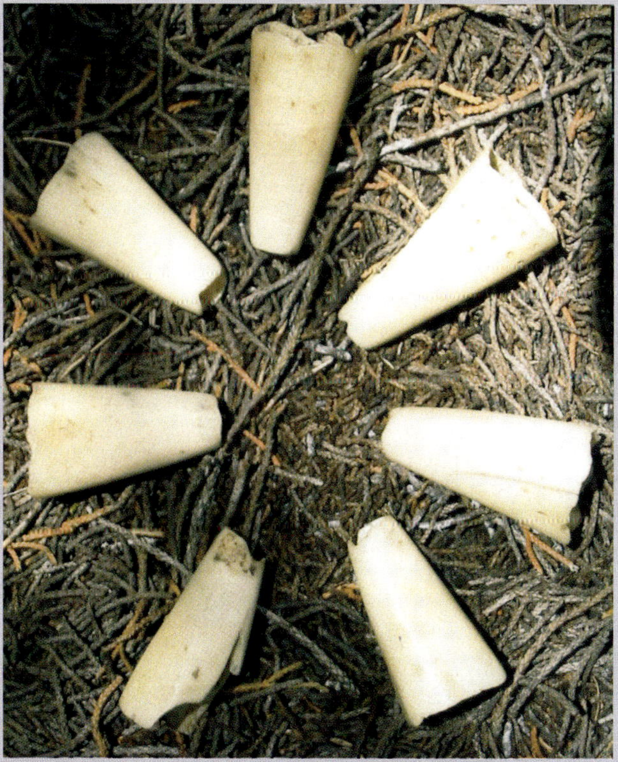

Gaming pieces, bone, average length is 1⅜". These are historic and Chippewa, probably from the Great Lakes region. John and Susan Mellyn collection, Texas. Each, **$35.00 – 50.00.**

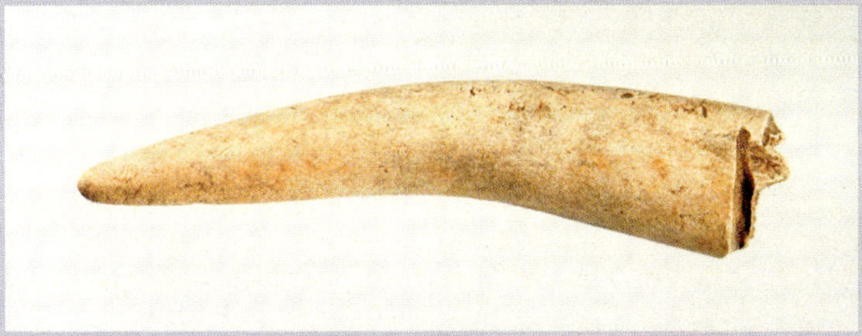

Antler tool, cut-marks still visible at base, 2¹⁵⁄₁₆" long. This is probably a flint-knapping tool. Ex-collection Hall, Wayne County, Kentucky. Private collection. **$12.00.**

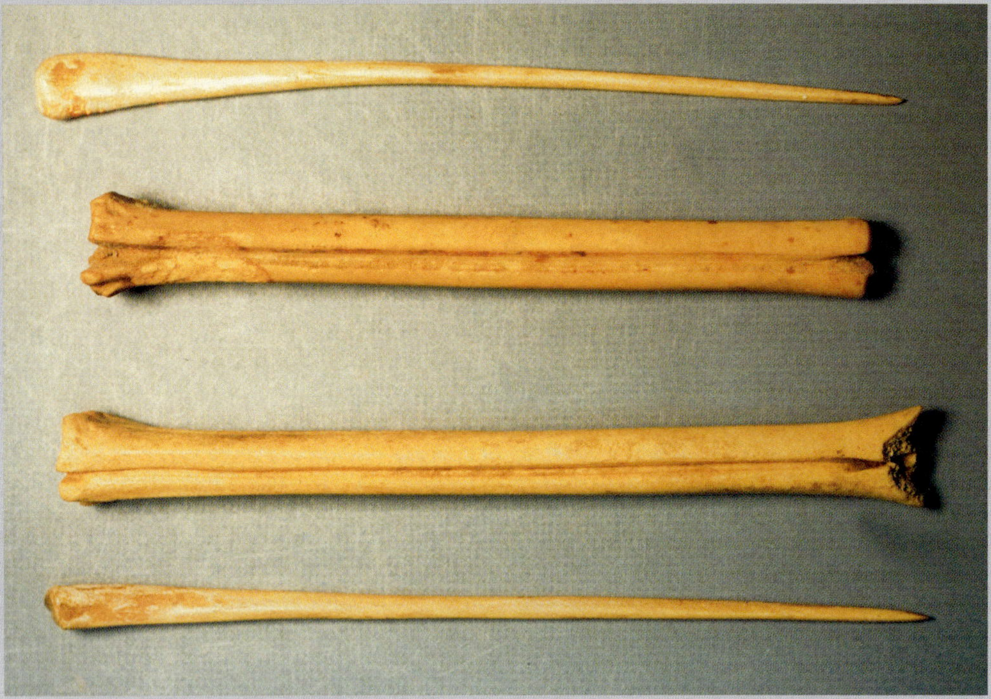

Bone artifacts, two hairpins(?) and two bones that have been grooved in preparation for making additional pins. The artifacts are 7 to 8¼" long, and all are ca. AD 1750. Morton County, North Dakota. Private collection. Pins, each **$125.00;** bone preforms, very unusual, **$200.00.**

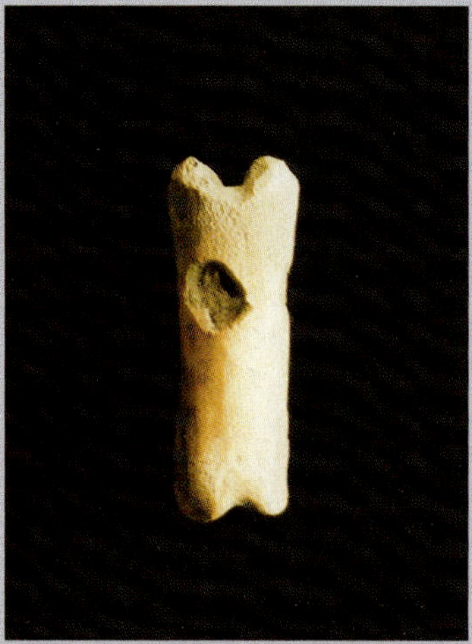

Jangle or decoration, deer toe bone with three drilled holes, historic Iroquois (Seneca), ca. AD 1675 – 1687. The artifact is 1½" long and was recovered near Victor, Ontario County, New York. Dave Summers collection, Victor, New York. **$20.00.**

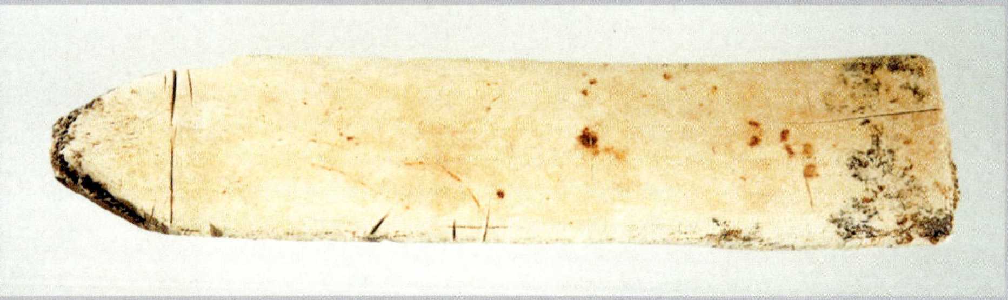

Ice glider, bison rib bone, historic, 1⅛ x 5⅝", ex-collection Sheild. Used with feathers in the base, the glider has some incised marks on the slightly incurvate top face. The bottom is white (compared with the creamy face shown) and highly polished from sliding on ice or crusted snow. South Dakota. Lar Hothem collection. **$75.00.**

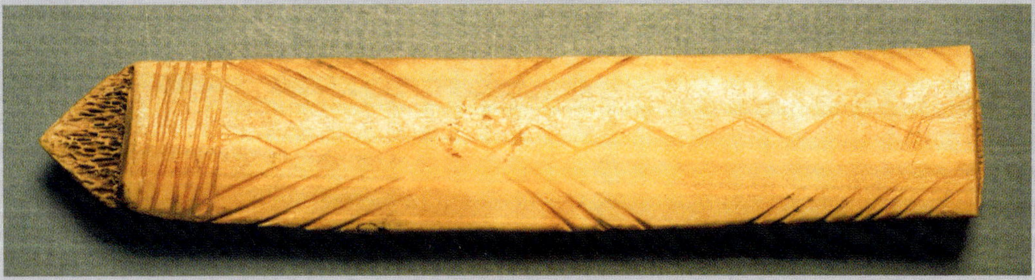

Ice glider, well-decorated, bison rib bone. It is 5" long, ca. AD 1750. In use, it had feathers inserted in the squared end. This is an excellent example, from Morton County, North Dakota. Private collection. **$150.00.**

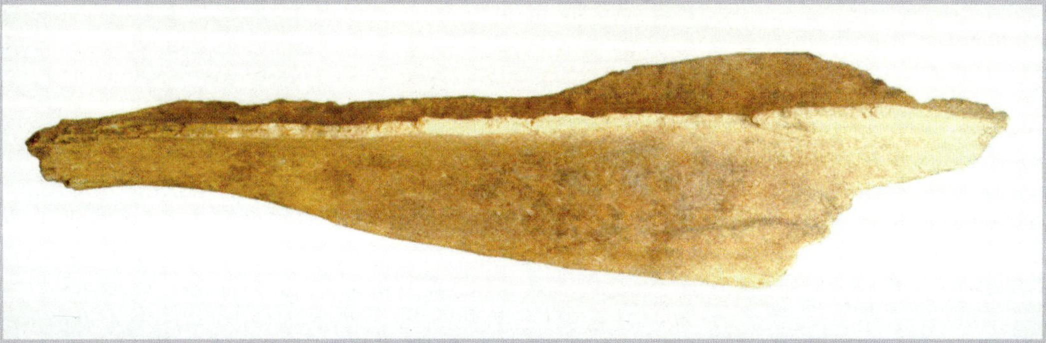

Bone knife, made from the scapula of what was likely an immature elk. It is large at 275mm long, and may have been used as a drawshave or hide-scraper. It was found in a pit at the Purdy Village site in Trumbull County, Ohio. Imaged by and in the collection of Thomas R. Pigott. Unlisted.

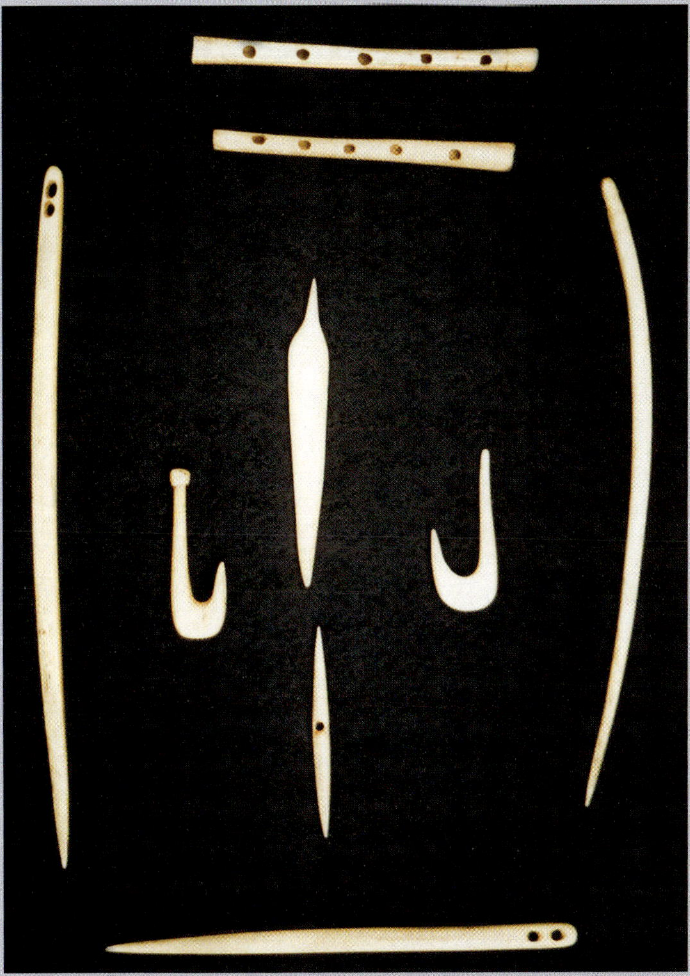

Bone artifacts, fishhooks and flageolets. The bone needles range in length from 5" (bottom) to 7" (at left), and the double drilled holes are of interest. The central projectile point is from Kentucky. The needles, ex-collection Ransbottom, are from Virginia. Bob Hess collection, Indiana. Projectile point, **$100.00;** needles, each **$175.00 – 250.00.**

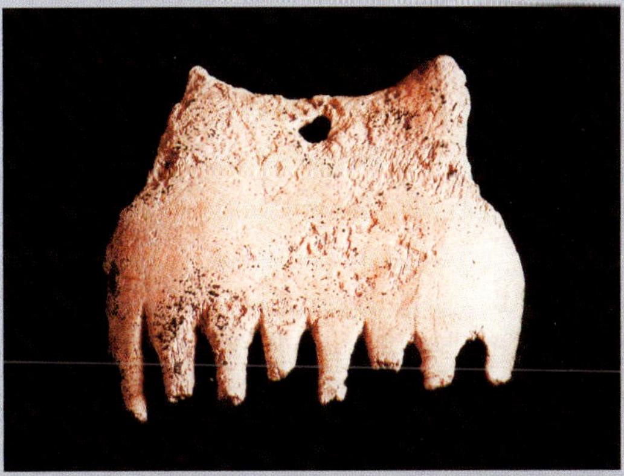

Bone comb, 2½" wide. Ex-collection Liehr, the find-location for this piece is unknown. John F. Wubker collection, Illinois. **$125.00.**

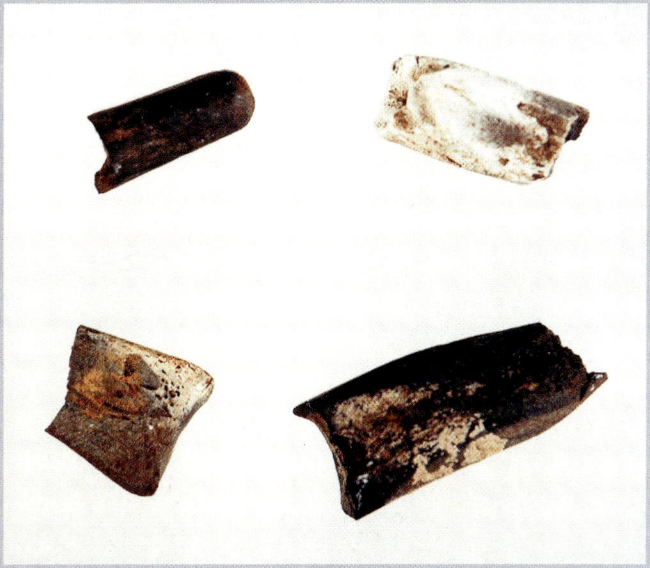

Midden debris, fired pieces of antler and bone, longest is 1½". Top left, tip of flint-knapping antler tool. Top right, carbonized antler fragment. Bottom left, blunt end of bone or antler hairpin. Bottom right, carbonized antler fragment. These came from a rock shelter in southern Tennessee. Private collection. Study value.

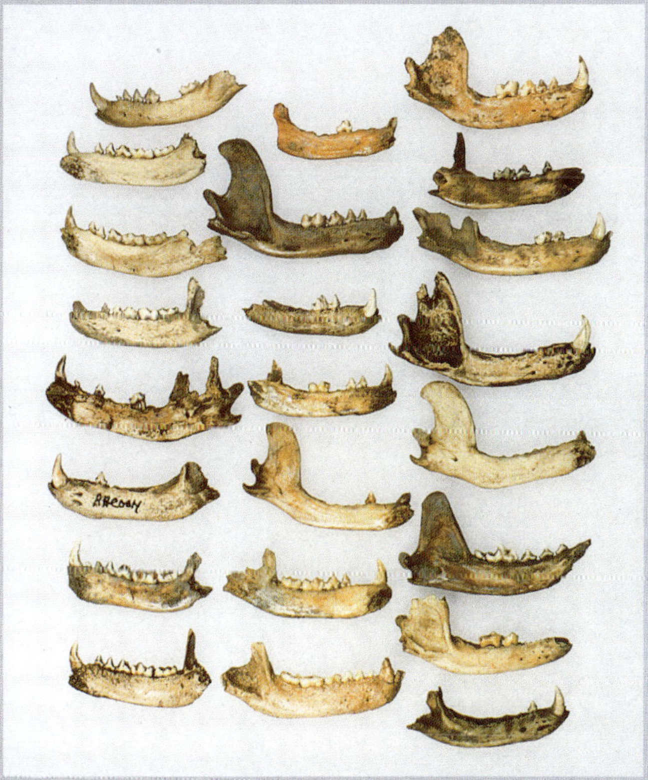

Ornaments or decorations, animal mandibles, longest is 3½", Woodland or Mississippian. Most are raccoon jawbones, some are notched for cord suspension. These are ex-collection Vietzen, from sites in Ohio and Kentucky. Private collection. Unlisted.

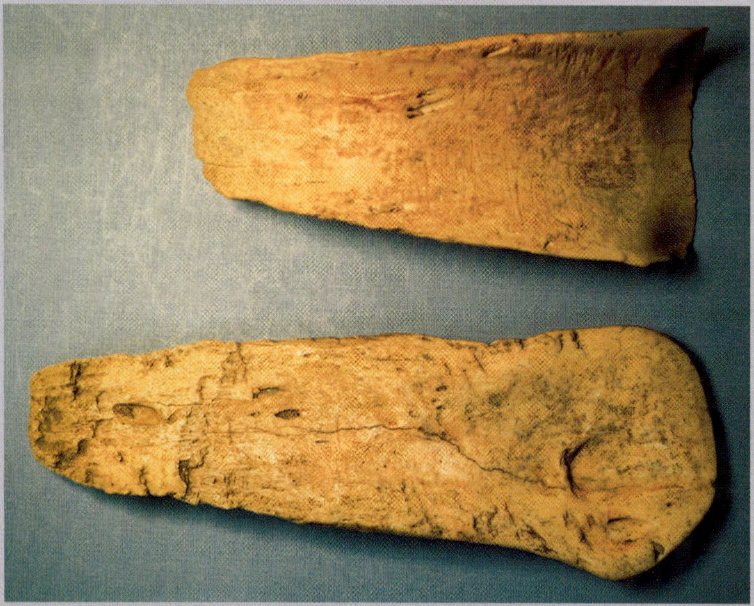

Elk antler hoes or scrapers, taken from the antler and skull area, longest specimen is 9½". They are ca. AD 1750, from Morton County, North Dakota. Private collection. Each, **\$150.00 – 175.00.**

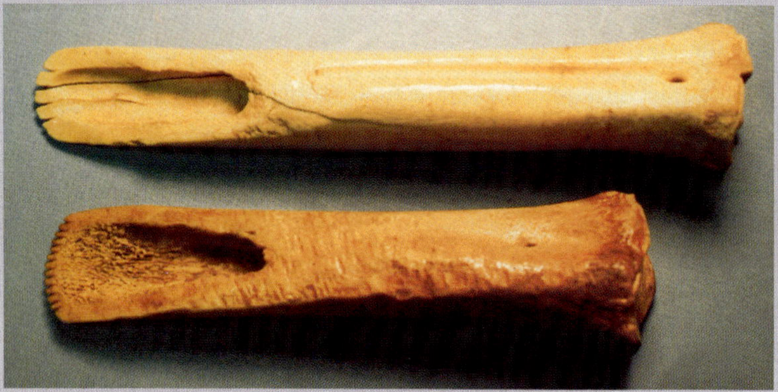

Fleshers, elk leg bones, serrated working edges, longest flesher is 8½". They are historic, ca. AD 1750, and were found in Morton County, North Dakota. Private collection. Each, **\$125.00 – 150.00.**

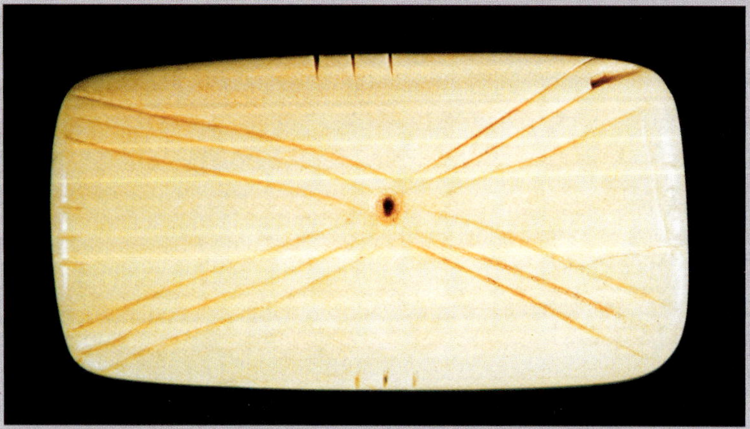

Gaming piece, probably bison bone, 1⅞ x 3⅝". This attractive artifact is smoothly polished and is decorated with incised lines and tally marks on the four sides. Historic period, the gaming piece was found in Morton County, North Dakota. Mike Fox collection, Iowa. **\$450.00.**

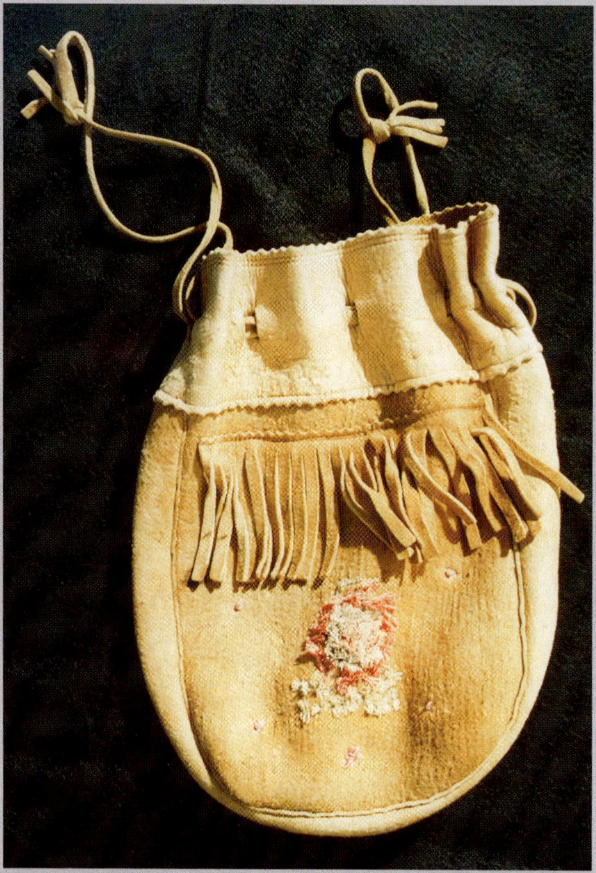

Moose hide bag with moose hair tufted floral design, Cree(?) Indian, ca. 1940, bag size is 8½ x 11". The origin of this piece is unknown. Dave Summers collection, Victor, New York. **\$150.00.**

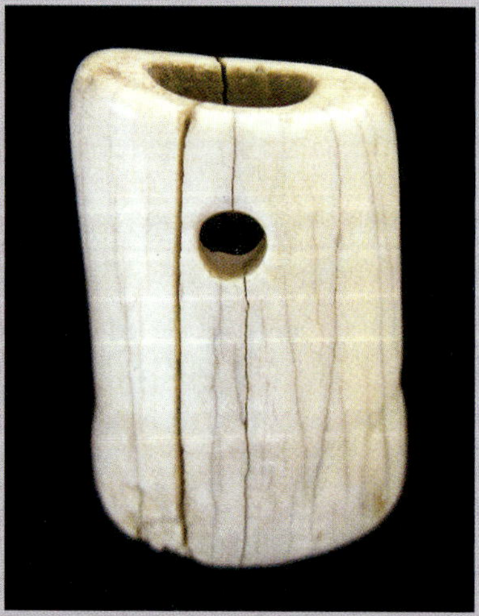

Bone ornament, 1½ x 2½", hollowed center with smaller side hole. Nicely shaped and finished, this piece is from California. Victor T. Trujillo collection, Nevada. **\$100.00.**

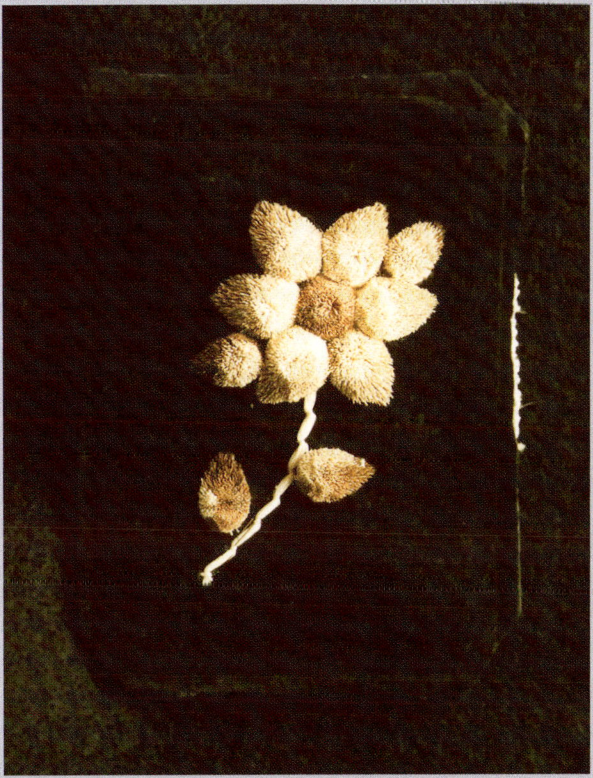

Moose hair floral design, organic material artifact, contemporary to recent, frame size is 4 x 5". This artwork is from Canada. Dave Summers collection, Victor, New York. **$100.00.**

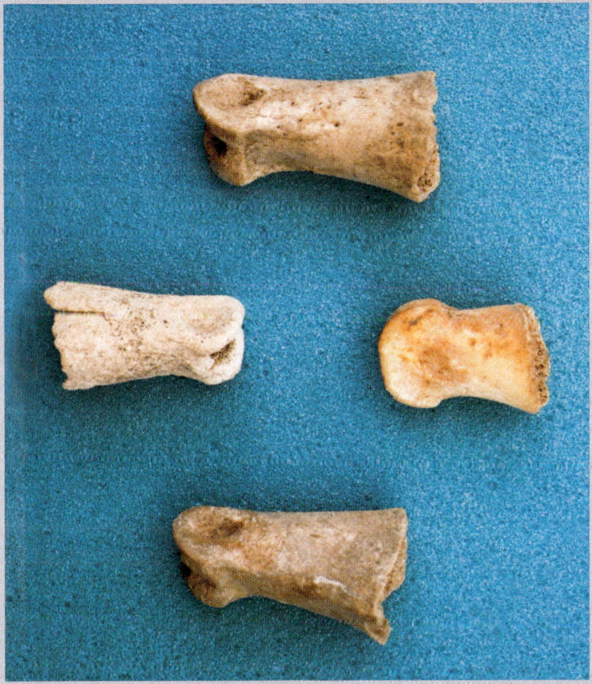

Beads, drilled deer toe bones, Woodland or later, largest is ¾ x 1½". Snyder found these between 1947 and 1958 in Polk County, Tennessee. Collection of, and photograph by, Gary Henry, North Carolina. Each, **$10.00 – 15.00.**

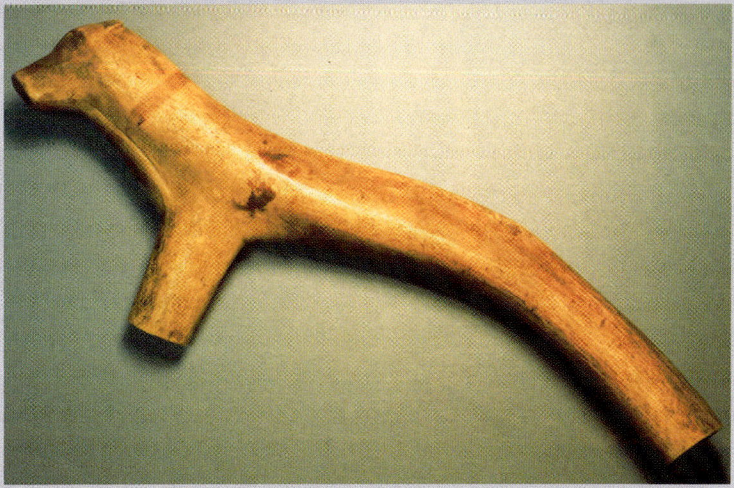

Elk antler club, so-called "Slave Killer" type, carved animal head, early nineteenth century, 16½" long. It is a rare artifact. Washington. Private collection. Museum quality.

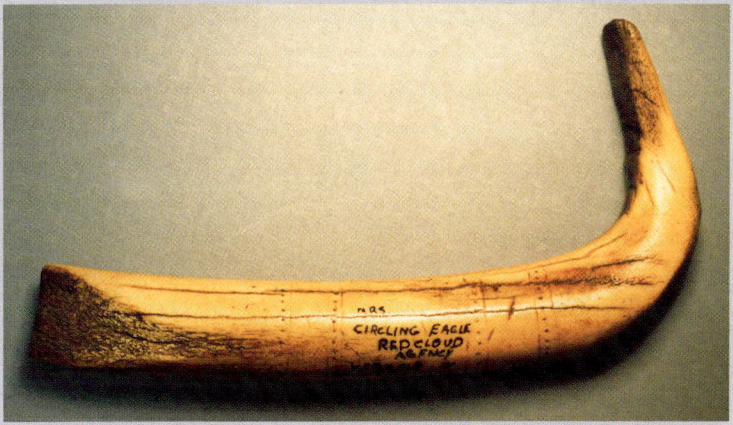

Elk antler hide-scraper, historic period, ca. AD 1850. Probably Sioux, it is 11" long and decorated with incised lines and dots. Red Cloud Agency, Dakota Territory. Private collection. Unlisted.

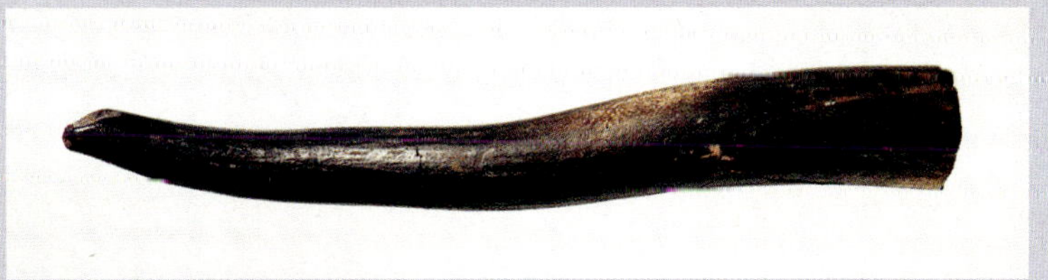

Antler knapper or punch, burned surface. This example, found in a rock shelter, is broken and glued. Southern Tennessee. Private collection. **$10.00.**

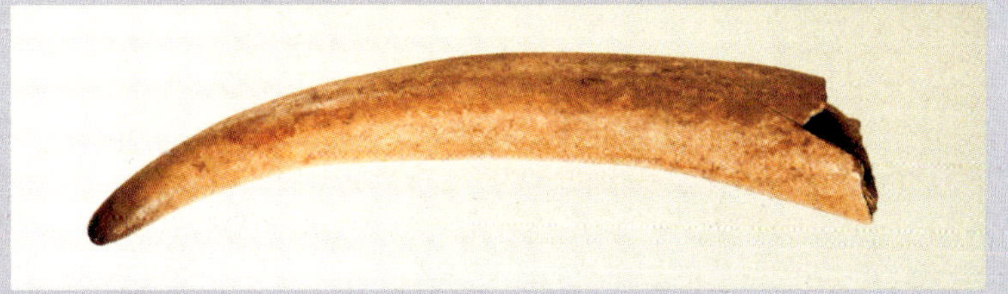

Deer antler tine, polished shaft, tip scorched, 2⅞" long. Probably a curved perforator or flint-knapping tool, it came from a rock shelter. Southern Tennessee. Private collection. **$7.00.**

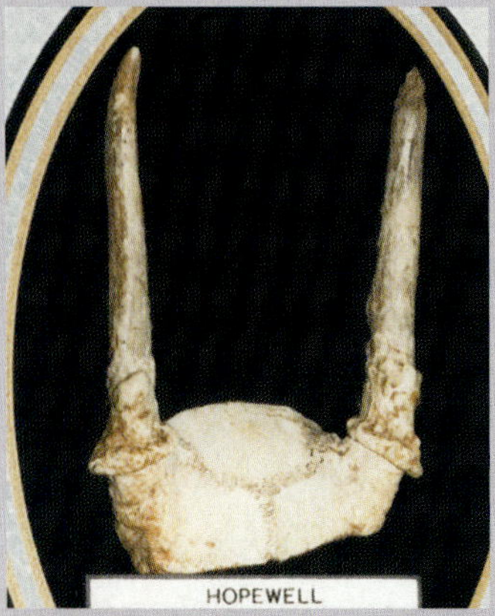

Deer antler headdress, highly unusual, 4¼ x 5¾" high. This was found in a rock shelter in Warren County, Tennessee. Back to Earth. Museum grade.

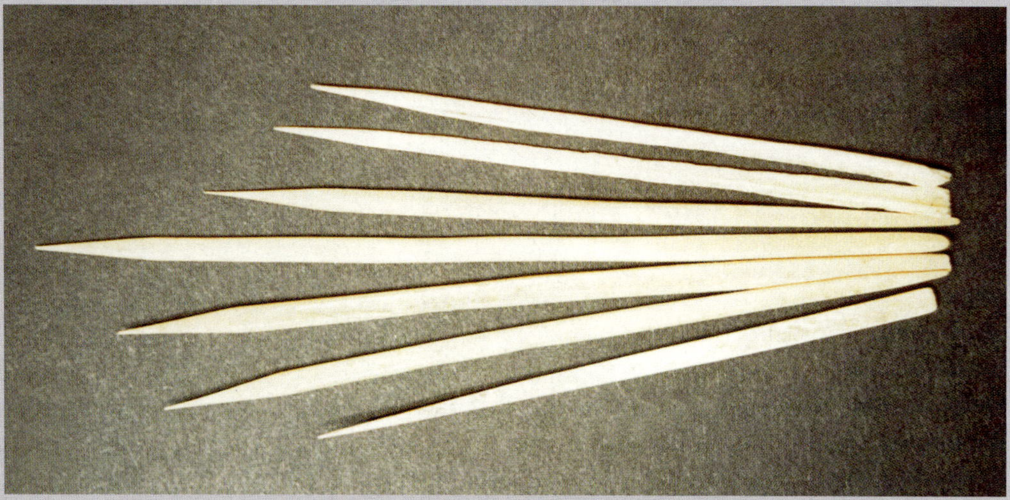

Bone needles, longest (at center) is 4½". They are historic period, from Morton County, North Dakota. Mike Fox collection, Iowa. Each, **$35.00 – 65.00.**

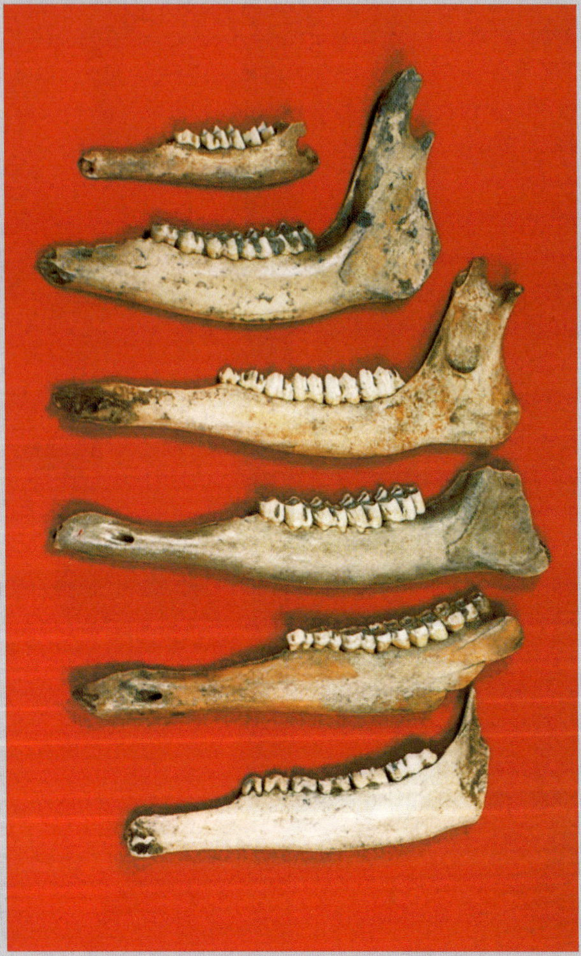

Deer jawbone artifacts, Woodland or Mississippian periods, longest is 8½". Ex-collection Vietzen, these were used as scrapers to remove corn from the cob. Note the handle polish on third example from the bottom. Ohio and Kentucky sites. Pete Timoch collection. Each, **$25.00 – 100.00.**

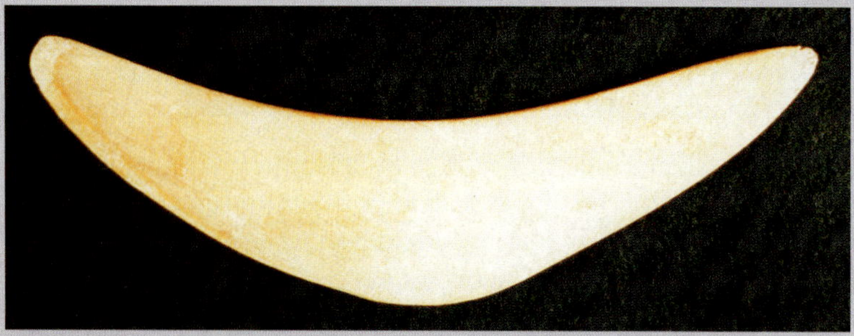

Bone squash knife, semi-lunate form, 5¼" long. It is historic period and was found near Pierre, South Dakota. Mike Fox collection, Iowa. **$275.00.**

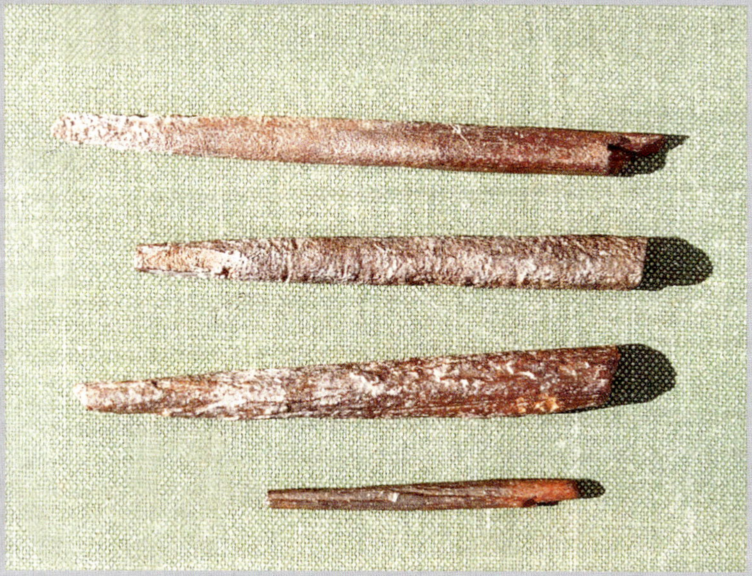

Pleistocene (Ice Age) bone tools, probably made by Paleolithic people, water-stained dark. They are from the Caloosahatchee River, Lee County, Florida. Dave Summers collection, Victor, New York. All four, **$250.00.**

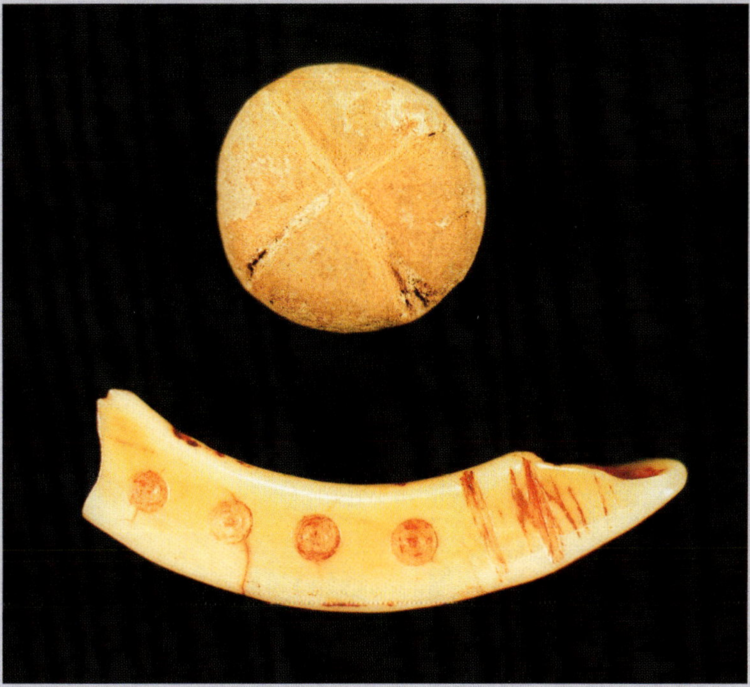

Gaming piece or marker, marmot tooth, 1⅛" long. It is accompanied by a smaller round piece with incised lines. Both are historic and were found in Campbell County, Wyoming. Mike Fox collection, Iowa. Marmot tooth, **$125.00;** other, **$75.00.**

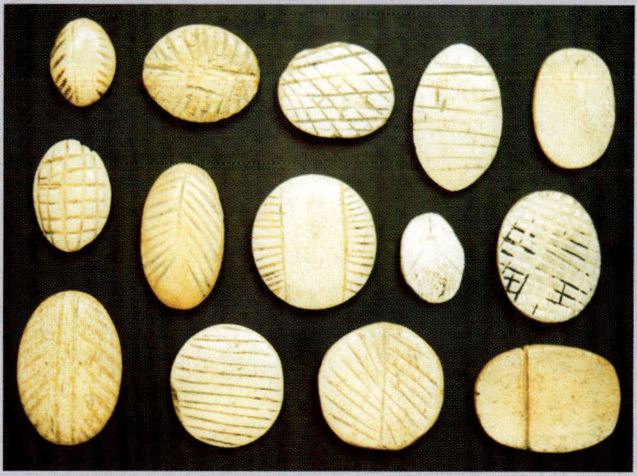

Gaming pieces, incised bones, largest center piece is 1" in diameter. These are historic period and all were found in Morton County, North Dakota. Mike Fox collection, Iowa. Each, **$75.00 – 100.00.**

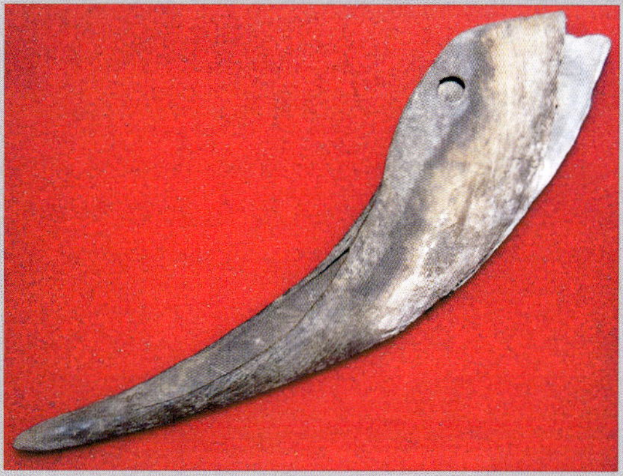

Bison(?) horn, center grooved or cut out, 9½" long, with suspension hole. This example is from the Great Basin, Nevada. Victor T. Trujillo collection, Nevada. Unlisted.

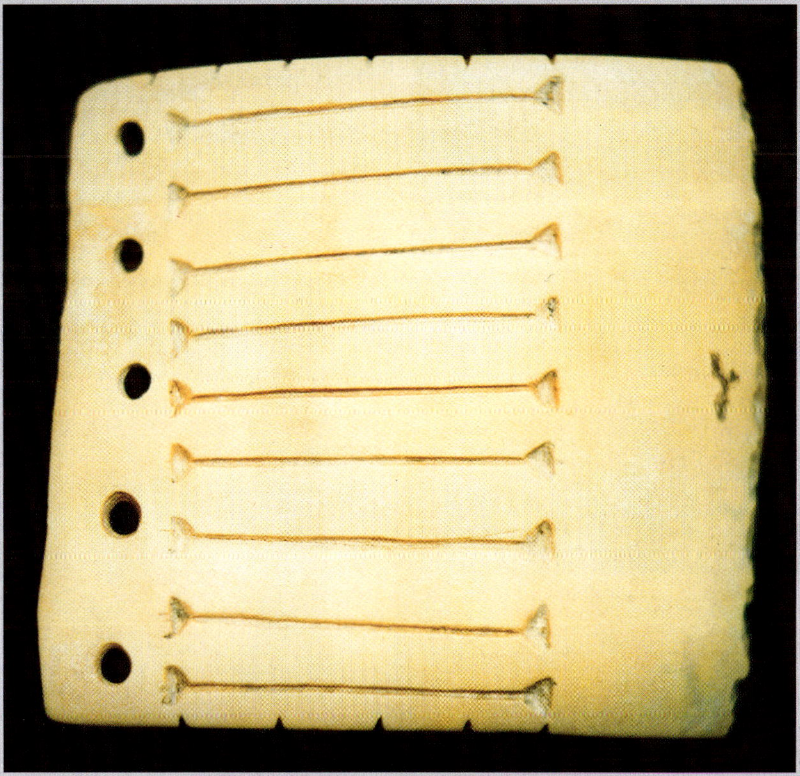

Bone wristguard, 3 x 3¼". Guards were used to protect the lower bow arm from bowstring snap. Historic period, the wristguard was found near Mobridge, South Dakota. Mike Fox collection, Iowa. **$425.00.**

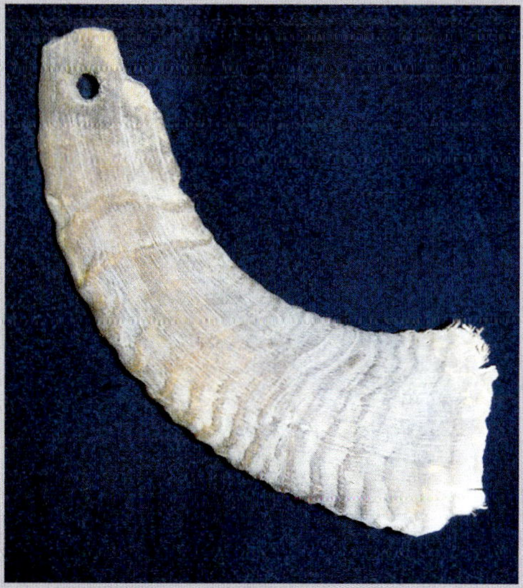

Shaft wrench, mountain sheep horn, 8¼" long. This tool was found in the Great Basin region, Nevada. Victor T. Trujillo collection, Nevada. **$300.00.**

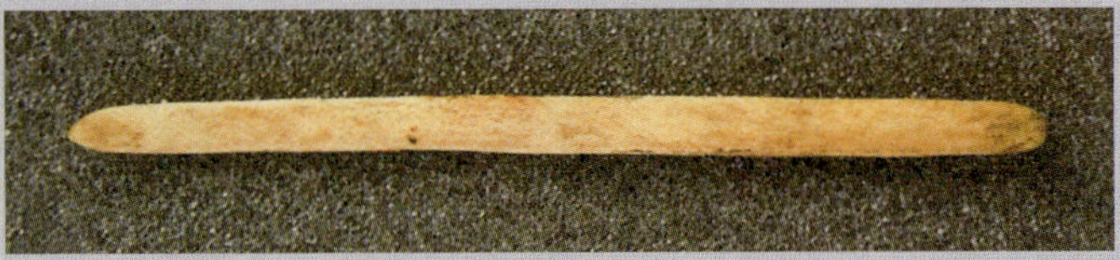

Bone hairpin, 3/16 x 4½" long. This artifact came from the Great Basin area, Nevada. Victor T. Trujillo collection, Nevada. **$90.00.**

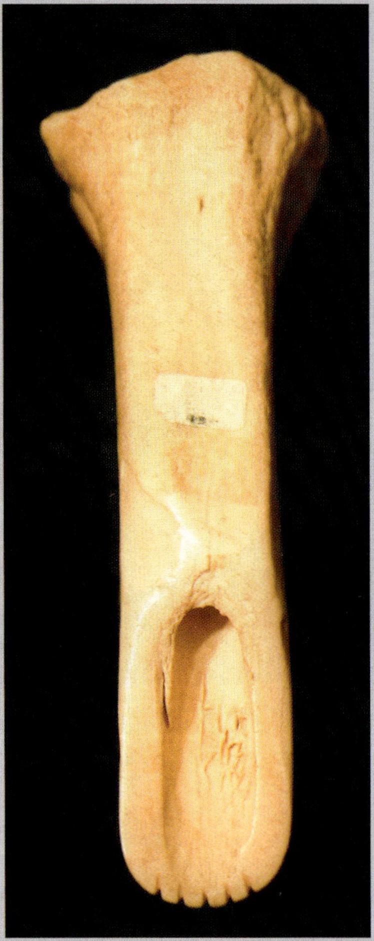

Bison bone flesher, 6" long, notched working edge with heavy polish. The flesher is marked "Mandan" which would place the artifact in the historic period. North Dakota. Tom Sekula collection, Pennsylvania. **$250.00.**

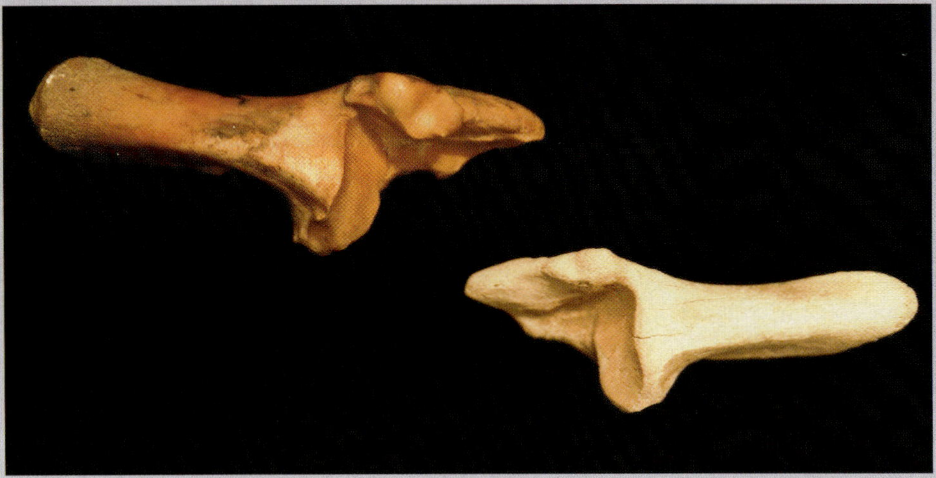

Animal bones, 3" long, found by the owner two years apart on an Archaic site. The head part of each bone has been reconfigured. Pennsylvania. Tom Sekula collection, Pennsylvania. Each, **$15.00 – 20.00.**

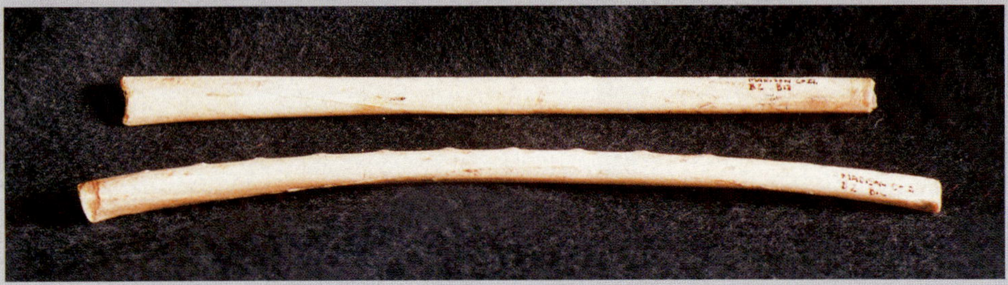

Bird bone artifacts, possibly pipe stems or bead preforms, 6½ and 7⅜" long. They were found in Madison County, Illinois. John F. Wubker collection, Illinois. Each, **$150.00.**

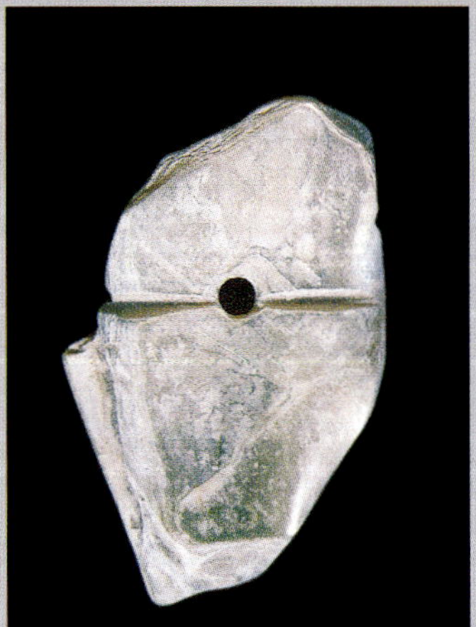

Abalone shell bead or pendant, 1¼" long, drilled and partially cut. It was found in the Great Basin region, Nevada. Victor T. Trujillo collection, Nevada. Unlisted.

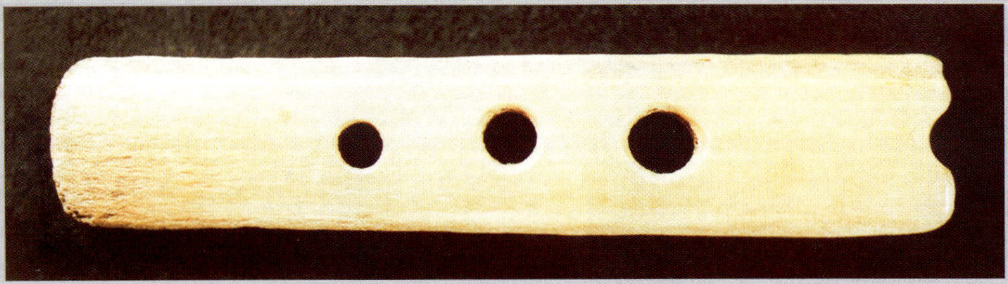

Bone shaft-straightener, 6¼" long. Probably made of bison bone, the smaller hole was used for sizing (diameter) and the two larger holes aided in bending and straightening wooden shafts. This artifact was found near Gettysburg, South Dakota. Mike Fox collection, Iowa. **$225.00.**

Tools to Make Tools

Some other artifacts are occasionally found on sites that have produced organic material objects. These tools were used in some stage of manufacture for the creation and maintenance of antler, bone, and shell artifacts.

Burins are often small and unimpressive objects unless their purpose is understood. Often made on the broken tips of points and blades, burins were formed by a special flint-knapping process (indirect percussion) that drove off long narrow flakes. Sometimes the flakes were used for boring tiny holes. The process also left behind a sharp, sturdy, jagged chisel-like edge. This edge could be used to score antler and bone. Thin channels might be made to isolate a bone strip that later became a needle or other artifact.

Blades and bladelets (long flake knives) were used both to whittle away excess antler and bone, and to prepare the material for breaking. To cut off a section, the sharp flint was used as a saw to encircle the material with a deep cut. The parts were then cleanly snapped apart. Bladelets, when first struck, have edges sharper than a surgeon's steel scalpel. Used as razor blades, they easily removed thin shavings.

Shapers were intermediate artifacts that ground and smoothed artifacts into a final shape. Sandstone or similar stones might be hand-held, or they could be large and part of the bedrock. Often, in or near rock shelters, grooves and channels in the rock indicate that antler and bone tools were shaped there.

Gravers are flint pieces with one or more short tips, and their probable purpose was to work antler, bone, shell, and wood. Gravers were suitable for grooving (like burins) and incising (for decoration.) Large examples were capable of boring holes.

Abraders were sandstone blocks with one or more narrow V- or U-shaped channels. These were used to sharpen needles, awls, and projectile point tips. Abraders were necessary to keep pointed bone tools in a serviceable condition.

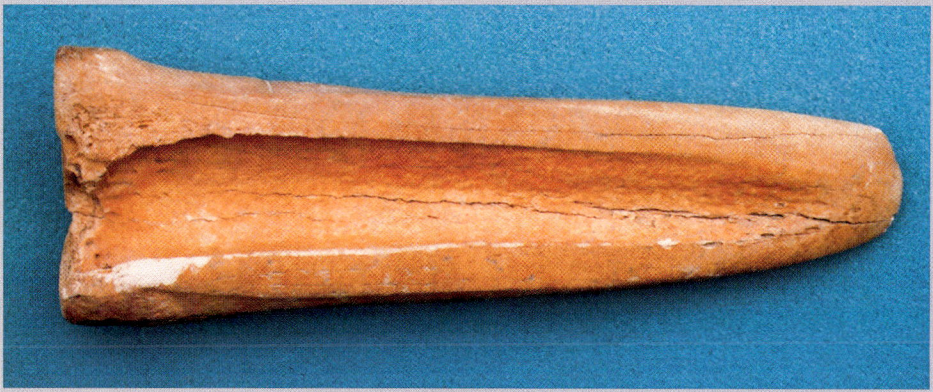

Elk bone wedge, prehistoric, 2¼ x 7¼", 1" thick. The artifact is ex-collections Woodcock and Hayden, and is probably Northwestern United States. Collection of, and photograph by, Gary Henry, North Carolina. **$50.00.**

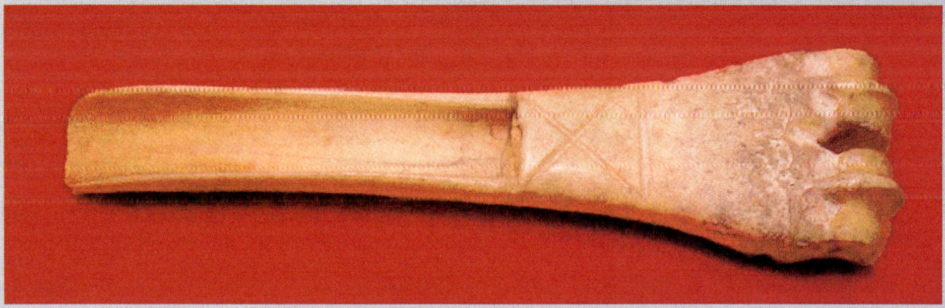

Bone scoop or gouge, 1⅛ x 4⅝", ⅝" thick. A wood plug closes the hollow of this decorated piece, probably made in historic times. This scarce artifact is in fine condition, provenance unknown. Michael F. Slasinski collection, Michigan. **$250.00.**

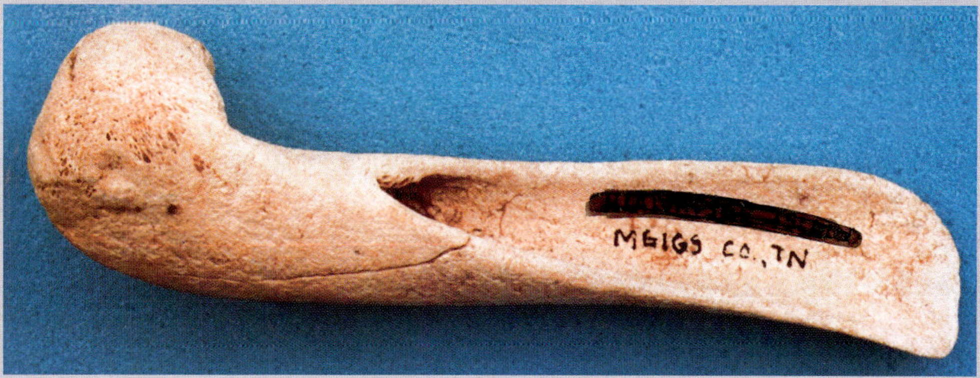

Bone gouge, black bear bone, 1½ x 6¼", 1½" thick. From the Mississippian period, this uncommon and heavy bone was ideal for tool use. Ex-collection Snyder, it is from Meigs County, Tennessee. Collection of, and photograph by, Gary Henry, North Carolina. **$150.00.**

Tools to Make Tools

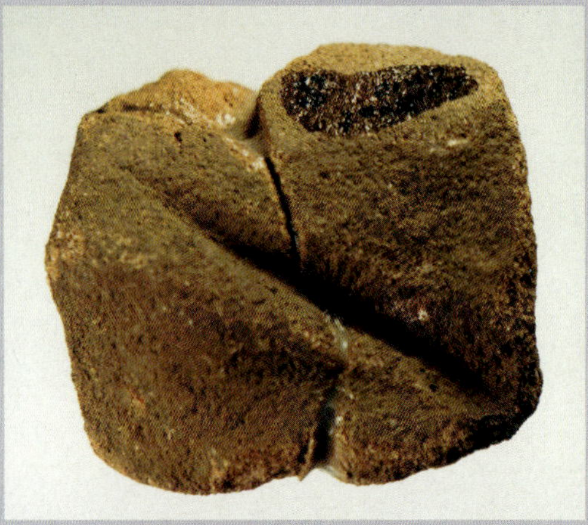

Sandstone awl or needle sharpener, Mississippian period, broken and glued, about 2¼" square. It is from southern Ohio. Private collection. **$15.00.**

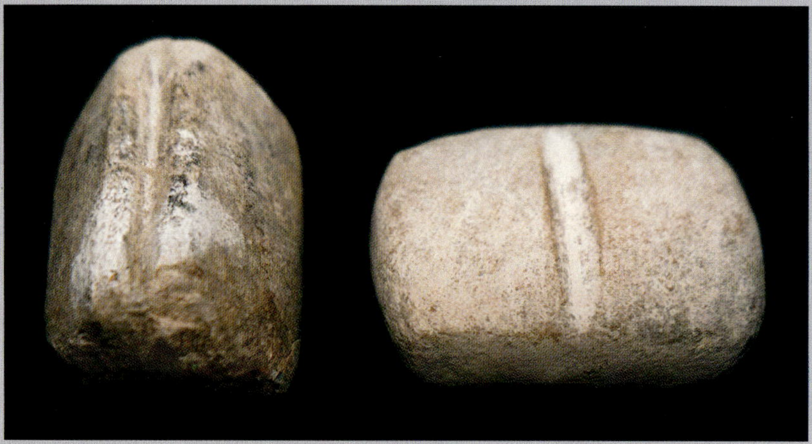

Tools for making tools, Left, awl- or needle-sharpener; right, shaft-straightener. Back to Earth. Unlisted.

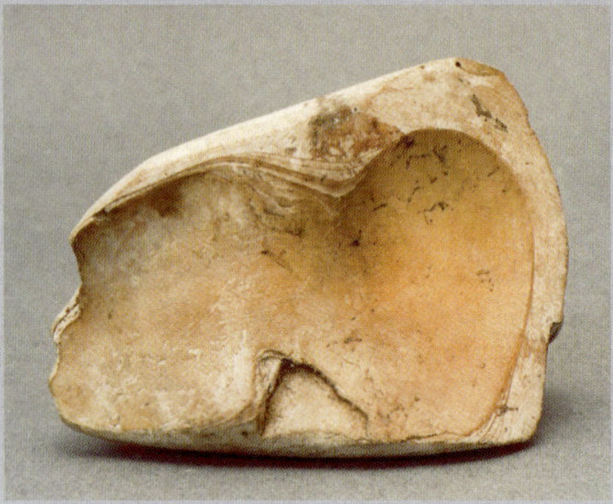

Shell adz blade, 1⅝ x 2⅜", made before AD 1400. Marine shell, the tool blade was found on Marco Island, Florida. H. B. Greene II collection, Naples, Florida. **$80.00.**

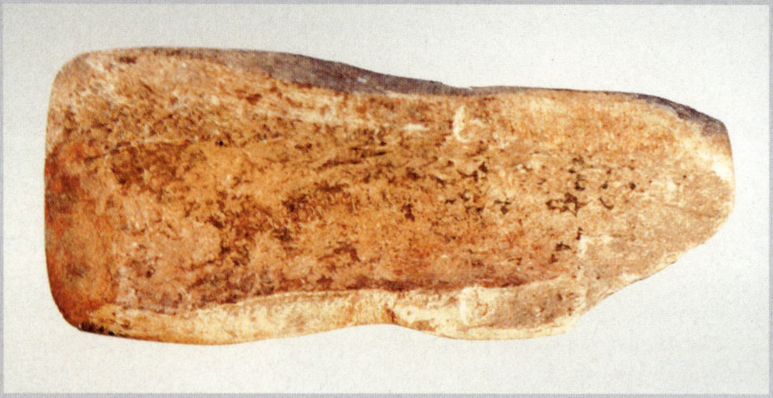

Elk antler adz, 4⅝" long. This is a scarce artifact, both in tool type and material. Fort Ancient, it is from southern Ohio. Fred Winegardner collection. **$150.00.**

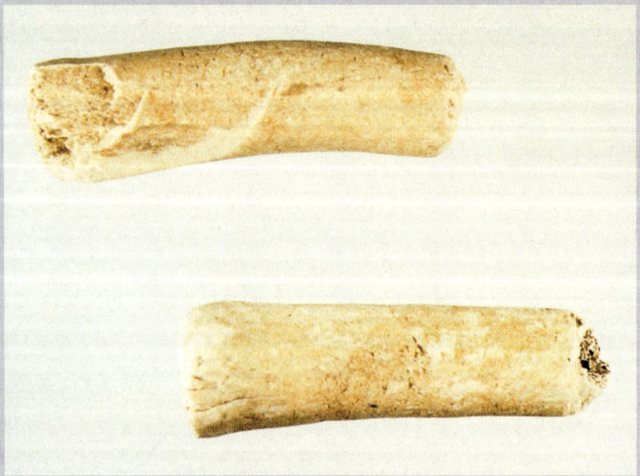

Antler flint-knapping tools or flakers, rounded at both large and small ends, probably Mississippian period. Each is 2⅝" long. Kentucky. Private collection. Each, **$12.00.**

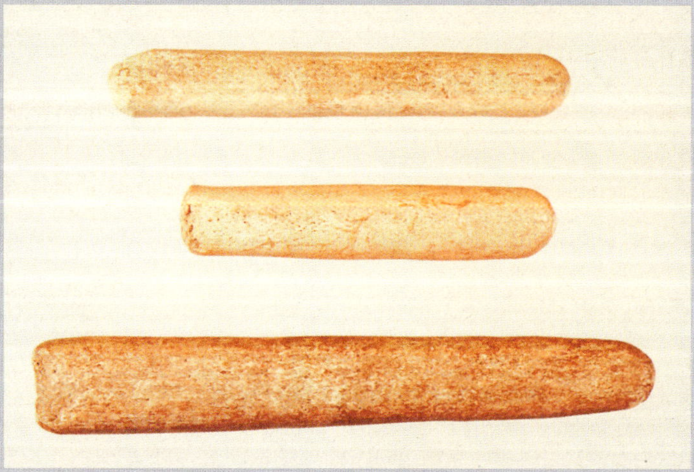

Antler drifts or flint-knappers, longest is 3⅝". They are from southern Ohio. Fred Winegardner collection. Each, **$15.00 – 30.00.**

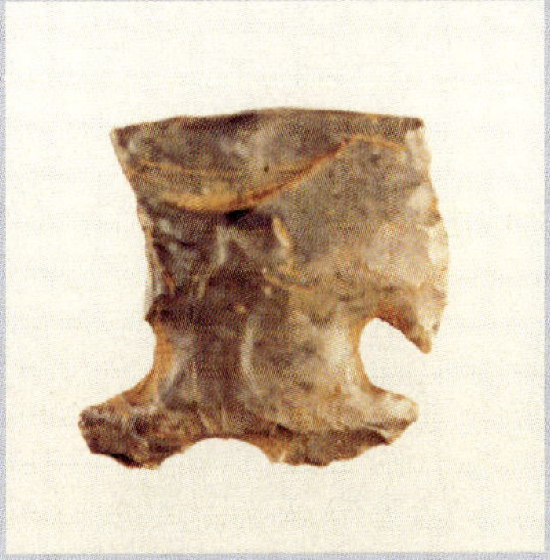

Burin, pale blue Upper Mercer flint, ⅞" long. This is a Jack's Reef type from Late Woodland times, and the upper left corner is the burin tip. Made from a point or blade, the artifact is from Ohio. Private collection. **$15.00.**

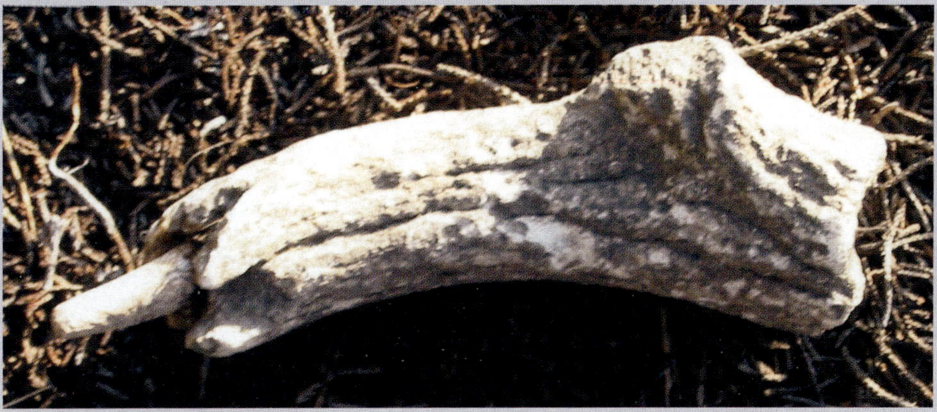

Antler flaking tool, 5" long. This unusual and scarce piece came from a dry cave, western Texas. John and Susan Mellyn collection, Texas. **$125.00.**

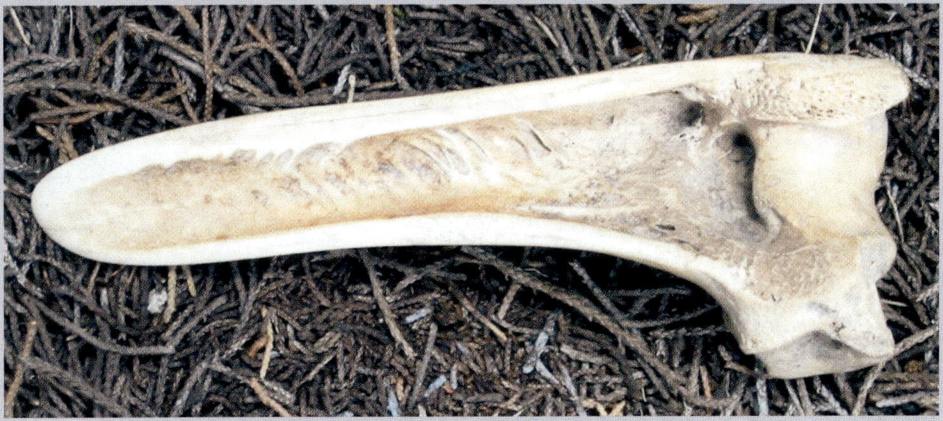

Adz blade, heavy animal bone, 4 9/16" long. It was found in the St. Johns area, Arizona. John and Susan Mellyn collection, Texas. **$100.00.**

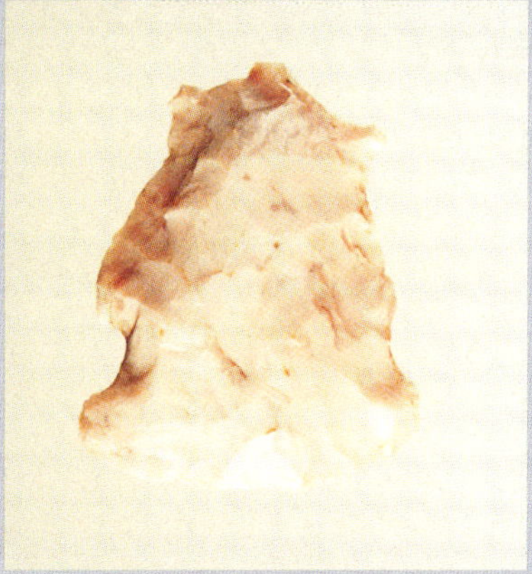

Graver, "coronet" or crown type, three graver tips. Made of pink Flint Ridge, it is 1⅛" long. Late Archaic, it is from Ohio. Private collection. **$25.00.**

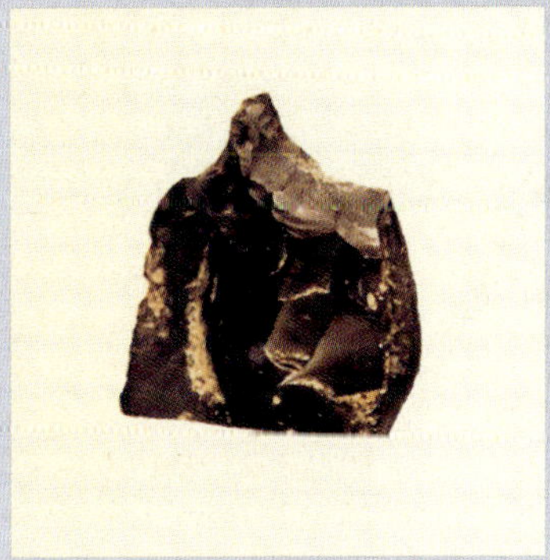

Graver, single tip, probably Late Woodland. It is ¾" long and made of blue Upper Mercer flint. Ohio. Private collection. **$10.00.**

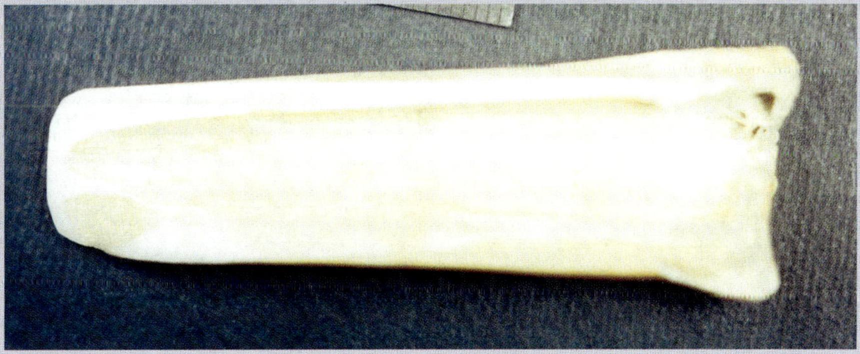

Bone gouge or adz blade, bison or elk bone. It is from near Chamberlain, South Dakota. Lee Hallman collection, Pennsylvania. **$75.00.**

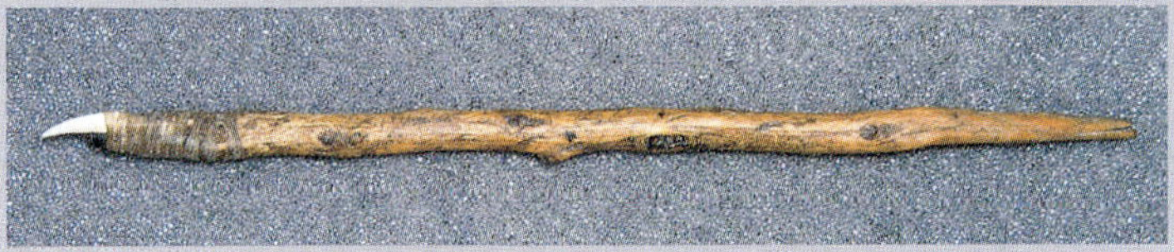

Perforator or flaker, 5" long, animal tooth tip, sinew-wrapped on greasewood shaft. Ex-collection Luke, it is from the Great Basin, Nevada. Victor T. Trujillo collection, Nevada. **$75.00.**

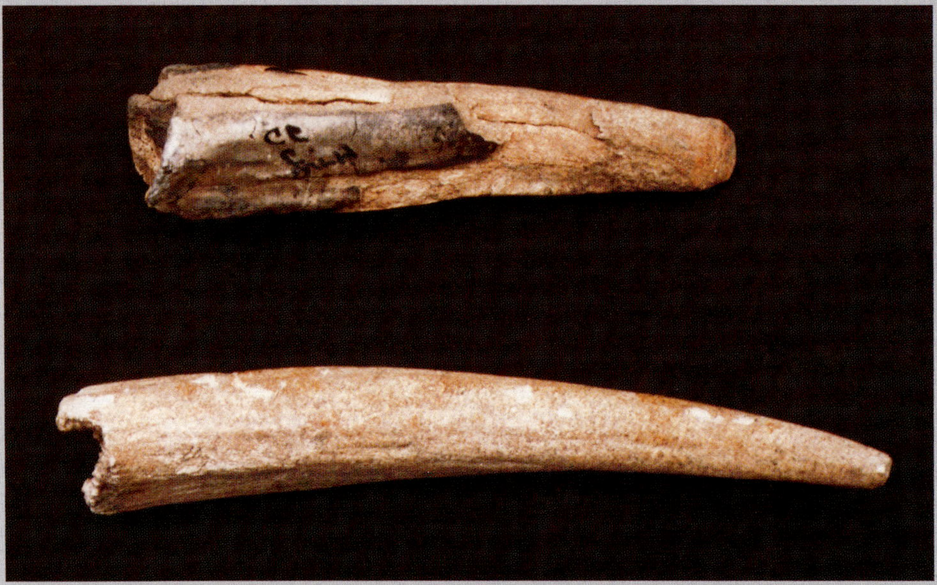

Deer antler flaking tools, Woodland or Mississippian, longest is ⅞ x 5$\frac{5}{16}$". Harwood found these between 1954 and 1982. Greene County, Tennessee. Collection of, and photograph by, Gary Henry, North Carolina. Each, **$8.00 – 10.00.**

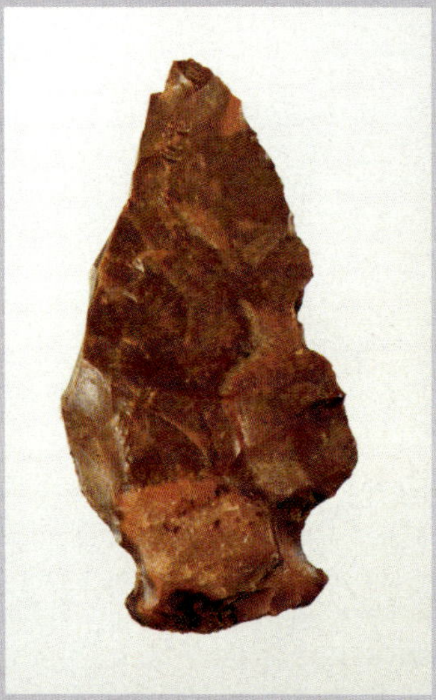

Graver, burin-flaked at tip and left edge, mixed brown unknown flint. This Archaic piece, 2" long, is from Delaware County, Ohio. Private collection. **$12.00 – 15.00.**

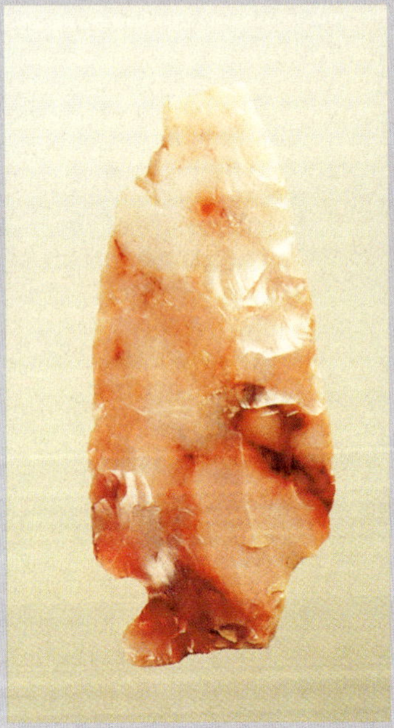

Burin, Archaic blade in translucent gem-quality Flint Ridge, 2¼". The burin tip is at top left and there are three overlapping burin scars with termination hinges. An excellent example, it is from Ohio. Lar Hothem collection. **$25.00.**

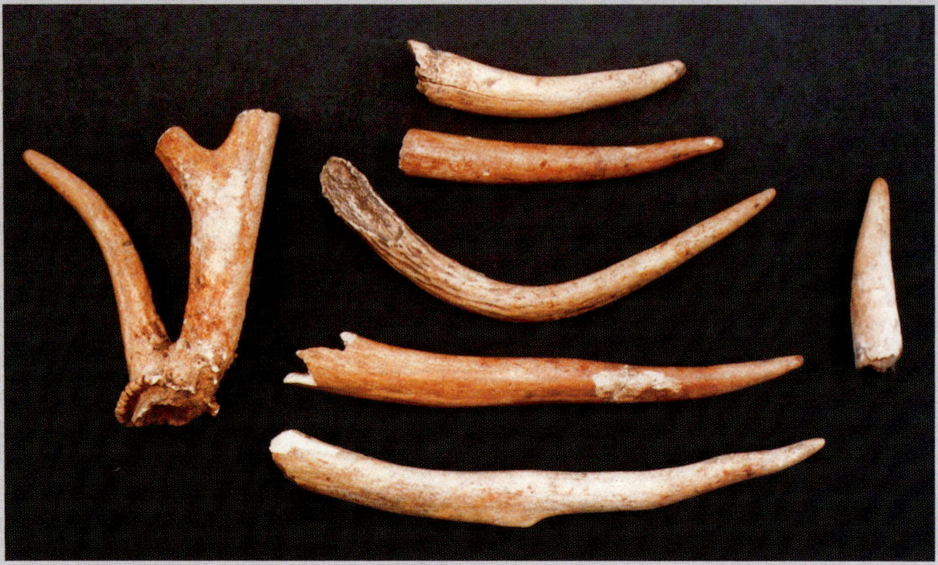

Antler flakers or drifts, Woodland or later in time, longest is ⅞ x 7⅝". These are ex-collection Snyder, from Meigs County, Tennessee. Collection of, and photograph by, Gary Henry, North Carolina. Each, **$10.00 – 25.00.**

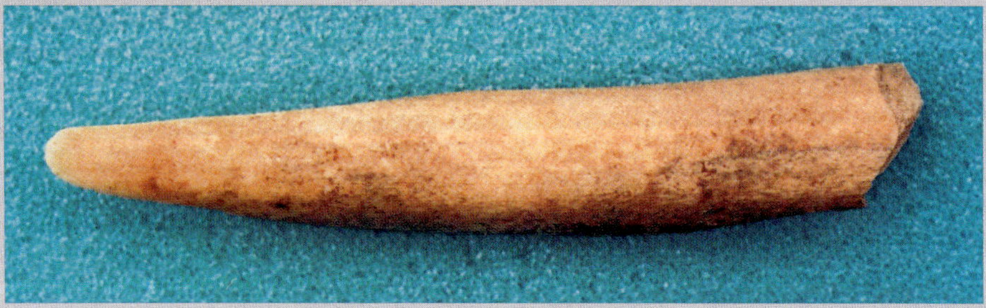

Bone flaker, ⅜ x 2⅜", Woodland or later. Harwood found it in 1957. Clay County, North Carolina. Collection of, and photograph by, Gary Henry, North Carolina. **$15.00.**

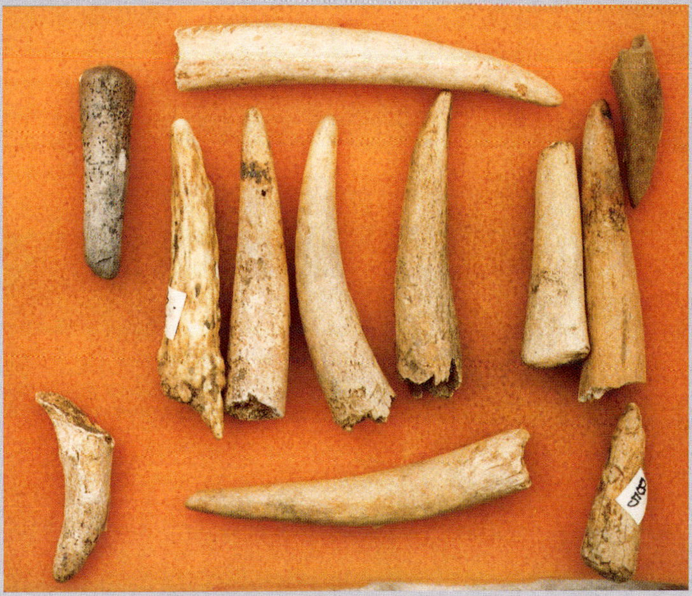

Flakers, antler and bone, Woodland or later, largest is ½ x 2⅞". These are ex-collection Snyder and were picked up in Meigs County, Tennessee. Each, **$10.00 – 15.00.**

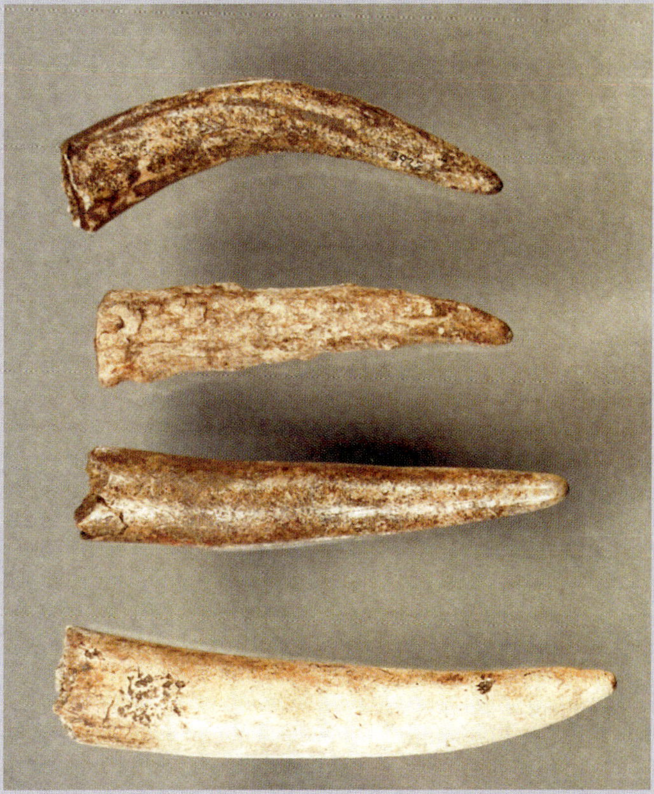

Antler flakers or flint-knapping tools, Riverton culture, Late Archaic period, 2¾ to 4" long. These were used in the final stages of chipping flint and chert. These artifacts were found in Crawford County, Illinois. John Smith collection, Illinois. Each, **$5.00 – 10.00.**

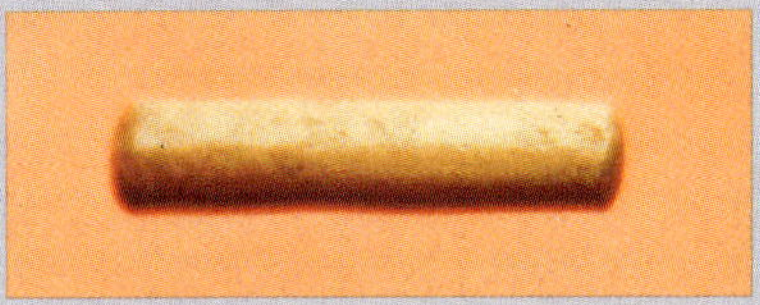

Flaker or drift, 1 7/16" long, Frontenac phase of the Late Archaic period. This flint-chipping tool was found in Cayuga County, New York. Dave Summers collection, Victor, New York. **$35.00.**

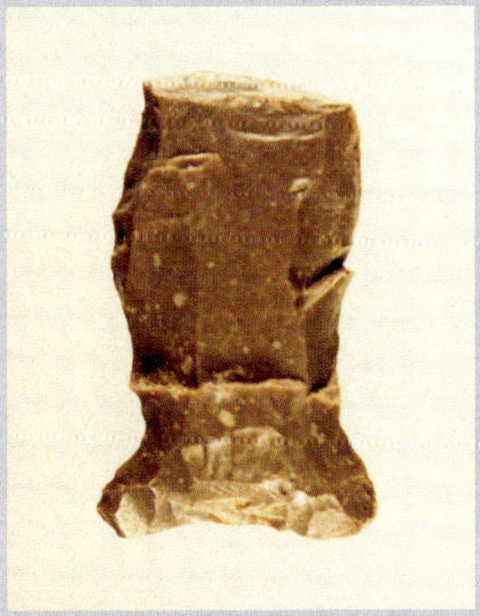

Burin tool, Fishspear type from the Late Archaic, brown Delaware County flint. It is 1½" long and has five broad to narrow burin scars on one face and both sides. All burin scars terminate abruptly and exactly at the hafting area. Ohio. Private collection. **$25.00.**

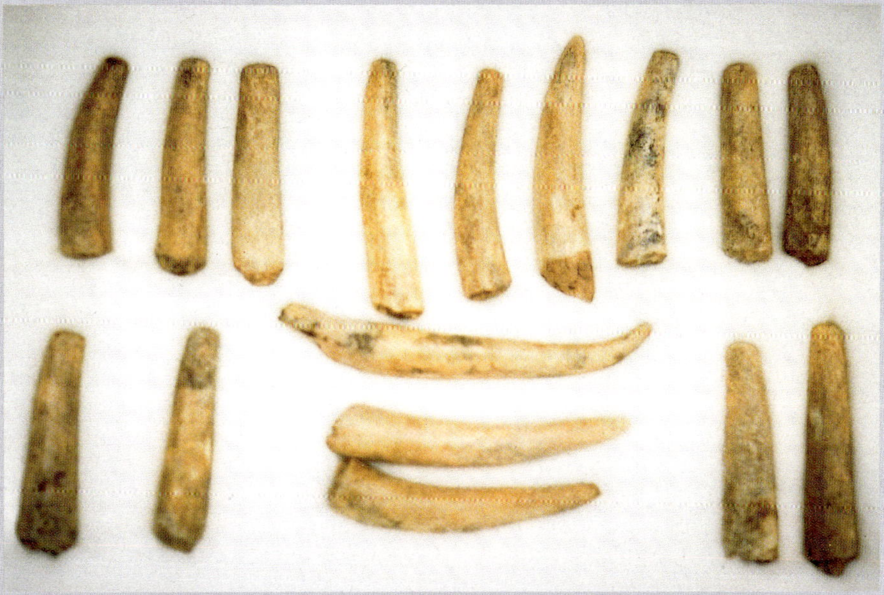

Antler flaking tools, 16 shown from a cache of 34, lengths range from 1¾ to 4". Mississippi County, Arkansas. Bob Hess collection, Indiana. Each, **$5.00 – 15.00.**

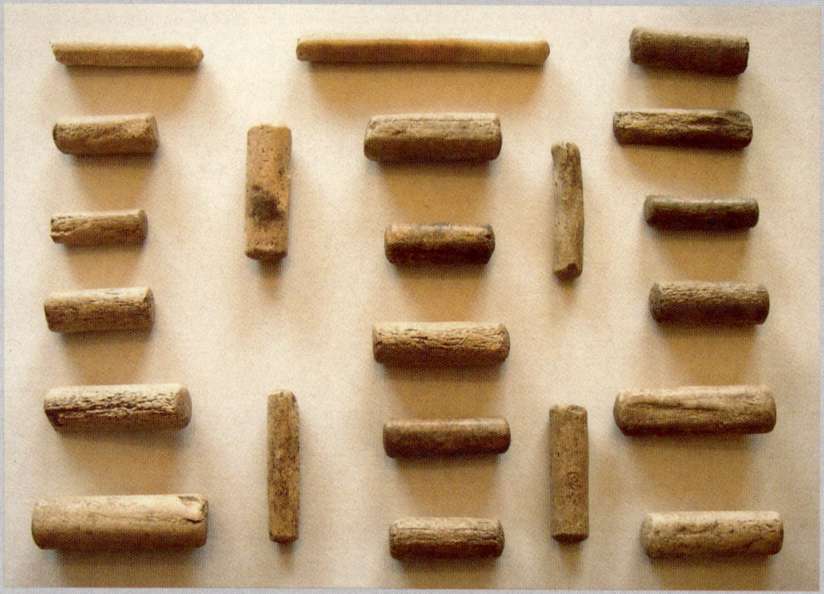

Antler flakers or drift pins, Mississippian, longest specimen is 2¾". These have the typical cylindrical form and rounded ends. All were found in the Ohio River Valley, Mason County, West Virginia. Private collection; Rodney Roberts photograph. Each, **$10.00 – 20.00.**

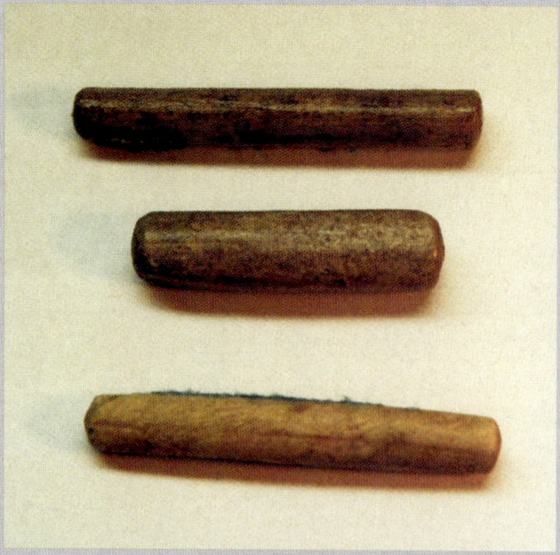

Deer bone drifts or flakers, longest is 2⅝". Commonly found on Mississippian-era sites, they were also made in earlier times. Fulton County, Illinois. Fred Smith collection, Illinois. Each, **$15.00 – 20.00.**

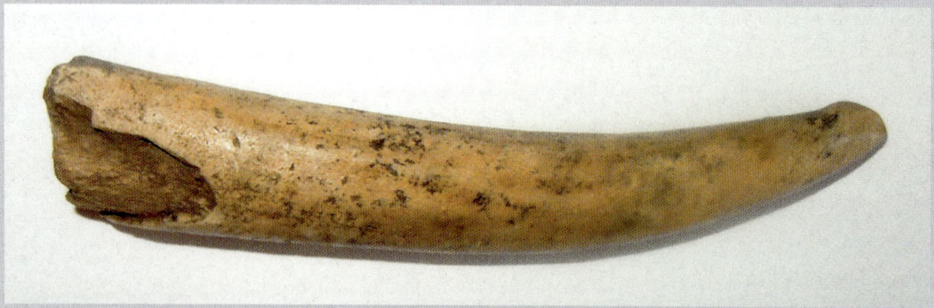

Antler chisel, Mississippian, with bit sharpened to a chisel edge. It is 4⅜" long and was found by the owner in April of 2003. Mason County, West Virginia. Private collection; Rodney Roberts photograph. **$35.00.**

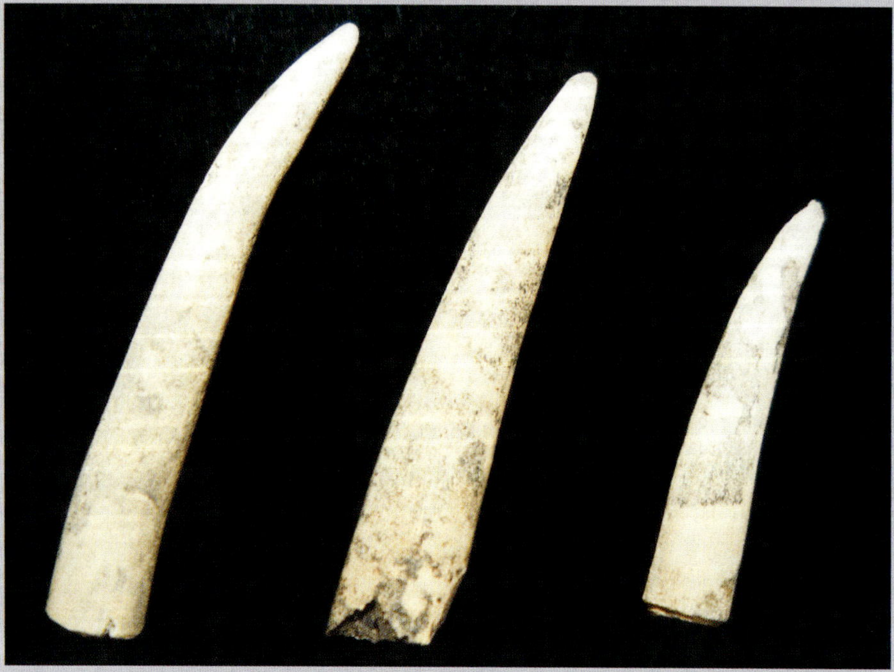

Antler flintknapping tools for pressure flaking, longest is 3¾". The three were personal finds by the owner. Mississippi County, Arkansas. Garvin collection. Each, **$15.00 – 25.00.**

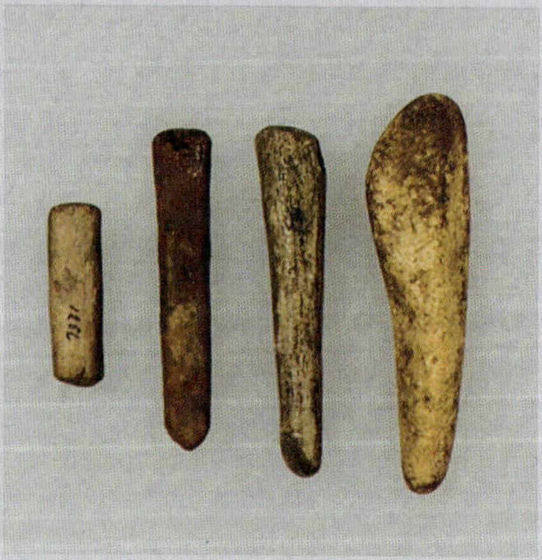

Antler flakers (also called punches or drifts), Mississippian period, longest is 3⅛". Used for knapping flint, they are rounded on the ends. Col. Vietzen found these in northern Ohio. Pete Timoch collection. Each, **$10.00 – 15.00.**

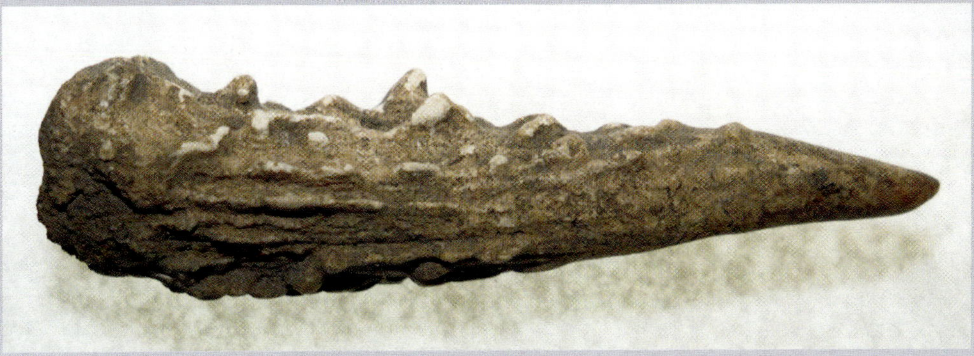

Antler flaking tool, spike buck, 4¼" long. It was found in a rock shelter in May of 2004. Robertson County, Tennessee. Garvin collection, Ohio. **$125.00.**

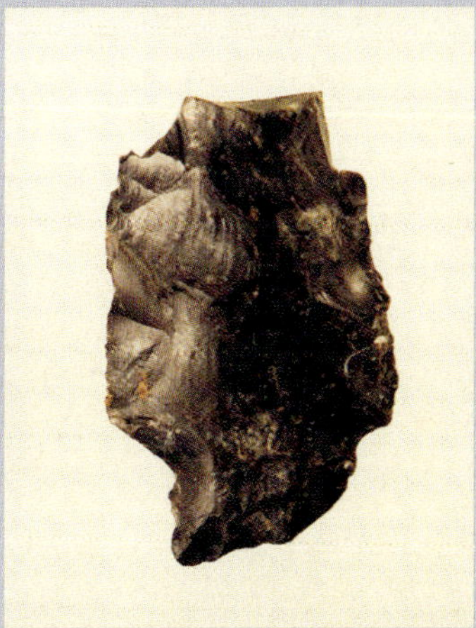

Burin, Archaic blade, 1¼" long. Made from a point or blade, there are burin tips at both corners of the break area. Dark blue Upper Mercer flint, it was found in Ohio. Private collection. **$20.00.**

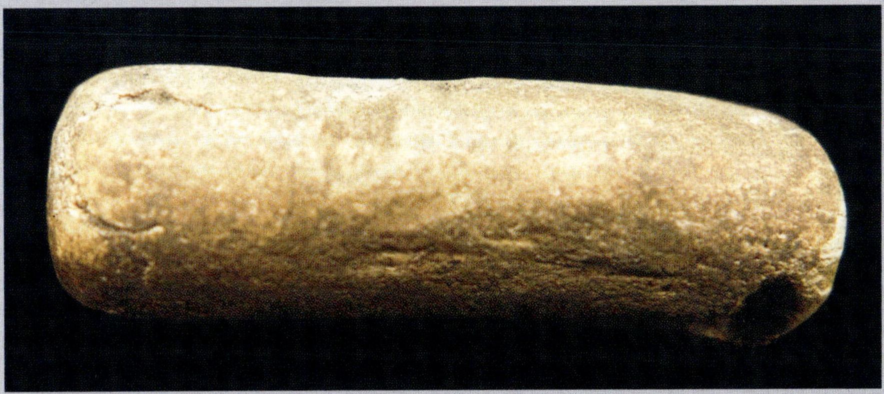

Bone drift or knapping tool, 2⅜" long, rounded ends. It was found in Mississippi County, Arkansas. Garvin collection. **$15.00 – 20.00.**

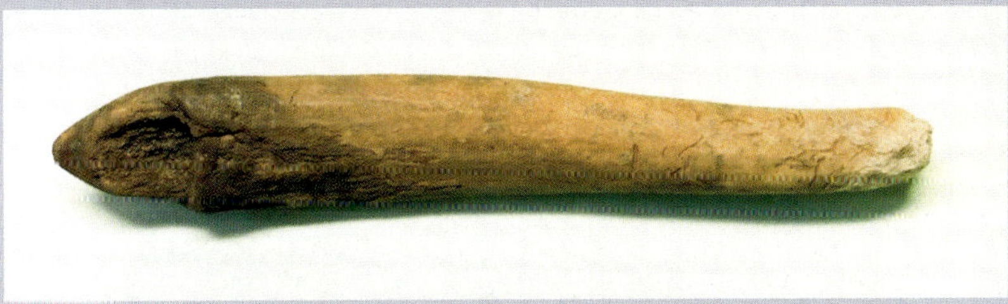

Antler tip flaking tool, mule deer, 1³⁄₁₆ x 5⁹⁄₁₆". One end has been split and ground to a wedge shape, possibly to produce notches in projectile points. Weber County, northern Utah. Dann Russell collection, Utah. **$50.00.**

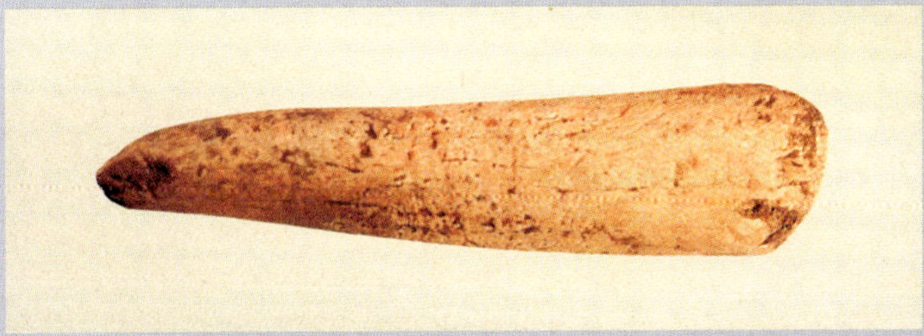

Flaker, deer antler section, cut and rounded base. The flaker is 2⅝" long, from Wayne County, Kentucky. Private collection. **$12.00.**

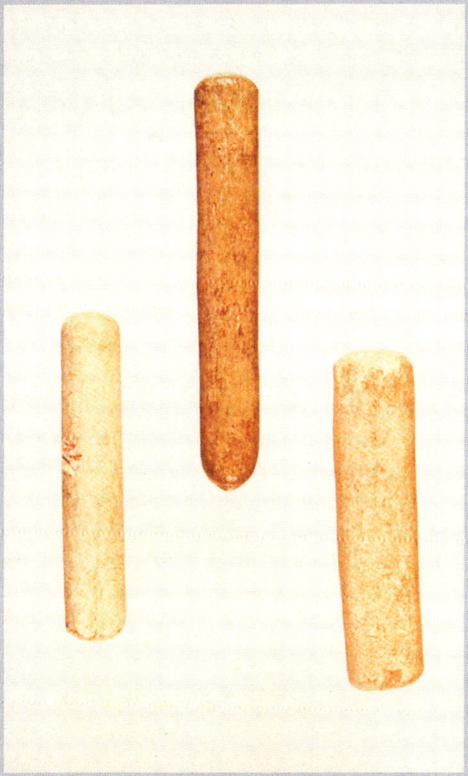

Antler drifts or flint-knapping tools, longest is 2". The polished examples came from southern Ohio. Fred Winegardner collection. Each, **$15.00 – 20.00.**

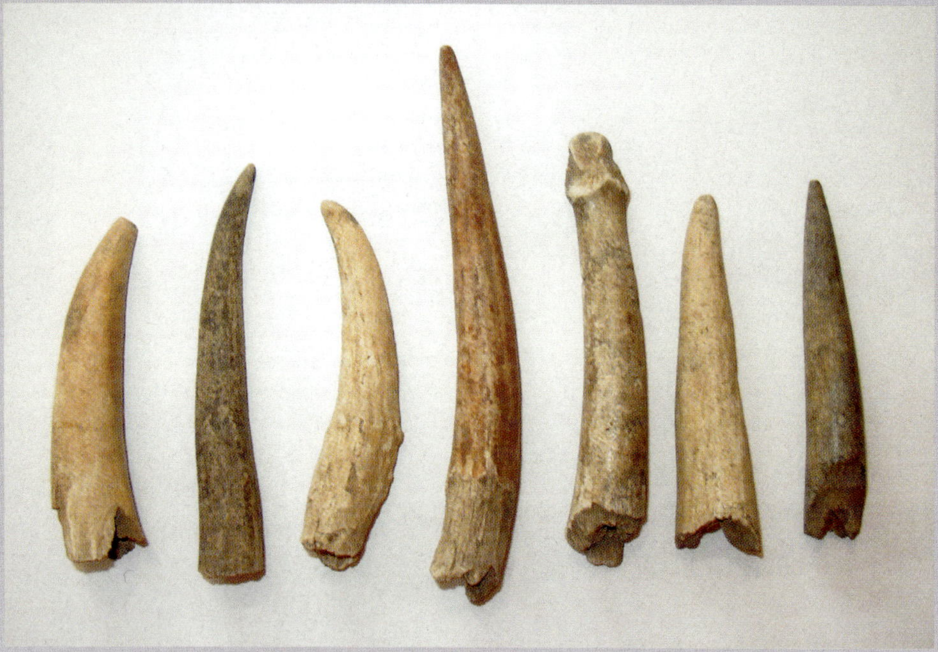

Antler flakers, Mississippian period, largest is 4⁷⁄₁₆" long. All were found in Mason County, West Virginia. Private collection. Rodney Roberts photograph. Each, **$20.00 – 30.00.**

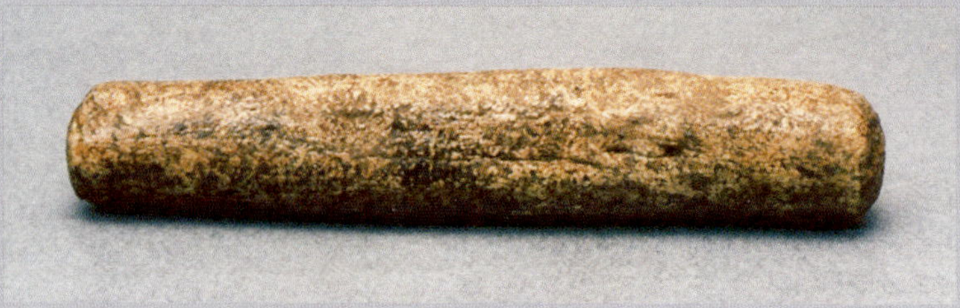

Bone drift or flint-knapping rod, 2⅞" long, ca. 2500 BC. It was found on an island in the Savanna River near Augusta, Georgia. H. B. Greene II collection, Naples, Florida. **$25.00.**

Antler handle, oval central hole, 3¾". The hilt end is highly polished as if from long-time use. Central Tennessee. Dwight Wolfe collection. **$125.00.**

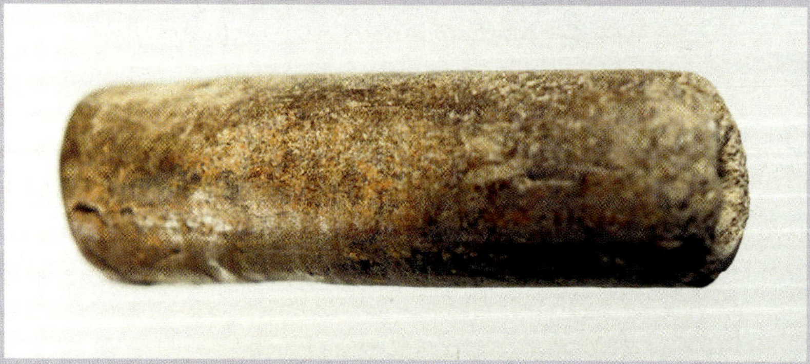

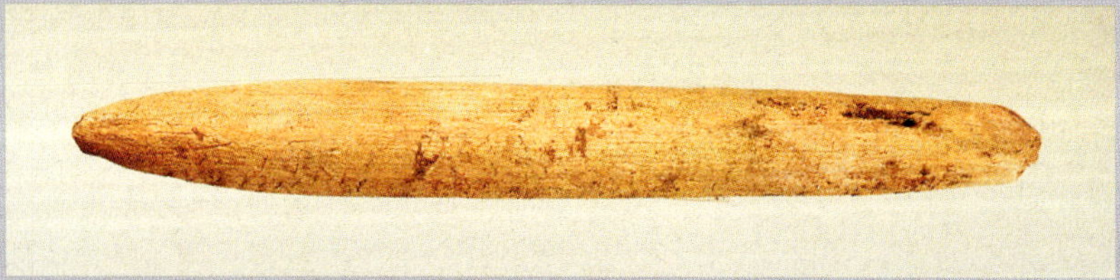

Bone flaker, unknown thick animal bone, 3¾" long. Origin unknown. Robin Fiser collection. **$25.00.**

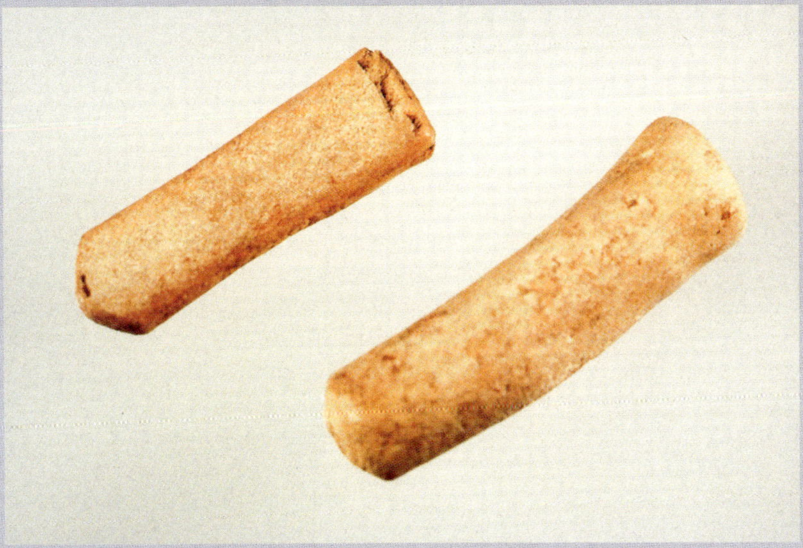

Bone flakers, longest is 2⅝". The smaller example has a rectangular cross-section and the flattened end is battered; it was perhaps used for indirect percussion knapping. West Virginia. Doug Hooks collection. Each, **$15.00 – 20.00.**

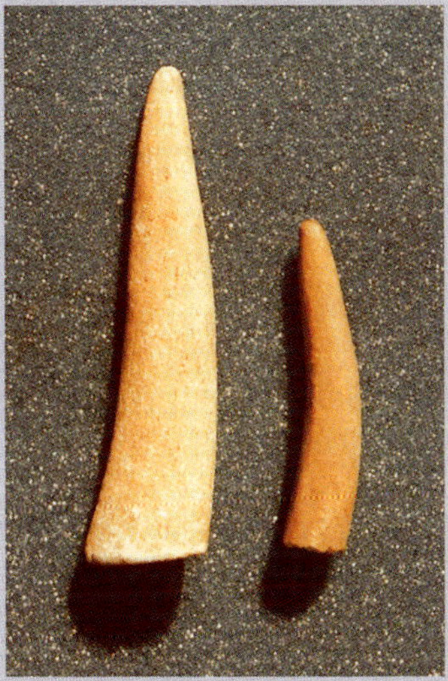

Flint-knapping tools, 2⅞ and 1⅞" long. Made of deer antler, they are historic Iroquois (Seneca), ca. AD 1650 – 1670. The knapping tools were recovered near East Bloomfield, Ontario County, New York. Dave Summers collection, Victor, New York. Larger, **$35.00;** smaller, **$15.00.**

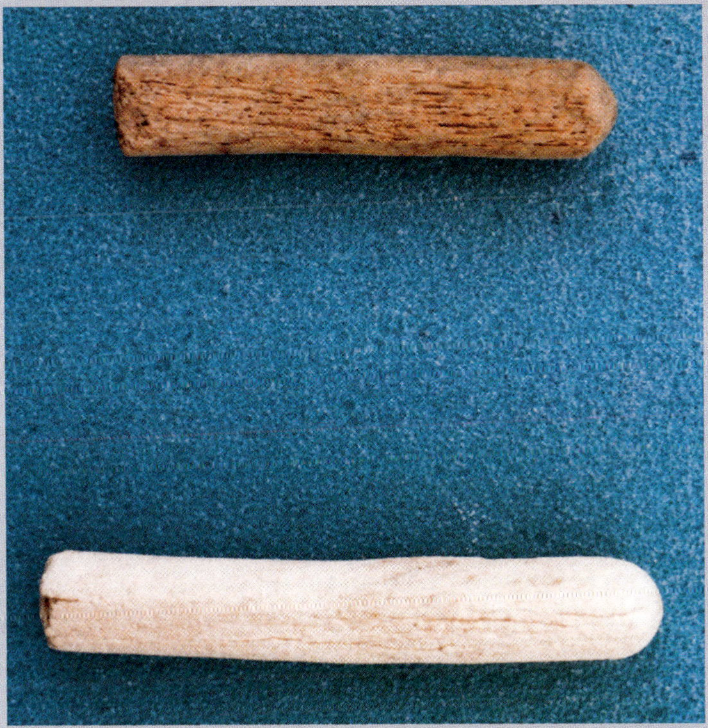

Bone flakers, Woodland or Mississippian, top example is 5⁄16 x 1 9⁄16" and bottom example is 9⁄16 x 1 15⁄16". These have the diagnostic rounded tip at one end, and flakers have also been called rods or drifts. Snyder found them between 1947 and 1958. Polk County, Tennessee. Collection of, and photograph by, Gary Henry, North Carolina. Each, **$15.00.**

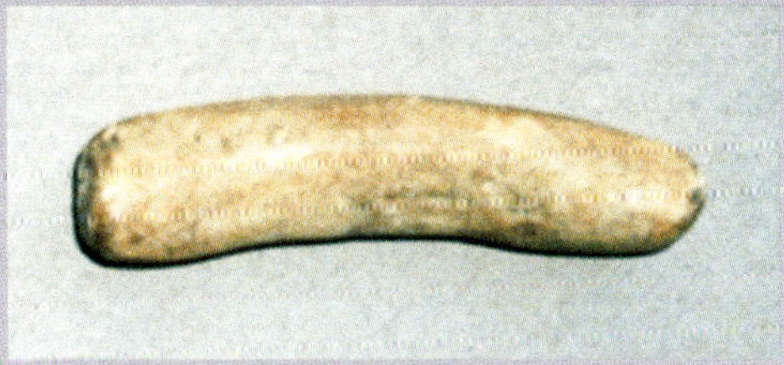

Antler drift or flint-knapper, polished shaft and rounded ends. It was found in Mississippi. Wilfred Dick collection, Mississippi. **$15.00.**

Facts About Artifacts

In the course of researching this book, I found many interesting accounts relating to antler, bone, and shell artifacts.

The more informative of these are in this chapter.

A rather strange incident involving bone artifacts took place years ago at Kentucky's King Mounds, later called Ancient Buried City. "One day, while excavating, I left my trowel for a moment. An old gentleman was curious to see what I had been digging, so he started to dig and, unfortunately, broke one of the handsomest bone tools that has been excavated. In his haste and excitement when he saw the tool projecting through the dirt, he dug frantically, and pop(!) went the artifact. It was the last of a cache of awls, needles, skivers, and a spatula. The artifact that was broken is highly polished, tapering to a point, 10" in length, and the artisan cleverly used the end of the deer bone out of which it was made for the handle, comparable to our paper knives." (King, Blanche Busey. *Under Your Feet*. Dodd, Mead & Company, New York, 1939, pp 158 – 159).

The columella (spiraled interior of large marine shells) was used for plummet-like pendants at Key Marco, Florida. Grooved or narrowed at the top, most were undecorated but one had three ridges. Most had smoothed surfaces. (Gilliland, Marion Spjut. *The Material Culture of Key Marco, Florida*. The University Presses of Florida, Gainesville, 1975, pp 173 – 175).

Bone fishhooks were made in several ways, and two are described here. "Phalanges (toe bones) of deer were split longitudinally, each half constituting a bone blank from which a hook could be cut. This produced a hook in one plane, with a sharp "elbow." Another form made from curved sections of long bone resulted in a broad hook which retained, on its face, the natural curvature of the long bone, and which had a broad, nearly square base and 'open elbow'." (Webb, William S. and David L. DeJarnette. *The Perry Site*. WPA/TVA, Alabama Museum Paper 25, 1948, pp 52 – 54).

A unique awl type from Tennessee suggests that the prehistoric users were highly skilled and had a sense of artistic perfection in their work:

"Delicate splinter awls may have been used for sewing skins, etc., the point being used to pierce the material for the thread. Several of these show an unusual treatment of the point which was narrowed to form slight shoulders to prevent the awl from passing through the material beyond that point and thus insuring the uniform size of the holes." (Lewis, Thomas M. N. and Madeline Kneberg. *Hiwassee Island – An Archaeological Account of Four Tennessee Indian Peoples*. The University of Tennessee Press, 1946, Knoxville, p 125, plate 78-B).

In the Central States region, bone points with sockets are found on Archaic, Woodland, and Mississippian sites. Those from the first two tend to be larger. Antler tines were commonly used, though an example made from a deer jawbone exists. The antler tine was drilled at the base for attachment to a shaft. (Wagers, Charlie. "Socketed Bone Points." *Central States Archaeological Journal*. Vol. 44 No. 1, January 1997, pp 14, 15).

One early report noted the varied condition of bone artifacts found in Ontario, Canada.

"Bone and Horn Articles, Also Those of Teeth – These articles constitute a very large percentage of artifacts found in ashbeds and around village sites. The acids of the ashes helped to preserve them in their pristine quality and shape. Some of these articles taken from undisturbed ashbeds look as if they were made the previous day, while others picked up on the surface of the ground are sometimes very fragile and chalky in nature, crumbling and splitting to the touch. Some of these bone and horn articles are of their natural color, others are charred or carbonized to a dark brown or black. Many fragments of burnt and broken bones occur. Some show traces of workmanship, such as cutting or sawing." (Laidlaw, Col. G. E. "Archaeological Notes on Victoria County, Ont." *The Archaeological Bulletin*. Vol. 6 No. 5. The international Society of Archaeologists, September-October 1915, pp 6, 8).

Tubular bone artifacts in prehistoric Arizona may have had several uses.

"The tubes of various sizes were cut from the shafts of long bones. Bones from the turkey and smaller birds, from rabbits and other small mammals furnished the material. It is not always possible to tell the source of the bone because of the removal of distinguishing features. The tubes were used as beads in necklaces, and in bracelets of the wrist-guard type, as bits for pipes, possibly as drinking tubes, and as handles for awls and other types of implements. Those with apertures in the side are usually classed as flageolets if there are several holes, and as whistles or bird calls if there is but one. The single-holed variety with the opening at approximately the center on one side is the only kind found during the Whitewater investigations. All of them are well polished and the edges of the apertures are carefully smoothed." (Roberts, Frank H. H. Jr. "Archaeological Remains in the Whitewater District / Eastern Arizona, Part II." *Bureau of American Ethnology*. Bulletin 126. Smithsonian Institution, Washington, 1940, pp 114, 115).

Based on textile materials found in dry Kentucky rock shelters, bone fishhooks would have had fishing lines made of several different materials. These could have been shredded bark, stems of grass, thin bark strips, strips of cornhusk, or leather cord. (Funkhouser, W. D. and W. S. Webb. "The So-Called 'Ash Caves' in Lee County, Kentucky." *Reports in Archaeology and Anthropology*. Vol. 1 No. 2, December 1929. University of Kentucky, Lexington, p 86).

Awls were present in the Early Woodland of the eastern Midwest, and some were quite large.

"The awl is a bona fide trait of Adena culture, although its identification value is somewhat lowered by the fact that it is found abundantly in other cultures... Those from the Adena Mound vary in length from 5 to 11", and are made of the shoulder blades of the elk and the Virginia deer. Those from Mound 53 were from 8 to 12½" long and were made from the metapodial bones of the elk." (Greenman, E. F. "Excavation of the Coon Mound and an Analysis of the Adena Culture," *Ohio Archaeological and Historical Quarterly*. Vol. XLI, No. 3, July 1932, pp 369, 457, 458).

The Late Woodland period (Kipp Island phase) of New York state had many bone artifacts. Besides typical awls and antler flakers, there were bone and antler harpoons (with up to 12 barbs), antler combs, antler handles with copper awls, perforated bear and lynx teeth, and antler armbands. (Ritchie, William A. *The Archaeology of New York State*. American Museum of Natural History, Garden City, 1965, pp 228, 230).

Occasionally bone artifacts were salvaged in prehistoric times and made into other, different artifacts. Examples were found at the Feurt site, (Mississippian period) in Scioto County, Ohio. Regarding an object made from a deer metapodial (lower leg bone):

"This specimen had formerly been made into a scraper used in dressing skins during the tanning process as were practically all of these bones. The heavy use to which these implements were subjected caused many of them to break at the center, rendering the implement useless. The distal end of the broken scraper was frequently made into a blunt awl." (Mills, William C. "The Feurt Mounds and Village Site." *Ohio Archaeological and Historical Quarterly*. Vol. XXVI No. 3, July 1917, p 406).

Several interesting items were found during explorations in Utah, one a club and one a paint container.

"A large elk horn found at Site 13 had been split and all the branches but one chopped off to give a sort of pistol grip, while the base was roughly pointed but showed no signs of wear. This would have been very serviceable for any purpose where a heavy pointed tool with a lot of weight behind it was desired.

"A small cup (from Site 27), 4" long, made from a ewe's (mountain sheep) horn, had been used as a receptacle for a red paint with a resinous base." (Morss, Noel. "Work in Horn and Bone." *The Ancient Culture of the Fremont River in Utah*. Peabody Museum of American Archaeology. Vol. VII No. 3. Cambridge, 1931, pp 59, 60).

The Dr. Stewart collection, Lock Haven, Pennsylvania, contained many thousand Indian artifacts. In this collection were "Bone combs, bone flakers, 80 bone awls, and several bone needles." (Landis, H. K. "Prominent Collections." *The Pennsylvania Archaeologist*. 1936/1987, Vol. 6 No. 2, p 39)

Some of the California coastal islands have produced bone artifacts.

"...in the same deposit, or accumulation of workshop debris, were a large quantity and variety of bone implements which, from their forms, may be named awls, knives, needles, perforators, and punches. Among these are perineal bones of the male seal, some of them sharpened to a point at the smaller end, and the ribs of the dog or wolf, and some of these are obtusely pointed and creased at the end evidently for flaking stone in making arrow-points." (Rust, Horatio N. "Prehistoric Relics from San Nicolas Island, California." *The American Archaeologist*. Vol. 2 Part 4. Columbus, Ohio, April 1898, p 101).

Mesa Verde, Colorado, is a major archaeological series of sites, and large numbers of bone artifacts were recovered there.

"Many bone implements were found during the excavation of Cliff Palace. They are of the bones of birds and small mammals, or, now and then, of those of antelope or bear, the latter furnishing the best material for large scrapers. These implements were evidently sharpened by rubbing on the stones of walls or on the face of the cliff, as grooves, apparently made in this way, are there visible in several places." (Fewkes, Jesse Walter. *Antiquities of the Mesa Verde National Park Cliff Palace*. Bureau of American Ethnology. Bulletin 51. Smithsonian Institution, Washington, 1911, pp 74, 75, plates 34, 35).

Bone artifacts in New England are generally scarce.

"From the fact that in the nature of things many objects made of material that could not withstand the vicissitudes to which, in the New England climate, they would be subject, have long since disappeared, we may be quite certain that bone and shell were much more commonly used in the manufacture of tools and ornaments than would appear from present finds. (...) Except near the coast, specimens made of bone are very rare throughout New England." (Moorehead, Warren K. *Prehistoric Implements*. The Robert Clarke Company, Publishers, Cincinnati, 1900, pp 92 – 93).

Handles for composite (separate parts) Atl-atls are occasionally encountered.

"The antler Atl-atl handle is found along the Tennessee River, the Green River in Kentucky, and in Indiana. It is constructed by cutting a short section of antler near the root and drilling it for attachment. The rough surface is sometimes left unmodified, but some examples give evidence of intentional shaping." (Kellar, James H. *The Atl-atl in North America*. Vol. III. No. 3. June 1955. Indiana Historical Society, pp 317 – 318).

The Iroquois in Canada (Ontario and Quebec)

"...were expert bone workers, bone and antler artifacts being more abundant than those of stone. (...) the arrow points are either solid, pointed pieces of bone with wedge-shaped, tapering, or notched bases; a few have both faces near the base grooved for insertion in the cleft end of the arrow shaft, or else they are hollow pieces of bone and antler, in some cases with barbed bases." Harpoon tips were also made.

"One type, made of bone and antler, is unilaterally barbed, having from one to four barbs on one edge only; the other is bilaterally barbed, having from one to five barbs on both edges, in a few cases more on one edge than on the other. Points of the second type are mostly more slender than points of the first. Only the unilaterally barbed points are perforated. Both types are found on the same sites, mostly those of the pre-European period. The bilaterally barbed specimens are the commoner at sites of this period; those barbed on one edge only are commoner at later sites." (Wintemberg, W. J. "Distinguishing Characteristics of Algonkian and Iroquoian Cultures." *Annual Report For 1929*. Bulletin No. 67. National Museum of Canada, Ottawa, 1931, pp 87, 88, plates XV, XVI).

Several authorities over the years have suggested that bone knives might not have served too well as actual cutting instruments. However, they would have been ideal for skinning animals. (Hothem, Lar. Various sources).

Deer bone at the Archaic period Anderson site in Tennessee provided 31% of all modified bone, and birds (including wild turkey, Canada goose, and trumpeter swan) provided 25%. Tools were antler flakers, bone Atl-atl hooks (7 complete examples), and antler Atl-atl weights (8). Fishhooks and fishhook parts (121) were made from four kinds of bone: deer, fox, raccoon, and wild turkey. Antler hide-scrapers, turtle-shell cups, needles, and awls (200 found, many more fragmentary) were recovered and these were sharpened bone splinters. A unique awl was made from a garfish jawbone. Bone pins, beads, and pendants were present, as were drilled mammal canines. Bone needles, made from splinters, had an eye near the blunt end. (Dowd, John T. *The Anderson Site: Middle Archaic Adaption in Tennessee's Central Basin*. Miscellaneous Paper No. 13. Tennessee Anthropological Association, Knoxville, 1989, pp 127 – 141).

One reason animal bones might not be found on some early historic sites is because the bones themselves could be a food source. There are accounts of animal skeletal parts being ground into bone meal as a food supplement. (Hudson, Charles. *The Southeastern Indians*. The University of Tennessee Press, 1976/1987, p 288).

In the Pacific Northwest, organic materials of several kinds were employed to make useful items in historic times. Ring and wand rattles had suspensions of puffin bills, and dishes were made of mountain sheep horn. Spoons were formed from either mountain sheep or mountain goat horns, and sometimes both were combined in the same spoon. Bone-handled and all-bone knives were also used. (Krause, Aurel. *The Tlinget Indians*. The University of Washington Press, Seattle, 1885/1956, pp 142, 143, 148).

The Atl-atl is a wooden (usually) device that, when propelling light lances or darts, extends the arm of the user and gives more distance to the dart. In ancient Europe they were often made of bone or ivory. Some Atl-atl hooks (which seated the end of the dart) carved from bone were found in Nevada. The handle of an Atl-atl found in an Oregon cave had a mountain sheep horn handle. (Strong, Emory. *Stone Age in the Great Basin*. Binfords & Mort, Publishers, Portland, 1969, pp 97 – 103, 211).

The Archaic people of Indian Knoll, Kentucky used bone for projectile points. These were made from deer cannon bone splinters and were pointed at each end. One end tapered to a point for penetration while the opposite end was more slender than the point midsection and was intended for seating in the shaft. At times this end still retained traces of asphaltum or tar adhesive, and some had circular scratches as if twisted into a socket. Other points shows signs of burning (discoloration) as if the bone tips had been fire-hardened. The average length of these Atl-atl points was a little over 3". (Webb, William S. *Indian Knoll / Ohio County, Kentucky*. The University of Tennessee Press, Knoxville, 1946/1974, p 294).

These brief comments add to the general knowledge about bone use in the Pacific Northwest: "Bone needles for sewing were scraped to a very sharp point. Large, blunt-pointed needles were used in making tule (bulrush plant) mats. Heavy, blunt ends (...) were used as a finishing tool in fine chipping work." (Seaman, N. G. *Indian Relics of the Pacific Northwest*. Binfords & Mort, Publishers, Portland, 1946/1956, p 54).

Several major sites at Brewerton, New York, accounted for very many artifacts made of animal material. Noteworthy was a large number of bone harpoons, with small barbs on one or both sides. Puzzling, however, was why so many harpoon heads were broken. "The extremely high incidence of breakage is difficult to explain." At Owasco, 17 harpoons were whole and 208 were broken parts tips, midsections, and bases. (There were more than a dozen broken for one complete example.) Of 42 Point Peninsula types, none were complete.

"At Jack's Reef, the only comparable site, the relative proportion of whole to fragmentary harpoons was higher, but here too broken implements far outnumbered whole ones. (...) Had the damage occurred during the use of the implement, (where function as a harpoon for spearing fish can hardly be doubted) and the shaft been retrieved for a new point, basal fragments would predominate on the site. The suspicion is inescapable that intentional breakage was practiced for some unknown reason." (Ritchie, William A. *A Stratified Prehistoric Site at Brewerton, New York*. Researches and Transactions of the New York State Archaeological Association, 1946, pp 1, 11, 12, 24, 26, plates 6, 9, 10).

Southern Illinois has provided many organic material artifacts associated with the great Hopewell culture of Middle Woodland times. Among them are cut and drilled animal jaws and bear teeth, flattened marine shell beads, conch shell dippers, copper awls with antler handles, bear teeth copied in bone, bone pendants, carved mussel shell spoons, antler spearheads, and carved turtle shell containers. (Hothem, Lar. Various sources).

Deer toe bones used for fishhooks have certain signs or hints that allow them to be identified.

"The hooks so made, are determined in length by the size of the deer toe bone. There is thus only a limited variation in size among such hooks. The stem side and pointed side of the hook have a fixed angle to each other, since the angle is determined by the conformation of the toe bone. Thus, near uniformity in overall size, and fixed angle between the two sides are characteristic of toe bone fish hooks. The rounded outer surface of the angle is also characteristic of this type of hook, which is a strong hook and rarely breaks at the angle, being a hard bone, with no natural tendency to split at that point. This type of hook was very plentiful in the shell mounds of Alabama on the Tennessee River...". (Webb, William S. "The Carlson Annis Mound / Butler County, Kentucky." *Reports in Archaeology*. Vol. VII No. 4. January 1950. University of Kentucky, Lexington, p 327).

Bone and ivory points believed to be from the Paleo period have been found across North America. Several came from Alaskan muck deposits, others from Klamath Lake, California. The Wakula Spring site in Florida produced some 600 points made of bone. (Haynes, Vance C. Jr. "Elephant-Hunting in North America." "Early Man in America." Readings from *Scientific American*. W. H. Freeman and Company, San Francisco, 1951/1973, pp 45, 48).

The Caribou Eskimo, as the name suggests, depended on caribou for many of their needs.

"...the caribou was well-nigh indispensable to all Eskimo, because its fur offered the most suitable clothing for extremely cold weather, its sinew provided thread for sewing and lines for sealing and fishing gear, and its bones and antlers could be worked into numberless articles ranging from harpoons and arrowheads to thimbles." (Jenness, Diamond. *The Indians of Canada*. National Museum of Canada, Bulletin 65, 2nd edition, 1934, p 408).

In Kentucky's Archaic period shell mounds, a chronology based on manufacturing method was noted for the gradual style change in fishhooks. The oldest (found deepest in the shell mound) was the type made of deer toe bones. Next oldest was a hook made by drilling a hole in a spatula-like bone, and grooves angled from the hole to the edges of the bone. The hole formed the inside crook of the V-shaped hook. Hollowing or grooving the interior of a long and flat bone formed the latest fishhook type (found highest in the shell mound). When only the sides remained, they were cut at the appropriate places to form a U-shaped hook. This left the original bone (which may have served as a fork-like artifact) with two short prongs. (Webb, William S. "The Carlson Annis Mound / Butler County, Kentucky." *Reports in Archaeology*. Vol. VII No. 4. January 1950. University of Kentucky, pp 329 – 335).

The Riverton people of southern Illinois (Late Archaic) had many bone tools. These were recovered at three sites, Riverton, Robeson, and Swan Island. Artifacts included: Conical antler projectile points, some with tally-like incised bars; cut garfish jaws; antler spoon; antler drifts and flakers; awls of antler and bone splinters; chisels of beaver and porcupine incisors; weaving shuttles; antler gouges; tubular beads; drilled ornaments of animal teeth; flutes; and, a box turtle shell rattle. (Winters, Howard D. "The Riverton Culture." *The Illinois State Museum Reports of Investigations No. 13*, and *Illinois Archaeological Survey No. 1*, 1969. Springfield, pp 13 – 21, plates 16 – 20, 24, 26 – 28, 33, 34, 36 – 38).

One type of soil, especially, seems to preserve bone. This is loess, wind-deposited, that contains calcium carbonates. This neutralizes the soil and protects bone and shell. (Perino, Gregory. "Points and Barbs." *Central States Archaeological Journal*. Vol. 48 No. 4, October 2001, pp 106 – 107).

Facts about Artifacts

Bone and shell were primary materials for artifacts in prehistoric California and the Channel Islands. Known artifacts are: Bone fishhooks, very curved and barbed; shell fishhooks, one example 2¾" long; bone harpoon points, single barb, one harpoon 9" long; awls or perforators or pins, one decorated with carved collars, and a smaller specimen "with remarkably sharp points at each end" in what may have been ivory; bone splinters with traces of asphaltum; cylindrical bone implements sharpened at one end; bone tubes and wedge-shaped objects; clubs or blunt-edged swords up to 15" long; eyed needles; and, bits of shell used as inlay for wooden artifacts. (Abbott, C. C. and F. W. Putnam. "Implements and Weapons Made of Bone and Wood." *Report Upon United States Geographical Surveys*. Vol. VII. Engineer Department / U. S. Army, Washington, 1879, p 222).

The site known as Belle Glade was in the Everglades near Lake Okeechobee, and bone artifacts were found there.

"Bone implements and ornaments are characteristic of the Belle Glade site. They are numerous and show a considerable diversity of form. The techniques of manufacturing apparently were cutting, grinding, and polishing. Presumably, stone and shell tools and hafted teeth were used for this work. Exact identification of the bones used for each artifact is impractical and impossible, but the general range can be stated. Long bones of deer and smaller mammals, such as the fox and raccoon, were commonly utilized. Large and small bird bones, alligator jaws, fish bones, turtle(?) bones, turtle shell, and porpoise and shark teeth are noted. As to be expected, the craftsman took advantage of the natural contours and articular surfaces of the bone in giving the implements or ornaments final form. Judging from numbers (496 bone or antler or tooth artifacts or fragments were found), bone points must have been the standard projectile for hunting and warfare. Bone pins were extremely common as ornaments.

"Deer antler was used almost as extensively as bone. The carving exhibited on some of the antler specimens, such as the ceremonial headdresses, is masterly and implies a long tradition of this work among the aboriginal inhabitants." (Willey, Gordon R. *Excavations in Southeast Florida*. Yale University Press, 1949, pp 19, 37 – 46, plates 7 – 10).

Projectile points made from small bird and animal bones were made in the Louisiana coastal region. A fairly direct method was used, whereby the bone was scored with a sharp implement, perhaps a deer tooth. Pressure and twist were then applied to the bone, which shattered and provided the points. (Davis, Dave D., et al. "Reduction Analysis of Simple Bone Industries – An Example From the Louisiana Coastal Zone." *Archaeology of Eastern North America*. Vol. 11, Fall 1983, pp 98 – 100).

Some bones worked for artifacts may have been processed in a fresh, or at least damp, state. This seems to soften the bone enough to make graving or cutting easier. It has even been suggested that perhaps bones were boiled to make the task easier. Old or dry bones are somewhat harder or more brittle. (Hothem, Lar. Various sources).

Dice, or thrown objects in games of chance, were used among some 130 historic tribes, and sometimes the dice were made of bone. Incising or painting marked the dice. Malecite Indians, New Brunswick, used disc dice an inch in diameter. The Arapaho Indians, Wyoming, had similar discs plus diamond-shaped, elongated oval, rectangular, and square dice. The Blackfeet, who also had rib-bone staves, used bone stick dice. Cheyenne Indians had diamond and oval bone dice, and Michigan members of the tribe used small bone animal and bird figures. Cree Indians (Saskatchewan) had bone dice in geometric shapes, while the Gros Ventre of Montana had triangular shapes. Bone discs, played by the Mic-mac of Nova Scotia, were button-like and had incised designs. The Mic-mac also had antler counting sticks. While dice made of stone or peach and plum pits were also widely used, bone remained a favored material across North America. (Culin, Stewart. "Games of the North American Indians." *Twenty-Fourth Annual Report of the Bureau of American Ethnology*. 1902 – 1903. The Smithsonian Institution, Washington, 1907, pp 29, 44 – 85).

Across North America, the large number of awls found may not necessarily mean more awls were made, but that more awls were protected and found.

"A larger percentage of bone awls have been recovered from village sites than of other objects in bone, excepting beads. The ash-pits of village sites preserved practically everything encompassed by them because of the preservative quality of ashes. Therefore, I have always believed that the proportion of bone awls to other things is no criterion as to the use of bone among the aborigines. (...) assuming that because of wars there were usually more women then men (...) the domestic arts were in excess of the other arts; and even if the persons engaged in domestic science were in the minority there would naturally be more cooking, garment-making, weaving, and general domestic science in vogue in a village or a cave or a cliff-dwelling than elsewhere. (...) An unknown number of bone effigies and bone tools that must have been made and used by the ancient people have disappeared, because as in the case of textile fabrics they were not preserved unless buried in ashes." (Moorehead, Warren K. *The Stone Age in North America*. Vol. II. Houghton Mifflin Company, Cambridge, 1910, pp 136 – 137).

A general comment made regarding bone artifacts, though made a century and a quarter ago, is worth repeating today:

"The range of variation in the forms of implements made of bone, wherever found, is much more limited than that of stone. As weapons, with few exceptions, they were not so effective as similar forms chipped from flint or obsidian. On the other hand, for certain purposes, bone was found particularly well adapted...". (Abbott, C. C. and F. W. Putnam. "Implements and Weapons Made of Bone and Wood." *Report Upon United States Geographical Surveys*. Vol. VII. Engineer Department / U. S. Army, Washington, 1879, p 222).

Artifacts made of animal teeth have long been noted in Canada.

"In all the ashbeds, teeth of various sorts turn up in varying numbers, and many of them show artificial workings. Bear teeth, canine, were formed into knives, shavers, and possibly borers by grinding laterally flat on the enamel, leaving sharp edges, which would cut wood as well as, if not better than, chipped flint. These same canine bear teeth are sometimes split longitudinally in half and the split side smoothed off. (...) Sometimes these teeth have the points ground off, leaving a flat circular surface, the use of which is problematic. The incisor teeth of beaver and porcupines were also made into tools, such as knives, chisels, and gravers. The knives were formed by splitting the teeth longitudinally and grinding the fractured side to an edge, either on the outside or inside of the tooth. The chisels and gravers have the top surface ground smooth, to a greater or less degree, forming a more acute angle with the cutting edge than the natural edge, and are generally the full width of the tooth." (Laidlaw, Col. G. E. "Archaeological Notes on Victoria County, Ont." *The Archaeological Bulletin*. Vol. 8 No. 5, 1915, p 11).

The ruins of Casa Grande near Florence, Arizona, produced some bone artifacts. One was a dirk or knife, while another was a bone with a mid-length hole, probably a whistle.

"Among the recognizable bones are those of the antelope, turkey, rabbit, and bear. Bird bones are the most common, but the specimens have been worked to so great an extent as to make identification impossible. Most of them are simply pointed, rarely decorated, but some are perforated for use as beads or needles." (Fewkes, Jesse Walter. "Casa Grande, Arizona." *Twenty-Eighth Annual Report of the Bureau of American Ethnology*. 1906 – 1907. The Smithsonian Institution, Washington, 1912, pp 33, 145, 146).

Grooved sandstone (sometimes claystone and mudstone) slabs or blocks are recognized as abraders, smoothers, or shapers for bone and antler artifacts. If two slabs are more or less paired, and obviously made to be placed together so that the grooves correspond to create a rounded hole, the artifact is a shaft-shaper or shaft-smoother. If only one slab is present and the groove is of uniform width and depth, it is considered another type of shaft-shaper. If the groove is tapered from wide to narrow and from deep to shallow, the artifact is called an awl- or needle-sharpener. (Hothem, Lar. Various sources).

At Pecos, New Mexico, 26 whole and 40 broken flutes or flageolets of bone were recovered. These were of two types, those with bone articular ends remaining, and those with the ends removed. Most were made from golden eagle ulnas, but one was an ulna from a whooping crane and another from a wild turkey. Lengths were from 4¾ to 10¼", though most were between 7½ to 8" long. Most had three finger holes. The first type is described:

"In preparing the bone, the proximal end was usually cut off at right angles, but so close to the joint as to leave a generous widening of the shaft. (...) At the distal end the shaft was generally opened by sawing away obliquely part of the articulation on the concave side of the bone. Each flageolet possesses a large stop near one end, and a set of smaller stops near the other. All the holes are in line, and they are always found on the concave side of the bone. They are usually very neatly drilled, less commonly produced by sawing and scraping. In number and in arrangement, the holes are very uniform. (...) There can be little doubt that the specimens of both subgroups were played from the end, and that they should, therefore, be identified as flageolets rather than as flutes." (Kidder, Alfred Vincent. "Objects of Bone." *The Artifacts of Pecos*. Robert S. Peabody Foundation for Archaeology, Yale University Press, New Haven, 1932, pp 248 – 252).

Split bone awl-like artifacts are widely found, and the manufacturing process at Stalling's Island, Georgia, was quite simple.

"If a split food bone was to be made into an awl, the point was carefully finished before any attention was paid to the rest of the object. It was evidently the practice to choose a section of split bone approximately the right length and work it down, beginning at the point, to its desired shape. There is no evidence of sawing the base, all unfinished objects having a roughly broken butt. The finishing of awls and needles was accomplished by scraping and rubbing, some sections of bone occasionally being split off before the rubbing stage.

"In conclusion, the workman of Stallings Island in shaping a bone tool first made sure that the bone could be made into the desired tool before spending time unnecessarily in finishing. The tools that he worked with were simple; a chipped knife hafted or unhafted, a piece of sandstone, and a small chipped scraper, presumably hafted, which be used as a chisel." (Claflin, William H. Jr. *The Stalling's Island Mound / Columbia County, Georgia*. Vol. XIV. No. 1. Peabody Museum, Harvard University, Cambridge, 1931, p 23).

Large tubular pipes made of steatite or serpentine, in the California region, usually had separate mouthpieces. These were made of bird bones and were secured to the pipe with asphaltum. Some of the bone mouthpieces were slightly curved so that the pipe bowl was more upright. (Abbott, C. C. "Smoking Pipes of Stone." *Report Upon United States Geographical Surveys*. Vol. VII. Engineer Department / U. S. Army, Washington, 1879, 125 – 127).

Fort Ancient people (Mississippian) made extensive use of bone artifacts throughout the Ohio River Valley. One assemblage included deer bone awls or perforators, a possible hairpin, flutes or whistles, pins, a fishhook, arrowpoints, and a gouge. (Editor. *Artifacts*. Vol. 10 No. 4, 1980, pp 112, 113).

At Arizona's Snaketown, a Hohokam settlement, "...shell objects were very abundant. Undoubtedly the chief reason for the emphasis on shell work was the proximity to the Gulf of California and the Pacific Coast, and the recognition that shell was admirably suited to carving. At the peak of their culture the Hohokam were indulging this knowledge to the limit." Artifacts included a carved shell needle with eye, several kinds of beads, pendants, carved bracelets, and finger rings. Some shell mosaic work was done, also shell painting and etching. Compared to shell, relatively few bone artifacts were found. "The only bone tools of a utilitarian nature found at Snaketown were awls, and these were far too few to supply the need for such instruments. It is probable that some of the hard desert woods, such as ironwood, were used instead." Some bone tubes had crosshatch incisings and other pieces were skillfully carved. Antler was painted red and black in geometric designs. (Gladwin, Harold S., Emil W. Haury, et al. "Shell." and "Bone." *Excavations at Snaketown / Material Culture*. The University of Arizona Press, Tucson, 1938/1975, pp 135 – 157).

In the American Southwest, some sites had mainly animal (antelope) bone artifacts while others were made mainly of bird bones. Many awls were shaped in a special way.

"As a rule, the bone of which they are made is so worked that the rounded end fits the palm of the hand and the sharpened extremity is continued to a needle-like point. These awls are made of the bones of different animals, of which the turkey is the most popular. They were probably used in ancient times in sewing or darning fabrics, possibly in weaving." (Fewkes, Jesse Walter. "Two Summers' Work in Pueblo Ruins." *Twenty-Second Annual Report of the Bureau of American Ethnology*. Part 1. 1900 – 1901. The Smithsonian Institution, Washington, 1904, pp 17, 93 – 95).

Blain Village, a Fort Ancient site located along the Scioto River south of Chillicothe, Ohio, contained some 257 bone tools. These were: 25 whole awls, mainly of deer bone; 4 awls of turkey bone; 13 awls made from split bone (11 mammal, 2 bird); 2 double-tipped pins or gorge hooks; 2 polished raccoon penis bones; 3 portions of polished elk or deer bones; 2 chisels of beaver teeth; 1 polished and split bird bone tube; 1 knife, deer scapula (shoulder bone); 6 partial or preform bone fishhooks; 36 whole or broken beamers, metatarsal bones from deer; 2 worked mountain lion metatarsals (foot bones); 8 perforated elk and deer phalanges (toe bones); 10 turtle shell cups or spoons; 2 flat needle fragments; 7 drilled canine teeth, 2 of them bear; 10 tubular beads, polished bird bone; 1 section of a decorated pin; 1 portion of a raven's beak (mandibula); 13 arrowpoints of antler, of which 3 were complete; 4 antler flakers; 3 antler punches; 1 antler spear point, broken, 72mm long; 1 antler scraper; 24 antler beams and tines with cutting marks; and, 29 miscellaneous pieces. (Prufer, Olaf H. and Orrin C. Shane III. *Blain Village and the Fort Ancient Tradition in Ohio*. The Kent State University Press, 1970, pp 3, 129 – 141).

Site excavators from regions as far apart as Arizona and Ohio have commented on the deer bones found. There was a definite lack of fawn or young deer bones compared with those of adult or near-adult deer. This can be interpreted in two ways. Indian hunters may, as an early form of conservation, spared the young animals so they could breed larger herds. Or, adult animals may have been preferred because they provided more meat (and larger, stronger bones) per animal. (Hothem, Lar. Various sources).

At the Riker site – a Mississippian-era village in Tuscarawas County, Ohio – many bone artifacts were found.

"Ulna bones of deer and elk were made into heavy awls and seldom is this bone found unworked. Shoulder blades made excellent knives and hoes although their thinness made them easily broken. Beaver teeth made excellent gravers and most specimens found had been cut or used for some purpose. Artifacts made of bone were almost endless in number and variety. (...) If you were to examine any ten bones taken from the kitchen midden, you would find at least one showing where man had cut, drilled, or shaped it for some purpose. Butchering marks are evident on many of the animal bones and others show where sections have been cut or split away to make awls, hide dressers, needles, and ornaments." (Vietzen, Raymond C. "The Riker Site, Sugar Creek Valley Chapter." *Archaeological Society of Ohio*. 1974, pp 115, 116).

When shell heaps along Puget Sound, Washington, were examined many bone artifacts were found. These were: A bone comb 1½" long with seven teeth; knives of bone 3 to 7" long and 1 to 2" wide; chisels and wedges, elk antler, 5 to 14" long; a bone awl; a "war club" made of whale bone; bone projectile points; bone hooks; and, bone gambling objects. (Editor. "Recent Intelligence." *The American Antiquarian*. Vol. IV No. 2, January 1882, pp 156, 157).

Cultural traits are not the only explanation for the presence or absence of bone artifacts at some prehistoric sites. For instance, at the Kincaid site (Mississippian) on the Ohio River in southern Illinois, the earth itself was a factor. "Objects of bone are rare at Kincaid due to acidity of the soil...". (Cole, Fay-Cooper. *Kincaid – A Prehistoric Illinois Metropolis*. The University of Chicago Press, Chicago, 1951, p 126).

Collectors need to keep in mind that prehistoric peoples might have made a far greater range of artifacts than it would appear today. The comments that follow, originating in Oregon, might apply nearly anywhere:

"A distorted perspective is apt to be formed of the furnishings of a typical Indian village because only the stone, and a few of the bone, articles are now found. Actually, stone implements were comparatively rare; bone or wood served to make nearly everything the natives used, especially on the lower river. For every stone piece found, hundreds of wood and bone articles have long since decayed away." (Strong, Emory. *Stone Age on the Columbia River*. Binfords & Mort Publishers, Portland, 1960, p 198).

Tube pipes in California, though usually made of steatite, also had parts made of organic materials. The pipes often had bone mouthpieces secured with asphaltum. This substance was also used to decorate the pipes, and bands of asphaltum may have had surfaces covered with crushed abalone shell. (Abbott, C. C. and Frederick W. Putnam. "Smoking-Pipes of Stone." *Report Upon United States Geographical Surveys*. Vol. VII. Engineer Department / U. S. Army, Washington, 1879, pp 128, 129).

Porcupine quillwork sometimes required the use of a specialized bone tool. "Among most tribes the awl was the only instrument used in quill-working. The Cheyenne, Arapaho, and Sioux (the principal quill-working tribes) had a specially shaped bone for flattening, bending, and smoothing." (Hodge, Frederick Webb. "Quillwork." *Handbook of American Indians*. Part 2. Bureau of American Ethnology Bulletin 30, 1910, p 341).

Daggers made of bone are sometimes found on prehistoric sites. "Daggers are large bone tools that are not socketed for hafting but have an integral handle. (...) Tools of this type are found in greater numbers on late prehistoric sites where they are preserved, and in states like Florida where chert was not as common a commodity as in other areas. (...) Bone daggers are sometimes mistaken for pins or other bone tools." (Perino, Gregory. *Selected Preforms, Points and Knives of the North American Indians*. Vol. I. Points and Barbs Press, 1985, p 42).

A number of antler and bone Hopewell artifacts were found at the Clear Lake site in Illinois. These included a long bone skewer, split bone tools, bones with chisel-like tips, needles or shuttles, antler projectile points, fish gorge hooks and fishhooks, plus antler flakers or drifts. (Fowler, Melvin L. "The Clear Lake Site." *Hopewellian Communities in Illinois*. Illinois State Museum, Scientific Papers Volume V, 1952, pp 131, 161 – 163).

Hogup Cave, in Utah's Great Salt Lake Desert, contained 269 antler, bone, horn, and shell artifacts. These were: Awls, made of antelope, deer and mountain sheep bones, and some bird bones; flakers, seven of antler and one of antelope horn core; two bone splinter needles with eyes; a bone net shuttle; nine bone game counters; 12 bones painted with hematite; 26 wapiti (elk) canine tooth pendants; disc and tubular beads; bone tubes, a bone pipe and a bone whistle; a wedge made of elk antler; bone sharp-pointed splinters; a flaked point with a rib-bone handle; two horn shaft wrenches; a paint horn containing red hematite pigment; a spatula, and various shell artifacts. (Aikens, C. Melvin. "Hogup Cave." *University of Utah Anthropological Papers*. No. 93, 1970, pp 1, 85 – 95).

The Fairport Harbor site (Lake County, northern Ohio), late prehistoric, contained a large number of animal bones, many of which were made into artifacts. Of the large mammals represented, three species were notable. Deer bones (1160 specimens) were made into awls, projectile points, and flakers. Elk remains (324 specimens) included teeth made into pendants and elk antler made into gouges and flakers. Black bear remains (285 specimens) included teeth made into pendants, a drilled claw, and artifacts made from bear penis bones. (Goslin, Robert M. "Animal Remains / Fairport Harbor Village Site." *Ohio State Archaeological and Historical Quarterly*. Vol. LII No. 1, January – March 1943, pp 45, 46).

Wedges, while scarce, were important tools.

"Horn and bone wedges are fairly easy to identify with certainty, though a few could have had other uses. When not too decayed or when 'green,' they often display obvious marks of pounding on the butts. The most complete range of wedges that have survived comes from the Yurok-Hupa cultures in northwestern California, where they were used into historic times." (Miles, Charles. *Indian and Eskimo Artifacts of North America*. Bonanza Books, 1963, p 71).

Awls were present across North America and had many uses.

"The awl was used to make perforations through which thread of sinew or other sewing material was passed when skins for moccasins, clothing, tents, etc., were sewed, and in quillwork, beadwork, and basket-work. Other uses for awls were for making holes for pegs in woodwork, as a gauge in canoe-making, for shredding sinews, for graving, etc. Various awl-like implements that were used by the Indians in weaving and making pottery, as pins for robes, as head-scratchers, pipe-picks, blood pins (for closing wounds in game to save the blood), marrow-extractors, forks, corn-huskers, etc., have sometimes been classed as awls." (Hodge, Frederick Webb. "Awls." *Handbook of American Indians*. Part 1. Bureau of American Ethnology Bulletin 30, 1907, p 120).

The Savannah River Focus of Archaic times, Southern U. S., had both common and atypical bone artifacts. Common were solid and sliver awls, flakers, chisels, eyed needles, and antler and bone projectile points. Atypical was a bone pin with a T-shaped base, and bone pins with painted or incised geometric designs. (Griffin, James B., Editor. *Archeology of Eastern United States*. The University of Chicago Press, 1952, illustrations / figure 168).

Eskimos have long been noted for artifacts made of organic materials.

"It was in working antler, bone, and, particularly, ivory, however, that the Eskimo most excelled. Arctic explorers have been astonished at the variety of articles they manufactured from these materials. The majority, it is true, were small, but they were made with great care and skill and in most cases served some useful purpose. Merely to list them all would fill several pages, for they ranged from parts of harpoons and arrows, ice-chisels, sled-shoes, toggles, and handles of various shapes and sizes, to needles and needle-cases, thimbles and thimble-holders, and a wealth of miscellaneous objects for everyday use, besides numerous toys and amulets. Some were carved into animal and human forms, others carried incised decorations. The latter were always geometrical in prehistoric times, but in Alaska, after the natives acquired iron tools, it blossomed into vivid scenes of daily life." (Jenness, Diamond. *The Indians of Canada*. National Museum of Canada, Bulletin 65, 2nd edition, 1934, p 408).

Historic Southeastern Indians used at least three different kinds of arrow points, two of them made of organic materials. According to an 1819 report, arrows made by the Powhatans were pointed "...with splinters of christall, or some sharpe stone, the spurres of a turkey, or the bill of some bird." (Holmes, William Henry. "Stone Implements of the Potomac – Chesapeake Tidewater Province." *Fifteenth Annual Report of the Bureau of Ethnology*. 1893 – 1894. The Smithsonian Institution, Washington, 1897, pp 13, 85).

The Naskapi Indians of the far north had many well-made artifacts of bone and antler. A sampling of such objects, some highly decorated, includes: Skinning tools or fleshers of bear bone, 3⅜, 5¾ and 6⅜" long; and, an awl with a caribou antler handle and an iron tip. (Editor. "Central Eskimo and Indian Dot Ornamentation." *Indian Notes*. Vol. 2 No. 3. July 1925. Museum of the American Indian, New York, p 165 figure 76).

A late prehistoric site near Blairsville, western Pennsylvania, produced the following bone and antler artifacts: Bone beads ¼ to 1" long and ¼ to ¾" in diameter (made from bird bones or deer cannon bones); worked bird bones 2¾ to 5¾" long (the beads were generally polished and had both ends smoothed); deer and elk scapula awls, with well-made tips and opposite ends unfinished; two fine awls about 5" long made from bear penis bones; deer and elk antler flakers or punches; a few antler arrowpoints; an elk antler chisel 6" long; a polished tube 5½" long made from bird bone; two fishhooks made of deer bone; turtle-shell cup fragments; mussel shell discs about ¾" in diameter; small shell beads made in imitation of elk teeth. (Dragoo, Don W. "Excavations at the Johnston Site." *Foundations of Pennsylvania Prehistory*. Harrisburg, Pennsylvania, 1971, pp 459, 460).

Oregon, in the Pacific Northwest, contributed bone artifacts to the archaeological record. Fort Rock Cave contained bone awls and a bone Atl-atl hook or spur, plus sagebrush bark sandals and a piece of twined basketry. Pointed Clovis-like bone tools came from the bed of Lower Klamath Lake, and the area of Upper Klamath Lake also had a beveled bone Clovis-like artifact. More Clovis-like bone shafts and a piece of serrated bone came from Lind Coulee. (Wormington, H. M. *Ancient Man in North America*. 4th edition. The Denver Museum of Natural History, Denver, Colorado, 1957, pp 184, 185).

One of the deadliest and most effective uses of bone was reported by early explorers in the Far North. There, in winter, some hunters killed wolves by using bait consisting of grease balls with bits of meat. Placed inside was a coiled strip of bone, pointed at each end. When the bait was eaten the fat dissolved and the bone strip slowly straightened, piercing the stomach or intestines, eventually killing the wolf. (Hothem, Lar. Various sources).

Since awls and awl-like artifacts are the single most common bone artifacts from most prehistoric sites in North America, a description of the types is of value. The noted archaeologist, Alfred V. Kidder, describes mammal leg-bone awls from Pecos, New Mexico, in the following ways, and the information would apply to many sites:

"Head of bone left intact – Numerically, this is a relatively small class. The awls are short, stout, and rather clumsy in appearance because of the disproportionately large size of their butts.

"Head of bone unaltered except by original splitting – Awls of this type (...) are stout and heavy-butted.

Almost all of them were produced by splitting a deer metapodial [lower leg bone] and using the resultant half, third or quarter of the articular end as a butt; the shaft had been tapered by grinding and the tip brought to a sharp, but seldom extremely keen, point.

"Head of bone partly worked down – This (...) comprises those awls which have a distinct butt provided by that part of the articular end which remained at the end of the shaft when the bone was originally split lengthwise. This bit of the joint has, however, been worked enough to obliterate any sharp projections or protruding lumps, and to leave a smoothed, swelled grip. (...) The points of these awls average sharper than do those of the preceding class, and the shafts show more careful work in the smoothing down of cut edges.

"Head of bone wholly or almost wholly removed – These are the most abundant, the finest, slimmest, and on the average the keenest-pointed, of the awls of mammal leg-bone. Many of the implements show no sign at all of the original shape of the bone, all surfaces and the butt having been worked perfectly smooth. In others a very slight swelling at one end, or cancellous remnants about the butt, indicate the former presence of the head of the bone. In still other cases, the only sign of the original shape is a groove down one side of the awl, representing the central cavity in the parent shaft. The finest examples are skewer-like and perfectly round in cross-section throughout their entire length; the butts are conical, the tips long, tapering and very keen.

"Splinter awls – These specimens, which form the third largest group, are fragments of long-bones whose shape happened to fit them for use after a little sharpening at the point. Raw material for such awls probably came from bones broken open for the extraction of marrow, or from the extra fragments produced when long-bones were being sectioned to make the more carefully shaped types. It is seldom possible to identify the bones employed, for the articular ends are never present, but from the general appearance of such parts of the shaft as remain, it would appear that a considerable variety of bones had been pressed into service.

"Minute awls – (These) are really in a class by themselves, for while they are not very much shorter than the shortest examples of the types described above, they are so slender and so carefully made that they must have had an entirely different function." (Kidder, Alfred Vincent. "Objects of Bone." *The Artifacts of Pecos*. Robert S. Peabody Foundation for Archaeology. Yale University Press, New Haven, 1932, pp 211 – 217).

A quite specialized tool was made from a bison horn case and adjoining section of skull, and the type has been found on Plains Village sites in Oklahoma and elsewhere. The horn case was split and an attached skull section had the edges sharpened. The tool may have been hafted or hand-held, and there is some information that the tool was used to slice pumpkins and squash into thin layers for drying and preservation. (Bell, Robert E. *Oklahoma Indian Artifacts*. Contributions from the Stovall Museum No. 4. University of Oklahoma, Norman, 1980, pp 76, 77).

Two pottery-producing sites in Pennsylvania also had organic material artifacts. These were box turtle shell cups or scoops (known from the Ohio Valley, Early Woodland to late prehistoric), beads of bird bone (eagle, hawk, owl, and turkey), and beaming tools for hide-working made from deer metapodial bones. Splint and joint-end bone awls, a long antler flaker, and a deer-jaw tool (probably for scraping corn) were found. (Witthoft, John and S. S. Farver. "Two Shenk's Ferry Sites in Lebanon County, Pennsylvania." *Foundations of Pennsylvania Prehistory*. Harrisburg, 1971, pp 459, 460).

Fox Field, Mason County, Kentucky, has long been known as a major Fort Ancient (Mississippian) village site. In 1895, the area was explored and among the many artifacts recovered were those of organic material. Animals represented were, black bear, Virginia deer, elk, wolf, raccoon, red fox, lynx, opossum, woodchuck, beaver, squirrel, wood rat, mink, weasel, great blue heron, wild turkey, duck, owl, eagle, turtles, and fish. Artifacts represented were, skin scrapers, awl-like tools, cylinders, needles, chisel-like implements, fishhooks, ring-and-pin game pieces or clothing pendants, fifes, whistles or animal calls, tubes and beads, antler arrowpoints, long and short antler objects, bear tooth pendants, pendants of elk, deer and wolf teeth, beaver tooth tools, clamshell spoons or scrapers, crushed clamshell used for tempering pottery, and marine shell beads, pendants, discs, and pins. (Smith, Harlan I. *The Prehistoric Ethnology of a Kentucky Site*. American Museum of Natural History. Vol. VI Part II, 1910, pp 177, 181, 182).

A late prehistoric site in Alberta, Canada, had flint, stone, and bone artifacts. "Work in bone is quite plentiful and includes awls, quill flatteners, shaft straighteners, and beads. Some beads were also made of shell." (Wormington, H. M. and Richard G. Forbis. *An Introduction to the Archaeology of Alberta, Canada*. Proceedings No. 11. Denver Museum of Natural History, Denver, 1965, p 140).

The Boley site, an historic Mandan Indian village in North Dakota, contained a large midden mound. It was excavated between 1952 and 1956, producing many artifacts made of bone. These were a split animal rib bone awl, a bone splinter awl, a large bird bone awl, awl or punch made from a catfish pectoral fin bone, beads made from fish spinal bones, short beads from bird bones, a bone effigy made from a solid animal bone, a bone fishhook grooved for the line, a fishhook preform on a flat bone slab, gaming pieces of antler, a knife or scraper made from a bison scapula (flattened shoulder bone), a bone hair pin, gouge or flaker of bison radius (lower leg bone), and a gouge or flesher of bison bone ground at an angle and with convex edge serrated. Other bone artifacts included knives, needles, digging sticks, flakers, bracelets, head ornaments, gouges, shaft-straighteners, whistles, hoes and shovels from bison shoulder-bones, abraders, and dangle ornaments. Animal teeth had been drilled, and elk, wolf, deer, and bison teeth were represented. Shell artifacts at the Boley site were beads and ornaments. The whistles were made from turkey and eagle bones. (Russell, Virgil Y. *Indian Artifacts*. 7th printing. Johnson Publishing Company, Boulder, Colorado, 1974, pp 38, 40 – 42).

Long-ago artifact dealers, such as F. M. Gilham, California, sometimes offered bone or ivory artifacts. "I have a large collection of over three hundred old ivory ancient pieces, from Alaska, consisting of wedges, sinkers, awls, knives, harpoons, etc. These are very rare and it is almost impossible to procure any more." (Editor. *The Archaeological Bulletin*. The International Society of Archaeologists, Vol. 6 No. 3, May – June 1915, Somerset, Kentucky, inside back cover).

The main difference between bone awls with eyes and needles with eyes is one of size and shape. Awls tend to be larger and thicker, and may be bigger at the end that contains the eye. Awls also usually retain much of the original bone shape. Needles, whether long or short, tend to be slender and have about the same diameter from one end to another. The eye of a needle can be located anywhere from near one end to near the center. Eyed needles, straight to curved, may be round to flattened in cross-section, and are often well polished. At times, combined characteristics make it difficult to determine if any one artifact is an awl or needle, and the division from one class to the other is often uncertain. In fact, if a true awl has an eye it might be considered an extra-large needle. Since we know little about how large needles with eyes and small awls with eyes were in fact used, the name designations may not have much meaning. In collector terminology, however, pointed bone artifacts with eyes are called needles and those without eyes are classed as awls. (Hothem, Lar. Various sources).

Certainly some of the finest and most extensive collections of bone artifacts came from Mandan sites in North Dakota. The bones of buffalo (bison), deer, and elk were used to make hide-scrapers, celts, elk-antler strip bracelets, shoulder-bone hoes and spades, and ornaments and effigies. The largest Mandan collection contained about 8000 items. (Moorehead, Warren K. *The Stone Age in North America*. Vol. II. Houghton Mifflin Company, Cambridge, 1910, pp 150 – 156).

Antler arrowpoints were made in large numbers, and many examples came from a large rock shelter in Christian County, Kentucky. Most of the points were made in certain ways that enhanced effectiveness in use.

"Some antler projectile points were cut square off and scraped down to a very sharp point. Others were cut off obliquely at the base and so scraped as to make the basal edge serve as a barb. In length, the points vary from two to four". Sockets for insertion of the wooden arrow shafts were usually drilled with a blunt flint drill as a tapered hole encouraged the point to split when the impact made by contact with a target caused the shaft to be driven into the taper much as a wedge. When tapered drillings were encountered we often discovered tapered ends on the shafts which were on occasion found charred and preserved. (...) Many antler projectile points found were split at the socket and several small grooves encircled them near their bases – these being made to hold sinew bindings used to retard further splitting and thereby prolong the life of the points. Many such examples prove these people to have been at times both practical and frugal." (Vietzen, Col. Raymond C. *The Saga of Glover's Cave*. Wahoo, Nebraska, 1956, p 197).

Archaic bone tools found in the Upper Ohio Valley included conical and cylindrical antler flakers, antler points, a bone splinter awl with notches toward the base, a barbed and perforated point that could be a harpoon, a cut and drilled bear jaw, and bone beads. (Mayer-Oakes, William J. *Prehistory of the Upper Ohio Valley*. Annals of Carnegie Museum, Vol. 34. Pittsburgh, 1955, pp 208, 209).

An interesting type of antler arrowpoint was found at the Mississippian-era Feurt site, Scioto County, Ohio. Besides the typical antler tip points with hollowed bases, the other type had a small hole drilled in the side near the base. Likely, this was for a string or peg for better attachment of the point to the end of the arrow shaft. (Mills, William C. "The Feurt Mounds and Village Site." *Ohio Archaeological and Historical Quarterly*. Vol. XXVI No. 3, July 1917, pp 426, 427).

Though somewhat romantic, these comments on bone use are still largely accurate.

"In the Mississippi Valley the most frequently occurring bone articles are awls and beads. Awls of the most massive sort were usually fashioned from the femurs of the larger animals, deer and even elk. They were used for perforating hides and well-tanned leather in the making of clothing and moccasins, and served in removing steaming food from the boiling pots. The larger specimens could very well have served as daggers to plunge into the enemy and the smaller ones as points for swiftly flying arrows." (Lilly, Eli. *Prehistoric Antiquities of Indiana*. Indiana Historical Society, Indianapolis, 1937, p 215).

Beaver incisor teeth, in the eastern Midwest and elsewhere, were used for cutting tasks. Basically natural chisels, the teeth were set in handles.

"The lower incisors are much more commonly used for this purpose as the curvature is less. The hard outer enamel of these teeth can be ground to a keen edge, and the tool is admirably adapted for making the smaller and more delicate objects of wood, bone, and antler. These blades were hafted in short handles, usually of wood or antler. Antler hafts, some of which were probably used with beaver tooth blades, are found on certain Ohio village sites, but none which could definitely be attributed to this use were obtained at Madisonville.

"All of the beaver-tooth cutting implements obtained during the Museum exploration were of the chisel type. None of the side-cutting knives, such as occur also with this form in New England and certain other sections, were found." (Hooton, Earnest A. *Indian Village Site and Cemetery / Near Madisonville, Ohio*. Peabody Museum, Vol. VIII No. 1, Cambridge, 1920, p 61).

Antler and bone were used for many purposes on the Great Plains. These uses included awls, fishhooks, needles, hoes, sickles, and rakes. (Zimerman, Larry J. *Peoples of Prehistoric South Dakota*. University of Nebraska Press, 1985, pp 43, 44).

Some California shell fishhooks had a peculiar shape, and the manufacture method is of interest.

"It is made of the thick portions of the shell of Haliotis, which are first cut into circular pieces of an inch or more in diameter, and then perforated, the margin of the hole forming ultimately the inside of the hook. This is then cut and rubbed into the required shape, and that portion of the shell, between what is to form the shank and the barb of the hook, is finally cut away, and the hook is made complete in all its parts by polishing." (Abbott, C. C. and F. W. Putnam. "Fish-Hooks." *Report Upon United States Geographical Surveys*. Volume VII. Engineer Department / U. S. Army, Washington, 1879, p 223).

Mississippian bone artifacts in the Upper Ohio Valley were made in a number of types. Such artifacts were antler tine points, antler flakers, an antler hoe, pins, deer and wild turkey awls, fishhooks, bone triangular points, a turtle shell cup, a tooth pendant, perforated teeth (including an imitation elk tooth), a bone flute, perforated deer and turkey bones, beamers, and a long bone chisel. (Mayer-Oakes, William J. *Prehistory of the Upper Ohio Valley*. Annals of Carnegie Museum. Vol. 34, Pittsburgh, 1955, pp 220 – 221).

The Lamoka people of New York state (Archaic period) had many classes of bone artifacts. Examples were fishhooks, small pointed bone pins (possibly used for fishing), gorge hooks, (possible leister points for fish spears), net-weaving tools, shaft-straighteners of antler, projectile points of bone, antler and bone daggers, bone knives, a great range of bone awls, whistles or flageolets, and perforated bones of several kinds, including fox and turtle. Universal were decorated antler pendant-like artifacts, some still with faint bands of red paint. (Ritchie, William A. *The Archaeology of New York State*. American Museum of Natural History, Garden City, 1965, pp 45 – 68).

Bone had many uses for artifacts, including some – as in the case of a Mandan warrior – that were usually made of wood. The artist, George Catlin, originally gave this account.

"His bow was of bone, and as white and beautiful as ivory; over its back was laid, and firmly attached to it, a coating of deer's sinews, which gave it its elasticity, and of course death to all that stood inimically before it. Its string was three stranded and twisted of sinews, which many a time had twanged and sent the whizzing death to animal and to human victims." (Palmer, Rose A. "Indians of the Plains." *The North American Indians*. The Smithsonian Series Volume Four, 1929/1944, p 163).

There are similarities in the form of some basic bone tools and they are relatively unchanged over time. "Such items as antler flaking tools, bone beads, and bone awls were used by most groups from the earliest Archaic time on." (Mayer-Oakes, William J. *Prehistory of the Upper Ohio Valley*. Annals of Carnegie Museum, Vol. 34, Pittsburgh, 1955, p 26).

A site in New York state had bone splinter awls of three types, and one had been manufactured from a catfish dorsal spine. There were also two leister points for fishing, very pointed at one end, and a flaker possibly made of bear's bone. (Tuck, James A. *Onondaga Iroquois Prehistory*. Syracuse University Press, 1971, pp 42, 43, plate 39).

Indians who engaged in whaling off the western coast of Canada often used a special harpoon head fastened to a wooden shaft 18 to 28 feet long. A long notched bone foreshaft was attached to the main shaft, and the oval-shaped harpoon head was attached to the foreshaft. The harpoon, with sharpened edges, was made of mussel shell and was connected to the foreshaft with a 3" bone section. The harpoon line was secured to this bone. (Jenness, Diamond. *The Indians of Canada*. 2nd edition. National Museum of Canada, Bulletin 65, 1934, p 59).

Shell mounds in Florida at times contained organic material artifacts of various kinds.

"Implements of bone were more frequent [than chipped artifact finds], but apparently limited to awls and piercers, an office for which bone, then and since, seems very generally reserved. Implements of shell, as might have been anticipated, were common, though very slightly if at all, varied in form, consisting of rectangular bits, ground down to edges on one side, forming an efficient scraper, cleaner, or bone wedge. Perforated shells, possibly used for ornament, are found near the upper surface of the mounds, and drinking cups made from the large univalve, Busycon perversa, are similarly found near the surface." (Gratacap, L. P. "Paleolithic Man in America." *The American Antiquarian*. Vol. IV No. 4, October 1882, pp 275, 276).

Bone artifacts in the Great Basin were both common and uncommon. Awls were shaped from the shoulder bone (scapula) of deer, antelope, or elk. A specimen of a thin bone awl with a wooden handle exists, as does a bird bone awl set in a larger bone handle. An elk bone wedge from an Oregon cave is known, as are bone gouges from the Klamath Lakes region. (Strong, Emory. *Stone Age in the Great Basin*. Binfords & Mort, Publisher, Portland, 1969, pp 93 – 95, 208, 209).

Some Atl-atls or wooden dart throwers had carved antler handles, and the eastern Midwest Adena Indians were one such group. The handles they made were rectangular in cross-section, ends were rounded and sides slightly incurvate. While only a few have been found, the average length was 6.33cm. (Dunnell, Robert C. "A Further Note on a Late Adena Atl-atl Handle Style." *The Best of 25 Years of the Central States Archaeological Journal*. 1954 – 1979, 1979, pp 150 – 152).

Bone artifacts from Arkansas and Missouri include awls, needles, handles, dice, and tubular beads from 1½" to 2" long. Shell artifacts include earspools, disc beads or gorgets, freshwater shell dippers, masks, earplugs, disc and tubular beads, and squared-corner one- and two-hole buttons. (Dethrow, James M. *Indian Relics of Northeast Arkansas and Southeast Missouri*. Jostens Publishing Company, Topeka, 1985, pp 54, 72 – 74).

Eskimos have long been noted for their detailed work on bone and ivory. "Carvings in walrus and fossil mastodon ivory were made both as ornaments and as toys. Etchings on ivory objects, such as pipes, bows for drills, etc., illustrate hunting and other scenes, and in some instances are records of important events." (Hodge, F. W. "Guide to the Museum / First Floor." *Indian Notes and Monographs*. Museum of the American Indian, New York, 1922, p 218).

Lindenmeier, the Folsom (Late Paleo) site in northeastern Colorado, contained bone artifacts. The bones of extinct animals and thousands of artifacts were recovered. Bone artifacts were awls, knives or fleshing tools, tube beads, and points that may have tipped spears. Two complete bone discs and one partial example had incised lines on the edges and may have been gaming pieces. (Wormington, H. M. *Ancient Man in North America*. 4th edition. The Denver Museum of Natural History. Denver, 1957, pp 31, 37).

The Reeves site in northern Ohio contained several artifacts of a scarce type. There were two antler harpoons, one with a single barb and two holes in the shaft, and a harpoon with three same-side barbs (one broken) and a notch on the shaft. In addition to the usual awls and fishhooks, this late prehistoric site also had tubular bone flutes or flageolets. (Vietzen, Col. Raymond C. *Indians of the Lake Erie Basin*. Ludi Printing Company, Nebraska, 1965, p 306).

New York state's Barnes site has been investigated since its discovery in 1929. Much bone was found, including: 59 bone awls; 2 awls or chisels; 46 complete or partial matting needles (rounded at ends, center-drilled); 4 flakers, 2 fishhooks; 1 leister point; 6 harpoons (lengths 15.2cm to 23.0cm), some made of bear bone; 1 disc; drilled animal teeth; deer and elk phalanx cones, polished; 2 perforated bear femora; 20 bird bone tubular beads; 1 complete polished bird bone; 1 antler maskette; and 10 beads of shell. (Tuck, James A. *Onondaga Iroquois Prehistory*. Syracuse University Press, 1971, pp 149, 157 – 160, plate 39).

Sites on the southern Oregon coast have been rich in bone artifacts. Double-ended points may have been parts of harpoons, and wood-splitting wedges were made of elk antler and whalebone. Bone fishhooks and spearpoints, and bone needles and awls came from various sites, as well as many shell beads and pendants. The Pistol River site, prehistoric to historic, had bone head-scratchers, ear and nose pins, and whalebone clubs. Of special interest were a bowl and a stool made from the vertebrae of a whale. (Aikens, C. Melvin. *Archaeology of Oregon*. U. S. Department of the Interior, Bureau of Land Management, Oregon State Office, 1984, pp 76, 77, 81, 82).

In 1938, a pottery-producing Plains Indian village, the Hagen site, was excavated in Montana. Complete or partial bone artifact finds totaled 252. Rib bones of bison or deer were made into flint-knapping tools.

"The usual form is flat and spatulate, the rib having been grooved along its anterior and posterior edges and split." Three awl types were encountered, and "In common with many other peoples, the metapodial [lower leg bone] of the deer was the most popular awl material, being the only identifiable bone used. This bone is well adapted for awls. It is of exactly the right texture to be worked into an excellent point. The natural grooves in the shaft made preliminary incising preparatory to breaking much easier...".

Bone scrapers with toothed ends were made of elk metapodials. "This is the typical Plains fleshing tool which is used in hide tanning. It is found throughout the Plains and in most of Canada east of the Rockies as well as sporadically in other regions of the United States." Shaft wrenches made of bison ribs had one or two holes. "These tools were probably used to straighten shafts for arrows. Arrow shafts were placed in the perforations and bent and twisted until they were more or less permanently straightened. These tools are very common on the plains and elsewhere. These tools were found at Pictograph Cave near Billings, Montana, as well as shafts which were being straightened, and show the characteristic indentations made by these implements." Other artifacts were wedges (bison tibiae), hooks, bracelets (split antler strips), beads, game counters, antler projectile points, picks, digging tools, knife handles, incised bones, and some worked shell pieces. (Mulloy, William. *The Hagen Site – A Prehistoric Village on the Lower Yellowstone*. The University of Montana Publications in the Social Sciences No. 1, WPA, Missoula, Summer 1942, pp 3, 63 – 84).

The buffalo or bison bone abrader is an unusual artifact. Made from a knee bone, the surface is quite rough. The tool was likely used like sandpaper, for shaping or finishing bone or wood. (Russell, Virgil Y. *Indian Artifacts*. 7th printing. Johnson Publishing Company, Boulder, Colorado, 1974, p 135).

Bone specimens from the Spoon River focus (Illinois) include: Turkey bone awl, 5" long; deer ulna awl, 4½" long; fishhook preform 2½" long; grooved-top fishhook, 1¼"; antler handle, 4¾"; hairpin, 12" long; portion of engraved bracelet; perforated deer phalanx; and an arrowpoint made of antler. Shell specimens include: Disc beads and beads in other shapes; marine shell pendants 3 and 6" long; rattles made of mussel shell and turtle shell; ladles or spoons, and hoes. (Cole, Fay-Cooper and Thorne Deuel. *Rediscovering Illinois*. The University of Chicago Press, 1937/1975, pp 127, 225, 226).

The Chucalissa site in Shelby County, Tennessee, Middle Mississippian in time, contained large numbers of animal bone and bone artifacts. Fish, amphibians, reptiles, birds, and mammals were represented, and the last included black bear, bobcat, mountain lion, and wolf. Artifacts consisted of many bone awls, antler flaking(?) tools, antler points, beamers, chisel-edged tool made from a mountain lion (cougar) radius, split bear canines, deer bone cube of unknown use, worked beaver incisor, dog bone radius awl, bone fishhook, fish bone (freshwater drum) with sharp tip, and worked and cut wild turkey bones. (Parmalee, Paul W. "Vertebrate Remains From the Chucalissa Site." *Ten Years of the Tennessee Archaeologist / Selected Subjects*. 1954 – 1963. Vol. XVI No. 2, pp 353 – 359).

In New York state the Geneva, Scottsville and Lamoka Lake sites provided ample evidence of bone tool use by their Archaic inhabitants. The artifacts were antler "pendant-like" bars (some of which were notched on the edges) up to 4½" long, with an engraved specimen and others painted. There were many awls, and one pin-like artifact, 9¼" long, was painted in wide, angled stripes. Bone double-pointed pins, fishhooks, whistles, flutes, perforated needles and shuttles, possible hairpins, bone knives, and miscellaneous bone items were recovered. (Ritchie, William A. "New Evidence Relating to the Archaic Occupation of New York." *Researches and Transactions of the New York State Archaeological Association*. 1936, pp 1, 2, plates VI – XII).

Regarding the use of antler and bone artifacts, both the Adena and Hopewell (Woodland period, eastern Midwest) had some traits in common. Both made awls from deer or elk cannon bones, and both had bone combs. The two cultural groups also had drilled small animal teeth plus cut animal jaws and antler or bone handles. (Webb, William S. and Charles E. Snow. *The Adena People*. The University of Kentucky, 1945/1988, p 155).

Col. Raymond Vietzen, Ohio author and archaeologist, provided a thorough review of eastern Midwest fishhooks based on his excavations and studies.

"Fishhooks found on the prehistoric sites in Kentucky are somewhat varied and represent seven distinct types: namely, the conventional hook without a barb, which is very common (found in Glover's Cave); the conventional hook with barb, this being rarely found; and the conventional type with a perforation for attachment of the line. This common fishhook form is also found with an enlarged knob or with a groove to retain the fishing line. Grooved specimens are common as are the plain forms which needed pitch or glue to hold the line. Fishhooks with enlarged knobs are rare on the Kentucky sites and but one was found in Glover's Cave. Gang hooks containing double and triple prongs were among the most unusual forms of fishhooks. A four pronged hook was found along the Cumberland River in Trigg County, Kentucky, which adjoins Christian County on the west. Fishhooks found in the cave were knobbed, grooved, or plain and contained but a single prong." (Vietzen, Col. Raymond C. *The Saga of Glover's Cave*. Wahoo, Nebraska, 1956, p 194).

The Point Peninsula lifeway, Late Woodland, had major bone artifact classes in New York state. Such objects included long bone harpoons with barbs on one side, a beaver incisor set crosswise in an antler handle, and a bone beamer similar to those used by later peoples in the Ohio Valley. (Griffin, James B., Editor. *Archeology of Eastern United States*. The University of Chicago Press, 1952, Illustrations / figure 6).

Ancient Buried City (formerly King Mounds) at the confluence of the Ohio and Mississippi Rivers, Wickliffe, Kentucky, was once a major tourist attraction. Occasionally duplicate or extra artifacts were sold, and an example is noted from a ca. 1939 flyer: "Whet Stones or tool sharpeners, from our excavations, $2.00 – 3.00." These were probably used for shaping and sharpening bone awls and needles. (Advertising flyer, *Ancient Buried City*. author's collection).

Ohio's Late Woodland site known as Raven Rocks contained 354 bone tools, some carefully and some casually made. In addition to the typical full and splinter bone awls (136) there were two awls made of deer jawbones and five miniature awls. Pseudo beamers (19) were present, which were beamers that did not quite compare (in manufacture) with well-made examples elsewhere and that did not evidence the same use-marks. Bone knives (65) and spatulates (15) were found, plus five turtle shell cups and three antler points. (Prufer, Olaf H. *Raven Rocks – A Specialized Late Woodland Rockshelter Occupation in Belmont County, Ohio*. Kent State Research Papers in Archaeology No. 1, 1981, pp 38 – 53).

Bone and ivory points from Paleo times have been found across North America, and there is now little doubt that such artifacts were used as lance or spear points. It was once thought that the large pins were a form of foreshaft, but their design – round, sometimes bipointed – suggests primary use as tips for pin-spears. Beveled and crosshatched ends on some suggest they were connected to make longer points for deeper penetration. One mammoth site in a Florida river produced over 80 bone points. (Painter, Floyd. "Pointed Weapons of Wood, Bone, and Ivory: Survival Tools of Early Man in North America." *Central States Archaeological Journal*. Vol. 33 No. 2, April 1986, pp 62 – 75).

The Upper Republican lifeway, Mississippian period, existed from Texas to Nebraska. This Plains people made wide use of bone for awls, fishhooks, and needles. Bodkins or pointed rods were part of their material cultural, also bison shoulder-blade hoes, holed bison rib shaft-straighteners, and antler handles. Bone cube-like objects may have been made for gaming. (Spencer, Robert F, et al. *The Native Americans*. Harper & Row, Publishers, 1965, pp 78, 79, 81).

Bone harpoons found at the famous Koster site in southwestern Illinois were 4 to 6" long, and made from the lower leg bones (metapodial) of deer. The bones were split and ground into shape using sandstone abraders. Final polish for the harpoons was probably done with dry soil and leather. (Struever, Stuart, and Felicia Antonelli Holton. *Koster – Americans in Search of Their Prehistoric Past*. Anchor Press / Doubleday, Garden City, New York, 1979, p 192).

Eskimo (Inuit) artifacts made of bone include, but are not limited to, the following: Maul handles and heads; horn dippers; whalebone cups; fossil ivory dippers; bone ladles; ivory belt-fasteners; labrets; ivory and antler combs; reindeer knife handles; ivory and bone crooked knives with small, curved iron or steel blades; ulu knife handles of walrus ivory; antler adz handles; bone adz-head sockets; bone adz blades; antler-handled chisels; deer scapula saw; ivory bows for drills; bone drill-tips; effigy bone drill-cord handles; ivory bag handles; bear bone daggers; antler bows; antler arrowpoints; antler stiffening rods for bow cases or quivers; bone wrist-guards for bow-strings; bone seal and bird dart (Atl-atl) heads; bone dart foreshafts; detachable harpoon heads; walrus harpoon parts; whale harpoon parts made of narwhale ivory; bolas with walrus tooth weights; antler handles for claw scratchers to decoy or call seals; ivory seal indicator rods set at breathing holes in ice; seal drags with ivory handles; bone snow goggles; ivory rod meat cache markers; antler pegs for deer snares; ivory harpoon holders; ivory fish lures; whalebone ice scoops; bone fish spear tips; bone-handled flint-flakers; ivory sinew twisters for backing bows; antler combs for deerskins; ivory and bone pickaxe heads; ivory snow knives; bone or antler netting needles and mesh spacers; bone net weights; bone needles; bone needle cases; and much more. (Murdoch, John. "Ethnological Results of the Point Barrow Expedition." *Ninth Annual Report of the Bureau of Ethnology*. Smithsonian Institution, Washington, 1892, pp 93 – 318).

Many observers have commented about the lack of barbs on North American fishhooks.

"The Indians were well acquainted with the barb, which they used on spears and harpoons; but they generally avoided it on fish-hooks, which in consequence served only for jigging or trolling. Their bait was either some part of a fish – the eye, or the skin from the belly – or else a bright bone, ivory, or even stone, often colored, and, among the Eskimo and Kutchin, carved to imitate a fish." (Jenness, Diamond. *The Indians of Canada*. Museum of Canada, Bulletin 65, 2nd edition, 1934, p 61).

Marine shell gorgets from the Archaic period in the eastern United States can be placed in three general classes. Each gorget type is named for a major site where the type was found. The Anderson (Tennessee) is small and rounded. The Chiggerville (Kentucky) is much larger and has a small hole near the center. The Indian Knoll (Kentucky) gorget has three holes, one near the center and two at the top or smaller end. The Anderson dates to 4000 – 3000 BC, the Chiggerville to c. 3000 – 2500 BC, and the Indian Knoll to the Late Archaic period, c. 3000

BC – 1800 BC. [In a personal communication, David Lutz notes that the Indian Knoll type eventually evolved into the well-recognized Glacial Kame (1200 BC – 900 BC) three-perforated gorget, giving the shell gorgets a timespan of about 3000 years.] (Lutz, David L. *The Archaic Bannerstone: Its Chronological History and Purpose From 6000 B. C. – 1000 B. C.* 2000, pp 39-43).

Sword-like bone artifacts were found in California and on nearby islands. They were made from porpoise lower jaw bones. One example, slightly curved as was the bone from which it was made, measured 17" long. (Abbott, C. C. and F. W. Putnam. "Swords." *Report Upon United States Geographical Surveys*. Volume VII. Engineer Department / U. S. Army, Washington, 1879, p 231).

Late prehistoric Fort Ancient Indians in the Ohio Valley are noted for the many artifacts made of organic materials. "This culture has a great variety of implements for the most part made of bone and horn [antler]. The fish hook is perhaps the most interesting and resembles the hooks of today, minus the barb. It is usually made from the wing bone of some large bird. The awls are numerous and for the most part made of the leg bones of the wild turkey, although the heavy awls are frequently made of the ulna and metapodial bones of the deer and elk. Needles [hairpins?] are in evidence practically in all tepee sites. They are from 5 – 10" in length, usually curved, and sharpened at one end with a small eye at the other." (Mills, William C. "Prehistoric Man in Ohio." *Hobbies – The Magazine for Collectors*. Chicago, August 1949, p 145).

Beamers – deer or elk long bones with a side strip cut away – sometimes were, or became, two different artifacts. Of all bone artifacts, beamers probably received the hardest use and most wear. It is thought they were used to process (deflesh and clean) hides and skins placed over a log or beam. Downward pressure was exerted from the ends, and the central cut portion acted as a drawknife. This portion received much pressure and abrasion. Wear-through and breakage was relatively rapid, and complete or unbroken beamers are not common. However, when they did break, one or both ends were sometimes reworked and recycled to become awls. (Hothem, Lar. Various sources).

West Coast Indians had several important uses for antler.

"The points of cutting instruments and other implements were made of elk horn, which was also used for spoons having rather flat bowls and carved handles. Most Californians dipped up their acorn gruel with their fingers, but the Yurok were more fastidious in their habits. Elk or deer horn was also used for making purses or money boxes, which were cylindrical in shape, like the large wooden boxes for valuables, but only six or seven" long, and would hold several folded strings of dentalia." (Palmer, Rose A. "West Coast Tribes." *The North American Indians*. The Smithsonian Series Volume Four, 1929/1944, p 196).

Astragalus or ankle bones from large mammals (especially deer and elk) were sometimes used to make artifacts. Dice were made, also an artifact of unknown purpose created by drilling a hole through the base center. Interestingly, for whatever reason, copies of these bones are known that are made of pottery and steatite. (Wagers, Charlie. "Astragalus (Ankle Bone Artifacts)." *Prehistoric American*. Vol. XXXII No. 1, 1999, p 7).

Bone was sometimes used as "background" for pictographs in historic times. Examples are bison skulls encountered by Major Long's expedition along the Platte River. The skulls were marked with red lines, providing information about the Pawnee Indians who had left them. Hidatsa Indians, upon vacating a camp, might leave behind a flat bone with charcoal or red lead markings. This would indicate the reason for the trip, as, an antelope sketch if that were the animal being hunted. Eskimo bone or ivory images sometimes were supplications for success in the hunt, and often had incised lines darkened with pigment or soot. A buffalo shoulder bone blade, found in Texas in Comanche territory, depicted a skirmish between Indians and Spaniards. (Mallery, Garrick. "Pictographs of the North American Indians." *Fourth Annual Report of the Bureau of Ethnology*. Smithsonian Institution, Washington, 1886, pp 59, 151, 192, 216).

Teeth from bears were highly prized in the New York region, probably both because of their size and also because of their obvious association with the animal itself.

"Bears' teeth unworked are frequent [finds]; and out of a great number of those used for ornament a few selections are here made. They occur on almost all village sites, and have a wider distribution than any other bone ornament in time and territory. Here there are three principal divisions; those grooved for suspension, those perforated, and those cut off for some other purpose." (Beauchamp, William M. *Horn and Bone Implements of the New York Indians*. Bulletin 50. New York State Museum, 1902, pp 276 – 277).

An excavator at a site in Nebraska expressed a belief that heat had been used to harden bone artifacts found in storage or refuse pits.

"All of the bone implements found in ruins of a similar character have been tempered by fire. This is easily discernable as they all are more or less covered by fire marks. At this day the bone implements are in splendid state of preservation, the cache being so protected that no water percolates into them. Even after a rain of several weeks the ashes with which they are packed are as dry as if just removed from a stove." (Gilder, Robert F. "The Ten Cache Ruin." *The Archaeological Bulletin*. Vol. I No. 3. The International Society of Archaeologists, 1910, p 62).

The Libben site near Oak Harbor, northern Ohio, produced an improbable artifact. This was a turtle bone about 2½" long with a naturally fringed or toothed end. It was likely used to incise decorative marks on pottery before firing. Technically, this was a non-artifact employed as an artifact. (Vietzen, Col. Raymond C. *From the Earth They Came*. White Horse Publishers, 1978, p 226).

Rattle parts were often made of organic materials, some of them unusual.

"On the North West coast, puffin beaks were strung on a frame composed of pieces of wood bent into two concentric rings and held together by crosspieces. From the Eskimo a similar rattle has been obtained in which the puffin beaks are replaced by bear claws. In the West, pecten shells were strung together to make rattles, while among some California tribes olivella shells took the place of the deer hoofs used by others. The Pueblos make rattles of conus and olivella shells, as well as of antelope hoofs, tortoise shells, and gourds. One Omaha rattle (...) was made of the molars of the elk." (Hodge, Frederick Webb. "Rattles." *Handbook of American Indians*. Part 2. Bureau of American Ethnology Bulletin 30, 1910, pp 355, 356).

One particular artifact made of deer antler may have had a special use.

"...a few years ago new light on the art techniques of the mysterious Hopewell people, the Mound Builders of the Middle West, came from the accidental discovery near Kansas City of an almost intact specimen of the instrument with which they made their intricate geometric and other designs on pottery.

"It was a deer horn, with notches [cut] out in its elliptical bottom, in the style of a roulette. By 'rolling' this over the unbaked clay vessel the Mound Builder artist was able to easily produce designs which would have been very difficult to make with a stamp." (Straley, Wilson. "Indian Relics." *Hobbies – The Magazine for Collectors*. December, 1946, Chicago, p 145)

An unusual patination has been seen on a few bone artifacts. The bone surface is generally dark, brownish-black, but the worked area (lower shaft and tip of an awl, for example) is the whitish or creamy tan color of old bone. These are not modern re-works, as the bone surface is uniform in surface treatment and patination, if present. The most likely explanation is that the unmodified bone was situated near a campfire, perhaps for some time, and then was retrieved and worked into an artifact. There is also the possibility that "green" bone was sometimes purposely fire-dried or seasoned for some reason. (Hothem, Lar. Various sources).

The Hohokam in the Southwest made shell beads, some in disc shape and others of entire shells with the ends removed. Shell bracelets also developed. Bone tubes were made, decorated with incised lines, and their purpose is not known. Hair ornaments were long bones with curved ends, sometimes depicting mountain sheep. (Wormington, H. M. *Prehistoric Indians of the Southwest*. The Denver Museum of Natural History, Popular Series No. 7, 1947/1973, pp 124, 137).

At the Koster site, Illinois, the extensive excavations revealed the presence of bone artifacts at Horizon 11, ca. 6500 BC. These artifacts were needles made from deer long bones and awls made from deer leg bones. The awls, with sharp tips, terminated in a rounded elbow joint. About 3000 years later, Koster people made engraved bone pins, probably used as hairpins or ornaments. Made from the lower leg bones of deer, the pins were 4 to 6" long, and ¼" in diameter. (Struever, Stuart, and Felicia Antonelli Holton. *Koster – Americans in Search of Their Prehistoric Past*. Anchor Press / Doubleday, New York, 1979, pp 192, 245).

Several historic tribes in the Labrador interior made fitted shirts, some with hoods, which they imprinted with designs in red. The designs were done with stamps made of antler or bone. (Jenness, Diamond. *The Indians of Canada*. 2nd edition. National Museum of Canada, Bulletin 65, 1934, p 272).

One artifact made of bone has long been somewhat of a mystery, and even after a century of study the use is uncertain.

"Punches and blunt implements: No precise use can safely be assigned to some articles with rounded or flattened ends. Those that are curved and slightly tapering were probably inserted in clubs. Others have purposely enlarged ends. If they had points, they might be considered pins, but usually these are lacking. It has been thought that some were used in decorating pottery, but a hollow bone seems the only bone article employed for this. In a general way it may be best to describe them simply as they are, unless there appear reasons for some special use." (Beauchamp, William M. *Horn and Bone Implements of the New York Indians*. Bulletin 50. New York State Museum, 1902, p 269).

Marks on bones, whether they are fragments or finished artifacts, leave a solid record of prehistoric activity.

"Few phases of stone-age craftsmanship can be reconstructed as satisfactorily as can the fashioning of bone. Specimens, to begin with, are abundant and ordinarily are well preserved (...) hence we find in the rubbish great quantities of unfinished pieces, fully illustrating all the methods used for roughing-out, for shaping, and for finishing. Bone, too, is a substance which, though it dries to stony hardness, is relatively soft when fresh, particularly at the surface, and it forms, therefore, a highly sensitive register of the marks of industry, every scratch and abrasion being clearly recorded." (Kidder, Alfred Vincent. "Objects of Bone." *The Artifacts of Pecos*. Robert S. Peabody Foundation for Archaeology, Yale University Press, New Haven, 1932, p 199).

Wild turkey bones were often used to make awls on late prehistoric sites in southern Ohio.

"[There were] twelve awls made from the tarsometatarsus of the wild turkey, six of which are decorated with notches cut upon the sides, and the other six plain. Awls made of this bone were very abundant in the village and several hundred in perfect condition were found. In practically every village site of this culture the awl made from this bone is present and very frequently exceed in numbers all other classes of awls." (Mills, William C. "The Feurt Mounds and Village Site." *Ohio Archaeological and Historical Publications*. Vol. XXVI. Columbus, 1917, p 410).

Two atypical uses of bone have been noted in historic times. "Champlain illustrates a game drive in which the drivers appear to be beating with bones upon clavicles of some large animal, and among the Plains tribes and the Pueblos a sort of saw-fiddle in which sometimes a scapula is drawn over a notched stick, or over another scapula, for keeping time in ceremonial dances, is employed." (Hodge, Frederick Webb. "Bone-work." *Handbook of American Indians*. Part 1. Bureau of American Ethnology Bulletin 30, 1907, p 160).

Antler and bone, though similar in some respects, was sometimes used for different purposes.

"Some readers might wonder why antler was used in preference to bone [for heavy-use tools]. A cutting or scraping edge on horn or antler is tougher and more effective than on bone; therefore the celts, gouges, and hide scrapers were made from basal portions of deer and elk antlers. Most bone would splinter and shatter under strain and shock encountered in operations performed with celts and gouges. Nature made the horns of animals tougher than the bones as the horns were exposed and to be used as weapons while the bones were encased and protected by skin, flesh, cords, and muscles to help cushion any excessive shocks. Primative man soon found antler and horn far superior to bone for the manufacture of projectile points, daggers, tool handles and celts. Bone was more suitable for slender needles and awls for which antler was of little or no use." (Vietzen, Col. Raymond C. *The Saga of Glover's Cave*. Wahoo, Nebraska, 1956, p 196).

In the Southwest, there is some evidence that slices of bone were used as rings for fingers.

"There was little indication in this district of the use of bone in the making of ornaments, excepting of course, the tubes made for beads. Pieces from two finger rings, fashioned from this material, were recovered from the refuse mound associated with the Great Pueblo ruins, but there were no traces of pendants, pins with carved heads, or hair ornaments such as are often found in Anasazi sites. Not enough remains of the rings to tell whether or not they were plain or, like some of those from the Chaco Canyon, were decorated with carved figures or insets of turquoise." (Roberts, Frank H. H. Jr. *Archaeological Remains in the Whitewater District, Eastern Arizona*. Part II, Bureau of American Ethnology Bulletin 126. Smithsonian Institution, Washington, 1940, p 116).

Eva, in Tennessee, was a major Archaic site that produced hundreds of bone, antler, and other artifacts. The 393 bone pieces consisted of awls, needles and fishhooks, plus probable flakers, tubes, and handles. The 275 antler pieces were scrapers, shaft-wrenches, projectile points, fishhooks, handles, pins, pendants, and a scoop. Drilled animal (bear and dog) teeth were found, plus beaver tooth tools, turtle shell rattles and a necklace made from snake vertebrae. (Lewis, Thomas M. N., and Madeline Kneberg Lewis. "Bone Artifacts." *Eva – An Archaic Site*. The University of Tennessee Press, 1961/1977, pp 75, 76, 87, 88, 91).

Some insightful observations have been made about bone fishhooks found in Kentucky. One is that complete fishhook finds are not frequent, because the hooks were seemingly used until they broke. Another is the kind of bone used for fishhooks.

"Very tiny hooks less than 1" long and ⅜" wide are made from bird bone spatulae. Large hooks more than 3" long, and 1" broad are made from large deer bones. When made from cylindrical long bones, the bone loop still holds the cylindrical curvature of the original bone, so that the hook also shows the same cylindrical curvature. As pointed out, hooks of this type may vary greatly in size, and are very numerous in Kentucky Shell Mounds. They apparently are not of long life. The bones from which they are made have a natural longitudinal structure, which cause the bone to split. Hooks are frequently found broken at the end of the loop, or in the angle." (Webb, William S. "The Carlson Annis Mound, Butler County, Kentucky." *Reports in Archaeology*. Vol. VII, No. 4, January 1950. University of Kentucky, pp 329 – 330).

There is a good description of antler points from Washington Borough in Pennsylvania, a late prehistoric site.

"The fact that the Susquehannock used antler projectile points was well established on this village site as several arrowheads in situ were recorded. They averaged between 1¼" and 2½" in length and were beautifully smoothed and pointed. At the proximal end they had one notched and pointed tang, and were hollowed out conically so the shaft of the arrow could be inserted. Three 'bunt' arrowheads, made of antler, were found. They had two, four, and six short pointed projections on the distal end, pointed on proximal end, and were probably stunning arrows taking small game or the property of children learning to use weapons. This type of antler point is still employed by Indians in the sub-Arctic." (Cadzow, Donald A. *Safe Harbor Report No. 2*. Publications of Pennsylvania Historic Commission, Vol. III, Harrisburg, 1936, pp 148, 149).

Hollow tubular bones, especially those of large birds, may have had multiple uses. Shorter tubes could be used as beads, or as whistles, by blocking one end and blowing sharply across the open end. Longer tubes may have served as drinking straws to obtain water from shallow pools. Thick hollow bones served as knife and tool handles, and also (possibly) as powdered paint containers. (Hothem, Lar. Various sources).

In Oklahoma (and elsewhere) deer cannon bones were often used to produce awls. The long bone was broken in half, and each half split so that four awls could be made from one cannon (between the knee and ankle) bone. The break areas were ground down and pointed, and the joint ends were left with little modification. (Bell, Robert E. *Oklahoma Indian Artifacts*. Contributions from the Stovall Museum, No. 4. University of Oklahoma, Norman, 1980, p 63).

Occasionally in early reports mention is made of the artifacts that were used to shape or maintain bone tools. One such relates to a Fort Ancient site in southern Ohio. "Polishing stones and whetstones used in the manufacture of bone awls were frequently met with in the tepee sites. They are mere slabs of waverly sandstone, showing great use, some having grooves worn into their faces from use in sharpening the bone into the desired shape." (Mills, William C. "The Feurt Mounds and Village Site." *Ohio Archaeological and Historical Publications*. Vol. XXVI, Columbus, 1917, p 405).

A cache of bone dice(?) was found in Poncho House, Arizona, and similar pieces were found elsewhere in the Southwest.

"This lot consists of eleven lenticular pieces averaging three-quarters of an inch in length by three-eighths of an inch in width; and four discoidal ones, three-eighths of an inch in diameter, all having one side rounded and the other side flat. The rounded side is polished, while the flat side is scored, and in most of them a cement-like substance [is] adhering to it. They were probably not dice, though the name best describes them." (Guernsey, Samuel James. *Explorations in Northeastern Arizona*. Papers of the Peabody Museum, Vol. XII No. 1, Harvard University, 1931, p 104 plate 24).

In 1925, the Museum of the American Indian in New York received a number of gifts from donors, and many relate to the topic of this book. The gifts included: Haida mountain goat horn spoon; alligator jaw, Florida; bone flute; neck chain of peccary teeth, British Guiana; very long elk horn spoon, California; bone comb, bone awl, and many shell beads, New York; shell disc beads, Idaho; small ivory carving, Alaska; long columella shell pendant, Florida; two horn spoons; deer bone game; dentalium shell necklace, North Dakota; oval clamshell artifact, Florida; 136 rectangular drilled shell beads, Peru; bone handles for Atl-atls, one animal effigy, and one a human face effigy, Peru; two bone needles, provenance unknown; old bone-handled knife, Washington; shell earplug, Tennessee; 17 bone pendants, Nevada; ivory toggle in shape of a seal, Alaska; bone bow, Greenland, and, purple and white wampum beads, New York. (Editor. "Recent Accessions by Gift." *Indian Notes*. Vol. 2 Nos. 1, 2, 3, & 4. 1925. Museum of the American Indian, New York).

Ancient Buried City, Wickliffe, Kentucky, once displayed numerous artifacts excavated there, and the bone tools are of special interest.

"Most bone implements found have been pale-white in color. The majority of those excavated here is the color of old ivory and has a lustrous polish and heavy patina, indicating long usage. Every day I am asked if we polish the bone implements. People can scarcely believe they have been in the ground for centuries and yet retain such a beautiful luster." (King, Blanche Busey. *Under Your Feet – The Story of the American Mound Builders*. Dodd, Mead & Company, 1939, New York, p 158).

At the Madisonville site, Ohio, many bone artifacts were found. The Fort Ancient village area produced numbers of beamers (skin-working tools made from deer cannon bones) and the manufacturing techniques could be determined.

"Fragments of several hundred of these were obtained. They were usually broken near the middle as this was the thinnest and most fragile point of the tool. Only a comparatively small number of unbroken ones were recovered. Among these are a few which are unfinished and clearly show the process of making. One method was to widen and deepen the natural longitudinal groove on the broad face of the bone, probably with the rounded edges of a flint scraper, until the required sharp edges upon either side were produced. Another was to cut a longitudinal slit through the wall and scrape away the bone upon either side until the proper edges were formed." (Hooton, Earnest A. *Indian Village Site and Cemetery Near Madisonville, Ohio*. Peabody Museum, Vol. VIII No. 1, Cambridge, 1920, p 53).

A description of eyed needles found at Pecos, New Mexico, might well apply to those found elsewhere.

"They are delicate little implements from 2 to 4½" long. Slivers, usually of bird-bone, were fashioned to the proper shape, with long tapering points and slightly swelling butts. The eyes were made by scratching a deep longitudinal groove (usually from the naturally convex side of the bone) into one side of the butt until it had cut through; or the groove was less deeply excavated and the final piercing was accomplished by drilling a small round hole." (When drilled, the hole had a diameter of about 1/32".) (Kidder, Alfred Vincent. "Objects of Bone." *The Artifacts of Pecos*. Robert S. Peabody Foundation for Archaeology. Yale University Press, New Haven, 1932, pp 222, 223).

Bone harpoons were made in a great number of forms.

"In some 30 specimens, principally from Alaska, belonging to the Peabody Museum, there are many varieties and sizes of barbed points of bone with their accompanying shafts; and in many instances the barbs are on one side only of the bone, though they are often several in number. These bone points vary much in size, and are from 1 to 6 or 7" in length. One bone implement (8" long), which evidently once fitted into a socket, has a hole at its base for the string, and is of special interest from the fact that it has three barbs on each side, and also has the point of the bone tipped by a sharp point of shell." (Abbott, C. C. and F. W. Putnam, "Implements Made of Bone." *Report Upon United States Geographical Surveys*. Volume VII. Engineer Department / U. S. Army, Washington, 1879, p 226).

The prehistoric popularity of awls and awl-like tools was illustrated at the Indian Knoll site in Kentucky. There, awls were made from 15 different kinds of bone. These were unidentified bone splinters, deer ulna, deer cannon bone, cannon bone ends, deer radius, deer tibia, scapulae, deer jawbones, bird bone shafts, shaft ends (mainly wild turkey), ulnae of small mammals (including dog), perforated flat bone, perforated and engraved bone, raccoon baculum, and fish-fin spines. (Webb, William S. *Indian Knoll, Ohio County, Kentucky*. The University of Tennessee Press, Knoxville, 1946/1974, pp 282 – 286).

Col. Raymond Vietzen excavated many late prehistoric sites in northern Ohio and Kentucky, and he wrote books about his archaeological and collecting activities. The Riker site, in Tuscarawas County, Ohio, contained many bone artifacts.

"Bone artifacts are the most numerous of all items made and used by the aborigines and culturally speaking it is almost impossible to classify such items. All cultures of man, and especially those of the Woodland and Mississippian groups, made and used similar bone tools, weapons, and ornaments, many of which look much the same when made by a Hopewell Indian as if made by a Fort Ancient or Iroquian craftsman.

"Bone awls, perforators, pins, needles and hair ornaments were produced by the Riker people. Fishhooks, gorges, spears, and projectile points were used in their daily chores. Bone knives, fleshers, digging tools and even bone ornaments were among the material recovered from the Riker site. The bone needles were found with eyes for sewing cord or with knobs and grooves to hold the thread.

"Antler was used as extensively as were the teeth and other parts of the animal skeletons. Little was wasted, as their very existence was dependent on utilizing whatever nature provided. Antler tines were used as projectile points, daggers, and digging tools. Flint chipping punches were cut and shaped from deer antler. Elk antler provided fleshing and digging tools and sometimes ornaments. The cannon bones (lower leg bones) of deer and elk were so cut out and sharpened as to make excellent hide scrapers somewhat resembling our draw knives. These were often broken in the center where worn thin and most were found fragmentary." (Vietzen, Col. Raymond C. *The Riker Site*. Sugar Creek Valley Chapter, Archaeological Society of Ohio, 1974, p 114).

In the northeastern U. S., Point Peninsula people of the Late Archaic – Early Woodland had some artifacts made of organic materials. These include antler harpoons with barbs on one or both sides, tools made of antler with a beaver incisor set at an angle, bone combs with engraving, antler flaking tools, antler projectile points, and cannon bone beamers. (Dragoo, Don W. *Mounds for the Dead*. Annals of Carnegie Museum Vol. 37, Pittsburgh, 1963 reprint, pp 264 – 265).

Bone artifacts of many kinds were found in the Indiana region. Common were tube beads, fishhooks, knapping drifts or rods, needles, pins, arrowpoints, awls, a flute or flageolet, and bone beamers. Uncommon was a flat drilled gorget, an Atl-atl hook, and a handle that may also have been for an Atl-atl. (Lilly, Eli. *Prehistoric Antiquities of Indiana*. Indiana Historical Society, Indianapolis, 1937, p 217).

Bone awls and flakers, while much alike in size and shape, in fact have some differences.

"Although some awls have relatively blunt points, and some of the awl-like implements which have been termed flakers have fairly sharp ones, the distinction between the two sorts of implements is, in general, well marked. The awls, even when blunted by long use, usually have tips that tend to taper gradually, while the flakers have stubby, rounded ends. (...) All tools, accordingly, whose points are apparently sharp enough to have been of use for perforating hides or for the manufacture of coiled basketry have been classed as awls. According to the material from which they were made, the awls fall into the following three main divisions: Mammal leg-bone, mammal rib, and bird bone." (Kidder, Alfred Vincent. "Objects of Bone." *The Artifacts of Pecos*. Robert S. Peabody Foundation for Archaeology, Yale University Press, New Haven, 1932, p 203).

Plains Indians used bone agricultural tools, among them hoes made of bison shoulder blades, horn-core and skull portions, and bison long bones. Elk bone fleshers, awls, gambling pieces, fishhooks, knives, quill-flatteners, bracelets, bow-guards, and shaft-straighteners were also created. (Perino, Gregory. "Mandan Artifacts from North Dakota." *Prehistoric Artifacts*. Genuine Indian Relic Society, Vol. XXI No. 3, 1987, pp 9 – 11).

Flakers or flint-knapping bone tools are frequent finds, and their probable origin is fascinating.

"The specimens about to be described are strongly suggestive of awls with blunt points; it seems probable indeed that most, if not all, of them were originally awls, and that they were put to secondary use after their ends in one way or another became unserviceable for perforating. The supposition that they were made from old awls is borne out by the fact that they occur in all the forms characteristic of mammal bone awls: with head unworked, partly worked, and entirely cut away. Interest, therefore, centers on their points, which, with few exceptions, are definitely rounded. The roundness appears to have been intentionally produced by grinding, rather than to have been acquired in service. This may seem a rather fine distinction, but careful examination of the worked ends of a long series of bone tools will show that where the principal use of a specimen has been in rubbing or polishing, the wear tends to become localized in flat, or flattish, polished, facet-like areas. The longer the tool remains in service the more strongly marked become the wear-facets. On the other hand, a tool which is deliberately worked to a blunt or rounded end exhibits general rather than localized abrasion, for in grinding it down the maker was evidently careful to keep turning it, in order that all sides might be evenly reduced. (...) Some are quite smooth, but the majority shows evident signs of hard use which has battered and even chipped them. The only industry with which we are familiar that could result in such markings is the chipping of flint." (Kidder, Alfred Vincent. "Objects of Bone." *The Artifacts of Pecos*. Robert S. Peabody Foundation for Archaeology, Yale University Press, New Haven, 1932, p 229).

Slender, well-shaped, and polished bipointed bone pins have come from different sites in Georgia. The pins exist in various colors, including red, black, and tan. (Editor. *Prehistoric Americans*. Genuine Indian Relic Society, Vol. XXX No. 2, 1996, p 17).

Professor Moorehead reported that bone artifacts were major implements on the West Coast.

"Bone implements are more numerous, perhaps, on the Pacific Coast than anywhere else in the United States, and are abundant in every part of this state [California]. Those of Central and Northern California have a much better appearance than those from the Islands and Southern counties. The bleached and weathered appearance of the latter is replaced in the former by a smooth, finished surface, yellowed with age. Occasionally a remarkably high polish remains. The most common form is the 'awl,' or perforator. These abound in all the mound and village sites, varying in size from 2 to 7". They were used in the construction of baskets, perforating any kind of skin or fabric which a woman would work, and during the regime of the Spanish missions in sewing up tallow in the hides of the slaughtered animals." (Moorehead, Warren K. *Prehistoric Implements*. The Robert Clarke Company, Cincinnati, 1900, p 269).

Bone artifacts from Canada are similar in many respects to those elsewhere in North America, although colder temperatures may have made a difference.

"The bone collections in Canadian and American museums are not as large as one would expect. (...) All the bone implements found in this province are taken from village sites or kitchen middens where the ashes from their winter fires had been deposited – the hardwood ashes acting as a preservative, and so great a preservative that after the lapse of many hundreds of years specimens have been taken from their ashy bed as perfect as the day they were made – the points of the awls so sharp, smooth, and glossy, one would think they had only left the maker's hand yesterday." (Editor. *Annual Archaeological Report*. The Legislative Assembly of Ontario, Toronto, 1911, p 65).

Large bear teeth found on prehistoric sites are sometimes without drilled holes, so were probably not ornaments. Wear and damage on the pointed end suggests they may have been flint-chipping tools. (Wagers, C. S. "Bear Tooth Flint Flakers." *Prehistoric Artifacts*. Genuine Indian Relic Society, Vol. XXII No. 3, 1988, p 19).

At the Franks site in northern Ohio, late prehistoric, a bone whistle was found that measured ⅜ x 5" long. Shell beads averaging ⅜ x ¾" were also recovered, and a large sandstone mortar with a long groove that might have been used to shape arrow-shafts or bone awls. A polished bone needle with incised lines was 6" long, and it had an eye at one end. Some shell beads had a covering of thin, beaten copper, an unusual find for the culture. There were drilled bear tusks, a fine mussel shell gorget, and an incised bone awl. A deer antler spearpoint 7½" long deserves a full description. "The original antler prong was scraped down to a very keen point and highly polished. A socket was drilled in the large end or base to accommodate a wooden handle. A small hole about one-quarter inch in diameter was drilled crosswise through this socket to enable the handle and spearhead to be fastened together by a pin of wood, bone or other material." Bone (not antler) arrowpoints ranged in length from 1 to 2¼", and these had tapered holes in the base. (Vietzen, Raymond C. *The Immortal Eries*. Wilmot Printing Company, Elyria, Ohio, 1945, pp 107, 110, 113, 114, 120, 121, 123, 124).

Wedge-like artifacts of antler and bone are sometimes seen, and the hard use they received no doubt contributed to their present scarcity.

"The antler wedge is an almost continent-wide tool. It appears from the Southeastern Archaic through adjacent areas to California and on up to Bering Straits. The implements themselves are as variable as different cultures and uses could make them but the basic functions remain the same. Trees were felled, split, and barked, and the wood was carved with these implements or their variants." (Osborne, Douglas. "Excavations in the McNary Reservoir Basin Near Umatilla, Oregon." *River Basin Survey Papers No. 8*. Bureau of American Ethnology Bulletin 166. Smithsonian Institution, Washington, 1957, pp 85, 86).

One early excavator of an Archaic site in Kentucky remarked about the unusual way deer bones had been broken.

"The preservation of bone material was exceptionally good due to the considerable lime content of the soil. Thus many artifacts were seemingly as sound as when they were first made. The midden yielded a great mass of deer bones, indicating that deer was an important item in the food supply. Such bones are rarely found complete. The type of breakage observed is not one of simple shear, which might cause a bone to break into two parts; the broken bones generally seem to have been subjected to a torque, which not only caused the bone to break, but split as well. This produced many long pointed rough splinters, often with the end of the bone remaining attached." (Webb, William S. *Indian Knoll – Ohio County, Kentucky*. The University of Kentucky, Reports in Anthropology and Archaeology, Vol. IV No. 3, Part 1, Lexington, 1946, p 281).

Certain conditions brought about by prehistoric activity (in addition to the well-known shell heaps) could preserve antler and bone artifacts.

"...mere camps did not produce sufficient ashes or carbonaceous matter to preserve perishable articles, while those of stone remained. They (...) must be sought where fires have long been in use. The dumping places, bordering most Iroquois villages, yield many, some of which are fine. Nothing preserves them so well as ashes, and these accumulated to a great depth where a fire burned for many years. (...) Where a village was edged with deep ravines, refuse was thrown down the banks, but sometimes a deep hole was found or formed and gradually filled. These have rich deposits." (Beauchamp, William M. *Horn and Bone Implements of the New York Indians*. Bulletin 50. New York State Museum, 1902, p 251).

Awls are usually the most common bone artifacts found anywhere in North America, and 131 examples were picked up at the proto-historic Schultz Farm site in Pennsylvania.

"Of all the artifacts recovered, awls and awl-like implements were the most numerous. They were fashioned from bones of various animals, birds, and fish. In size they varied from 1½" to 8½" in length. (...) Although generally termed awls by archaeologists, these useful implements were employed for many purposes. Their points varied considerably, some were sharp, others blunt, and many chisel and gouge shaped. The limb bones of small mammals and the wing bones of birds, some retaining the natural articular end, were favored. The bird radii and fish bones required very little sharpening and were probably employed also as pins. The natural joints of small animals and birds were also cut off and used for awl handles. One with an iron awl in place was recovered." (Cadzow, Donald A. *Safe Harbor Report No. 2*. Publications of Pennsylvania Historic Commission, Vol. III, Harrisburg, 1936, pp 170, 171).

Bone was a favored material for gaming devices. "Bones also were largely used in the making of dice and tubes for gambling purposes. The Huron-Iroquois, during the long winter nights, spent much of their leisure time playing games of chance, and, like their European successor, made dice their favorite form of gambling. In most cases the counting was done numerically, using pieces of bone or pebbles." (Editor. *Annual Archaeological Report*. The Legislative Assembly of Ontario, Toronto, 1911, p 65).

The Mogollon people in the Southwest had a cultural awl type. It was made of bone and was notched on one side, just below the larger end. (Wormington, H. M. *Prehistoric Indians of the Southwest*. The Denver Museum of Natural History, Popular Series No. 7, 1947/1973, pp 155, 162).

The simple beauty of shells made them valuable to prehistoric artisans.

"Shell was a favorite material with the aborigines all over America for the manufacture of implements, utensils, and ornaments; and shells in their natural state or merely notched or perforated for attachment were, on account of their beauty of form and color, extensively used for personal embellishment. Among the tribes north of Mexico, clam and mussel shells served for cups and spoons, were hafted for scraping and digging, and worked up into fishhooks, knives, and other minor implements. The large conchs were used as drinking vessels after the interior portions had been removed, and in Florida they were hafted as clubs and picks. In many sections the thick walls were cut up to be shaped by tedious processes of scraping, grinding, and drilling with stone tools into celts, adzes, gouges, scrapers, and plummets. Ornaments of shell were exceedingly varied in form, and the clam, unio, conch, and many of the larger shells in the East, and like forms, and more especially the beautiful abalone of the Pacific coast, were cut up, trimmed, ground, and polished and perforated for beads, pins, pendants, and breastplates or gorgets." (Hodge, Frederick Webb. "Shell / Shellwork." *Handbook of American Indians*. Part 2. Bureau of American Ethnology Bulletin 30, 1910, p 539).

Among the bone and antler artifacts found at a Tennessee Archaic site were Atl-atl hooks. The Eva type was short and cylindrical, with a small projection for engaging the dart butt. In comparison, the Indian Knoll (Kentucky) type was larger and the projection longer. (Lewis, Thomas M. N., and Madeline Kneberg Lewis. "Antler Artifacts." *Eva – An Archaic Site*. The University of Tennessee Press, 1961/1977, pp 92, 95, 96).

The importance of bone and other organic materials is illustrated by the following observation:

"The use of bone and related materials, including antler, ivory, horn, whalebone, turtle-shell, and the teeth, hoofs, beaks, and claws of many creatures, was almost universal among Indian tribes. The hardness and toughness of these materials made them desirable for many kinds of implements and utensils, and their pleasing color and capacity for high polish caused them to be valued for personal ornaments." (Hodge, Frederick Webb. "Bone-work." *Handbook of American Indians*. Part 1. Bureau of American Ethnology Bulletin 30, 1907, p 159).

Large pointed shafts from Paleo times, made of bone or ivory, have been found on early sites across North Americ. An example from Canada, though broken, was over 8" long. Several came from Blackwater Draw, Texas, and three were found at Lind Coulee, in Washington state. A bone point was excavated in the northern Great Basin, which had a pointed end and a beveled end. (Wilmeth, Roscoe. "A Fossilized Bone artifact From Southern Saskatchewan." *American Antiquity*. Vol. 33 No. 1, January 1968. The Society for American Archaeology, pp 100, 101).

Manufacturing methods for bone artifacts found at Clark's Pond, Massachusetts, are described here. "Bone was reduced in size by sawing or splitting or by sawing and breaking. Implements were further formed by scraping and finished by grinding or polishing." Awls and spatulate artifacts were recovered, also harpoon-like barbed bone points. Antler flakers and beads of bird bone were present, also three worked beaver incisors. (Bullen, Ripley P. *Excavations in Northeastern Massachusetts*. Papers of the Robert S. Peabody Foundation for Archaeology, Phillips Academy, Andover, 1949, pp 95, 125, 126, plate XIX).

Deer, turkey, and elk bones were used to make tools at Hardin Village in Kentucky. This Mississippian site had 114 awls, of which 64 were made of bone splinters. Beads were barrel, tube, and animal teeth that had been drilled. Antler and beaver incisor chisels, bone pendants, antler and bone punches, antler points, bone pins and fishhooks, flakers, gaming bones, gouges and beamer fragments, and flutes or whistles were all recovered. Shell artifacts included beads, hoes, pendants, and gorgets. (Hanson, Lee H. Jr. *The Hardin Village Site*. University of Kentucky Press, Studies in Anthropology No. 4, 1966, pp 141 – 165).

Comments about the use of shell in New York state are of interest.

"The later Iroquois loved shell ornaments, such as beads, perforated shells, runtees and disks, maskettes, and variously formed effigies, but they did not have them in any abundance until the coming of the white man. Shell beads of spherical shape, cylindrical, or even discoidal appear on early sites, most of them made from the columella of the conch. Perforated periwinkles also were used but only a few beads small enough to be similar to the wampum of the colonial period have been found, compared with the abundance that later appeared. Large conch shells have been found on certain Neuter [Neutral] sites, especially in Erie and Genesee counties. Now and then a clam shell is found used possibly as a potter's tool. The fresh-water Unio valve was frequently employed for this purpose and they are sometimes found in pits filled with clay scraped in shaping a pot." (Parker, Arthur C. *The Archaeological History of New York*. Part I. New York State Museum Bulletin, Authors Edition #89/200, 1922, pp 108, 110).

Bone artifacts are of highest interest, but even unworked animal bones provide good information. While the following comments apply to one site in New Mexico, the general observations have validity anywhere.

"Unmodified Refuse Food Bones – This class, of course by far the largest, comprises the enormous quantities of animal and bird bones which, picked of their flesh, found their way into the rubbish heaps. Such specimens are of value because they indicate what species were used by the Pecos Indians for food, and in what proportion they depended upon each. The bones of species not indigenous to the region give hints as to travel and hunting expeditions; while those of such animals as were introduced by the Spaniards provide our surest and most abundant evidence for separating prehistoric from historic deposits." (Kidder, Alfred Vincent. "Objects of Bone." *The Artifacts of Pecos*. Robert S. Peabody Foundation for Archaeology, Yale University Press, New Haven, 1932, p 195).

A site on Marco Island, Florida, had much Gulf of Mexico shell, and many pieces were made into tools. The heavy shell was used for anvils, hammers, and gouges, and some had cutout sections where material had probably been removed to make gorgets and pendants. The shell came from the conch and whelk families. (Meyer, Charles D. "Shell Factory?" *Central States Archaeological Journal*. Vol. 32 No. 1, January 1985, pp 21 – 23).

Based on knowledge from prehistoric times, it has long been thought that at least some awls were used for tattooing in the prehistoric era. "The usual method was to pass an awl under the skin and draw through the puncture a thread of sinew covered with charcoal or soot." (Jenness, Diamond. *The Indians of Canada*. Museum of Canada, Bulletin 65, 2nd edition, 1934, p 79).

Only a very few smoking pipes may have been made of antler and bone.

"It is barely possible, but hardly probable, that pipes of bone and horn may sometimes have been used in prehistoric times. These materials are combustible in a limited degree, and the burning tobacco would certainly have had a new flavor in a bone pipe, while the latter would soon have lost form and substance. This difficulty was obviated, at a later day, by lining the bowl with a thin sheet of metal." (Beauchamp, William M. *Horn and Bone Implements of the New York Indians*. Bulletin 50. New York State Museum, 1902, p 288).

Elk or wapiti (*Cervus canadensis*) are massive animals compared to deer, and once roamed most of North America below Hudson's Bay and above Mexico. They can weigh up to one thousand pounds, and both antlers (as much as 25 pounds each in winter prime) and bones are large and heavy. These materials were used by prehistoric Indians for tools and weapons; in some cases, both were probably obtained from dead (not killed) animals. This is because there were always fewer elk to hunt (again compared to deer) and elk were dangerous to attack. At breeding (rutting) time the male animals were very aggressive. Too, elk bones and antlers, due to the size, may have been too large for some uses or they at least required much more work to make them suitable for the usual artifacts. (Hothem, Lar. Various sources).

Bone materials found at the Chucalissa site, Tennessee, included those of black bear, bobcat, mountain lion, and wolf, plus the more usual deer and smaller mammals. Of birds represented, the most common was wild turkey, followed by blue or snow goose and sandhill crane. Representative artifacts were bone splinter awls, antler flakers, antler tips with drilled bases, a chisel-edged tool, drilled bear teeth, and a probable bone fishhook. Turkey bone awls were made from lower leg bones of the birds. (Parmalee, Paul W. "Vertebrate Remains from the Chucalissa Site." *Tennessee Archaeologist*. Tennessee Archaeological Society, Vol. XVI No. 2, Autumn 1960, pp 84 – 90).

In Georgia, the Stalling's Island site contained a range of bone and antler artifacts. These were awls and needles, antler flakers, knife or awl handles, rounded-end bones or punches, arrowpoints, and fishhooks. [Three larger hooks, thought to be for net making, are now known to be Atl-atl hooks]. (Claflin, William H. Jr. *The Stalling's Island Mound, Columbia County, Georgia*. Peabody Museum, Harvard University, Vol. XIV No. 1, Cambridge, 1931, pp 21 – 26).

A comparison has been made about the effectiveness of Iroquois flint and bone arrowpoints.

"Pointed with a head of flint chipped down to a sharp edge, and propelled from a tautly strung bow, such an arrow could easily bring down the deer, the wildfowl, or an enemy. Sometimes the tips were of horn or bone, which, although not so hard as the flint, could be given longer points and were therefore more dangerous." (Palmer, Rose A. "A League of Five Nations: The Iroquois." *The North American Indians*. The Smithsonian Series Volume Four, 1929/1944, p 77).

A rock shelter in Jackson County, Ohio, had a number of artifacts in it, including some of bone. An area in front of the shelter contained so many pieces of bone that it was known to area residents as the "bone yard." (Mills, William C. "Archaeological Remains of Jackson County." *Certain Mounds and Village Sites in Ohio*. Vol. 2 Part 2, Columbus, 1912, p 74).

San Miguel Island, California, had a great variety of bone and shell artifacts.

"...the ancient inhabitants of San Miguel turned to bone rather than to stone for the manufacture of implements, doubtless due in part to the fact that suitable materials for many kinds of stonework are not found on this island. The collection presents a large variety of forms in bone, including among others, beads, pendants, ornamental pins, awls, needles, points for arrows or spears, whistles, and flageolets. Especially worthy of notice are the mortar made of a whale's vertebra; the long pointed bone object, probably a hairpin, to the large end of which a quartz crystal has been attached with asphaltum; the cylindrical box of deerbone, with a shell disc set in one end...". (Hodge, F. W., Editor. "Guide to the Museum, Second Floor." *Indian Notes and Monographs*. Museum of the American Indian, New York, 1922, pp 217, 218).

While many animals were used to make bone artifacts, in the eastern Midwest, bison (buffalo) bones are generally absent before about AD 1500. It is possible that bison gradually appeared after that date in response to prairies being burned for agricultural use, which caused a retreat of forest land. (Struever, Stuart and Felicia Antonelli Holton. *Koster – Americans in Search of Their Prehistoric Past*. Anchor Press/Doubleday, Garden City, New York, 1979, p 155).

Near Lovelock, Nevada, Leonard Rockshelter contained some organic material artifacts. A 1936 find was made of an Atl-atl dart and 30 shell beads; the beads originated on the California coast. In 1937 pieces of wooden Atl-atl foreshafts were found. At the same site, 1950 excavations produced more shell beads and cordage nets. In the early 1950s, Fishbone Cave, Nevada, produced extinct animal bones and netting, matting, and basket pieces. An awl, possibly made from the foot bone of an extinct horse, was recovered. Many of the animal bones had been split and burned. (Wormington, H. M. *Ancient Man in North America*. 4th edition. The Denver Museum of Natural History, Denver, 1957, pp 190 – 192).

A report by an explorer (Sagard) in 1636 recounts an experience with historic Indian fishhooks and the manner in which they were discovered. "We found in the bellies of several large fish hooks made of a piece of wood and a bone, so placed as to form a hook, and very neatly bound together with hemp; but the line being too weak for drawing on board such large fishes, the result was the loss of labor of the fisherman, and of the hooks thrown into the sea by them...". (Willoughby, Charles C. *Antiquities of the New England Indians*. Peabody Museum, Cambridge, 1935, p 218).

Rock shelters in Kentucky are sometimes the source for much organic material.

"Another characteristic of the home of the cliff-dweller is the peculiar type of kitchen-midden. Apparently the easiest way in which to dispose of refuse in a rock shelter was to sweep it over the side of the cliff and as a result the accumulation of debris is found at the base of the cliff directly beneath the shelter. Here it is to be found piled up in a talus [debris slope]. These trash-piles are often very rich in artifacts, probably because it often happened that objects fell over the side of the cliff which were not intended to be thrown away. We have found some of these heaps of refuse so large and so full of bones and other animal matter that the farmers in the neighborhood were hauling it away and spreading it over the fields to enrich the land, a purpose to which it was well adapted." (Webb, William Snyder, and William Delbert Funkhouser. *Ancient Life in Kentucky*. The Kentucky Geological Survey, Frankfort, 1928, p 145).

Bone artifacts can be many colors as a result of their surroundings and other factors. Alaskan bone from permafrost and beaches is sometimes a rich amber color. Bone from ashpits and shell middens can retain much of the original color or may be off-white to ivory to tan. Some bone has shaded to a yellowish-brown, which might be considered a typical color, at least in much of the Midwest. In the Southeast, bone from large springs and clear rivers may be whitish-gray, while staining in slow-moving rivers and in lakes may produce deep brown to black. (Hothem, Lar. Various sources).

An Early Woodland site in Tennessee, excavated in 1954 – 1955, had more than 500 bone specimens. The finds included over 300 awls of wild turkey leg bones, deer cannon bone ends, halves or splinters; awls of raccoon baccula and a bear bacculum; deer cannon bone fishhooks; perforated or grooved bear canines; cut bear and cut deer jaws, one each; pendant made of turkey leg with spur remaining; necklaces of perforated elk teeth; turtle carapace bowl; two carapace spoons; two tubes, large bird bones; antler flakers, three engraved; chisels; antler handles with sockets; two antler projectile points; elk antler comb, engraved; and an engraved antler pin, 10" long. Shell artifacts from marine mollusks were disc and cylindrical beads; and, circular shell gorgets. (Lewis, T. M. N. and Madeline Kneberg. "The Camp Creek Site." *Ten Years of the Tennessee Archaeologist / Selected Subjects*. 1954 – 1963, Vol. XIII No. 1, pp 101, 109 – 115).

In addition to many other artifacts, some 39 workers at the late prehistoric Riker site (Tuscarawas County, Ohio) also recovered antler and bone objects. There were 401 bone beads, 61 bone awls, 365 other bone tools, 18 bone needles, 42 antler points, 2 bone flutes, 8 antler scrapers, and 25 bone beamers. (Vietzen, Raymond C. *The Riker Site*. Sugar Creek Valley Chapter, Archaeological Society of Ohio, 1974, pp 170 – 171).

A Paleo tool in Arctic regions combined the use of burins, microblades, and bone or antler. Burins (small, chisel-like chert pieces) were used to make slots in antler, and long antler sections were then broken away. These were triangular in cross-section. They were then rounded, and broken pieces of microblades (bladelets) were then set in slots along the sides. The final result was a pointed weapon tip with razor-like sides, quite suitable for hunting. (Anderson, Douglas D. "A Stone Age Campsite at the Gateway to America," *Avenues to Antiquity, Readings from Scientific American*. W. H. Freeman and Company, San Francisco, 1976, pp 93 – 96).

Among the uses of deer jawbones were sickles, corn-shellers, and picks. Wear-patterns on existing examples indicate the primary tasks for which they were used. (Editor. *Central States Archaeological Journal*. Vol. 25 No. 1, January 1978, p 19).

In the Northeast, especially in well-drained shell deposits, many artifacts of organic materials survived.

"Bone and antler were extensively used in making many types of implements. These materials occupied an intermediate place between stone and wood. They were fairly easy to work, and were very serviceable. Bone was preferred for most of the smaller objects, antler being reserved for certain types which from their form or size made it preferable, and it was easier to work than bone, especially after being boiled. Leg bones of the deer and moose were commonly used in making the larger bone implements, the metacarpal and metatarsal, commonly called cannon bones, being favorites. The bone was split lengthwise by cutting a deep groove upon opposite sides with sharp flints and breaking it apart. Suitable pieces for making harpoon points, awls, bodkins, etc., were obtained by again grooving and breaking off pieces and cutting and grinding them into the desired shape. Excellent examples of grooved and split bones and antler showing the processes followed are found in most of the larger shellheaps." (Willoughby, Charles C. *Antiquities of the New England Indians*. Peabody Museum, Cambridge, 1935, p 214).

While surviving Paleo artifacts are almost always made of chipped cryptocrystalline materials, a few were made of bone. "Bone dart points were made from Clovis times to historic times. Clovis-period bone points are large, rounded, and bipointed. They are made of solid bone, presumably from large animals." (Perino, Gregory. *Selected Preforms, Points and Knives of the North American Indians*. Vol. I. Points and Barbs Press, 1985, p 41).

Toggle-head harpoon tips are well known from the Arctic, but they have also been found in much of the northern U. S. and Canada. Wisconsin has produced a number of examples made from deer antler. Toggle heads have a hole about mid-length, and a hollowed base to receive the end of a shaft. One part of the base edge has a protrusion that serves as a barb. These harpoon types are from the Middle Woodland, although other types date to the Middle Archaic, ca. 3500 BC. (Mason, Ronald J. "Wisconsin Middle Woodland Toggle Head Harpoons." *The Michigan Archaeologist*. Vol. 11 Nos. 3 – 4, Sept – Dec 1965, pp 156 – 158).

Very little has been published about true daggers made of bone, but there is some coverage of specimens found in Canada.

"Daggers are made from the large leg bones of the deer, etc., and are similar to the larger awls or piercers, but are very much larger and heavier at the butt. One 10½" long, 1 inch wide, and of a triangular cross-section tapering gradually to a point, and well-polished, has a pattern of incised lines on one side not unlike some pottery markings, which covers a space of about 5½" in length. Other daggers are plain. The proximal end, ending in the point of the bone, makes a convenient knob." (Laidlaw, Col. G. E. "Archaeological Notes on Victoria County, Ont." *The Archaeological Bulletin*. Vol. 8 No. 5, 1915, p 9).

There are time and regional differences in the basic form of antler Atl-atl hooks. The basic sequence of Atl-atl hook styles was not well understood until David Lutz, after many years of research, identified and named each of its major types as they passed through time. The identifying traits are briefly listed here; each listing includes a major site where the type was found and which provided the type name in the first three cases. This time progression is from early to late. Eva (Tennessee, c. 4800 – 3800) is short and has a small projecting tip that seats the lance base. The Black Earth (Illinois, c. 3800 – 3200 BC) hook is longer, with a knobbed end and a raised hook tip. The Indian Knoll hook (Kentucky, c. 3200 – 2000 BC) is long, slender, and tapered. Slotted hooks (Terminal Archaic into Early Woodland) have a base that is slotted to receive the Atl-atl shaft. (Lutz, David L. *The Archaic Bannerstone: Its Chronological History and Purpose From 6000 B. C. to 1000 B. C.* 2000, pp 44, 45, 47 – 49).

The Ripley site, New York state, contained scrapers made of deer jaws, and their typical use is explained:

"It is perhaps not customary to rank deer jaws as implements. Nevertheless, the Seneca up to within the last ten years have used them when they could obtain them, for scraping corn from the green cob. The sharp teeth were raked over the kernals to break and cut the hulls and then the hold on the jaw changed and the milk and meat scraped out with the sharp edge that is nearest the chin." (Parker, Arthur C. *The Archaeological History of New York*. Part I. New York State Museum Bulletin, Author's Edition #89/200, 1922, pp 108, 110).

Facts about Artifacts

The Stalling's Island site in Georgia contained nearly 500 bone artifacts in all states of manufacture, and materials most frequently used were deer leg bones and antlers. The method of obtaining pieces of antler was a groove sawed around the antler prong, done anywhere from the base to 2" from the base. The groove was deepened until the hard outside of the antler was cut through and the softer interior was reached. This lessened the possibility of splitting, and the section was then broken off. "In some cases the final cutting was evidently done with a small chisel-shaped object, the marks of such a tool existing on the hard covering of the antler just outside the pithy center and extending into the pithy core." (Claflin, William H. Jr. *The Stalling's Island Mound, Columbia County, Georgia*. Peabody Museum, Harvard University, Vol. XIV No. 1, Cambridge, 1931, pp 21 – 22).

Whalebone sword-like clubs with knobbed effigy handles and expanded and rounded blades were made along the British Columbia coast. Examples were from 19 to 24" long. "A general type of paddle-shaped club with carved handle knob is found on the north Pacific coast of America, from Alaska to Columbia river, but chiefly on western Vancouver island where the type is most uniform." (Smith, Harlan I. *An Album of Prehistoric Canadian Art*. Victoria Memorial Museum Bulletin No. 37, June 1, 1923, Ottawa, pp 62, 63, 68).

Bone was of major importance to the Iroquois in what is now New York state. "Their weapons were simple at first. An ungrooved stone ax, a long bow and arrows, defensive armor including a shield at times, a club with bone or stone inserted at the head, a knife of stone or bone and afterward of steel, furnished all that was needed in war. Nets and bone harpoons were used in fishing, and more rarely lines with bone hooks. Weirs and hurdles were also employed, but in shallow waters spearing was the favorite mode. Arrows were tipped bone, iron, or stone, and the use of metal changed the material but not the form." (Beauchamp, William M. *A. History of the New York Iroquois*. New York State Museum, Bulletin 78, 1905, p 140).

Shell hoes are commonly found on Mississippian sites, and some turned up at the Cahokia Mound Group in Illinois. "Shell Hoes – These pieces are made from the large, heavy-ribbed mussel shells known locally as washboard shells. Fragments of the hoes are more or less common on the village sites, and there are eight fairly complete specimens in this series. Of these, seven were found together in a refuse pit, and the eighth was found in the loose dirt scattered from the Powell Mound.

"Each is perforated by an irregular, circular hole in the body near the larger end, varying from 5⁄8" to 1" in diameter, and also has a shallow notch near the hinge. The largest piece is 5⅞" long and 4" wide, and the smallest is 3⅝" by 3¾"." (Titterington, P. F. *The Cahokia Mound Group and Its Village Site Materials*. St. Louis, 1938, p 9).

Aricara (late prehistoric) sites in South Dakota have produced an unusual knife form. Set in the end side of a long bone handle, the blades were made of kettle brass or chipped from flint. The blades themselves were rectangular or elongated, with one cutting edge and one edge inset in a handle slot. The middens also produced other bone artifacts including serrated points, awls, and well-made fishhooks. (Editor. *Artifacts*. Vol. 14 No. 1, 1984, p 12).

Dentalia shells, on the northern Pacific Coast, were valued both for decoration and as money. The following quotation is from a 1903 publication written by Goddard: "The individual shells are measured and their value determined by the creases on the left hand. The longest known shells were about 2½" long. One of them would reach from the crease of the last joint of the little finger to the crease on the palm opposite the knuckle joint of the same finger. The value of such a piece in early days was about $5. Shells of this length were called *dinket*. The next smaller shells were called *kiketukutxoi*, and measured about 2⅜" They were worth about $1.50 each. A shell about 1⅛" long was called *tcwolahit*. Their value was from 25 to 50 cents. Shells smaller than these were not rated as money and had no decoration." (Hodge, Frederick Webb. "Media of Exchange." *Handbook of American Indians*. Part 1. Bureau of American Ethnology Bulletin 30, 1907, pp 446, 447).

One does not usually think of Indian artifacts from New York City, but the historic Siwanoy once lived in what is now the Bronx. "The implements are of the general Algonkian type. Many bone awls were found, also arrowpoints and flakers made of antler. Pendants made of animal teeth and a shell bead were to be expected, but the presence of two cups made of shell is unusual...". (Hodge, F. W., Editor. "Guide to the Museum / Second Floor." *Indian Notes and Monographs*. Museum of the American Indian, New York, 1922, pp 118, 119).

Harpoons in North America (except in the Far North) are more scarce than are barbed projectile points, and they are generally found more in some regions than in others.

"It is not difficult to explain the preponderance of harpoons in the North and the scarcity of them in the South. They are essentially a cold-climate implement. In the St. Lawrence region, where they abound, nets and traps cannot be used save during summer and fall. The winter sets in early and the spring is late. While fish were harpooned when on the spawning-beds, yet most of the harpooning was done in the winter." (Moorehead, Warren K. *The Stone Age in North America*. Vol. II. Houghton Mifflin Company, Cambridge, 1910, pp 137 – 138).

Rare fishhooks not constructed of bone have been encountered in the eastern Midwest. "Fish hooks made from the teeth of deer or elk are found occasionally, and in a fair state of preservation. These are very carefully worked and show much ingenuity." (Webb, William Snyder, and William Delbert Funkhouser. *Ancient Life in Kentucky*. The Kentucky Geological Survey, Frankfort, 1928, p 189).

The Southwestern U. S. is noted for both quality and quantity of bone artifacts.

"In the Southwest, bone tool-making became a fine art in prehistoric times. The prehistoric inhabitants used the bones of birds, rodents, and mammals for artifacts. In many cases it is not possible to identify the animal from which the tool was made because working and polishing have removed the distinguishing characteristics. In the Southwest, prehistoric peoples used bone to manufacture workday implements, musical instruments, ornaments, charms, and ceremonial objects. Next to stone, bone is one of the most durable substances known." (Britt, Claude Jr. "Colorado Bone Tools." *The Redskin*. The Genuine Indian Relic Society, Vol. X No. 3, 1975, pp 86, 87).

In the interior of Canada's British Columbia, elaborate and artistic objects were made of bone and antler. Such objects were decorated gambling bones, sap-scrapers of antler, decorated bone head-scratchers or hairpins, antler digging stick handles with one large hole, carved animal heads, antler dog harness toggles, and carved elk tooth pendants. (Smith, Harlan I. *An Album of Prehistoric Canadian Art*. Victoria Memorial Museum Bulletin No. 37, June 1, 1923, Ottawa, pp 85 – 95).

Bone so-called rasps or sounding-sticks are sometimes found, and those from Pecos, New Mexico, might be considered typical.

"These are of two sorts: deer-scapulae; and long, narrow bones such as the ribs and leg bones of large animals. Both kinds are provided with deep, close-set notches so cut into them that a stick or another bone rubbed along the series of indentations produces a resonant, rattling sound much like that made by drawing a stick across the palings of a wooden fence. (...) In each case the notches are greatly abraded by the friction of the rasping stick, and there is little doubt that the specimens served as rattles rather than as tally bones." (Kidder, Alfred Vincent. "Objects of Bone." *The Artifacts of Pecos*. Robert S. Peabody Foundation for Archaeology, Yale University Press, New Haven, 1932, p 252).

Many aboriginal groups used ornaments of organic materials in historic times. "Hunting peoples naturally tend to adorn themselves with trophies of the chase. The Eskimo attached bear teeth and bear claws to their clothing, several Indian tribes wore bear-claw necklaces, and some Pacific Coast natives used bear-claw headdresses on ceremonial occasions. The Slaves and Dogribs of the Mackenzie basin delighted in headbands of leather embroidered with porcupine quills, and embellished with animal claws and the white skins of the ermine. The plains' Indians wore bracelets of antelope teeth, the Carrier of northern British Columbia attached the claws and teeth of both the caribou and the beaver to their clothing, and wore necklaces of split and dyed antler, while their neighbors, the Tsimshian, and other coastal tribes, sewed fringes of jingling caribou claws or puffin bills to their dancing aprons." (Jenness, Diamond. *The Indians of Canada*. Museum of Canada, Bulletin 65, 2nd edition, 1934, pp 77, 78).

Flint chips with saw-tooth edges are found in a limited region of eastcentral Arizona and westcentral New Mexico. From Mogollon sites dating c. AD 1000 – 1350, the saws "...were most likely used in the manufacture of highly polished bone rings, almost invariably found on the same sites." (Britt, Claude Jr. "Flint 'Saws' From New Mexico." *The Redskin*. Genuine Indian Relic Society, Vol. V No. 1, January 1970, pp 22, 23).

Heat and exposure to air (or at least removal from the original site) seem to have an effect on bone artifacts, as exemplified by a bone awl 3⅝" long. "It is broad near the center, regularly tapering to a sharp point at one end, and to a narrow rounded base at the other. It is nearly flat, but with rounded edges. Its polished surface has been beautifully mottled by fire, making it very attractive in appearance. A recent inspection showed that in two years [since the finding] its rich hues had greatly faded from exposure." (Beauchamp, William M. *Horn and Bone Implements of the New York Indians*. Bulletin 50. New York State Museum, 1902, p 262, plate 2 figure 19).

Four terms are sometimes used to describe artifacts made of organic materials, especially bone and ivory, sometimes antler. The terms are petrified, fossilized, mineralized, and preserved. Something petrified has had its structure replaced (all or part) with dissolved minerals to become stone-like. An example is petrified trees. Fossils are traces or parts of something from a former geological age, like dinosaur bones. Something mineralized has been impregnated or supplied with minerals (inorganic materials). The basic structure has been added to, but has not been replaced. Some artifacts are in this category, and examples are "fossilized" ivory from Alaska and other northern regions. Preserved objects are those that were somehow prevented from decaying, like animal bones in California's tar pits or surviving organic material artifacts from many locations including the bones of ice-age mammals. Technicalities and word definitions aside, in North America it is not that uncommon for artifacts to be made from petrified and fossilized materials. Some artifacts have been made from mineralized material, or if old enough and under certain conditions they might themselves have become mineralized to some extent. Any early artifact that normally would not last long but that now exists is preserved, though the word preservation might imply some chemical treatment to prevent any further deterioration. (Hothem, Lar. Various sources).

Reed Fort, a pottery-producing site in New York state, contained many artifacts of organic materials. Approximately one-third of the artifacts known to have probably been found are listed here: Pointed bone awls, 384; blunt point awls, 72; bone punches, 56; bone arrow points, 6; bone fishhooks, 26; bone harpoons, 9; bone beads, 708; pierced bone pieces, 28; whole or partial bone combs, 7; bone needles, 24; bone draw shaves [beamers], 9; bone ceremonial object, 1; worked deer antler, 63; hairpins, 3; tally bones, 2; perforated bear teeth, 62; unperforated bear teeth, 44; perforated elk teeth, 29; unperforated elk teeth, 7; and moose, wolf, and dog teeth, 43. (Parker, Arthur C. *The Archaeological History of New York*. Part I. New York State Museum Bulletin, Author's Edition #89/200, 1922, pp 203, 204).

Tennessee has long been noted for the many shell artifacts made and used there in prehistoric times.

"Of the marine shells, the Busycon perversum, or conch, is found in the greatest numbers. Thousands of them must have been used in manufacturing the various utensils, ornaments, and implements discovered. The interior columns were utilized in making pins, beads, and other articles; the outside remaining shells formed useful and convenient vessels and cups. The cassis, the strombus, the oliva, and other univalves were also used. The main supplies, however, came from the more convenient unio, or mussel shells of the rivers. They were pounded into powder to temper the fine clays in the manufacture of pottery. They were utilized as spoons, forks, paint cups, knives, and mechanical and gardening tools. Thousands of them were cut into beads and ornaments." (Thruston, Gates P. *The Antiquities of Tennessee*. Robert Clarke & Co., Cincinnati, 1890, p 310).

Artifact Finds

Far fewer antler, bone, and shell artifacts (compared with flint and stone artifacts) are found on the average surface hunt. This is largely because the soil in agricultural areas has been churned for many years, breaking the objects and permitting access to water. This, combined with acidic soils, has largely destroyed anything made of organic materials. Under optimal conditions, antler and bone can survive for thousands of years. Under poor conditions, they can last less than a century.

This chapter contains accounts of artifacts that have managed to survive in some way. They give us at least an idea of the great wealth of tools, weapons, and ornaments that enriched life in North America long ago.

At the Abbott Farm site in New Jersey (Middle Woodland period) bone and antler artifacts were found. These were splinter awls, a needle, cylindrical antler flakers or drifts, punches or flakers, pins, and chisels. Artifacts with points were shaped or sharpened on stone. (Cross, Dorothy. "The Abbott Farm Site: Middle Woodland Summary." *Foundations of Pennsylvania Prehistory*. Harrisburg, Pennsylvania, 1971, pp 324, 326).

Bone artifacts were found at Key Marco, Florida, some of them made of atypical material. Points were made of stingray spines and woodworking tools were fashioned from barracuda jaws. Shark teeth provided the cutting edge for tools and weapons. Sawfish teeth were also mounted for tool use. (Gilliland, Marion Spjut. *The Material Culture of Key Marco, Florida*. The University Presses of Florida, Gainesville, 1975, pp 205 – 207).

Finely styled and highly engraved bone hairpins from the Southeast were made of deer metapodials. Found in prehistoric middens or refuse deposits, the pins generally have one pointed end and one thick end, with the wider portion covered with geometric designs. The pins are up to 8" long. (Peck, Rodney. "The Ogeechee River Bone Pins." *Prehistoric Artifacts*. Genuine Indian Relic Society, Vol. XX No. 1, 1986, p 5).

The Dallas component at Hiwassee Island, Tennessee, had musical or rhythmic instruments made from box turtle shells. The tops and bottoms were drilled to tie the rattles together, and they contained either pebbles or the teeth of drumfish. (Lewis, Thomas M. N. and Madeline Kneberg. *Hiwassee Island – An Archaeological Account of Four Tennessee Indian Peoples*. The University of Tennessee Press, 1946, Knoxville, pp 126, 127).

A mound in Pennsylvania near McKees Rock contained many Early Woodland bone tools. These were long antler flakers, awls made from cannon and scapula bones, and gouges. The 1896 excavations also resulted in finding conch tubular beads, disc beads, and freshwater pearl beads. (Mayer-Oakes, William J. *Prehistory of the Upper Ohio Valley*. Annals of Carnegie Museum Vol. 34, Pittsburgh, 1955, pp 130, 146, 149).

Among the bone artifacts from the Feurt site in Scioto County, Ohio, were large gouges and chisels, some nearly 6" long. A probably unique artifact was a chipping rod made from a mountain lion leg bone. (Editor. *Ohio Archaeologist*. Vol. 10 No. 4, October 1960, p 122).

Two kinds of bone needles were found in a Kentucky overhang shelter. One was the conventional kind with an eye at the wider end. Another form was made of hollow bird bone with an eye at the joint and with a bevel-sharpened tip. The sewing cord ran through the hollow center (actually being enclosed) and emerged at the needle tip. (Vietzen, Col. Raymond C. *The Saga of Glover's Cave*. Wahoo, Nebraska, 1956, p 38).

One of the largest shell gorgets recovered came from Trigg County, Kentucky. Incised with a stylized rattlesnake design, the gorget had two suspension holes. Its greatest diameter was 7¼". (Young, Col. Bennett H. *The Prehistoric Men of Kentucky*. Filson Club Presentations No. 25, Louisville, 1920, pp 238, 241).

A highly unusual artifact was used at Key Marco, Florida, cut from turtle plastrons. Rectangular in shape, many were worked so that the natural shell divisions separated the shells into six sections. These may have been used as game counters or playing pieces. Apparently they were made in uniformly different sizes. (Gilliland, Marion Spjut. *The Material Culture of Key Marco, Florida*. The University Presses of Florida, Gainesville, 1975, pp 205 – 207).

A one-of-a-kind artifact came from the Middle Woodland period in Illinois. This was a bear canine tooth, hollowed to serve as a knife sheath. A tiny handled knife, of bone or tooth, fit into the sheath. (Throop, Addison J. *Mound Builders of Illinois*. East St. Louis, 1928, p 52).

Beamers or skin-scraping tools at a Fort Ancient village site were usually made of deer bones. However, and surprisingly, many beamers were made from bison (buffalo) bones. (Bison apparently came into the region in late prehistoric times.) Such beamers or drawshaves were large, from 11 to 16" long. A few beamers of elk bone were found, plus one made from the femur of a mountain lion. (Hooton, Earnest A. *Indian Village Site and Cemetery Near Madisonville, Ohio*. Peabody Museum, Vol. VIII No. 1, Cambridge, 1920, p 53).

A cave or rock shelter in Wisconsin contained pictographs and a few artifacts, one of them a large bone tool.

"In the third [sand and ash layer], more elaborately wrought pottery, the newest kind found in mounds; with numerous fragments and whole sides of Mississippi river bivalve shells, and a bodkin of bone, 7" long. This, according to the opinion of old hunters, was of the 'hock-bone' of an elk. It was in dry, white sand and is quite sharp and smooth with use, and in a perfect state of preservation, even retaining the glassy polish of wear and handling, as if used yesterday." (Brown, Rev. Edward. "The Pictured Cave of La Crosse Valley, Near West Salem, Wisconsin." *The American Antiquarian*. Vol. II No. 4, April – June 1880, pp 258, 259).

A mix of bird and animal bones provided artifacts on Late Mississippian sites in Tennessee. In addition to shell ear-pins, spoons and beads, there were bone combs, projectile points, fishhooks, pins, perforators, chisels, and a spearpoint [or dagger] with a side fastening hole. Animal teeth included a wolf-tooth pendant and a beaver incisor perhaps used as a chisel blade. (Chapman, Jefferson. *Tellico Archaeology*. The University of Tennessee Publications in Anthropology No. 41 / TVA, 1985, p 88).

A notched point with a turkey bone handle found in Monroe County, Kentucky, may have been secured in a special way. Notches on the handle end may have anchored rawhide cords, which when dried would have pulled the blade tightly into the handle. (Wagers, Charles. "Hafting Techniques." *Prehistoric American*. Genuine Indian Relic Society, Vol. XXVI No. 1, 1992, p 12).

Portions of deteriorated bone from Wyoming's Colby site (Paleolithic) were possible tools. One object was probably made from a deer or mountain sheep. (Frison, George C. and Lawrence C. Todd. *The Colby Mammoth Site*. University of New Mexico Press, Albuquerque, 1986, pp 100 – 103).

The Reckner pottery-bearing site, near Confluence, Pennsylvania, had numerous bone artifacts: Beads of bird bones, 52; bone awls, 13; unfinished fishhook, 1; large bones that may have been used as tobacco pipes, 2; pressure flakers, 2; bone pin, 1; drilled bear tooth pendant, 1; cut and polished bear teeth, 3; drilled elk tooth pendant, 1; perforated needle (bird bone), 1; and, black shell effigy of a bear tooth, 1. (Augustine, Edgar E. "Recent Discoveries in Somerset County." *The Pennsylvania Archaeologist*. 1938/1987, Vol. 8 No. 1, pp 6, 8).

A fine, long bone hairpin came from San Miguel Island, California. Tapered and polished, the thicker end was grooved "...to hold the cords by which feathers and shell ornaments were attached." The artifact was 9½" long. (Moorehead, Warren K. *Prehistoric Implements*. Robert Clarke Co., Cincinnati, 1900, p 236).

Bone tools and other objects were found at McNeeley Lake Cave or rock shelter, Jefferson County, Kentucky. Late Archaic into Fort Ancient, the artifacts included awls, projectile points, flakers, and a whistle. There were in addition 4066 pieces of bone or antler, and 117 pieces of shell. (Hockensmith, Charles D., et al. *Paleoindian and Archaic Research in Kentucky*. Kentucky Heritage Council, 1988, pp 180, 187, 189).

The historic period Sarf cache was a buried container made of two top-to-top brass kettles. This doubled container held a leather pouch with 16,967 glass and shell beads, six brass tube beads, and 24 shell artifacts. From the Wyoming Valley, Pennsylvania, the cache was discovered in 1964 when topsoil was being removed. There were 6667 purple shell beads and 5475 white shell beads. The shell artifacts were carved bird and animal figures and runtees. (Kent, Barry C. "An Unusual Cache From the Wyoming Valley, Pennsylvania." *American Antiquity*. Society for American Archaeology, Vol. 35 No. 2, April 1970, pp 185 – 192).

Several rare tools made of walrus tusks were found near Brewerton, New York. "It is curved, angular, and has been ground to a broad point at one end. The actual dimensions are 16" of length and 1½" of thickness, being nearly as wide throughout as at the thickest part. With it were found large bones and other relics, and a gouge of walrus tusk broken in two." (Beauchamp, William M. *Horn and Bone Implements of the New York Indians*. Bulletin 50. New York State Museum, 1902, p 288).

Arrowpoints in some cases existed in both antler and flint at the same time. A Kentucky overhang shelter produced a bow and a quiver with 19 arrowpoints. There were 13 points made of antler and six of flint. (Vietzen, Col. Raymond C. *The Saga of Glover's Cave*. Wahoo, Nebraska, 1956, pp 42, 46).

Two unusual artifacts were found near Pelican Rapids, Minnesota. A conch shell with two holes was picked up, and an elk antler knife 8 to 9" long was also present. They came from what had once been a glacial lake. (Wormington, H. M. *Ancient Man in North America*. 4th edition. The Denver Museum of Natural History, Denver, 1957, pp 232, 233).

The Watson site in West Virginia (Middle Woodland) had some bone artifacts. A 1939 excavation uncovered 30 splinter bone awls and broken bowls made of freshwater turtle shells. A 1953 exploration contributed another five bone splinter awls. (Dragoo, Don W. "The Watson Site, Hancock County, West Virginia." *Foundation of Pennsylvania Prehistory*. Harrisburg, Pennsylvania, 1971, pp 287, 314).

A grooved needle with cord still attached provided a glimpse into how bone awls or needles were actually used in prehistoric times. Discovered in a Rowan County rock shelter in Kentucky, the cord was twisted and probably made of plant fiber. (Editor. *Artifacts*. Vol. 9 No. 4, 1979, p 102).

Bone, antler, and horn artifacts came from Ventana Cave, southern Arizona, during excavations from 1940 to 1942. Bone items were 111 awls, 17 flakers, 1 flesher, 3 scrapers, 2 spoons, 9 tubes (both bird and mammal), 1 gaming(?) die, 1 painted bone, 4 rodent jaws with cord wraps, and 1 perforated bone. Horn items were 4 artifacts that may have been awl handles, 5 hammers, 31 flakers, 6 spoons, and 1 spatula. (Haury, Emil W. *The Stratigraphy and Archaeology of Ventana Cave*. The University of Arizona Press, 1950 / 1975, pp 374 – 390).

The handle for a knife found in Catlow Cave, Oregon, narrow and with medium curve, was made of mountain sheep horn. It was hollowed at the end to receive a knife blade. Two other knife handles found were made of wood. (Aikens, C. Melvin. *Archaeology of Oregon*. U. S. Department of the Interior, Bureau of Land Management, Oregon State Office, 1984, p 18).

One of the finest bone artifacts from Archaic times was found at Kentucky's Indian Knoll site. Probably a hairpin, it was 10⅜" long, decorated with undulating narrow grooves, and had a small perforation near the wide end. In overall shape it was like a large awl with a tapered tip. (Moore, Clarence B. "Some Aboriginal Sites on Green River, Kentucky." Reprinted from *Journal of The Academy of Natural Sciences of Philadelphia*. Vol. XVI, 1916, p 452).

The Casas Grandes ruins, in northern Mexico, had some caches of probable trade goods inside pottery vessels. One vessel, in the form of a fish, contained 12 obsidian points, 5 bracelets made of shell, 182 shell beads, 9 bone beads, 5 coral beads, and a small crushed copper bell. (Britt, Claude Jr. "A Fish Effigy Cache Pot." *The Redskin*. Genuine Indian Relic Society, Vol. VI No. 1, 1971, pp 10, 11).

In the Woodland period, Kipp Island artifacts included large antler harpoons with barbs on only one side. Examples ranged from 6 to 12" in length. (Ritchie, William A. *The Archaeology of New York State*. American Museum of Natural History, Garden City, 1965, p 244).

California, probably due to the availability of bones from sea mammals, has produced some very large tools or weapons. "Bone knives and daggers are not uncommon. They are from 4 to 18" in length and among the finest specimens of the kind ever brought to light." (Moorehead, Warren K. *Prehistoric Implements*. Robert Clarke Co., Cincinnati, 1900, p 271).

Rock shelters are known for preserving normally perishable materials, and an account of a long ago excavation is of interest.

"The whole of this material [ashes and dirt] was filled with evidences of the occupancy of the place as a human residence – pottery, bones, shells, and stone implements. In the deposit of these there was no sudden transition; the bones near the top were in a good state of preservation, those that had not been changed by the fire not blackened but colored yellow by the lapse of time. This became darker and less abundant as the excavation was carried deeper, and substantially disappeared before the bottom of the excavation was reached, showing that the earliest occupancy was so long ago that the deposited bones in the dry shelter had been consumed by time." (Read, M. C. "Exploration of a Rocky Shelter in Boston, Summit County, Ohio." *The American Antiquarian*. Vol. II No. 2, October – December 1879, pp 203, 204).

Found in Ontario County, New York, a fine antler comb was just over 5½" long. Two human effigy figures were at the top, and the comb had 21 long, narrow teeth. (Vietzen, Col. Raymond C. *Sittin' On a Stump*. 1968, p 120).

A site in Morton County, North Dakota, held some extraordinary bone artifacts. Triangular side-notched bone knives were as long as 8½", and a single-barb Mandan harpoon was 5" long. Of four bone knife handles, three had blades (two were made of copper) set in the side of one handle end. (Editor. "The Boley Site Artifacts." *Prehistoric American*. Genuine Indian Relic Society, Vol. XXX No. 1, 1996, pp 6, 7).

Though broken along the shaft, an effigy (deer head?) bone hairpin was found in Calloway County, Missouri. Taken from a refuse pit located on a terrace, the pin was 2½" long. (Editor. *Central States Archaeological Journal*. Vol. 15 No. 3, July 1968, p 116).

Site 23PL43 in Missouri contained a Hopewell deer antler tool, probably used for making roulette designs on pottery. The artifact had the larger antler end slightly rounded and the edge notched in a regular pattern. (Chapman, Carl H., Editor. *Missouri Archaeological Society Research Series*. Number 5, December 1967, Columbia, pp 74, 75).

A highly different bone artifact came from a cave in Hardin County, Kentucky. About 5¾" long, it was a torch holder made from a bear bone. (Editor. *Prehistoric Artifacts*. Genuine Indian Relic Society, Vol. XXIII No. 1, 1989, p 28).

In historic times [and with White-supplied blades], Indian-made knife handles were common. Broad dagger or stabber blades often had bone or horn handles. One knife example was 13" long overall. (Feder, Norman. *Art of the Eastern Plains Indians*. The Brooklyn Museum, 1964, pp 53, 56).

Adena bone combs (Early Woodland, eastern Midwest) were made in a special way and may have had specific uses. "These combs are well made, deeply carved from sections of very heavy animal bone. To obtain greater breadth, two bone sections were very exactly fitted together edge to edge and parallel. They seem to have been bound together in this position. The purpose of these bone combs is not certain. The study of certain textiles may indicate that bear's wool was spun into thread. It has been suggested that these combs may have been carding tools used in the preparation of textiles." (Webb, William S. and Charles E. Snow. *The Adena People*. The University of Kentucky, 1945/1988, pp 96, 97).

Perhaps the most unusual find of antler artifacts in the Northeast was the discovery of Iroquoian pipes in Pennsylvania at the Washington Borough site. There, "One very fine finished antler pipe and two in preparation..." were found. (Cadzow, Donald A. *Safe Harbor Report No. 2*. Publications of Pennsylvania Historic Commission, Vol. III, Harrisburg, 1936, pp 148, 149).

At the well-known Pecos site, New Mexico, a cache of small shell beads was uncovered. "The largest single find of Olivellas was made in Kiva XVI, a chamber dating from post-Columbian times, where, in a subfloor cist or repository, was a large waterworn stone of peculiar shape, about which had been wound many times a string of nearly one thousand shells measuring thirty-eight feet in length." (Kidder, Alfred Vincent. "Objects of Shell." *The Artifacts of Pecos*. Robert S. Peabody Foundation for Archaeology, Yale University Press, New Haven, 1932, pp 185 – 186).

A very large early bone artifact was found over half a century ago. It was made from a mammoth or mastodon fibula [outer and smaller hind leg bone] and was 17" long. One end was worked to a point. A farmer in Manitoba, Canada plowed up the tool. (Wormington, H. M. *Ancient Man in North America*. 4th edition. The Denver Museum of Natural History, Denver, Colorado, 1957, pp 99 – 100).

Some very distinctive bone artifacts came from a New York state site. Antler sockets may have held stone celts for insertion into a wood handle, while a bear jawbone 7" long, was a knife or scraper. A bone tool handle and an antler chisel were both polished to a glossy finish. Most interesting was a ladle made from the skull of a deer. (Ritchie, William A. *A Prehistoric Fortified Village Site at Canandaigua, Ontario County, New York*. Rochester Museum of Arts and Sciences, 1936, pp 46, 47, plate X).

Two bone artifacts were found in dry caves or rock shelters in Kentucky. An engraved Archaic pendant, 4½" long (Todd County), and a carved and engraved harpoon, also 4½" long (Logan County). (Editor. *Central States Archaeological Journal*. Vol. 13 No. 2, April 1966, p 57).

Antler and bone drifts or flakers were widely used in prehistoric America. "The shaping of stone by fracture processes is one of the earliest as well as one of the most important arts of primitive men. Two distinct classes of processes, as well as two widely differing classes of implements, are employed. Fracture by percussion is accomplished by means of hammers of stone or other hard material [like elk antler], and fracture by pressure employs a number of devices, perhaps the most usual among the northern tribes being bits of hard bone, antler, or ivory, somewhat resembling an awl in shape and often set in handles of wood or other suitable material." (Hodge, Frederick Webb. "Flaking Implements." *Handbook of American Indians*. Part 1. Bureau of American Ethnology Bulletin 30, 1907, p 465).

During the construction of a pond in 1977, the bones of a mastodon were uncovered in Washington state. One of the skeletal parts had a bone projectile point embedded, and there was other evidence that the mastodon had been butchered. Carbon 14 dating of nearby peat placed the age of the find at 9000 BC to 12,000 BC. Most North American finds of large bones from Paleo times involve mammoths, not mastodons. (Oppenheimer, Betty. "Donation Preserves 'Manis Mastodon' Site." *The Sequim Gazette*. August 7, 2002, Washington, pp A-1, A-4).

One method of mass-producing bone beads was indicated by a specimen found on a Fort Ancient (Mississippian period) site in Mason County, Kentucky. A long bone was deeply grooved at regular intervals around the circumference, and the sections were then broken apart. (Editor. *Artifacts*. Vol. 9 No. 1, 1979, p 8).

The find circumstances for a superb bone artifact are quite unusual. From Massachusetts, this was a moose-bone harpoon, about 11¾" long, pointed at each end and with a row of barbs down one side. "This interesting specimen, showing fine workmanship, was drawn up with the anchor of a fishing vessel at the mouth of Vinalhaven harbor in 1888...". (Willoughby, Charles C. *Antiquities of the New England Indians*. Peabody Museum, Cambridge, 1935, pp 214, 215).

Hines Cave in Kentucky, first explored in 1922, contained many normally perishable items. "A few of the artifacts represented rare and valuable types. Among these was a remarkable pendant of bone, most artistically fashioned and highly polished with the hole drilled horizontally through a flat projection at the top." (Webb, William Snyder, and William Delbert Funkhouser. *Ancient Life in Kentucky*. The Kentucky Geological Survey, Frankfort, 1928, p 133).

Late Woodland people in some areas of Missouri made extensive use of bone for artifacts. Numerous polished bone tools, some having an awl-like and others a spatula-like appearance, were found in the deposits left by these people. Certain shapes and polish suggest the use of bone as weaving tools...". (Marshall, Richard A. *Prehistoric Indians at Maramec Spring Park*. University of Missouri, 1966, p 17).

A very long, two-hole, bone gorget was found in Spencer County, Indiana. Round-ended, it was smoothly shaped and 9" in length. (Editor. *Central States Archaeological Journal*. Vol. 44 No. 3, July 1997, p 143).

Shell was frequently used for ornaments on the West Coast of the United States. "In California, some of the showiest primitive jewelry artifacts occur in great numbers in varied and often quaint shapes made from iridescent abalone shells. In their pristine form, they must have been colorful in the extreme. Much fewer but equally artistic as jewelry are carved shells, some of which are found in the Southwest and some among the mounds of the East." (Miles, Charles. *Indian and Eskimo Artifacts of North America*. Bonanza Books, 1963, p 135).

Many bone fishhooks were found on a Late Archaic site in Clark County, Indiana. Dating to about 2500 BC, the hooks were U-shaped, rounded, or squared. Most were either knobbed or had a small extension at the shaft top for line attachment. Only a few complete hooks were found, while large numbers were apparently broken in use. (Matthews, James J. "Remains of a Shell Mounder's Fishing Tackle." *Artifacts*. Vol. 9 No. 4, 1979, p 99).

Some of the largest fishhooks in North America apparently were made in Canada. "Several completed hooks have been found in ashbeds, also some incompleted ones. These fishhooks are up to 5½" long, 1 inch across bend, and length of barb up to 1½". The shank has a knob at end to attach the line to." (Laidlaw, Col. G. E. "Archaeological Notes on Victoria County, Ont." *The Archaeological Bulletin*. Vol. 9 No. 5, 1915, p 9).

Conch shell was the material used for a Mississippian gorget with two small suspension holes, found in Gordon County, Georgia. It had a stylized rattlesnake design, and the gorget was 4¾" wide and 4¼" high. (Editor. *Central States Archaeological Journal*. Vol. 35 No. 4, October 1988, p 229).

Found with an effigy pot in Hickman County, Kentucky, a flat bone tool may have been used to shape the features. The tool was long and tapered, with the small end rounded. (Editor. *Prehistoric American*. Vol. XXXVI No. 4, 2002, p 19).

Bone artifacts from a river in Ontario, Canada, included an awl 7⅜" long. There were also harpoon heads with three, five, and seven barbs respectively; smaller awls; and a hammer made of elk antler. (McLeod, Edward. "Underwater Finds." *The Redskin*. Genuine Indian Relic Society, Vol. VII No. 3, 1972, pp 94, 95).

Bone flakers have been found in many shell heap sites, including several on Martha's Vineyard, Massachusetts. "The implements that are called flakers are all made of antler tines. One may have been cut from the antler, the others have fractured butts. All the flakers show scars on the surface and one exhibited a definitely artificial blunted end. The term 'flaker' may be a misnomer for it implies that these tools were used in chipping stone. It cannot be denied at present that these tools may have been used for some other purpose, opening molluscs for instance." (Byers, Douglas, and Frederick Johnson. *Two Sites on Martha's Vineyard*. Vol. 1 No. 1. Phillips Academy, Andover, 1940, p 53).

Some of Mesa Verde's numerous spectacular cliff dwellings (Colorado) have names derived from a notable feature, such as Square Tower House and Spruce Tree House. Of interest for this book, due to the large number of awls found, is Bone Awl House. (Gladwin, Harold Sterling. *A History of the Ancient Southwest*. The Bond Wheelwright Company, Portland, Maine, 1957, p 274).

Measuring 9" long, an antler harpoon was a surface find in Pickaway County, Ohio. Pointed at both ends, one side had seven short back-angled barbs. (Editor. *Ohio Archaeologist*. Vol. 11 No. 4, October 1961, p 111).

Twenty bird-bone whistles were found at Pecos, New Mexico: "...each of which is pierced by a single hole, usually at or near the middle of the shaft. Aside from the above-mentioned hole, they are precisely like the very abundant tubular beads and, indeed, some of the shorter ones may perhaps actually have been beads cut from broken flutes. The majority, however, were probably whistles or bird-calls...". (Kidder, Alfred Vincent. "Objects of Bone," *The Artifacts of Pecos*. Robert S.

Peabody Foundation for Archaeology, Yale University Press, New Haven, 1932, p 252).

A bone awl or knife found in Mason County, Tennessee, had a handle wrapped in deerskin and secured with a cord made of plant fiber. The entire artifact was about 6" long. (Editor. *Central States Archaeological Journal*. Vol. 41 No. 1, January 1994, p 45).

Long ago, in the Valley of Mexico at Tequixquiac, a unique bone effigy was found. In 1870 the carved sacrum (lower vertebrae, part of the pelvis) from an extinct form of llama was discovered 40 feet below the ground surface. Possibly carved to represent a coyote head, holes had been drilled to represent the nostrils. (Wormington, H. M. *Ancient Man in North America*. 4th edition. The Denver Museum of Natural History, Denver, Colorado, 1957, pp 199 – 201).

A 1992 cache from Gibson County, Indiana, consisted of four highly developed anchor pendants and a number of bone and shell artifacts. Three engraved mink jawbones were present, also two chipped blades, and 40 drilled conch shell beads. (Editor. *Prehistoric American*. Genuine Indian Relic Society, Vol. XXXVI No. 3, 2002, p 41).

Found as a cache, a total of 34 river otter baculum bones came from Tennessee. The bones were drilled for suspension at one end and averaged about 3½" in length. (Editor. *Central States Archaeological Journal*. Vol. 28 No. 4, October 1981, p 210).

Bone whistles or single-note musical instruments are found across North America. A hollow bone was used and the end opposite the mouth-hole was closed with some object or substance, and the shaft had a single hole that was either drilled or cut. Some large examples, found in California and on Santa Cruz Island, ranged in length from 3⅗ to 6½". Instruments with more than a single hole are considered flutes or fifes. A few paired or double whistles were found. (Abbott, C. C. "Musical Instruments Made of Bone." *Report Upon United States Geographical Surveys*. Vol. VII. Engineer Department / U. S. Army, Washington, 1879, pp 234 – 237).

A long, triangular bone knife (or spearpoint) was collected in Morton County, North Dakota. The artifact, with narrow side notches, was 8½" long. (Editor. *Artifacts*. Vol. 13 No. 1, 1983, p 11).

Middlesex County, Ontario, Canada, was the region that produced the following bone knife. Made from an animal bone, the knife was black and polished. Probably late prehistoric, the knife was 1¼" wide and 8½" long. (Wolfe, Brian. "An Unusual Bone Knife From Ontario." *The Redskin*. Genuine Indian Relic Society, Vol. VII No. 2, 1972, p 76).

An exceptional shell gorget was found in southcentral Kentucky. Picked up in 1985, the gorget measured 5 x 8¾". (Cooper display advertisement. *Prehistoric Antiquities and Archaeological News Quarterly*. February 2004, Vol. XXIV No. 1, p 25).

A small cache of bone artifacts was unearthed in a rubbish deposit at Pecos, New Mexico. Included were the ulna (8" long) of a golden eagle, five polished eagle-bone tubes (5 to 5⅞" long), and two beads (one turkey, one small mammal). The objects had been bundled and placed in an oval hole. (Kidder, Alfred Vincent. "Objects of Bone." *The Artifacts of Pecos*. Robert S. Peabody Foundation for Archaeology, Yale University Press, New Haven, 1932, p 264, 266).

One of the most unusual bone necklaces was found in Washington County, Virginia. Dozens of bones were used, and all were tips from wild turkey wings. (Editor. *Central States Archaeological Journal*. Vol. 16 No. 1, January 1969, p 39).

Some bone projectile points were found at the Clark's Pond (shell heap) site in Massachusetts. "All five barbed bone points came from the southwestern part of the excavated area where fish bones were very common. Unfortunately, the bases of the multi-barbed points are missing so that it is impossible to tell whether they were points for spears, harpoons, or leisters. Single-barbed bone points show two different types of bases. In the first, sawing transversely, and then breaking, made the base. This point could have been at the side to a piece of wood or bone to form a compound fishhook. The other point, highly polished and missing part of the barb, has a wedge-shaped base. A short facet on the barbed side and a long facet on the other side form this base. The longer facet, which is the more finished of the two, presumedly represents a contact surface for attachement or for lashings." (Bullen, Ripley P. "The Collections." *Excavations in Northeastern Massachusetts*. Phillips Academy, Vol. 1 No. 3, Andover, 1949, p 126).

At a Folsom bison kill-site in eastern Wyoming, the bones of perhaps five bison were found. In addition to three Folsom points, three other projectile points were made of splintered bone. (Ebeling, Walter. *Handbook of Indian Foods and Fibers of Arid America*. University of California Press, 1986, p 21).

North of the Platte River in Nebraska an early investigator found numerous bone artifacts in storage pits. "In one of these lodges I have found ten caches extending into the ground an average depth of 11 feet from the present surface. There was an outer row inside the rim or outer edge of the circle and another row three feet nearer the center of the ruin. These caches were placed alternately, not opposite each other.

"From these caches I have taken a great variety of objects [including] fish hooks of bone; nine complete bone hoes formed from the shoulder blades of bison; a long bead from the hinge of a sea shell (not a mussell shell); scores of bone needles, punches, and awls; [and] a half dozen arrow-shaft straighteners(?) of antler and bone. (Gilder, Robert F. "The Ten Cache Ruin." *The Archaeological Bulletin*. Vol. I No. 3. The International Society of Archaeologists, 1910, pp 59 – 61).

In 14 feet of layered deposits, Danger Cave near the Bonneville Salt Flats held many specimens of basketry, mats, netting, and artifacts made of bone, hide, shell, and wood. Food animal bones were from antelope, deer, and [mountain] sheep. (Wormington, H. M. *Ancient Man in North America*. 4th edition. The Denver Museum of Natural History, Denver, Colorado, 1957, p 193).

The Snyders site in Illinois produced many bone and antler artifacts. Some of the more interesting were imitation bear teeth (some drilled) that were actually made from split and polished deer bone. (Fecht, William G. "The Snyders Site / Calhoun County, Illinois." *Central States Archaeological Journal*. Vol. 16 No. 2, April 1969, pp 62 – 75).

Large marine shell beads were made by the Adena (Early Woodland) in the eastern Midwest. "Enough have been found to demonstrate that Adena used marine shell forms for bead manufacture, and that the columella of large gastropoda were cut and worked down into cylindrical beads. They were not so completely worked down, a portion of the spiral whorl of the columella still showed on the beads." (Webb, William S. and Charles E. Snow. *The Adena People*. The University of Kentucky, 1945/1988, p 99).

A series of antler flaking tools came from the Reeves site in Ohio. Most examples were polished cylinders with flattened ends, and the average size was ½ x 2". (Vietzen, Col. Raymond C. *Indians of the Lake Erie Basin*. Ludi Printing Co., Wahoo, Nebraska, 1965, p 304).

Horn was sometimes used to make utensils in historic times.

"The animals supplying the most materials for spoons, dippers, and ladles were the mountain sheep and mountain goat. All the tribes living in the habitat of these animals utilized their horns for this purpose, and the manufactured products were distributed widely in trade among neighboring tribes. Specimens have been gathered among the Pueblos, Havasupai, Ute, Cheyenne, and Sioux, the Salishan and northern Algonquian tribes, and the North West Coast and Athapascan tribes. Among the southern Rocky Mountain Indians these utensils were rude, but the northern tribes made them works of art, softening the horn and bending and shaping it over forms by means of heat, and carving and inlaying the material with great skill. Spoons were also made from the horns of the buffalo. After cattle were introduced, their horns were substituted, especially among the Plains tribes, for those of the disappearing wild animals." (Hodge, Frederick Webb. "Spoons and Ladles." *Handbook of American Indians*. Part 2. Bureau of American Ethnology Bulletin 30, 1910, pp 625, 626).

Two bowls made of desert tortoise shells were found in Nevada's Gypsum Cave. One was 5⅜" long, the other 6½". Both had been modified for use. (Harrington, Mark Raymond. *Gypsum Cave, Nevada*. Southwest Museum Papers No. Eight, Los Angeles, 1933/1963, p 89).

One of the largest, unilaterally barbed, antler harpoons was found in New York state. With 12 barbs on one side and a tapered base, it was about 13" long. The Kipp Island people made the harpoon. (Ritchie, William A. *The Pre-Iroquoian Occupations of New York State*. Rochester Museum Memoir No. 1, Rochester, 1944, p 136).

The Shaffer site, near Worthington, Greene County, Indiana, produced Find 21 which apparently was a set of flint-working tools. These "...consisted of 14 unworked antler tips, 5 antler punches or flakers, [and] 2 metapodial bone flakers...". (Black, Glenn A. *The Archaeology of Greene County*. Vol. X No. 5. Indiana History Bulletin, Indianapolis, 1933, p 276).

Among the bone artifacts found in a rock shelter were three common awls that had additional artifacts or artifact parts with them. One awl, 2½" long, was associated with a cylindrical bone point protector. Another bone awl had a handle-like padding of yucca fiber around the base. And a long bone awl had a fitted skin or leather sheath, for carrying or storage of the awl. (Guernsey, Samuel James. *Explorations in Northeastern Arizona*. Papers of the Peabody Museum, Vol. XII No. 1, Harvard University, 1931, p 84 plate 56).

Antler was associated with the Atl-atl in three ways. Spurs or hooked tips were often set at the distal end, and antler handles have been found from Archaic and Woodland times. More unusual are Atl-atl balance weights made from a thick section of antler and drilled in the center like a bannerstone. Many of these weights, from 3 to 6" long, have been found in the Southeast from Kentucky to Florida. (Hothem, Lar. Various sources).

Old-Time Dealer Listings

It is fascinating to look back and see how artifacts made of antler, bone, and shell were once advertised and sold. To some extent, the advertising emphasis given to such items certainly reflected collector demand. If so, these artifacts years ago took somewhat of a secondary position behind flint and stone artifacts. Of course this has changed and today the better pieces are both highly respected and avidly collected.

"Wampum [shell beads] – Assortment of 15 wampum, $1.85. Ten wampum from Seneca tribe, New York, $1.60. Ten different wampum, Oklahoma, $1.60. String of Seneca wampum about 3 feet long, very nice and rare, New York, $16.80." (*Heike's Hobby Catalogue*. R. Heike, Wenona, Illinois, 1950).

"Alaska horn spoon, 6" long, very cheap, $2.25. Alaska huge horn totem spoon, over 10" long, finely carved and polished, very rare specimen, very fine indeed, price $7.00. Ivory cribbage board, length 15", carved from large walrus tusk, with incised polar bear, whale, men, and scenery. Must be seen to be appreciated. Price of this fine specimen $12.50." (Descriptive circular No. 32, N. E. Carter, Elkhorn, Wisconsin, Spring 1914).

"Beads, saucer shape, ancient shell, large size, string, $1.00. Ancient shell beads, ½ x 1 inch and larger, each $0.25. Ancient shell disk beads, small size, about ¼" string, $1.00. Old shell beads, all cut square, string, $1.00. Ancient tubular shell beads, string, $1.00. Pendant, old shell, one hole, $0.50. Pendants, mostly round, two or more holes, some are engraved, each $0.50 - 1.25. Ancient shell ceremonial, 1 x 1½", toadstool shape, very fine, $1.00. Ancient shell bead, 1¼ x 5⅕", rare size, very fine, $2.50. Ancient shell awl, ⅝ x 6¾", rare size, fine, $2.25. Ancient shell plummet, ⅝ x 3¾", groove around tip, very fine, $3.00." (Catalog, A. D. Grutzmacher, Mukwonago, Wisconsin, 1940, p 31).

"Large California shell bead strand, heavy beads, polished, 18", $5.00. Small California shell bead strand, smaller unpolished, 24", $3.50. Shell beads, strand, Oklahoma, flat long type, 28 beads, 21", $15.00. Shell beads strand, heavy oval, outstanding quality, 7", $15.00. Shell beads strand, small alternating hour glass and round type, 12", $20.00. Curved bone Alaska ice pick with wood handle, $10.00. Old Alaska ivory shuttle, and, spacing tool, both $10.00. Bird or small game snare, Alaska, bone slides, $2.00. Old Alaska bone harpoon or fishing points, barbed, each $2.00. Bone awl-like piece, Alaska, $3.00. Small, bone weaving shuttle, Alaska, $3.00. Decorated Alaska bone needle case complete with tiny ivory needles and drawstring, $10.00. Feathered arrows with long, bone, Alaska point, $7.50. Old Alaska ivory fish-shaped fishing lure, $7.50. Small Alaska curved old ivory bow, etched figures, 16", $12.50. Shuttle-type Alaska fishing tool, 16", still contains some fishing line and hooks, fine, $15.00. Ivory tusk gouge-like implement, Alaska, 15", $7.50. Old Alaska bone harpoon head, with socket and transverse hole and split ends, 10", $5.00. Old fish-killer club of walrus bone, 25", $15.00. Polished small hollow bone needle case, Alaska, ends missing, $2.00. Solid bone ulu knife, knobbed handle top, black spot decorations, $12.50. Ivory lip plug, $3.00. Alaska bone comb, $2.00. Old Alaska bone knife handle, rusted blade section, for dressing skins, $4.00. Old bone sled runner, 11", $5.00. Old Alaska bone handle with metal saw-like blade inserted full-length, $7.50. Indian four-piece bone cup-and-pin game pieces, pin with beaded string, $8.50. Fine swirled shell hair pin, perforated end, $5.00. Long dark brown bone awl, 8", $3.00. Sioux elk antler hide-dressers, $10.00." (Catalog, *Tilton Indian Relics*. Topeka, Kansas, 1958, pp 77, 87 – 91).

"String of rare shell beads, Le Flore County, Oklahoma, $0.75. Fifty tiny disc wampum, Le Flore County, Oklahoma, $0.25. One hundred mixed wampum, tubes, ball, disc, etc., only $0.50. Ten fine shell wampum, Sacramento County, California, $0.10. Disc shell bead, extra large, $0.10. Dentalium or tooth shell wampum, rare, 3 for $0.10. Elk tooth pendants, each $1.00." (Catalog, H. T. Daniel, Hot Springs, Arkansas, 1938, p 14).

"Sioux bone breast plate, three rows, 84 bone tubes, $18.00. Necklace, black bear claws, 20 claws with beads between, $4.00. Necklace, wolf claws, beads and shell pendant, $2.50. Necklace, 68 beads plus glass(?) beads, $2.50." (Price lists, Fred M. Smith, Chicago, Illinois, 1913).

"Five old shell disc wampum, five assorted up to the size of a five-cent nickel, large perforation, $0.75. Six shell wampum, Genesee County, New York, cylinder shape, perforated, $0.25. Two oblong shell beads, large and small, Gila River, Arizona, $0.25. Pearl beads, drilled, with much of original luster, two for $0.75. Tubular beads (historic), bison horn, ¾" long, well preserved, each $0.35." (Catalog, J. R. Nissley, Mansfield, Ohio, ca. 1911, p 7).

"Wampum beads, red and black, per string, $0.75 – 2.00. Wampum beads, strings of little shell discs, $1.00 – 2.50. Bone awls, $0.40 – 1.50. Odd shell plummets, rare, $3.50 – 5.00." (Catalog, L. W. Stilwell, Deadwood, South Dakota, 1911, p 20).

"Buffalo horns, mounted, buffalo hide between, Cree, Montana, $35.00. Deerhorn dance wand, eagle feather pendants, Ute, near Pine River, Colorado, $10.00. Bone and sinew tubular pipe, Kiowa, near Washita River, Oklahoma, $17.00. Bone war-whistle, Sioux, Upper Missouri River, North Dakota, $15.00. Turtle shell paint cup, Arapaho, near Canadian River, Oklahoma, $3.00. Perforated bear's foot bone and needle game, Sioux, South Dakota, $7.25. Turtle shell and animal hoof rattle, Pueblo, New Mexico, $12.00. Buffalo horn pouch, quilled, near Wind River, Wyoming, $7.50. Animal teeth necklace, metal pendants, Cree, near Red River, Manitoba, $4.25. Halibut hook, wood frame, bone hook, Haida, Queen Charlotte's Island, British Columbia, $3.50. Bone knife, Eskimo, Cook Inlet, Alaska, $4.00. Bone knitting needle, Eskimo, Cook Inlet, Alaska, $1.50. Mountain sheep horn spoon, Sioux, near White River, South Dakota, $20.50. Mountain goat horn spoon, Massett, Vancouver Island, British Columbia, $12.00. Elk antler hide-scraper, Sioux, Upper Missouri River, North Dakota, $16.00. Whalebone scraper, Bella Coola, Vancouver Island, British Columbia, $18.00. Bone scraper, buffalo(?), San Juan Pueblo, New Mexico, $5.00. Bear claw necklace, Gros Ventre, Upper Missouri River, North Dakota, $60.00. Bear foot bone necklace, Sioux, near White River, South Dakota, $18.25. Bead and turtle leg necklace, Cheyenne-Arapaho, near Canadian River, Oklahoma, $12.00. Shell wampum necklace, turquois pendants, Zuni Pueblo, New Mexico, $50.00. Shell ear ornaments, Sioux, near Rapid City, South Dakota, $4.50. Gaming bones, Cheyenne, near Canadian River, Oklahoma, $3.45." (Catalog No. 2, A. H. Gottschall, Harrisburg, Pennsylvania, 1909).

"Abalone shell pendant, fine, $1.00. Camp site shell beads, 100, $1.50. Bone tube beads, 3" long, each, $0.75. Bone spades, 9 to 10", fine, $8.00. Bone knives, 6 to 8", fine, $5.00. Joint bone awls, very fine, $2.00 to $5.00. Joint bone chisel or gouge, $2.50 to $6.00. Bone awls, $0.25 – 2.00. Bone flaking tools, $0.50 – 1.00. Antler flaking tools, $1.00 – 2.00. Bone knife handles, $1.00 – 2.50. Bone needles, approx. 3 in. long, $4.00. Bone fishhooks, small, good, $1.50; larger, fine, $4.00. Bone lance head, $2.00. Bone pendants, $2.00. Bone awls, short, about good, $0.35; three for $1.00. Large elk antler hide-fleshers with metal blade tied on, $9.00. Small elk antler hide-fleshers, $7.50. Grooved awl sharpeners, $0.50. Eagle leg bone war whistle, fine, $3.00 – 5.00. Horn spoons, $1.50 – 3.50. One cloth vest, shell-covered, $22.50." (Advertising flyer, Allen Brown, Chicago, Illinois, ca. 1952).

"I have a great lot of beads on hand – something like one hundred thousand, from Le Flore County, Oklahoma. They are strung on strings from 100 to 600 each. I have only one string of fresh water pearls, which I will sell for $15.00. I have five strings of mother-of-pearl, about 50 to the string, $4.00 per string. Two strings of finger bone type shell beads, $4.00 – 5.00. I have many thousands of the little disc bone beads at $1.50 a string, in good condition. Many thousands of little disc beads, $0.25 per 100, about 600 to the string. I have several hundred of the large shell beads at $3.50 per string of 50." (Catalog No. 1, G. E. Pilquist, Dardanelle, Arkansas, 1937, p 9).

In *Hobbies* magazine, the October 1936 issue, there was an advertisement for artifacts from the famous Edward W. Payne collection. Among the items listed were "Bone Needles and Awls @ 50 cents to $2.00 each." (Editor. *Artifacts*. Vol. 5 No. 4, 1975, p 30).

Author's notes – Some of the necklace strands were likely made up of various individual pieces the dealer (other than collector-dealers like Gottschall) had in stock. While the separate artifacts were probably authentic, the complete necklace (as offered for sale) was not necessarily the original item as used by Indians.

Also, the purchase of certain animal and bird parts is no longer legal under federal laws regarding endangered and some migratory species. As an example, possession of eagle bones, talons, and even feathers is no longer permitted except in certain cases.

Auction Results

Sale figures are a good way to determine recent artifact values, for these represent actual buying activity. Special thanks are due Jan Sorgenfrei, Manager-Owner of Old Barn Auction (10040 SR 224 West, Findlay, Ohio, 45840 / #419-422-8531) for permission to reproduce auction results in this chapter.

Each antler, bone, or shell listing has the artifact type, a brief description, and the auction date. The winning bid amount includes a 10% buyer premium.

Bone awls, four, longest 4", found in West Virginia.	17 May 2003	$60.50
Awl, polished deer bone, 4⅛", Hocking County, Ohio.	9 Mar 2002	$55.00
Knife, bone-handled, 6¼" long, from Alaska.	28 Apr 2001	$286.00
Shell beads, strand 36" long, Le Flore County, Oklahoma.	8 May 2004	$385.00
Bone fishhooks, two, one broken and glued, Virginia.	15 Mar 2003	$165.00
Deer leg sinew-wrapped pipe, 6¾", Cheyenne, ca. 1880s.	12 June 2004	$88.00
Bone awl, with eye, 10" long, Hamilton County, Ohio.	15 Jun 2002	$1,100.00
Knife, 14½", elkhorn handle, ca. 1880s, probably Western.	22 Nov 2003	$88.00
Horsehair quirt, 25¼", Sharp's Trading Post, early 1940s.	12 June 2004	$412.50
Seal effigy, bone or ivory, 1½", St. Lawrence Island.	9 Feb 2002	$60.50
Tool, bone, expanded tip, 4¾", Hocking County, Ohio.	9 Mar 2002	$110.00
Duck effigy, bone or ivory, 1¼", Eskimo.	9 Feb 2002	$198.00
Cribbage board, bone, 14¼", human head at end, Northwest Coast.	16 June 2001	$132.00
Ivory gaming sticks, two, 4⅞", Eskimo.	9 Feb 2002	$88.00
Leather bag, abalone and shell beaded drops, 13½", ca. 1890s.	12 June 2004	$550.00
Scraper, bone handle, 5¼" long, Alaska.	4 Nov 2000	$55.00
Necklace, shell beads, strand 38" long, Tennessee.	15 June 2002	$302.50
Three ivory harpoon heads, longest 5 1/16", St. Lawrence Island.	12 June 2004	$440.00
Pendant, circular, shell, 3⅜" diameter, Boone County, Kentucky.	21 Sep 2002	$220.00
Axe, ivory, tourist item ca. 1940s, 7¼", Alaska.	22 Nov 2003	$82.50
Gorget, shell, 5¼", two suspension holes, Tennessee.	25 Aug 2001	$1,375.00
Knife, ulu-type, bone handle and slate blade, 3½", Alaska.	23 Dec 2002	$121.00
Bone harpoon head, 1⅛ x 11½", "Terra del Fuego / 1844."	12 June 2004	$330.00
Mask, shell, 6 x 8", collected in 1931, Bell County, Kentucky.	26 Oct 2002	$247.50
Ivory scrimshaw cribbage board, 16¼", seals.	12 June 2004	$770.00
Purse, shell, elk antler, inlays, 5¼", Tlingit.	16 June 2001	$357.50
Shell bead strand, 36", Le Flore County, Oklahoma.	8 May 2004	$440.00
Shaft wrench, desert sheephorn, 9½", Jemez Pueblo, New Mexico.	27 Oct 2001	$154.00
Engraved pin, ivory, with hole, 6¾", Eskimo.	16 June 2001	$154.00
Duck effigy, bone, 2¼", St. Lawrence Island.	9 Feb 2002	$231.00
Dance club, buffalo horns, 20½", ca. 1890 – 1910.	12 June 2004	$770.00
Awls, two, 7" long, one engraved, Kentucky.	26 Oct 2002	$247.50
Sandal sole gorget, shell, broken, 7½", Hamilton County, Ohio.	16 June 2001	$3,850.00
Walrus oosik with ivory polar bear head, 20" long, Eskimo.	27 Oct 2001	$330.00
Shell decorative artifacts, frame of twenty, California.	26 Oct 2002	$495.00

Sheephorn ladle, 9¼", southwest Alaska.	12 June 2004	$176.00
Bone needle with eye, curved, 5⅝", Hocking County, Ohio.	9 Mar 2002	$165.00
Bone hide flesher, 11½", Plains Indian.	12 June 2004	$302.50
Scrimshaw board, carved ivory, incised, 10⅞" long.	16 June 2001	$330.00
Beads, deer bone, 113 in strand, patinated, West Virginia.	17 May 2003	$1,292.50
Flesher, buffalo bone, 13" long, metal blade, Plains region.	11 Jan 2003	$423.50
Awl, deer bone, 6", Christian County, Kentucky.	9 Mar 2002	$55.00
Shell beads, strand 35" long, Le Flore County, Oklahoma.	8 May 2004	$467.50
Ivory comb, 1800s, 7½" high, Eskimo.	16 June 2001	$341.00
Gouge, deer bone, 5" long, West Virginia.	17 May 2003	$27.50
Human figurine, bone or ivory, 2" high, Eskimo.	9 Feb 2002	$330.00
Shell mask, Fort Ancient, 4½" high, Scioto County, Ohio.	15 Feb 2003	$385.00
Scraper, bone, stone bit, 3⅞" long, Eskimo.	9 Feb 2002	$66.00
Fishhook, bone, 2" long, Hamilton County, Ohio.	17 Mar 2003	$121.00
Bone snow goggles, carved, with strap, Eskimo.	15 Mar 2003	$412.50
Hairpin, bone or antler, crane effigy, 4½", New York state.	9 Feb 2002	$440.00
Beads, deer bone, patinated, 31" strand, West Virginia.	17 May 2003	$302.50
Harpoon socket, ivory, whale head effigy, 9" long, Eskimo.	16 June 2001	$495.00
Fishhook, bone, 1¾" long, find-location unknown.	18 May 2002	$275.00
Fishing lure, bone or ivory, 3⅞" long, St. Lawrence Island.	9 Feb 2002	$352.00
Effigy awl, 7½" long, bear head, drilled, New York state.	21 June 2003	$1,210.00
Hairpin, bone, 6½", tapered shape, Kentucky.	18 May 2002	$71.50
Ivory engraved cribbage board, seal, duck, kayak, 13½".	12 June 2004	$550.00
Shell bead strand, 30" long, Le Flore County, Oklahoma.	8 May 2004	$880.00
Polar bear oosik with seal heads, 6" long, Eskimo.	27 Oct 2001	$159.50
Awl or hairpin, bone, slender, 7⅛", find-location unknown.	9 Mar 2002	$352.00
Sled yoke, curved, 17¾", bone and iron, 1800s, Alaska.	23 Aug 2003	$715.00
Awl, bone, human head effigy with seed bead eyes, 4¾", Plains.	27 Jan 2001	$176.00
Scrimshaw antler knife, 9", effigy faces, Eskimo.	12 June 2004	$357.50
Beamer, deer bone, 7¾", from Old Town on Harbeth River.	18 May 2002	$137.50
Ivory human figure, 3¼", Alaska.	25 Aug 2001	$1,155.00
Hairpin, curved rib bone, 6⅞", glued, Hocking County, Ohio.	18 May 2002	$60.50
Charm, seal tooth, wood and sinew, 3½", Eskimo.	12 June 2004	$121.00
Bone awls, two, 7¼", polished shafts, Ohio.	8 Dec 2001	$264.00
Hairpin, weathered bone, 10⅛", find-location unknown.	9 Mar 2002	$82.50
Hidescraper, bone, 13", ca. 1870s, dot-engraved.	12 June 2004	$330.00
Tool, bone handle and steel bit, 8½", Eskimo.	16 June 2001	$220.00
Fishhooks, four, bone, 1⅜", Scioto County, Ohio.	23 Aug 2003	$302.50
Scraper, bone handle, 11½", St. Lawrence Island.	4 Nov 2000	$66.00
Shell beads, strand 34" long, Le Flore County, Oklahoma.	8 May 2004	$495.00
Awls, group of seven in Winegardner wood frame, Kentucky.	20 July 2002	$187.00
Harpoon head, bone, 10", incised lines, Alaska.	24 June 2000	$60.50

Auction Results

Shell beads, 24" strand, Ex-Morast, Smyth County, Virginia.	15 Mar 2003	$302.50
Womens' choker, dentalia shells, 18", Plains.	12 June 2004	$935.00
Child's boat, ivory, 5" long, Eskimo.	28 Apr 2001	$187.00
Pendant, marine shell, 7¼", ex-Morast, Oklahoma.	15 Mar 2003	$440.00
Hide-scraper, Sioux, buffalo bone, 11¾", engraved.	21 June 2003	$192.50
Ivory effigy of man, 6⅛", engraved, Alaska.	28 Apr 2001	$1,320.00
Awl, bone with engraving, 2¾", Hocking County, Ohio.	9 Mar 2002	$99.00
Buffalo horn spoon, turtle effigy handle, 10¼", ca. 1890s.	12 June 2004	$550.00
Bone flute, 3⅛", four holes, find-location unknown.	18 May 2002	$302.50
Whale effigy, whalebone, 4½", Alaska.	28 Apr 2001	$187.00
Projectile point, antler, conical, 1⅞" long, Hocking County, Ohio.	18 May 2002	$132.00
Bone flute, three holes, 3½", Hamilton County, Ohio.	24 June 2000	$242.00
Needle holder, walrus effigy, ivory, 4¾", Eskimo.	25 Aug 2001	$660.00
Bone whistle, effigy form 4⅜", Virginia.	16 June 2001	$110.00
Buffalo horns, beaded, 14", c. 1880s, ex-Sharp Museum.	12 June 2004	$660.00
Shell bead strand, 34", Le Flore County, Oklahoma.	8 May 2004	$313.50
Necklace, shell and dog tooth beads, 26", Sioux.	12 June 2004	$99.00
Ivory handle with three brass rivets, 2½", Eskimo.	22 Nov 2003	$38.50
Tubular beads, bone, strand about 40", Scioto County, Ohio.	15 Mar 2003	$165.00
Celt, 7¼", old ivory, St. Lawrence Island.	21 June 2003	$357.50
Bone flute, 3" long, Fort Ancient aspect, West Virginia.	21 Sept 2002	$187.00
Maskette, whalebone, 6¾", rare, Yakitat, Alaska.	16 June 2001	$7,150.00
Projectile point, antler, 2⅛", tapered, find-location unknown.	9 Mar 2002	$33.00
Bone scraper, 13" long, Plains, c. 1890s.	12 June 2004	$275.00
Bone tool frame, Alaskan, variety of forms, 20 in all.	15 Mar 2003	$148.50
Bone-handled hide-scraper, Plains, steel blade, 13" long.	8 Dec 2001	$110.00
Shell mask, Weeping Eye design, 3⅛", Tennessee.	25 Aug 2001	$385.00
Bone ring, 1¼" in diameter, pierced holes, West Virginia.	21 Sept 2002	$275.00
Handle, ivory, engraved, 7½" long, Arctic Coast.	8 Dec 2001	$440.00
Fishhooks, three, bone, 1¾", Scioto County, Ohio.	23 Aug 2003	$275.00
Eskimo sealskin mask, 11¼" high, Alaska.	12 June 2004	$110.00
Bone needle with eye, 8" long, Lorain County, Ohio.	24 June 2000	$385.00
Shell beads, strand 30", Le Flore County, Oklahoma.	8 May 2004	$577.50
Bone tools, one frame of 11 pieces, Eskimo.	15 Mar 2003	$220.00
Fishhook preform, bone, 2" long, Hocking County, Ohio.	18 May 2002	$247.50
Hide-flesher handle, bone, 13½", Plains region.	22 Nov 2003	$214.50